THE CLINICAL PRACTICE OF
Neurological and Neurosurgical Nursing

THE CLINICAL PRACTICE OF

Neurological and Neurosurgical Nursing

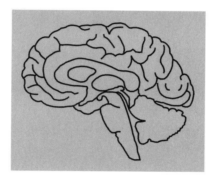

FOURTH EDITION

JOANNE V. HICKEY
PhD, RN, CS, ANP, CNRN, FAAN
Professor of Clinical Nursing
The University of Texas–Houston
Houston, Texas

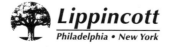 **Lippincott**
Philadelphia • New York

Acquisitions Editor: Lisa Stead
Assistant Editor: Brian McDonald
Project Editor: Sandra Cherrey Scheinin
Production Manager: Helen Ewan
Production Coordinator: Patricia McCloskey
Design Coordinator: Doug Smock
Indexer: Maria Coughin

Edition 4th

9 8 7 6 5 4 3 2 1

Library of Congress Cataloging-in-Publications Data

The clinical practice of neurological and neurosurgical nursing /
   [edited by] Joanne V. Hickey.—4th ed.
       p.   cm.
   Rev. ed. of: The clinical practice of neurological and
neurosurgical nursing/Joanne V. Hickey. 3rd ed. ©1992.
   Includes bibliographical references and index.
   ISBN 0-397-55319-6
   1. Neurological nursing.   I. Hickey, Joanne V.   II. Hickey,
Joanne V.   Clinical practice of neurological and neurosurgical
nursing.
   [DNLM: 1. Nervous System Diseases—nursing.   2. Neurosurgery—
nursing.   WY 160.5 C641 1997]
RC350.5.H52   1997
610.73'68—dc20
DNLM/DLC
for Library of Congress   96-24963
                                                                    CIP

Care has been taken to confirm the accuracy of the information presented and to describe generally accepted practices. However, the authors, editors, and publisher are not responsible for errors or omissions or for any consequences from application of the information in this book and make no warranty, express or implied, with respect to the contents of the publication.

The authors, editors and publisher have exerted every effort to ensure that drug selection and dosage set forth in this text are in accordance with current recommendations and practice at the time of publication. However, in view of ongoing research, changes in government regulations, and the constant flow of information relating to drug therapy and drug reactions, the reader is urged to check the package insert for each drug for any change in indications and dosage and for added warnings and precautions. This is particularly important when the recommended agent is a new or infrequently employed drug.

Some drugs and medical devices presented in this publication have Food and Drug Administration (FDA) clearance for limited use in restricted research settings. It is the responsibility of the health care provider to ascertain the FDA status of each drug or device planned for use in their clinical practice.

As always . . . it is you, my family—my husband Jim, daughter Kathan, and son Christopher—who have given my life meaning, direction, and purpose through your continued love, support, encouragement, understanding, interest, and assistance. Our family has expanded to include a wonderful daughter-in-law, son-in-law, and now, grandchildren. It is family that is the most precious of gifts and the substantive denominator of life.

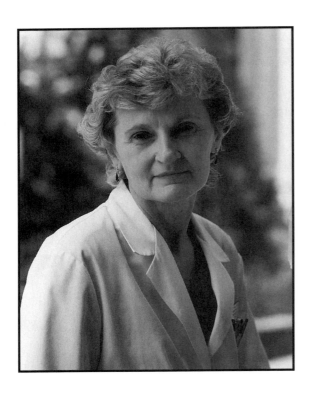

About the Author

Dr. Hickey received her diploma in nursing from Roger Williams General Hospital School of Nursing in Providence, Rhode Island; her BSN from Boston College, Massachusetts; her MSN from the University of Rhode Island, Kingston, Rhode Island; her MA in counseling from Rhode Island College, Providence, Rhode Island; her PhD from the University of Texas at Austin; and her post-master's certificate as an adult nurse practitioner from Duke University, Durham, North Carolina. She is certified in neuroscience nursing (CNRN) by the American Board of Neuroscience Nursing, and as an acute care nurse practitioner (CS) by the American Nurses Credentialing Center. She is also a fellow in the American Academy of Nursing (FAAN).

Dr. Hickey has focused her career on education, practice, research, and publications in the neurosciences and neuroscience patient populations. She has had clinical appointments at Massachusetts General Hospital in Boston and at Duke University Medical Center, where she was Attending Nurse, Neuroscience Nursing. She has been a faculty member in a number of nursing schools. At Duke, she developed and directed the university's first acute care nurse practitioner program. Dr. Hickey's neuroscience research interests include cerebrovascular problems and increased intracranial pressure. She was an American Foundation of Nursing Research Scholar in 1992 for research on preparing family caregivers for recovery from stroke.

The Clinical Practice of Neurological and Neurosurgical Nursing, now in its fourth edition, has received the American Journal of Nursing (AJN) Book of the Year Award, and has been repeatedly cited in the Brandon Hill list of recommended books in nursing. The text has been translated into Japanese. Dr. Hickey is also senior editor of *Advanced Practice Nursing: Changing Roles and Clinical Applications* published in 1996 by Lippincott-Raven Publishers and co-edited by Ruth Ouimette and Sandra Venegoni. She serves on a number of editorial and advisory boards including *Heart and Lung* and *The Journal of Neurovascular Disease.*

Dr. Hickey is a member of the American Nurses Association, the American Association of Critical Care Nurses, the American Association of Neuroscience Nurses, and the Society of Critical Care Medicine. She serves on a number of national boards and commissions including the American Nurses Credentialing Center Board on Certification for Acute Care Nurse Practitioners. Dr. Hickey is a frequent national and international speaker and consultant on topics in neuroscience patient management, neuroscience nursing practice, and advanced practice nursing.

Contributors

Terri Armstrong, MSN, RN, ANP, OCN
Brain Tumor Center
Emory University
Atlanta, Georgia
Chapter 25: Brain Tumors
Chapter 26: Spinal Cord Tumors

Rosemary Brown, MSN, RN, CNRN
Clinical Nurse Specialist, Neurosurgery
Rex Medical Center
Raleigh, North Carolina
Chapter 19: Management of Pain

Deidre M. Buckley, BSN, RN
Nurse Coordinator, The Brain Aneurysm/AVM Center
Massachusetts General Hospital
Boston, Massachusetts
Chapter 29: Arteriovenous Malformations and Other
*   Cerebrovascular Anomalies*

Sherry W. Fox, MS, RN, CNRN
Neuroscience Clinical Nurse Specialist
Medical College of Virginia Hospitals
Richmond, Virginia
Chapter 33: AIDS: Neurological Manifestations

Stephen W. Janning, PharmD
Pharmacy Supervisor
Duke University Medical Center
Durham, North Carolina
Chapter 11: Pharmacological Management
*   of Neuroscience Patients*

Timothy F. Lassiter, MS
Pharmacist
Duke University Medical Center
Durham, North Carolina
Chapter 11: Pharmacological Management
*   of Neuroscience Patients*

Donna Nayduch, MSN, RN
Trauma Clinical Nurse Specialist
Duke University Medical Center
Durham, North Carolina
Chapter 20: Multiple Trauma

Mary L. Ryan, BSN, RN
Assistant Head Nurse, Neuro ICU
Duke University Medical Center
Durham, North Carolina
Chapter 28: Cerebral Aneurysms

Jane T. Settle, MS, RN, CS, FNP
Infectious Disease Clinic
Medical College of Virginia Hospitals
Richmond, Virginia
Chapter 33: AIDS: Neurological Manifestations

Christine Willis, MSN, RN, ANP, CS
Nurse Practitioner, Cystic Fibrosis Clinic
Duke University Medical Center
Durham, North Carolina
Chapter 12: Respiratory Management of Neuroscience Patients

Reviewers

Terry Armstrong, MSN, RN, ANP, OCN
Brain Tumor Center
Emory University
Atlanta, Georgia
Chapter 25: Brain Tumors
Chapter 26: Spinal Cord Tumors

Catherine Browkowski Benoit, MSN, RN,C, CNRN
Nurse Practitioner/Neurosurgery
Beth Israel Hospital
Boston, Massachusetts
Chapter 23: Back Pain and Intervertebral Disc Injuries

Deidre M. Buckley, BSN, RN
Nurse Coordinator, The Brain Aneurysm/AVM Center
Massachusetts General Hospital
Boston, Massachusetts
Chapter 29: Arteriovenous Malformations and Other
* Cerebrovascular Anomalies*

Jane Castle, MSN, RN
Doctoral Student
Boston College
Chestnut Hill, Massachusetts
Chapter 4: Ethical and Legal Issues in Neuroscience
* Nursing Practice*

Helen A. Cook, MSN, RN
Advanced Staff Nurse, Neuro ICU
Duke University Medical Center
Durham, North Carolina
Chapter 21: Craniocerebral Injuries

Carolyn J. Graham, MSN, RN, PhD (candidate)
Rehabilitation Clinical Nurse Specialist
Duke University Medical Center
Durham, North Carolina
Chapter 14: Rehabilitation of Neuroscience Patients

Nanette H. Hock, MSN, RN, CCRN, CNRN
Nurse Coordinator
Stanford University Stroke Center
Palo Alto, California
Chapter 27: Stroke and Other Cerebrovascular Diseases

Gail Levy, MSN, RN, CS
Formerly Psychiatric Clinical Nurse Specialist
Massachusetts General Hospital
Boston, Massachusetts
Chapter 13: Behavioral and Psychological Responses to
* Neurological Illness*

Donna Nayduch, MSN, RN
Trauma Clinical Nurse Specialist
Duke University Medical Center
Durham, North Carolina
Chapter 20: Multiple Trauma

Mary L. Ryan, BSN, RN
Assistant Head Nurse, Neuro ICU
Duke University Medical Center
Durham, North Carolina
Chapter 28: Cerebral Aneurysms

John Sampson, MD, PhD (candidate)
Department of Neurosurgery
Duke University Medical Center
Durham, North Carolina
Chapter 24: Peripheral Nerve Injuries
Chapter 32: Selected Infections of the Nervous System
Chapter 35: Cranial Nerve Diseases

Patti Osborne Shafer, MSN, RN
Epilepsy Nurse Specialist, Comprehensive Epilepsy Center
Beth Israel Hospital
Boston, Massachusetts
Chapter 31: Seizures and Epilepsy

Julie C. Stoops, MS, RD
Dietitian
Duke University Medical Center
Durham, North Carolina
Chapter 9: Nutritional Support for Neuroscience Patients

Richard Tim, MD
Department of Neurology
Duke University Medical Center
Durham, North Carolina
Chapter 34: Selected Degenerative Diseases
* of the Nervous System*

Marilyn Bell Wagner, RN, CCSW
Coordinator, Spinal Cord Injuries
Duke University Medical Center
Durham, North Carolina
Chapter 22: Vertebral and Spinal Cord Injuries

Roberta M. Wallace, MSW
Clinical Social Worker
Duke University Medical Center
Durham, North Carolina
Chapter 15: Transitions in Care and Discharge Planning

Preface

Since the publication of the third edition of *The Clinical Practice of Neurological and Neurosurgical Nursing,* neuroscience practice and health care have changed significantly. What has endured, and what I remain committed to, are the goals, purposes, scope, and intended audience of the text as discussed in the preface of the third edition. That is, the text continues to be focused on the care of *adult* neuroscience patients and is intended to be a ready reference and reliable resource for practicing nurses in beginning and advanced practice roles, for nursing students, and for other health professionals. What has changed and continues to change is how we practice in a predominantly cost-controlled, outcomes-focused, and managed-care environment, and the scientific and technological advances in the neurosciences.

This edition will not only be useful through the end of this "decade of the brain," but it will also prove to be invaluable as we move into the 21st century. These landmarks are the temporal context for quantum leaps in the basic understanding of the neurosciences and applications to clinical practice which include substantive and fundamental new knowledge about the nervous system, injury, recovery, and overall management of patients. More progress has been made in this decade than in any other decade, thus far. Changes in patient management both emphasize and de-emphasize the use of technology. Hospitals are environments in which the physiologically unstable, technologically dependent, or fragile-vulnerable patients receive acute care. New and refined technology provides sophisticated diagnostics and physiological monitoring data for complex clinical reasoning and decision making. "High-tech" therapies are the means for survival and quality of life for many persons who would have had a shortened life span just a few years ago. On the other end of the spectrum of health care is the growth of community based care and home care for many neuroscience problems. In some instances, the use of technology in the home provides the means for home discharge for persons previously destined for life-long institutional care. Many neurological conditions are chronic health problems that require equally powerful but "low-tech" strategies such as assessment and modification of risk factors, health promotion, disease prevention, and symptom management strategies for optimal health and quality of life. The cornerstone of management is patient education for lifestyle changes and self-management. The empowerment of patients and families with knowledge and active decision making roles regarding their own health care is perhaps one of the most effective cost-saving and quality-promoting approaches in health care that needs to be further developed and expanded.

From the health care providers' perspective, managed care and cost containment are demanding that health professionals examine every aspect of care to determine its efficacy and contribution to measurable outcomes. The goal of research-based practice forces an examination of all management components in regard to what is in the scientific literature, and it also highlights the need for much more clinical research to fill the many gaps in the knowledge base of practice. There is sufficient data in some areas for clinical guidelines, protocols, algorithms, and clinical care maps to be written to guide clinical practice decisions based on the most up-to-date knowledge and professional consensus. The Agency for Health Care Policy and Research of the United States Public Health Service, specialty practice organizations, and individual institutions all contribute to this work. Ongoing update of content should reflect new research findings and practice changes.

This edition of *The Clinical Practice of Neurological and Neurosurgical Nursing* is the result of extensive revision of content to reflect the growth of knowledge and current practice changes in the management of neuroscience patients. What became apparent to me during this process was that much controversy related to practice standards and treatment protocols still remains. There is, however, a trend toward critically evaluating the efficacy of treatments based on scientific and research knowledge, recognizing that specific treatment needs to be targeted to the underlying pathophysiological processes, and to subgroups within a clinical diagnosis, such as those with severe head injury who would benefit from a particular treatment, and recognizing prime time points in a disease process when one can expect an optimal response to a particular treatment.

Six new chapters have been added that address the complexity of health care systems, clinical reasoning, pharmacology, respiratory management, pain, and acquired immunodeficiency syndrome (AIDS). A number of experts have contributed new chapters to this edition, and I have invited other well known clinical experts to share authorship with me on other chapters. These new chapters are mentioned below in a review of each section in the book, and authorship for all chapters is noted on the title page of each chapter.

Section One, Neuroscience Nursing Practice: A Perspective on Practice, provides a current perspective of changes in neuroscience nursing practice, and forecasts trends as we move into the 21st century. Models of practice with interdisciplinary collaboration are being developed to maintain continuity along the continuum of care. "Seamless" care for populations is now the focus of care. Nurses need to understand models of practice and health care systems so they can develop "system savvy" to navigate complex systems and access the services that patients need to meet their health care needs. Also, clinical reasoning is addressed because of the increased interest in how nurses make complex clinical decisions related to patient care. The chapter on ethics has been rewritten to reflect the development of the ethical dimensions in practice.

Section Two, Assessment and Evaluation of Neuroscience Patients, begins with expansion of the content on anatomy and physiology of the nervous system. Other chapters on assessment and evaluation of neuroscience patients have been expanded and updated with the details of patient assessment.

Section Three, General Considerations in Neuroscience Nursing, updates several chapters on general considerations in neuroscience nursing practice such as nutritional support, fluid and electrolyte management, behavioral and psychological responses, and rehabilitation. Two new chapters are included in this section. Overall pharmacological management of neuroscience patents is addressed in Chapter 11 to provide the reader with an overview of practical information related to drug therapy. Respiratory management is critical to the delivery of adequate cerebral oxygenation delivery, therefore principles and methods of supporting oxygen and ventilation are discussed in detail in Chapter 12. Another completely revised chapter is "Transitions in Care and Discharge Planning." Moving patients along the continuum is important in optimizing patient outcomes and cost containment. These considerations are discussed in this extensively revised chapter.

Section Four, Special Considerations in Neuroscience Nursing, addresses management of the unconscious patient, intracranial pressure, and perioperative care in extensively updated chapters. A chapter has been added on management of pain, a problem that is often seen on the neurosurgical service. This chapter has been coauthored by a nurse with a clinical focus in pain management. Pain is the most basic of human experiences, and there are many approaches to pain management that are discussed.

Section Five, Nursing Management of Patients with Injury to the Neurological System, focuses on patients with injury to the brain, spinal cord, and peripheral nerves. Multiple trauma and back pain are also discussed. Again, chapters have undergone major revision with the addition of more information on underlying pathophysiological processes and relation to therapeutics.

In Section Six, Nursing Management of Patients with Tumors of the Neurological System, nursing management of patients with nervous system tumors is discussed. A nurse expert in management of patients with neoplasms of the nervous system is the coauthor, and she helps to refocus the chapter on the changes in practice and treatment protocols for this population.

Cerebrovascular problems are addressed in Section Seven, Nursing Management of Patients with Cerebrovascular Problems. A paradigm shift has occurred from management alone to a strong emphasis on prevention of strokes. Recent research based information on pathophysiological alterations and changes in management practices are reflected in the completely revised chapter on stroke. Neuroprotective drug protocols are assuming a more prominent role in patient management, and are sure to play an even more important role in the future. The chapters on cerebral aneurysms and arteriovenous malformations are also updated and revised.

Finally, Section Eight, Nursing Management of Patients with Headaches, Seizures, Infections, Degenerative Processes, and Cranial Nerve Diseases, addresses these special neurological problems. Chapters in this section have been significantly revised and updated to include more community based care such as is evident in the chapter on seizures. In addition, newer classification systems of particular diseases are found in the chapters. Because AIDS is such an important health problem with nervous system manifestations, a chapter, written by two expert nurses who care for these patients, has been included.

Nurses engaged in practice at different levels in intensive care units, emergency departments, neuroscience specialty units, and other units that provide care to neuroscience patients should find this text a helpful and reliable reference. Throughout *The Clinical Practice of Neurological and Neurosurgical Nursing*, pathophysiology is correlated with nursing management to provide a rationale for care and to identify patient outcomes. Summaries of common nursing diagnoses, nursing interventions, and expected outcomes for nursing management are included and have been expanded.

Caring for patients with neurological problems and disabilities requires special knowledge and skills to support the optimal functional level, quality of life, and patient outcomes. This book is written in an effort to respond to the diverse needs of the many committed nurses who provide compassionate, quality care to patients and their families.

Joanne V. Hickey

Acknowledgments

Writing is a demanding and often difficult process that competes with other commitments for time, creative energy, and academic rigor. Yet, somehow, major writing projects like *The Clinical Practice of Neurological and Neurosurgical Nursing* are completed. Many wonderfully supportive and helpful people have sustained me during the writing of this book and have challenged me to think new things and find new ways to capture the essence of clinical practice. These people, along with my clinical experience and the patients and families with whom I have worked, have influenced my thinking over the years about neuroscience patient management and neuroscience nursing care.

There are so many people to whom I am indebted. Prior to coming to the University of Texas in Houston, I held a joint appointment at Duke University Medical Center that included being Attending Nurse, Neuroscience Nursing. I thank my physician colleagues and friends, Cecil O. Borel, MD, Director of the Neuro Intensive Care Unit; Carmelo Graffagnino, MD, Codirector of the Neuro Intensive Care Unit; and Allan H. Freidman, MD, neurosurgeon and professor extraordinare; for all that they have contributed to my knowledge of patients and caring. Myra Williams, MSN, RN, was an exceptionally talented nurse manager who set a climate for unit self-governance and professional growth in the Neuro Intensive Care Unit that supported a highly developed professional and outstanding nursing staff. I also maintained contact with my many friends at Massachusetts General Hospital in Boston who are as close as e-mail or the telephone; they were great resources for all kinds of information. So many other nurses, physicians, other health care providers, students, patients, and families have shaped and expanded my thinking and understanding over the years. My thanks and appreciation to all of you.

There are a number of people to whom I would like to express a special thanks:

To my husband and best friend, Jim Hickey, who continues to help me refine my ideas, serves as the in-house editor, and provides ongoing support and encouragement.

To Diana Intenzo, now retired from Lippincott-Raven Publishers, with whom the book was born and nurtured through three editions; and now Lisa Stead, the editor for the fourth edition, who continues the stewardship with the same commitment and standards.

Finally, I would like to gratefully acknowledge and thank the contributors and the many reviewers who shared their expertise and ideas with me. All are listed elsewhere in this book.

Contents

Section 1

NEUROSCIENCE NURSING: A PERSPECTIVE ON PRACTICE

Section 2

ASSESSMENT AND EVALUATION OF NEUROSCIENCE PATIENTS 33

CHAPTER 6

Diagnostic Procedures and Laboratory Tests for Neuroscience Patients 81
Joanne V. Hickey

CHAPTER 7

The Neurological Physical Examination 103
Joanne V. Hickey

CHAPTER 8

Neurological Assessment 133
Joanne V. Hickey

Section 3

GENERAL CONSIDERATIONS IN NEUROSCIENCE NURSING 163

CHAPTER 9

Nutritional Support for Neuroscience Patients 165
Joanne V. Hickey

CHAPTER 10

Fluid and Electrolyte Management in Neuroscience Patients 179
Joanne V. Hickey

Section 4

SPECIAL CONSIDERATIONS IN NEUROSCIENCE NURSING   275

Section 5

NURSING MANAGEMENT OF PATIENTS WITH INJURY TO THE NEUROLOGICAL SYSTEM 373

Section 6

NURSING MANAGEMENT OF PATIENTS WITH TUMORS OF THE NEUROLOGICAL SYSTEM
499

Section 7

NURSING MANAGEMENT OF PATIENTS WITH CEREBROVASCULAR PROBLEMS
541

Section 8

NURSING MANAGEMENT OF PATIENTS WITH HEADACHES, SEIZURES, INFECTIONS, DEGENERATIVE PROCESSES, AND CRANIAL NERVE DISEASES
595

Section 1

Neuroscience Nursing: A Perspective On Practice

CHAPTER 1

Neuroscience Nursing: Moving into the 21st Century

Joanne V. Hickey

NEUROSCIENCE NURSING PRACTICE: COMING OF AGE

Neuroscience nursing has come of age as a fast-growing specialty practice. The explosion of new knowledge in the neurosciences, from basic research, clinical medical research, and nursing research, has fostered significant development of neuroscience nursing practice within the profession of nursing. These developments in neuroscience nursing interact with significant new developments in the nursing profession as a whole, and in health care in general. What emerges from this melding of influences are forces producing powerful trends affecting neuroscience nursing practice.

Tremendous strides have been made in the basic neurosciences and in clinical neurology, neurosurgery, neuropharmacology, and neuropsychology. Concurrent with the addition of new treatment options come questions about access, efficacy, cost, and ethical implications. Progress is also reflected in the increased complexity of the knowledge base now required for neuroscience nurses. Meanwhile, health care trends are encouraging many neuroscience nurses to become specialists in the care of particular populations of neuroscience patients and to assume new roles as advanced practice nurses.

Practice, theory development, and research are the interrelated cornerstones of professional nursing practice. Questions raised in clinical practice lead to the development of theories which are then tested as research questions. When validated by research, theory-based knowledge is applied to explain clinical phenomena and improve patient management.

Neuroscience nurses have applied a number of theoretical and conceptual models to the care of neuroscience patients. Some theories may be more effective than others for particular patient populations and practice settings. More of this important work needs to be done and the results disseminated in the literature and at conferences so that nurses can incorporate this information into their practices. Neuroscience nurses also need to increase their use of new knowledge from other biological and psychosocial disciplines to provide quality care to patients and their families.

Nursing research is the foundation for building a scientific knowledge base for practice. The establishment of the National Center for Nursing Research (NCNR) has been a monumental step forward in setting research priorities and supporting nursing research efforts on a national level. A number of NCNR research priorities apply to neuroscience patients. Many other organizations provide small grants for nursing research. As the many nurses who are contributing to neuroscience nursing by conducting clinical research have learned, neuroscience practice is a fertile area for independent nursing research and for collaborative research projects on a variety of neuroscience patient populations. The neurosciences are the fastest-growing life science field in the United States, a growth reflected in neuroscience nursing practice. Research opportunities beckon to those willing to seize them.

THE DECADE OF THE BRAIN

By declaration of Congress, the 1990s have been designated the decade of the brain. This declaration recognizes the immense potential of basic and clinical research in the neurosciences and focuses attention on the planning and program initiatives of the National Institute of Neurological Disorders and Stroke.[1] If one views the 1990s as a decade of transition to the 21st century, this may be interpreted as national recognition of the pivotal role that the neurosciences are expected to play in the health care arena well into the next century.

Being a neuroscience nurse has always been challenging and stimulating. With the dedication of this decade to the brain, neuroscience nursing is poised to enjoy a new level of prominence and attention. The opportunity to shape neuroscience nursing practice in the waning years of the 20th century and in the 21st century is compelling. This evolution is closely tied to changes in the American society, in the health care delivery system, and in the nursing profession.

A THIRD WAVE SOCIETY

We are living at a time when the world's developed nations are being transformed into what the futurist Alvin Toffler calls Third Wave societies.[2] The First Wave, the agricultural revolution, occurred over thousands of years and transformed humankind from nomadic hunter-gatherers to cooperative communities of farmers relying on the soil, a strong extended family, and community networks for support. Health care was provided by the family in the home, sometimes with the assistance of a midwife or doctor.

The Second Wave of change, the rise of the industrial civilization, began with the 19th century and was well under way in the middle 1800s. Jobs shifted from the farms to the city factories where a variety of industries were manufacturing products that the general population craved. The urban population shift accounted for the major societal change in family structure from an extended to a nuclear family and created a need for radically different social, political, economic, and health care structures and services. Rampant communicable diseases and deplorable workplace conditions posed major health problems restricting average life expectancy to less than 50 years. Extended families were not available to care for sick family members; health care shifted to hospitals.

The Third Wave of change brought in the information society, in which we are now living. This wave began to take hold about 1955 with white-collar workers outnumbering blue-collar workers and the widespread introduction of computers, national–international jet travel, and easy communications. Because of the scientific and technological knowledge which had been accumulating for many years, common communicable diseases have been held in check, and there has been a phenomenal growth of medical knowledge resulting in people living longer, but with chronic illnesses. Workplaces are becoming smaller due to the growth of information businesses and the easy access to information through computer technology and the information superhighway.

Colliding waves of change cause conflict and tension. The fiber of American culture is undergoing radical changes as the current political, economic, and societal structures that were erected to support an industrial-wave economy are being reformed to meet the needs of an information society. The health care industry is undergoing major changes as it struggles to align itself with the needs and demands of contemporary society. The only thing certain for the future of health care is more fundamental change in how and where health care is delivered.

MAJOR CHANGES IN THE HEALTH CARE DELIVERY SYSTEM

Health care delivery can be conceptualized as a triad of cost, access, and quality. An understanding of each component of the triad and how these interrelated components affect each other provides a framework for understanding how the entire health care delivery system responds to societal pressures and demands.

The cost of health care in the United States now consumes approximately 15% of the gross national product. Assuming an efficient health care system, access to care and quality of care will be reduced if the revenues available to health care are constrained. Experience in the United States indicates that the response to cost control efforts is an increasingly uneven distribution of health care services, with some clients enjoying state-of-the-art care, many receiving suboptimal care, and others receiving no care. Consumers, third-party reimbursers, and health care authorities agree that the cost of health care must decrease. They maintain that cost can be reduced while providing quality care and access for all. How to achieve this goal is hotly debated.

The inevitability of change is a cliché, but the rate and magnitude of change in health care delivery in the mid-1990s has been unprecedented and promises to accelerate as we go into the next century. Despite the failure of national health care reform legislation in 1994, health care delivery is being radically restructured from within, fueled by the uncompromising goal to control cost while increasing access to care for all and insuring quality. Quality is best evaluated through the use of predetermined measurable outcomes. Practice guidelines, care maps, and standards of care are being used as criteria for evaluating quality of care. Multidisciplinary models of practice with greater emphasis on prevention and health promotion are being implemented to address quality and control cost. Health care is being offered in a variety of convenient settings to increase access to care. Reformation of national health care is being shaped by a number of societal trends which are discussed briefly in the next section.

TRENDS SHAPING HEALTH CARE DELIVERY

Powerful political, economic, demographic, sociological, and technological trends are shaping the health care delivery system as the nation struggles to meet the growing health needs and expectations of its diverse people. These trends are summarized in Chart 1-1. They are discussed briefly below to provide a framework for understanding their impact on the health care system. Due to the overlapping nature of trend categories, some of the discussion relates to more than one category. For efficiency, discussions of particular impacts have been placed in the category that seems most logical.

Political Trends

To some extent, national political trends reflect long-term and deeply held attitudes of the country's middle-class electorate. However, these attitudes are filtered through the prisms of

CHART 1-1
Trends Influencing Reshaping of the Health Care Delivery System

Political

Power and lobbying
Impact of government regulations

Economic

Cost containment
Financing and reimbursement practice

Demographic

Graying of America
Immigration and consequent cultural diversity

Sociological

Consumer activism in health care
Lifestyle changes
Women's movement
AIDS
Quality of life
Caregiver stress

Technological

Proliferation of scientific knowledge
Computer technology
Information superhighway
Influence of trauma centers and specialized units
Increased specialization in medical and nursing practice
Increased emphasis on rehabilitation

multitudes of special interest groups that lobby politicians. The policies, laws, and regulations that result from this process have tremendous impact on economic, demographic, sociological, and technological trends. For this reason, we should be aware of the importance of the political process in promoting or retarding general trends in society.

POWER, SPECIAL INTEREST GROUPS, AND THE BALANCE OF POWER

Politics is the art and science concerned with guiding or influencing policy. It is also the art and science concerned with winning and holding control over a government or an organization. Politics has to do with *power* and who has the power or assumes the most central position to influence, control, and shape the outcome of decisions. Regardless of how small or large the group or organization is, a struggle for power is a dynamic force underlying the relationship and how it develops. Power struggle, power balance, and the exchange of power are ongoing processes that make the world go round.

Being elected or appointed to public or private office provides the holder with power that, if seized, can be used as the bearer sees fit. Health care as a major industry in the United States involving billions of dollars annually is a potent reservoir of power. There are those within the industry who wield tremendous power and represent the special interests of insurers, hospital corporations, health providers such as nurses and physicians, and manufacturers of equipment and supplies. There are also consumer groups that express the views and the special interests of consumers. Elected and appointed persons make laws and rules governing health care; their decisions are influenced by the lobbying of diverse special interest groups that try to exert their influence on decisions regarding health care. In this ongoing process, the key players and pivotal issues can change rapidly under the influence of local and national events and media coverage.

IMPACT OF REGULATIONS

Currently, there is a broad political consensus with regard to health care for the nation: comprehensive, affordable, quality health care for all Americans. The struggle for political power revolves around how "comprehensive," "affordable," and "quality" are ultimately defined from among a wide range of interpretations. For example, the Joint Commission on Accreditation of Healthcare Organizations (JCAHO) defines quality as measurable, prescribed patient care outcomes that require documentation. For the consumer, quality is often defined by the friendliness of the staff or a positive outcome of surgery.

Cost of care continues to rise, largely because of requirements mandated by Medicare, Medicaid, and other entitlement programs whose regulations prescribe certain activities and proscribe others, thus stifling flexibility and creativity. There is an increasing public sentiment to decrease the burdensome requirements of the entitlement programs, to allow states to try different approaches to cost containment, and to require able people to work rather than depend on government-funded health care. These and other controversial issues will be decided in a variety of political arenas. These power struggles will establish the latest political trends shaping the American health care system.

Economic Trends
COST CONTAINMENT

Cost containment and affordability continue to be driving forces affecting all aspects of health care delivery. The cost containment strategies of the 1980s, including diagnosis related groups (DRGs) and utilization review, have had mixed results. Increases in hospital acuity levels and paperwork requirements tended to offset any real cost savings accomplished. The cost control strategies for the 1990s are being spearheaded by managed care and large health networks. In 1993, for the first time, more than half of all Americans whose employers provided health insurance coverage were enrolled in managed-care plans.[3] In managed care environments, there are, theoretically, savings because primary care physicians act as gatekeepers to more expensive specialists such as neurologists and neurosurgeons. What is not clear are the long-term implications for costs if optimal patient outcomes have not been achieved and patients eventually require even more expensive care. Of primary importance are the criteria by which patients are triaged to specialists and the competence of those performing the triage functions. These are complex questions for which there are no simple answers.

Among the promising trends emanating from the cost containment dilemma is the emergence of community based care. There is growing interest in reimbursement for home health care, hospice care, and various outpatient services that can be justified on the basis of cost savings. Another strong trend with cost-saving implications is reimbursement for preventive, health promotion, and rehabilitative services. Preventive and health promotion measures keep people healthy or identify problems in the early, less costly intervention stage. Rehabilitation assists people to be as functional and as independent as possible, thus limiting disuse syndromes, disabilities, and other problems requiring more expensive care.

FINANCING AND REIMBURSEMENT PRACTICES

Fees for health care services in the United States are largely set by formulas promulgated by the federal and state governments for Medicare (elderly) and Medicaid (poor), and by third-party insurers for group and individual insurance. Current estimates indicate that approximately 37 million people in the United States have no medical insurance and little or no ability to pay for services. The cost for their care must be absorbed by the system, mostly through nonprofit hospital emergency rooms. The younger cohorts of the population, together with their employers, are balking at the dramatic increases in Medicare and health insurance costs that they must bear.

People are being asked to choose intelligently among a large assortment of health care plans and health care packages. They are also being required by their employers to assume a greater portion of health care premiums. A more ominous trend is that many employers are no longer offering health care benefits as a condition of employment. Rather than hiring permanent employees, they now fill positions with "temporary help" who are not given health care benefits. These economic trends are central to the health care delivery debate and place pressure for reform squarely in the political arena.

DEMOGRAPHIC TRENDS

There are two major demographic trends impacting on health care in the US: the graying of America associated with the baby boom phenomenon and increasing life span for many, and increasing cultural diversity associated with increased immigration.

The Graying of America. Many believe that the changing age profile of America will be the greatest force shaping health care for the next 40 years. The nation's baby boomers, those 76 million born between 1946 and 1964, will drive the nation's health care consumption curve up steeply as they enter the age spectrum where the manifestations of chronic illness predominate. By the year 2000, people aged 45 to 54 years will number 36 million, and the onslaught of their increased health

care needs should be well under way. By the year 2030, those who are 65 years and older will account for 20% of the population, a greater percentage than children.[4] The groups of people over 75 years and even over 85 years are the fastest-growing segments of the population.

The graying of America is occurring not only because the absolute numbers entering these age groups are growing, but also because a larger percentage is surviving to older ages. Life expectancy has been increasing steadily for several decades, largely as a result of (1) improved economic conditions for older Americans, coupled with improved access to affordable, quality health care; (2) strides made in the treatment of many diseases of old age, especially cancer and heart disease, which have extended life significantly; and (3) a new appreciation for the benefits of a healthy lifestyle, including diet, personal habits, exercise, and stress reduction. Nevertheless, with aging eventually comes an overall increase in chronic illnesses such as coronary artery disease, osteoarthritis, and Alzheimer's disease. The greatly increased prevalence of these diseases and others will impose an increased burden on the system and require a redirection of scarce societal resources toward these needs. While management of chronic illness is causing a major shift in health care to meet the needs of people who are living longer, it is apparent that at some point, the common good may require that some of the resources devoted to elder care be allocated to other segments of society.

Related ethical decision making is likely to focus on the care provided for the growing number of chronically ill elderly who have a substantially decreased quality of life. It is well documented that the use of health care resources is the highest during the last year of life and that these resources are often expended with little, if any, gain in quality or quantity of life. The underdevelopment of less costly community based care and support services to assist the elderly and their families in managing their needs in their homes has led to utilization of the high cost alternative, hospital care. Independent healthy elderly, on the other hand, need help with continued health promotion and preventive measures to keep them healthy and independent. There is a growing realization that the impending stress posed by the graying of America on the health care system has serious consequences for the future health of all sectors of the U. S. economy.

Immigration and Consequent Cultural Diversity. The second major demographic trend to shape and increase the need for health care into the 21st century is the greatly increased infusion of multiple ethnic and culturally diverse groups into the United States. This reality is changing the economics, process, and structure of health care delivery. The primary migration from Western Europe in the first half of the century has been replaced by an influx of people from Asia, Africa, and Central and South America. Smaller but growing numbers are coming from the Moslem countries of the Middle East and the newly configured countries of the former Soviet Union. A relatively small number come through the traditional and legal immigration channels. Many now come through special immigration programs for political refugees.

The problems accompanying the illegal influx of millions of uneducated and poor immigrants from Mexico and Central and Latin American countries have become a source of great political and economic stress in the border states affected. Intolerant border-state taxpayers argue that this influx is over-burdening schools, health care facilities, and other institutions while placing an unfair tax burden on them. This economic burden has raised the cry for the federal government, which has been unsuccessful in curbing the illegal migration, to absorbed the cost of all these services.

Immigrant groups bring with them ethnic and cultural values that include belief–value systems about health and illness throughout the life cycle. The values and rituals of Western medicine are often held suspect by members of these groups and may be rejected in favor of their own ethnic and folk medicine. Health care professionals must nevertheless understand and respect their cultural values and strive to develop cultural competence and implement programs that are culturally sensitive as well as effective. Education of both health care providers and health care recipients with the goal of easing the transition from native culture to American culture is necessary if mutual needs are to be addressed.

Sociological Trends

Unlike temporary fads and fashions, deep-rooted trends in attitude and values develop over generations in reaction to our shared experiences on community, national, and global levels. These long-term trends, therefore, have a tremendous impact on the ways in which we shape and interact with institutions of society. Of the numerous sociological trends influencing society in general and the course of health care in particular, the following few are discussed briefly because of their relevance in neuroscience practice: consumer activism, lifestyle changes, the women's movement, acquired immunodeficiency syndrome (AIDS), quality of life, and caregiver stress.

CONSUMER ACTIVISM IN HEALTH CARE

Our values and attitudes toward our health, as indeed toward all matters, are formed by the information to which we are exposed. As more and more information has become widely available, consumers have become more active in choosing, evaluating, and criticizing the products and services available to them. The health care delivery system has been tremendously affected by this growing activist trend in the age of information.

Broadcast and print media are still the principal sources of consumer information about health care; cable television, books, video tapes, and computer networks in particular are growing in importance, especially among the better-educated segments of society. For example, Medline and on-line computer health bulletin boards are now easily accessible by the public, and people are using them in greater numbers to become well educated and informed about their health and medical problems. As a result, many consumers demand to be actively involved in making decisions about their health and health care options. They no longer do what they are told to do by the health provider without question or input into selection of alternatives for care. They are also interested in alternative, nontraditional health care such as massage therapy, homeopathic treatment, and relaxation therapies. Advance directives are becoming more common. The demand for information and involvement in decision making has created a new industry of educational material for the consumer.

LIFESTYLE CHANGES

Despite sending sometimes confusing signals, widely disseminated information about the health implications of smoking, alcohol abuse, drug abuse, diet, exercise, stress, and sexual practices has had an enormous impact on the behavior of many individuals, leading to lifestyle changes that are decreasing disease frequency and severity. Failure to heed, however, continues to be a serious public health dilemma. For example, adult obesity continues to increase and smoking in certain segments of the female population continues to increase while smoking in general declines. With so many serious chronic diseases associated with smoking and obesity, these are ominous trends. As women have become more engaged in high-stress occupations, negative lifestyle factors such as poor diet, infrequent exercise, and increased stress are afflicting them as grievously as they have been afflicting men. Positive lifestyle changes are also apparent. Exercise, weight control, low-fat and low-cholesterol diets, and stress reduction are all health promotion and disease prevention basics embraced by a large and growing number of Americans. The outcome of these conflicting trends in terms of mortality and morbidity is uncertain. Either way, they will be felt in practice settings.

THE WOMEN'S MOVEMENT

An important social and political trend labeled "feminism" or "equal rights for women" has been steadily growing in the united states for the last three decades and has gradually changed the role of women in society. In line with this trend, women's health is being recognized as a legitimate specialty practice, more programs designed to meet the special health needs of women across the life cycle are being established, and more health providers are practicing in this specialty area. In addition, research funds are being earmarked to support women's health issues such as breast cancer screening and treatment. Coronary artery disease in women, previously neglected because of a gender bias in medical thinking, is now receiving the attention it deserves on the basis of the prevalence and severity of the disease in women.

AIDS

Perhaps the most dramatic sociological phenomenon to impact on the health care system in recent years is AIDS. Because of its communicability and its current incurability, AIDS presents issues that extend to every segment of health care. Of the issues involved, legal, ethical, and caregiver safety concerns predominate. AIDS offers a good example of how priorities can be skewed by effective political activism so that a disproportionate amount of governmental funding and health care system resources are targeted toward one problem at the expense of other health problems. As with many modern diseases, AIDS is almost exclusively a behaviorally related condition which is theoretically susceptible to preventive lifestyle change. As with other such preventable diseases, efforts to change behavior are likely to continue to be met with mixed results.

QUALITY OF LIFE

In many cases, technology now allows for extension of life indefinitely even though the quality of that life may be minimal or nonexistent. With regard to these cases, there is passionate debate on the humanity of and entitlement to high-tech care. Patients and family members have become more attuned to factoring quality of life into their decisions about health care and extraordinary means of maintaining life. How these issues, which are addressed in Chapters 4 and 15, are resolved has tremendous implications for the future cost of health care, personal and clinical decision making, and the way health professionals practice.

CAREGIVER STRESS

The role of caregiver has increasingly been assumed by family members who must care for another family member at home. Caring for a person with multiple deficits and needs for 24 hours a day is now recognized as an overwhelming responsibility for anyone to assume. The successful resuscitation of trauma victims and patients experiencing acute neurological events results in survival, but with multiple deficits. Improved management of patients with chronic neurological diseases, such as stroke, multiple sclerosis, Parkinson's disease, and others, has resulted in longer survival. Such patients have needs that can place a tremendous burden on the family caregiver. The public outcry for recognition of the stresses and needs of family caregivers has resulted in increased community support services for both the patient and family caregiver. Support groups and lobbying efforts of organizations such as the National Head Injury Foundation and Alzheimer's disease groups have helped to focus attention and secure funds for the care of persons with neurological deficits. There are many groups with worthwhile goals competing for limited resources to fund programs for special patient populations. As a result, there are great opportunities for neuroscience nurses to develop programs that address the special needs of patients and their family caregivers.

Technological Trends

The information society in which we live is characterized by a proliferation of information about world, national, and local issues, all of which are rapidly communicated to anyone able to read a newspaper, watch television, or turn on a computer. Computer technology has changed how we live, work, and learn. Computers provide access to information superhighways to more and more people. Moreover, the information is disseminated so rapidly that today's sensational product is obsolete by tomorrow. Even a casual reader of the scientific literature cannot help but be amazed by the discoveries and new technologies that are emerging in almost every area of scientific study.

The various areas of impact of this great technology explosion have already been mentioned in the previous sections. Diseases are being diagnosed at an earlier stage, new interventions have been developed for previously untreatable diseases (notably, genetically based diseases), more interventions are noninvasive, and more precise and effective interventions with fewer complications and residual effects are becoming available for common medical problems.

To cope with these events, medicine and nursing continue to become more specialized as the time and practice requirements to become expert in certain procedures and equipment become more demanding. Interventional neuroradiology and interventional cardiology are recent examples. At the same time, health care settings are becoming more specialized. The new, experimental, and highly advanced interventions of the future will only be available at a relatively few, highly specialized centers. Technology is also having a dramatic effect on rehabilitation. Development of new, high-tech prosthetic devices, as well as the opportunity that new interventions offer for saving and restoring function, will have a profound effect on the quality of life of many patients who have sustained trauma or who are dealing with chronic disease.

NATIONAL AGENDAS FOR HEALTH

A number of initiatives have been undertaken by governmental, private, and professional organizations in an attempt to influence the future direction of health care in the nation. Three of the more ambitious and promising initiatives are *Healthy People 2000,* Patient Outcomes Research Teams, and Prevention Guidelines.

Healthy People 2000

The quintessential document outlining a comprehensive plan for the health care of the nation is *Healthy People 2000,* an unprecedented cooperative effort bringing together a wide spectrum of interests including government and business, voluntary and professional organizations, and private individuals. The report urges the following broad public health goals: (1) increase the span of healthy life for Americans; (2) reduce health disparities among Americans; and (3) achieve access to preventive services for all Americans. To meet these goals by the year 2000, 300 specific objectives were identified and organized around 22 priority areas. Measurable targets were set for improvements in health status, risk reduction, and service delivery. The national objectives are organized under the three broad categories of health promotion, health protection, and preventive services.[5] An additional priority, surveillance and data systems, addresses the need for systematic collection, analysis, interpretation, dissemination, and use of health data to understand the health status of the nation and to plan effective prevention programs.[6] The challenge of *Healthy People 2000* as stated in the document is

. . . to use the combined strength of scientific knowledge, professional skill, individual commitment, community support, and political will to enable people to achieve their potential to live full, active lives. It means preventing premature death and preventing disability, preserving a physical environment that supports human life, cultivating family and community support, enhancing each individual's inherent abilities to respond and to act, and assuring that all Americans achieve and maintain a maximum level of functioning.[7]

The reader is encouraged to review the entire publication to appreciate the magnitude of this national health agenda.

Patient Outcomes Research Teams (PORTs)

Medically effective research relating clinical practices and their costs to measurable improvements in patients' health is a mandate of the Agency for Health Care Policy and Research (AHCPR). This mandate is being funded through PORTs. The purpose of the PORT program is to fund multidisciplinary teams of investigators to identify effective care for a variety of common medical and surgical health problems.[8] The ultimate goal of this program is to disseminate the findings of these studies to the clinical community in the form of clinical practice guidelines as a means of establishing effective standards of care.[9] Examples of topics that have been the focus of PORT studies are type II diabetes, management of cancer pain, and stroke rehabilitation. Once clinical practice guidelines are made available through the AHCPR Publications Clearinghouse, they become the standards of care for health professionals. These guidelines are exceptional resources for nurses to incorporate into their practice. Headache treatment will be the next addition to the guidelines.

Prevention Guidelines

The United States Public Health Services has taken a major step in enhancing the delivery of preventive care in primary care practice with the campaign called "Put Prevention Into Practice." The *Clinician's Handbook of Preventive Services: Put Prevention Into Practice,* published by the American Nurses Association, is part of a set of published materials created for dissemination to primary care clinicians as a practical and comprehensive reference on clinical preventive services.[10] Included are health screening schedules for the early detection of disease, immunizations and prophylactics to prevent disease, and counseling to modify risk factors that lead to disease. The book provides concise, brief descriptions of current, targeted, age-specific preventive interventions and strategies recommended for preventive care. This outstanding, up-to-date reference, which also lists educational resources on preventive care for health professionals, patients, and their families, is now the gold standard for preventive care in the United States.[11] Neuroscience practitioners will find this book helpful as they assume more responsibility for prevention. Stroke, for example, is a common neurological problem that has risk factors, such as hypertension and high cholesterol, that can be controlled. Specific information about modification of risk factors is included in this book.

Primary care has become a central component of federal, state, local, and private initiatives to reorganize health care, highlighting preventive care as a component within the context of primary care. The term *primary care,* introduced in the 1960s from Europe, traditionally specified four main components: the provision of first-contact care, person-focused care over time, comprehensive care, and coordinated care. In the 1990s, the traditional definition seemed inadequate for the contemporary complexities in health care delivery and the more multidisciplinary, collaborative models of practice. As a result, the Institute of Medicine (IOM) refined the definition of primary care in a report entitled *Defining Primary Care: An Interim Report.*[12] In that report, primary care is defined as "the provision of integrated, accessible health care services by clinicians who are accountable for addressing a large majority of personal health care needs, developing a sustained partnership with patients, and practicing in the context of family and community."

What is going to happen to specialty practice?[13] Those of us in specialty practice, in considering the holistic needs of our neuroscience patients, will interface with primary care providers and work collaboratively to achieve optimal outcomes for our patients.

REFORMATION OF HEALTH CARE AND IMPLICATIONS FOR NEUROSCIENCE PATIENTS AND NEUROSCIENCE NURSING PRACTICE

Reformation of the Health Care System

The health care system and how health care professionals practice is changing and will continue to change significantly into the 21st century.[14] This fundamental reform of health care will have a major impact on both neuroscience patients and neuroscience nursing practice.

Three terms commonly used to provide a framework for understanding health care reform are restructuring, reengineering, and redesigning. *Restructuring* means to rebuild, reorganize, reconfigure, reconstruct or change the *structure* of an organization or system; in the context of health care, restructuring refers to the reconfiguring of the organization or institution and is usually diagrammatically noted on the organization chart. *Reengineering* is the fundamental rethinking and radical redesign of *processes* to achieve dramatic improvements in critical, contemporary measures of performance such as cost, quality, service, and speed;[15] in health care, it is "starting over" and rethinking all of the processes involved in providing care. *Redesigning* is a term focusing on the revision in appearance, function, or content of *what people in an organization do*; in health care it is redesigning that answers the question who does what in providing care and services to patients. Redesigning of practice has utmost impact on nurses and nursing practice.

RESTRUCTURING OF HEALTH CARE

Dramatic and innovative changes are underway in the structuring of health care facilities as they attempt to respond to the forces and trends of the marketplace. Some hospitals have closed after realizing that they could not offer quality care amidst the new economic realities. Those tertiary hospitals that remain are giant intensive care units (ICUs). Hospital stays are shorter and patients are going home "quicker and sicker" with needs that extend beyond the walls of the hospital into the community.

Most hospitals are either downsizing, often called "right-sizing," or merging with other health care organizations. Mergers allow independent facilities to work collaboratively to capture a mutually profitable market share of patients rather than compete on an independent basis for a limited pool of patients. In many mergers, services that were previously duplicated in the independent facilities are consolidated or reapportioned to eliminate duplication. This is true not only for medical services but also for administrative, purchasing, janitorial, and other nonmedical functions. Some mergers and buyouts are designed to create major comprehensive regional health care networks to provide a continuum of care from primary preventive care through centralized tertiary care. Large regional networks are forming and serve both rural and urban areas. These networks use sophisticated systems of communication and transportation for consultations and referrals to health providers who schedule periodic clinics in facilities located where the patients live. Comprehensive care networks also offer community based care (home care, hospice care), ambulatory clinics, short stay hospitalization, and tertiary care centers.

As restructuring is apparent in the changed mix of facilities and services being offered by providers, it is also apparent in their altered organizational charts. Decentralization, begun in the 1980s, continues, and the business concepts of a matrix structure and product lines are being added to better delineate responsibility and accountability for managers. New product line categories, such as "hotel services," are now included in the organizational structure, reflecting the new emphasis on creature comforts of patients and their families. Health care facilities are striving to become user-friendly, comfortable environments that meet the needs of their patients rather than inflexible structures requiring conformity of patients and their families.

Restructuring: Implications for Neuroscience Patients and Practice. A paradigm shift from an acute care model to a chronic care model is occurring in health care and will dictate how health care is delivered into the 21st century. In this context, it is significant that so many neurological problems are either chronic in nature, such as with Parkinson's disease and multiple sclerosis, or result in chronic, long-term functional disabilities, such as with head injury, spinal injury, and stroke. The needs of patients with chronic illness are quite different from those with acute problems. Home care is more desirable for most neurological patients and their families. It is also less expensive than institutional care. To meet these realities, the structures for chronic illness management within the health care system and health networks need to be better defined, developed, and expanded.

For neuroscience patients who need acute care management, it is available in hospital Neuro ICUs and other specialty units. As already noted, hospitals are becoming giant ICUs. Neuro ICUs especially are becoming high-tech environments filled with computers, complex patient support and monitoring equipment, and highly skilled staff with very specialized training. Other specialty units, such as Acute Stroke Units, focus on supporting early recovery from stroke, often with the use of neuron-protective drugs and thrombolytic therapy for ischemic strokes. The intermediate units of hospitals are shrinking in size. In all units, stays are shorter with patients being discharged often with major rehabilitative and other needs. One concern with health care reform is whether patients will be able to efficiently access specialists and specialty units for care. Currently, given the cost containment environment, the question of how effectively patients are being triaged to specialty care within their managed care plans is of major concern.

REENGINEERING OF HEALTH CARE

Health care reengineering focuses on the processes involved in providing care and services to patients and their families. According to Hammer and Champy, reengineering begins with asking "why do we do what we do? and why do we do it in the way we do?"[16] Particularly in health care, the answer is often "that's the way we have always done it here," or "that's our policy. . . ," discussion closed! Practitioners can point to countless ways of conducting business that appear mindless and idiotic, but traditions live on. How we develop standards of care or care maps; how we develop and regulate visiting hours, admission, discharges, and transfers; and how we teach patients and families are examples of processes that can be conducted in many ways, some more reasonable, sensible, and successful than others.

Many confusing and imprecise terms are used to describe health care reform. Often, they refer to new processes in the delivery of care intended to increase efficiency through coordination, collaboration, cost control, and refinement of whatever measurable outcomes seem appropriate at the time. Managed care, a key concept in health care reform, is an example. Other process-focused reengineering initiatives intended to control cost are managed competition, health alliances, and capitation. One could argue that health alliances are also new structures within health care and therefore are examples of restructuring. While it is true that they may be viewed as conceptual structures, the primary purpose of alliances is a reengineering of business processes, and for that reason, they should be considered a reengineering rather than a restructuring initiative.

Reengineering: Implications for Neuroscience Patients and Practice. Most patients, including neuroscience patients, will receive care under managed care contracts. Patients will receive all of their care from prevention, health promotion, acute and chronic illness management, and rehabilitative services through giant health care networks. Nurses caring for neuroscience patients will work collaboratively with case managers to expeditiously provide the care patients and families need using care maps. Nurses will be responsible and accountable for achieving predetermined measurable outcomes for patients. More and more health services will be shifted from the relatively high-cost institutional arena to community settings.[17] Community based care will grow tremendously, and this will include further development of home care for neurological patients.

Multidisciplinary care maps will guide neuroscience practice with achievement of measurable outcomes as the goal. Additional guidelines for practice will be introduced as national and hospital groups study specific processes of care to determine efficacy and cost. For example, hospitals will publish guidelines and criteria on when to intubate and when to extubate. Neuro drug formularies will be developed which will indicate drugs that should be used for sedation of agitated patients based on literature reviews and efficacy studies as well as costs. Practitioners will have less latitude to choose from a wide array of interventions available, but instead will be expected to use those interventions that have proven quality outcome measures and are cost effective.

Traditional policies and procedures will be examined. More services will be provided for the comfort of patients and families as health care organizations compete for patients. Settings of care will be reexamined. More patients will receive high-tech care in the home and in community based facilities rather than in hospitals. Patients and families will assume more responsibility for care. In addition, health care will focus on disease prevention and health maintenance in all health care services rendered. Neuroscience nurses should be an integral part of teams making these critical decisions about care and should be in the vanguard of those reaching out to provide community and home-based care for neuro patients.

REDESIGNING OF HEALTH CARE

Redesigning of health care refers to who does what. The optimum staff mix for a unit has been a matter of debate for many years, regardless of whether the unit under discussion is within a hospital, a clinic, or a community based program. From the nursing perspective, the 1980s saw the trend to an all-RN staff intermingled with the optimistic goal of requiring a BSN degree for all members of the nursing staff. A substantial portion of an operating budget is devoted to RNs' salaries, and the question is raised whether an RN must personally execute all of the activities that are commonly performed directly and indirectly for patients. The informal nursing communication network, as well as the nursing literature, has long discussed the inappropriate utilization of professional nurses and the need to assign tasks based on educational preparation.

With the new focus on redesign, many health care organizations have engaged consultants to examine which types of activities are best performed by professional nurses and other nonlicensed staff and how much time is spent performing each activity. Transport of some patients, restocking equipment, and answering the telephone are examples of activities that could be assumed safely by nonlicensed persons at a savings in cost. It is these concerns that are the basis for proposed changes of the unit staff mix and for the redesign of roles and responsibilities. Proponents of redesign also argue that redistributing non-nursing functions to nonlicensed personnel will improve the job satisfaction of nurses. Many health care organizations begin redesign with a nurse to non-nurse staff mix of around 70/30. A common goal of redesign is to reduce this mix to at least 50/50. The effects of this effort in redesign are apparent nationwide, with some new graduates and experienced nurses unable to find nursing positions.

Embedded within the above redesign process is the unresolved issue of what is the appropriate differential practice for nurses educationally prepared at the associate, baccalaureate, and graduate levels. Integrative tri-level models of professional practice have been proposed by Newman, but there has been little success over the years to clearly differentiate roles in nursing practice based on educational

preparedness.[18] Moreover, both master's-prepared and doctorally prepared nurses have traditionally been lumped together for purposes of describing nurses with graduate education. Some of the current discussion on redesign centers on the need for graduate preparation of nurse practitioners and on the appropriate role for clinical nurse specialists who have been traditionally prepared at the master's level. The debate seeks to resolve the issues surrounding educational preparation and the clinical roles of those nurses considered "advanced practice nurses."

Redesigning: Implications for Neuroscience Patients and Practice. Who should do what for patients is central to redesign. As roles, responsibilities, and accountability for neuroscience practice is redesigned, neuroscience practice will continue to evolve. This is true for physicians as well as nurses and other health professionals. Redistribution of roles and responsibilities will occur depending on education, experience, and the environment. In the early 1900s, the blood pressure cuff, heralded as a cutting-edge innovation, was introduced in the United States. Taking a blood pressure was the sole responsibility of the physician. Now, nurses and some nonlicensed personnel take and record blood pressure. While giving up responsibility for some activities, physicians assume new responsibilities; this is also true of nurses.

As staff-mix changes occur, nurses will be responsible for supervising nonlicensed personnel. Nurses must be involved in decisions regarding the use of nonlicensed personnel including identification of activities to be safely assumed and under what circumstances they can be assumed; educational requirements to safely and competently execute assumed duties; and requirements for supervision and monitoring of personnel to assure quality and accuracy. For example, nonlicensed personnel can safely assist a neurological patient with eating if the patient has been assessed for swallowing and found to have no difficulty. However, if the patient is at high risk for aspiration, then the nurse should attend to the patient. Neurological patients can change rapidly and the nurse must assume responsibility for making ongoing decisions about delivery of safe care.

Advanced practice nurses (APNs) are assuming new roles in neuroscience practice as nurse practitioners in tertiary settings on Neuro ICUs, intermediate units, neuro clinics, rehabilitation programs, and community based programs such as home care. These nurses are assuming responsibility for diagnosing some neurological problems and for prescribing treatment plans. Many chronic neurological problems can be well managed by APNs who combine a holistic nursing framework with a medical framework. This trend is expected to grow in the United States as medical residents in specialty practice decrease due to a shift to primary care. Furthermore, there is the realization that differentiation of roles for nurses is key to providing cost effective, quality care.

Neuroscience nurses working at the bedside will find that they are being cross trained in other clinical areas so that they can move between areas as staffing needs increase and decrease. Fewer RNs will be practicing in hospitals; however, this will be balanced by a growing need for nurses with neuroscience skills in community based care, especially home care. A discussion of changing models of practice is found in Chapter 2.

LIVING IN THE PRESENT WHILE PREPARING FOR THE FUTURE

Professional life on the brink of the 21st century involves dealing with a rapidly changing present while preparing for future change which may come quickly and frequently. No longer can a nurse depend on his or her basic training to prepare for years of practice. This creates ongoing challenges and stresses. Neuroscience nurses need general knowledge and skills that will provide them with the tools to function effectively now, to anticipate future change, and to confidently ease themselves into the future. The bank of information grows exponentially each year. Perhaps the most useful and versatile tools for practice in the future environment are critical thinking skills and computer literacy.

No one can know everything, but through critical reasoning one can decide which information is necessary and where to find it. Critical reasoning applied to clinical practice is called *clinical reasoning* or *diagnostic reasoning*. Reasoning skills help us to analyze clinical situations and choose an appropriate plan of care. Critical thinking and clinical reasoning skills can be learned and developed. They are discussed further in Chapter 3.

Computer literacy is already vital if one wishes to access information efficiently. It will become essential in the future. The information highway is not just a marketing phrase: it describes a system that will provide easy access to libraries, databases, bulletin boards, and countless other resources in the world—a system that will become every bit as integral to society as the interstate highway system. Without the necessary driving skills, one will be living in the equivalent of horse-and-buggy America without the basic tools to sustain a viable professional life. Critical thinking skills and computer literacy are the keys to surviving into the 21st century and beyond.

References

1. Goldstein, M. (1990). The decade of the brain: An era of promise for neurosurgery and a call to action. *Journal of Neurosurgery, 73,* 1–2.
2. Toffler, A. (1980). *The third wave.* New York: Bantam Books.
3. Gabel et al., 1994.
4. Kennedy, P. (1993). *Preparing for the twenty-first century.* New York: Random House.
5. United States Public Health Service. (1990). *Healthy people 2000* (DHHS Publication No. PHS 91-50213). Washington, DC: U.S. Government Printing Office, p. 6.
6. Ibid., p. 79.
7. Ibid., p. 60.
8. Greene, R., Maklan, C. W., & Bondy, P. K. (1994). The national medical effectiveness research initiative. *Diabetes Care, 17*(Suppl. 1), 45–49.
9. Greenfield, S., Kaplan, S. H., Sillman, R. A., Sullivan, L., Manning, W., D'Agostino, R., Singer, D. E., & Nathan, D. M. (1994). The uses of outcomes research for medical effectiveness, quality of care, and reimbursement in type II diabetes. *Diabetes Care, 17*(Suppl. 1), 32–39.
10. American Nurses Association. (1994). *Clinician's handbook of preventive services: Put prevention into practice.* Washington, DC: Author.
11. Ibid., p. xi.
12. Donaldson, M., Yordy, K., & Vanselow, E. (Eds.). (1994). *Defining primary care: An interim report.* Washington, DC: National Academy Press.
13. Kassirer, J. P. (1994). Access to specialty care. *New England Journal of Medicine, 331*(17), 1151–1152.
14. Lundberg, G. D. (1994). An overview of health system reform. *JAMA, 271*(17), 1368, 1374.
15. Hammer, M., & Champy, J. (1993). *Reengineering the corporation.* New York: Harper Business, p. 32.
16. Ibid., p. 32.
17. Hash, M. (1988). Structuring and financing of community health services. In *Nursing practice in the 21st century.* Kansas City, MO: American Nurses Association.
18. Newman, M. A. (1990). Toward an integrative model of professional practice. *Journal of Professional Nursing, 6*(3), 167–173.

CHAPTER 2

The Continuum of Care and Models of Practice

Joanne V. Hickey

After several decades of relative stability, the health care system has been changing dramatically in recent years. In response, neuroscience nursing practice is transforming itself to adjust to the new realities of health care going into the 21st century. Neuroscience nurses, regardless of their practice settings, are rethinking their roles and responsibilities to patients, to families, and to their employers. All health professionals are being encouraged to expand the scope of practice to include disease prevention activities such as early screening, counseling on modification of risk factors, and promotion of healthy lifestyles. For neuroscience nurses, who care for patients along the continuum of care from intensive care units to home care, managed care environments are forcing more global thinking about health care delivery and scope of practice. The purpose of this chapter is to explore the implications of these changes for neuroscience nursing.

THE CONTINUUM OF CARE

It used to be that the term *continuum of care* (not to be confused with *continuity of care*, which will be discussed later in this chapter) referred to providing patients with an appropriate level of care in the hospital setting as they progressed toward recovery from an acute illness. Thus, the concept was narrowly focused on units of acuity within hospitals such as intensive care, intermediate, and outpatient settings. After tertiary hospitalization, some patients were admitted to rehabilitation or long-term care facilities, but the ultimate endpoint of care was always return to the community and home. Information about what happened in the community was scant and often was a tangential and disjointed piece of the patient's health history if they were readmitted to a health care facility.

As the health care system evolves both *structurally* and *in the processes* of providing care, continuum of care is becoming a less exact and more comprehensive concept which is contin-

ually undergoing refinement and redefinition. Three major forces—restructuring, redesigning, and reengineering—are reshaping the concept of continuum of care.

The restructuring and downsizing of predominantly institutional care has placed a new emphasis on community based care leading to accelerated growth in this care setting. Institutional care refers to care provided in facilities such as hospitals and nursing homes where patients are admitted for a period of time on a 24-hour-a-day basis until they are discharged to another type of institution, to community based care, to their homes, or to die. Within hospitals, more specialty units have developed, such as chronically critically ill units, ventilatory dependent units, stroke step-down units, and collaborative care units, all designed to meet the needs of special populations efficiently and cost-effectively.

Community based care refers to care that is provided in a community setting, usually the community where the patient resides. Care is provided in the home or at a site where the patient goes for care and then the patient returns home at the end of the day. Community based care is generally less expensive than institutional care, and is often preferable and more convenient to the patient and family. The cost savings is particularly attractive to third party payers. More and more high-tech care, traditionally provided only in institutions, is becoming available in the community. Home health care, in particular, is being used more often and has expanded services to include more infusion therapy, ventilatory support, rehabilitation, and other services traditionally associated with institutional care. This phenomenal growth of services in the community has led to corresponding organizational structures to support community based care.

The second major force affecting changes in the continuum of care is the redesigning of care, that is, "who does what," which is an issue that will continue to be renegotiated in all care settings. As certain responsibilities are relinquished by middle-level care providers, other health professionals will assume new responsibilities and accountabilities within the rapidly changing health care system. Further discussion of roles and responsibilities is found within the section on collaboration.

A third major force, the reengineering of the processes of care, that is, "how" care is delivered and "what" care is delivered, is also affecting the continuum of care. The shift of focus from sick care to health care is apparent as emphasis in processes of care shift to primary care. The provisional definition of primary care adopted by the Institute of Medicine (IOM) is as follows:

Primary care is the provision of integrated, accessible health care services by clinicians who are accountable for addressing a large majority of personal health care needs, developing a sustained partnership with patients, and practicing in the context of family and community.[1]

According to the IOM report, primary care is *comprehensive care*, that is, care of any and all health problems at a given stage of a person's life. It includes ongoing care of patients in various care setting such as hospitals, nursing homes, clinicians' offices, community sites, schools, and homes.[2] The assumption was made by the committee that primary care is the logical foundation of an effective health care system because primary care can address a large majority of the health problems of the population.[3] The diagnosis and treatment of some neurological problems will be managed exclusively by primary care physicians or collaboratively with neurologists and neurosurgeons. This positions the primary care physician as the gatekeeper for care including referrals for specialty neurological care. Within the context of primary care, disease prevention, health promotion, and health maintenance are major focuses.

DISEASE PREVENTION, HEALTH PROMOTION, AND HEALTH MAINTENANCE

Three levels of prevention are generally recognized for disease and disability:[4]

1. *Primary prevention*: any intervention that prevents a pathological process from occurring. Examples include immunization or identification and control of risk factors such as smoking with the ultimate goal of preventing vascular disease such as stroke.
2. *Secondary prevention*: intervention after a pathological process has been initiated, but before symptoms occur. For example, prescription of acetylsalicylic acid in patients who have significant plaque formation in one or both carotid arteries may prevent stroke.
3. *Tertiary prevention*: prevention of progressive disability or other complications in individuals with established disease. For example, community management of patients with Parkinson's disease or multiple sclerosis is designed to include prevention of complications such as injury due to falls and decreased levels of mobility.

Health promotion and health maintenance are related terms that refer to the advocacy and provision of programs and strategies that have been demonstrated through research and practice to be beneficial in maintaining optimum health and preventing disease and disability. For instance, we now know that there are many factors related to diet, exercise, and personal habits that are essential for all people to live healthy and productive lives.

As primary care physicians become more involved in managing care of neurological patients, there will be increased emphasis on maintaining and promoting health so there will not be an exacerbation of neurological conditions due to problems with other systems, or conversely, an effect on other systems due to poorly managed neurological conditions.

New partnerships between primary care physicians and neuroscience health professionals are being forged in the new health care system. Patients with complex neurological problems and those requiring acute care management or hospitalization or long-term management of chronic illness will continue to need neurological specialists to assume a leadership role in their care. The neurological specialist assuming this role may be a physician or an advanced practice nurse.

The efficient and economical movement of patients along the continuum of care will grow in importance as the transformation in health care continues. The criteria for deciding when patients should be moved from one stage to another will come from new research initiatives focusing on the key indicators of transition points of diseases and illnesses and on measurable outcomes to be expected at various stages. Transitions in health status and the consequent changing need for health care services are occurring more rapidly. The health care system must be able to respond quickly and efficiently to provide transitional care and control costly delays in services. Transitions in care and transitional care will be discussed in Chapter 15.

KEY CONCEPTS IN PROVIDING HEALTH CARE

Chapter 1 discusses the difficulty of both providing increased access to health care and reducing health care costs while still maintaining quality care. The success of individual efforts toward these seemingly contrary goals depends strongly upon how well three key interrelated concepts in providing care are implemented. These concepts, which are the cornerstones of health care for the mid-1990s and 21st century, are coordination of care, continuity of care, and accountability for care.

Coordination of care implies that there is an active and effective coordinator who identifies specific patient needs, initiates actions to meet those needs, and integrates these actions to promote *appropriate and timely* use of resources and services for the patient and family. Services can include laboratory services, support services, and specialty consultative services. Essential components of effective coordination are (1) the positioning of the coordinator to be able to envision the "big picture"; and (2) the coordinator's ability to communicate proper information to the appropriate people (*e.g.*, patient, family, service providers) regarding what is specifically needed, why it is needed, and the expected measurable outcome to be achieved. The person responsible and accountable for coordination must also be effective in follow-up to monitor the progression of activities and be able to identify when course modification or implementation of an alternative plan is necessary to achieve optimal outcomes.

Continuity of care is a concept that describes the ideal result of well-coordinated care throughout a person's illness and across health care settings. It is the expeditious process of providing uninterrupted, cohesive, continuous care that is maintained throughout the transition points of illness including transition from institutional care to community based care.

Accountability for care, as defined by the IOM, includes the following: measuring outcome against standards for quality of care; providing information to allow for informed decision making by patient, family, and health professionals; accountability for appropriate and efficient use of services and care; high standards of ethical and moral behavior; and patient satisfaction.[5]

These concepts apply equally to the models for management of patients with acute and chronic neurological problems discussed later in this chapter.

Financing and Delivering Health Care

Over the last 40 or 50 years, the United States has evolved a complex system of delivering and financing health care. Health insurance companies, the so-called "third party payers," have become the universal vehicles through which health service providers are paid. This creates a discontinuity between the receivers and providers of health services which limits an individual's ability to search out and select the most cost-effective provider. Health policy authorities often identify this as a major source of the health care financing crisis.

As health insurance has evolved, benefit packages have become increasingly comprehensive, another basis for increasing costs. Copayments required of subscribers have tended to remain modest and many services are often completely reimbursed. While few people can afford complete fee-for-service care, it has become increasingly obvious that the system cannot be sustained without greater cost assumption from the consumers.

Those without health care insurance and with very low financial assets and income receive reasonably adequate care free of charge through Medicaid, the governmental program for the poor. Others without health insurance who do not qualify for Medicaid receive limited and sporadic care on a "catch as catch can" basis, often through hospital emergency departments with the cost transferred to the health insurance system. The effect that providing equal access to comprehensive care through a federally financed system has on health costs and quality has been hotly debated. For the foreseeable future, it appears that other remedies will be sought. Among the most popular is the concept of managed care.

MANAGED CARE

One might ask, if we are in the era of "managed care," was what came before "unmanaged care?" There are those who would argue that it was and, in many cases, still is. However, "managed" in this context is intended to convey the concept of a close attention to every detail of a person's care to ensure not only that the care is effective and appropriate but also that it takes advantage of the least expensive alternatives and that those providing care have a stake in keeping costs low.

Managed care is formally defined as a system that integrates the financing and delivery of health care through contracts with selected health providers and hospitals that provide comprehensive health care services to enrolled members of a health care plan.[6] The provider network is the single most important feature distinguishing a managed care from an indemnity (fee-for-service) plan.[7] This means that managed care subscribers must choose from among the plan's designated health providers and hospitals for their care.

In comparing health plans, the following are key dimensions of performance:

- Utilization (*e.g.,* hospital admission rates, average length of stay, ambulatory care visits, use of expensive tests and procedures)
- Expediters for each type of health services utilization
- Use of preventive tests, exams, and procedures
- Quality of care including health outcomes
- Enrollee satisfaction
- Enrollee out-of-pocket expenditures
- Level and rate of growth of health care expenditures and premiums

Managed care plans boast that they compare favorably to other approaches based on these criteria. Specifically, they claim lower hospital utilization (admission rates and length of stay); greater use of less costly procedures and tests; greater emphasis on disease prevention and screening; comparable quality of care; and greater enrollee satisfaction with cost. However, some report that enrollee satisfaction with the care they receive lags behind that of other plan options.[8] The following characteristics are central to managed care environments: projected length of stay designations, care managers, care maps, and approval/documentation requirements. Projected length of stay designations are guided by diagnosis related groups (DRGs) and the experience of the insurer. Hospital use is minimized by providing for as many of the patient's needs as possible on an outpatient basis before admission to the hospital. The concept relies heavily on care managers assigned for each patient who work with the health care team and patient and must approve care and specific utilization of resources before implementation.

CARE MAPS

To promote efficient utilization of services in a managed care facility, managed care plans depend upon what is commonly called a *care map*. A care map is a multidisciplinary plan of care written for a specific diagnosis or procedure which outlines a timeline for the particular care and services that a patient should receive to expeditiously progress to discharge. The purpose of a care map is to maintain continuity and coordination of care through timely and appropriate use of personnel and resources. Timelines are associated with critical pathways through which a patient with a particular diagnosis is projected to pass. Appropriate personnel from interdisciplinary health teams and other necessary resources are scheduled to optimize their utilization at appropriate points in the timeline. The goal is consistent, efficient, and effective coordination to achieve high-quality patient care outcomes for a particular diagnosis.

Many care maps use a daily timeline to map care, but care maps may be hourly timelines in such areas as the emergency department, where patient status may be projected to change rapidly for some diagnoses. Care maps include designation of measurable outcome criteria which assist in quality assurance management. Most patients (about 80%) will progress according to the care map. For those patients who do not follow the care map due to complications or other events, the care map may need to be revised or written on a daily basis by a case manager.

CARE MAPS AND NEUROSCIENCE PATIENTS

For patients with some neuroscience diagnoses, writing care maps is difficult. This is partially due to the lack of predictability associated with some diagnoses. For example, many patients with a subarachnoid hemorrhage due to a cerebral aneurysm bleed are at high risk for vasospasm. How long should they be maintained in the Neuro ICU? Other difficulties concern the lack of availability of special units (e.g., Neuro ICUs, step-down units) with consequent inappropriate levels of care available on step-down and intermediate units (e.g., use of vasopressors) and widely varying physician preferences in treatment plans.

Care maps for trauma patients (severe head injury and cervical spinal cord injury) are also very challenging because of the variety of courses experienced due to multisystem involvement or complications. Important questions for constructing care maps become difficult to answer. What is the profile of the "average" patient? How many days should be included on the care map? Should all of these patients be case managed? Other neurological diagnoses follow more predictable plans of care (e.g., a patient admitted for steroid therapy to manage an exacerbation of multiple sclerosis). While continuing to dedicate our best effort to developing care maps, we should recognize that changes in technology and treatment options will necessitate a frequent revision schedule. A number of care maps are included in this text to assist the reader in providing care.

MODELS OF PRACTICE

Nurses use models to guide their thinking about patient care and to place their practice in the context of the overall organizational structure in which they function. As a theoretical or conceptual framework that guides practice, a model can be so broad as to describe the philosophy, purposes, and values of a profession such as nursing. Practice models can also be narrowly focused to guide thinking and actions with regard to a specific phenomenon such as intracranial pressure, chronic illness, health promotion, or caregiver stress. Models are often presented as diagrammatic representations of relationships among key components of a phenomenon. Nursing models will continue to be developed and refined through practice-based research.

A hallmark of professional nursing is its holistic model of care. Holistic care implies comprehensive care across settings to the patient and the family. How nurses shape holistic care depends on the circumstances and needs of the patient and family and on the educational background and experience of the nurse. Nurses prepared at the graduate level as advanced practice nurses (APNs) are prepared to implement an advanced model of practice with substantial autonomy and independence.

The following describe how neuroscience nurses provide holistic care to patients with a variety of neurological problems across various settings and levels of acuity.

INTENSIVE/CRITICAL CARE MANAGEMENT

Patients are admitted to neuroscience intensive care units for physiological stabilization and vigilant monitoring. Neuroscience nurses possess the knowledge and skill to monitor and interpret the various physical assessment and computerized physiological data, to adjust drips, and to perform other technological interventions to support all body systems. In addition, they possess the communication and counseling skills to provide emotional and psychological support to the patient and family through the uncertainties related to outcomes from catastrophic acute neurological illness. Once physiologically stabilized, the patient moves to a subacute care unit for continued holistic management. Recovery may be complete or the illness may become a chronic condition.

SUBACUTE CARE

The term subacute care (average length of stay, 5 to 30 days) is frequently discussed in the literature and is a growth area in health care delivery. Subacute care is the area of care between intensive care and recovery or home care. Candidates for subacute care are those patients who do not require surgery or invasive procedures but do require frequent assessment and longer patient stays. Subacute care provides coordinated services to patients from an interdisciplinary team of nurses, physicians, specialized rehabilitative therapists (e.g., physical, occupational, speech, respiratory, recreational), social workers, dieticians, and other professionals. Lines between disciplines are blurred because all disciplines work closely together to achieve the same goals through an interdisciplinary approach. This is accomplished through frequent team conferences and informal ongoing communications. In addition, subacute units work toward creating a home-like environment for patients.

The International Healthcare Association outlines four categories of subacute care:[9]

1. *Transitional subacute care units* (average length of stay, 5 to 30 days). Patients require 5.5 to 8 hours per day of nursing care. These types of units or facilities serve as a hospital step-down unit and can significantly reduce high-cost acute care hospitalization by substituting less costly care. Patients include those who may need ventilator weaning (Guillian-Barré syndrome), those recovering from stroke or head injury; and those with medically complex conditions. The goal of care is discharge home or to less expensive care such as long-term care or an assisted living arrangement.

2. *General subacute care units* (average length of stay, 10 to 40 days). The major difference between the general subacute and transitional unit is patient acuity. Patients need approximately 3.5 hours of nursing care and 1 to 3 hours of rehabilitation therapies per day. Some patients may require IV therapy or dressings. The goal of care is the same as for transitional subacute care.

3. *Chronic subacute care units* (average length of stay, 60 to 90 days). These units provide care for patients with little hope of recovery or functional independence such as unweanable ventilator-dependent patients, long-term comatose patients, and those with progressive neurological disease. Patients need approximately 3.5 hours of nursing care and 1 to 3 hours of therapies per day. The goal of care is stabilization so patients can go home or to a long-term care facility or have a peaceful death.

4. *Long-term transitional subacute facilities* (average length of stay, 25 days or more). These facilities are usually licensed as long-term hospitals rather than as nursing facilities. Typical patients include acute–ventilator-dependent patients and those with medically complex conditions who require 6.5 to 9 hours per day of nursing care. The goal of care is stabilization of medical conditions with possible discharge to complex home care or continued long-term care.

How illness is viewed shapes care. A key transition point in illness comes when a patient moves from an acute care model to a chronic illness model, thus redefining the illness and necessary care. The *chronic illness trajectory model*, proposed by Corbin and Strauss, is particularly helpful for understanding the nurse's role in symptom management, in rehabilitation, in education and support, and as an advocate for the patient and the family.[10] This model is based on the fundamental idea that chronic conditions have an illness course that changes over time but that can be shaped and managed. While shaping may not change the direction of the illness, the course of the illness can be extended and stabilized, and symptoms can be controlled and managed. The shaping process is complicated by the use of technology, which has a potential impact on the patient's personal identity, well being, and activities of daily living. Chronic illness also has a profound influence on the family unit and quality of life.

Technology and advances in medical science are salvaging people who formerly would have died. Many of these survivors are left with chronic conditions that must be managed for their life spans. How they are managed directly influences the quality of life for both the patient and family. With the growth of community based care and home care, more nurses will be caring for patients with chronic illnesses not only in acute hospitals but also in subacute care units and in the home.

COMMUNITY BASED CARE

Patients with neurological conditions have always been managed in the community. The changing environment for neuroscience community care has to do with the greatly increased numbers who will be managed in this setting and the complexity of the interventions involved in their care. A typical neuroscience patient can be managed in the community with follow-up by neuroscience health professionals providing periodic monitoring and fine tuning of drug therapy and other interventions. Day care programs for cognitively impaired adults offer cognitive retraining programs to improve the client's quality of life and functional level. Another example of community care involves a weekly exercise program for persons with Parkinson's disease to improve muscle strength, balance, and education. High-tech care for neurological problems, such as ventilatory support, is increasingly available in the home but requires high-level support by appropriately skilled health professionals to make it work.

Collaboration and Collaborative Models of Practice

As traditional practice models in health care delivery give way to more efficient and cost-effective alternatives, the concept of what constitutes effective collaboration among members of a health care team is changing. In their excellent text on collaboration, Siegler and Whitney note that no definition can convey the rich variety and complexity of collaboration in health care.[11] However, they cite the following definition by Shortridge, McLain, and Gilliss as insightful:

. . . a reciprocal relationship wherein the [providers] assume the greatest responsibilities for patient care within the framework of their respective fields. Although there are areas of overlap . . . the majority of the services provided . . . are complementary. . . . A collaborative practice emphasizes joint responsibility in patient care management, with a bilateral process of decision making based on each practitioner's education and ability.[12]

Models of practice can be viewed from the perspective of structure, process, and outcomes. Three models of collaborative practice have been cited:[13]

1. *Hierarchical model*: characterized by unidirectional communications with the physician in the highest position as leader; contact between patient and physician is limited.

2. *Collaborative practice model, type I*: characterized by bidirectional communications among providers; the physician is still the leader; contact between patient and physician is limited.

3. *Collaborative practice model, type II*: patient centered; all providers work both with each other and with the patient; no provider is dominant.

The distinction between multidisciplinary teams and interdisciplinary teams is also made. A **multidisciplinary team** refers to any team that has *more than one discipline* in its membership. The core multidisciplinary team members may include physicians (attending, resident, intern), nurses (care nurse, nurse practitioner, clinical nurse specialist, nurse manager), respiratory therapist, pharmacist, nutritionist, physical therapist, speech therapist, occupational therapist, social worker, and chaplain. Other health professionals may be included as needed. An **interdisciplinary team** is one in which there is *collaborative interaction* between members of the different disciplines; the team works for mutual goals and outcomes. It is what goes on in the group (process) that is key to differentiating group type. Therefore, not all multidisciplinary teams are interdisciplinary.

Multidisciplinary care maps are used to provide quality care. Interdisciplinary team work characterized by effective ongoing communications, cost consciousness, mutual goals, and measurable outcomes are the hallmarks of the collaborative practice model of the 21st century.

Collaborative Practice in Neuroscience Patient Care

Many factors influence the manner in which patient-centered care is provided. These include type of patient population, availability of human and material resources, availability of support services, and the focus of care. With a neuroscience population, the consciousness and cognition of the patient add special dimensions to the model of practice. Because of a diminished level of consciousness or altered cognition, it may not be possible to exchange information directly with the patient, and a family member may assume the role of surrogate decision maker for the compromised patient. In this situation, the interdisciplinary team of physician and nurse assumes an advocacy role for the patient to assure that decisions made on the patient's behalf by the family member and health team are, to the best of everyone's knowledge, the decisions that the patient would make if he or she were able. Although the communications may be directed toward the family, care is still patient centered.

Many neurological problems affect the personhood, activities of living, and independence of the patient. To assist the patient achieve optimal outcomes, the most successful approach is through patient-centered interdisciplinary collaboration applied across settings and across transitions in illness and care.[14] At one major medical center, an interdisciplinary collaborative model of practice begins in the Neuro ICU. The cornerstone of this collaboration is interdisciplinary collaborative rounds conducted every morning during which time each patient is reviewed by system (neurological, cardiovascular, respiratory, etc.) and parameters and goals are set for the day. The interdisciplinary team includes physicians, nurses, pharmacist, nutritionist, and respiratory therapist.

The attending intensivist, as team leader, guides the review of the patient. The nurse caring for the patient provides a complete assessment based on current data and compares these data with previous data to highlight changes. The acute care nurse practitioner works collaboratively with the physician and care nurse to assess the patient, plan care, and select interventions. The pharmacist makes recommendations on the appropriateness of drug therapy, monitors drug levels, advises on possible drug interactions and side effects, and outlines any special drug administration parameters. The respiratory therapist reports respiratory and ventilatory data, assesses respiratory mechanics, recommends ventilator setting adjustments, and advises on extubation or intubation. The nutritionist calculates target nutritional requirements and monitors albumen, magnesium, and other indicators of nutritional status. Communication is open throughout the patient review, during which questions are raised and discussed and opinions are shared. After a review of the data, the team enters the patient room and the physician examines the patient. When the examination is completed, the goals for the day are summarized and orders written. Discharge criteria are set that must be met before the patient can be transferred from the ICU to intermediate care.

Once the patient is moved to intermediate care, the structure and processes of the interdisciplinary collaborative model are reformatted to meet the changing acuity needs of the patient. Rounds become briefer and a greater emphasis is placed on rehabilitation and discharge planning. Transition to the community or other levels of care is planned to be appropriate to maintain quality of care, as well as to be cost conscious (see Chap. 15). The hallmarks of interdisciplinary collaborative care are that each patient is valued as a unique individual, care is individualized, and care is patient centered.

Summary

This chapter has presented a brief discussion of the realities of practice now and into the 21st century. Change has been rapid and substantive. Caring for neuroscience patients in this health care culture is also being reshaped and redefined. The merit of future changes must be measured by the gold standard of patient-centered care that meets the health care needs of all populations.

References

1. Donaldson, M., Yordy, K., & Vanselow, E. (1994). Defining primary care: An interim report. Washington, DC: National Academy Press.
2. Ibid., p. 23.
3. Ibid., p. 6.
4. Barker, L. R. (1991). Distinctive characteristics of ambulatory medicine. In L. R. Barker, J. R. Burton, & P. D. Zieve (Eds.), *Principles of ambulatory medicine* (3rd ed.). Baltimore: Williams & Wilkins, p. 14.
5. Donaldson, Yordy, & Vanselow, p. 31–32.
6. Iglehart, J. K. (1994). Physicians and the growth of managed care. *New England Journal of Medicine, 331*(17), 1167–1171.
7. Miller, R. H., & Luft, H. S. (1994). Managed care plans: Characteristics, growth, and premium performance. *Annual Review of Public Health, 15,* 437–459.
8. Ibid., p. 451.
9. Griffin, K. M. (1995). What is subacute care? *AACN News,* April, p. 6.
10. Corbin, J. M., & Strauss, A. (1988). *Unending word and care: Managing chronic illness at home.* San Francisco: Jossey-Bass.
11. Siegler, & Whitney. (1994).
12. Shortridge, L. M., McLain, B. R., & Gilliss, C. L. (1986). Graduate education for family primary care. In M. D. Mezey & D. O. McGivern (Eds.), *Nurses, nurse practitioners: The evolution of primary care* (pp. 120-134). Boston: Little, Brown.
13. Siegler, E. L., & Whitney, F. W. (Eds.). (1994). *Nurse-physician collaboration: Care of adults and the elderly.* New York: Springer.
14. Counsell, C. M., Guin, P. R., & Limbaugh, B. (1994). Coordinated care for the neuroscience patient: Future directions. *Journal of Neuroscience Nursing 26*(4), 245–250.

CHAPTER 3

Clinical Reasoning and Neuroscience Nursing Practice

Joanne V. Hickey

In Chapter 1, we discussed how the economics and technological complexities of the changing medical marketplace are producing a wholesale restructuring of the health care environment. If nurses want to remain a relevant part of this dynamic process, they must recognize that "business as usual" will no longer be adequate for survival in this new technocratic age of cost-conscious health care. Nursing education is only now beginning to recognize and implement the changes necessary to prepare nurses to take advantage of trends and opportunities. In today's fast-moving health care culture, a failure of nursing educators to change with the times will not only be lethal for those nurses undergoing the educational process, but will also be devastating for the nursing profession as a whole.

What changes are needed in the educational process? To explore answers to this question, this chapter (1) examines the nursing process as a framework for nursing practice; (2) explores the importance of critical thinking and clinical reasoning skills in nursing practice; and (3) discusses the essential relationship between critical thinking skills and providing optimal patient outcomes in a cost-efficient manner. Critical thinking skills are of paramount importance if nurses are to provide quality care in the new health system. Nurses must be willing to consciously strive to examine, develop, and refine their critical thinking skills to provide quality care to patients and their families.

NURSING PRACTICE IN THE INFORMATION AGE

The demands on the intellect to function in a fast-paced technocratic society can often seem overwhelming. Nurses are surrounded by complex technologies which are invariably controlled by computers and connected to exquisite da-

tabases. The technologies are constantly being upgraded through software and hardware enhancements. Patient assessment and treatment often involves interfacing with a computer. Sophisticated physiological monitoring systems provide an integration of waveforms and digital values for a number of cardiopulmonary and cerebrovascular variables. Decision making software identifies deviations from set parameters and offers diagnostic and management suggestions. More and more technology is found in home care. The nurse receives data from a myriad of sources to interpret, validate, and process. This complex process requires well-developed critical thinking skills, broad-based scientific knowledge, and communication skills.

Leaders in nursing have underscored the role of the nurse as provider of holistic care to patients and their families. As a result, the emphasis in nursing curricula has been on psychosocial aspects of care. While not neglecting the psychosocial aspects, it is now apparent that nurses need a stronger foundation in the biological sciences. For nurses to be able to function in the current health care system, they must gain a more detailed understanding of the effects of disease on the body and the various diagnostic and treatment options.

To provide this knowledge, nursing curricula need to include more extensive coverage of physiology, pathophysiology, immunology, genetics, and pharmacology. The revolutionary new knowledge in diagnosis and treatment coming from molecular biology and research at the cellular level must be presented so that nurses will be comfortable dealing with procedures and data based on these fields. In order for the nurse to understand patient care and collaborate with the health team to achieve optimal patient outcomes, the nurse must possess a broad knowledge base in biological and behavior sciences along with nursing theory. The same knowledge is needed to provide effective education and anticipatory guidance to patients and their families. But knowledge is not enough. What one does with knowledge and information is critical to patient outcomes. Critical thinking skills will be the most valuable tool in nursing practice. The practice arena is changing rapidly and nurses need to examine the adequacy of their knowledge and skills for contemporary practice.

NURSING PROCESS

The nursing process, first proposed by Yura and Walsh in the 1970s, provides a unidimensional cognitive model of thinking that includes the five steps of assessment, analysis, planning, implementation, and evaluation. Nursing process is a systematic method of decision making modeled after the scientific method of problem solving. The goal of the nursing process is to identify patient problems using nursing diagnosis and prescribe appropriate nursing interventions.

Development and refinement of the North American Nursing Diagnosis Association taxonomy of nursing diagnoses has been in progress for over 10 years. A nursing diagnosis is defined as "a clinical judgment about an individual, family, or community response to actual or potential health problems/life processes which provide the basis for definitive therapy toward achievement of outcomes for which the nurse is accountable" (Carpenito, 1991, p. 65). Most of the health professions have their diagnostic categories which are discipline specific. In nursing, discipline-specific factors such as basic education, knowledge base, language, diagnostic categories, role expectations, and relationships influence diagnoses and treatment (Carnevali & Thomas, 1993, p. 143).

The single model of nursing process for practice has been embraced in nursing education and nursing practice as the common denominator and standard for conceptualizing nursing practice and patient care. It has found its way into every nursing textbook as well as the test construction blueprint for state board licensure examinations.

In the past few years, the adequacy of nursing process to guide nursing practice has been challenged. Although nursing process has provided a context for nursing practice, it is narrow and restrictive and does not capture the essence or complexity of professional practice in the 1990s or beyond. The nursing process does not incorporate all of the cognitive and intuitive processes that Benner (1985) described in *Novice to Expert*, a description of how nurses think about patients and patient care. Jones and Brown (1993) state that the nursing process and problem solving are subsumed under critical thinking.

CRITICAL THINKING AND NURSING PRACTICE

The need for nurses with well-developed critical thinking skills has never been more apparent than in the current health care system. Cost containment initiatives and managed care have resulted in shortened hospital stays with patients who are going home or to less expensive care settings sicker and with more complex needs. More and more care is being provided in the community and through home care. In order to move patients through the various levels of care expeditiously

and efficiently, nurses are assuming more responsibility and accountability for patient outcomes within compressed time frames. Care is often complex and requires the collaborative effort of a coordinated multidisciplinary team for transitions in illness and care.

The critical thinking skills of nurses drive nursing practice and directly influence the achievement of optimal outcomes for patients. The foundation of professional nursing practice, critical thinking involves a philosophical perspective toward thinking and cognitive processes characterized by reasoned judgment and reflective thinking. Nurses can be taught the principles of critical thinking beginning in basic nursing programs and on through graduate and continuing education programs. However, these skills are only properly honed in clinical practice where the nurse must have the intellectual openness and curiosity to question the status quo and accepted explanations and display the courage to rigorously explore new possibilities and explanations.

Critical Thinking Defined

Critical thinking is a broad concept that can be applied to all aspects of life. The terms *critical thinking, clinical reasoning,* and *diagnostic reasoning* are sometimes used interchangeably in the literature and need to be distinguished. Much discussion has been directed at defining the elusive concept of critical thinking, and many narrow and comprehensive definitions currently exist. However, most experts believe that there are key conceptual elements to critical thinking. Jones and Brown (1993) state that critical thinking is not a single way of thinking but a multidimensional cognitive process that demands the skillful application of knowledge and experience in making judgments and evaluations. Critical thinking involves a healthy, reflective skepticism in which complex meanings are analyzed, solutions critiqued, alternatives explored, and contingency-related value judgments are made (Jones & Brown, 1991). The critical thinker does not accept conclusions but rather analyzes and evaluates reasons and evidence. Assumptions are made explicit, and unwarranted and irrelevant inferences are rejected. Apparent contradictions are reconciled (Jones & Brown, 1993). The best and most encompassing evidence is cited. Conclusions are the result of reasoned evaluative judgment (Paul, 1990).

As an example of definitions, the National Council for Excellence in Critical Thinking Instruction defines **critical thinking** comprehensively as "the intellectually disciplined process of actively and skillfully conceptualizing, applying, analyzing, synthesizing and evaluating information gathered from or generated by observation, experience, reflection, reasoning, or communication as a guide to belief and action" (1992, p. 2). Woods (1993) notes that in this definition, the Council suggests two components to critical thinking: (1) a set of information and beliefs *and generating and processing skills and abilities;* and (2) application of those skills and abilities to guide behavior.

Critical thinking is an active process directed toward guiding behavior in every aspect of one's personal and professional life. In nursing, critical thinking is the crux that guides professional practice and patient care. The definition cited also recognizes the importance of the nurse's observation, experience, and reflection to provide context and meaning to information, and reasoning to analyze and synthesize information to make judgments and reach conclusions.

Clinical reasoning is all the thinking and reasoning about patient care and management questions one considers in providing care in clinical practice. It is a special type of critical thinking and has been pioneered in medical education. Kassirer and Kopleman define clinical reasoning as the essential function of the physician in which optimal patient care depends on keen diagnostic acumen and thoughtful analysis of the trade-offs between the benefits and risks of tests and treatments (1991, p. 2). They point out that optimal patient outcomes cannot be achieved if reasoning skills are deficient. Excellence in clinical reasoning as applied to nursing practice is also key for nurses to achieve optimal patient outcomes.

Diagnostic reasoning, a subheading of clinical reasoning, refers to the reasoning that takes place in relation to arriving at a diagnosis. In medicine, the processes of diagnosis and decision making about patient management follow five steps: generation of diagnostic hypotheses, refinement of hypotheses, diagnostic testing, causal reasoning, and diagnostic verification (Kassirer & Kopleman, 1991, p. 3). Nursing uses the five-step nursing process for diagnosing patient problems.

Many advanced practice nurses such as nurse practitioners have followed the five-step diagnostic reasoning model in diagnosing and treating patients. For nurses not involved in advanced practice roles, will the concepts of clinical reasoning and diagnostic reasoning be incorporated into nursing practice and, if so, how will they be adapted for nursing practice? Answers to these questions are important for the further development of the profession of nursing.

Application to Neuroscience Nursing Practice

What does this all mean for neuroscience nurses? The ramifications of neurological disease and illness have far-reaching implications for the patient, family, and health team. Neuroscience nurses are integral members of the team and work independently and collaboratively to achieve optimal patient outcomes. Neuroscience nurses cannot be limited by narrow models of processing information and thinking. Critical thinking skills will provide the tools to sustain the lifetime practice of nurses in an ever changing practice environment. These skills need to be promoted and valued.

Bibliography

Bates, B. (1995). *A guide to physical examination and history taking*, (6th ed.) Philadelphia: J. B. Lippincott Co., pp. 635–648.

Benner, P. (1985). *From novice to expert: Excellence and power in clinical nursing practice.* Menlo Park, CA: Addison-Wesley.

Carnevali, D. L., & Thomas, M. D. (1993). *Diagnostic reasoning and treatment decision making in nursing.* Philadelphia: J. B. Lippincott.

Carpenito, L. (1991). The NANDA definition of nursing diagnosis. In Carroll-Johnson, R. M. (Ed.), *Classification of nursing diagnoses: Proceedings of the ninth conference.* Philadelphia: J. B. Lippincott, pp. 65–71.

Facione, N. C., & Facione, P. A. (1996). Externalizing the critical thinking in knowledge development and clinical judgment. *Nursing Outlook, 44*(3), 129–136.

Jones, S. A., & Brown, L. N. (1991). Critical thinking: Impact on nursing education. *Journal of Advanced Nursing, 16,* 529–533.

Jones, S. A., & Brown, L. N. (1993). Alternative views on defining critical thinking through the nursing process. *Holistic Nursing Practice, 7*(3), 71–76.

Kassirer, J. P., & Kopleman, R. I. (1991). *Learning clinical reasoning.* Baltimore, MD: Williams & Wilkins, pp. 1–46.

Paul, R. (1990). *Critical thinking: What every person needs to survive in a rapidly changing world.* Rohnert Park, CA: Center for Critical Thinking and Moral Critique.

Woods, J. H. (1993). Affective learning: One door to critical thinking. *Holistic Nursing Practice, 7*(3), 64–70.

Yura, A., & Walsh, M. (1978). *The nursing process: Assessing, planning, implementing, and evaluating* (3rd ed.). New York: Appleton-Century-Crofts.

CHAPTER 4

Ethical and Legal Issues in Neuroscience Nursing Practice

Joanne V. Hickey

Ethical and legal dimensions of conduct in professional practice are especially compelling and complex in many situations faced by the neuroscience nurse. The primary focus of this chapter is clinical ethics in neuroscience nursing practice. **Clinical ethics** is primarily concerned with the ethics of clinical practice and the ethical problems that arise in the care of patients. The discussion of legal dimensions is included when judicial decisions have influenced standards of practice. The three main areas discussed in this chapter are (1) the basis for ethical and legal dimensions of practice; (2) a framework for ethical decision making; and (3) selected ethical issues that commonly arise in neuroscience nursing practice.

AN ETHICAL AND LEGAL PERSPECTIVE OF NEUROSCIENCE PRACTICE

Unique ethical challenges are presented to neuroscience nurses by patients with neurological illnesses or impairments. These patients cross the lifespan, and frequently, they experience damage to their personhood that compares with no other illness. Neuroscience nurses must be prepared to care for the young victim of trauma who is left with irreversible paralysis or in a persistent vegetative state, for the adult in midlife who is newly diagnosed with a progressive neurological disease, and for the elderly person with dementia caused by multiple infarcts from small strokes. Recovery almost never means a return to the pretrauma or pre-illness functional level. These patients may experience complete personality changes or, in other tragic cases, lose the ability to comprehend or communicate information. Although the specific issues involving ethical questions such as determining patient capacity in decision making or decisions about withholding or withdrawing

treatments are similar in theory to those identified with many other patients who are seriously ill, the *context* in which these questions arise for the neurologically compromised patient is often very different and usually even more complex.[1]

Use of the term *ethical and legal* is avoided in this chapter to diminish the confusion of the ethical and legal perspectives and avoid the suggestion that ethics and legality are more synonymous than distinctly different. An **ethical perspective** addresses the moral duties and obligations to provide optimal care for patients and families. A **legal perspective** speaks to the minimal standards of care set forth in the judicial system to which health care providers must adhere. Simply relying on legal precedents does not necessarily imply that ethically grounded care is being provided. However, many issues, including decisions about withholding or withdrawing treatment or surrogate decision making, require addressing both the ethical dimensions and legal precedents, such as those set forth in the Quinlan and Cruzan cases, for a comprehensive understanding of the complexity of clinical situations.

A generally recognized phenomenon in the health care arena is the unprecedented development and rapid implementation of new technologies. The appropriate use of technology and its impact on human life are usually secondary, de facto considerations; the lag time between implementation of a new technology and recognition of its broader impact is often the foundation for the associated ethical dilemmas. The dynamics involved in this adjustment process are often played out in the judicial system—the wrong institution to resolve ethical issues. As a result, there has been an uncomfortable uncertainty about the legalities surrounding many ethical issues, leaving the practitioner to sort them out at the bedside.

The lack of clarity in how to proceed in ethical dilemmas and how to interpret personal wishes and laws has created further problems for the health care system. Before the advent of technology in medical practice, the failure of one or more body system usually limited life long before cognitive capacity was affected. Now, technology is available to keep patients "alive" indefinitely. This includes patients in a persistent vegetative state, in which the "organ of reason" is rendered permanently nonfunctional and unable to make informed consent decisions. This care is very costly and uses a disproportionate amount of scarce health care dollars. How does one reconcile the concepts of fair distribution of scarce resources, cost–benefit ratio, and quality of life in these clinical situations?

ETHICS, MORALITY, AND LEGALITY

Ethics

According to Webster's dictionary, *ethics* is variously defined as the "discipline dealing with moral duty and obligation, a set of moral principles or values, and the principles of conduct governing an individual or a group." Ethics has also been defined as the inquiry into the nature of morality or moral acts and the search for the morally good life.[2] Ethics dates back to the beginning of human civilization, when mores and laws were developed to allow groups of people to live together. Most ethical principles represent cultural and religious values of groups of people and, therefore, differ from culture to culture and from religion to religion. Even within cultures, there are subcultures that differ significantly in some aspects of their ethics and, therefore, in their standards of behavior.

When the concept of ethics is applied to professional practice, there are basic principles that govern how health care professionals practice within a culture. These principles are usually stated within a code, such as the *Code for Nurses,*[3] which proclaims to the public the guidelines that will govern how the professional nurse will practice.

Morality

Within the definition of ethics is the word *morality.* **Morality** is variously defined as having to do with human activities that are looked upon as good/bad or right/wrong; conforming to the accepted rules of what is considered right (virtuous, just, proper conduct); having the capacity to be directed by an awareness of right and wrong; and pertaining to the manner in which one behaves in relationships with others. Morality implies the making of judgments about what is right in given circumstances and the guidance of one's conduct by reason.[5] It suggests doing what seems right while giving equal weight to the interests of each individual who will be affected by one's conduct.

Four moral principles that are of particular importance in nursing practice are autonomy, beneficence, justice, and fidelity.

Autonomy is the act of self-governing, self-determining, or self-directing; it involves independence from the will of others, as well as the right to make and follow one's decisions.

The principle of autonomy affirms the nurse's duty to respect the decisions of the patient and the family and to assume the role of a patient/family advocate when necessary.

Beneficence is the charge to do good; it implies the principle of **nonmaleficence,** which is the duty to prevent or avoid doing harm. Many believe that upholding the principle of nonmaleficence is more binding than the duty to do good. For example, although the nurse cannot change the medical diagnosis or injuries incurred, secondary injuries and pain can be controlled.

Justice is defined as fairness, correctness, and impartiality in the application of principles of rightness and of sound judgment. The nurse must treat patients fairly based on their needs and the situation. It suggests an obligation for nurses to distribute their time, expertise, and resources as fairly as possible among patients assigned to their care.[4]

Fidelity is the obligation to be truthful and to keep promises. This principle supports the practice of obtaining informed consent and being honest and genuine in interactions with the patient and family.

Principles are guidelines and, as such, are not absolute in their application to situations. This is also true of moral and ethical principles. It is not uncommon to have more than one principle applicable to a situation simultaneously. Someone must determine which principle takes precedence in the given situation and why. These dilemmas are what make ethical decision making so difficult at times.

Legality

Legality has to do with lawfulness or the obligations imposed by law to bind certain behaviors within a society. The professional nurse, licensed to practice in a particular state, is bound by the laws within that state. Each state has its own Nurse Practice Act that defines professional nursing practice within that state. In addition, there are other laws and legal decisions related to health care issues that set a precedent for practice within that state and, often, within other states. An example of a precedent-setting decision is the Karen Quinlan case.[6] In this well-known case, a young woman suffered unexplained apnea and did not receive immediate ventilatory support. She was subsequently placed on a ventilator and remained in a persistent vegetative state. The family petitioned the court to allow the ventilator to be removed so that she could die. Permission was granted. Unexpectedly, she began to breathe spontaneously, and she lived in a persistent vegetative state for a number of years. This case established the precedent that a ventilator could be removed even when the consequence might be death.

Laws and legal precedents related to health care matters may originate at the state or federal levels. The judicial system is divided into municipal, state, and federal courts. The right to appeal to a higher court is provided as a safeguard to protect individual and group rights. Some cases related to health care have reached the U.S. Supreme Court. Laws reflect the values and beliefs of society, and thus are subject to review and to change. Although a law is legal, it may not seem moral to some individuals or groups. In a rapidly changing society such as that of the United States, challenges to current laws are common. With respect to health care issues, the changing and competing values and beliefs of a heterogeneous society, along with the unprecedented development of technology, account for the number of health-related issues that end up in the courts.

FRAMEWORK FOR ETHICAL DECISION MAKING

Decision Making in General

Decision making involves distinct, logically organized steps that involve choosing among alternative courses of action. These steps include collecting relevant data, analyzing data, proposing alternative solutions, identifying the pros and cons of each alternative, and selecting the best alternative based on established criteria.

Framework for Ethical Decision Making

Ethical decision making is a dynamic process requiring reflection, discussion, and evaluation. Like decision making in general, it should follow the same basic steps. Ethical decisions, as they apply to health care issues, can be unique in that they involve obligations, responsibilities, duties, rights, and values affecting life-and-death situations. The highly emotional nature of these issues often makes it difficult to separate feelings from facts. It is, therefore, of critical importance for the decision makers to separate personal attitudes, beliefs, and feelings from the factual data that are relevant to the particular situation. Without this separation, objectivity is lost.

Many ethical decisions require the input of a variety of disciplines and of people to provide a broad, comprehensive perspective of the issues at hand. Members of the collaborative team must be knowledgeable about the fundamental principles of ethical decision making to guide their analysis of complex decisions. The unique input of each of the team members will reflect their collaborative roles.

Collecting Relevant Data. The data collected should include medical information and preferences for treatment. Determination of an accurate diagnosis and prognosis, made by the physician, is critical to the database. In cases of coma, a diagnosis detailing the type of brain damage and the likelihood of recovery is important in planning care. The most important information about treatment preference comes from the patient if he or she is an adult and is mentally capable of making decisions. Consulting the patient in this regard recognizes the patient's right to autonomy and to define quality of life for himself or herself. If the patient is incapable as a result of coma, cognitive deficits, or other causes, then information regarding treatment preferences may be found in a living will or the expression of wishes made to the family or significant other while he or she was well. A surrogate decision maker may be necessary to represent the patient's wishes. The family's preference for treatment is also explored and established. Other data collected include information on state laws, hospital policies, and professional codes related to the particular situation. In some situations, it may be necessary to seek advice from the institutional ethics committee or hospital attorney.

Analyzing Data. Once all relevant data have been collected, they are then analyzed. One can apply the question, "What are the duties, rights, and responsibilities of all persons involved?" The moral principles of autonomy, beneficence, justice, and fidelity must be a part of this determination.

Proposing Alternative Solutions. Considering the diagnosis, prognosis, treatment preferences of the patient, laws, policies, and other relevant data, alternative actions are then identified.

Identifying the Pros and Cons of Each Alternative. The consequences and benefits of each alternative action are weighed and considered on the bases of treatment preferences, laws, and policies.

Selecting the Best Alternative Based on Established Criteria. Finally, an alternative or action is selected on the basis of treatment preferences, laws, and policies, and with acceptance of the consequences and benefits of that action. The decision must be based on accepted ethical standards and with due consideration of treatment preferences. Physicians, however, are not morally obliged to fulfill patients' requests for actions that they consider ethically objectionable. They have the right to be removed from the care of such patients, though they have the obligation to arrange for another physician to care for the patient.[7] When there are questions or disagreements about the best course of action or treatment for a patient, most hospitals consult their institutional ethics committee. The purpose of an ethics committee is to review cases impartially and make recommendations. A statement, often written by the chairperson, summarizes the recommendations of the committee as it relates to the best interest of the patient within the context of the situation.

Process of Ethical Decision Making

Ethical decision making is an integral part of medical and nursing practice, regardless of the setting, and includes both the independent role and the collaborative role of professional practice.

INDEPENDENT ROLE OF THE NURSE

The independent role of the nurse as it relates to ethical decision making generally involves the following:

- Establishing a database, making nursing diagnoses, establishing outcomes, and developing a plan of care
- Orienting the family to the unit and unit policies (*e.g.*, visiting hours)
- Identifying a family spokesperson and providing for scheduled updates regarding the patient's condition or progress
- Providing information about the patient's nursing care and response to nursing care
- Seeking information about the patient's or family's care preferences
- Reassuring the family that the patient is receiving sensitive, compassionate care and is comfortable
- Respecting the patient's/family's decisions regarding care
- Supporting the patient or family in the grieving process
- Making appropriate referrals to clergy, psychiatric clinical nurse specialists, social workers, or other support resources as necessary

• Documenting the information and support given, other interventions, and patient or family responses

INDEPENDENT ROLE OF THE PHYSICIAN

Bernat presents both general and specific guidelines for the physician who must make decisions about terminating care in patients with severe, irreversible brain damage.[8] These guidelines are applicable for most neurological and all comatose patients. According to Bernat, the role of the physician as it relates to a specific comatose patient includes:

• Making a diagnosis of the patient's medical condition and of brain damage (*e.g.*, brain death, persistent vegetative state)
• Making a determination of prognosis based on all available data and the physician's professional experience
• Identifying the patient's preference for treatment, if possible
• Identifying the family's preference for treatment
• Selecting the level of care appropriate for the patient
• Making referrals to other physicians, clergy, and other resources as necessary
• Documenting the plan of care and interactions with family

COLLABORATIVE ROLES

The **collaborative role** of the nurse and physician is based on open, honest, and respectful communications. Ongoing communication with the family is a shared responsibility. The family must be given information and frequent updates regarding the patient's condition and prognosis in a caring, gentle manner. Nurses should know what information has been given to the family because they may need to clarify and reinforce what has been said. People in high-stress situations often do not absorb all the information given and need repetition. Questions raised by the family with the nurse may need to be referred to the physician. The nurse is responsible for notifying the physician of family concerns and the possible need for a family meeting. Depending on the situation, the assistance of other professionals, such as clergy, social workers, or psychiatric or mental health professionals, may be requested to provide support to the patient and family. Discussions with other collaborators can be very helpful in clarifying related issues, not only to the patient and family, but also to the health professionals involved.

The database established by the physician related to the medical diagnosis and prognosis of a patient provides information that is necessary to the nurse's ethical decision making process. Likewise, information collected by the nurse regarding the patient, as derived from periodic neurological examinations, patient's or family's preferences or responses, and other sources, assists the physician. This information provides a current database for ethical decision making.

Documentation. Written documentation of communications with the family and the decisions made is important to validate that the ethical and legal dimensions of care have been met. The written documentation of both the nurse and the physician helps to keep the professional staff aware of what has transpired in the decision making process and what issues need to be addressed. The physician has the responsibility to provide data about the patient's condition and documentation of decisions for the plan of care. In special situations, such as with "do not resuscitate" (DNR) orders, hospital policy often dictates the frequency of documentation and inclusion of data.

DECISION MAKING CAPACITY AND ADVANCE DIRECTIVES AND LIVING WILLS

Patient's Capacity to Make Decisions

Discussion about the appropriate use of "competency" has been raised. According to *Guidelines on the Termination of Life-Sustaining Treatment and the Care of the Dying*, the use of competence and incompetence should be restricted to situations in which a formal judicial determination has been made.[9] Under the law, until such time as a judicial determination of incompetence has been made, individuals are presumed competent to manage their own affairs. The report goes on to promote the use of the notion of decision making capacity.[10] **Decision making capacity** refers to a patient's functional ability to make informed health care decisions in accordance with personal values. A person can be legally competent and nonetheless lack the capacity to make a particular treatment decision and vice versa.

Valid consent or refusal assumes adequacy of information provided, absence of coercion, and capacity to make decisions. The accepted standards in designating a patient's decision making capacity were put forth in the President's Commission report on *Deciding to Forego Life-Sustaining Treatment*.[11] The criteria include that the patient must be able to (1) understand all information relevant to the decision; (2) communicate with caregivers about the decision; and (3) possess the ability to reason about relevant alternatives against a background of "reasonably stable personal values and life goals."

When cognitive abilities are compromised so that informed consent is no longer possible, the patient is not capable to make decisions. The health team members then look to a designated family member or significant other as the surrogate to make decisions on behalf of the patient. The decisions made should be guided by the patient's previous expressions of wishes regarding treatment decisions (see discussion later of the substitute judgment standard) and an understanding of the patient's life goals, values, and beliefs and not those of the surrogate. Some states recognize living wills (discussed later).

In neuroscience nursing practice, "the organ of reason" is often the organ of injury or deficit, so that cognitive function is often compromised. The nurse then becomes the patient's advocate to ensure that adequate care is provided within the context of the expressed wishes of the patient as best as they can be determined. There are times when the patient is admitted to a facility in a comatose state, and the nurse has no idea of what the wishes of the patient would be if he or she could convey them. As patient advocates, the health team is obliged to seek this information as it has been expressed in the past to family members or is found in written documents.

Advance Directives and Living Wills

Advance directives are often misunderstand by the lay person and health professionals. Formalized advance directives are **written documents** by a competent person outlining the extent and form of care in the event of subsequent inability to participate in decision making. A **living will** is an advance directive specifying that, if the person is incapable of participating in decision making, life-sustaining treatments to postpone death should not be used in the event of a terminal illness.[12] The living will is a provision under a state's "Natural Death Act" or "Terminal Care Document." The problem with a living will is that it fails to provide the detailed instructions necessary for care and only applies when the patient is unable to communicate his or her wishes, and then only if death is imminent. It does not imply that the patient wishes to be designated DNR. It lacks the specifics to make decisions from many treatment options. A more useful directive is the **Durable Power of Attorney for Health Care** (DPAHC), and it is available in all states. The DPAHC permits adults to authorize a person to make surrogate medical decisions on his or her behalf if he or she becomes incapable of making decisions.[13]

The Patient Self-Determination Act of 1990 supports proxy statutes specifically for health care.[14] It also requires that health care providers elicit and clarify patients' preferences for care and treatment options. This information may be elicited through conversations with the patient or surrogate about the patient's beliefs, values, and life goals.

States have different titles for advance directives, living wills, and durable power of attorney. For example, in North Carolina a living will is called "A Declaration for the Desire for a Natural Death." The formalized designation of a surrogate decision maker for health care decisions is titled "Designation of a Health Care Power of Attorney" in some states and "Durable Power of Attorney for Health Care" in others. Nurses need to be familiar with the relevant documents and statutes in the state in which they practice.

In the absence of any advance directives, the principles of nonmaleficence and best interest become operative. Medicare and Medicaid nursing home certification requires inpatient assessment to determine the status of advance directives and durable power of attorney in those settings.

SELECTED ETHICAL ISSUES COMMON IN NEUROSCIENCE NURSING PRACTICE

Although there are many major and minor ethical decisions that the nurse makes daily regarding care, there are a few situations and issues that are particularly common to the practice setting of neuroscience nurses. Those selected for discussion in this section include levels of care, removal of ventilatory support, removal of enteral support, brain death criteria, and donor organs.

Levels of Care

Medical care can be organized according to hierarchical levels of aggressiveness involving (1) technology (*e.g.,* ventilators); (2) medications; (3) hydration and nutrition; and (4) basic care (*e.g.,* basic hygiene and comfort measures).[15] When the level of care is downgraded, the most aggressive therapy is withdrawn first.

There are three general indications for writing DNR orders: no medical benefit; poor quality of life after CPR, and poor quality of life before CPR.[16] A DNR decision means that mechanical ventilation or cardiac defibrillation will not be used in the event of a cardiopulmonary arrest, nor will CPR be performed. Medications, hydration/nutrition, and basic care will still be provided. In hopeless cases, the decision may be made to discontinue other, less aggressive treatment. In such cases, the physician would probably avoid the use of all technology and most medications. Vasopressors, antibiotics, steroids, and other drugs would likely be discontinued. Although most physicians would not treat an infection with antibiotics in such an instance, some physicians might continue an order for antipyretics to treat an elevated temperature, considering this a comfort measure. The Joint Commission for Accreditation of Healthcare Organizations (1992) requires that hospitals, psychiatric facilities, and nursing homes have policies regarding withholding of resuscitate services.

Discontinuation of hydration and nutrition is more ambiguous. Hydration and nutrition provided by an artificial means is considered a medical treatment, although some have challenged this concept. Further, some clinicians even differentiate between tube feeding and hydration (water), arguing that, although tube feeding is an "extraordinary measure," hydration is an "ordinary" measure and should be provided. Others argue that, without hydration/nutrition, the patient will feel pain and will suffer as a result of starvation. The American Academy of Neurology has published a position paper on various aspects of the care and management of patients who are in a persistent vegetative state and guidelines for clinicians.[17,18] In their position paper, it is stated that the diagnosis of a persistent vegetative state "can be made with a high degree of medical certainty" and "that these patients are incapable of experiencing pain or suffering because of the loss of cerebral cortical functioning."[17] (Every nurse is encouraged to read these important papers.)

Regardless of the gravity and hopelessness of the diagnosis, the fourth level of care—basic hygienic care and comfort measures—is always provided. The rationale for this steadfast care is based on respect for the sanctity of the human body, the dignity of the person, and the right to a peaceful death.

Removal of Ventilatory Support

When a ventilator is provided, it can legally be removed from either a patient who is capable or one who is incapable of making decisions. Two cases illustrate this point. The first case, *Satz v. Perlmutter,* pertains to a fully capable patient, Mr. Satz, who was 73 years old and ventilator-dependent as a result of amyotrophic lateral sclerosis. He wanted the ventilator to be removed even though he knew death would result. The Florida court ruled that, because Mr. Satz was a competent adult with no minor children, he had a right to refuse life-sustaining treatment if all affected family members consented. The ventilator was discontinued, and he died within a short period of time.

The second case, cited previously, is the Karen Quinlan case, in which the patient was comatose and, therefore, incapable of making decisions. Her father, the court-appointed legal guardian, petitioned the court to allow removal of the ventilator based on the assumption that she was brain dead. The court denied this request because she did not meet brain death criteria. However, the request to remove the ventilator was granted based on the irreversibility of her condition, as well as statements attributed to the patient prior to her illness that indicated an unwillingness to be maintained on life support indefinitely if there was no hope for quality of life.

Removal of Enteral Support

The position paper of the American Academy of Neurology clearly describes the persistent vegetative state and the fact that nutrition and hydration via the enteral route is a medical therapy that can be discontinued. However, the Cruzan case continued in the courts even after the position paper was published.

Nancy Cruzan was a victim of a motor vehicle accident in 1983, and had been in a chronic vegetative state since the accident. She was confined to a Missouri state hospital with no hope of recovery. Her parents petitioned the state courts for permission to terminate her enteral nutrition and hydration after hospital employees refused to do so without court approval. The family petitioned on the basis of the standards of "substitute judgment" and "best interest."

The **substitute judgment** standard conveys the idea that a surrogate, such as family member or the court, can determine what he/she believes a person would have chosen if he/she could participate in the decision. (*Note:* In situations in which there is disagreement within the family, or between the family and physician, a family member does not have legal authority over an adult patient unless he or she is the court-appointed guardian.[19])

The **best interest** standard directs the surrogate decision maker to consider what the patient would have wanted if he/she had been able to make the decision. The surrogate decision maker is obliged to protect the patient's welfare, such as relief of suffering, preservation or restoration of function, protection of worldly assets, and quality of life.[20]

Permission was granted by the Missouri Trial Court based on Nancy's testimony to a friend concerning her wish not to continue her life unless she could have a reasonable quality of life.[21] However, on appeal, the Missouri Supreme Court reversed the lower court decision, rejecting Nancy's statement to her friend as unreliable and rejecting her parent's request for termination of treatment. They concluded that no one else can make that choice for an incompetent person in the absence of either a formal document of a living will or "clear and convincing evidence" of the patient's wishes. A distinction was also made by the Missouri Supreme Court between initiation and discontinuation of medical treatment.[12,15]

The case was appealed to the U.S. Supreme Court, which upheld the decision of the Missouri high court. In this decision, the U.S. Supreme Court concluded that the states have the right to adopt their own standards to determine a patient's wishes regarding treatment. It also ruled that states are not required to recognize the right of a family to make decisions for the incompetent patient.[22,23]

On November 1, 1990, the case was again heard by the original lower court in Missouri. The testimony of three witnesses was heard; they recounted specific conversations with Nancy in which she stated that she would not wish to live "like a vegetable." The judge reaffirmed his decision to allow the feeding tube to be pulled. The family directed hospital authorities to remove the tube on December 14; Nancy died 2 weeks later.

Brain Death Criteria

The concept of brain death is an artifact of our technological society. Because of unprecedented advances made in the ability to support multiple body systems, the traditional earmarks of life—the heart beat and respiratory pattern—can be maintained even though the brain is nonfunctional.

The definition of brain death and the criteria for making the diagnosis are not universally agreed upon. Variations in definition and criteria are based on cultural, moral, religious, and legal differences. The definitive criteria for brain death currently followed in the United States were proposed in 1981 by the President's Commission for the Study of Ethical Problems in Medicine and Biomedical and Behavioral Research.[24] According to the commission, brain death is defined as "irreversible cessation of all functions of the entire brain including the brain stem."[25] The bases for demonstrating brain death are absence of brain stem reflexes, absence of cortical activity, and demonstration of the irreversibility of the state.[26] Usually, brain death criteria assessment is conducted two times with an interval of hours (*e.g.*, 6 to 8 hours) elapsing between examinations.

ABSENCE OF BRAIN STEM REFLEXES

Cranial nerves III through XII attach themselves to the central nervous system (CNS) beginning at the midbrain and extending to the lower medulla. Cranial nerve function is a recognized, sensitive indicator of brain stem function. The brain stem reflexes that are assessed include pupillary reaction to light, corneal reflex, gag reflex, and oculovestibular reflex.

In diagnosing brain death, the most important brain stem sign is apnea.[27] The current method, which is considered reliable for testing respiratory drive, is the apnea test. The steps involved in the apnea test, which is conducted by a physician, include the following:[28]

- The patient is preoxygenated with 100% oxygen for 5 minutes.
- The patient is disconnected from the ventilator.
- Immediately upon disconnection, 100% oxygen is delivered via endotracheal tube at 8 to 12 L/min.
- The PCO_2 is allowed to rise to 55 to 60 mm Hg, a level sufficient to trigger the respiratory drive. (A PCO_2 rise of 2.5 torr/min is expected in brain-damaged persons.)
- The chest is observed and palpated for evidence of spontaneous respirations.
- Arterial blood gas measurements are done periodically.
- The patient is reconnected to the ventilator.

If, after a given period of time off the ventilator, the PCO_2 exceeds 50 mm Hg, the pH is acidotic, and there is no evidence of respiratory effort, apnea is considered to have been proven.

ABSENCE OF CORTICAL ACTIVITY

In the United States, the electroencephalogram (EEG) is one test used to establish brain death. In the comatose patient who is unresponsive to painful stimuli (no evidence of withdrawal or posturing to painful stimuli), a flat (isoelectric) EEG is considered a necessary criterion of brain death.

IRREVERSIBILITY

In the United States, establishing irreversibility is based on the following criteria:

- A neurological diagnosis adequate to produce brain death
- A neurological examination that demonstrates the absence of brain stem function that is reproducible
- An absence of confounding factors that might account for loss of neurological function, such as:
  Drug overdose from barbiturates or other CNS depressants, or high levels of barbiturates as a result of barbiturate coma
  Drug toxicity (*e.g.,* neuromuscular blockers, antibiotics)
  Hypothermia (core body temperature ≤ 90° F)
  Local disease involving the eye or ear (cataracts, eye trauma)
  Shock
- Elapse of a period of observation of at least 24 hours without clinical neurological change

In the case of children, special considerations are observed.

OTHER TESTING

Other tests and procedures have been suggested as part of the criteria to establish brain death. They include nuclide brain scanning, blood flow studies, and evoked potentials. No test alone can establish brain death conclusively. Once brain death has been determined, it is mandatory for the patient to be pronounced brain dead and all treatment stopped.[29] The time of death is when the second set of brain death criteria are met.[30] The organs may be supported for a short period of time if organ harvest is planned.

Organ Procurement

One important result of declaring brain death is the possibility of organ donation. Although kidneys are the most common organs to be donated, other organs, such as the cornea, skin, bone, liver, and heart valves, may be given. When organ donation is considered, donor criteria must be followed meticulously. Donor criteria will vary depending on the particular organ to be given, but criteria include a specified age range, no history of malignant neoplasms, absence of sepsis or transmittable diseases, and procurement of the organ within 12 to 24 hours of death. In addition, the medical team involved in the declaration of brain death and the organ harvest team must be kept separate to avoid any special interests.

Once brain death has been declared, blood pressure, hydration, and ventilation are supported to provide adequate organ perfusion and oxygenation until surgery. Use of a ventilator, and sometimes vasopressors, is necessary to maintain the patient.

The nurse conveys sensitivity and caring for the patient and family by keeping the patient clean and comfortable-looking. Provisions must be made to support the family in their decision for or against organ donation. In addition, the family needs time and privacy to say their good-byes to their loved one.

FOSTERING PROFESSIONAL GROWTH IN ETHICAL DECISION MAKING

Professional Development and Ethical Caring

Exploring the ethical dimensions of professional practice is necessary to understand the duties and obligations in providing care. It also may be uncomfortable because it forces us to examine fundamental and personal life–death issues and personal values as moral beings. According to the Joint Commission on Accreditation of Healthcare Organizations Standards, facilities are required to provide a "mechanism to assist in the resolution of ethical problems in patient care."[31] All clinicians are also encouraged to become familiar with the mechanisms that exist within their own institutions. There are a number of resources and opportunities that foster growth.

For those nurses engaged in neuroscience nursing, there are a number of ethical issues that arise in everyday practice that can be sources of confusion and discomfort. It is important for the nurse to examine these situations, identify the type of problem that exists, identify the underlying ethical principles that impact on the situation, and sort out the components of the clinical situation to arrive at a sense of understanding that will guide clinical practice.

Professional development in ethical care can be supported by departments of nursing and health care institutions in several ways. institutional ethics committees, ethics rounds, and ethical educational programs and discussion groups are helpful in responding to individual patient situations and needs of health professionals.

INSTITUTIONAL ETHICS COMMITTEE

Many health care facilities have some form of an institutional ethics committee. Committee membership is multidisciplinary to represent broad views. Often, community representation is sought and may include an ethicist, lawyers, and lay persons. The committee's purposes include education; development of institutional guidelines and standards; concurrent case review; and retroactive case review. Many of the substantive issues center on neurological patients.[29]

ETHICS ROUNDS

Ethics rounds can be conducted on patient care units periodically (*e.g.,* once a month). These rounds have a clinical focus, and are usually directed by a group leader with an interest and background in ethics and clinical decision making. Particular patient situations can be reviewed to examine ethical components of care and the bases for decision making. Ethics rounds help to examine and clarify what is being done to address the ethical aspects of care and the rationale for those actions. Other resources can also be identified that may be helpful in resolving ethical matters when there is a need for assistance.

ETHICS EDUCATIONAL PROGRAMS AND DISCUSSION GROUPS

Educational programs with a focus in ethics are important to promote growth of the staff. They may be focused on the review of new guidelines or patient care scenarios. Ethics discussion groups are an informal method for discussion of topics of interest related to the ethical dimension of practice. The discussion may or may not address a currently active clinical situation in that facility. Cases reported in the press, recent legal opinions rendered, or the ethical dimensions of a new technology may be among the topics discussed. This forum provides the opportunity to consider a proactive approach to a potential problem. Other issues that may be addressed include clinical situations within the facility that were not adequately resolved in the past and that deserve a fresh review.

Application of the Ethical Dimension to Clinical Practice

Ethical and legal dimensions of nursing practice cut across all clinical areas of practice. For those nurses practicing in neuroscience nursing, the complexity of ethical practice is further compounded by the fact that the "organ of reason" is often involved, thus creating questions about the patient's capacity in decision making, autonomy, and best interest. Many of the clinical situations that confront the neuroscience nurse are life-and-death situations in which there are no second chances to undo previously made decisions. This places a tremendous burden of responsibility to do the "right" thing. Some situations precipitate an ethical dilemma for the practitioner. It is, therefore, important to prepare oneself for this awesome responsibility through ongoing professional development.

References

1. Castle, J. (1995). Personal communication. June 7.
2. Angeles, P. A. (1981). *Dictionary of philosophy.* New York: Barnes & Noble.
3. Pryor-McCann, J. M. (1990). Ethics in critical care nursing. *Critical Care Nursing Clinics of North America,* 2(l), 1–13.
4. Angeles, P. A. (1981). *Dictionary of philosophy.* New York: Barnes & Noble.
5. Rachels, J. (1986). *Elements of moral philosophy.* New York: Random House.
6. *In re Karen Quinlan,* 70 N.J. 10, 335 A. 2d 647 (1976).
7. Nelson, W. A., & Bernat, J. L. (1989). Decisions to withhold or terminate treatment. *Neurologic Clinics,* 7(4), 759–773.
8. Bernat, J. L. (1988). Ethical aspects of withdrawing treatment from patients with severe brain damage. In A. H. Ropper & S. F. Kennedy (Eds.). *Neurological and neurosurgical intensive care* (2nd ed.) (pp. 345–350). Baltimore: Aspen.
9. *Hastings Center Report.* (1987). Guidelines on the termination of life-sustaining treatment and the care of the dying. Bloomington, IN: Indiana University Press, p. 131.
10. Ibid., p. 132.
11. President's Commission for the Study of Ethical Problems in Medicine and Biomedical and Behavioral Research. (1983). *Deciding to forego life-sustaining treatment: A report on the ethical, medical, and legal issues in treatment decisions.* Washington, DC: U.S. Government Printing Office, p. 121.
12. Hoffinan, N. (1992). Ethical considerations and quality of life. *Cardiovascular Clinics,* 22(2), 243–251.
13. Nelson, W. A., & Bernat, J. L. (1989). Decisions to withhold or terminate treatment. *Neurologic Clinics,* 7(4), 759–773.
14. Emanuel, E. J., & Emanuel, L. L. (1992). Proxy decision making for incompetent patents: An ethical and empirical analysis. *Journal of the American Medical Association,* 267(15), 2067–2071.
15. Cranford, R. E. (1984). Termination of treatment in the persistent vegetative state. *Seminars in Neurology,* 4, 36–44.
16. Hoffinan, N. (1992). Ethical considerations and quality of life. *Cardiovascular Clinics,* 22(2), 243–251.
17. American Academy of Neurology. (1989). Position of the American Academy of Neurology on certain aspects of the care and management of the persistent vegetative state patient. *Neurology, 39,* 125–126.
18. American Academy of Neurology. (1989). Guidelines on the vegetative state: Commentary on the American Academy of Neurology statement. *Neurology, 39,* 123–124.
19. Bleck, T. P., & M. C. Smith. (1989). Diagnosing brain death and persistent vegetative states. *Journal of Critical Illness,* 4(11), 60–65.
20. President's Commission for the Study of Ethical Problems in Medicine and Biomedical and Behavioral Research. (1983). *Deciding to forego life-sustaining treatment: A report on the ethical, medical, and legal issues in treatment decisions.* Washington, DC: U.S. Government Printing Office, pp. 132–136.
21. *Cruzan, by Cruzan v. Harmon,* 760 S.W. 2d 408 (Mo. banc 1988); affirmed in *Cruzan, by Cruzan v. Director, Missouri Department of Health, et al.* 497 U.S. 261 (1990).
22. Quigley, F. M. (1990). The incompetent patient: What will the Cruzan decision mean? *Focus on Critical Care,* 17(5), 410–411.
23. Quigley, F. M. (1990). Withdrawing treatment. *Focus on Critical Care,* 17(6), 464–468.
24. President's Commission for the Study of Ethical Problems in Medicine and Biomedical and Behavioral Research. (1981). *Defining death: Medical, legal, and ethical issues in the determination of death.* Washington, DC: U.S. Government Printing Office.
25. President's Commission for the Study of Ethical Problems in Medicine and Biomedical and Behavioral Research. (1981). President's Commission medical consultants on the diagnosis of death for the study of ethical problems in medicine and biomedical research. *JAMA,* 246, 2184–2186.
26. Black, P. M. (1978). Brain death. *New England Journal of Medicine,* 299, 330–344, 393–401.
27. Black, P. M. (1988). Guidelines for the diagnosis of brain death. In A. H. Ropper & S. F. Kennedy (Eds.). *Neurological and neurosurgical intensive care* (2nd ed.) (pp. 323–333). Rockville, MD: Aspen.
28. Ropper, A. H., Kennedy, S. K., & Russell, L. (1981). Apnea testing in the diagnosis of brain death: Clinical and physiological observations. *Journal of Neurosurgery* 55, 942–946.
29. Cranford, R. E. (1989). The neurologist as ethics consultant and as a member of the institutional ethics committee. *Neurologic Clinics,* 7(4), 697–713.
30. Bernat, J. L. (1989). Ethical issues in brain death and multiorgan transplantation. *Neurologic Clinics,* 7(4), 715–728.

31. Joint Commission on Accreditation of Healthcare Organizations. (1992). *Comprehensive accreditation manual for hospitals.* Oakbrook Terrace, IL: Joint Commission on Accreditation of Healthcare Organization.

Bibliography

Beresford, H. R. (1989). Legal aspects of termination of treatment decisions. *Neurologic Clinics, 7*(4), 775–787.

Foley, J. M. (1991). Ethical issues in the management of cerebrovascular disease. *Clinics in Geriatric Medicine, 7*(3), 631–636.

Gaylin, W. (1994 May/June). Knowing good and doing good. *Hasting's Center Report,* 36–41.

Gert, B., Nelson, W. A., & Culver, C. M. (1989). Moral theory and neurology. *Neurologic Clinics, 7*(4), 681–696.

Howe, E. G. (1995). Impossible choices: When patients and care providers face impossible decisions. *Journal of Clinical Ethics, 6*(10), 3–13.

Jecker, N. S., & Schneiderman, L. J. (1995). When families request that "everything possible" be done. *Journal of Medicine and Philosophy, 20,* 145–163.

Kapp, N. O. (1994). Futile medical treatment: A review of the ethical arguments and legal holdings. *Journal of General Internal Medicine, 9*(March), 170–177.

Kopelman, L. M. (1995). Conceptual and moral disputes about futile and useful treatments. *Journal of Medicine and Philosophy, 20,* 109–121.

Latimer, E. J. (1991). Ethical decision-making in the care of the dying and its applications to clinical practice. *Journal of Pain and Symptom Management, 6*(5), 329–336.

Lynn, J. (1992). Procedures for making medical decisions for incompetent adults. *Journal of the American Medical Association, 267*(15), 2082–2084.

Weber, L. J., & Campbell, M. L. (1996). Medical futility and life-sustaining treatment decisions. *Journal of Neuroscience Nursing, 28*(1), 56–60.

Wocial, L. D. (1996). Achieving collaboration in ethical decision making: Strategies for nurses in clinical practice. *Dimensions of Critical Care Nursing, 15*(3), 150–159.

Section 2

Assessment and Evaluation of Neuroscience Patients

CHAPTER 5

Overview
of Neuroanatomy
and Neurophysiology

Joanne V. Hickey

The purpose of this chapter is to provide an overview of essential neuroanatomy and neurophysiology as a quick reference to assist the reader in understanding the underlying principles of neurological function and dysfunction as a basis for nursing management. Further discussion of anatomy and physiology is presented in Chapters 7 and 8 to clarify information about neurological assessment.

The recent phenomenal increase in knowledge about the nervous system has been extraordinary. The most exciting new knowledge about the nervous system is a result of molecular biological research such as cellular and neuroendocrine function. Neuroanatomy and neurophysiology texts should be consulted if more detail is desired.

EMBRYONIC DEVELOPMENT OF THE NERVOUS SYSTEM

The human brain is composed of billions of cells. The nervous system is one of the first recognizable features in embryonic development. From a simple longitudinal invagination on the dorsal portion of the ectodermal layer, a neural groove and neural tube form at about 3 weeks. At the cranial end of the neural tube, rapid and unequal growth occurs, giving rise to the three primary vesicles of the brain. These vesicles, in turn, become five cerebral areas: the telencephalon, the diencephalon, the mesencephalon, the metencephalon, and the myelencephalon (Table 5-1). By 7 weeks, the brain and spinal cord are apparent. At 12 weeks, the brain is the size of a large pea.

Concurrently, the cells of the neural tube form two types of cells: the spongioblasts, which give rise to the neuroglia (glia) cells, and the neuroblasts, which give rise to the nerve cells (neurons). Processes from the neuroblasts form the white matter of the brain. Some of these processes leave the brain and spinal cord to form the fibers of the cranial and ventral roots of the spinal nerves.

Throughout the prenatal period, there is further growth and refinement of the nervous system. All of the neurons that a person will ever have are present at birth. These highly specialized cells do not have mitotic capacity and, therefore, are not replaceable. At birth, the brain is about one quarter the size of an adult brain.

CELLS OF THE NERVOUS SYSTEM

From the ectodermal layer, two types of cells develop: neurons and neuroglia cells. **Neurons** are the basic anatomical and functional unit of the nervous system. **Neuroglia cells** provide a variety of supportive functions for the neurons.

Neuroglia Cells

The term *glia* comes from a Greek word meaning "glue" or "holding together." In this regard, the glia cells provide structural support, nourishment, and protection for the neurons of the nervous system. There are 5 to 10 times more neuroglia cells than there are neurons. About 40% of the brain and spinal cord is composed of neuroglia cells.

From a clinical viewpoint, neuroglia cells are important because they can divide by mitosis and are the major source of primary tumors of the nervous system. In the central nervous system (CNS), glia are subdivided into four main types: astrocytes, oligodendrocytes, ependymal cells, and microglia. In the peripheral nervous system, Schwann cells form myelin sheaths.

TABLE 5-1
Development of the Primary Vesicles

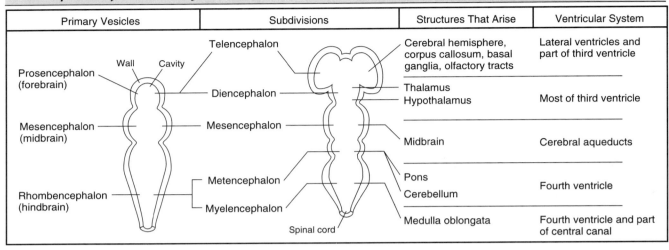

Primary Vesicles	Subdivisions	Structures That Arise	Ventricular System
Prosencephalon (forebrain)	Telencephalon	Cerebral hemisphere, corpus callosum, basal ganglia, olfactory tracts	Lateral ventricles and part of third ventricle
	Diencephalon	Thalamus / Hypothalamus	Most of third ventricle
Mesencephalon (midbrain)	Mesencephalon	Midbrain	Cerebral aqueducts
Rhombencephalon (hindbrain)	Metencephalon	Pons / Cerebellum	Fourth ventricle
	Myelencephalon	Medulla oblongata	Fourth ventricle and part of central canal

Astrocytes have multiple processes extending from the cell body that give it a starlike appearance. Some astrocytic processes may terminate as swellings called end-feet on neurons and blood vessels. Functions attributed to astrocytes include providing nutrition for neurons; regulating synaptic connectivity; removing cellular debris; and controlling movement of molecules from blood to brain (part of the blood–brain barrier).

On microscopic examination, **oligodendrocytes** have few branching processes. Oligodendrocytes produce the myelin sheath of the axonal projections of neurons in the CNS. An individual cell can maintain the myelin sheaths of several axons.

Ciliated **ependyma cells** line the ventricular system and the choroid plexuses. They aid in the production of cerebrospinal fluid (CSF) and act as a barrier to foreign substances within the ventricles, preventing them from entering cerebral tissue.

Microglia are minute cells that are scattered throughout the CNS and have a phagocytic function. They remove and disintegrate the waste products of neurons.

Schwann cells function similarly to oligodendrocytes, forming the insulating myelin sheaths around axons to facilitate saltatory conduction of impulses in the peripheral nervous system.

Neurons

Neurons vary from 5 to 100 μm in diameter. As the basic anatomical and functional unit in the nervous system, the neuron has a number of functions: responding to sensory and chemical stimuli, conducting impulses, and releasing specific chemical regulators.

Neurons are classified as unipolar, bipolar, or multipolar. **Unipolar neurons** possess only one process or pole. This process divides close to the cell body. One branch is called the peripheral process and carries impulses from the periphery toward the cell body. The other branch, called the central process, conducts the impulse toward the spinal cord or the brain stem. **Bipolar neurons** are found only in the spinal and vestibular ganglia, the olfactory mucous membrane, and in one layer of the retina. The anatomical structure is peculiar to the organ in which it is found. Most neurons in the nervous system are **multipolar.** These neurons consist of a cell body, one long projection (the **axon**), and one or more shorter branches (the **dendrites**).

There are three major components of a neuron: a **cell body,** which constitutes the main part of the neuron; a **single axon,** or **axis cylinder,** which consists of a long projection extending from the cell body; and **several dendrites,** which are thin projections extending from the cell body into the immediate surrounding area. The axon carries impulses **away** from the cell body, whereas the dendrites direct impulses **toward** the cell body.

COMPONENTS OF THE CELL BODY

The main organelles of the neuronal cell body include the nucleus, the cell membrane, and the cytoplasm. There are organelles within each of these structures that are important and will be mentioned briefly.

The **nucleus** is a double-membrane structure that contains chromatin and a prominent nucleolus. **Chromatin** is the threadlike structures in the cell nucleus consisting primarily of **deoxyribonucleic acid (DNA)** and protein. DNA contains genes and the genetic code or information about the cell. The **nucleolus** contains **ribonucleic acid (RNA).** RNA is the "messenger" from the genes of the nucleus; it contains the code for synthesis of specific cellular protein.

The **cell membrane** is a triple external membrane primarily consisting of lipoproteins. The cell membrane creates the parameters of the cell body, enclosing the cytoplasm within its border. The main purpose of the cell membrane is to control the interchange of material between the cell and its environment.

The **cytoplasm** contains smooth and rough endoplasmic reticula, Nissl bodies, Golgi apparatus, mitochondria, lysosomes, neurotubules, and neurofibrils. The **endoplasmic reticulum** of the cytoplasm is a network of tubular, membranous structures. There are two types of endoplasmic reticulum, smooth and rough. The smooth endoplasmic reticulum serves as the site for enzyme reactions. **Nissl bodies** are masses of granular (rough) endoplasmic reticulum with ribosomes, which are the protein-synthesizing machinery of the neuron. The endoplasmic reticulum system connects with the nucleus at that portion of the reticulum called the Golgi apparatus. Substances formed in different parts of the cell are transported throughout the cell by means of this system. The **Golgi apparatus** provides for two interrelated functions: (1) further modification of protein by adding carbohydrates and temporary storage; and (2) separation of protein types depending on their function and destination. It is also responsible for the formation of substances important for the digestion of intracellular material.

Mitochondria are structures that serve as the site for production of most of the cellular energy. Cell nutrients are oxidized to produce carbon dioxide and water. The energy released is used to produce adenosine triphosphate (ATP). **Lysosomes** isolate the digestive enzymes of a cell from the cytoplasm to prevent cell destruction. They are involved in digestion of phagocytosis products and worn-out organelles.

The elongated axons or dendrites can extend a meter or more from the cell body. These fibers require protein and other substances produced in the cell body which must be transported from the cytoplasm by a process called axoplasmic flow. **Neurotubules** carry out part of axoplasmic transport. **Neurofibrils** are delicate threadlike structures within the cytoplasm and the axon hillock that assist in the transport of cellular material.

CELL PROCESSES: THE AXON AND DENDRITES

Axons and dendrites constitute the cell processes. Dendrites usually extend only a short distance from the cell body and branch profusely. By contrast, an axon can extend for long distances from the cell body before branching near the end of the projection.

Many axons in the peripheral nervous system are covered by a myelin sheath composed of a white, lipid substance that acts as an insulator for the conduction of impulses. Nerve fibers enclosed in such a sheath are referred to as **myelinated;** those without the myelin sheath are referred to as **unmyelinated** (Fig. 5-1). As a rule, larger neuron fibers are myelinated, whereas smaller fibers are unmyelinated.

The **myelin sheath** is formed by Schwann cells that encircle the axons. When several **Schwann cells** are wrapped around an axon, their outer layer (sheath of Schwann) encloses the myelin sheath. This outer layer is called the **neurolemma** and is said to be necessary for the regeneration of axons. The myelin sheath itself is a segmented, discontinuous layer that is interrupted at intervals by the **nodes of Ranvier.** The distance from one node to the next is called an **internode.** Each internode is formed by, and surrounded by, one Schwann cell. At the junction between each of the two successive Schwann cells along the axon, a small non-insulated area remains where ions can easily flow between the extracellular fluid and the axon. It is this area that is known as the node of Ranvier. In the CNS, the oligodendroglial cells provide the myelination of the neurons, similar to the role of the Schwann cells in the peripheral nervous system.

PHYSIOLOGY OF NERVE IMPULSES

Resting Membrane Potential of the Neurons. Although a resting neuron is not conducting an impulse, it is considered to be a charged cell. The difference in electrical charge on either side of the membrane is called the **potential difference** and is related to the unequal distribution of potassium and sodium on either side of the membrane. Normal resting potential of -70 mV is maintained by the various concentrations of ions in the fluid on either side of the cell membrane.

The cell membrane is both semipermeable and selectively permeable. The area outside the cell is called the interstitial space; the area inside the cell is called the intracellular space. Sodium ions (Na^+) and chloride ions (Cl^-) are found in much greater concentrations in the interstitial space than in the cell. The sodium ion gradient is caused by the powerful sodium pump that continually pumps sodium out of the cell. The potassium ion (K^+) and organic protein material are found in high concentrations within the cell. Potassium is also pumped back into the cell by the potassium pump. The concentration of dissolved ions in a solution is a potential source of energy to drive cellular processes.

Action Potential of the Neuron. The fluid and ions in the intracellular space create a highly conductive solution. The large diameter (10 to 80 μm) allows for unrestricted conduction of impulses from one part of the interior of the cell to the other. A variety of stimuli can change the permeability of the cell membrane to certain ions, resulting in alterations in the membrane potential (Fig. 5-2). The stimuli must be of sufficient magnitude to conduct an impulse and thus create an **action potential.** An action potential is the fundamental unit of signaling in the nervous system.

Many simultaneous discharges at the synaptic junction must occur to create a sufficient effect on the cell membrane. The membrane potential reverses, and the intracellular surface becomes positive (approximately $+20$ to $+40$ mV). When the action potential is realized, there is a sudden reversal of the sodium and potassium relationship across the cell membrane of the axon. This event is called **depolarization.** The neuron receives an influx of sodium and loses potassium to the interstitial space; the time required is only a few milliseconds. With the change in polarity, an impulse is conducted from one neuron to the next at the same amplitude and speed. The cell repolarizes and returns to its resting membrane potential. This sequence of events occurs during the conduction of an impulse in an unmyelinated nerve.

Saltatory Conduction. In myelinated nerves, the action potential hops from one node of Ranvier to the next as a means of rapidly conducting an impulse. This is called **saltatory con-**

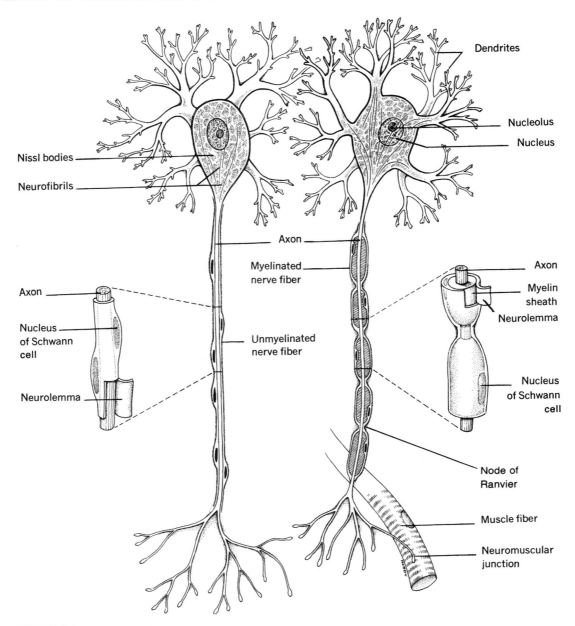

FIGURE 5-1
Typical efferent neurons: unmyelinated fiber (*left*); myelinated fiber (*right*). (From Chaffee, E. E., and I. M. Lytle. [1980]. *Basic physiology and anatomy.* Philadelphia: J. B. Lippincott.)

duction. Although ions cannot flow out through the myelin sheath of myelinated nerves, the break in the myelin sheath at the nodes of Ranvier (see Fig. 5-1) provides a perfect route of escape. At this point, the membrane is several times more permeable than many unmyelinated nerves. Impulses are conducted from node to node rather than continuing along the entire span of the axon, as is the case in unmyelinated nerves. Saltatory conduction is advantageous because it increases the velocity of an impulse and conserves energy (because only the nodes depolarize). The velocity of an impulse depends on both the thickness of the myelin and the distance between the in-

ternodes. As these two factors increase, the velocity of the impulse also increases.

Synapse. The junction between one neuron and the next where an impulse is transmitted is called the **synapse.** There are three anatomical structures that are necessary for an impulse to be transmitted at a synapse. These include the presynaptic terminals, the synaptic cleft, and the postsynaptic membrane (Fig. 5-3).

The **presynaptic terminals** are either excitatory or inhibitory. An excitatory presynaptic terminal secretes an excitatory

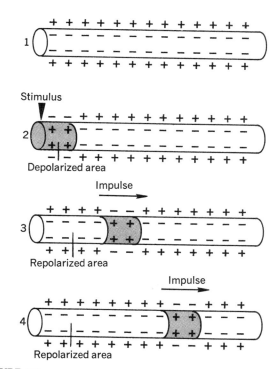

FIGURE 5-2
Diagram of membrane potentials. (*1*) Resting membrane potential—the outer surface bears a positive charge and the inner surface bears a negative charge. (*2*) Action potential, first stage—stimulation of fiber results in depolarization; that is, the outer surface becomes negative and the inner surface becomes positive. (*3*) Action potential, second stage—repolarization occurs as the resting potential is restored. (*4*) Propagation of the impulse continues in the direction of the arrow. (From Chaffee, E. E., and I. M. Lytle. [1980]. *Basic physiology and anatomy.* Philadelphia: J. B. Lippincott.)

substance into the synaptic cleft, thereby exciting the effector neuron. The inhibitory presynaptic terminal secretes an inhibitory transmitter which, when secreted into the synaptic cleft, inhibits the effector neuron. The excitatory or inhibitory transmitter secretions arise from the **synaptic vesicle** in the presynaptic terminal of the axon. Mitochondria in the axon supply the ATP to synthesize new transmitter secretions. The **synaptic cleft** is the microscopic space (200 to 300 angstroms) between the presynaptic terminal and the receptor area of the effector cell. The **postsynaptic membrane** is that part of the effector membrane that is proximal to the presynaptic terminal.

When an action potential spreads over the presynaptic terminal, the membrane depolarizes, emptying some of the contents of the presynaptic vesicles into the synaptic cleft. The released transmitter changes the permeability of the subsynaptic membrane. This results in either excitation or inhibition of the neuron, depending on the type of transmitter substances secreted into the synaptic cleft.

Neurotransmitters. Chemical substances found in the CNS that excite, inhibit, or modify the response of another cerebral cell or cells are called **neurotransmitters.** The presynaptic terminals of one neuron release the chemical that affects particular postsynaptic cells of another neuron. Generally, each neuron releases the same transmitter at all of its separate terminals. Over 30 neurotransmitters have been identified. They include specific **amines** (acetylcholine, serotonin), **catecholamines** (dopamine, epinephrine, and norepinephrine), **amino acids** (GABA, glutamic acid, glycine, and substance P), and **polypeptides** (endorphins and enkephalins). Table 5-2 summarizes the major neurotransmitters.

Postsynaptic Membrane—Excitation and Inhibition. The postsynaptic membrane (the dendrite cell body region of the effector neuron) initiates its response to stimuli by decremental conduction through the synapse; that is, the impulse becomes progressively weaker the more prolonged the period of excitation. Stimulation of the effector cell at the dendrite cell body can create an action potential. For the action potential to be fired, however, the intensity of an impulse must be sufficient to fire the initial segment of axon (just distal to the axon hillock), where the action potential is initiated. It is said that any factor that increases the potential inside the cell body at any given point also increases the potential throughout the cell body.

Because of differences in the cell membrane and shape of the cell, the intracellular voltage necessary to elicit an action potential will vary at different points on the cell membrane. The most sensitive point is the initial segment of the axon, but the impulse must be of sufficient magnitude to depolarize the axon. **Excitation** is the response of the subsynaptic membrane to the neurotransmitter substance that lowers the membrane potential to form an **excitatory postsynaptic potential** (EPSP) (Fig. 5-4, *top*). The potential is a small depolarization that conducts itself by decrement. The cell membrane is made more permeable to sodium, potassium, and chloride. Sodium ions rush into the neuron, while potassium ions leave the cell through the postsynaptic membrane.

Inhibition acts upon a cell so that it is more difficult for it to fire. The inhibitory neurotransmitters increase permeability to only potassium and chloride ions at the synaptic membrane. The membrane potential is raised to form the **inhibitory postsynaptic potential** (IPSP) (see Fig. 5-4, *bottom*).

Presynaptic Inhibition. Another type of inhibition, **presynaptic inhibition,** results from inhibitory knobs being activated on the presynaptic terminal fibrils and synaptic knobs of an axon. When the inhibitory knobs are activated, they secrete a neurotransmitter substance that partially depolarizes the terminal fibrils and excitatory synaptic knobs. As a result, the velocity of the action potential that occurs at the membrane of the excitatory knob is depressed. This action greatly reduces the quantity of excitatory neurotransmitter released by the knob and suppresses the degree of excitation of the neuron.

FUNCTIONS AND DIVISIONS OF THE NERVOUS SYSTEM

The nervous system controls the motor, sensory, autonomic, cognitive, and behavioral functions of the body. It is divided into a hierarchy with three major functional units:

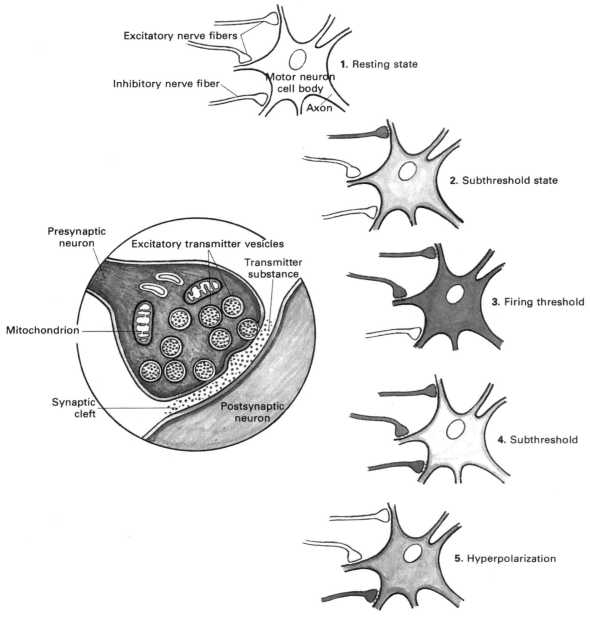

FIGURE 5-3
Conduction at synapses. *Left,* enlarged view of liberation of chemical transmitter substance at a synapse; *right,* diagrams illustrating how a neuron may be excited or inhibited by transmitter substances liberated by presynaptic nerve fiber endings. Two excitatory and one inhibitory fiber are shown: *1,* resting state; *2,* subthreshold state; impulses from only one excitatory fiber cannot cause the postsynaptic neuron to fire; *3,* firing threshold is reached by the addition of impulses from a second excitatory fiber; *4,* subthreshold state is restored by impulses from an inhibitory fiber; *5,* when the inhibitory fiber alone is carrying impulses, the postsynaptic neuron is in a state of hyperpolarization and is unable to fire.

- Spinal cord level—the lowest functional level; controls automatic motor responses such as reflexes
- Brain stem and subcortical level—the second functional level; controls blood pressure, respirations, equilibrium, and primitive emotions
- Cortical level—the highest level; responsible for cognition (storage of information, thinking, memory, and abstraction)

The nervous system is also divided into the CNS and the peripheral nervous system. The CNS is composed of the brain and spinal cord. The peripheral nervous system includes the following: (1) the 12 pairs of cranial nerves; (2) the 31 pairs of spinal nerves; and (3) the autonomic nervous system, which subdivides into the sympathetic and parasympathetic nervous systems.

TABLE 5-2
Neurotransmitters: Source and Action

NAME	SECRETION SOURCE	ACTION
AMINES		
Acetylcholine (ACh)	Neurons in many areas of brain	Usually excitatory
First neurotransmitter identified	Large pyramidal cells (motor cortex)	Inhibitory effect on some of parasympathetic nervous system (*e.g.*, heart by vagus)
Chief transmitter of parasympathetic nervous system (NS)	Some cells of basal ganglia	
	Motor neurons that innervate skeletal muscles	
	Preganglionic neurons of autonomic NS	
	Postganglionic neurons of parasympathetic NS	
	Postganglionic neurons of sympathetic NS	
Serotonin (5-HT)	Nuclei originating in the median raphe of brain stem and projecting to many areas (especially the dorsal horns of the spinal cord and hypothalamus)	Inhibitor of pain pathway cord; helps to control mood and sleep
Controls body heat, hunger, behavior, and sleep		
CATHECHOLAMINES		
Dopamine (DA)	Neurons on the substantia nigra; many neurons of the substantia nigra send fibers to the basal ganglia that are involved in coordination of skeletal muscle activity	Usually inhibitory
Affects control of behavior and fine movement		
Norepinephrine (NE)	Many neurons whose cell bodies are located:	Usually excitatory, although sometimes inhibitory
Chief transmitter of sympathetic nervous system	In brain stem and hypothalamus (controlling overall activity and mood)	
	Most postganglionic neurons of sympathetic NS	Some excitatory and some inhibitory
AMINO ACIDS		
Gamma-aminobutyric acid (GABA)	Nerve terminals of the spinal cord, cerebellum, basal ganglia, and some cortical areas	Excitatory
Glutamic acid	Presynaptic terminals in many sensory pathways; cerebellum mossy fibers	Excitatory
Glycine	Synapses in spinal cord	Inhibitory
Substance P	Pain fiber terminals in the dorsal horns of the spinal cord; also, the basal ganglia and hypothalamus	Excitatory
POLYPEPTIDES		
Enkephalin	Nerve terminals in the spinal cord, brain stem, thalamus, and hypothalamus	Excitatory to systems that inhibit pain; binds to the same receptors in the CNS that bind opiate drugs
Endorphin	Pituitary gland and areas of the brain	Binds to opiate receptors in the brain and pituitary gland; excitatory to systems that inhibit pain

NS = nervous system; ANS = autonomic nervous system; CNS = central nervous system.

CRANIAL AND SPINAL BONES

The purpose of the skull and vertebral column is to protect the most vulnerable parts of the nervous system—the brain and spinal cord.

Skull

The **skull** is the bony framework of the head; it is composed of the 8 bones of the cranium and the 14 bones of the face. Knowledge of the anatomy of both the external and internal surfaces of the bones (Figs. 5-5 and 5-6) is helpful in understanding the pathophysiology of craniocerebral trauma.

The **cranium** is defined as that part of the skull that encloses the brain and provides a protective vault for this vital organ. The bones that compose the cranium are the frontal, occipital, sphenoid, and ethmoid, as well as the two parietal and temporal bones.

The **frontal bone** forms the forehead and the front (anterior) part of the top of the skull. The supraorbital arches form the roofs of the two orbits. Frontal sinuses are also located in this bone. The inner table of the frontal bone has a highly irregular bony surface.

The **occipital bone** is the large bone at the back (posterior) of the skull that curves into the base of the skull. The significant markings include (1) the large hole (foramen magnum) in the base of the skull and (2) the occipital condyles located on either side of the foramen magnum that fit into depressions on the first cervical vertebra.

The **sphenoid bone** is a wedge-shaped bone alleged to resemble a bat's wings. The significant bone markings include a body, lesser wings, greater wings, pterygoid process, the

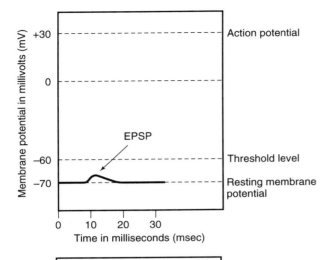

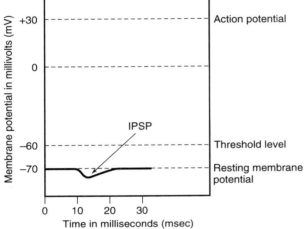

FIGURE 5-4
Comparison of excitatory and inhibitory postsynaptic potentials. (*Top*) Excitatory postsynaptic potential. (*Bottom*) Inhibitory postsynaptic potential. (From Tortora, G. J., and N. P. Anagnostakos. [1987]. *Principles of anatomy and physiology.* [5th ed.]. New York: Harper & Row.)

sella turcica (also known as the "Turk's saddle"), and the clivus. The **clivus** is the slanted dorsal surface of the body of the sphenoid bone between the sella turcica and basilar process of the sphenoid bone. The hypophysis (pituitary gland) is located in the region of the sella turcica.

The **ethmoid bone,** largely hidden between the two orbits, contains both a perpendicular and horizontal plate, as well as two lateral masses. The horizontal plate, also called the cribriform plate, forms part of the base of the skull through which the olfactory nerves (first cranial nerves) travel. The perpendicular plate forms part of the nasal septum, whereas the lateral masses are part of the ethmoid sinuses.

The **temporal bones** are situated at the sides and base of the skull and consist of three anatomical divisions: the squamous, mastoid, and petrous portions. The temporal bone is highly irregular, both on the internal and external surfaces.

The **squamous portion** is very thin just above the auditory meatus. It contains the zygomatic process externally; internally, there are numerous eminences and depressions to accommodate the contour of the cerebrum. Two well-marked internal grooves are evident for the branches of the middle meningeal artery, a common point of trauma with head injury.

The **mastoid portion** is perforated by many foramina, including a larger foramen, the mastoid foramen, which contains a vein that drains the lateral sinus and a small artery to supply the dura mater. The mastoid process is also contained in this portion of the temporal bone.

The **petrous portion** is so named because it is extremely dense and stonelike in its hardness. There is a pyramidal process that is directed inward and is wedged at the base of the skull between the sphenoid and occipital bones. The internal plate of the petrous portion of the temporal bone is proximal to the branches of the middle meningeal artery.

The **parietal bones,** which fuse on the top of the skull, form the sides of the skull. Externally, they are smooth and convex; internally, the surface is concave with some depressions to accommodate the convolutions of the cerebrum and the grooves for the middle meningeal artery. With these exceptions, the bone has a regular inner surface.

SUTURES OF THE SKULL

The bones of the skull join at various places, known as suture lines. The four major sutures of the skull include the following (see Fig. 5-5):

Sagittal suture—the midline suture formed by the two parietal bones joining on the top of the skull
Coronal suture (frontoparietal)—connecting the frontal and parietal bones transversely
Lambdoidal suture (occipitoparietal)—connecting the occipital and parietal bones
Basilar suture—created by the junction of the basilar surface of the occipital bone with the posterior surface of the sphenoid bone.

Spine

The spine is a flexible column formed by a series of bones called **vertebrae**, each stacked one upon another to support the head and trunk. The vertebral column is made up of 33 vertebrae: 7 cervical vertebrae, 12 thoracic or dorsal vertebrae, 5 lumbar vertebrae, 5 sacral vertebrae (fused into one), and 4 coccygeal vertebrae (fused into one) (Fig. 5-7). Each vertebra consists of two essential parts, an anterior solid segment or **body,** and a posterior segment or **arch.** Two **pedicles** and two **laminae** supporting seven processes (four articular, two transverse, and one spinous) make up the arch (Fig. 5-8).

The cervical vertebrae are smaller than those in any other region of the spine. The first cervical vertebra is called the **atlas,** whereas the second cervical vertebra is known as the **axis.** Each of these two vertebrae is unique in appearance. The axis has a perpendicular projection called the **odontoid process** upon which the atlas sits (Fig. 5-9).

The thoracic or dorsal vertebrae are intermediate in size, becoming larger as they descend the vertebral column. The lumbar vertebrae are the largest segments in the spine (see Fig. 5-9).

The vertebral bodies are the largest part of the vertebrae, above and below which flattened surfaces are found for attachment of fibrocartilage. There are apertures for spinal nerves,

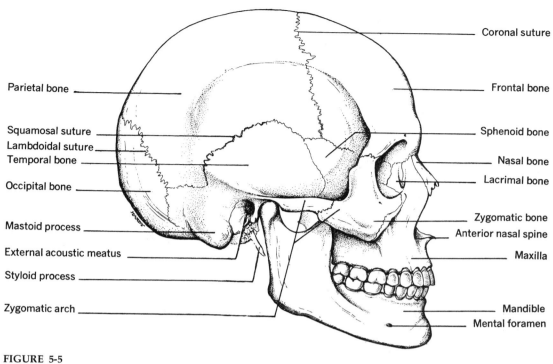

Coronal suture

Parietal bone

Frontal bone

Squamosal suture

Sphenoid bone

Lambdoidal suture

Nasal bone

Temporal bone

Lacrimal bone

Occipital bone

Zygomatic bone

Anterior nasal spine

Mastoid process

Maxilla

External acoustic meatus

Styloid process

Zygomatic arch

Mandible

Mental foramen

FIGURE 5-5
Lateral view of the skull.

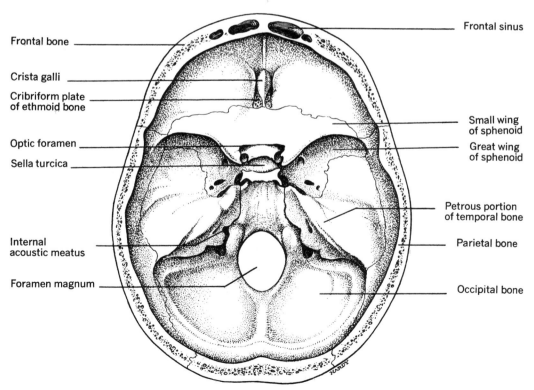

Frontal sinus

Frontal bone

Crista galli

Cribriform plate
of ethmoid bone

Small wing
of sphenoid

Optic foramen

Great wing
of sphenoid

Sella turcica

Petrous portion
of temporal bone

Internal
acoustic meatus

Parietal bone

Foramen magnum

Occipital bone

FIGURE 5-6
View of the base of the skull from above, showing the internal surfaces of some of the cranial bones.

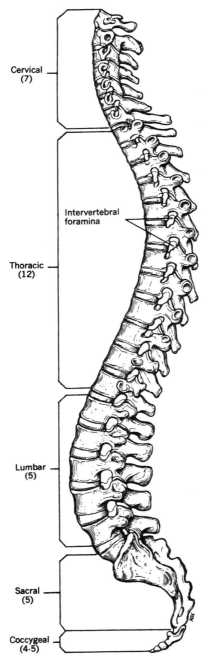

FIGURE 5-7
Lateral view of the adult vertebral column.

Cervical (7)

Intervertebral foramina

Thoracic (12)

Lumbar (5)

Sacral (5)

Coccygeal (4-5)

veins, and arteries. The vertebrae are connected by means of the articular processes and the intervertebral fibrocartilage.

The arch of the vertebrae is composed of two pedicles, two laminae, a spinous process, four articular processes, and two transverse processes. The two **pedicles** are short, thick pieces of bone. The concavity above and below the pedicles creates the intervertebral notches from which the spinal nerves emanate. The two **laminae** are broad plates of bone. They complete the neural arch by fusing in the midline and enclose the spinal foramen, which protects the spinal cord. The upper and lower borders are rough in order to allow for the attachment

of the ligamenta subflava. The **spinous process** projects backward from the laminae and serves as the attachment for muscles and ligaments. The four **articular processes** (two on either side) provide stability for the spine. The two **transverse processes** provide stability for the spine and serve as points of attachment for muscles and ligaments.

LIGAMENTS OF THE SPINE

The most important ligaments of the vertebral column are the anterior and posterior longitudinal ligaments and the ligamenta flava. The **anterior longitudinal ligament** consists of longitudinal fibers firmly attached to the anterior surface of the vertebral bodies and intervertebral discs. The **posterior longitudinal ligament** is attached to the posterior surface of the vertebral bodies within the spinal canal. The **ligamenta flava** consists of yellow elastic fibers that connect the laminae of adjacent vertebrae. The attachment pattern is unique in that the attachment is from the lower margin of the anterior surface of the superior lamina to the posterior surface of the upper margin of the inferior lamina.

The **supraspinous ligament** joins the spinous process tips from C7 to the sacrum. The **interspinal ligaments** connect adjacent spinous processes from their tips to their roots. The interspinals fuse with the supraspinals posteriorly and with the ligamentum flavum anteriorly. Such an arrangement controls vertebral movement to prevent excessive flexion. If violent force in any direction occurs, these ligaments can be ruptured, possibly causing injury to the vertebrae and spinal cord (see Chaps. 22 and 23).

INTERVERTEBRAL DISCS

The **intervertebral discs** are fibrocartilaginous, disc-shaped structures located between the vertebral bodies from the second cervical vertebra to the sacrum. They vary in size, thickness, and shape at different levels of the spine. The purpose of the intervertebral disc is to cushion movement. The central core, the **nucleus pulposus,** is surrounded by a fibrous capsule called the **annulus fibrosus.** As a result of aging and trauma, discs lose their water content and the tissue is more prone to injury.

MENINGES

Meninges cover both the brain and spinal cord. The layers, from the outermost layer inward, are called the **dura mater,** the **arachnoid,** and the **pia mater** (Figs. 5-10 and 5-11).

The **dura mater** is a double-layered, whitish, inelastic, fibrous membrane that lines the interior of the skull. The outer layer of the dura is actually the periosteum of the bone. The inner layer is the thick membrane that extends throughout the skull and creates compartments. The dura lines various foraminae that exit at the base of the skull. Sheaths for the nerves passing through these foraminae are also formed by the dura.

Four folds of dura (see Fig. 5-11) are situated within the skull cavity to support and protect the brain. They include the following:

1. **Falx cerebri,** a double fold of dura, descends vertically into the longitudinal fissure between the two hemi-

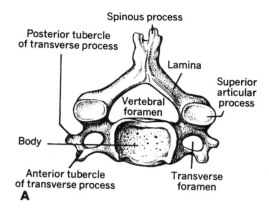

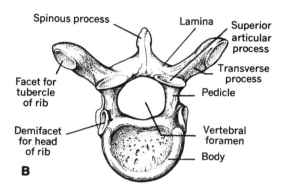

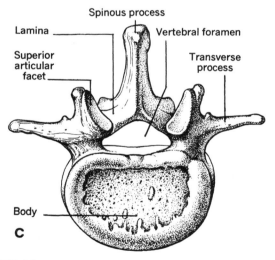

FIGURE 5-8
Views of three types of vertebrae. (*A*) Fourth cervical vertebra, superior aspect. (*B*) Sixth thoracic vertebra, superior aspect. (*C*) Third lumbar vertebra, superior aspect.

spheres of the brain and partially divides the frontal lobe into a left and right side.
2. **Tentorium cerebelli** is a tentlike double fold of dura that covers the upper surface of the cerebellum, supports the occipital lobes, and prevents them from pressing upon the cerebellum. The falx cerebri attaches midline to the tentorium. (The tentorium is an important anatomical point to note. The area above the tentorium is termed **supra-**

tentorial, whereas the area below it is called **infratentorial.** The nursing care given differs based on these two classifications, as discussed in Chap. 18.) In addition, the opening in the tentorium from which the brain stem emerges is called the tentorial notch. Herniation through this opening is called uncal herniation.
3. **Falx cerebelli** is found between the two lateral lobes of the cerebellum.
4. **Diaphragma sella** is a horizontal process that forms a small circular fold, thus creating a roof for the sella turcica.

The spinal dura is a continuation of the inner layer of the cerebral dura. The outer layer of the dura terminates at the foramen magnum, being replaced by the periosteal lining of the vertebral canal. The spinal dura encases the spinal roots, spinal ganglia, and spinal nerves. The spinal dural sac terminates at the second or third sacral level.

The second meningeal layer, the **arachnoid membrane,** is an extremely thin and delicate layer that loosely encloses the brain. The subdural space separates the dura mater from the arachnoid layer. Bleeding within this space (subdural hemorrhage) can occur with head injury. The subarachnoid space is not really a clear space because there is much spongy, delicate connective tissue between the arachnoid and pia mater layers. CSF flows in the subarachnoid space. The cisterna magnum is a space between the hemispheres of the cerebellum and the medulla oblongata. The arachnoid layer of the spinal meninges is a continuation of the cerebral arachnoid (Fig. 5-12). The arachnoid is a delicate, gossamer network of fine, elastic, fibrous tissue; it also contains blood vessels of varying sizes, which may be damaged by lumbar or cisternal puncture, resulting in hemorrhage.

The innermost layer of the meninges is called the **pia mater.** It is a meshlike, vascular membrane that derives its blood supply from the internal carotid and vertebral arteries. The pia mater covers the entire surface of the brain, dipping down between the convolutions of the surface. Because the pia covers the gray matter, the vascularity increases and minute perpendicular vessels extend for some distance into the cerebrum. The pia mater of the spinal cord is thicker, firmer, and less vascular than that of the brain.

Spaces of the Meninges

Three spaces located within the meninges are important to note. The **epidural** or **extradural space** is a potential space located between the skull and outer layer of the dura layer of the brain. In the vertebral column, the epidural space is between the periosteum and the single dural layer. The **subdural space** is between the inner dura mater and arachnoid layer. This is a narrow space and is the site of subdural hemorrhage with certain injuries. The third space is the **subarachnoid space,** which is between the arachnoid and pia mater layers and contains CSF.

CEREBROSPINAL FLUID

CSF is normally a clear, colorless, odorless solution that fills the ventricles of the brain and the subarachnoid space of the brain and spinal cord. The purpose of the CSF is to act as a

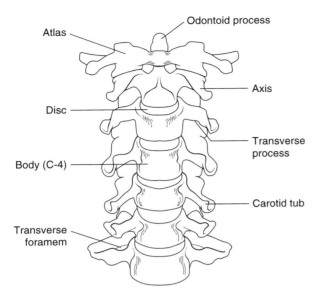

FIGURE 5-9
The cervical spine.

shock absorber, cushioning the brain and spinal cord against injury caused by movement. The specific gravity of CSF is 1.007 (see Chart 6-2 for CSF normal values). CSF differs from other extracellular fluids in the percentage of composition of various factors. It is composed of water, a small amount of protein, oxygen, and carbon dioxide. The electrolytes—sodium, potassium, and chloride—and glucose, an important cerebral nutrient, are also present. An occasional lymphocyte may be present. Normally, CSF pressure is in the range of 60 to 180 mm of water pressure in the lateral recumbent position, which is the position assumed for a lumbar puncture. In the sitting position, a normal lumbar puncture will register 200 to 350 mm of water pressure. Fluctuation in pressure occurs in response to the cardiac cycle and respirations. The amount of CSF in adults is approximately 125 to 150 ml.

Formation of Cerebrospinal Fluid

CSF, which is produced by active transport and diffusion, is formed from three different sources. The major source of CSF is the secretions from the choroid plexus, a cauliflower-like structure located in portions of the lateral, third, and fourth ventricles (Fig. 5-13). The **choroid plexus** is a collection of blood vessels covered by a thin coating of ependymal cells. CSF is constantly secreted from these surfaces. It is estimated that the amount of CSF produced daily by the choroid plexus is about 500 ml, or 25 ml per hour. A lesser proportion of CSF is secreted from the second source, the ependymal cells, which line the ventricles and blood vessels of the meninges. Finally, CSF is also produced by the blood vessels of the brain and spinal cord. The amount produced from this source is very small.

Ventricular System

The two **lateral ventricles,** one on either side of the midline, are located in the lower and inner parts of the cerebral hemisphere. Each lateral ventricle consists of a **central cavity** or **body** and

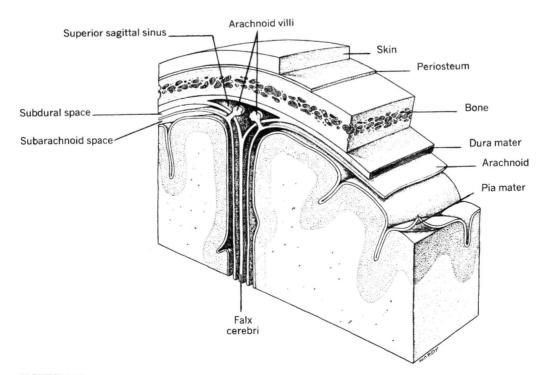

FIGURE 5-10
The cranial meninges. The arachnoid villi shown within the superior sagittal sinus are one site of passage of cerebrospinal fluid into the blood. (From Chaffee, E. E., and I. M. Lytle. [1980]. *Basic physiology and anatomy.* Philadelphia: J. B. Lippincott.)

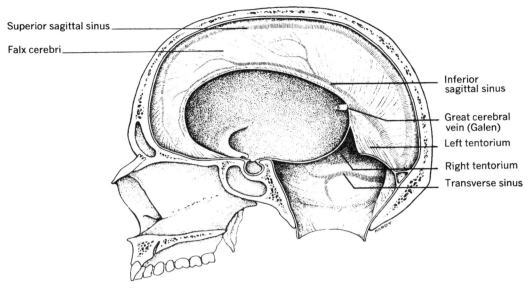

FIGURE 5-11
Cranial dura mater. The skull is depicted open to show the falx cerebri and the right and left portions of the tentorium cerebelli, as well as some of the cranial venous sinuses. (From Chaffee, E. E., and I. M. Lytle. [1980]. *Basic physiology and anatomy*. Philadelphia: J. B. Lippincott.)

three **horns.** The central cavity is located in the lower part of the parietal lobe. The **anterior horn** curves forward and outward into the frontal lobe; the **posterior horn** curves backward and inward into the occipital lobe; and the **middle or lateral horn** descends into the temporal lobe. The curved corpus callosum forms the undersurface of the central cavity and the roof of the anterior, middle, and posterior horns.

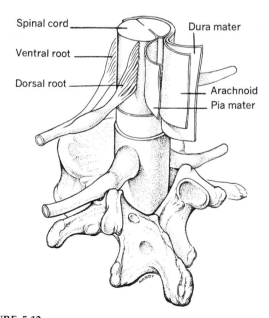

FIGURE 5-12
Spinal cord and meninges. (From Chaffee, E. E., and I. M. Lytle. [1980]. *Basic physiology and anatomy*. Philadelphia: J. B. Lippincott.)

The singular **third ventricle** is a midline inner brain cavity structure. The two optic thalami form the side walls. The floor is formed by the tuber cinereum (infundibulum, pituitary), corpora albicantia, and crus cerebri. The ventricle is bounded by the fornix in the front and pineal body in the back. The singular, diamond-shaped **fourth ventricle** is laterally bounded by the pons and the superior cerebellar peduncles. The roof is formed by the superior cerebellar peduncles and medulla. The floor of the fourth ventricle is continuous with the central spinal canal.

Flow of Cerebrospinal Fluid

CSF circulation has been termed the "third circulation." It is a closed system. Fluid formed by choroid plexuses in the two lateral ventricles passes into the third ventricle by way of the two foramina of Munro. The single cerebral aqueduct or aqueduct of Sylvius connects the third and fourth ventricles. CSF flows through the two lateral foramina of Luschka and midline through the foramen of Magendie to the cisternal magnum. At this point, the CSF enters the subarachnoid space. The foramen of Magendie allows CSF to circulate around the cord, whereas the foramen of Luschka directs the CSF around the brain (Fig. 5-14).

Expanded areas of the subarachnoid space are called **cisterns.** CSF may be aspirated from some of these areas for analysis. The major cisterns are the cisterna magnum, between the medulla and cerebellar region, and the lumbar cistern, between vertebrae L-2 and S-2.

Cerebrospinal Fluid Absorption

Most of the CSF produced daily is reabsorbed into the **arachnoid villi,** which are projections from the subarachnoid space into the venous sinuses of the brain (see Fig. 5-13). CSF drains

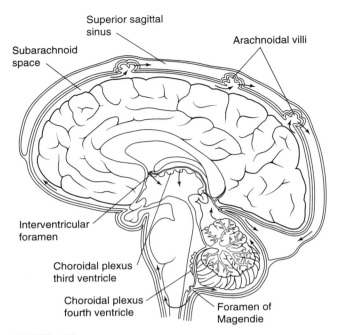

FIGURE 5-13
Diagram of the flow of cerebrospinal fluid from the time of its formation from blood in the choroid plexuses until its return to the blood in the superior sagittal sinus.

into the superior sagittal sinus. Arachnoid villi are very permeable and allow CSF, including protein molecules, to exit easily from the subarachnoid space into the venous sinuses. CSF flows in one direction through the arachnoid villi (most of which are located in the subarachnoid space of the cerebrum), which have been compared to pressure-sensitive valves. When CSF pressure is greater than venous pressure, CSF leaves the subarachnoid space. As pressures are equalized, the valves close.

CEREBROVASCULAR CIRCULATION

The blood vessels that supply the nervous system form an extensive capillary bed, particularly in the gray matter of the brain. About **20% of the oxygen** consumed by the body is used for the oxidation of glucose to provide energy. The brain is totally dependent on glucose for its metabolism. A lack of oxygen to the brain for 5 minutes can result in irreversible brain damage.

The brain receives **approximately 750 mL/min of blood, or 15% to 20% of the total resting cardiac output.** These figures remain relatively constant because of various control systems affecting the brain. Blood flow rates to specific areas of the brain correlate directly to the metabolism of the cerebral tissue. The brain is supplied by two pairs of arteries: the two internal carotid arteries and the two vertebral arteries. Cerebral circulation is also divided into the anterior and the posterior circulation. The **anterior circulation** refers to the common carotids and their distal branches including the internal carotid arteries, the middle

cerebral arteries, and the anterior cerebral arteries. The **posterior circulation** refers to the vertebral arteries, the basilar artery, and the posterior arteries.

Internal Carotid Arteries

The internal carotid arteries originate from two different vessels: the **left common carotid,** which originates directly from the aorta; and the **right common carotid,** which arises from the **innominate artery** also originating from the aorta. The common carotids branch to form the external and internal carotid arteries. The external carotid artery supplies the face, scalp, and other extracranial structures. The internal carotid artery enters the cranial vault through the foramen lacerum in the floor of the middle cranial fossa. As the internal carotid passes through the bone and dura at the base of the skull and approaches the upper brain, it passes forward through the cavernous sinus just lateral to the pituitary fossa. It curves sharply several times and roughly forms an S, called the **carotid siphon.** Most of the hemispheres, excluding the occipitals, the basal ganglia, and the upper two thirds of the diencephalon, are supplied by the internal carotid arteries.

The first intracranial branch from the internal carotid artery is the ophthalmic artery. The terminal branches of each carotid include the posterior communicating artery, the anterior cerebral artery, and the middle cerebral artery (Fig. 5-15).

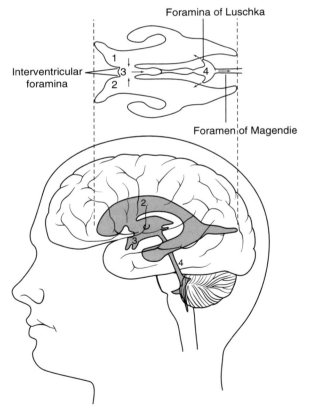

FIGURE 5-14
The ventricles of the brain—the ventricles are outlined, and the arrows indicate the direction of flow of CSF (*above*) and their relation to the brain as a whole (*below*).

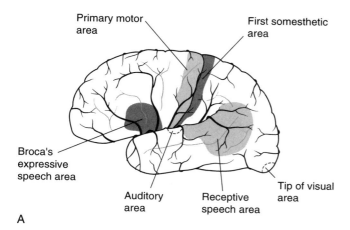

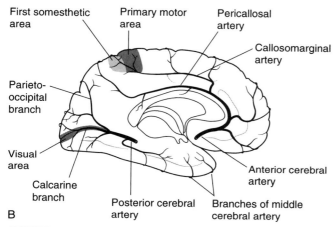

FIGURE 5-15
(*A*) Distribution of the middle cerebral artery on the lateral surface of the cerebral hemisphere. (*B*) Distribution of the anterior and posterior cerebral arteries on the medial surface of the cerebral hemisphere. (From Barr, M. L., and J. A. Kiernan. [1988]. *The nervous system.* [5th ed.]. Philadelphia: Harper & Row.)

Table 5-3 summarizes the major branches of the carotid arteries and the areas supplied.

CHARACTERISTICS OF THE CEREBRAL CIRCULATION

The following lists the outstanding characteristics of cerebral circulation:

1. Cerebral arteries have thinner walls than arteries of comparable size in other parts of the body. Cerebral arteries have an internal elastic tissue and scanty smooth muscle.
2. The veins (other than sinuses) have even thinner walls in proportion to their size and lack a muscle layer.
3. The veins and sinuses have **no** valves.
4. The venous return does not retrace the course of corresponding arteries but follows a pattern of its own.
5. The dural sinuses are unique to cerebral circulation.

6. The distribution of the arteries with rich surfaces (arteries anastomosed by localized "end-artery" distribution of branches penetrating the nervous tissue) is distinctive.

Vertebral Arteries

The **vertebral arteries,** originating from the **subclavian arteries,** enter the skull through the foramen magnum, ventrolateral to the spinal cord. The two vertebral arteries unite at the level of the pons to become the singular **basilar artery** (Fig. 5-16). The basilar artery subdivides into the two posterior cerebral arteries that supply part of the cerebrum.

In general, the vertebral arteries and their branches supply the cerebellum, the brain stem, the spinal cord, the occipital lobes, the medial and inferior surfaces of the temporal lobes, and the posterior diencephalon.

Before they begin to supply blood to the brain, the vertebral arteries give off recurrent branches that anastomose with the anterior and posterior spinal arteries and with a posterior meningeal branch. In its intracranial course, the vertebral arteries give rise to direct bulbar arteries to the medulla, the anterior spinal artery, the **posterior inferior cerebellar artery (PICA),** sometimes the posterior spinal artery, and small branches to the basal meninges. The first branch off the basilar artery is the **anterior inferior cerebellar artery (AICA).** The basilar artery is also the origin of the pontine arteries, the internal auditory arteries, the superior cerebellar arteries, and the posterior cerebral arter-

TABLE 5-3
Major Internal Carotid Arterial Branches and the Cerebral Areas They Innervate

ARTERY	AREA SUPPLIED
Ophthalmic	Orbits and optic nerves
Posterior communicating (Pcom)	Connects the carotid circulation with the vertebrobasilar circulation
Anterior choroidal	Part of choroid plexuses of lateral ventricles; hippocampal formation; portions of globus pallidus; part of internal capsule; part of amygdaloid nucleus; part of caudate nucleus; part of putamen
Anterior cerebral (ACA)	Medial surfaces of frontal and parietal lobes; part of cingulate gyrus and "leg area" of precentral gyrus
Recurrent artery of Heubner	Special branch of ACA, penetrates the anterior perforated substance to supply part of basal ganglia and genu of internal capsule (also called medial striate artery)
Middle cerebral (MCA) (has several branches)	Entire lateral surfaces of the hemisphere except for the occipital pole and the inferolateral surface of the hemisphere (supplied by posterior cerebral artery)
Lenticulostriate (from MCA)	Part of basal ganglia and internal capsule
Anterior communicating (Acom)	Connects the two ACAs

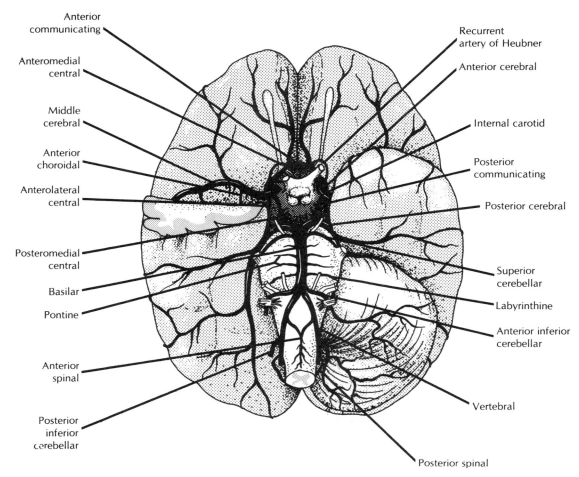

FIGURE 5-16
The blood supply of the brain, as seen on the ventral surface. (The right cerebellar hemisphere and the tip of the right temporal lobe have been removed.) (From Barr, M. L., and J. A. Kiernan. [1993]. *The human nervous system.* [6th ed.]. Philadelphia: J. B. Lippincott.)

ies. Table 5-4 summarizes the major branches of the vertebral arteries and the areas supplied.

Circle of Willis

The circle of Willis, which is located at the base of the skull, is divided into anterior (carotid portion) and posterior (vertebrobasilar portion) circulation (see Fig. 5-16). The composition of each portion includes these elements:

- Middle cerebral arteries, the anterior cerebral arteries, and the anterior communicating artery which connects the two anterior cerebral arteries
- Two posterior cerebral arteries; two posterior communicating arteries connect the middle cerebral arteries with the posterior cerebral arteries, thus uniting the internal carotid system with the vertebral–basilar system

The circle of Willis encloses a very small area that is little more than one square inch in diameter, or approximately 6 cm². Functionally, the carotid circulation and the posterior circulation usually remain separate. At one time, the circle of

Willis was thought to be a protective mechanism by which blood was shunted to compensate for alterations in cerebral blood flow or pressure. However, collateral circulation through the circle depends on the patency of its components. The vessels of the circle of Willis, particularly the communicating arteries, may be anomalous. Nevertheless, in *favorable instances,* the circle does permit an adequate blood supply to reach all parts of the brain, even after one or more of the four supplying vessels has been ligated.

Venous Drainage

Unlike venous drainage in other parts of the body, which closely follows the arterial pattern, the cerebral venous drainage is chiefly managed by vascular channels created by the two dural layers called **dural sinuses.** There are no valves in dural sinuses. A few dural sinuses deserve mention; these are included in Table 5-5 along with the areas they supply (Fig. 5-17). **Emissary veins** join extracranial veins with the venous sinuses. **Bridging veins** connect the brain and dural sinuses and are often the cause of subdural hemorrhage. Cerebral veins empty into the dural sinuses

TABLE 5-4
Major Vertebral Arterial Branches and the Cerebral Areas They Innervate

ARTERY	AREA SUPPLIED
VERTEBRAL BRANCHES	
Anterior spinal (only one artery)	Anterior two thirds of spinal cord
Posterior spinals	Posterior one third of spinal cord
Posterior inferior cerebellar (PICA)	Undersurface of the cerebellum; medulla; and choroid plexuses of 4th ventricle
BASILAR ARTERY BRANCHES	
Posterior cerebral (PCA)	Occipital lobes, medial and inferior surfaces of the temporal lobes, midbrain, and choroid plexuses of 3rd and lateral ventricle
Posterior choroidals (from PCA)	
Medial posterior choroidal	Tectum, choroid plexus of 3rd ventricle, and superior and medial surfaces of the thalamus
Lateral posterior choroidal	Penetrating the choroidal fissure and anastomosing with branches of the anterior choroidal arteries
Anterior inferior cerebellar (AICA)	Undersurface of the cerebellum and lateral surface of the pons
Superior cerebellar (SCA)	Upper surface of the cerebellum and midbrain
Pontine	Pons

which, in turn, empty into the **jugular veins,** which return the blood to the heart.

Meningeal Blood Supply

The meninges are supplied with arterial blood by the anterior, middle, and posterior meningeal arteries. The main route for the arterial supply of the dura mater is through the middle meningeal branches of the external carotid artery. Each vessel ascends through a foramen in the base of the skull and is then situated between the dura mater and the skull. These vessels may be torn as a result of a head injury, thereby causing an epidural hematoma, which requires immediate medical attention.

Blood Supply to the Spinal Cord, Spinal Roots, and Spinal Nerves

The upper cervical cord receives its arterial blood supply from the vertebral arteries via recurrent branches. Below this region, the spinal cord receives its arterial blood supply, in part, from the anterior spinal artery and the two posterior spinal arteries, which arise from the vertebral arteries. The **anterior spinal artery** runs the full length of the cord midventrally, whereas the two **posterior spinal arteries** run full length along each row of the dorsal roots. As these three vessels pass down the cord, they receive feeders from deep cervical, intercostal, lumbar, and sacral arteries.

Additional blood supply comes from **radicular arteries** (supply blood to only one nerve root) and **radiculospinal arteries** (supply blood to about six spinal cord segments). The large **artery of Adamkiewicz** originates from the aorta and enters the cord at about the second lumbar (L2) ventral root level (range T10 to L2) and supplies most of the caudal third of the cord.

The venous system of the spine includes an intradural and extradural system. The intradural veins follow the pattern of the arteries, whereas the extradural intravertebral veins form a plexus extending from the cranium to the pelvis and having many communications along the way with veins of the neck, thorax, and abdomen.

BLOOD–BRAIN BARRIER

For the CNS to function normally, a very stable environment must be maintained within that body system. The so-called blood–brain barrier is a descriptive term for the network of endothelial cells (cells that compose the walls of capillaries) and the projections from the astrocytes located in close proximity to the neuron. Astrocytes are large stellate cells with numerous radiating cytoplasmic processes. Extensions of astrocytes called **perivascular feet** surround the brain capillaries.

Capillaries in the brain, unlike those in other areas, do not have pores between adjacent endothelial cells. Therefore, the brain cannot derive molecules from blood plasma by a nonspecific filtering process. Instead, molecules within cerebral capillaries are transported through the endothelial cells by active transport, endocytosis, and exocytosis. This creates a highly selective blood–brain barrier that guards the entrance into neurons. Before molecules in the blood can enter neurons in the CNS, they pass through both the capillary endothelial cells and the astrocytes. The tight junctions between the endothelial cells and the astrocytes are largely responsible for

TABLE 5-5
Major Sources of Venous Drainage of the Cerebral Circulation and the Areas Drained

VENOUS STRUCTURE	AREA DRAINED
Superior longitudinal (sagittal) sinus	Superior cortical veins of the convexity of the brain; drains CSF
Inferior longitudinal sinus	Medial surface of the brain
Straight sinus	Joins the superior longitudinal sinus; the vein of Galen drains into the straight sinus
Transverse sinus	Area of the ears; collects blood from superior longitudinal and straight sinuses and drains it into the internal jugular vein
Cavernous sinus (contains several cranial nerves and internal carotid artery)	Inferior surface of the brain, including the orbits

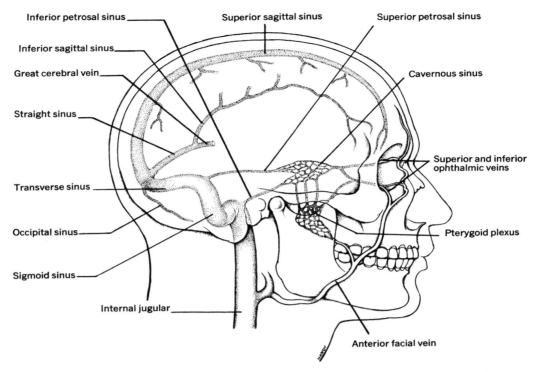

FIGURE 5-17
The cranial venous sinuses. The sigmoid portion of the transverse sinus continues as the internal jugular vein. (From Chaffee, E. E., and I. M. Lytle. [1980]. *Basic physiology and anatomy.* Philadelphia: J. B. Lippincott.)

the blood–brain barrier. Because of this barrier, most drugs are prevented from affecting the brain and spinal cord.

The movement of substances into the brain depends on particle size, lipid solubility, chemical dissociation, and the protein-binding potential of the drug. In general, drugs that are lipid-soluble and undissociated at body pH will rapidly enter both the brain and the CSF. When compared with other body organs, the CNS is very slow in its uptake of dyes and both organic and inorganic anions and cations (*e.g.,* sodium, potassium, glutamic acid) from the circulating blood. The barrier is very permeable to water, oxygen, carbon dioxide, other gases, glucose, and lipid-soluble compounds.

BRAIN (ENCEPHALON)

The brain constitutes approximately 2% of body weight. The average weight of the brain of a young adult male is about 1,400 g. The brains of older people weigh less, with the average weight being about 1,200 g.

The brain is divided into three major areas: the cerebrum, the brain stem, and the cerebellum (Fig. 5-18). The **cerebrum** is composed of the cerebral hemispheres, thalamus, hypothalamus, and the basal ganglia. In addition, the olfactory and optic nerves (cranial nerves I and II) are located in the cerebrum. The **brain stem** includes the midbrain, pons, and medulla. The midbrain, which contains the cerebral peduncles and corpus quadrigemina, is a short segment between the hypothalamus and the pons.

Another means of subdividing the brain is by fossae. The **anterior fossa** contains the frontal lobes; the **middle fossa** contains the temporal, parietal, and occipital lobes; and the **posterior fossa** contains the brain stem and cerebellum.

Cerebrum

The cerebrum comprises **two cerebral hemispheres** that are incompletely separated by the great longitudinal fissure. A **fissure,** also called a **sulcus,** is a large, predictable separation in the cerebral hemisphere. The following are some important fissures that are landmarks in studying the gross anatomy of the brain:

1. The **great longitudinal fissure** is a midsagittal fissure that separates the cerebral hemispheres into a left and right side. The hemispheres are joined at the bottom of the fissure by the corpus callosum.
2. The **lateral fissure of Sylvius** separates the temporal lobe from the frontal and parietal lobes.
3. The **central fissure of Rolando** separates the frontal lobe from the parietal lobe.
4. The last major fissure is the **parieto-occipital fissure,** which separates the occipital lobe from the parietal and temporal lobes (Fig. 5-19).

The surface of the hemispheres consists of numerous "wrinkles," or **gyri** (also called **convolutions**). The gyri fold in upon one another, thereby substantially increasing the sur-

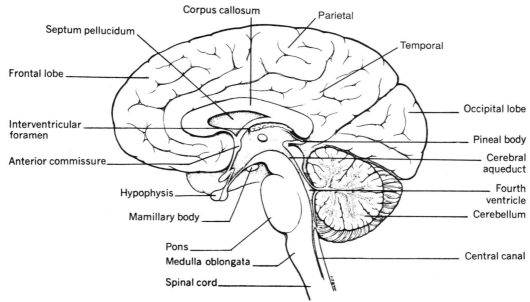

FIGURE 5-18
Midsagittal section of the brain. (From Chaffee, E. E., and I. M. Lytle. [1980]. *Basic physiology and anatomy.* Philadelphia: J. B. Lippincott.)

face area of the brain. Each hemisphere is covered by a cerebral cortex of gray matter that is 2- to 5-mm thick and contains billions of neurons.

Under the cerebral cortex is **white matter,** which serves as an association and projection pathway. The white matter of the cerebral hemispheres contains nerve fibers and neuroglia of various sizes. Three types of myelinated nerve fibers comprise the center of the hemisphere. They are the transverse fibers, the projection fibers, and the association fibers (Fig. 5-20).

- **Transverse (commissural) fibers** are tracts of fibers that interconnect corresponding parts of the *two* hemispheres. The

corpus callosum is the largest commissure. It is an arch-shaped structure that crosses the great longitudinal fissure.
- **Projection fibers** connect the cerebral cortex with the lower portions of the brain and spinal cord.
- **Association fibers** connect various areas within the *same* hemisphere.

The cerebral hemispheres are composed of pairs of frontal, parietal, temporal, and occipital lobes. **Brodmann** is credited with mapping the cortical areas of the brain based on slight histological differences of the cells. Almost 100 different areas of the cerebral cortex have been identified. This method

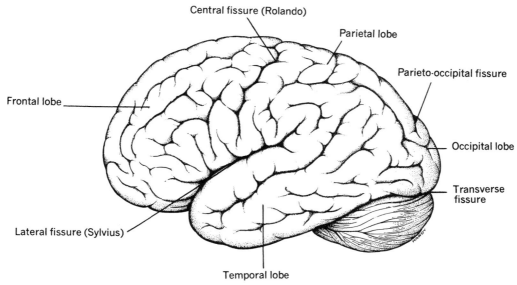

FIGURE 5-19
Lateral aspect of the left cerebral and cerebellar hemispheres.

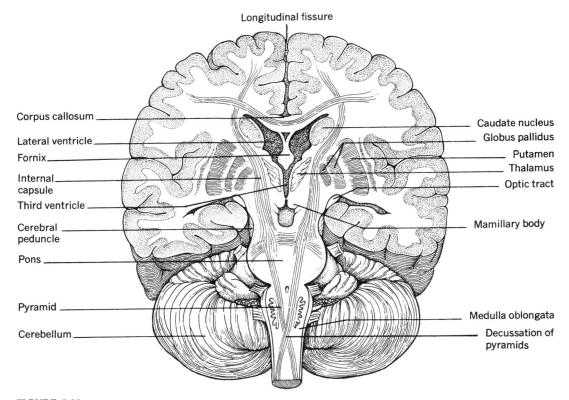

FIGURE 5-20
Oblique coronal section through the cerebrum and brain stem. (From Chaffee, E. E., and I. M. Lytle. [1980]. *Basic physiology and anatomy.* Philadelphia: J. B. Lippincott.)

of classification provides a basis for the discussion of functional areas of the brain (Figs. 5-21 and 5-22). The following are some Brodmann areas along with their functional classifications:

- **Area 4**—primary motor cortex or primary motor strip
- **Areas 1, 2, and 3**—primary somatic sensory areas
- **Areas 41 and 42**—primary receptive areas for sound
- **Area 17**—primary receptive area for vision

The primary sensory and motor areas perform highly specialized functions.

Other areas of the brain that do not perform primary functions are called **association areas.** Functions of the association areas are more general but nonetheless important. Functional loss of a sensory association area greatly reduces the ability of the brain to analyze characteristics of sensory experience. It should be mentioned that the cerebral cortex is closely associated, both anatomically and functionally, with the thalamus. Many afferent and efferent pathways connect with specific parts of the thalamus to perform various complex functions.

GENERAL FUNCTIONS OF THE CEREBRAL CORTEX ACCORDING TO LOBES

Frontal Lobe. The major functions of the frontal lobes are to

- Perform high level cognitive functions such as reasoning, abstraction, concentration, and executive control

- Provide for storage of information (memory)
- Control voluntary eye movement
- Influence somatic motor control of activities such as respirations, gastrointestinal activity, and blood pressure
- Motor control of speech in the dominant hemisphere (usually the left hemisphere)

The **motor cortex (area 4),** located anterior to the central fissure, contains giant Betz cells or pyramidal cells that control voluntary motor function. The various muscles are spatially arranged on the strip so that the feet are located in the area of the longitudinal fissure and the muscles of the face are located at the opposite end of the motor strip. Note the large area allocated to the hand (Fig. 5-23).

Areas 6 and 8 of the cortex are called **motor association areas,** or the premotor cortex. There is a connection between these areas and the oculomotor, trochlear, abducens, glossopharyngeal, vagus, and spinal accessory cranial nerves. Stimulation of the lateral portion of area 6 results in massive generalized movements, such as the turning of the eyes and head, movement of the trunk, and flexion and extension of the extremities, particularly the hands. Area 8 is concerned with the eye field and coordinates eye movement.

Broca's area (areas 44 and 45), located at the inferior frontal gyrus, is classified as an association area because it is critical for motor control of speech. Damage to this area in the dominant hemisphere results in the inability of the patient to express his or her thoughts (non-fluent aphasia).

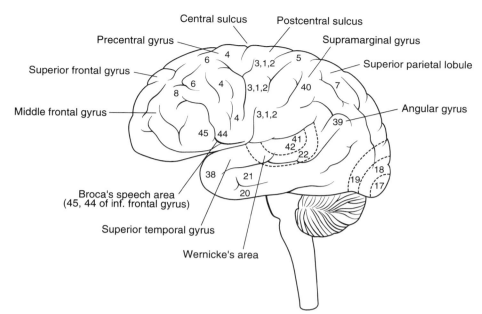

FIGURE 5-21
Lateral view of the brain depicting the
most significant areas of Brodmann.

Parietal Lobe. Posterior to the central fissure is the **primary sensory cortex (areas 1, 2, and 3)**, which is arranged in the same topographic scheme as the motor strip—that is, the feet are controlled by an area in the longitudinal fissure, and the muscles of the face are controlled by the temporal region. Area 1 receives fibers responsible for cutaneous and deep sensibility sensations. The fibers in area 2 are concerned with deep sensibility, whereas those in area 3 interpret the cutaneous sensations of touch, position, pressure, and vibration.

Input from the thalamus also reaches the primary sensory cortex. The purpose of the primary sensory cortex is to analyze only gross aspects of sensation and send the results of its interpretation to the thalamus and other cortical areas. It is the function of the **sensory association areas (areas 5 and 7)** to analyze the specific characteristics of sensory input.

In the parietal lobes, sensory input is interpreted to define size, shape, weight, texture, and consistency. Sensation is localized, and modalities of touch, pressure, and position are identified. In addition, a person's awareness of the parts of his or her body are parietal lobe functions. The nondominant parietal lobe processes visual–spatial information and controls spatial orientation, whereas the dominant lobe is involved in ideomotor praxis.

Temporal Lobe. The **primary auditory receptive areas (areas 41 and 42)** are located in the temporal lobes. The **auditory association area** occupies a part of the superior temporal gyrus (**area 22**) and is also known as **Wernicke's area.** This area is usually largest in the dominant hemisphere. If Wernicke's area is damaged in the patient's dominant hemisphere, words are heard, but they are meaningless to the person (fluent aphasia). Thus, affected persons would be able to verbalize but would unknowingly make many errors in content because of a failure to comprehend what has been said by others or by themselves.

A very important area, called the **interpretive area,** is located in the supramarginal and angular gyri of the temporal lobe. This area is at the junction of the lateral fissure where the temporal, parietal, and occipital lobes meet. It provides an

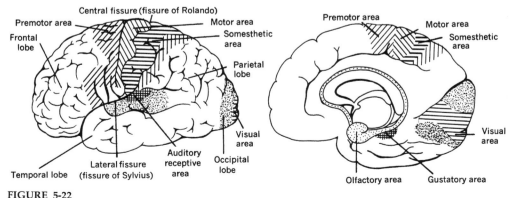

FIGURE 5-22
Diagram of the localization of function in the cerebral hemisphere. Various functional areas are shown in relation to the lobes and fissures—lateral view (*left*) and medial view (*right*).

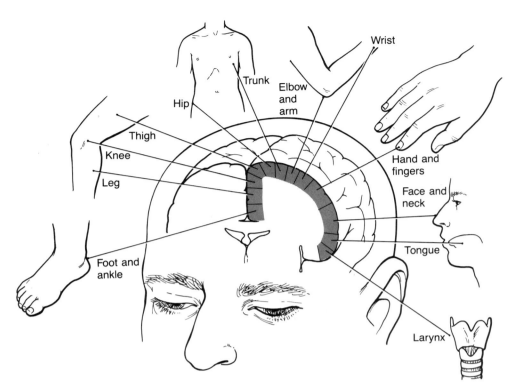

FIGURE 5-23
Areas of the brain that control specific areas of the body. Size indicates relative distribution of control. (From Bullock, B. L. [1996]. *Pathophysiology: Adaptations and alterations in function.* [4th ed.]. Philadelphia: Lippincott-Raven.)

integration of the somatic, auditory, and visual association areas and plays an important role in visual, auditory, and olfactory perception; learning; memory; and emotional affect. Types of thoughts that might be experienced are greatly detailed memories of past experiences, conversations, artwork, music, and taste. Memory that requires more than one sensory modality is stored, in part, in the angular gyrus of the temporal lobe. Any destruction of the **dominant temporal lobe** and angular gyrus in an adult will result in great impairment of intellectual ability.

Occipital Lobe. The **primary visual cortex** is **area 17** of the occipital lobe. The **visual association areas** are **18** and **19.** Neurons of the **lateral geniculate bodies** give rise to fibers that form the geniculocalcarine tract (optic radiation) to the cortex of the occipital lobes. The major functions of the occipital lobes are visual perception, some visual reflexes (*i.e.,* visual fixation) and involuntary smooth eye movements (smooth pursuit system).

DOMINANCE OF A CEREBRAL HEMISPHERE

Cerebral dominance is an important consideration. It is generally accepted that most people have one cerebral hemisphere that has become more highly developed than the other. At birth, both hemispheres have an equal capacity for development. As a child develops, the attention of the mind is directed to one specific hemisphere, which develops rapidly in relation to the other side. Left hemispheric dominance is found in 90% of the population; these are right-handed people. Surprisingly, most, but not all, left-handed people also have a dominant left cerebral hemisphere. Many "split brain" studies have been conducted on the left and right hemispheres of the brain. The left side of the brain controls language, whereas the right side is the nonverbal or perceptual hemisphere.

CORPUS CALLOSUM

The **corpus callosum,** as mentioned previously, is a thick area of nerve fibers directed transversely, through which every part of one hemisphere is connected with the corresponding part of the other hemisphere. When the fibers of one hemisphere pass into the opposite hemisphere, they permeate the hemisphere in all directions, terminating in the gray matter of the periphery. As a result of this connective process, the two hemispheres are intricately linked.

BASAL GANGLIA

The **basal ganglia** are the several masses of subcortical nuclei located deep in the cerebral hemispheres. Their anatomical parts include the **lenticular nucleus** (composed of the **globus pallidus** and **putamen**), the **caudate nucleus,** the **amygdaloid body,** and the **claustrum.** The lenticular nucleus and the caudate nuclei are collectively called the **corpus striatum.** The lenticular nuclei and the caudate nucleus are closely related functionally to the thalamus, subthalamus, substantia nigra, and red nucleus. These structures compose the basal ganglia system for motor control of fine body movements, particularly of the hands and lower extremities.

DIENCEPHALON

The **diencephalon,** a major division of the cerebrum, is divided into four regions: the thalamus, hypothalamus, subthalamus, and epithalamus. The thalamus and hypothalamus are the major areas of importance. These four areas will be discussed along with the internal capsule and hypophysis (pituitary gland), which are located in this region.

Thalamus. The **thalamus** consists of a pair of egg-shaped masses of gray matter located in the ventromedial part of the hemispheres that has connections to multiple areas of the brain. The thalamus is divided into anterior medial and lateral groups, and each group includes specific nuclei. The lateral border of the thalamus is the posterior limb or the internal capsule, and the third ventricle lies medially to the thalamus. The thalamus is the last station where impulses are processed before they ascend to the cerebral cortex. All sensory pathways (with the exception of olfactory pathways) have direct afferent and efferent connections with the thalamic nuclei. The thalamus plays a role in conscious pain awareness, in focusing of attention, in the reticular activating system, and in the limbic system.

Epithalamus. The **epithalamus** is the most dorsal portion of the diencephalon. It is composed of the pineal body, which is thought to have a role in growth and development. The epithalamus is also involved in the regulation of the primitive "food-getting" reflex.

Hypothalamus. The **hypothalamus** is located in the basal region of the diencephalon, forming part of the walls of the third ventricle. The optic chiasma, the point at which the two optic tracts cross, is located at the rostral area of the hypothalamic floor. The stalk of the pituitary, **infundibulum,** connects the hypophysis with the hypothalamus. The hypothalamus regulates important physiologically based drives such as appetite, sexual arousal, and thirst. It is the center for the autonomic nervous system, particularly the sympathetic portion. The hypothalamus controls

Temperature, by monitoring the blood temperature that flows through the hypothalamus and then sending afferent impulses to the sweat glands, peripheral vessels, or muscles (for shivering)
Water metabolism, through the regulation of antidiuretic hormone
Hypophyseal secretions (*e.g.,* growth hormone, follicle-stimulating hormone)
Visceral and somatic activities, by many excitatory–inhibitory functions of the autonomic nervous system (*e.g.,* heart rate, peristalsis, pupillary dilation and constriction)
Visible physical expressions in response to emotions, such as blushing, dryness of mouth, and clammy hands
Sleep–wakefulness cycle

Subthalamus. The **subthalamus** is located below the thalamus and is closely related to the basal ganglia in function.

INTERNAL CAPSULE

Many nerve fibers coming from various parts of the cerebral cortex converge at the brain stem, forming the corona radiata. As the fibers enter the thalamus–hypothalamus region, they are collectively termed the **internal capsule.** The internal capsule is a **massive bundle of sensory and motor** fibers connecting the various subdivisions of the brain and spinal cord. Although it includes only a small area of tissue, it is a critical anatomical area which controls major sensory and motor function. It is part of the white matter of the cerebrum and contains both radiation and projection fibers. The internal capsule is formed by fibers of the crus cerebri, with additional fibers from the corpus striatum and optic thalamus laterally.

All afferent sensory fibers going to the cortex pass through the internal capsule in the following succession: the brain stem to the thalamus to the internal capsule to the cerebral cortex. All efferent motor fibers leaving the cortex for the brain stem pass through the internal capsule according to the following schemata: cerebral cortex to the internal capsule to the brain stem.

HYPOPHYSIS (PITUITARY GLAND)

The **hypophysis,** also called the **pituitary gland,** is a small gland that is located in the sella turcica at the base of the brain and is connected to the hypothalamus by the **hypophysial stalk** (also called the **infundibulum**). The hypothalamus controls pituitary secretions. The hypophysis is divided into two lobes, the anterior and the posterior. The anterior lobe secretes six major hormones related to metabolic function of the body: (1) **growth-stimulating hormone** (GSH), (2) **adrenal-stimulating hormone** (adrenocorticotropin, ACTH), (3) **thyroid-stimulating hormone** (TSH), (4) **prolactin,** (5) **follicle-stimulating hormone** (FSH), and (6) **luteinizing hormone** (LH).

The posterior lobe produces **vasopressin,** also called **antidiuretic hormone** (ADH), and **oxytocin.** ADH controls the rate of water secretion into the urine, thereby controlling the water content of the body. Commonly, abnormal secretion of ADH accompanies intracranial surgery, a pituitary adenoma, or cerebral trauma.

Relationship Between the Hypothalamus and Hypophysis in Neuroendocrine Control. The control center for the autonomic nervous system and the neuroendocrine system is the **hypothalamus.** The following two pathways of hypothalamic connection to the hypophysis enable hypothalamic influence of the endocrine glands: (1) nerve fibers that travel from the supraoptic nuclei and paraventricular nuclei to the posterior lobe of the hypophysis (**hypothalamohypophysial tract**); and (2) long and short portal blood vessels that connect sinusoids in the median eminence (portion of the hypophysis) and the infundibulum with the capillary plexuses in the anterior lobe of the hypophysis (**hypophysial portal system**) (Fig. 5-24).

Hypothalamohypophysial Tract. The precursors of the hormones vasopressin and oxytocin are synthesized in the nerve cells of the **supraoptic** and **paraventricular nuclei.** The precursor material then passes along the axons and is released at the axon terminals, where it is absorbed into the capillaries of the posterior hypophysial lobe. **Vasopressin** is produced mainly in the nerve cells of the supraoptic nucleus. The functions of vasopressin are to increase water absorption in the kidney's distal convoluted tubules and to initiate vasoconstriction. The other hormone, **oxytocin,** is

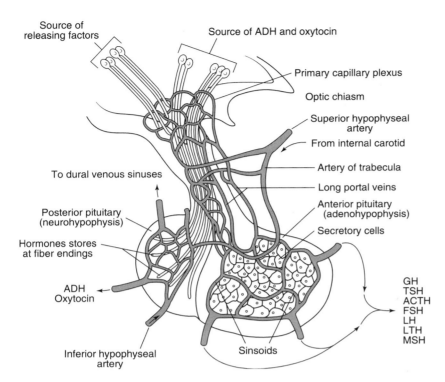

FIGURE 5-24

Diagrammatic and schematic representation of hypophysial nerve fiber tracts and the portal system. Releasing factors produced by cell bodies in the hypothalamus trickle down axons to the proximal part of the stalk where they enter the primary capillary plexus and are transported via portal vessels to sinusoids in adenohypophysis for control of secretions. Antidiuretic hormone (ADH) and oxytocin, produced by other cell bodies in the hypothalamus, trickle down axons for storage in the neurohypophysis until needed.

produced mainly in the paraventricular nucleus and is responsible for uterine contraction and for stimulating the growth of those cells of the mammary glands responsible for milk production.

Hypophysial Portal System. The hypophysial portal system is derived from the superior hypophysial artery. Upon entering the median eminence and dividing into capillaries, the capillaries drain into long and short descending vessels that terminate in the anterior lobe of the hypophysis. The release-stimulating hormones and release-inhibiting hormones are delivered to cells of the anterior hypophysis so that the appropriate releasing or inhibiting hormone is synthesized and secreted (*e.g.,* TSH, FSH). Feedback systems from afferent fibers in the hypothalamus, as well as from the target organ, help to regulate the level of the various hormones.

Brain Stem (Midbrain, Pons, and Medulla)

The second major subdivision of the brain is the brain stem (Fig. 5-25). Many significant anatomical parts are found in the brain stem and are discussed in relationship to the three major divisions, the midbrain, pons, and medulla.

MIDBRAIN

The **midbrain** is a small, 1.5-cm segment of the upper brain stem lying between the diencephalon and the pons. The midbrain can be divided into the tectum (the roof), the tegmentum (the posterior portion), and the crus cerebri (the peduncle). The anterior surface extends from the mamillary bodies of the diencephalon to the pons. The **crus cerebri** consists of two

ropelike bundles of fibers separated by a deep **interpeduncular fossa.** The ropelike bundles include the corticospinal and corticobulbar tracts centrally and are flanked by corticopontine fibers. Many small penetrating blood vessels emanate in the floor of the interpeduncular fossa. The optic tracts are noted just above the crus cerebri.

The base of the midbrain, also called the **basis pedunculi,** consists of the **cerebral peduncles** (comprising the corticospinal, corticobulbar, and corticopontine tracts) and the substantia nigra. The crus cerebri and tegmentum are collectively called the **cerebral peduncles.** The **substantia nigra** lies between the crus cerebri and peduncles. Because of melanin pigment in the substantia nigra cell bodies, the neurons appear brownish.

On the posterior part of the tectum are four rounded masses: two superior colliculi (optic system) and two inferior colliculi (auditory system). Collectively, the superior and inferior colliculi are called the **corpus quadrigemina.** The **superior colliculi** process visual stimuli and also integrate visual and auditory motor reflexes. The **inferior colliculi** are nuclei to relay auditory information.

The **superior cerebellar peduncles** are efferent fibers coming from the dentate nucleus of the cerebellum passing rostrally and near the posterior surface of the midbrain. The crossing of the tracts to the opposite side is called the point of **cerebellar decussation.** The fibers then proceed to the red nuclei and the thalamus.

The **red nuclei** are globular gray masses located at the anterior-central tegmentum. Crossed fibers from the cerebral cortex and superior cerebellar peduncles enter the red nuclei or pass around its edges. The **rubrospinal** and **tectospinal tracts** emanate from this area. They form a relay station for many of the efferent cerebellar tracts. On the lateral surface of the midbrain are the **medial geniculate bodies,** which are the

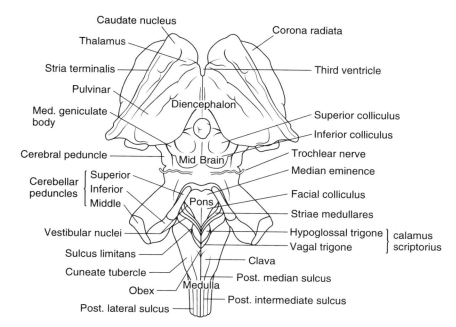

Caudate nucleus
Thalamus
Stria terminalis
Pulvinar
Med. geniculate body
Cerebral peduncle
Cerebellar peduncles {
Superior
Inferior
Middle
Vestibular nuclei
Sulcus limitans
Cuneate tubercle
Obex
Post. lateral sulcus

Corona radiata
Third ventricle
Diencephalon
Superior colliculus
Inferior colliculus
Mid Brain
Trochlear nerve
Median eminence
Facial colliculus
Pons
Striae medullares
Hypoglossal trigone } calamus
Vagal trigone } scriptorius
Clava
Post. median sulcus
Medulla
Post. intermediate sulcus

FIGURE 5-25
Dorsal view of the brain stem.

auditory–sensory relay centers. Functionally, the midbrain serves as the pathway for the cerebral hemispheres and the lower brain and as the center for auditory and visual reflexes. Cranial nerves III and IV nuclei are located in the midbrain. The midbrain contains the aqueduct of Sylvius.

PONS

The **pons,** about 2.5 cm long, is the bridge between the midbrain and the medulla. The anterior surface of the pons is composed of a band of thick, transverse fibers. The **basal sulcus,** a midline furrow, matches the course of the basilar artery. The anterior area is called the **basis pontis** and is composed of crossing fibers of the middle cerebellar peduncles. The **tegmentum** contains spinothalamic tracts, the lateral lemnisci, the medial longitudinal fasciculi, and part of the reticular formation (regulates consciousness). A number of tracts cross through the pons. The inferior, middle, and superior cerebellar peduncles are pathways for the corticospinal tract, and they also connect to the cerebellum. Many other pathways pass through this region connecting higher cerebral regions with the lower levels of the nervous system. The pons contains the fourth ventricle and some control of respiratory function.

Four cranial nerves, V through VIII, have nuclei in the pons. Cranial nerve V exits laterally from the midpons. At the pontomedullary junction, cranial nerve VI exits medially and cranial nerves VII and VIII exit laterally. About 70% of the neurons of cranial nerve VI are motor neurons located in the floor of the fourth ventricle; they innervate the lateral rectus muscle. The remanding 30% of neurons are internuclear neurons, whose axons cross midline, ascend in the **medial longitudinal fasciculus (MLF)**, and connect with the medial rectus motor neurons on the opposite side. The abducens is the center for conjugate horizontal gaze. Cranial nerve VI has the

longest intracranial course and is, therefore, more vulnerable to injury and dysfunction.

MEDULLA

The **medulla oblongata,** also approximately 2.5 cm long, is continuous with the spinal cord and level with the foramen magnum and rootlet of the first cervical nerve; it connects with the pons rostrally. On the posterior surface, the point of division between the pons and medulla is an imaginary transverse line that passes between the caudal margins of the middle cerebellar peduncles. Part of the fourth ventricle is located in the medulla. Anteriorly, the pyramidal (corticospinal) tracts decussate or cross; the pyramidal tracts from the left cross to the right side (and vice versa). The point of decussation forms a ridge on either side of the **median fissure.** In the caudal medulla rostral to the pyramidal decussation, axons from the nucleus gracilis and cuneatus loop anterior-medially around the central gray matter as the **internal arcuate fibers.** These fibers cross the midline to the opposite side and continue as the **medial lemniscus.** Laterally, the **olive** is a prominent oval swelling of convoluted bands that includes the inferior olivary nuclei; they receive fibers from the dentate nucleus of the cerebellum, red nucleus, basal ganglia, and cerebral cortex. Axons from the inferior olivary nuclei form the **olivocerebellar tract** (goes from the inferior cerebellar peduncle to the opposite cerebellar hemisphere). The dorsal the spinocerebellar tract is found in a ridge called the **tuberculum cinereum.**

The **MLF** is located in the paramedian area dorsal to the medial lemniscus. The MLF extends rostrally from the cervical cord to the upper midbrain level. It transmits information for the coordination of head and eye movement. In addition to motor and sensory tracts, there are also cardiac, vasomotor, and respiratory centers in the medulla.

Cranial nerves IX through XII emanate from the medulla. Cranial nerves IX, X, and XI exit the brain stem in the post-olivary fissure, whereas cranial nerve XII exits from the pre-olivary fissure.

Cerebellum

The **cerebellum**, located in the posterior fossa, is attached to the pons, medulla, and midbrain by the three paired cerebellar peduncles. The organization of the cerebellum allows it to be conceptualized in many ways. The cerebellum consists of three major layers: (1) the cortex, which is the outer gray covering; (2) the white matter, which forms the connecting pathways for efferent and afferent impulses joining the cerebellum with other parts of the CNS; and (3) four pairs of deep cerebellar nuclei.

The cerebellum can also be divided from side to side and anteriorly to posteriorly. From the anterior to posterior direction, the cerebellum is composed of an **anterior lobe, a posterior lobe,** and a **flocculonodular lobe.** Approaching it from side to side, it is divided into midline structures and lateral structures. The midline of the anterior and posterior lobes is called the **vermis,** and the lateral portions are the **cerebellar hemispheres.** The midline of the flocculonodular lobe is the **nodulus;** the lateral portion is the **flocculus.**

The **anterior lobe** uses impulses from the spinocerebellar proprioception to regulate postural reflexes. The **posterior lobe** controls coordination of voluntary muscle activity and muscle tone. The **flocculonodular lobe** is the primary connection with the vestibular apparatus for coordination of location in space and movements. Afferent and efferent nerve fibers are found in the **inferior, middle,** and **superior cerebellar peduncles.** The **cerebellar peduncles** receive direct input from the spinal cord and brain stem and convey it to the deep cerebellar nuclei (**dentate, globose, emboliform,** and **fastigial nuclei**) and cerebellar cortex. The result is both an excitatory and inhibitory influence on the cerebellar nuclei; the excitatory influences predominate. An excitatory effect on the brain stem and thalamic nuclei maintains a tonic discharge to the motor system.

The cerebellum is integrated into many connective efferent and afferent pathways throughout the brain, thus providing muscle synergy throughout the body. All sensory modalities are circuited through the cerebellum, which provides information about muscle activity. Impulses to provide "corrections" are sent after sensory data are evaluated. In other words, there are many feedback loops in which cerebellar function is the center of the circuit receiving and sending impulses to maintain muscle activity. In summary, the cerebellum controls fine movement, coordinates muscle groups (agonist and antagonist muscles), and maintains balance through feedback loops.

SPECIAL SYSTEMS WITHIN THE BRAIN

Two systems that entail anatomical structures throughout the various levels of the brain should be mentioned. These include the reticular formation and the reticular activating system. The brain stem and portions of the diencephalon include neurons collectively known as the **reticular formation (RF).** There are motor and sensory neurons scattered throughout the system that provide information concerning muscle activity. As a result, both facilitory and inhibitory impulses from the RF affect the bulboreticular facilitory and inhibitory area. The function of the RF is continuous impulse input to the muscles to support the body against gravity.

The **reticular activating system (RAS)** is a diffuse system that extends from the lower brain stem to the cerebral cortex, from which it disperses (Fig. 5-26). The RAS controls the sleep–wakefulness cycle; consciousness; focused attention; and sensory perception that might alter behavior. The brain stem and thalamic portion of the RAS have different functions. Stimulation of the brain stem portion results in activation of the entire brain. Wakefulness is controlled by the brain stem. Stimulation of the thalamic portion relays facilitory impulses, causing generalized activation of the cerebrum and cognition. Stimulation of selective thalamic areas activates specific areas of the cerebral cortex. This selective stimulation plays a role in directing one's attention to certain mental activities.

Limbic System

The **limbic system** is a group of subcortical nuclei and fiber tracts that form a border around the brain stem. The system includes the **hypothalamus,** the **cingulate gyrus,** the **fornix,** the **hippocampus,** the **anterior nucleus of the thalamus,** the **uncus,** and the **amygdaloid nucleus** (a part of the basal ganglia). Connections exist with the mamillary bodies, olfactory tract, and the upper RF of the midbrain (Fig. 5-27). The major connections of the limbic system are called the circuit of Papez.

The complex function of the system involves basic instinctual and emotional drives, such as fear, sexual drive, hunger, sleep, and short-term memory. These emotional reactions are expressed through endocrine, visceral, somatic, and behavioral reactions via neural pathways that connect with the hypothalamus, brain stem, spinal cord, and hypophysis.

SPINAL CORD

The spinal cord is an elongated mass of nerve tissue that occupies the upper two thirds of the vertebral canal and usually measures 42 to 45 cm in length in the adult. The spinal cord extends from the upper borders of the atlas (first cervical vertebra) to the lower border of the first lumbar vertebra (Fig. 5-28). As the cord reaches the lower two levels of the thoracic region, the cord becomes tapered and is called the **conus medullaris.** A nonneural filament called the **filum terminale** continues caudally until it attaches to the second segment of the coccyx. The three meninges surround the spinal cord for protection.

Spinal Nerves

Spinal nerves are part of the peripheral nervous system. There are 31 pairs of spinal nerves exiting from the spinal cord (Fig. 5-29), including 8 cervical, 12 thoracic, 5 lumbar, 5 sacral, and 1 coccygeal. Each spinal nerve has a dorsal root by which afferent impulses enter the cord and a ventral root by which efferent impulses leave. The first pair of cervical spinal nerves leaves the cord above the C-1 vertebra, and spinal nerves of C-2 through C-7 leave by way of the intervertebral foramina,

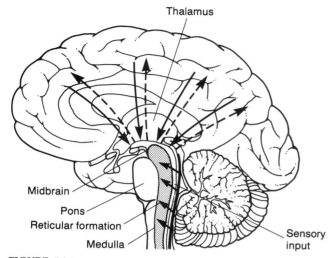

FIGURE 5-26
The anatomical components of the reticular activating system.

above their corresponding vertebrae. Since there are seven vertebrae and eight pairs of spinal nerves, the C-8 spinal nerve leaves the cord by way of the intervertebral foramina below the C-7 vertebra. All spinal nerves from T-1 to the caudal end of the cord leave by way of the foramina immediately below the corresponding vertebrae.

In the cervical region, the spinal nerves are almost on a horizontal plane with the corresponding vertebra; however, since the spinal cord is shorter than the vertebral column, the spinal nerves become increasingly oblique as they descend the spinal cord. The lumbar and sacral spinal nerves develop long roots, collectively referred to as the **cauda equina.**

There are two enlargements in the spinal cord to accommodate innervation to the extremities. The cervical (**brachial**) enlargement innervates the upper extremities and extends from the C-5 to the T-1 spinal levels. The lower extremities are innervated by the **lumbosacral** enlargement, which extends from the L-3 to the S-2 levels.

DORSAL (SENSORY) ROOTS

The **dorsal roots (posterior roots)** convey sensory input (afferent impulses) from specific areas of the body known as **dermatomes** (Fig. 5-30). There is considerable peripheral overlap between one dermatome and another so that no demonstrable sensory deficit will be found unless the sensory component of two or more spinal nerves is interrupted. Interruption of one sensory nerve root may result in paresthesia or pain in that dermatomal area.

Afferent impulses are directed from the dermatomal area by way of the dorsal root to the dorsal root ganglia, in which the cell bodies of the sensory component are located. The sensory fibers are of two types:

1. **General somatic afferent** (GSA) fibers, which carry sensory impulses for pain, temperature, touch, and proprioception from the body wall, tendons, and joints
2. **General visceral afferent** (GVA) fibers, which carry sensory impulses from the organs within the body (Table 5-6)

VENTRAL (MOTOR) ROOTS

The **ventral roots** convey efferent impulses from the spinal cord to the body. The motor fibers are of two types:

1. **General somatic efferent** (GSE) fibers, which innervate voluntary striated muscles and have axons originating from the alpha and gamma motor neurons of lamina IX
2. **General visceral efferent** (GVE) fibers, include the preganglionic and postganglionic autonomic fibers that innervate smooth and cardiac muscle and also regulate glandular secretion

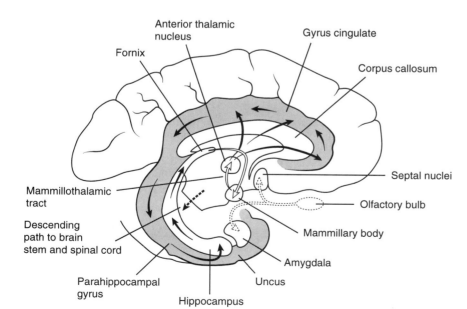

FIGURE 5-27
Papez circuit (*arrows*) is depicted in this schematic view of the limbic system. The solid arrows represent the hypothetical circulation of impulses during the experiencing of emotions. The thick dotted arrow indicates the descending path to the brain stem and spinal cord for the expression of emotions. The olfactory afferent fibers (*lightly dotted arrows*) are also shown.

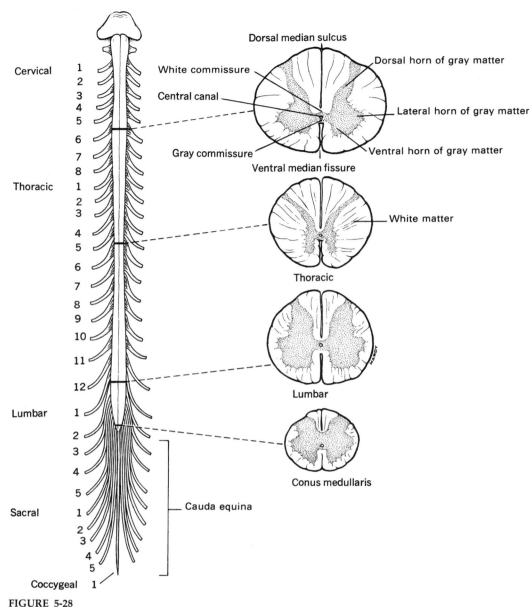

FIGURE 5-28
Cross-sectional views of the spinal cord showing the regional variations in the gray matter. (From Chaffee, E. E., and I. M. Lytle. [1980]. *Basic physiology and anatomy*. Philadelphia: J. B. Lippincott.)

Impulses to the motor end-plate of voluntary muscle fibers are conveyed by **alpha motor neurons**; impulses to the motor end-plates of intrafusal muscle cells of the neuromuscular spindles are conveyed by **gamma motor neurons.** These motor neurons (alpha, gamma) are called lower motor neurons. Table 5-7 provides a list of myotomes, which are areas of motor innervation to specific muscle groups.

CLASSIFICATION OF NERVE FIBERS

Nerve fibers can be classified by various criteria, including the diameter of the fiber, thickness of the myelin sheath, and speed of conduction of the impulse. Large fibers conduct impulses quickly, and the thicker the myelin sheath, the faster the speed of the impulse conductivity.

Sensory fibers are classified into groups I through IV, depending on their conduction velocities. Group I fibers are the quickest to conduct impulses, whereas group IV fibers have the slowest velocity. Group I is further divided to include I_a fibers (spindle primary afferent) and I_b fibers (from Golgi tendon organs). Group II conveys sensation from the myelinated skin and joint receptors (spindle secondary afferent). Groups III and IV convey impulses from unmyelinated fibers. Another system uses the capital letters A, B, and C to classify both sensory and motor fibers. Type A is either a small, lightly myelinated sensory fiber for touch, pressure, pain, and temperature or alpha or gamma motor neurons of lamina IX. The greatest diameter and velocity are characteristic of type A fibers. Type B fibers have a smaller diameter and are lightly myelinated preganglionic motor fibers. Type C fibers have a small diameter and are unmyelinated. They include motor postganglionic fibers and sensory fibers for pain and temperature.

Plexuses

A **plexus** is a network of interlacing nerves. Sometimes a plexus is formed by the primary branches of the nerves, such as the cervical, brachial, lumbar, and sacral plexuses. Other plexuses are formed by the terminal funiculi at the periphery. The following are the major plexuses:

1. The **cervical plexus** is formed from the ventral branches of the first four cervical nerves of the spine. The resulting branches innervate the muscles of the neck and shoulders. This plexus also gives rise to the **phrenic nerve,** which supplies the diaphragm.
2. The **brachial plexus** is composed of the ventral branches of the lower four cervical and first thoracic spinal nerves. Important nerves that emerge from this plexus are the radial and ulnar nerves.
3. The **lumbar plexus** originates from the ventral branches of the 12th thoracic and the first 4 lumbar nerves. The femoral nerve arises from this plexus.
4. The **sacral plexus** arises from the ventral branches of the last two lumbar and first four sacral nerves. The sciatic nerve arises from this plexus.

The Spinal Cord in Cross Section

When viewed in cross section, the spinal cord appears to be a gray *H* surrounded by white matter. The **gray matter** consists of cell bodies and neuronal projections (axons and dendrites). The **white matter** includes longitudinally running fiber tracts, some of which are myelinated. Each **funiculus** (column) contains ascending and descending tracts (Fig. 5-31). There are two midline sulci, the **anterior median sulcus** and the **posterior median sulcus.** The lateral surface contains both a **posterolateral** and an **anterolateral sulci** that serve to divide the white matter into the anterior, lateral, and posterior funiculi.

Cross sections of the cord at various levels show striking differences in the shape and extent of gray and white matter. The gray matter of the cord contains the **posterior (dorsal)** and **anterior (ventral) horns. Lateral horns** are smaller in the thoracic and upper lumbar segments because the muscle mass of the trunk is less than that of the extremities, and these horns are made up largely of cell bodies of neurons that innervate skeletal muscles. In the lumbosacral region, the anterior horns are larger than those of the cervical area because of the greater muscle mass in the lower extremities. There is more white matter, as compared with gray matter, in the cervical region than in the lumbosacral region. This difference exists because the white matter in the cervical region is made up of connecting fibers that span the entire spinal cord and the brain, whereas the white mat-

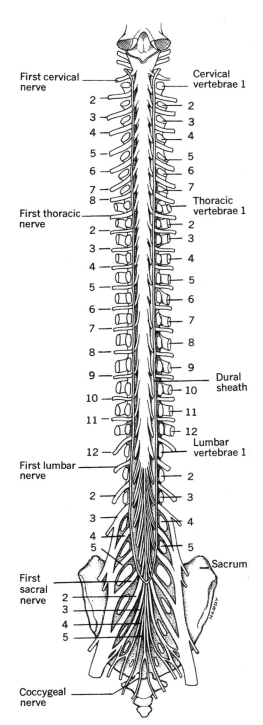

FIGURE 5-29
The spinal cord lying within the vertebral canal. Spinal nerves are numbered on the left side, and the vertebrae are numbered on the right side. (From Chaffee, E. E., and I. M. Lytle. [1980]. *Basic physiology and anatomy.* Philadelphia: J. B. Lippincott.)

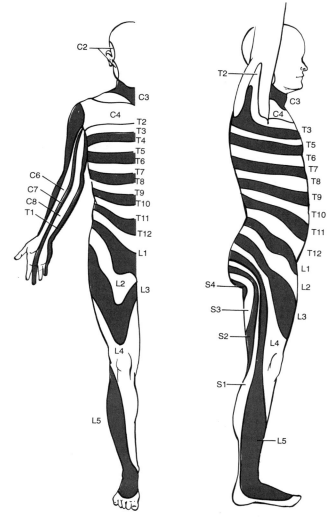

FIGURE 5-30
Cutaneous distribution of the spinal nerves (dermatomes). (From Conn, P. M. [1995]. *Neuroscience in medicine.* Philadelphia: J. B. Lippincott.)

ter of the lumbosacral cord contains only fibers serving the caudal end of the cord.

On cross section, the gray matter of the spinal cord is divided into sections I through X, called the **laminae of Rexed** (see Fig. 5-31). Each lamina extends the length of the cord. Numbering of the laminae begins at the most dorsal point of the posterior horn; lamina IX is located at the most ventral point of the anterior horn. Therefore, the posterior horn contains laminae I through VI. Cells receive and send information about sensory input from the spinal nerve. Lamina VII is located in the intermediate gray zone and extends into the anterior horn. Within this area are the nucleus dorsalis and the intermediolateral gray columns. The anterior horn contains laminae VIII and IX. Lamina VIII contains neurons that send commissural axons to the opposite side of the cord. Lamina IX contains alpha and gamma motor neurons that innervate skeletal muscles. The area surrounding the central canal is the site of lamina X.

MOTOR SYSTEM

Movement is the result of complex higher-level structures, descending spinal cord tracts, segmental spinal cord circuits, and muscles. The major higher-level structures involved in movement are the cerebral cortex, basal ganglia, cerebellum, brain stem, spinal cord, and final common pathway (Fig. 5-32).

Nearly all voluntary muscle activity originates from the corticospinal tract (motor cortex, area 4). Other fibers originating in areas 4 and 6 do not initiate voluntary muscle activity, but act as inhibitors or suppressors of the lower motor neurons (LMN). Without these controls, LMNs would fire excessively in response to reflex stimuli or discharge spontaneously, resulting in hyperreflexia or spasticity. Other tracts originate in the brain stem and also modify muscle function. The basal ganglia exert an inhibitory effect on LMNs by synapses with the reticular formation. Damage to the basal ganglia results in increased motor tone. The cerebellum's role in movement is indirect via its effect on the vestibular nuclei, red nucleus, and basal ganglia. The tracts affected by these structures include the vestibulospinal, rubrospinal, and reticulospinal tracts. These tracts, in turn, affect the LMNs.

Descending Motor Pathways: Upper Motor Neurons and Lower Motor Neurons

Descending motor pathways are divided into **upper motor neurons (UMNs)** and **lower motor neurons (LMNs)**. UMNs are the facilitory and inhibitory descending supraspinal pathways that modify LMNs and are located entirely in the CNS. UMNs include the neurons and their fibers within the corticospinal tract and corticobulbar tracts originating in the cerebral cortex; the rubrospinal and tectospinal tracts originating in the midbrain; and the reticulospinal and vestibulospinal tracts emanating from the pons and medulla. **LMNs** are located in both the CNS and peripheral nervous system (PNS). Voluntary striated muscles are innervated by alpha and gamma neurons and are the **final common pathway** or final linkage between the CNS and voluntary muscles. The LMNs are the GSE components of the spinal nerves and of cranial nerves III, IV, VI, and XII and the special visceral efferent components of cranial nerves V, VII, IX, X, and XI.

Voluntary muscle activity is the sum of neural control of the alpha and gamma motor neurons of muscle and motor components of the cranial nerve nuclei (Fig. 5-33). Final neural pathways influence the muscle by way of the myoneural junction. A summary of the major descending motor tracts is found in Table 5-8.

SENSORY SYSTEM

Sensory receptors, which are located throughout the body, convey afferent impulses for interpretation of stimuli. Sensory input may be integrated into spinal reflexes or it may be relayed to the higher centers of the brain by way of ascending pathways. The impulses are analyzed and can influence unconscious and conscious activities by way of efferent responses. There are various types of receptors that convey spe-

TABLE 5-6
Sensory Nerve Roots and the Areas They Innervate (Dermatome)

SPINAL NERVES	DERMATOME
C-2	Back of head (occiput)
C-3	Neck
C-4	Neck and upper shoulder
C-5	Lateral aspect of shoulder
C-6	Thumb; radial aspect of arm; index finger
C-7	Middle finger; middle palm; back of hand
C-8	Ring and little finger; ulnar forearm
T-1–T-2	Inner aspect of arm and across shoulder blade
T-4	Nipple line
T-7	Lower costal margin
T-10	Umbilical region
T-12–L-1	Inguinal (groin) region
L-2	Anterior thigh and upper buttocks
L-3–L-4	Anterior knee and lower leg
L-5	Outer aspect of lower leg; dorsum of foot; great toe
S-1	Sole of foot and small toes
S-2	Posterior medial thigh and lower leg
S-3	Medial thigh
S-4–S-5	Genitals and saddle area

cific types of stimuli: **exteroceptors** are stimulated by touch, light pressure, pain, temperature, odor, sound, and light; **proprioceptors** convey a sense of position, movement, and muscle coordination; **interoceptors** provide visceral information concerning pain, cramping, and fullness; and **chemoreceptors** are stimulated by chemicals (*e.g.,* lactic acid).

Pain and Temperature. The pain and temperature pathways are so closely related throughout the body that they are treated collectively as one system. The **anterolateral system** is made up of the **anterior spinothalamic, lateral spinothalamic,** and **spinoreticulothalamic** tracts. These are the major tracts that convey pain and temperature sensation. The afferent impulse enters the cord by way of the **posterolateral tract of Lissauer** and crosses to the opposite side of the spinal cord. Impulses ascend the cord to terminate in the thalamus, with synapsing occurring within the reticular formation of the brain stem.

Proprioception. The posterior funiculus is totally enveloped by two ascending tracts—the **fasciculus gracilis** and **fasciculus cuneatus.** These tracts ascend the cord uncrossed until they reach the area of decussation in the medulla. After the fibers decussate in this area, they proceed initially to the thalamus and then to areas 1 through 3 of the cerebral cortex. These are the major tracts that convey the sensation of **proprioception,** which includes position and movement, vibration, two-point discrimination, deep pressure, and touch.

Coordination of Muscle Contraction. The anterior and posterior spinocerebellar tracts convey impulses of proprioception for the coordination of locomotion in the lower extremities. The fasciculus cuneatus and spinocerebellar tracts convey sim-

ilar information from the upper half of the body. A summary of the major ascending sensory tracts is found in Table 5-8.

AUTONOMIC NERVOUS SYSTEM

The **autonomic nervous system** (ANS), part of the peripheral nervous system, is made up of only motor neurons, collectively called the GVE system. The ANS regulates the activities of the viscera, which includes all smooth (involuntary) muscles, cardiac muscles, and glands (Fig. 5-34). The purpose of the ANS is to maintain a relatively stable internal environment for the body. Two major subdivisions of the ANS are the sympathetic and parasympathetic systems.

The **sympathetic system** is activated during stress situations such as fright, fight, or flight phenomena. During these stressful periods, the heart rate and blood pressure increase, and there is vasoconstriction of the peripheral blood vessels.

The **parasympathetic system** stimulates those visceral activities associated with conservation, restoration, and maintenance of a normal functional level. The parasympathetic system decreases heart rate and increases gastrointestinal activity (Table 5-9).

Both divisions of the ANS, which function in an antagonistic relationship, innervate most body organs. The ANS is activated primarily by centers located in the spinal cord, brain stem, and hypothalamus. A two-neuron chain is characteristic of the ANS. The cell bodies and their fibers are classified into the following two categories: (1) the **preganglionic neuron,** which is the primary neuron and is located in the brain stem or cord (intermediolateral gray column in the thoracic cord); and (2) the **postganglionic neuron,** which is the postsynaptic or secondary neuron located in the ganglia and innervating the end-organ.

TABLE 5-7
Motor Nerve Roots (Myotomes) and Areas They Innervate

SPINAL NERVES	MUSCLES
C-1 to C-4	Neck (flexion, lateral flexion, extension, rotation)
C-3–C-5	Diaphragm (respirations)
C-5–C-6	Shoulder movement and flexion of elbow
C-5–C-7	Forward thrust of shoulder
C-5–C-8	Adduction of arm from front to back
C-6–C-8	Extension of forearm and wrist
C-7, C-8, T-1	Flexion of wrist
T-1–T-12	Control of thoracic, abdominal, and back muscles
L-1–L-3	Flexion of hip
L-2–L-4	Extension of leg; adduction of thigh
L-4, L-5, S-1, S-2	Abduction of thigh; flexion of lower leg
L-4–L-5	Dorsal flexion of foot
L-5, S-1, S-2	Plantar flexion of foot
S-2, S-3, S-4	Perineal area and sphincters

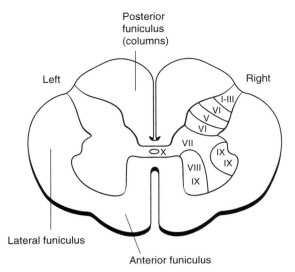

FIGURE 5-31
The three funiculi of the spinal cord.

Sympathetic Nervous System

The sympathetic nervous system is also called the **thoraco-lumbar system** because its preganglionic fibers emerge from cell bodies in the **intermediolateral nucleus of lamina VII.** The sympathetic nervous system extends through the thoracic and upper two lumbar levels (T-1 through L-2). These preganglionic fibers leave the spinal cord with the motor fibers of the ventral roots. After traveling less than 1 cm, the sympathetic fibers pass into the **white rami communicantes**—a branch of the spinal nerve—which, in turn, enters the **sympathetic chain** or trunk. (The sympathetic chain consists of a chain of ganglia located on either side of the spinal cord that extends from the base of the skull to the coccyx. These ganglia are all interconnected by longitudinal fibers, thus forming a continuous chain.) In the sympathetic chain, the fibers may synapse immediately with postganglionic fibers located in the chain at the level of entry (**paravertebral ganglia**), travel up or down the trunk to synapse in one of the chain ganglia above or below the point of entry, or pass on to synapse with a postganglionic neuron in an outlying sympathetic ganglia (**prevertebral ganglia**).

Some fibers from the postganglionic neuron in the sympathetic chain return to the spinal nerve by way of the **gray rami communicantes** at all levels of the spinal cord. Each spinal nerve receives a gray ramus, which controls the blood vessels, sweat glands, and piloerector muscles of the hairs.

Sympathetic fibers leave the spinal cord to enter the sympathetic chain in only the thoracic and upper lumbar regions; none of the fibers enter the chain in the cervical, lower lumbar, or sacral regions. Sympathetic innervation to the head is supplied by sympathetic fibers extending from the thoracic chain. In this way, the neck and all structures of the head are innervated. Sympathetic fibers also pass downward from the sympathetic chain into the lower abdomen and legs.

The sympathetic outflow is distributed in the following way: T-1 to T-5 innervate the head, creating three ganglia (superior cervical, middle cervical, and cervicothoracic stellate). Of those sympathetic fibers directed to the head, those from T-1 and T-2 innervate the eye for pupillary dilation; T-2 through T-6 innervate the heart and lungs; and T-6 through L-2 innervate the abdominal viscera through the thoracic and lumbar splanchnic nerves. The thoracic splanchnic nerves carry the preganglionic fibers to the prevertebral ganglia of the abdomen. The celiac, superior mesenteric, and aorticorenal ganglia arise in this area. The lumbar splanchnic nerves terminate in the inferior mesenteric and hypogastric ganglia.

The preganglionic sympathetic nerve fibers pass directly to the adrenal medulla without synapsing. These fibers are

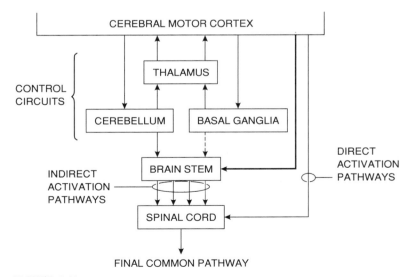

FIGURE 5-32
Outline of the motor system. (Adapted from *Medical neurosciences*, Westmoreland, B. F. et al., Copyright © 1994 Published by Little, Brown and Company)

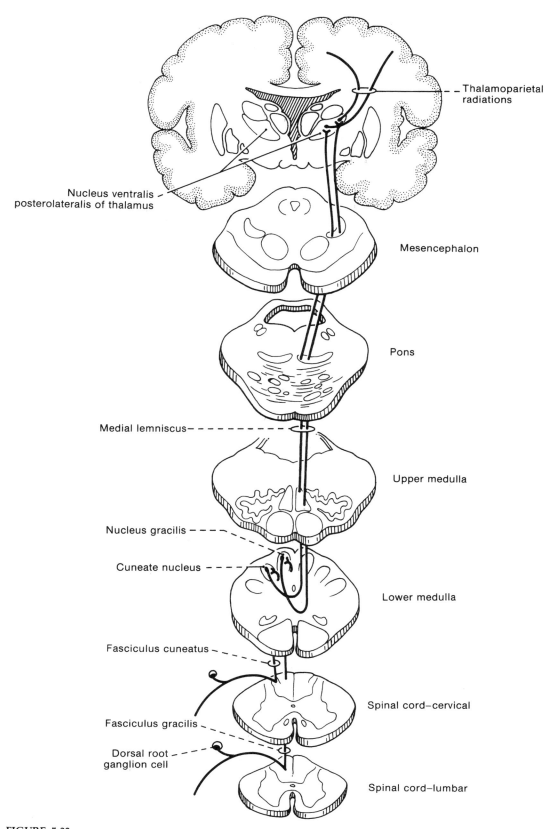

Thalamoparietal radiations

Nucleus ventralis posterolateralis of thalamus

Mesencephalon

Pons

Medial lemniscus

Upper medulla

Nucleus gracilis

Cuneate nucleus

Lower medulla

Fasciculus cuneatus

Spinal cord–cervical

Fasciculus gracilis

Dorsal root ganglion cell

Spinal cord–lumbar

FIGURE 5-33

Diagram of the motor pathways. (From Haerer, A. F. [1995]. *DeJong's the neurologic examination.* [5th ed.]. Philadelphia: J. B. Lippincott.)

TABLE 5-8
Major Spinal Cord Tracts

NAME	ORIGIN	TERMINATION	CROSSED	FUNCTION	DYSFUNCTION
ASCENDING TRACTS					
Fasciculus gracilis	Spinal cord at sacral and lumbar level	Medulla → thalamus → cerebral cortex (sensory strip)	Yes	Conscious proprioception, fine touch,* and vibration sense from lower body	Lower body Astereognosis Loss of vibration sense Loss of two-point discrimination Loss of proprioception
Fasciculus cuneatus	Spinal cord at thoracic and cervical levels	Medulla → thalamus → cerebral cortex (sensory strip)	Yes	Conscious proprioception, fine touch,* and vibration sense from upper body	Upper body Astereognosis Loss of vibration sense Loss of two-point discrimination Loss of proprioception
Posterior spinocerebellar	Posterior horn	Cerebellum	No	Conduction of sensory impulses from muscle spindles and tendon organs of the trunk and lower limbs from one side of the body to the same side of cerebellum for the subconscious proprioception necessary for coordinated muscular contractions	Ipsilateral uncoordinated postural movements
Anterior spinocerebellar	Posterior horn	Cerebellum	Some	Conduction of sensory impulses from muscle spindles and tendon organs of the upper and lower limbs from both sides of the body to the cerebellum for the subconscious proprioception necessary for coordinated muscular contractions	Ipsilateral uncoordinated postural movements
Lateral spinothalamic	Posterior horn	Thalamus → cerebral cortex	Yes	Interpretation of pain and temperature	Loss of pain and temperature sensation contralaterally below the level of the lesion
Anterior spinothalamic	Posterior horn	Thalamus → cerebral cortex	Yes	Conduction of sensory impulses for pressure and crude touch† from extremities and trunk	Because one branch of the first neuron immediately synapses with a second, which ascends ipsilaterally for many levels; cord injury rarely results in complete loss of pressure and crude touch sensation
DESCENDING TRACTS					
Lateral corticospinal	Motor cortex (area 4) → internal capsule → midbrain → pons → medulla	Anterior horn; all spinal levels in laminae IV through VII and IX	80%–90% cross at the medulla	Controls voluntary muscle activity	Voluntary muscle paresis/paralysis
Anterior corticospinal	Motor cortex (area 4) → internal capsule → midbrain → medulla →	Anterior horn (at each level of cord, axons cross to other side)	Not at medulla; synapse with cells of lamina VIII	Controls voluntary muscle activity	Voluntary muscle paresis/paralysis

(continued)

TABLE 5-8
Major Spinal Cord Tracts Continued

NAME	ORIGIN	TERMINATION	CROSSED	FUNCTION	DYSFUNCTION
Anterior corticospinal *continued*	anterior funiculus of the cervical and upper thoracic levels				
Corticobulbar	Areas 4, 6, and 8 of cortex → internal capsule → brain stem	Brain stem; connects with cranial nerves V, VII, IX, X, XI, and XII	Yes	Controls voluntary head movement and facial expression	Because of bilateral innervation, facial expression is usually not affected
Rubrospinal	Midbrain (red nucleus)	Anterior horn	Yes	Facilitates flexor alpha and gamma motor neurons and inhibits extensor motor neurons; also influences muscle tone and posture, particularly of the arms	Altered muscle tone and posture

Reticulospinals
  Pontine reticulospinal
  Medullary reticulospinal
	Reticular formation (brain stem)	Anterior horn	No	Facilitates extensor motor neurons, particularly of the legs; input to gamma motor neurons	Altered muscle tone and posture

Vestibulospinals	Reticular formation (brain stem)	Anterior horn	No	Conveys autonomic information from higher levels to preganglionic autonomic nervous system neurons to influence sweating, pupillary dilatation, and circulation	Altered muscle tone and sweat gland activity
Lateral vestibulospinal			No	Facilitates extensor alpha motor neurons and inhibits flexors	Altered muscle tone and postural equilibrium
Medial vestibulospinal			No	Inhibits fibers to upper cervical alpha motor neurons; influences extraocular movements and visual reflexes	Altered muscle tone and equilibrium in response to head movement

* Fine touch is the ability to identify various objects (e.g., a key) that are placed in the hand while the eyes are closed.
† Crude touch refers to light touch, and may be tested with a wisp of cotton placed in the hand while the eyes are closed.

cholinergic and end directly on the special cells of the medulla that secrete epinephrine and norepinephrine.

SYMPATHETIC NEUROTRANSMITTER

The neurotransmitter released by the postganglionic fibers is **norepinephrine** (noradrenaline). This is why the sympathetic system is termed **adrenergic.** Acetylcholine is secreted at the preganglionic terminal and quickly deactivated by cholinesterase. (There are few exceptions in the postganglionic neurons in the sympathetic nervous system.) Some blood vessels in skeletal muscles and most sweat glands in the palms of the hands have adrenergic postganglionic neurons.

Parasympathetic Nervous System

The parasympathetic system is also called the **craniosacral system** because its preganglionic fibers emerge with cranial nerves III, VII, IX, and X. The specific parasympathetic innervation to these cranial nerves includes the following:

- Oculomotor (III)—supplies the ciliary muscles for accommodation and constrictor sphincter muscles of the pupil
- Facial (VII)—innervates many glands of the head, such as lacrimal, submandibular, sublingual, nasal, oral, and pharyngeal areas
- Glossopharyngeal (IX)—innervates the parotid glands

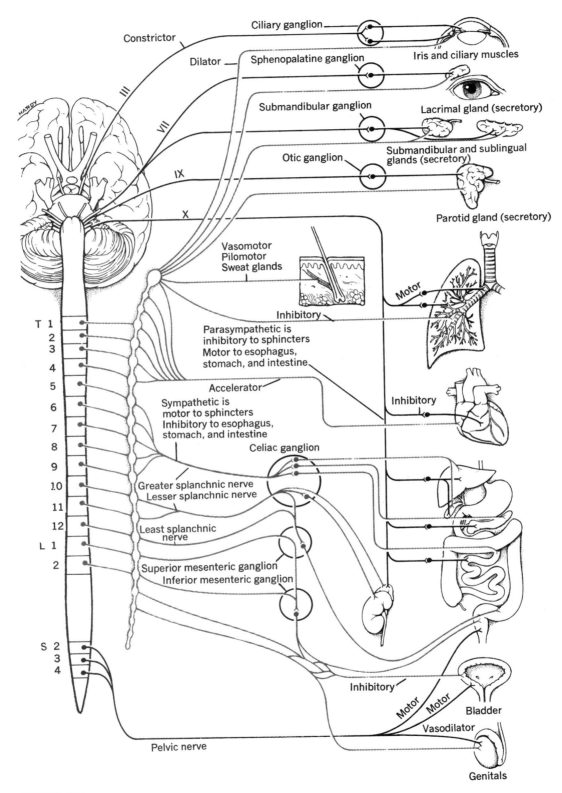

FIGURE 5-34

Diagram of the autonomic nervous system, including the parasympathetic or craniosacral fibers and the sympathetic or thoracolumbar fibers. Note that most organs have a double nerve supply. (From Chaffee, E. E., and I. M. Lytle. [1980]. *Basic physiology and anatomy*. Philadelphia: J. B. Lippincott.)

TABLE 5-9
Autonomic Effects of the Nervous System

STRUCTURE OR ACTIVITY	PARASYMPATHETIC EFFECTS	SYMPATHETIC EFFECTS
PUPIL OF THE EYE	Constricted	Dilated
CIRCULATORY SYSTEM		
Rate and force of heartbeat	Decreased	Increased
Blood vessels		
In heart muscle	Constricted	Dilated
In skeletal muscle	*	Dilated
In abdominal viscera and the skin	*	Constricted
Blood pressure	Decreased	Increased
RESPIRATORY SYSTEM		
Bronchioles	Constricted	Dilated
Rate of breathing	Decreased	Increased
DIGESTIVE SYSTEM		
Peristaltic movements of digestive tube	Increased	Decreased
Muscular sphincters of digestive tube	Relaxed	Contracted
Secretion of salivary glands	Thin, watery saliva	Thick, viscid saliva
Secretions of stomach, intestine, and pancreas	Increased	*
Conversion of liver glycogen to glucose	*	Increased
GENITOURINARY SYSTEM		
Urinary bladder		
Muscular walls	Contracted	Relaxed
Sphincters	Relaxed	Contracted
Muscles of the uterus	Relaxed; variable	Contracted under some conditions; varies with menstrual cycle and pregnancy
Blood vessels of external genitalia	Dilated	*
INTEGUMENT		
Secretion of sweat	*	Increased
Pilomotor muscles	*	Contracted (gooseflesh)
MEDULLAE OF ADRENAL GLANDS	*	Secretion of epinephrine and norepinephrine

No direct effect.
(From Chaffee, E. E., & I. M. Lytle. (1980). *Basic physiology and anatomy* (3rd ed). Philadelphia: J. B. Lippincott.)

- Vagus (X)—synapses with terminal ganglia located adjacent to, or within, the various viscera throughout the body

The sacral portion of the parasympathetic system arises from cell bodies in the intermediate gray matter of sacral segments S-2 through S-4. These fibers pass through the pelvic splanchnic nerve to synapse in the terminal ganglia with the postganglionic neurons, which innervate the descending colon, rectum, bladder, lower ureters, and external genitalia. The parasympathetic system is involved with the mechanisms of bladder and bowel evacuation and, unlike the sympathetic system, is designed to respond to a specific stimulus in a localized area for a short period of time.

PARASYMPATHETIC NEUROTRANSMITTERS

The parasympathetic system secretes **acetylcholine** at the postganglionic neuron. This is why the parasympathetic system is termed **cholinergic.** Acetylcholine is also secreted at the preganglionic synapse and is quickly deactivated by **cholinesterase.**

Spinal Reflexes

A **reflex** is a stereotypical response, mediated by the nervous system, to a particular stimulus of sufficient magnitude. The simplest type of stereotypical neural pathway is called a **reflex arc.** There are five components to a reflex arc, including the following (Fig. 5-35):

Receptor—specific sensory fibers that are sensitive to the stimulus
Sensory (afferent) neuron—relays the impulse via the posterior root to the CNS
Interneuron—an association or connecting neuron located within the CNS
Motor (efferent) neuron—relays the impulse via the anterior root to the effector organ
Effector—a specific organ that responds

Reflexes can be classified by the extent of the regional involvement of the spinal cord. This classification includes **segmental, intersegmental,** and **suprasegmental reflexes.**

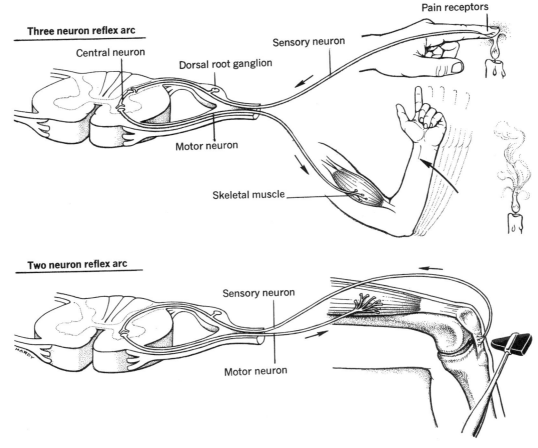

FIGURE 5-35
Diagram of a flexor reflex (*top*) and a stretch reflex (*bottom*). (From Chaffee, E. E., and I. M. Lytle. [1980]. *Basic physiology and anatomy.* Philadelphia: J. B. Lippincott.)

A reflex whose arc passes through only one anatomical segment is called a **segmental reflex.** A knee-jerk reflex is an example of both a segmental and a simple or monosynaptic reflex. A monosynaptic reflex includes an afferent limb that synapses directly with an efferent limb. Most reflexes, however, are more complex and polysynaptic.

An **intersegmental reflex** involves several spinal segments. A flexor or withdrawal reflex is an example of an intersegmental reflex.

A **suprasegmental reflex** involves interaction between the brain centers that regulate cord activity and the segments of the cord itself. An example of a suprasegmental reflex is extension of the legs in response to movement of the head.

Another classification system useful in clinical practice divides reflexes into stretch, cutaneous, and pathological reflexes.

Muscle stretch reflexes, also called deep tendon reflexes (DTRs), are elicited by striking a tendon that stretches the neuromuscular spindles of the muscle group. The knee-jerk reflex, a stretch reflex, results in contraction of the quadriceps and extension of the leg in response to tapping the patellar tendon. Other common stretch reflexes involve the biceps, triceps, and ankle.

Cutaneous reflexes, also termed superficial reflexes, are initiated when the skin or mucous membrane is stimulated by light stroking or scratching, resulting in a specific response in a muscle or muscle group. The withdrawal reflex, which is a flexor reflex, is an example of a cutaneous reflex that is a protective reflex. In response to a noxious cutaneous stimulus to the fingers, the hand is flexed and withdrawn (see Fig. 5-33). Another cutaneous reflex is contraction of the superficial abdominal muscles in response to light, rapid stroking of the skin on the abdomen.

Pathological reflexes are those reflexes that should not be present and indicate organic interference with CNS function. The method of eliciting these reflexes usually involves stimulation of the skin in a particular area. Presence of a Babinski sign is a common pathological reflex.

Micturition

Micturition, also called voiding or urination, is the process of evacuating urine from the bladder. In the infant and young child, micturition is a simple reflex initiated by distention of the bladder by urine. Between 2 and 3 years of age, the maturation of spinal cord segments, along with the conscious inhibitory ability of the cerebral cortex, results in voluntary control of micturition. The average capacity of the urinary bladder is 700 to 800 cc. Stimulation of the stretch receptors by a volume of 200 to 300 cc of urine will trigger the micturition reflex and a concurrent conscious desire to void.

Two main anatomical parts constitute the smooth muscle urinary bladder: (1) the body, which is the **detrusor muscle;** and (2) the **trigone,** a small, triangular area at the base of the bladder that includes the bladder–ureter junction, the urethra, and the external sphincter (a voluntary skeletal muscle). The external sphincter is located at the opening of the bladder and is normally contracted to prevent dribbling.

Micturition is primarily a parasympathetic function. The micturition reflex is mediated by S-2, S-3, and S-4 spinal segments, from which the preganglionic parasympathetic fibers synapse within the ganglia located in the bladder wall by way of the pelvic splanchnic nerves (Fig. 5-36). Short postganglionic parasympathetic fibers innervate both the detrusor muscle and internal sphincter. Parasympathetic stimulation that is caused by the stretching of the bladder wall results in contraction of the detrusor muscle and relaxation of the internal sphincter. Although there is some sympathetic innervation to the bladder, its role is not certain. Micturition is primarily a parasympathetic function.

The external sphincter is under voluntary control and is mediated by the pudendal nerve. It can be voluntarily contracted, but it relaxes by reflex action when urine is released from the internal sphincter.

Defecation

The act of evacuating the large bowel is called **defecation.** Several physiological mechanisms are involved in defecation. **Peristalsis** is the wavelike movement of smooth muscles within the wall of the large intestines. There are a two important reflexes related to defecation. The gastrocolic and duodenocolic reflexes that result from distention of the stomach and duodenum after eating facilitate peristalsis and mass movement along the gastrointestinal tract toward the rectum.

There are also two defecation reflexes. The first, the **intrinsic defecation reflex,** is triggered by feces entering the rectum. Pressure on the rectal wall sends afferent impulses through the **mesenteric plexus** to initiate peristaltic waves in the descending colon, sigmoid, and rectum, forcing feces toward the anus. The peristalsis relaxes the internal anal sphincter, and if the external anal sphincter is also relaxed, defecation occurs. The intrinsic defecation reflex is a weak reflex and

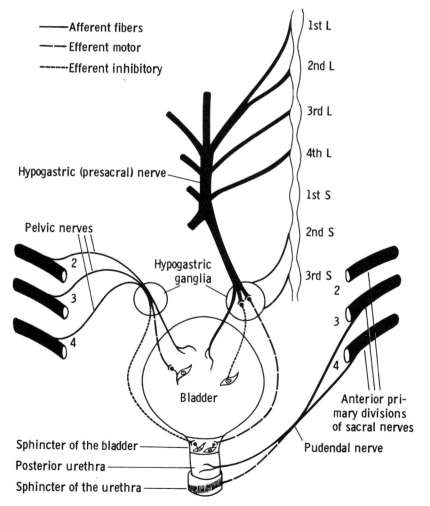

—— Afferent fibers
— — Efferent motor
----- Efferent inhibitory

1st L
2nd L
3rd L
4th L
1st S
2nd S
3rd S

Hypogastric (presacral) nerve

Pelvic nerves

2
3
4

Hypogastric ganglia

2
3
4

Bladder

Anterior primary divisions of sacral nerves

Sphincter of the bladder

Posterior urethra

Sphincter of the urethra

Pudendal nerve

FIGURE 5-36
Diagrammatic representation of the innervation of the bladder and urethra. (From Chaffee, E. E., and I. M. Lytle. [1980]. *Basic physiology and anatomy.* Philadelphia: J. B. Lippincott.)

must occur in combination with another reflex for defecation to occur.

This second reflex, the **parasympathetic defecation reflex,** involves the sacral segments (S-3, S-4, S-5) of the spinal cord. Stimulated afferent fibers in the rectum send signals to the spinal cord, and signals are sent back to the descending colon, sigmoid, rectum, and anus via the parasympathetic nerve fibers in the pelvic nerves. The parasympathetic signals do three things: intensify peristalsis, relax the internal anal sphincter, and augment the intrinsic defecation reflex. A powerful bowel evacuation can occur if the external anal sphincter is relaxed.

CONSCIOUS CONTROL OF DEFECATION

During infancy, defecation is a purely reflex action. However, in early childhood, voluntary control is learned so that defecation can be postponed until a socially acceptable place to evacuate the bowel is found. Voluntary consciousness now controls the external anal sphincter. If the sphincter is relaxed, defecation can take place. If contraction of the sphincter prevents defecation, the defecation reflexes soon cease, remaining inactive for several hours until more feces enter the rectum and once again initiate the defecation reflexes. The frequency of defecation among people varies from once per day to two or three times per week.

CRANIAL NERVES

The 12 pairs of cranial nerves are part of the peripheral nervous system. Besides having a name, each cranial nerve is also numbered in Roman numerals. The number is based on the descending order in which the cranial nerves and their nuclei attach to the CNS. Cranial nerve I connects to the brain in the cerebral hemispheres, whereas cranial nerve XII attaches at the lower medulla (Fig. 5-37). There are three pure sensory cranial nerves (I,

II, and VIII), five pure motor cranial nerves (III, IV, VI, XI, and XII), and four mixed cranial nerves (V, VII, IX, and X).

The anatomical locations of connection of the cranial nerves are as follows: I and II are in the cerebral hemispheres; III and IV are in the midbrain; V, VI, VII, and VIII are in the pons; and IX, X, XI, and XII are in the medulla. There are a few exceptions to the schemata: cranial nerves VII and VIII have dual citizenship in both the pons and, to a lesser degree, in the medulla. Cranial nerve V, primarily associated with the pons, also has branches in the midbrain and medulla (Fig. 5-38).

As a rule, cranial nerves do not cross in the brain (with the exception of cranial nerve IV). There are three sensory cranial nerves (I, II, and VIII), five motor cranial nerves (III, IV, VI, XI, and XII), and four cranial nerves with mixed functions (V, VII, IX, and X).

Classification of nerve fibers is similar to spinal nerves in some cases and dissimilar in other instances. Cranial nerves that have functions similar to those of spinal nerves are categorized as **general**; those with specialized functions (olfactory and gustatory) are **special**. The GSA, GVA, GSE, and GVE fibers are similar to spinal nerves of those categories and have already been discussed with spinal nerves. Fibers that are specific to cranial nerves include **special somatic afferent** (SSA), **special visceral afferent** (SVA), and **special visceral efferent** (SVE). SSA fibers convey sensory impulses from the special sense organs in the eye (vision) and ear (hearing and balance). SVA fibers convey impulses from the olfactory and gustatory receptors. SVE fibers innervate striated skeletal muscles from the branchial arches (jaw muscles, facial expression muscles, and muscles of pharynx and larynx).

Olfactory (I) Nerve (Sensory)

The olfactory nerve is a pure SVA nerve for the sense of smell. The receptors for smell are located in the superior nasal mucosa of each nostril. The **olfactory** nerve is composed of multiple small fibers from bipolar chemoreceptor cells called olfactory cells. The

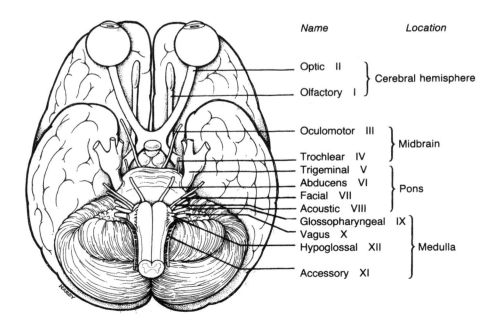

FIGURE 5-37
Diagram of the base of the brain showing entrance or exit of the cranial nerves. The eyeballs are shown schematically in relation to the optic nerves. The right column indicates the anatomical location of the connection of each cranial nerve to the central nervous system.

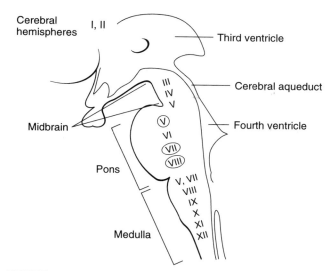

FIGURE 5-38
Lateral view of sites of cranial nerves and their nuclei within the cerebral hemispheres and brain stem (midbrain, pons, or medulla).

axons penetrate the skull through the cribriform plate to terminate in the **olfactory bulb.** From the bulb, the **olfactory tract** continues backward to the base of the frontal lobes where the two principal areas—the medial olfactory area and the lateral olfactory area—are located. The **medial olfactory area** is located anteriorly and superiorly to the hypothalamus (septum pellucidum, gyrus subcallosus, paraolfactory area, olfactory trigone, and medial part of the anterior perforated substance). The **lateral olfac-**

tory area is composed of the prepyriform area, the uncus, the lateral part of the anterior perforated substance, and part of the amygdaloid nucleus.

Optic (II) Nerve (Sensory)

The **optic nerve,** another pure SSA nerve, arises from the retina of the eyeball and is a part of the visual system. The **fundus** or **optic disc** represents the point where the optic nerve joins the retina and can be visualized by using the ophthalmoscope (it is the only cranial nerve that can be visualized). The optic disc is a natural blind spot because it does not contain any rods or cones. The **macula** is a 3-mm circular area on the retina, located near the posterior pole of the orbit, that is the point of clearest vision. The **scotoma** is an expected blind spot on the retina.

Vision is complex not only because many steps are involved in the process, but also because the visual tracts cut through all the lobes of the cerebral hemispheres. Therefore, visual deficits are common with many intracranial problems.

The **rods and cones** of the retina are the photoreceptors that are stimulated by light, thereby initiating nerve impulses that are conducted to the cerebral cortex (Fig. 5-39). Each **optic nerve** (4.5- to 5.0-cm long) runs posteriorly until it meets the optic nerve from the other side at the **optic chiasma.** The **visual pathways** posterior to the retina include a number of structures. The optic nerves come together at the optic chiasma, above the sella turcica. A partial decussation takes place at the chiasma whereby the nasal half of each optic nerve crosses to the other side. The **optic tracts** proceed laterally and posteriorly to terminate in the **lateral geniculate bodies** (a flat-

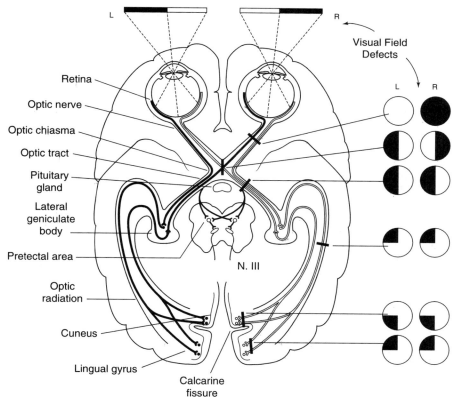

FIGURE 5-39
Fields of vision.

tened area in the posterolateral surface of the thalamus). Before reaching the lateral geniculate body, a few fibers leave the optic tract to go to the pretectal areas. These fibers become the afferent limb of the light reflex.

The **lateral geniculate body** is the terminal point of the optic tract; the geniculocalcarine tract originates from the cells of the geniculate bodies. The **geniculocalcarine tract** passes through the retrolenticular part of the internal capsule and forms the **optic radiations.** The upper fibers of optic radiations pass posteriorly in the *parietal lobe* and terminate in the superior portion of the calcarine cortex (occipital lobe); the lower fibers (**Meyer's loop**) loop anteriolaterally around the temporal horn of the *temporal lobe* and terminate in the inferior calcarine cortex. The **calcarine cortex,** also called the **primary visual cortex,** is organized such that the upper part of the visual field terminates in the inferior calcarine cortex and the lower visual field terminates in the superior cortex. The primary cortex (area 17) is located in the walls of the calcarine fissure and receives primary visual stimuli. The **visual association areas** (areas 18 and 19) are located in the **peristriate cortex** of the temporal and occipital lobes, lateral to the primary cortex. The visual association areas are necessary for visual impressions, recognition of colors and formed objects, and visual memory. In addition, eye movements activated by visual stimuli are controlled by the association areas.

THE VISUAL SYSTEM

When the visual system is considered it includes not only the optic nerves, visual pathways, and visual cortex, but also eye movement. Eye movement is addressed here to complete the discussion of the visual system.

Conjugate gaze and eye movement are complex processes for which the following areas have specific functions:

Brainstem for premotor conjugate gaze and vergence eye movement (**vergence** movements are both eyes moving medially to look at a near object or laterally to look into the distance)

Thalamic-midbrain centers for vertical gaze and vergence

Paramedian pontine reticular formation of the pons for horizontal eye movement.

Five subsystems are identified to enable the fovea to find and fixate on a target, stabilize an image on the retina, and maintain binocular focus during head or target movement (Lavin & Weissman, 1991, pp. 628–629). These systems are the

Saccadic system: (a **saccade** is a rapid, refixational eye movement) saccades may be voluntary or involuntary

Pursuit system: provides for eyes to track slowly moving targets

Vestibular system (semicircular canals): maintains a stable image on the retina during head movements

Optokinetic system: enables stabilization of images on the retina during sustained head rotation such as spinning

Vergence eye movement system: allows the eyes to move convergently and divergently to maintain binocular fixation on a target moving toward or away from the subject

The frontal-parietal gaze center (posterior portion of middle frontal gyrus, area 8; and ventral parietal lobe, area 7a)

and the occipital gaze center (areas 18 and 19) are important. The **frontal gaze center** is responsible for rapid (saccadic) voluntary control of conjugate gaze to a point of interest. Its fibers pass through the anterior internal capsule to the pons and connect with the lower centers. The **occipital gaze center** controls involuntary slow-tracking eye movement or visual pursuit. The center is responsible for fixing the eyes on an object and maintaining that visual fixation as the object moves through the visual field. Its fibers pass medially to the optic radiations and down through the posterior portion of the internal capsule, connecting with the conjugate eye movement centers in the midbrain and pons.

The **MLF** extends from the thalamic–midbrain region to the anterior horn cells of the spinal cord; it coordinates the eye and the neck movement pathways for gaze. The MLF connects and integrates fibers from the following areas of eye movement: brainstem oculomotor, trochlear, and abducens nuclei; fibers from the synapse of cerebellar nuclei and the semicircular canals; and the horizontal gaze center of the pons. Convergence of the eyes is not well understood and seems to be mediated by pontine and medullary structures, but not by the MLF (Westmoreland et al., 1994, p. 440). Divergence is controlled by centers located near the abducens nuclei.

The **paramedian pontine reticular formation (PPRF)** is located in the pons and receives fibers from the superior colliculus, the vestibular nuclei, and other parts of the reticular formation. The PPRF is known as the lateral gaze center. It sends fibers to the ipsilateral abducens nucleus (lateral movement) and through the MLF to cells of the contralateral oculomotor nucleus that supply the medial rectus muscle thus coordinating horizontal movement (Barr & Kiernan, 1993, pp. 127–129). Therefore, the descending pathways for horizontal conjugate gaze include the PPRF and the MLF. Much less is known about vertical movement. The oculomotor and trochlear nuclei, located in the brain stem, are involved in vertical eye movement: vertical and torsional saccadic innervation arise in the midbrain; the vertical gaze-holding impulses are integrated in the midbrain; and the vestibular and pursuit impulses ascend to the midbrain from the lower brain stem.

Oculomotor (III) Nerve (Motor)

The oculomotor nerve innervates four of the six extrinsic muscles responsible for movement of the eye. These muscles are the medial, superior, and inferior recti and the inferior oblique; they are controlled by GSE fibers. The eyes are rotated by these muscles in the following manner: medial recti—inward (medially); superior recti—upward and inward; inferior recti—downward and inward; and the inferior oblique—upward and outward (Table 5-10).

The oculomotor nerve has two other functions. First, it innervates the levator palpebrae superioris, which is responsible for elevating the upper eyelid (also GSE fibers). Second, it provides motor innervation to the intrinsic smooth muscles of the iris for pupillary constriction and to the muscles within the ciliary body for lens accommodation (both GVE functions).

The eye is innervated by both parasympathetic and sympathetic fibers to control pupillary size. Parasympathetic innervation is responsible for **pupillary constriction.** The parasympathetic preganglionic fibers arise in the **Edinger-Westphal nucleus** (the visceral nucleus of cranial

TABLE 5-10
Cranial Nerve Function Relative to Eye Movement

CRANIAL NERVE	MUSCLE	MOVEMENT OF EYEBALL
Oculomotor (III)	Medial rectus	Inward or medially on the horizontal plane
	Superior rectus	Upward and outward
	Inferior rectus	Downward and outward
	Inferior oblique	Upward and inward
Trochlear (IV)	Superior oblique	Downward and inward
Abducens (VI)	Lateral rectus	Outward or laterally on the horizontal plane

Note that the eye muscles function in pairs: the superior and inferior recti turn the eye upward and downward when the eye is looking outward (temporally); the inferior and superior obliques turn the eye upward and downward when the eye is looking inward; and the medial and lateral recti turn the eye inward (nasally) and outward (temporally) on the horizontal plane.

* *The oculomotor nerve also innervates the levator palpebrae oculoris muscle, which elevates the upper eyelid and the muscles that control the iris and ciliary body.*

(Figure from Bates, B. (1980). A guide to physical examination. Philadelphia: J. B. Lippincott.)

nerve III) and then proceed in cranial nerve III to the ciliary ganglion. Here, the preganglionic fibers synapse with post-ganglionic parasympathetic neurons that send fibers through the ciliary nerves into the eyeball. These nerves excite the ciliary muscles and the pupillary sphincter of the iris, resulting in pupillary constriction.

Pupillary dilation is the result of sympathetic innervation of the pupil originating in the intermediolateral horn cells of the first segment of the spinal cord. Proceeding from here, sympathetic fibers enter the sympathetic chain and pass upward to the superior cervical ganglion, where they synapse with postganglionic neurons. These fibers radiate along the carotid artery and smaller arteries until the eye is reached. Here, the sympathetic fibers excite the radial fibers of the iris and cause pupillary dilation.

Accommodation is the mechanism by which an automatic adjustment or accommodation of the curvature of the lens is made to focus images on the retina for visual acuity. Accommodation results from the contraction or relaxation of the ciliary muscles of the eye. Contraction of the smooth muscle fibers of the ciliary body causes the **suspensory ligaments** to relax and the lens to become thicker. Relaxation of the **ciliary body's** smooth muscle fibers results in tension of the suspensory ligaments and elongation of the lens.

Trochlear (IV) Nerve (Motor)

The trochlear nerve, a GSE nerve, supplies the superior oblique muscle. It is responsible for moving the eye downward and inward. The **trochlear nucleus** is located immedi-

ately caudal to the oculomotor nucleus at the level of the inferior colliculus in the midbrain. It exits the brain stem dorsally, the only cranial nerve to exit from the dorsum (posterior part) of the brainstem. Small bundles of fibers curve around the periaqueductal gray matter and decussate in the superior medullary velum; the trochlear emerges caudal to the inferior colliculus. The superior oblique muscle is supplied by crossed fibers.

Trigeminal (V) Nerve (Mixed)

The trigeminal is unique in that its main components are located in the pons with additional components in the midbrain and medulla. The trigeminal nerve has both GSA and SVE components. Pain, temperature, and light touch are conveyed from the entire face and scalp, the paranasal sinuses, and the nasal and oral cavities by the GSA component. The SVE motor component supplies the muscles of mastication which arise from the branchial arches.

The GSA fibers arise from the cell bodies in the **trigeminal ganglion.** The sensory components of the trigeminal nerve are divided into three sensory branches: **ophthalmic, maxillary,** and **mandibular** (Fig. 5-40). Axons travel centrally from the ganglion to enter the lateral aspect of the pons. Fibers for touch synapse directly on the **main sensory nucleus of V** which is located in the dorsolateral tegmentum of the pons. Pain and temperature fibers follow a different course. They turn caudally and descend via the dorsolateral medulla and upper three or four segments of the cervical spinal cord as the **spinal tract of the trigeminal**

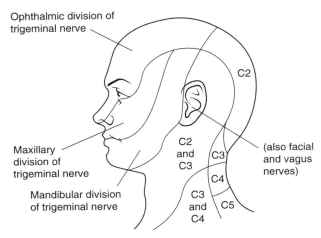

FIGURE 5-40
Cutaneous innervation of the head and neck. The boundaries between the territories supplied by the three divisions of the trigeminal nerve do not overlap appreciably, as do the boundaries between spinal dermatomes. (From Barr, M. L., and J. A. Kiernan. [1988]. *The human nervous system.* [5th ed.]. Philadelphia: J. B. Lippincott.)

nerve. The peripheral path followed by sensory fibers after the trigeminal ganglion is as follows:

1. The **ophthalmic division (V1)** passes through the superior orbital fissure to innervate the upper face.
2. The **maxillary division (V2)** exits the skull via the foramen rotundum to innervate the midface.
3. The **mandibular division (V3),** joined by the motor root, exits the skull via the foramen ovale to innervate the lower face.

The SVE fibers that innervate the muscles of mastication arise from cell bodies in the **motor nucleus of V,** which is located medial to the main sensory nucleus in the pons. The axons follow a ventrolateral path and exit from the lateral surface of the pons.

Abducens (VI) Nerve (Motor)

The abducens is a GSE nerve that innervates the lateral rectus muscle and rotates the eye laterally on the horizontal plane. The abducens nerve arises from the **abducens nuclei** that is located in the floor of the fourth ventricle of the midpons. Axons follow an anterior course through the tegmentum and basis pontis to the pontomedullary junction. The abducens then ascends to the pontine base through the cavernous sinus and exits the cranium through the superior orbital fissure to the lateral rectus muscle.

Facial (VII) Nerve (Mixed)

The facial nerve has its nucleus primarily in the pons, but also has connections to the medulla. It has SVE, GVE, and SVA components. The **facial nucleus** is located in the pons and has two branches: SVE fibers (arise in one branch and innervate

the muscles of facial expression), and GVE and SVA fibers. The SVE branch is responsible for closing the eye, smiling, whistling, showing the teeth, wrinkling the nose, and grimacing. The parasympathetic GVE fibers originate in the superior salivatory nucleus and control tearing and salivation of the lacrimal, sublingual, and submandibular glands. The sensory fibers originate in the **geniculate ganglion**; these SVA components mediate taste to the anterior two thirds of the tongue and sensation from the skin lining the external auditory meatus.

The SVE innervation of the muscles of facial expression can be divided into the muscles of the lower part of the face and the muscles of the upper part of the face. **Crossed fibers** project from the cerebral cortex to the facial nuclei that supply the contralateral lower part of the face (the area below the eye). **Crossed and uncrossed fibers** project to motor cells that innervate the upper part of the face. Movement of the upper face (*e.g.,* wrinkling the brow) comes from bilateral input from the cortex to the facial nerve nucleus. Because the upper facial muscles receive both crossed and uncrossed fibers, the upper part of the face is spared with central cerebral injury such as in stroke. The upper motor lesion results in a paralysis that is limited to muscles of the contralateral lower face (below the eye). If the facial nerve is injured, the entire side of the face (upper and lower face) would be affected. Therefore, the deficits on the affected side would include an "ironed out" forehead, an inability to close the eye, and a flattening of the nasolabial fold.

Acoustic (VIII) Nerve (Sensory)

The acoustic nerve is divided into two branches: the cochlear, which is concerned with hearing; and the vestibular, which influences balance, maintenance of body position, and orientation in space. Because these branches are two distinct systems, they are discussed separately.

In the **auditory system,** the **acoustic nerve** has SSA fibers that carry impulses from the cell bodies in the spiral ganglion of the cochlea. Vibrations proceed through the tympanic membrane and activate the three small bones of the middle ear (malleus, incus, and stapes). These vibrations then continue to the cochlea of the inner ear where the basilar membrane with the **organ of Corti** (hairlike mechanoreceptors) send fibers to the spiral ganglion of the cochlea. The spiral ganglion contains the bipolar cells of the cochlea (dorsal and ventral cochlear nuclei) that connect to the brain stem. The primary auditory receptive areas of the cortex are 41 and 42. From here, the impulses proceed to the auditory association area where recognition of the particular sound takes place.

In the **vestibular system,** the **vestibular nerve** has SSA fibers. The vestibular receptor end-organs in the vestibular system include the three cristae ampullares, one located in each of the semicircular canals, and the maculae of the utricle and saccule. All of these structures are sensitive to movement in a particular direction. The vestibular ganglion of the vestibular nerve receives input from the vestibular receptors and the cerebellum. The vestibular nuclei have projections into the following areas: spinal cord, by way of the lateral and medial vestibular spinal tracts (inhibitory and facility influence to extensor muscle tone and spinal reflexes); cerebellum; reticular formation; and, via the medial longitudinal fasciculus, the nuclei of cranial nerves III, IV, and VI.

Glossopharyngeal (IX) Nerve (Mixed)

The glossopharyngeal nerve is a mixed nerve with SVE, GVE, GSA, GVA, and SVE fibers. The vagus nerve is closely related, both anatomically and physiologically, to the glossopharyngeal nerve. The glossopharyngeal nerve has five branches, all of which penetrate the skull via the jugular foramen. The glossopharyngeal nerve innervates the stylopharyngeus of the pharynx (SVE); taste receptors from the posterior third of the tongue (SVA); parasympathetics of the parotid gland (GVE); sensation from the back of the ear (GSA); and sensation from the pharynx, tongue, eustachian tube, carotid sinus, and carotid body (GVA).

The SVE fibers of the stylopharyngeus muscle originate in the nucleus ambiguus. The GVE fibers carry parasympathetic fibers to the parotid gland and terminate in the otic ganglion. The cell bodies for sensory innervation are located in the inferior and superior petrosal ganglia.

Vagus (X) Nerve (Mixed)

The vagus nerve is also a mixed nerve with SVE, GVE, GSA, GVA, and SVE fibers. It branches into several segments. The functions include innervation of the striated muscles from the branchial arches (soft palate, pharynx, and larynx [SVE]); the parasympathetic innervation of the thoracic and abdominal organs (GVE); sensory innervation from the external auditory meatus (GSA); sensory innervation from the pharynx, larynx, and thoracic and abdominal viscera (GVA); and sensory innervation from the taste receptors of the posterior pharynx (SVA).

The SVE fibers (soft palate, pharynx, and larynx) come from the nucleus ambiguus found in the lateral medullary region dorsal to the inferior olive. The GVE components include preganglionic parasympathetic fibers coming from the dorsal motor nucleus to supply the thoracic and abdominal viscera. Preganglionic vagal neurons from the nucleus ambiguus innervate the heart. The preganglionic fibers synapse with the postganglionic neurons in the cardiac, pulmonary, esophageal, or celiac plexuses or within the visceral organs. The cell bodies for sensory innervation are dispersed throughout the body in a number of ganglia.

Spinal Accessory (XI) Nerve (Motor)

This spinal accessory nerve is an SVE nerve that innervates the sternocleidomastoid and upper portion of the trapezius muscle, allowing one to shrug the shoulders and rotate the head. The two roots of the spinal accessory nerve originate in the lower medulla and the upper five cervical cord segments. It ascends in the spinal canal and enters the skull via the foramen magnum, where it is joined by the minor accessory component originating in the nucleus ambiguus; the spinal nerve leaves the cranial cavity through the jugular foramen to innervate the sternocleidomastoid and trapezius muscles.

Hypoglossal (XII) Nerve (Motor)

The hypoglossal nerve is a GSE nerve that innervates the intrinsic muscles of the tongue to permit normal speech and swallowing. The paramedian area of that caudal medulla in the floor of the fourth ventricle is the location of the hypoglossal nucleus. The fibers exit from the ventral medulla, between the medullary pyramids and the olive. The fibers then pass through the hypoglossal canal in the occipital condyle and innervate the striated muscles of the tongue.

Bibliography

Barr, M. L., & Kiernan, J. A. (1993). *The human nervous system: An anatomical viewpoint* (6th ed.). Philadelphia: J. B. Lippincott.

Conn, P. M. (Ed.). (1995). *Neuroscience in medicine.* Philadelphia: J. B. Lippincott.

Garoutte, B. (1994). *Survey of functional neuroanatomy* (3rd ed.). Mill Valley, CA: Mill Valley Medical Publishers.

Gilman, S., & Winans, S. A. (1992). *Manter and Gatz's essentials of clinical neuroanatomy and neurophysiology* (8th ed.). Philadelphia: F. A. Davis.

Guyton, A. C. (1991). *Basic neuroscience: Anatomy and physiology.* Philadelphia: W. B. Saunders.

Guyton, A. C. (1991). *Textbook of medical physiology* (8th ed.). Philadelphia: W. B. Saunders.

Jennes, L., Traurig, H. H., & Conn, P. M. (1995). *Atlas of the human brain.* Philadelphia: J. B. Lippincott.

Lavin, P. J., & Weissman, B. (1991). Neuro-ophthalmology. In W. G. Bradley, R. B. Daroff, G. M. Fenichel, & C. D. Marsden (Eds.), *Neurology in clinical practice: Principles of diagnosis and management,* vol. 1 (pp. 627–654). Boston: Butterworth-Heinemann.

Watson, C. (1995). *Basic human neuroanatomy: An introductory atlas* (5th ed.). Boston: Little, Brown.

Westmoreland, B. F., Benarroch, E. E., Daube, J. R., Reagan, T. J., & Sandok, B. A. (1994). *Medical neurosciences: An approach to anatomy, pathology, and physiology by systems and levels* (3rd ed.). Boston: Little, Brown.

CHAPTER 6

Diagnostic Procedures and Laboratory Tests for Neuroscience Patients

Joanne V. Hickey

Diagnostic procedures and laboratory tests for neuroscience patients are becoming more sophisticated and specific. Development of diagnostic technologies has resulted in a cadre of highly specialized health professionals skilled in the techniques of testing and the interpretation of the findings.

More and more diagnostic procedures that formerly required hospital admission are now scheduled as outpatient procedures. This change in practice has been driven by the need for cost containment, the recognition that many procedures can be safely conducted on an outpatient basis, and patient convenience. On the day of the procedure, patients report to a special hospital area (*e.g.,* 23-Hour Unit, Ambulatory Center) or the procedure site, undergo the procedure, and recover in a special unit; they are then discharged home without an overnight hospital stay. In other instances, diagnostic procedures are ordered during the patient's hospitalization.

The variations of entry points for diagnostics create special challenges for patient and family education related to the procedure, preparation, and postprocedure care. Previously, patient teaching was usually the responsibility of the nurse. Now the nurse may not see the patient until arrival for the procedure, or there may not be a nurse present at all. When outpatient procedures are scheduled, written information about the procedure and preparation is often mailed to the patient. This precludes time for discussion or questions. Nurses need to recognize the realities of how patient teaching is conducted in their environments and that the responsibility for teaching is now shared with others. This sensitivity must be incorporated into their interactions with patients and families to assure patient/family understand and opportunities for questions.

PATIENT AND FAMILY TEACHING

Community Based Education

Neurological diagnostic procedures are performed in a variety of settings including the radiology department, special procedure areas, and patient care units. The large number of people undergoing diagnostic procedures on an outpatient ambulatory basis presents special challenges for education and preparation of patients. Education may be provided through a patient–nurse conference. Reading material such as a written description and a set of instructions, booklets, and illustrated pamphlets may be given or sent to the patient before the procedure. Literacy, reading level, and level of comprehension must be assessed and matched to the patient. Videotapes can provide another effective medium for education; the tape may be sent as a "loaner" for review and return, or it may be given to the person. With more and more people becoming computer literate, nurses may soon be sending e-mail/Internet information to patients. Regardless of which media are selected to dispense information, there is always need for follow-up to answer questions and clarify information. This may be done with a telephone call or electronic media.

Focus of Patient Teaching

Patients undergoing a diagnostic procedure need a general explanation of the procedure with special emphasis on what to expect and their role as participants. For example, patients who are about to undergo a brain computed tomography scan should be told that they must remain very still while the scan is being taken to ensure accuracy and quality graphics. For a more thorough briefing, information can be expanded to describe the procedure according to the patient's level of understanding and desire for information. Patients should know where the procedure will take place and where they will be taken upon its completion.

If a patient's level of consciousness has been altered sufficiently to affect attention span, comprehension, understanding, and appreciation of causal associations, the nurse should provide a simple explanation. Repetition and reinforcement of information may be necessary because the patient may have difficulty comprehending and remembering. He or she may also be very anxious or fearful.

The following nursing diagnoses are common in neurological patients undergoing diagnostic work-up; they require special consideration when preparing and teaching the patient about a scheduled diagnostic procedure. These nursing diagnoses include the following:

Altered thought processes related to:
  Altered consciousness (confusional state)
  Memory deficits
  Limited cognitive functions (concentration, reasoning)
  Effects of drugs
  Anxiety or fear
Sensory–perceptual alterations (visual, auditory, kinesthetic, or tactile) related to:
  Altered, impaired, or distorted vision, hearing, touch, or position sense
Knowledge deficit related to:
  Cognitive deficits
  Decreased level of consciousness
  Anxiety state
  Impaired communication
Anxiety and/or fear related to:
  Hospitalization
  Mutilation/death
  Unknown diagnosis

OUTPATIENT PROCEDURES

For outpatient procedures, nurses must be knowledgeable about procedures and hospital protocols and be sensitive to the anxiety or fear related to the diagnostic process. Patients and families are often aware that the purpose of the procedure is to rule in or rule out certain diagnoses and treatments. As a result, they are often anxious and fearful and need emotional support and education.

HOSPITALIZED PATIENTS AND PROCEDURES

For hospitalized patients, the care nurse or someone that he or she supervises prepares the patient for the procedure; a unit nurse or other personnel may accompany the patient to the diagnostic procedure. Sometimes, it is an absolute necessity that a nurse accompany the patient to the procedure, for example, when the patient requires frequent suctioning or is hemodynamically fragile and needs frequent monitoring. For the patient with impaired cognitive function or a high anxiety

level, the nurse may make the difference between success or failure of the diagnostic procedure. It is often necessary for the patient to cooperate, lie quietly, or follow instructions. The familiar nurse is often able to gain the patient's cooperation. Judicious use of sedation before and during the procedure is also useful and sometimes necessary.

Other times, the unit care nurse completes certain aspects of preprocedural preparation in the clinical unit. The patient is then taken to the designated area by someone responsible solely for patient transport. Once the patient arrives at the procedure site, technicians and/or the physician are the principal personnel involved. Therefore, it is most important that a proper explanation of the procedure and what to expect be provided to the patient beforehand.

INFORMED CONSENT

Written consent is required for many diagnostic procedures; there may be some variation among institutions. The nurse should adhere to institutional policies and procedure manuals. If patients have an altered level of consciousness, cognitive deficits, or other impairments that will affect their ability to give informed consent, a family member must provide written consent and it must be witnessed. It is usually the physician's responsibility to obtain written consent after explaining the procedure to the patient and family and answering their questions.

X-RAYS OF THE HEAD AND VERTEBRAL COLUMN

Skull/Facial X-Rays

Skull films are ordered infrequently because computed tomography and magnetic resonance neuroimaging provide much more anatomical information including information generally available from skull films. If a computed tomography scan is ordered, the need for skull films is eliminated. One of the most frequent reasons for ordering skull films is to determine whether a skull fracture is present. When skull films are ordered, they usually include anteroposterior and lateral radiographic views (Fig. 6-1). Other angles may be included in the series to provide information about specific areas such as the orbits or paranasal sinuses. Films provide information about the presence of a skull or facial fracture; unusual calcification or presence of air; the size and shape of skull or facial bones; and bone erosion, particularly of the sella turcica.

When skull films are reviewed, certain landmarks are identified to determine the presence of abnormalities. For example, the pineal body, normally calcified in the adult, is a midline structure. If it appears to be skewed to one side, it suggests that pressure from a space-occupying lesion is responsible for the deviation from the midline. Abnormal calcification raises suspicion of a calcified component located within a tumor; bone erosion suggests the presence of an intracranial lesion close to bone. The following are key points in understanding skull film reports:

- Fractures through the base of the skull or paranasal sinuses may produce pneumocephalus or air in the temporomandibular joint.

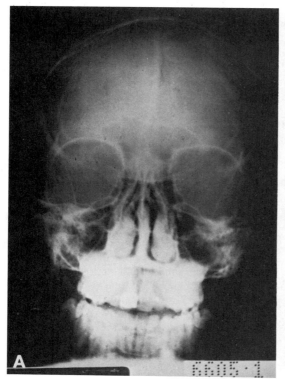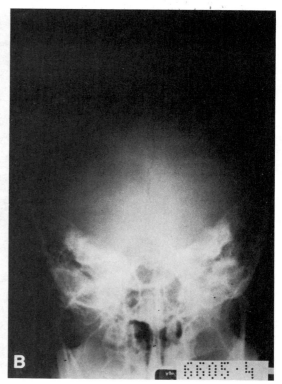

FIGURE 6-1
Anterior (*A*) and posterior (*B*) radiographic views of the skull.

- A skull fracture with a depression of more than 0.5 cm will result in an underlying contusion.
- Most depressed skull fractures require surgical debridement.

PATIENT MANAGEMENT

Other than encouraging the patient to lie still for the few moments necessary to take the films, no preparation or postprocedure care is required.

Spinal X-Rays

Spinal films are simple x-rays of various regions of the spine: cervical (Fig. 6-2), thoracic, lumbar, or sacral. The most commonly obtained views are the anterior–posterior (AP) and the lateral. Because the vertebrae are highly irregular anatomical structures, it is easy to overlook fractures of these bones. This is why lateral films, along with anterior and posterior views, are necessary to rule out the possibility of fracture. Indications for spinal films include trauma to the back or vertebral column or conditions in which the patient experiences pain or motor or sensory impairment.

In the emergency department, AP and lateral films of the cervical region are taken to rule out cervical fracture. To view the seventh cervical vertebrae, it is often necessary to pull the shoulders down. To view the odontoid process to determine fracture or instability of C1 and C2 vertebrae, an open-mouth view is necessary. Flexion–extension films are often used to

evaluate the presence of spinal injury. When ordered, the patient must be cooperative and cognitively intact to be able to report pain or neurological symptoms. These films are taken under the direct supervision of the physician. A magnetic resonance or computed tomography scan may replace or follow a spinal x-ray for more detailed information.

Abnormal findings found on spinal films may include wedging or compression of a vertebra; bone decalcification (osteoporosis); irregular bone calcification (osteophyte/spur); narrowing of the vertebral canal; vertebral fractures and/or dislocations; and spondylosis.

PATIENT MANAGEMENT

Other than encouraging the patient to lie still for the few moments necessary to take the films, there is no preparation or postprocedure care required.

ANATOMICAL IMAGING TECHNIQUES OF THE BRAIN

Computed tomography (CT) and magnetic resonance imaging (MRI) are the anatomical imaging cornerstones of the diagnostic workup for neurological and neurosurgical patients and are readily available technologies (Fig. 6-3). These technologies have made many previously ordered procedures obsolete.

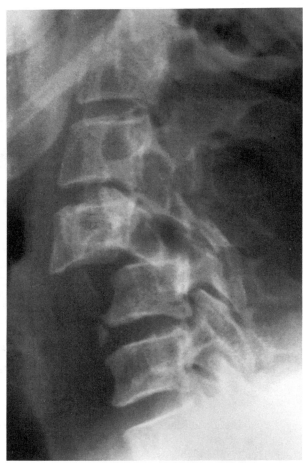

FIGURE 6-2
Radiograph showing an abnormality of the cervical spine. (From Errico, T. J., R. D. Bauer, and T. Waugh. [1991]. *Spinal trauma.* Philadelphia: J. B. Lippincott.)

Computed Tomography

Since its introduction by Hounsfield in England in 1972, refinement in CT technology has reduced scanning time and complexity of computations needed and improved the quality of anatomical image resolution. CT scans can be done with or without radiocontrast media. Use of a radiopaque medium increases the sharpness of the image.

During a CT scan, the head is scanned in successive layers by narrow x-ray beams that pass through the head and are absorbed and/or transmitted, depending on the density of tissue. The thickness of a scanner layer, called a slice, can vary from 1.5 to 10 mm; slices are taken at a slightly angled horizontal plane. The ionized radiation transmitted from the tissue is detected by an array of scanners that convert the transmitted radiation into light photons in proportion to its energy and intensity. The photons are, in turn, converted to electrical signals that are digitized and stored in a computer. The digitized information can then be manipulated by computer programs to reproduce images representing the various slices of the cranium or brain; films of the various cuts are then made.

The digitized conversion of the image results in anatomical visualization (in gray tones) which correlates to tissue den-

sity. The denser structures, such as bone, appear as relatively whiter areas. Cerebrospinal fluid (CSF) and air are less dense and, therefore, appear as black areas. Brain tissue appears as various shades of gray. When the radiologist reviews a CT scan, changes in tissue density; displacement of structures; and abnormalities in size, shape, or location of structures are noted (Fig. 6-4).

PROCEDURE

The patient lies on a movable x-ray table with his or her head carefully positioned and immobilized. The head of the x-ray table is then rolled several feet into the scanner. A movable circular frame (gantry) encircles the head and revolves around it, making a clicking sound while taking radiographic readings. Periodic slight adjustments are made to the machine. The head is scanned numerous times at different angles to collect data.

If contrast enhancement is desired to improve anatomical image clarity, iodinated radiopaque material will be administered intravenously. Some scanning may be done before the contrast medium is injected. CT scanning can begin 10 seconds after the beginning of the contrast infusion. If a contrast medium is used, a capital "C" will be noted somewhere on the films. The entire CT scanning procedure lasts 15 to 20 minutes. The patient must remain motionless, as movement can cause artifacts within the image that will affect the clarity of the pictures. Agitated or uncooperative patients require sedation or anesthesia to ensure the quality of the pictures.

DIAGNOSTIC APPLICATIONS TO NEUROLOGICAL DISEASE

The CT scan is most useful to identify hemorrhage (*e.g.,* hematomas, subarachnoid hemorrhage); ventricular size (*e.g.,* enlarged as a result of hydrocephalus, reduced because of the effects of a mass); cerebral atrophy; and larger space-occupying lesions (tumors). Serial CT scans can be used to follow the resolution or onset of acute cerebral disorders (*e.g.,* hemorrhage, edema).

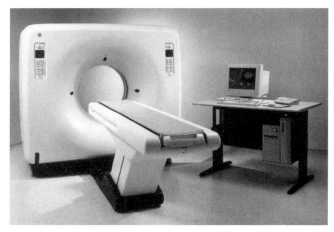

FIGURE 6-3
General Electric computed tomography system. (Courtesy of GE Medical Systems, Waukesha, WI)

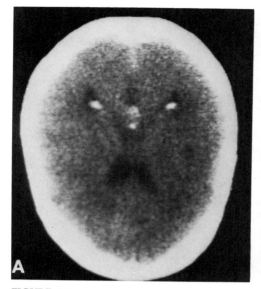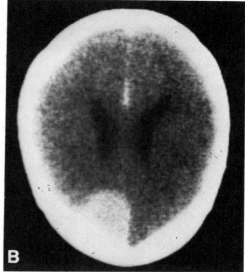

FIGURE 6-4
Computed tomography (CT) scan of the brain. (*A*) Normal scan. (*B*) Scan showing a large mass in the left frontal lobe.

SUMMARY OF ADVANTAGES AND DISADVANTAGES

Advantages. CT is a painless, safe, readily available procedure that can be performed on both conscious and unconscious patients and inpatient or outpatient populations. The cost is relatively reasonable (MRI costs significantly more) and has drastically reduced the need for more dangerous and expensive diagnostic tests. Radiation exposure is relatively low and comparable to that of skull films.

Disadvantages. CT scans have decreased sensitivity in detecting lesions adjacent to bone or small soft-tissue lesions. Criteria are being refined to help clinicians determine whether CT scanning or MRI is most appropriate for a particular patient (Chart 6-1).

PATIENT MANAGEMENT

Preparation. All jewelry, eyeglasses, and hair clips or pins should be removed from the head and neck. Unless a contrast medium will be administered, there are no dietary restrictions before the procedure. The specific routine of the physician and the hospital should be followed. The blood urea nitrogen and creatinine levels should be checked for adequate kidney function.

CHART 6-1
Comparison of Indications for CT Scans and MRIs

CT Scan	MRI
• Pacemaker in place*	• Allergy to contrast medium
• Metal prosthesis in place*	• Subacute/chronic cerebral trauma
• Uncooperative patient*	• Pituitary tumors
• Acute craniocerebral trauma	• Posterior fossa tumors (*e.g.,* acoustic neuroma)
• Acute subdural, acute epidural, or acute intracerebral hemorrhage	• Demyelinating disease (*e.g.,* multiple sclerosis)
• Predicting cerebral vasospasm	• Cerebral atrophy
• Aneurysm clipping with metal*	• Seizure disorders when CT scan yields normal results
• Hemorrhagic stroke	• Spinal cord tumors (primary and metastatic)
• Subarachnoid hemorrhage	• Spinal cord trauma
• Ischemic stroke (48–72 hours old)	• Intervertebral disk disease when myelographic results are normal
• Supratentorial enhancing tumors	
• Hydrocephalus	

*MRI contraindicated

Before the radiopaque contrast medium is administered, a skin test is done to check for an allergic reaction. If a contrast medium is planned, many protocols require nothing by mouth for 4 to 8 hours before the test. Some patients experience flushing or a feeling of warmth, transient headache, a salty taste in the mouth, nausea, or vomiting when the contrast medium is administered; patients should be prepared for these possible reactions.

Premedication such as diazepam (Valium) or lorazepam (Ativan) may be administered orally before the procedure to anxious patients. For agitated patients, short-acting intravenous sedation may be necessary. The procedure and equipment used are briefly explained to the patient, and reassurance is given that the procedure is painless. No motion will be felt, and a clicking sound of the machine is to be expected. Even though the technician and radiologist are outside the room, they can see the patient at all times. Oral communication between the patient and staff is maintained through an intercom system. The need to remain perfectly still should be emphasized.

Postprocedural Care. Patients who have received contrast media should be observed for signs and symptoms of delayed allergic reactions such as hives, skin rash, itching, nausea, or headache. If symptoms are severe, antihistamines may be administered. Intravenous hydration or encouragement of fluids to help clear the dye from the body is important. Kidney failure can result from inadequate hydration; older patients are at higher risk for kidney problems.

Magnetic Resonance Imaging

MRI, now readily available at most medical and imaging facilities, is a painless diagnostic procedure that can be used to image all parts of the body. In neuroscience practice, MR images of the head and spinal column provide images that are unmatched for exquisitely detailed cross sections of anatomical structures.

MRI scanners are located in specially constructed, copper-lined rooms that provide shielding from the strong magnetic fields associated with MRI equipment. The physics of the nuclear magnetic resonance phenomena on which MRI technology is based is complex. Through the use of a strong magnetic field, the nuclei of hydrogen atoms in tissues under study are aligned. These nuclei, which are like bipolar magnets and can spin, are then subjected to computer-programmed bursts of radio frequency (RF) waves which set them rotating about their axes in a uniform manner. This effect is known as **resonance**. When the nuclei seek to return to the imposed alignment, an effect known as **relaxation**, they give off tiny RF signals with the frequency, amplitude, and phase characteristics of electromagnetic waves. These signals are detected and converted to data which are stored and analyzed by sophisticated computer programs. Various mixtures of signals can be obtained by manipulating the RF characteristics of the bursts and other control elements of the equipment. The protocol chosen is intended to optimize the images possible for the type of tissue under study and the type of pathology of interest.

MR images of the human body take advantage of the following unique properties of the hydrogen atom and its differential distribution in tissues of the body:

- Hydrogen atoms have single-proton (odd number) nuclei.
- These ions resonate under specific conditions.
- The hydrogen ion is the most abundant chemical in human tissue.

By providing different RF wave patterns that "tickle" the hydrogen ions, different images are produced. Some images are based on the amount of time that it takes for the hydrogen protons to relax to their prior magnetic state after they have been turned 90 or 180 degrees by the RF pulses. This so-called **relaxation parameter** is called "T1." T1 depends on the tissue density (hydrogen ion density) in specific tissue (*e.g.*, white and gray matter) which differs greatly for various tissue types.

A second important relaxation parameter, called "T2," is based on the interaction of the perturbed magnetic fields of hydrogen atoms with each other. The RF pulse pattern causes hydrogen protons to gyrate in unison initially, so that each proton generates its own tiny magnetic field. Because of complex interactions among the magnetic fields, some protons accelerate while others decelerate. Various tissues have characteristic differences in their T2 relaxation patterns due to slight differences in tissue biochemistry. These differences can be correlated to the inception of disease processes, which can often be detected long before any structural changes have occurred.

Contrast media may be used in MRI studies; gadolinium is the usual drug used for enhancement. Careful analysis of preenhancement and postenhancement images may help to reveal the precise location of a lesion in situations in which precision is critical.

The interpretation of MRI images is heavily dependent upon the choice of images expected to provide the best contrast for the diagnostic evaluation under study. Three types of images dependent upon the type of RF pulse sequence employed are in general use: proton density images; T1-weighted images; and T2-weighted images. Initial evaluations for tumors need to include all three types to be complete. Each type has distinct advantages and disadvantages in terms of ability to detect pathology at certain tissue interfaces and potential for false positive information which should be evaluated in light of information obtained from the other sequences. T1 scans are superior in demonstrating general brain anatomy while T2 scans are superior in demonstrating areas of tissue pathology such as multiple sclerosis plaques or areas of infarction.

To determine if an MRI is a T1 or T2 image, look at the color of the cerebrospinal fluid (CSF). In the T1-weighted image, the CSF appears very dark; gray matter is lighter and white matter is bright. In the T2-weighted image, the CSF appears very bright and there is a poor color discrimination between gray and white matter.

Magnetic resonance angiography (MRA) is an exciting new application which attempts to take advantage of various relaxation-time and phase-shifting techniques to enhance the appearance of blood and CSF and measure its rate of flow through vessels and tissue.

PROCEDURE

After removing all metal objects and credit cards, the patient lies on a padded stretcher that slides into a tunnel-like chamber. The head is placed in a plastic helmet-like structure; the arms are at the side of the body and are held in place with Velcro straps.[1] The head of the x-ray table is then rolled several feet into the scanner. The scanner tube has a restricted opening; it has been compared to the opening of a trash can or large pipe (Fig. 6-5). During the scan, loud noises are caused by the pulsating RF waves that resemble a jackhammer or drill. The patient must be prepared for this and the absolute requirement to remain motionless for the scan, which lasts about 35 to 45 minutes. Although the patient is alone in the room, voice contact is maintained with the technician via an intercom. If contrast enhancement is desired to improve anatomical image clarity, iodinated radiopaque material will be administered intravenously.

DIAGNOSTIC APPLICATIONS TO NEUROLOGICAL DISEASE

Although MRI technology has diagnostic applications to several body systems, only its application to the nervous system will be considered here. Because MR images are not obscured by bone, MRI is excellent in detecting soft-tissue changes which may be impossible to detect with x-ray. These include necrotic tissue, oxygen-deprived tissue, small malignant tumors (as little as .3 mm in size), and degenerative diseases within the central nervous system (CNS) such as multiple sclerosis. It is also efficient in identifying cerebral and spinal cord edema; CNS ischemic-infarcted areas; hemorrhage; arteriovenous malformations; CNS tumors, particularly in the difficult-to-visualize areas of the brain stem, basal skull, and spinal cord; degenerative diseases (*e.g.,* multiple sclerosis, Alzheimer's disease); and congenital anomalies. The superb sharpness and precision of detail are superior for diagnosis and location of lesions.

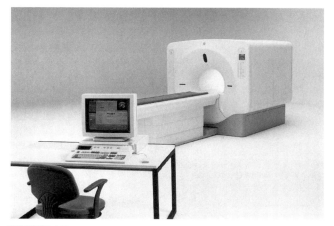

FIGURE 6-5
General Electric magnetic resonance system. (Courtesy of GE Medical Systems, Waukesha, WI)

SUMMARY OF ADVANTAGES AND DISADVANTAGES

The following are advantages of MRI:

- Provides detailed sagittal (right-to-left side); axial (top to bottom of the head) and coronal (front to back of the head) images for precise lesion assessment and location
- Does not use ionizing radiation, thus eliminating that risk
- Provides better differentiation than CT of water, iron, fat, and blood using physical and biochemical characteristics of tissues imaged
- Higher level of gray–white matter contrast obtainable as compared to CT
- Provides higher-resolution detail of the posterior fossa, skull base, and orbits as compared to a CT scan

Disadvantages of MRI include its higher cost relative to CT scan and the need to exclude of a number of patients who could be adversely affected by the procedure because the strong magnetic field can move or dislodge metallic material and cause injury to body tissue. The contraindications for MRI include the following:

- Patients with metallic devices, such as artificial pacemakers, prosthetic devices (*e.g.,* metallic hip replacements, orthopedic pins), artificial limbs, respirators, and other metallic equipment
- Patients with older metal intracranial aneurysm clips or metal bullet fragments in the brain
- Agitated or uncooperative patients (must lie perfectly still)
- Obese patients who cannot fit into the MRI tube
- Claustrophobic patients who cannot tolerate the closeness of the tube to their face
- Patients who have back pain and cannot lie flat and immobilized for 45 minutes

In the last few years, new MRI-friendly materials from the manufacturers of neurological and orthopedic equipment have become available. It is imperative to accurately screen patients for the presence of any devices that are contraindications for MRI **before** scheduling the procedure.

PATIENT MANAGEMENT

Preparation. Carefully question and screen for the presence of any metal implants. For the patient who is vague about this possibility, x-ray screening may be necessary. The patient should be counseled about the necessity to remain still for up to 45 minutes in very close quarters. Antianxiety medication may be ordered for some patients. All jewelry, eyeglasses, and hair clips or pins and any other metal objects should be removed. Credit cards should not be in the room because the magnetic field will erase the card. Unless a contrast medium will be administered, there are no dietary restrictions before the procedure. The specific routine of the physician and the hospital should be followed. The blood urea nitrogen and creatinine levels should be checked for adequate kidney function.

Before a radiopaque contrast medium is administered, a skin test is done to check for an allergic reaction. If the use of a contrast medium is planned, many protocols require nothing by mouth for 4 to 8 hours before the test.

Postprocedural Care. There are no special aftercare requirements.

PHYSIOLOGICAL IMAGING TECHNIQUES OF THE BRAIN

The major studies for *physiological neuroimaging* are positron emission tomography (PET) and single photon emission computed tomography (SPECT). These techniques rely on radiopharmaceuticals and principles of tracer kinetic techniques to observe and measure local biochemical processes in the brain. PET uses positron-emitting radionuclides and SPECT uses single photon radioisotopes.

Positron Emission Tomography

PET scanning is a sophisticated technique to measure regional physiological functions such as glucose uptake and metabolism, oxygen uptake, and cerebral blood flow patterns. Its elegance of detail is unmatched for demonstration of hypometabolic and hypermetabolic regions of the brain. It is the gold standard for all other physiological imaging techniques. In neuroscience research, PET is a developing technology that is providing new information in understanding epilepsy, dementia (*e.g.*, Alzheimer's disease), cerebrovascular disease, cerebral trauma, and mental illness. It is used in a limited number of patients for diagnostic purposes.

The technology is based on the use of an on-line cyclotron or linear accelerator to create positron-emitting radionuclides. The patient is injected with a compound that has been labeled with a positron-emitting nuclide "tag" (carbon 11, fluorine 18, oxygen 15, glucose or its analog F-fluorodeoxyglucose [FDG]). Once inside the body, the compound selected concentrates in the area of clinical interest and emits positrons. As the positrons decay, they emit photons that move in diametrically opposite directions and are recorded by detectors located on either side of the body. Multiple scanners detect and code these data into a computer which reconstructs cross-sectional images of the tissue containing the labeled compounds.[2]

PROCEDURE

After 6 to 12 hours NPO, the patient is placed on a stretcher in the imaging center and prepared. An arterial line may be inserted to draw blood samples for measurement of cerebral metabolic rates. The radiopharmaceutical agent of choice is injected via venous access. The patient rests quietly in a dimly lighted room for about 45 minutes while uptake of the radiopharmaceutical occurs. Only the head is placed inside the scanner for the procedure. The scanning portion of the procedure takes about 45 minutes. If blood samples are required, they are drawn quietly by the technician without disturbing the quiet environment created for the study. The entire procedure takes about 2 to 3 hours.

SUMMARY OF ADVANTAGES AND DISADVANTAGES

A major advantage of PET is the clarity of images produced. The major drawbacks of PET are the following:

- An on-line cyclotron or linear accelerator is necessary to manufacture the short-lived isotopes on site; this equipment is found only in major research centers and thus limits access.
- It is an expensive study.
- It is used for diagnostic purposes for only a limited number of patients.

PATIENT MANAGEMENT

Preparation. Maintain NPO status for 6 to 12 hours before the procedure. No glucose solution intravenous infusions should be used.

Postprocedural Care. After completion of the study, fluids should be encouraged to clear the body of the radioisotopes.

Single Photon Computed Emission Tomography

SPECT scans are physiological imaging studies which measure blood perfusion of the brain. This approach evolved from PET technology. The difference is that a SPECT scan is conducted using a rotating gamma camera, an instrument currently available in many nuclear medicine departments.

The radioactive tracers used in SPECT scans are commercially prepared and therefore do not require an on-line cyclotron. The most commonly used tracers are lipid soluble N-isoptopyl 123 I-p-iodooamphetamine (IMP), which diffuses across the blood–brain barrier with almost complete extraction during a single pass through the cerebral circulation, reflecting regional blood flow.[3] SPECT tracks the single photons resulting from radioactive decay using the gamma camera, which collects data from multiple angles to reconstruct regional blood flow. It is a useful study to demonstrate cerebral blood flow in focal and diffuse cerebral disorders in dementia, cerebral trauma, and cerebrovascular disease. It is believed that the SPECT scan will be the major diagnostic procedure for dementia in the future.

PROCEDURE

The patient lies quietly on a padded stretcher and the isotope is administered. The isotope decays in about 1 hour so the scan must be conducted within that window of time. The patient must lie quietly for the scan. The entire study takes about 1 to 2 hours.

SUMMARY OF ADVANTAGES AND DISADVANTAGES

The major advantages of SPECT are the widespread availability of the technology within many nuclear medicine departments and the excellent information it provides on cerebral perfusion to specific areas of the brain. The major disadvantage of SPECT is its cost, about as much as a CT scan.

PATIENT MANAGEMENT

Preparation. No special preparation is required other than the usual explanation of the procedure to the patient.

Postprocedural Care. No special care is required.

CEREBROSPINAL FLUID AND SPINAL PROCEDURES

Lumbar Puncture

A lumbar puncture involves the introduction of a hollow needle with a stylet into the lumbar subarachnoid space of the spinal canal using strict aseptic technique. In the adult, the needle is placed between L-3 and L-4 or L-4 and L-5. This location is a safe distance from the end of the spinal cord, which terminates at L-1.

The indications for lumbar puncture can be divided into diagnostic and therapeutic purposes. The diagnostic indications include measurement of CSF pressure; examination of CSF for the presence of blood; collection of CSF for laboratory study; radiological visualization of parts of the nervous system by injection of air, oxygen, or radiopaque material; and evaluation of spinal dynamics for signs of blockage of CSF flow. Chart 6-2 details the characteristics of CSF. The therapeutic indications of lumbar puncture include the introduction of spinal anesthesia for surgery; intrathecal injection of antibacterial or other drugs; and removal of CSF in benign intracranial hypertension (formerly called pseudotumor cerebri).

CONTRAINDICATIONS

The contraindications for lumbar puncture are relative and require careful medical judgment, weighing benefits against risks. When clinical evidence indicates a substantial increase in intracranial pressure, caution is advised. Increased intracranial pressure can be found in patients with any space-occupying lesions, such as brain tumors. Performing a lumbar

---

CHART 6-2
Characteristics of Cerebrospinal Fluid (CSF)

Parameter	Normal Value	Abnormal Findings
Volume	About 150 cc	↑ with hydrocephalus
Specific gravity	1.007	↑ with blood cells and infections
Pressure	76–200 mm H_2O	↑ with ↑ intracranial pressure
Color	Crystal clear	*Xanthochromia* (discoloration) of CSF; usually due to breakdown of RBCs from previous intracranial hemorrhage; appears yellow, orange, or brown. (See also Chart 6-3). *Turbidity* (cloudiness): due to ↑ WBCs or ↑ protein from microorganisms in CSF
Protein count	16–45 mg/dL	Mild ↑ with viral meningitis, subdural hematoma, brain tumor, and multiple sclerosis. Moderate/high ↑ with bacterial or TB meningitis, cerebral hemorrhage, brain and spinal cord tumors, and GBS (Guillain Barré Syndrome)
White cells count	0–5 cells/mm³	*10–200 cells mostly lymphocytes:* viral meningitis, multiple sclerosis, CNS tumor and late neurosyphilis
		200–500 cells mostly lymphocytes: TB meningitis, herpes infection of CNS, and meningovascular syphilis
		>500 cells, mostly granulocytes: acute bacterial meningitis
Glucose	40–80 mg/dL (50%–80% of blood value)	↑ has specific significance; ↓ often seen with all meningitis and subarachnoid hemorrhage
Lactate	10–20 mg/dL	↑ indicates ↑ glucose metabolism often associated with bacterial or fungal meningitis

puncture in a patient with drastically increased intracranial pressure may result in brain stem compression, herniation through the foramen magnum, and, ultimately, death.

Cutaneous or osseous infection at the site of the lumbar puncture is an absolute contraindication for lumbar puncture. Additionally, patients who are receiving anticoagulation therapy should be considered carefully because of the added risk of hemorrhage.

PROCEDURE

The lumbar puncture is usually done at the patient's bedside or in an outpatient facility. A lumbar puncture set is prepared. The patient assumes a lateral recumbent position along the edge of the bed, arching the back so that the knees are flexed on the chest with the chin touching the knees (Fig. 6-6). This position allows maximal separation of the vertebrae, thereby facilitating insertion of the lumbar needle and reducing the degree of trauma. The nurse may be called upon to assist the patient if this position cannot be assumed independently.

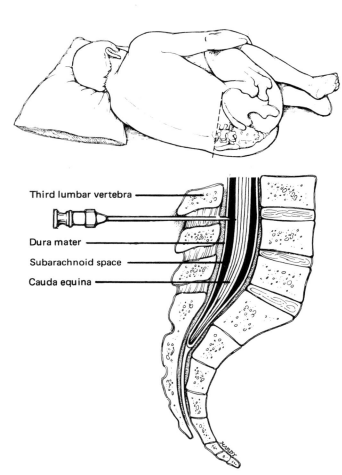

FIGURE 6-6
Technique of lumbar puncture. The interspaces between the spines of L-3 and L-5 are just below the line joining the anterosuperior iliac spines. (From Smeltzer, S., and B. Bare [1996]. *Brunner and Suddarth's textbook of medical-surgical nursing.* [8th ed.]. Philadelphia: Lippincott-Raven.)

Before any attempt is made to insert the lumbar needle, the lumbar site is aseptically prepared, draped, and locally anesthetized with an intradermal injection of procaine (Novocaine). Strict aseptic technique is essential. After the lumbar needle is successfully introduced into the subarachnoid space, the stylet is removed and a manometer is affixed to measure and record entrance pressure of CSF. Once this measurement is obtained, the manometer is removed and samples of CSF are collected into sterile test tubes for visual and laboratory examination. The physician may choose to record the exit pressure, for which the manometer would again be necessary. If the lumbar puncture is done solely for the purpose of instilling contrast medium or medication, recording the CSF pressure or collecting CSF specimens is not necessary.

When the procedure is completed, the lumbar needle is removed and a bandaid is applied over the puncture site.

Complications. It is important to know when a lumbar puncture has resulted in trauma. A traumatic tap causes trauma to the tissue at the lumbar puncture site with subsequent bleeding. In this instance, the initial sample of CSF would contain blood. Such bleeding could be misinterpreted as resulting from subarachnoid hemorrhage. However, in the case of a traumatic tap, the CSF clears progressively in successive samples. If there has been hemorrhage into the subarachnoid space from intracranial bleeding, successive samples of CSF would continue to be just as bloody as the first specimen. Other characteristics that differentiate a traumatic bloody tap from CNS hemorrhage are summarized in Chart 6-3.

In addition, some patients have a severe headache due to leakage of CSF from the puncture side. A "blood patch" is used to seal the site of leakage with good results.

PATIENT MANAGEMENT

Preparation. Ask the patient to empty his or her bladder immediately before the procedure. Usually, no dietary restriction or preprocedural medication is warranted.

Postprocedural Care. The care of a patient who has undergone lumbar puncture includes the following:

- Have the patient lie flat in bed 6 to 12 hours following the procedure, depending on physician preference, hospital policy, and continued signs of headache.
- Frequently monitor neurological and vital signs.
- Force fluids.
- Administer analgesics (for headache) prn.

Following lumbar puncture, a mild to severe headache may occur, caused by leakage of CSF at the puncture site or by irritation of the meninges. Acetaminophen (Tylenol), 650 mg p.o. every 4 hours, is used for mild headaches, whereas methylmorphine (codeine phosphate), 30 mg p.o. may be ordered for severe headaches. Because headaches are aggravated by an upright position, the patient is advised to lie flat in bed to relieve the pain. A blood patch may be used as discussed above. Other possible symptoms that can occur after lumbar puncture include backache or spasms in the lower

CHART 6-3
Lumbar Puncture: Traumatic Tap Versus Central Nervous System (CNS) Hemorrhage

Characteristics	Traumatic Blood Tap	CNS Hemorrhage
Color	Clears with successive collection of samples	Bloody in all samples
Coagulation	Often clots	Rarely clots
Supernatant fluid after centrifuge	Clear	
Supernatant		Xanthochromic
Appearance of RBCs	Normal	Crenated

back or thighs; transient voiding problems; nuchal rigidity; and slight rise in temperature.

Myelography

Myelography is a diagnostic procedure ordered to visualize the lumbar, thoracic, or cervical area, or the whole spinal axis, for diagnosis of a spinal cord tumor, a herniated intervertebral disk, or a ruptured disk. Any partial or complete obstruction that hinders the flow of the contrast medium will be visualized on the films. Many physicians order an MRI first for patients with back pain; if this inconclusive, then a myelogram is ordered.

PROCEDURE

A lumbar puncture is performed and approximately 10 mL of CSF is removed. A water-soluble contrast medium (Isovue or Amipaque) is then injected into the subarachnoid space and x-ray films are taken of the spinal cord and vertebral column.

Contrast Media. A few points need to be made about radio-paque media. In the past, oil-based media were used. Since the introduction of water-soluble contrast media, use of oil-based media has ceased. Once the water-based contrast medium is injected into the CSF, it diffuses upward through the CSF and penetrates into the nerve root sleeves, nerve rootlets, and narrow areas of the subarachnoid space. Upward diffusion occurs regardless of the position of the patient. The head is kept elevated about 30 degrees at all times and the patient is kept quiet to reduce the rate of upward dispersion of the contrast medium. Upward dispersion is controlled to prevent the contrast medium from entering the cranial vault, which could easily result in seizures.

Special precautions should be followed in postprocedure care to prevent seizures. In addition, confusion, hallucinations, depression, hyperesthesia, chest pain, and arrhythmias can occur from the contrast medium.

PATIENT MANAGEMENT

Preparation. The patient should be well hydrated. Omit the meal prior to the myelogram. Explain the need to force fluids (3 L) for the first 24 hours after the procedure, and keep the head elevated 16 to 30 degrees at all times.

Postprocedural Care. The patient should be transported back to his or her room or the recovery area with the head of the stretcher elevated 30 degrees. In addition, the following points should be followed (there may be slight variations among institutional practice guidelines):

- Keep the patient on bedrest for 4 hours with the head of the bed elevated 30 degrees
- Keep the patient quiet and still for 24 hours after the procedure
- Head must be elevated (chair or bed) for a total of 12 hours
- Force oral fluids immediately upon return from the procedure to 2,400 to 3,000 cc per 24 hours
- Monitor neurological and vital signs
- Maintain an intake and output record
- After 4 hours, resume diet as tolerated if there is no nausea or vomiting
- Do not give any phenothiazine derivatives for 48 hours (increase possibility of seizures)
- Observe the patient for untoward signs and symptoms such as back pain, spasms, elevated temperature, difficulty voiding, nuchal rigidity, nausea, and vomiting
- Treat nausea with trimethobenzamide hydrochloride (Tigan) 200 mg IM q 6 hour prn
- Treat headache with analgesics prn

CEREBROVASCULAR STUDIES

Cerebrovascular studies are broadly classified as noninvasive and invasive. Major strides have been made in the last few years with noninvasive transcranial Doppler technology.

Ultrasonography and Noninvasive Cerebrovascular Studies

The fastest area of development of diagnostics for carotid and intracranial cerebrovascular assessment is with noninvasive ultrasonography technology. The technology is being refined and now has broader applications to include intracranial vessels rather than only extracranial vessels. Clinicians are learning how to use and interpret data for the managemen of patients with cerebrovascular disease. It is relatively inexpensive, noninvasive, and can be done at the bedside is a short period of time.

Ultrasound technology uses the transmission of ultrasonic pulses through tissue and the reflection of the sound at tissue interfaces. The amplitude of the reflected sound waves depends on the orientation of the reflecting surface. The amplitude is maximal when the transmitted sound wave is at right angles to the surface.

Doppler Ultrasound. Doppler ultrasonography is based on a change in the frequency of sound whenever there is a relative motion between the source of a sound and the detector. Doppler ultrasound detects this frequency change in the echoes returning to the transducer (frequency shift). Frequency change is directly related to change in velocity, and in the carotid arteries the frequency shift detected is that of the red blood cells traveling through the lumen of the vessel. When the lumen of a blood vessel is narrowed, there is increased flow velocity of the blood through the stenosis. Concurrently, there is disturbance of the normal flow of blood in the vessel upstream, resulting in turbulence in the lumen distal to the stenosis. With Doppler ultrasound, this event would result in an increased velocity of the red blood cells as they accelerate through the stenosis.

Doppler technology is developing rapidly and is now the cornerstone of noninvasive carotid testing. Clinical use has expanded to diagnosis of carotid artery stenosis or occlusion (atherosclerotic changes) of the common carotid (CCA), internal carotid, and external carotid arteries to include intracranial vessels. A Doppler ultrasonic probe (which sends high-frequency sound waves) is placed on the skin over the CCA or on the skull. The sound waves reflect back the velocity of the blood flow. These data are amplified, and graphic recordings of the wave forms common to each vessel, as well as sound recordings of the blood flow, are produced. The test takes 15 to 45 minutes.

Transcranial Doppler. Transcranial Doppler (TCD) is a portable, noninvasive technology that allows assessment of the intracranial cerebral circulation at the bedside. TCD is used in evaluating patients with vasospasm, transient ischemic attack, headache, subarachnoid hemorrhage, head injury, and arteriovenous malformation. Serial studies may be conducted to monitor changes over time such as the evolution or resolution of vasospasm. TCD may also be used during surgical procedures such as cardiopulmonary bypass or carotid endarterectomy to monitor blood flow. It is now being used experimentally to monitor embolic stroke. TCD does not provide an actual image of the vessel or measure cerebral blood flow; rather, it determines velocity and direction of the moving column of blood in a major artery.

The newer models of TCD provide patient reports that include colored printouts and descriptive data about the waveforms and identify the blood vessel.

B-Mode Imaging. B-mode (brightness-modulated) imaging, or real-time ultrasonographic angiography, offers visualization of the structural detail of both the vessel walls and atherosclerotic plaques by recording the reflection of ultrasonic waves introduced through a probe. Two-dimensional images of a pulsating blood vessel in longitudinal and transverse sections allow visualization of most of the vessel's circumference. The image is reflected on a display screen in tones of gray. A photograph of the image can be taken to provide a permanent record. The purpose of the procedure is to detect minimal plaque formation and stenosed carotid vessels. Poor-quality images can result if the patient has a short, thick neck because the carotid bifurcation is high in the neck and difficult to scan. The procedure takes approximately 30 to 45 minutes.

Duplex Scanning. Duplex scanning of the carotids is based on the combination of two modalities: (1) high resolution, real-time, two-dimensional, cross-sectional imaging which demonstrates detailed anatomical images of the vessel, and (2) pulsed Doppler ultrasound which evaluates the physiological properties of red blood cell velocity movement in the vessel. This dual modality allows a Doppler cursor to be placed into any specific area of a two-dimensional image to collect data; data about the lumen of selected blood vessels can be collected at various points along the vessel.[4]

PATIENT MANAGEMENT

Preparation. Patient management is the same for all noninvasive carotid studies. Regardless of the test to be performed, the patient should be given an explanation of what to expect. All of the noninvasive carotid studies just presented are painless. For all of these tests, the patient will be asked to remain still. Beyond these points, there is no other patient preparation.

Postprocedural Care. Other than washing away any gel used as a conductor in Doppler studies, there is no specific aftercare required for patients in whom noninvasive carotid studies have been performed.

Cerebral Blood Flow Studies: Xenon-133

There are a number of cerebral blood flow (CBF) study methods available; the method chosen will determine the range of normal and pathological values, the anatomic specificity or resolution, and the set of assumptions necessary for interpreting the data.[5] The conceptual basis for the measurement of brain tissue perfusion was developed by the seminal work of Kety and Schmidt in 1945. Current CBF techniques are based on their work. A frequent choice is xenon-133 as a radioactive tracer for cerebral perfusion and CBF either as an inhaled gas or an intra-arterial injection. After administration of the tracer, the cerebral washout is followed with external scintillation counters placed over the skull, making it possible to perform regional determination of CBF. The rate of washout is proportional to CBF.

Xenon-Enhanced Computed Tomography. Xenon may also be used with rapid sequential CT scanning to quantify CBF. CBF studies are useful to determine viability of cerebral tissue globally and regionally and as part of brain death criteria.

PATIENT MANAGEMENT

Preparation. No special preparation is required.

Postprocedural Care. No special care is required.

Cerebral Angiography

Cerebral angiography is the definitive diagnostic procedure for aneurysms, arteriovenous malformations, and other cerebrovascular abnormalities. The lumen of the blood vessels can be visualized to determine patency, narrowing or stenosis, thrombosis, vasospasm, and displacement of cerebral vessels. Causes of displacement include space-occupying lesions such as hematomas, cysts, tumors, and abscesses. Cerebral angiography can be performed using local anesthesia or as part of a surgical procedure if the patient is undergoing general anesthesia. For example, cerebral angiography can be obtained during an aneurysm clipping to check the position and integrity of the clip.

PROCEDURE

The patient is placed in a supine position on the x-ray stretcher. A wide area around the puncture site is shaved. A local anesthetic is usually administered; procaine (Novocaine) is often the drug of choice. The puncture site is aseptically cleansed. After local injection with Novocaine, the contrast medium is either injected directly into the carotid arteries (rare) or introduced by the indirect route, through catheterization of the carotid or vertebral arteries using the femoral, brachial, subclavian, or axillary artery as a point of entry (the femoral route is the most common). X-ray films are then taken at various time intervals after injection for visualization of the intracranial and extracranial blood vessels (Fig. 6-7). When the examination is completed, direct manual pressure is applied to the puncture site for 5 to 10 minutes to prevent bleeding into the subcutaneous space.

Possible complications following cerebral angiography include allergic reactions to contrast media, seizures, stroke, pulmonary emboli, thrombosis, symptoms of carotid sinus

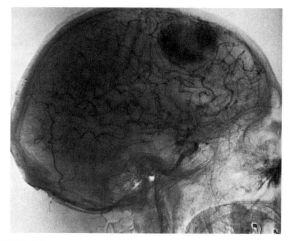

FIGURE 6-7
Cerebral angiogram showing an abnormal, large, space-occupying lesion at one o'clock.

sensitivity (hypotension, syncope, and bradycardia), aphasia, and visual difficulty.

PATIENT MANAGEMENT

Preparation. The skin is shaved at the puncture site; this may be ordered on the evening preceding the procedure or immediately before the procedure. The patient should be told that, during injection, a burning sensation may be felt for a few (4 to 6) seconds behind the eyes or in the jaw, teeth, tongue, and lips. Even the fillings in the teeth may feel warm. Moreover, the physician should explain the possibility that the procedure may precipitate a stroke, although this is unlikely. A consent form outlining risks is signed by the patient. The need to lie still during the procedure is emphasized to the patient.

Preoperative medication is usually administered half an hour before the procedure. The choice of drugs used varies from physician to physician and may include any of the following: pentobarbital (Nembutal); atropine sulfate, IM, to protect against the effect upon the carotid sinus; diazepam (Valium); and meperidine (Demerol), IM. Preparation for the examination is similar to that for any operative procedure. Dentures and eyeglasses are removed. Most physicians prefer that the patient not have anything by mouth for 6 to 8 hours before the examination. Baseline vital and neurological signs are recorded.

Postprocedural Care. When the procedure is completed, the patient is returned to his or her room. Nursing responsibilities include the following:

- Maintain the patient on complete bedrest for 8 hours.
- If the puncture site was through the femoral artery, immobilize the patient's upper leg for 8 hours (a sandbag may be helpful) to prevent rebleeding.
- Observe the puncture site (pressure dressing) frequently for bleeding.
- Monitor vital signs and neurological signs frequently. After the initial period of monitoring every 15 to 30 minutes, check these signs every 1 to 4 hours for a 24-hour period.
- Check pedal pulses in the affected leg if a femoral puncture was performed; also check the color and temperature of the extremity.
- Maintain an accurate intake and output record.
- Force fluids to clear the dye (a toxic response may include kidney shut-down to dye).
- Apply an ice bag to the puncture site to promote comfort.

Digital Subtraction Angiography

In evaluating the carotid arteries, invasive digital subtraction angiography (DSA) is a complementary procedure to the non-invasive carotid testing previously discussed. DSA is a computer-assisted radiographic procedure for visualization of the carotids and other cerebral vessels. The image produced is made more distinct by the elimination of surrounding and interfering anatomical structures. This is accomplished by recording images before and after injection of contrast medium and subtracting the first image from the second.

The purposes of DSA include assistance in the diagnosis of the following conditions:

- Atherosclerotic disease (stenosis, occlusions, ulcerations)
- Vascular lesions (arteriovenous malformations, aneurysms, carotid cavernous fistulas)
- Postoperative evaluation of endarterectomy, aneurysm clipping, arteriovenous malformation repair, and anastomosis

PROCEDURE

The antecubital area, usually of the right arm, is cleansed and lidocaine is injected locally so that the antecubital vein (usual approach) or the brachial artery can be incised. A catheter is advanced into the superior vena cava, and contrast medium is injected. Selected vessels are visualized with an image-intensifier video system that displays vessels on a monitor. Pictures are taken and stored on magnetic tape. The images, which are collected before contrast injection, are received by the computer and are then subtracted from those taken after injection so that the image of the desired area is enhanced. The remaining contrast-enhanced images can be manipulated by the computer to focus on specific problems that might otherwise not be visualized.

Upon completion of the procedure, which takes from 30 to 45 minutes, the catheter is removed. Pressure is applied to the puncture site for several minutes, and a sterile dressing is applied.

PATIENT MANAGEMENT

Preparation. The procedure should be explained to the patient. Oral intake is withheld for 2 hours before the procedure. During the procedure, patients are required to hold their breath on command, remain motionless, and lie in the supine position on the x-ray table. Prior to conducting the study, the patient should be questioned about any history of allergic reaction to iodine or contrast media.

Postprocedural Care. Vital signs should be checked and the patient observed for the unlikely occurrence of stroke, allergic reaction, or hemorrhage and hematoma at the injection site. Fluids should be forced, with up to 2,000 to 3,000 mL being given in the ensuing 24 hours to facilitate excretion of the contrast medium. Other possible rare complications are venous thrombosis and infection.

Temporal Artery Biopsy

For patients who experience facial pain and nonspecific neurological symptoms, a temporal artery biopsy may be considered. After administration of local anesthesia, a small incision is made over the superficial temporal artery. A small piece of temporal artery is then removed. The specimen is examined for evidence of temporal arteritis.

In preparing the patient, explain the procedure. A surgical permit may need to be signed depending on hospital policy. Medication for sedation may be ordered before the procedure. After the procedure, observe the dressing for bleeding. Vital signs and neurological signs should be monitored.

NERVOUS SYSTEM ELECTRICAL ACTIVITY AND CONDUCTION

Electroencephalography

An electroencephalogram (EEG) is a diagnostic procedure that measures the physiological activity of the brain (brain waves) using multiple scalp electrodes and records each tracing on graph paper for interpretation (Fig. 6-8). Neuronal electrical

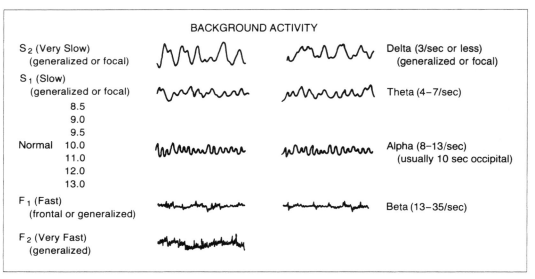

FIGURE 6-8
Electroencephalogram classifications.

signals from the cerebral cortex are about 1% as strong as those from the heart. Signals are picked up from surface cerebral cortex neurons and amplified one million times for an acceptable recording to be made. The EEG provides complementary data to anatomical imaging studies such as CT and MRI to document abnormal functions that are not associated with detectable anatomical alterations in cerebral tissue. The EEG is rarely specific to a cause because a variety of conditions can produce similar EEG changes. Although pattern changes are nonspecific, some changes are highly suggestive of specific conditions such as particular types of epilepsy, herpes simplex encephalitis, and dementia disorders. The EEG is useful in following patients with altered states of consciousness and is an important criterion in the determination of brain death.

PROCEDURE

Once a patient is oriented to the test environment, he or she is made comfortable in an easy chair or on a stretcher. Cooperation is very important to the quality of the test data. A series of small electrodes (16 to 21) are symmetrically affixed to the scalp in standard locations with a pastelike substance. The recording electrodes are interconnected in chains. Extra electrodes (*e.g.,* nasopharyngeal and sphenoidal) are available to record activity from the undersurface of the temporal lobes. Routinely, brain waves are recorded at rest, after hyperventilation, with photic stimulation, and during drowsiness or sleep. Hyperventilation and photic stimulation may precipitate abnormal focal or generalized diagnostic changes in brain waves which would otherwise not be detected. Wave types vary with activity and specific stimulation.

A baseline recording at rest is taken of spontaneous brain wave activity; this takes about 30 minutes. The patient is asked to hyperventilate for 2 to 3 minutes. The blowing off of CO_2 raises the serum pH to approximately 7.8 from the normal range of 7.35 to 7.45, at which time another recording is obtained. Nerve excitability is increased, and this may trigger seizure activity in a susceptible patient. The recording is continued to determine how long it takes to reestablish the baseline. Next, photic stimulation is applied by focusing a flickering light (strobe light) on the closed-eyed patient and a recording is taken. The last recording phase is that of drowsiness or sleep. An EEG takes 45 to 60 minutes and produces about 100 pages of recording paper.

A **sleep deprivation** technique is often used to demonstrate suspected abnormalities that are not evident on routine EEG. The patient is kept awake for most of the night before the EEG. Sleep deprivation stresses the brain and, therefore, may evoke abnormal waves not seen in the normal state. An all-night EEG is useful in studying sleep problems.

For patients who have intractable seizures that cannot be controlled well by drug therapy, continuous EEG monitoring and videotaping may be ordered. This provides continuous data about cerebral electrical activity and behavioral changes which can be correlated to determine the type and characteristics of the seizure activity. It often helps to identify epileptogenic areas in the brain. If this is unsuccessful, electrodes can be inserted surgically into the cerebral cortex. This approach allows for better localization of epileptogenic foci in the brain which may be excised surgically to provide better control of seizures.

PATIENT MANAGEMENT

Preparation. The nurse should explain what will be required of the patient during the EEG. Preparation is very important to ensure patient cooperation and also to allay anxiety. Anxiety can block alpha waves and produce head and neck muscle tension, resulting in recording artifacts. The procedure is painless, and there is no possibility of electrical shock.

Because anticonvulsants, stimulants, tranquilizers, and depressants can alter brain wave activity and mask or suppress abnormal brain waves, the physician may withhold selected medications for 24 to 48 hours prior to the EEG. Coffee, tea, colas, and chocolate are withheld from the regular diet to exclude dietary stimulants. To promote sleep during the EEG, the patient should go to sleep late and arise early. Napping prior to the test is discouraged. If a sleep deprivation study is required, the patient should be prevented from sleeping the night before the EEG. The patient's hair should be clean and no oils, sprays, or lotions should be used prior to the test.

Postprocedural Care. The hair is washed to remove the electrode-affixing paste. Any drugs that were withheld specifically for the EEG are resumed.

CLASSIFICATION OF BRAIN WAVES

Classification of brain waves is based on the number of cycles per second (cps), which are recorded in hertz (Hz) units. Four frequency bands are identified for EEG interpretation:

Alpha rhythms (8 to 12 Hz) are most prominent in the occipital leads. Alpha waves can be blocked by opening of the eyes, mental effort, anxiety, apprehension, and sudden noise or touch.

Beta rhythms (13 to 35 Hz) are most prominent in the frontal and central areas. Beta waves are triggered by opening of the eyes, mental activity, anxiety, or apprehension. They are especially prominent in patients receiving barbiturates and benzodiazepine drugs.

Theta rhythms (4 to 7 Hz) originate from the temporal lobes; there may be a very small amount of delta waves over the temporal regions in normal adults. Theta activity increases slightly in persons over the age of 60 years.

Delta rhythms (1 to 3 Hz) are not normally present in awake adults; normally seen in stages 3 and 4 of sleep (slow wave sleep).

NORMAL ELECTROENCEPHALOGRAPHIC ACTIVITIES

Different areas of the cerebral cortex generate relatively distinctive potential fluctuations, and different patterns also characterize waking and sleep states. In most *normal adults*, the waking pattern of EEG activity consists primarily of alpha waves (8 to 12 Hz) occurring mostly over the occipital area and beta waves (greater than 12 Hz) occurring over the frontal areas. Delta waves are not present in awake adults. Theta and delta waves are seen in sleep; their amount and amplitude correlate with the depth of sleep.[6]

Common Abnormal Electroencephalographic Abnormalities

An EEG is considered abnormal not when it lacks normal patterns but when it contains epileptiform activities, slowing of normal rhythms, abnormalities of amplitude, or variations from age-specific patterns.

Artifacts. Artifacts are abnormal pen deflections on the graphic recording that are not caused by cerebral activity but rather by other physiological activities, such as eye movement, muscle contraction, or heart action.

Epileptiform Activities. Epileptiform activities appear as single or repetitive focal spikes on the EEG that resemble epilepsy. These can be divided into focal, multifocal, and generalized events. For example, the patient with temporal lobe seizures will have characteristically abnormal electrical discharges over one anterior temporal lobe, whereas absence epilepsy is evidenced by widespread, bilateral, synchronous 3 Hz discharges. The normal EEG includes a range of variations which must be differentiated from a true form of epilepsy and abnormal activity related to cerebral lesions (Fig. 6-9).

Slow Wave Abnormalities. Slow wave (defined as 1 to 7 Hz) findings are classified as either focal or diffuse abnormalities.

1. **Focal slow waves** may be related to gray or white matter dysfunction in a localized area that is secondary to a tumor, hemorrhage, or other space-occupying lesion. Focal lesions directly involve either the cerebral cortex or the thalamocortical projection pathways. The finding of a fo-

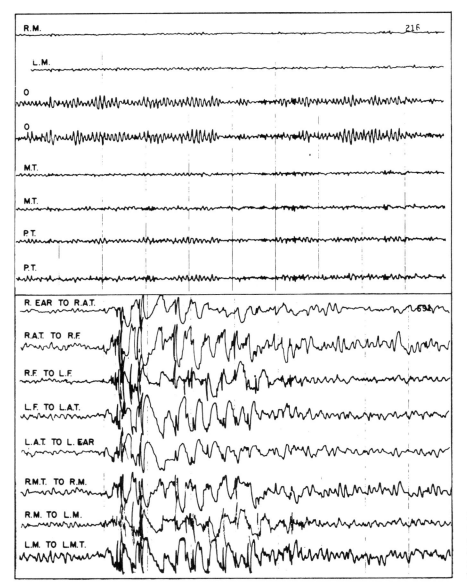

FIGURE 6-9
Comparison of a normal electroencephalogram (*top*) with that of an epileptic patient during a tonic–clonic seizure (*bottom*). Note the sharp, spiky waves recorded during the seizure.

cal abnormality indicates the need for further diagnostic testing, such as a CT scan or MRI. As the lesion increases in size and affects the diencephalon, the slow waves can become diffuse.

2. **Diffuse slow waves** are usually seen with toxic (drug), metabolic (*e.g.,* hepatic), degenerative (*e.g.,* Alzheimer's disease), infectious (*e.g.,* encephalitis), or postictal conditions. Generally, a pattern of diffuse slowing does not point to a specific diagnosis but only provides collaborative diagnostic information. A few forms of dementia, however, do have a characteristic wave pattern.

Flat EEG, or Electrocerebral Silence. The "flat" EEG indicates the absence of brain waves and is one finding seen in brain death (others include absence of brain stem function, loss of brain stem reflexes). Brain death is never declared on the basis of a flat EEG only.

Related Patterns Associated With Age. Age-related EEG characteristics are categorized as follows: children and teenagers (younger than 20 years of age); adults (20 to 60 years of age); and older adults (older than 60 years of age). In the older-than-60-years group, EEG results are similar to those in the 20- to 60-year group with a few exceptions: alpha waves are slower; beta waves are more prominent; there are more sporadic, generalized slow waves; and some intermittent temporal slow waves are evident. Thus, age-related data are considered in the interpretation of EEGs.

Electromyography (EMG) and Nerve Conduction Velocity Studies

Electromyography (EMG) and nerve conduction velocity (NCV) are electrophysiological studies usually ordered together to diagnose and differentiate between peripheral nerve and muscle disorders.

PROCEDURES

Electromyography. Recordings of muscle activity at rest, during voluntary movement, and with electrical stimulation are made by inserting small needle electrodes into the muscle. Patient cooperation is necessary; some discomfort is to be expected. An EMG may be ordered for patients who are thought to have myasthenia gravis, Eaton-Lambert syndrome, or peripheral nerve injury or disease (lower motor neuron disease) or when it is unclear whether the primary problem is muscle or nerve. It can also differentiate among lesions of the anterior horn cell, root, plexus, and specific nerves and muscles.

Nerve Conduction Velocity Studies. NCV studies measure the conduction time and amplitude of electrical stimulation along two or more points of a peripheral nerve using a cathode (negative electrode) and an anode (positive electrode). The recorded response has a simple, biphasic waveform with initial negativity and maximal amplitude. The routine measurements recorded include

- Amplitude from baseline to the negative peak or between negative and positive peaks

- Duration from onset to the negative or positive peak or to the final return to baseline
- Latency from stimuli artifact to onset of negative response

The results are then compared to standardized norms. For example, normal motor conduction speeds are 50 to 60 m/sec for the ulnar and median nerves and 45 to 55 m/sec for the lateral popliteal nerve. Values below these ranges suggest neuropathy. NCV studies are conducted when nerve damage is suspected because of clinical symptoms of motor weakness or atrophy. They are helpful in the diagnosis of neuropathies (*e.g.,* those induced by diabetes, alcoholism, or nutritional deficiencies and compression of or trauma to the peripheral nerves).

PATIENT MANAGEMENT

Preparation. Explain the procedure to the patient, emphasizing the importance of cooperation. The patient should be informed of the discomfort accompanying the procedure.

Postprocedural Care. There is no aftercare required except to wash any gel out of the hair.

Evoked Potentials

Evoked potentials (EPs) are a noninvasive means of applying a specific sensory stimuli and recording the minute electrical potentials that are subsequently created. Using a computerized averaging program, the stimulus is repeated several times, allowing a return to the resting state between stimuli. Each evoked response is measured and the data are stored in the computer. After a number of potentials have been stored (100 to 200), the computer then calculates the average curve.

EPs are used as a complementary procedure in the battery of testing conducted for problems that are not well demonstrated clinically or easily diagnosed. EPs are classified into three categories based on the type of stimulus provided and the sensory system stimulated. Each system stimulated produces a characteristic wave formation. The three sensory systems used in EPs are the visual, auditory, and somatosensory pathways.

VISUAL EVOKED POTENTIALS

In visual evoked potentials (VEPs), the stimuli provided are patterned, most often by reversing checkerboard patterns and flashing lights. The retina is stimulated, allowing the pathways to the occipital cortex to be evaluated. Each eye is tested separately. The response is recorded with electrodes over the occipital region. If the patient wears eyeglasses, they should be worn during the procedure. The cooperation of the patient is necessary during testing. VEPs are used in the diagnosis of optic neuropathies (*e.g.,* optic neuritis) and optic nerve lesions (*e.g.,* tumors). Optic neuritis is usually related to multiple sclerosis.

BRAIN STEM AUDITORY EVOKED RESPONSES

Brain stem auditory evoked responses (BAERs) are primarily used to evaluate brain stem function. The stimuli for measuring BAERs are provided, via headphones, as a series of clicks that vary in rate, intensity, and duration. Five wave formations, based on the site of origin, are recorded: wave I from the acoustic nerve, wave II from the cochlear nucleus, wave III from the superior olivary complex, wave IV from the lateral lemniscus, and wave V from the inferior colliculus.

BAER testing can be conducted on alert or comatose patients. It is helpful in diagnosing brain stem lesions in multiple sclerosis, acoustic neuroma, brain stem lesions related to coma, and hearing loss (especially in infants). BAERs are also used intraoperatively to monitor the eighth cranial nerve for surgical injury.

SOMATOSENSORY EVOKED RESPONSES

Somatosensory evoked responses (SSERs) can measure peripheral nerve responses in the upper (median nerve) or lower (posterior tibial nerve) extremities. SSERs are helpful in evaluating spinal cord function, sensory dysfunction associated with multiple sclerosis, and nerve root compression.

TESTING OF THE SPECIAL SENSES

Electronystagmography

Electronystagmography (ENG) measures and graphically records the electrical potentials emitted by eye movements precipitated by spontaneous, positional, or calorically evoked nystagmus. Interpretation of these data can provide information on the frequency, intensity, and maximum speed of the slow and fast components of the nystagmus. The purpose of ENG is to diagnose the underlying etiology of nystagmus or vertigo related to dysfunction of the vestibular branch of the eighth cranial nerve.

PROCEDURE

Electrodes are placed on either side of the eye in the direction of the plane to be recorded. The basic principle underlying ENG is the difference in voltage between two dipole structures, the cornea (+) and retina (−). At least a 1-mV difference normally exists between the two poles. Any changes in potential caused by eye movement are collected, amplified, and recorded. Data are collected during tracking, fixation on points in either plane, and caloric stimulation. The patient is positioned at various angles for data collection. One advantage of ENG is that it enables nystagmus to be recorded behind closed eyelids and in the dark. ENG is contraindicated in patients with a pacemaker in place.

PATIENT MANAGEMENT

Preparation. The procedure is explained to the patient, noting that some vertigo may be experienced. Usually, the patient receives nothing by mouth for at least 8 hours before the test. Antivertigo drugs, tranquilizers, depressant drugs, alcohol, and stimulant drugs and foods (*e.g.*, cola, coffee, tea) are usually withheld for 24 to 48 hours before testing. The physician should be consulted about withholding any medication.

Postprocedural Care. The patient should lie down until any vertigo, dizziness, nausea, or vomiting has subsided. An antiemetic will probably be ordered by the physician. A normal diet is resumed when the patient is able to tolerate it.

Audiometric Studies

Audiometric testing assesses the auditory branch of the eighth cranial nerve for type and cause of hearing loss. Testing is divided into pure-tone audiometry and speech audiometry. The basis for *pure-tone audiometry* is that the louder the sound stimulus (pure or musical tone) necessary before the patient perceives it, the greater the hearing loss. The decibel (dB) is the unit of measure of loudness. *Speech audiometry* is based on the ability of the patient to understand and discriminate between sounds of the spoken word. In testing, a soundproof room and earphones are used to screen out ambient noise. A graphic representation of testing results is interpreted to differentiate between conduction and sensorineural hearing loss. **Conduction loss** results from outer ear or middle ear dysfunction or impairment to both structures. The inner ear is not involved. In such cases, a hearing aid is helpful. **Sensorineural loss** occurs in diseases of the inner ear or nerve pathways. This type of hearing loss is characterized by loss of sensitivity to and discrimination of sounds. Hearing aids are not very effective with this form of hearing loss.

Hearing loss in the neuroscience patient is usually related to head injury, meningitis, acoustic neuroma, or drug toxicity.

Caloric Testing

Caloric testing is a diagnostic procedure designed to evaluate the vestibular portion of the eighth cranial nerve and the presence or absence of the oculovestibular reflex. The underlying principle of the procedure is that thermal stimulation of the vestibular apparatus (the balance-sensing mechanism in the inner ear) with cold water will elicit the oculovestibular reflex. The test is contraindicated in patients with a ruptured tympanic membrane or cervical injury.

PROCEDURE

Once the physician has confirmed that the tympanic membrane is intact and the cervical neck is stable, the patient's head is tilted backward at a 60-degree angle from the horizontal plane to allow maximal stimulation of the lateral semicircular canal, the canal which is most responsible for reflex lateral movement. The external auditory canal is slowly irrigated with 10 cc of ice-cold water. The cold irrigation causes convection currents in the endolymph of the labyrinths, resulting in a change in the baseline firing of the vestibular nerve and slow conjugate deviation of the eyes toward the stimulated ear (Fig. 6-10).

In the normal waking state with an intact oculovestibular reflex, there is an initial conjugate eye movement (lasting 30 to 60 sec) toward the side being irrigated with the cold water (slow phase). This is controlled by the brain stem. The eye deviation is corrected shortly by a rapid component of nystagmus (occurring within 20 to 30 sec), which pulls the eyes toward the opposite side, back to the midline (fast phase). The rapid component is controlled by the cerebral cortex.

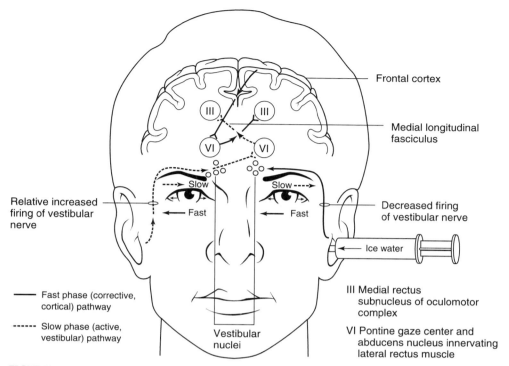

FIGURE 6-10
Physiology of the oculovestibular reflex (vestibulo-oculare reflex, cold calorics). Infusion of ice water into the ear of a comatose patient will elicit the oculovestibular reflex if both the cerebral hemisphere and brain stem are intact. With an intact brain stem, a signal passes through pathways from the medulla to the midbrain, generating a slow movement of the eyes to the side of the ice water infusion. This is followed by a rapid corrective movement of the eyes, generated by an intact ipsilateral side of the cerbral hemisphere. The ice water infusion test can be repeated in the other ear of the comatose patient to test the integrity of the other side of the brain stem.

As a patient becomes lethargic, the fast component becomes less pronounced. Deterioration into obtundation and semicoma results in loss of the fast component because the cerebral cortex is depressed. If the patient slips into a deep coma, the tonic deviation toward the side of irrigation (slow component) may be lost. This indicates that the oculovestibular reflex, a reflex controlled by the brain stem, is absent. Absence of brain stem function is a poor prognostic indicator.

Warm water irrigation produces reversal of endolymphic flow. This results in conjugate eye deviation with the slow phase away from the stimulated ear and normal correction phase toward the irrigated ear. The type of nystagmus is named by the direction of the fast phase. The mnemonic **COWS** (Cold Opposite, Warm Same) refers to the **fast phase** of nystagmus. It is also possible to irrigate both ear canals simultaneously with cold water, which results in slow downward deviation; simultaneous warm water irrigation results in slow upward deviation.

RESPONSES TO CALORIC TESTING

Nausea, vomiting, or dizziness can be precipitated by caloric testing in normal patients. Patients with diseases involving the vestibular branch of the eighth cranial nerve, such as an acoustic neuroma or Meniere's disease, will not have the eye move-

ments normally associated with caloric testing; instead, these movements will be diminished or absent.

PATIENT MANAGEMENT

Preparation. In conscious patients, an order for nothing by mouth should be maintained for at least 8 hours before the procedure. In the unconscious patient this is not a problem.

Postprocedural Care. Bedrest should be maintained until nausea, vomiting, vertigo, or dizziness have subsided. A normal diet can be resumed when the patient feels ready.

CALORIC TESTING IN THE EMERGENCY DEPARTMENT

In some instances, such as when a comatose patient has just been admitted to the emergency department, assessment of the patient may be facilitated by establishing whether brain function is intact. After inspecting the tympanic membrane to ensure that it is intact, cold water irrigation may be initiated. If there is tonic deviation of the eyes toward the side being irrigated, brain stem function is intact. This is considered a positive prognostic sign. With a brain stem lesion, the caloric reflex will be absent or the ocular movement will be dysconjugate. Absence of the reflex is associated with a poor prognosis.

NEUROPSYCHOLOGICAL EXAMINATION

A neuropsychological examination is a comprehensive assessment of the brain achieved by studying its behavioral products. A licensed neuropsychologist conducts the examination. The purposes of a neuropsychological examination include the following:

- To assist in diagnosis by determining the presence or absence of cognitive deficits
- To determine whether brain dysfunction is localized (focal) or diffuse
- To plan, manage, and evaluate an individualized rehabilitation program
- To determine competency for self-care and decision making
- To document disability for insurance purposes
- To provide information about competency for legal matters such as the need for a guardian
- To conduct research

Lezak conceptualizes behavior as three functional and integrated systems: *cognition*, the information aspect of behavior; *emotionality*, the feelings and motivation of behavior; and *executive functions*, how behavior is expressed.[7] Performance skills are examined in great depth and detail to determine cerebral function. A major benefit of this extensive testing is that subtle changes may be discovered that would not be detected with less refined testing methods or anatomical imaging studies. The extent of the examination is reflected in the time required for testing, which is approximately 6 to 10 hours.

Components of a Neuropsychological Evaluation

The examination is tailored to the patient's needs, abilities, and limitations. The specific tests included in a neuropsychological evaluation will vary depending on the age of the patient, the nature of the problem, the deficits present, the specific questions asked by the physician in the referral note, and the ability of the person conducting the testing. Information about the type of neurological insult, premorbid function and personality, personal and family history, and data from other diagnostic tests are correlated with data from the neuropsychological examination.

Components of the examination will evaluate the following cognitive functions:

Attention: vigilance (the ability to sustain attention over a period of time, concentration), self-regulation, and screening out of distracting environmental stimuli

Visual perception and visual reasoning: picture completion, picture arrangement, judgment of line orientation, visual search

Memory and learning: short term, immediate, long term; new learning such as remembering word lists; verbal and nonverbal memory. Testing includes sentence repetition, serial digit learning, auditory–verbal learning tests.

Language: understanding of single words and sentences; reading; speaking; and auditory discrimination

General intelligence: verbal and nonverbal; includes information, comprehension, and similarities; naming objects; arithmetic calculations

Constructional ability: drawing to command; drawing to copy; block designs; visual organization of a picture and its parts; right–left orientation; clock setting

Map orientation: being able to read a map

Conceptualization: metaphors and proverbs

Abstraction: verbal and nonverbal abstract reasoning

Perceptual motor speed: ability to plan ahead and shift from one concept to the other

Emotional status: assess for depression, suicidal ideation, anxiety, paranoia, and other abnormal responses

A depression inventory or other inventories of emotional status may be administered in some situations.

Common Deficits Associated With Organic Brain Disease

Many patients with organic brain dysfunction develop cognitive and behavioral deficits as a result of head trauma, stroke, CNS degenerative disorders (*e.g.*, Alzheimer's disease), and CNS infections (*e.g.*, encephalitis, meningitis). Common deficits include a decreased ability to concentrate, increased irritability, emotional lability, decreased ability to screen out irrelevant information, decreased ability to solve problems, inability to sequence complex actions correctly, inability to learn new tasks, deficits in memory, deficits in logical reasoning, perceptual deficits, and general slowing of all cognitive functions.

These cognitive and behavioral deficits cause serious difficulty in the social and vocational readjustment of the patient into the family, community, and work setting. Diagnosing the specific deficits and developing a plan for rehabilitation are necessary to help the patient achieve the highest possible level of function and independence.

Because of the focus and time required for neuropsychological evaluation, patient selection is important. The patient must be alert, be able to actively participate, and have the physical endurance and stamina to complete the examination. The physician should be specific in explaining why neuropsychological evaluation is desired.

There is some natural recovery that occurs over time after cerebral insult. Seeking neuropsychological evaluation too soon after the insult does not allow sufficient time for spontaneous improvement to occur. In addition, natural recovery can be so rapid that findings on the examination from one day may be negated with spontaneous improvement evident on the next day. Many physicians postpone evaluation for approximately 3 to 6 months after insult to allow for natural recovery. In some instances, a modified version of the evaluation may be requested.

SUMMARY

The major diagnostic procedures commonly used with a neurological patient population have been discussed. Some laboratory studies specific to a condition will be included in the related chapter. In caring for patients, the nurse must view the patient holistically and recognize that stabilization and recovery require close monitoring of a number of laboratory data such as electrolytes, glucose, blood urea nitrogen, creatinine, complete blood count and differential, coagulation panel, arterial blood gases, creatinine phosphokinase, liver function studies, thyroid function studies, plasma cortisol levels, serum osmolality, and drug and toxicology screening. Other tests specific for a particular neurological problem will be discussed in the respective chapters.

References

1. Souder, E., & Alavi, A. (1995). A comparison of neuroimaging modalities for diagnosing dementia. *Nurse Practitioner, 20*(1), 66–67.
2. Bradley, W. G., Daroff, R. B., Fenichel, G. M., & Marsden, C. D. (Eds.). (1991). *Neurology in clinical practice: Principles of diagnosis and management*, vol 1. Boston: Butterworth-Heinemann.
3. Ibid., p. 500.
4. Ibid., p. 501.
5. Young, W. L., & Ornstein, E. (1994). Cerebral and spinal cord blood flow. In J. E. Cottrell & D. S. Smith (Eds.), *Anesthesia and neurosurgery* (3rd ed.) (pp. 33–36). St. Louis: Mosby-Year Book.
6. Bradley et al., op. cit., p. 430.
7. Lezak, M. D. (1995). *Neuropsychological assessment* (3rd ed.). New York: Oxford University Press.

Bibliography

Adelstein, W. (1994). Confirmation of brain death using 99m Tc HM-PAO. *Journal of Neuroscience Nursing, 26*(2), 118–120.

Bell, T. E., LaGrange, K. M., Maier, C. M., & Steinberg, G. K. (1992). Transcranial Doppler: Correlation of blood velocity measurement with clinical status in subarachnoid hemorrhage. *Journal of Neuroscience Nursing, 24*(4), 216–219.

Fearson, M., & Rusy, K. L. (1996). Transcranial Doppler: Advanced technology for assessing cerebral hemodynamics. *Dimensions of Critical Care Nursing, 13*(5), 241–248.

Herzag, R. J. (1991). Selection and utilization of imaging studies for disorders of the lumbar spine. *Physical Medicine and Rehabilitation Clinics of North America, 2*(1), 7–59.

Mason, P. J. B. (1992). Neurodiagnostics testing in critically injured adults. *Critical Care Nurse, 12*(6), 64–73, 75.

Stubris, R. S. (1993). Nuclear medicine cerebral perfusion imaging. *Applied Radiology, 22*(6), 33.

Wilson, J., & Wyper, D. (1992). Neuroimaging and neuropsychological functioning following closed head injury: CT, MRI, and SPECT. *Journal of Head Trauma Rehabilitation, 7*(2), 29–33.

CHAPTER 7

The Neurological Physical Examination

Joanne V. Hickey

The neurological physical examination is conducted to determine whether nervous system dysfunction is present, to diagnose disease of the nervous system, and to localize disease within the nervous system. Although diagnosis of disease is usually the responsibility of the physician, advanced practice nurses and other health professionals also may conduct the neurological examination. Therefore, the neurological physical examination is included in this text for several reasons. First, the neurological physical examination provides a comprehensive database of critical information about the patient's neurological function. As part of the patient's record, it is available for the nurse and other health professionals to review. Second, a review of these data by the nurse may be helpful in identifying areas of special consideration in neurological assessment, as well as special observations to be made and documented. These should be noted in the patient's individualized care plan. Third, potential nursing diagnoses may be suggested by the dysfunction identified. For example, a patient with ataxia, a symptom of cerebellar dysfunction, also will have problems with balance and coordination and should be supervised when ambulating. The potential for falls and injury should be considered by the nurse and noted on the care plan. Finally, although the nurse establishes a database of information about the patient's neurological function independently, a collaborative relationship suggests a sharing of information so that each participant understands the basis upon which other participants are operating.

Nurses involved in advanced practice may conduct a complete neurological physical examination. The nursing purposes of this examination are to determine whether nervous system dysfunction is present and to determine the human responses to actual or potential health problems precipitated by the dysfunction. It is the purpose of the data collection that differentiates medical practice from nursing practice. Nurse practitioners may overlap with physicians in the purpose of the examination. More information about specific findings in

the neurological examination is included in the nursing neurological assessment in Chapter 8.

THE NEUROLOGICAL EXAMINATION

Purpose

Physical examinations are often classified as screening and extended examinations. A **screening examination** refers to a complete medical history and physical examination for persons who come for a general assessment and may or may not have complaints. An **extended examination** is an extension of the screening examination whereby the examiner follows leads from specific symptoms or abnormal findings. A **problem-focused examination** is a subset of an extended examination because it confines itself to a specific system or region that has specific complaints or signs and symptoms.

This chapter focuses on an extended examination of the neurological system. It also further explores specific areas of the nervous system that require more refined techniques to determine dysfunction. This chapter also includes the elements of a neurological screening examination of the nervous system that all practitioners will include in any comprehensive examination of any patient.

The medical purpose for conducting a neurological examination is to determine the presence of nervous system dysfunction. A skilled examiner knows the appropriate technique for testing function and is familiar with the expected normal responses to such testing. Deviation from these norms indicates dysfunction which may or may not be a part of a disease process. Diagnosis of disease is based on identification of a constellation of signs and symptoms constituting critical elements of a disease. Based on the findings of the neurological examination, other diagnostic procedures may be indicated. However, the goal of the diagnostic phase is to establish a working diagnosis so that treatment can be prescribed. Finally, because the nervous system is composed of highly specialized cells with unique functions, it may be possible to localize and pinpoint the site of dysfunction and disease within the nervous system.

Role of the Nurse During the Examination

The nurse may be present during the neurological examination. The role of the nurse is to be supportive of the patient by providing brief explanations, emotional support, and physical support and assistance as needed.

Sometimes, the examiner may prefer to examine the patient alone, particularly if the patient is easily distracted by the presence of another person in the room. Also, some patients tend to reveal more information to the examiner when the exchange is one-to-one.

Equipment

The usual equipment necessary to conduct a neurological physical examination includes the following:

- Ophthalmoscope
- Pointed instrument: pin or broken wooden applicator, key
- Stethoscope
- Reflex hammer
- Tongue blade
- Wisp of cotton or fluffed cotton swab
- Tuning fork
- Flashlight
- Tape measure
- Snellen or Rosenbaum eye chart

Approach

The neurological examination is preceded by a complete history and general physical examination. The neurological examination is conducted in a systematic, hierarchical, stepwise approach that proceeds from the highest level of function (cerebral cortex) to the lowest (reflexes) and from the general integrated functions to areas of specific functions. The examination encompasses a review of mental state; the cranial nerve, motor system, sensory system, and cerebellar system; and reflexes. By approaching the patient with a mental framework for the examination, no parts of the examination will be forgotten. The examiner may decide to defer certain parts of the examination. What parts can be deferred is difficult to say. It is the judgment and experience of the examiner that will guide these decisions.

Circumstances of the Neurological Examination

The circumstances surrounding the neurological examination of a patient can vary greatly. Patients may be seen in the physician's office, in an ambulatory care center, or in a hospital emergency room. At the time of the examination, patients may be alert, oriented, and conversant, or they may have an altered

level of consciousness with significant neurological deficits. After reviewing the patient's medical record, a history of the neurological problem is obtained before the neurological examination is begun. It is advisable to start from scratch in collecting the complete medical history even though this has already been documented by another practitioner. An explanation to the patient will help in gaining cooperation. For example, one can say, "I know that you have answered some of these questions before. However, I like to start from scratch and collect this information without being influenced by what is in your chart so I can make an unbiased assessment of you." Often an experienced examiner with a neurological focus will delve into areas that were not considered in a general screening examination. This information may be critical in making a diagnosis.

The patient's condition and ability to cooperate will influence the physician's ability to collect a complete database. The examiner may need to elicit some information from a reliable family member or significant other, whereas other areas of inquiry may not be pursued until the patient's condition improves.

MENTAL STATUS EXAMINATION

Many parts of the **mental status examination** are integrated into the history-taking portion of the interview. This context provides a natural way of collecting information without creating an artificial test setting that could make the patient uncomfortable or anxious. There may be some slight differences in allocation of areas of testing between the screening and extended examination. This chapter follows the Bates (1995)[1] model in organizing this content.

The following areas should be evaluated in a **screening examination**: orientation; appearance and behavior; mood; speech pattern; and thought and perceptions. An **extended examination** is warranted if abnormalities are found on the screening portion. Additional examination components are added.

ORIENTATION AND LEVEL OF CONSCIOUSNESS

In order to conduct a mental status examination, the patient must be awake, alert, able to understand questions, and able to respond. If the patient does not respond to simple questions, try to establish eye contact and speak louder. If this is not effective, you may need to touch the patient on the shoulder or arm or even gently shake him or her. If the patient does not respond to these stimuli, then you cannot proceed with this portion of the examination. Proceed to examination of the patient with an altered level of consciousness.

APPEARANCE AND BEHAVIOR

Attire, grooming, and personal appearance should be appropriate for the setting and the patient's age. A neat and clean appearance reflects good grooming and good personal hygiene habits. An unkempt appearance, on the other hand, might suggest depression or chronic organic brain disease. **Posture and motor conduct** contribute to the examiner's general impression about the patient. A slumped posture coupled with slow movements suggests depression, whereas pacing suggests anxiety. **Facial expression** should be assessed for appropriateness and variations in expression depending on topics under discussion. Finally, **affect and manner** provide a composite of the openness, approachability, and response to the environment and other people.

MOOD

Ask about the patient's perception of his or her mood. Questions that are helpful include "How are your spirits?" "What makes you angry?" and "What makes you sad?" Reactions to the topic being discussed and to the people around should also be noted. Abnormal responses might include hostility, evasiveness, anger, tearfulness, or depression. If depression is suspected, a depression scale can be administered to further evaluate the patient. Of special concern is any suggestion related to thoughts about suicide. Any hint about contemplating suicide should be taken seriously. A direct inquiry can be made. One can ask "Have you ever thought of killing yourself?" or "Do you ever feel that life is not worth living?" Special observation, supervision, and further evaluation are warranted if suicidal tendencies are suspected. The reports of family or friends can be very helpful in evaluating changes in mood.

SPEECH PATTERN

Although the substance of a verbal response and fluency (use of language) are important, the examiner should also listen to the sound and flow of the words. Quality, quantity, pace, tone, and spontaneity should be noted.

THOUGHT AND PERCEPTION

Thought processes, thought content, perception, insight, and judgment are evaluated throughout the interview for deviations from normal. **Thought processes** refer to the subjective responses to life experiences and how they are verbally expressed. Indicators of thought processes are coherence, relevance, logic, and organization of the patient's thoughts. Be alert for flight of ideas, incoherence, confabulation, perseveration, echolalia, and other disorders in thought processes.

Thought content refers to abnormal themes in content. By active listening, reflecting, and exploring the answers offered, the examiner can evaluate the presence of any of the following themes or flaws in thought content: compulsive behaviors (obsessions, phobias, or repetitive thinking about issues); indecision; feelings of unreality, depersonalization, persecution, or control by others; delusions or illusions; or hallucinations.

Perception is a person's subjective interpretation of real or perceived stimuli. Does the patient hear voices? Is there any evidence of illusions or hallucinations? Explore any suggestions of these disorders to determine specifics of the experience.

Insight is the act of seeing the inner nature of things or of seeing intuitively. "What seems to be the problem?" and "Why are you here today?" are good questions that uncover insight into a situation. A person might say that he or she is here because of certain signs and symptoms that are appropriate for the problem at hand. Or a symptomatic patient might say that there is nothing wrong, but the patient's spouse insisted on the visit. The later suggests a lack of insight due to denial or being unaware of the relationship of symptoms to illness.

Judgment is the process of forming an opinion or evaluation about something. The examiner can evaluate a patient's judgment by asking questions such as "How are you going to manage at home after hospitalization?" or "What activity limitations do you need to follow?" The examiner can determine how accurate and reasonable judgments are based on the patient's age and condition.

The presence of abnormal findings in the screening examination may indicate depression, mental illness, or organic disease which needs further evaluation and an extended examination.

Cognitive Functions

For an **extended examination**, cognitive functions, sometimes called higher-level functions, should be evaluated. Cognitive functions include several areas of higher-level intellectual ability. In the examination, the examiner proceeds from general cognitive functions to special cognitive functions. The following areas are included:

General Cognitive Functions

- Orientation to time, place, and person
- Attention and concentration
- Memory (new learning, recent, remote)
- Calculations
- General fund of information
- Abstract thinking

Special Cognitive Functions

- Naming objects
- Three-step command
- Construction ability
- Language

ORIENTATION

The three areas to be tested are **time, place,** and **person**.

Time: the time of day, day of the week, month, season, date, and year, as well as any possible upcoming holiday or one in the immediate past
Place: present location, home address, city, state
Person: ability of the patient to give his or her own name

Carefully phrased questions, when asked in the context of the interview, can help when evaluating orientation. For example, asking a patient his or her name and address, the names of family members, and specific dates of significant life events will provide insight into awareness of time, place, and person. For some patients, however, a more direct approach, using specific questions (*e.g.*, "What day is it today?") is indicated.

ATTENTION AND CONCENTRATION

Attention and concentration can be tested by reading a series of digits to the patient and then asking him or her to repeat the numbers in turn.

Number Series. The series should start with a short list, with each digit being enunciated clearly and paced at 1-second intervals. Number series can begin with two digits then progress to a maximum of six digits (*e.g.*, 7, 2; 9, 5, 2). Avoid consecutive numbers or digits that form easily recognizable combinations, such as the date 1776. If the patient makes an error in repeating the digits, the patient should be given a second chance with another series of digits of similar length. Stop after two consecutive failures in a series of any length. In the second part of this test (beginning with the shortest list of digits), the patient is asked to repeat a series in reverse order. Normally, a person should be able to repeat correctly at least five digits forward and four in reverse order.

Serial 7s. Another common exercise is to ask the patient to count backward from 100 in decrements of 7. Normally, patients should be able to complete this exercise with few errors in 90 seconds. In practice, if a patient can accurately complete five subtractions, this is usually sufficient. Patients unable to do serial 7s should be instructed to complete serial 3s in a similar manner.

Spelling Backwards. Say a five-letter word and ask the patient to spell it backwards. The word commonly used is W-O-R-L-D.

MEMORY

Memory can be subdivided into remote (long-term) memory and recent (short-term) memory. New learning evaluates retention and immediate recall.

Remote Memory. Ask about birthdays, anniversaries, or previous residences.

Recent Memory. Ask about the weather or how the patient came to the clinic or hospital. In both remote and recent memory, be sure that you can validate the information supplied by the patient.

New Learning. Give the patient three unrelated words to remember (*e.g.*, lilies, courage, and screwdriver). Ask the patient to repeat each word after you. Then ask the patient to tell you those three words. Instruct the patient to remember those three words because you will be coming back to them in a few minutes. Go on with the examination. In 3 to 5 minutes, ask the patient to tell you what those three words are. Normally, the patient should be able to remember the three words.

CALCULATIONS

Serial 7s give some indication of subtraction ability. In addition, simple calculation problems should be asked, such as

- How much is a quarter, a dime, and a nickel?
- How much is 3×9?
- How much is $11 + 7$?

GENERAL FUND OF INFORMATION

To evaluate the patient's general knowledge, consider the patient's educational level. Ask about current events or general information that you would expect an average adult to know who lives in the area. Examples of questions are

- Who is the president of the United States?
- Name the last five presidents from the current president back.
- What is the capital of England?

ABSTRACT THINKING

The ability to think abstractly can be evaluated through the use of proverbs and similarities. Ask the patient what is meant by the following **proverbs**:

- All that glitters is not gold.
- People who live in glass houses should not throw stones.
- Rolling stones gather no moss.

A literal, concrete interpretation may indicate organic brain disease, mental illness, mental retardation, or simply limited education.

In evaluating ability to recognize **similarities**, ask the patient to explain how two given objects are alike, such as the following:

- A rose and a carnation
- A piano and a violin
- Silk and linen

Cortical Integrative Functions

There are three high-level cognitive skills that require cortical integration of a few areas of the brain. They are recognition of objects through the senses, skilled motor acts, and communications skills.

NAMING OBJECTS

One of the special cognitive abilities is to recognize objects through the senses (vision, hearing, and touch). Most often, the patient is evaluated for identification of objects by sight. The ability to name objects by sight can be easily evaluated by pointing to common objects and asking the patient to identify those objects. Examples of common objects in the environment include

- Ring
- Pen

- Stethoscope
- Watch
- Stem on a watch
- Lapels on lab coat
- Tie
- Desk
- Mirror

A deficit in identifying common objects by sight is called **visual agnosia**.

If the examiner wishes to test for ability to identify common sounds, the patient can be asked to identify the sound of a ringing telephone or the honking of an auto horn. A deficit in identifying common sounds is called **auditory agnosia**. A lesion in a portion of the temporal lobe is usually the cause of this form of auditory agnosia.

To evaluate the ability to identify common objects by touch, ask the patient to close his or her eyes and place a common object in the patient's hand for identification. A key, closed safety pin, or coin can be used. A deficit in identifying common objects by touch is called **tactile agnosia**. A parietal lobe lesion is the usual cause of tactile agnosia.

There are also some special forms of agnosia. **Autotopagnosia** is the inability to identify body parts or understand the relationships of body parts. This condition results from a lesion in the posteroinferior region of the parietal lobe. **Anosognosia** is defined as a lack of awareness of or a denial of a deficit in physical function. It is seen most often in patients with left hemispheric lesions. In this case, the patient is unaware of the right side of his or her body.

THREE-STEP COMMAND

A skilled motor act is a complex act requiring cortical integration. To evaluate this ability, ask the patient to perform a three-step command such as "When I snap my fingers, touch your right ear with your left hand." Including "left" and "right" in the command also evaluates left–right discrimination. Inability to perform a skilled act in the absence of motor deficits is called **apraxia**.

To perform a skilled motor act, a person must understand what the act entails, remember the steps long enough to complete the act, and possess normal motor strength. For example, if handed a comb and told to comb his hair, a patient must pick up the comb, lift his arm to his head, and pass the comb through the hair from top to bottom. If he cannot carry out such a skilled act in the absence of paralysis, the term **apraxia** is applied.

Performing a skilled act on demand requires an integrated function of several areas of the cerebral cortex. Three steps are necessary to execute a purposeful, skilled act successfully, as detailed in Table 7-1. Certain forms of apraxia are caused by lesions in the parietal lobe of the nondominant hemisphere, producing a group of one-sided neglect syndromes. For instance, **dressing apraxia** is characterized by neglect of one side of the body in the process of dressing and grooming. For example, the patient may wash only one side of his or her face.

CONSTRUCTION ABILITY

The ability to **reproduce figures** or draw a figure on command can be assessed easily if the patient has motor function in his or her writing hand. To evaluate copying skill, draw two five-sided figures that overlap to form a four-sided figure. This is the figure that is included for copying in the Mini Mental Status Examination, a commonly used instrument to assess mental status function.

The second method to assess construction ability is to ask the patient to **draw on command** a clock with all the numbers and to set the clock at a given time. (A variation for the clock is drawing a daisy.) Patients with a neglect syndrome would not draw one side of the clock or flower. **Constructional apraxia** is the inability to reproduce geometric figures. It is characterized by an inability to copy a complex figure, draw a clock with the numbers on it, or draw a daisy. In the case of the clock or daisy, only one side of the figure will be drawn.

LANGUAGE ABILITY

The ability to communicate is a complex process. Normally, a person can understand the spoken and written word and also express thoughts verbally and in writing. The following outlines how language skills can be tested.

- **Understanding the spoken word**: Ask the patient to follow commands such as "close your eyes" or "show me your thumb."

TABLE 7-1
Purposeful Motor Acts and Apraxia

STEPS	ACTIVITY	DEFICITS	APRAXIA TYPE
1	Comprehend concept or idea Remember long enough to accomplish the act	General suppression of cerebral function, rather than a lesion in one specific area	Ideational apraxia
2	Formulate an organized plan to accomplish the task Create a mental image of the action	Lesion at the junction of the frontal, temporal, parietal, and occipital lobes	Ideokinetic or ideomotor apraxia
3	Actually execute the detailed plan	Lesion involving premotor frontal cortex The disability is usually limited to one extremity without weakness or loss of movement	Kinetic apraxia

- **Understanding the written word**: Tell the patient that you are going to write some instructions on a piece of paper that you want him or her to follow. Write a simple command such as "point to the door"; observe for accuracy in execution.
- **Expressing thoughts verbally**: The examiner may become aware of difficulty in expressing ideas in the course of the interview. The examiner can ask the patient to describe the kind of work he or she does. Do not ask questions that can be answered by a "yes" or "no" response. A more formal way of assessing the patient is to give him or her a card with a picture and ask him or her to describe what is happening in the picture. Observe for difficulty with word finding, hesitation, and flow of words and ideas.
- **Expressing thoughts in writing**: Provide paper and pencil; ask the patient to write a sentence describing the weather or something else that can be validated by the examiner.

A language disorder is called **aphasia**. Aphasia can be subdivided into **nonfluent aphasia** and **fluent aphasia**. Specific types of aphasia are listed in Table 7-2, along with their respective areas of involvement.

Most patients with neurological deficits have some communication function left intact even though certain functions have been greatly diminished because of a disease process. Carefully evaluating the complex communication system can aid in localizing the lesion.

CRANIAL NERVE EXAMINATION

The next part of the neurological examination focuses on the cranial nerves. There are twelve pairs of cranial nerves. Each cranial nerve has a left and a right nerve; each side must be evaluated separately. There may be dysfunction on one side or both sides. Findings from each side are compared for symmetry. This chapter is organized to include details of testing, discussion of findings, and abnormal findings. See Chapter 5 for a review of the anatomy and physiology of cranial nerves.

TABLE 7-2
Types of Aphasia
With Anatomical Correlation

EXPRESSIVE DEFICITS: NONFLUENT APHASIA
- *Broca's aphasia* (sometimes called nonfluent aphasia or expressive aphasia)—lesion involving Broca's area of the frontal lobe
- *Agraphia* (writing aphasia)—lesion involving the posterior frontal area

RECEPTIVE DEFICITS: FLUENT APHASIA
- *Wernicke's aphasia* (sometimes called fluent aphasia or receptive aphasia)—lesion involving Wernicke's area of the temporal lobe
- *Alexia* (reading aphasia)—lesion involving the parieto-occipital area
- *Global aphasia* (a form of aphasia that involves both expressive and receptive aphasias)—extensive lesions involving Broca's area, Wernicke's area, the parieto-occipital area, and the posterior frontal area

Olfactory (I) Nerve (Sensory)

Testing of the olfactory nerve is usually deferred unless an anterior fossa tumor is suspected. The sense of smell is tested by obstructing one nostril while testing the other. A piece of cotton that has been saturated with a common, odoriferous, nonirritating substance is placed under the unobstructed nostril. Camphor, coffee, lemon oil, and peppermint are possible odors that patients should be able to identify if cranial nerve I is intact.

Anosmia indicates an inability to smell. There are several causes of anosmia, some of which are attributable to neuropathological conditions. Common neurological causes of anosmia include tumors of the base of the frontal lobe or pituitary area, fractures of the anterior fossa, atherosclerotic/cerebrovascular syndromes, meningitis, hydrocephalus, and posttraumatic brain syndrome. Common nonneurological causes of anosmia include the common cold, inflammation of the nasal cavity, and congenital defects.

The **Foster-Kennedy syndrome** is a special syndrome involving the olfactory nerve that is caused by a tumor or abscess at the base of the frontal lobe. Signs and symptoms of this condition include ipsilateral blindness and anosmia, ipsilateral atrophy of the olfactory and optic nerves, and contralateral papilledema. The frontal mass is on the same side as the atrophy.

Optic (II) Nerve (Sensory)

Each eye is evaluated individually. Testing encompasses an evaluation of visual acuity and visual fields and a funduscopic examination.

Visual acuity can be evaluated informally by asking the patient to read from printed material, such as a newspaper. A standard Snellen chart is available in office or clinic settings for more formal testing. Each eye is checked individually. The patient is asked to read the line on the chart with the smallest letters that they are able to read at a distance of 20 feet. The number beside each line of letters signifies the number of feet at which the letters can be read by a person with normal vision. This becomes the denominator in recording vision. Normal vision is 20/20. When vision is defective, the patient may only be able to see the larger letters at 20 feet. For example, persons with 20/40 vision are able to see at 20 feet what those with normal vision can see at 40 feet.

An adaptation of the Snellen chart, the Rosenbaum Pocket Vision Screener, is designed for quick bedside use. The chart is held at a distance of 14 inches from the patient. Normal vision in this instance is 14/14. The ratio is calculated in the same manner as for the Snellen test.

A **visual field** normally extends 60 degrees on the nasal side, 100 degrees on the temporal side, and 130 degrees vertically. A rough evaluation of visual field can be made by using the **confrontation test**, in which the examiner confronts or faces the patient at a distance of 2 feet. The patient covers one eye lightly and looks at the examiner's eye directly opposite. The examiner then closes one eye, superimposing the examiner's visual field on the patient's field. A pencil or a moving finger is then introduced from the periphery into the patient's field of vision; each quadrant (upper and lower) is checked. The patient is asked to indicate when the object is first seen.

The examiner uses himself or herself to establish the norm for comparison.

The confrontation test is designed to reveal only gross defects of the visual fields. If any defects are found, the visual fields should be plotted by an ophthalmologist using the standard **perimetric test** or a **tangent screen.**

Visual field tests can reveal disturbances in function anywhere along the visual pathway (retina, optic nerve, optic tract, lateral geniculate body, geniculocalcarine tract, or occipital lobe). The defects noted are associated with particular lesions along the visual pathway (Chart 7-1). Table 7-3 summarizes common visual defects.

The **funduscopic examination** is conducted with an ophthalmoscope. The ophthalmoscope contains a special lens that is used to visualize the inside of the eyeball by shining a beam of light directly into the eye. The room must be darkened and the examiner must sit directly opposite the subject. To examine the patient's right eye, the examiner holds the ophthalmoscope in the right hand and looks through the instrument with the right eye while the patient focuses on an object straight ahead (Fig. 7-1). The diopter is adjusted to visualize the optic disc (fundus), macula, and blood vessels (Fig. 7-2). The termination of the optic nerve, visible as a prominent, tubelike structure at the back of the eyeball, is called the **optic disc.** As one views the optic disc, small blood vessels can be visualized as they exit and enter the eye. The normal disc is round or slightly oval with sharply defined margins.

The four main pairs of blood vessels exiting and entering the optic disc are examined to compare the diameters of the arteries and veins and to determine whether the veins are tortuous. Normally, the veins are about 30% larger than the arteries; however, tortuous veins are present in certain clinical conditions in which intracranial pressure is increased. Another area of the retina is the **macula,** which has the highest density of visual receptors. The center of the macula, called the **fovea,** represents the point of greatest visual acuity. As the retina is examined, any abnormalities, such as hemorrhage, swelling, and exudate, should be noted. Table 7-4 presents a summary of common abnormal optic disc findings.

Oculomotor (III), Trochlear (IV), and Abducens (VI) Nerves (All Motor)

Cranial nerves III, IV, and VI are tested together because all three nerves supply the extraocular eye muscles (see Fig. 7-3 and Table 5-10). In addition, the oculomotor nerve controls the levator palpebrae superioris, which raises the upper eyelid, and the parasympathetic innervation to the pupil.

Injury to an extraocular muscle compromises the corresponding eye movement. Injury to the oculomotor nerve can result in an inability to focus the eyes medially on the horizontal plane, upward and outward, downward and outward, and upward and inward. In addition, a droopy eyelid (**ptosis**) or a dilated pupil with a loss of accommodation may also be present. A damaged trochlear nerve results in compromised downward and inward movement of the eye, whereas injury to the abducens causes loss of lateral movement on the horizontal plane. Trochlear nerve dysfunction is rare. The abducens nerve has the longest intracranial course and is frequently involved with neurological disease.

Extraocular eye movement is evaluated by asking the patient to follow the examiner's finger or a pencil through the six cardinal directions of gaze in an ''H'' sequencing (Fig. 7-3). When both eyes move in the same direction, at the same speed, and maintain a constant alignment, the gaze is termed **conjugate gaze.** If there is a lack of parallelism between the two visual axes, it is called **dysconjugate gaze** or **strabismus.** Extraocular deviation is often limited to a specific direction of gaze. Double vision, **diplopia,** will be present in a particular direction of gaze if the eye cannot be moved conjugately in that direction. The **oculocephalic reflex** (doll's eye response) and the **oculovestibular reflex** (cold calorics) can be tested in the unconscious patient (see Chap. 6).

The loss of normal function to any of the muscles responsible for extraocular movement may be attributable to damage to the muscles themselves or injury to the cranial nerve nuclei located in the midbrain and pons. **Ophthalmoplegia** is the term used to describe paralysis of one or more muscles. Table 7-5 summarizes the common ophthalmoplegias.

The **position of the eyeball** is noted. This is determined by looking at the position of the eyeball from frontal and lateral views, as well as by looking down from above the patient's head. Abnormal protrusion of one or both eyeballs is termed **proptosis** or **exophthalmos.** Abnormal recession of an eyeball within the orbit is termed **enophthalmos.**

In assessing the **upper eyelid,** the patient is asked to look straight ahead. The width of the palpebral fissure in each eye is noted and a comparison is made. The **palpebral fissure** is the space between the upper and lower eyelids. The term for a drooping upper eyelid is **ptosis.** Ptosis is also seen in Horner's syndrome. Edema of the eyelid, if present, should be noted. Edema can result from trauma to the orbit and may occur in the upper eyelid, the lower eyelid, or both. Next, the position of the eyelids in relation to the pupil and the iris in each eye is noted and compared.

Severe injury to the peripheral portion of the cranial nerve can result in nerve fiber degeneration, followed by unpredictable regeneration. Because of the proximity of other cranial nerves, the regenerating fibers from one nerve can be misdirected, resulting in innervation of other adjacent nerves. Such atypical regeneration is called the **misdirection syndrome.** Frequently, the oculomotor nerve is misdirected toward cranial nerve IV or V. Other examples of the misdirection syndrome include the pseudo-Graefe lid sign and Gunn's syndrome. The **pseudo-Graefe lid sign** is an atypical connection between cranial nerves III and IV. With this condition, any attempt to look downward is followed by upper eyelid retraction. **Gunn's syndrome** involves cranial nerves III and V. As the mouth is opened and the jaw moves to one side, ptosis of the eyelid changes to lid retraction.

ABNORMALITIES IN GAZE

In evaluating the visual system (see Chap. 8), an important consideration is gaze. **Gaze** is the act of focusing in a particular direction. It is a combination of coordinated eye and head movements and is the result of a complex interaction between the visual and vestibular systems. The following are various abnormalities in gaze.

CHART 7-1
Visual Field Defects Produced by Selected Lesions in the Visual Pathways

Visual Pathways

Visual Fields

Blackened Field Indicates Area of No Vision

Blind Right Eye (right optic nerve)
A lesion of the optic nerve and, of course, of the eye itself, produces unilateral blindness.

Bitemporal Hemianopia (optic chiasm)
A lesion at the optic chiasm may involve only those fibers that are crossing over to the opposite side. Because these fibers originate in the nasal half of each retina, visual loss involves the temporal half of each field.

Left Homonymous Hemianopia (right optic tract)
A lesion of the optic tract interrupts fibers originating on the same side of both eyes. Visual loss in the eyes is therefore similar (homonymous) and involves half of each field (hemianopia).

Homonymous Left Upper Quadrantic Defect (optic radiation, partial)
A partial lesion of the optic radiation may involve only a portion of the nerve fibers, producing, for example, a homonymous quadrantic defect.

TABLE 7-3
Common Vision Defects

TYPE	DESCRIPTION	CAUSES
Scotomas	Abnormal blind spots on the visual fields	Localized lesions, hemorrhage, glaucoma, or neuritis
Amblyopia	Dim vision that results in compromised visual acuity	Hereditary or acquired
Amaurosis	Complete blindness; amaurosis fugax is temporary blindness	Cerebral lesion, retinal or optic nerve disease, or heredity
Photophobia	Sensitivity of the eyes to light; often seen in meningitis and subarachnoid hemorrhage	Etiology is unclear
Diplopia	Commonly known as double vision; note if double images are side by side or one above another; special testing can be done using a red glass or a Maddox rod test	Paralysis of movement of the eyeball in a particular direction; involves extraocular muscles

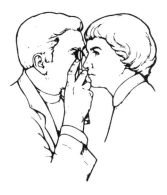

FIGURE 7-1
Technique for the proper use of the ophthalmoscope. The examiner holds the ophthalmoscope with the **right** hand and uses the **right** eye to look into the patient's eye. The index finger is used to adjust the lens for proper focus. For a **myopic** (nearsighted) patient, turn the lens control counterclockwise to the minus diopter; for a **hyperopic** (farsighted) patient, turn the lens control clockwise to the plus diopter.

Horizontal Gaze

- With a **destructive hemispheric lesion**, both **eyes deviate toward** the side of the lesion; that is, if the right side is destroyed, the eyes will deviate toward the right.
- With an **irritative hemispheric lesion**, such as a hemorrhage, both **eyes deviate away from** the side of the irritation. The deviation lasts only minutes or hours and is replaced by paralysis of conjugate gaze.
- With a **destructive pontine lesion**, the **eyes deviate away from** the lesion.
- A lesion in the lateral midbrain tegmentum will cause a horizontal gaze palsy **away from** the lesion (opposite side to the lesion) by interrupting the cerebral pathways for conjugate gaze before their decussation.

Vertical Gaze

Abnormalities of vertical gaze imply a lesion of the rostral interstitial nucleus of the medial longitudinal fasciculus (riMLF) in the midbrain. A unilateral lesion of the riMLF results in a mild defect in vertical saccades; bilateral lesions result in deficits in vertical eye movements. Lesions of the interstitial nucleus of Cajal (INC) result in impaired vertical gaze-holding. Normally, elderly persons have upward gaze abnormalities with no apparent underlying disease. Paralysis of upward gaze is most often caused by destruction at the pretectal and posterior commissural area at the midbrain–diencephalic junction.

Bilateral lesions of the MLF produce abnormalities in upward gaze and impair vertical vestibular and pursuit movement but spare vertical saccades (Evinger, Fuchs, & Baker, 1977)[2].

An additional vertical gaze abnormality is Parinaud's syndrome (see Table 7-5).

Medial Longitudinal Fasciculus

A lesion of the MLF between the III and VI nuclei causes **internuclear ophthalmoplegia (INO)**. The signs and symptoms of INO include a deficit in adduction (medial rectus) of the ipsilateral eye, overshooting (dissociated nystagmus) of the abductor (lateral rectus) of the contralateral eye, and retention or loss of convergence. The lesion is very small and occurs with a number of brain stem disorders; it is also seen as an area of demyelinization in multiple sclerosis or as a small vascular lesion from diabetes mellitus. As mentioned above, bilateral lesions of the MLF produce abnormalities in upward gaze.

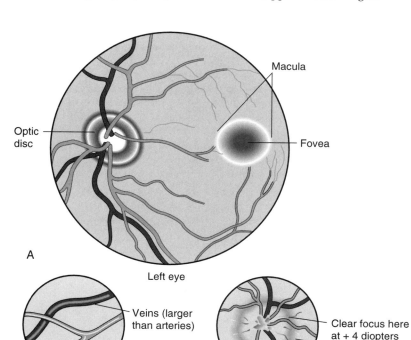

FIGURE 7-2
The retina as seen through the ophthalmoscope. The ophthalmoscope is capable of visualizing only a portion of the retina at any one time. In examining the retina (*A*) identify the disc; ascertain the sharpness of the disc margins; identify the macula and fovea (bright reflection in the center); (*B*) compare the diameters of the veins to the arteries; follow the vessels in each quadrant from the disc to the periphery; and note any exudate, hemorrhagic areas, or abnormalities present. **Measurements within the eye.** Lesions are recorded in relationship to the optic disc as **disc diameters.** For example, in *A*, the macula is about 2 disc diameters from the disc. (*C*) For an elevated optic disc due to pilledema, note the **differences in diopters** measurement of the two lenses used to focus clearly on the disc and on the uninvolved retina.

TABLE 7-4
Common Abnormal Optic Disc Findings

TYPE	DESCRIPTION	CAUSES
Papilledema (choked disc)	Margin of the disc is distorted and swollen; the disc has a reddish hue because of congestion	Increased intracranial pressure; pseudotumor cerebri
Optic atrophy	Paleness (the disc is light pink, white, or gray owing to decreased blood supply); visual acuity is decreased	Primary causes: tabes dorsalis and multiple sclerosis Secondary causes: neuritis or prolonged increased intracranial pressure
Retrobulbar neuritis	Inflammatory lesion of the posterior portion of the optic nerve; no swelling of disc	Hemorrhage, diabetes, or retinitis
Optic neuritis	Inflammation of the disc; associated with loss of vision secondary to a central scotoma	Inflammatory process
Cotton wool patches (seen during fundus examination)	Whitish or grayish oval lesions that look like cotton balls; smaller than disc	Hypertension

Other Gaze Abnormalities

Skewed deviation (Hertwig-Magendie vertical divergence ocular position) is a condition in which one eye looks downward and the other looks upward. It is caused by a lesion in the pons on the same side as the downward eye. (The MLF receives cerebellar innervation.) Skewed deviation can also be a symptom of posterior fossa or cerebellar disease; it is one of the four cardinal symptoms of cerebellar disease.

Roving-eye movement is characterized by spontaneous, slow, and random deviation. It is seen in comatose patients with intact brain stem oculomotor function. Absence of roving-eye movement indicates brain stem dysfunction.

Ocular bobbing is characterized by episodic, intermittent, usually conjugate, downward, brisk eye movement followed by a return to the resting position by a "bobbing action." It is seen in severe destructive lower pontine lesions, pontine hemorrhage, or infection.

Nystagmus. **Nystagmus** is a common, involuntary, rhythmic to-and-fro oscillation of the eyes that may be horizontal, vertical, rotary, or mixed in direction. The tempo of the movements can be regular, rhythmical, pendular, or jerky, with a noted fast and slow movement component.

With normal eye movement, there may be three or fewer beats at the extremes of eye position; this finding is disregarded. True nystagmus is a pathological condition caused by a central or peripheral lesion in the visual perceptual pathways, the inner ear vestibular system, and portions of the proprioceptive system and their brain stem and cerebellar connections. This complex system normally keeps the eyes in a constant relationship with their environment. Specific types of nystagmus can be caused by lesions in particular areas of the system. Therefore, it is important to describe the characteristics of the nystagmus in the patient's record. The following are a few specific types of nystagmus, along with the related anatomical area:

- **Retraction nystagmus**—irregular jerks of the eyes backward into the orbit, precipitated by an upward gaze; midbrain tegmental damage
- **Convergence nystagmus**—slow, spontaneous, drifting, ocular divergence with a final quick, convergent jerk; midbrain lesion
- **See-saw nystagmus**—a rapid, pendular, dysconjugate see-saw movement accompanied by deficits of visual fields and visual acuity; proximal optic chiasmal lesion
- **Downbeat nystagmus**—irregular jerks precipitated by downward gaze; lower medullary damage
- **Optokinetic nystagmus**—a rapid, alternating motion of the eyes normally noted when the eyes try to fixate on a moving target; presence of optokinetic nystagmus indicates physiologic continuity of the optic pathways from the retina to the occipital cortex. Because it is involuntary, a positive response provides reliable verification of intact vision in a patient feigning blindness.
- **Vestibular nystagmus**—a mixed nystagmus that can be horizontal, rotational, or both, resulting from vestibular disease

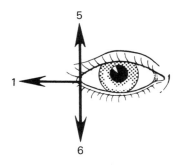

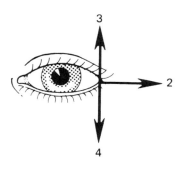

FIGURE 7-3
Sequence of eye-testing movements. (*Note:* Numbers indicate the appropriate sequence of movement.)

TABLE 7-5
Types of Ophthalmoplegias

TYPE OF OPHTHALMOPLEGIA	DESCRIPTION
External	Paralysis of one or more of the extraocular muscles
Internal	Paralysis of one or more intraocular muscles
Nuclear	Paralysis caused by a lesion involving the nuclei of the motor nerves of the eye (III, IV, or VI)
Internuclear	Paralysis caused by injury or a lesion of the medial longitudinal fasciculus located within the brain stem
Supranuclear	Paralysis caused by injury or a lesion to the conjugate eye movement centers located in the frontal, frontal-parietal, and occipital lobes
Parinaud's syndrome or dorsal midbrain syndrome	A type of supranuclear ophthalmoplegia; conjugate upward gaze paralysis; caused by a lesion in the dorsal midbrain

• **Toxic nystagmus**—induced with certain drugs at toxic levels such as phenytoin (Dilantin), barbiturates, and bromides

PUPILS

The oculomotor nerve (III) controls pupillary function. To assess the pupils, the patient should be directed to focus on a distant object located straight ahead. With a comatose patient, the pupils are examined as they are found. The pupils are examined for size, shape, and equality. The normal diameter of a pupil is 2 to 6 mm, with an average diameter of 3.5 mm. When the pupils are compared with each other, their diameters should be equal; however, about 12% to 17% of the normal population has discernible unequal pupil size (**anisocoria**) in the absence of a pathological condition.

The shape of the pupils is also noted and compared. Normally, the pupils are round; however, in patients who have had cataract surgery, the pupils assume the keyhole shape. An ovoid pupil indicates pupillary dysfunction; it may be seen in early uncal herniation.

Sensitivity to light or **photophobia** may be noted when checking the pupils, or the patient may complain of this problem. The etiology is unclear, but is usually associated with increased intracranial pressure.

Pupillary Reflexes. A few important reflexes relating to pupillary responses and eye movement can be tested.

DIRECT LIGHT REFLEX. The direct light reflex refers to the constriction and dilation of the pupil when a light is shone into that pupil and withdrawn (Fig. 7-4). Each pupil is tested individually and the results are compared. Response to light is recorded as:

• **Brisk:** (very rapid constriction when light is introduced)
• **Sluggish:** (constriction occurs, but is slower than expected)
• **Nonreactive or fixed:** (no constriction or dilation is noted)

Normally, pupillary constriction is brisk, although age may affect the degree of reaction. Pupils in younger people tend to be larger and more responsive than those in older people. Withdrawal of light should result in dilation.

In addition to the constriction of the pupil that occurs with direct light stimulation (direct light response), there is a somewhat weaker constriction of the nonstimulated pupil. This is called the **consensual light reflex**, which occurs as a result of fibers that cross both the optic chiasma and the posterior commissure of the midbrain.

The sensory receptors for the light reflex are the rods and cones of the retina. Afferent impulses follow the normal visual pathway as far as the lateral geniculate bodies. Rather than entering the geniculate body, sensory impulses enter the pretectal area (near the superior colliculus). Con-

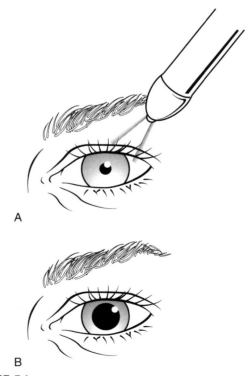

A

B

FIGURE 7-4
Direct light reflex. (*A*) A bright light is introduced from the temporal area; the pupil normally rapidly constricts when exposed to the light. (*B*) The pupil rapidly dilates when the light is removed.

necting neurons synapse in the **Edinger-Westphal nucleus** (oculomotor nucleus) located in the midbrain. From here, the parasympathetic fibers proceed to the ciliary ganglion. The postganglionic parasympathetic fibers contract the pupilloconstrictor fibers of the iris, causing the pupil to constrict. When the light is withdrawn, the pupil normally dilates because of sympathetic stimulation. Sympathetic innervation originates in the **intermediolateral horn cells** that pass to the superior cervical ganglion. The postganglionic sympathetic fibers synapse with the pupillodilator muscles, resulting in pupillary dilation.

NEAR-POINT REACTION. In testing the near-point reaction, patients are asked to focus on the examiner's finger, which is positioned 2 to 3 feet directly ahead of them, and to follow it with their eyes as it is rapidly moved closer to their face. Three reflex responses normally occur:

- **Convergence**—the medial recti muscles contract, thus directing both eyes toward the midline. This occurs so that the image in each eye will remain focused on the fovea; without this reflex, diplopia would occur.
- **Accommodation**—to sharply focus the image on the fovea, the lenses thicken as a result of tension in the ciliary muscles; the ciliary muscles are innervated by the postganglionic parasympathetic neurons in the ciliary ganglion.
- **Pupillary constriction**—the pupils constrict as an optical adjustment to regulate depth of focus. (This pupillary constriction does not depend on light and is regulated separately from the light reflex).

A summary of abnormal pupillary responses is found in Table 7-6.

Trigeminal (V) Nerve (Mixed)
SENSORY COMPONENT

The three sensory vectors of the face are tested (Fig. 7-5). The **ophthalmic division** innervates the frontal sinuses, the conjunctiva and cornea, the upper lid, the bridge of the nose, the forehead, and the scalp as far as the vertex of the skull. The **maxillary division** innervates the cheek, the maxillary sinus, the lateral aspects of the nose, the upper teeth, the nasal pharynx, the hard palate, and the uvula. The **mandibular division** innervates the chin, the lower jaw, the anterior two thirds of the tongue, the gums and floor of the mouth, and the buccal mucosa of the cheek.

With the patient's eyes closed, **light touch** is tested by touching the forehead, cheek, and jaw with a wisp of cotton. The patient is instructed to respond every time the skin is touched. **Pain perception** is evaluated with the "picky" and dull ends of a wooden applicator or by the pinprick method. After demonstrating the difference between sharp and dull, the skin is touched with the sharp end and occasionally with the dull end. The patient is asked to respond "sharp" or "dull." **Temperature** is only evaluated if abnormalities are found in pain perception. Two test tubes, one with cold water and one with hot water, are individually placed on the skin and patients are asked to respond "hot" or "cold." In practice, many people use a tuning fork instead of test tubes for testing.

The tuning fork is occasionally placed on the face and the patient is asked to respond "warm" or "cold." Accuracy of response and a comparison between findings on each side of the face is made.

MOTOR COMPONENT

Next, the muscles of mastication are evaluated. The strength of the masseter and temporal muscles is evaluated by palpating them when the jaw is clenched. Differences in muscle tone or atrophy should be noted.

Facial (VII) Nerve (Mixed)
SENSORY COMPONENT

The sense of taste on the anterior two thirds of the tongue is controlled by the facial nerve. Testing of this function is often deferred. However, if tested, each side of the protruded tongue is tested separately. There are four basic modalities of taste: sweet (tip of tongue), sour (sides of tongue), salty (over most of tongue but concentrated on the sides), and bitter (back of tongue; controlled by cranial nerve IX). The patient is asked to identify the taste of sugar placed on the tip of the tongue, after which a sip of water is given. The same procedure using sour and salty substances is used. If bitter is tested on the posterior third of the tongue, it should be recognized that it is innervated by the glossopharyngeal nerve. Sensation to the external ear is also supplied by the facial nerve.

MOTOR COMPONENT

The motor component is tested by observing the symmetry of the face at rest and during deliberate facial movements, such as smiling, showing the teeth, whistling, pursing the lips, blowing air into the cheeks, wrinkling the nose and forehead, and raising the eyebrows. Note the nasolabial folds for symmetry. In addition, ask the patient to close the eyes tightly. The examiner should not be able to open the patient's eyes. The facial nerve also controls tearing and salivation.

When weakness is noted, it is important to observe whether the entire side of the face or just the lower face (below the eyes) is affected. There are two types of weakness. If the lower portion of one side of the face is involved, the lesion is said to be central (involves the central nervous system) or an **upper motor neuron lesion** (as seen with a stroke). In this instance, the corticobulbar tracts are involved, resulting in contralateral weakness of the lower face with normal function of the upper face. Wrinkling of the forehead is left intact because of bilateral innervation of the upper face from the corticobulbar fibers. The lower face, by contrast, has only unilateral contralateral cortical innervation. The patient is unable to retract the corner of his or her mouth in a smile. The second type of facial weakness involves the total face with ipsilateral facial muscle involvement. The lesion is said to be peripheral (involves the peripheral nervous system) or a **lower motor neuron lesion**. In addition to muscle weakness, note any evidence of spasms, atrophy, or tremors of the facial muscles.

TABLE 7-6
Abnormal Pupillary Responses

CONDITION/RESPONSE	CHARACTERISTICS

AMAUROTIC PUPIL (BLIND EYE)

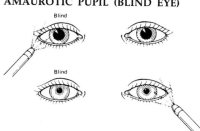

Blindness in one eye secondary to disease of the retina or optic nerve results in loss of the sensory limb of the light reflex arc. As long as the oculomotor nerve (the motor limb of the arc) is intact, a light directed into the good eye produces normal direct and consensual reactions. Blindness in one eye may be confirmed by

- No direct light response in the blind eye
- No consensual response to light in the intact eye
- A direct light response in the intact eye
- A consensual response in the blind eye (from light shone into the intact eye)
- A near pupillary response in both eyes

MARCUS-GUNN PUPIL (SWINGING FLASHLIGHT SIGN OR AFFERENT PUPILLARY DEFECT)

This condition accompanies optic atrophy or retinal pathology. A bright light must be used. There is a normal bilateral response (constriction) when the intact eye is illuminated, but pupillary dilation occurs when the flashlight is quickly switched to the diseased eye.

OCULOMOTOR NERVE COMPRESSION

The ipsilateral pupil is dilated and fixed as a result of uncal herniation compressing the oculomotor nerve (parasympathetic fibers for pupillary constriction) against the tentorium and/or posterior cerebral artery. Related to rising intracranial pressure or cerebral edema.

HORNER'S SYNDROME

This syndrome is characterized by a unilateral, small pupil that reacts to direct light and demonstrates accommodation; ptosis of the eyelid; and possibly, loss of sweating on the affected side. It is caused by a lesion involving the descending sympathetic fibers in the ipsilateral brain stem or upper cord, or the ascending sympathetic fibers in the neck or head. The result is unilateral interruption or complete loss of sympathetic innervation to the pupil.

HIPPUS PHENOMENON

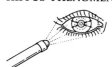

An alternating pupillary dilation and constriction in response to light is typical of hippus. This may be considered normal if the pupil is being observed under high magnification. This finding also occurs in early uncal herniation when there is pressure on the oculomotor nerve.

ADIE'S PUPIL (TONIC PUPIL)

This abnormality is usually confined to one side. The pupil is large and regularly shaped and reacts very slowly to light; it accommodates slowly. The pupil also dilates slowly in darkness. This condition may be associated with diminished knee and ankle reflexes. It is attributable to postganglionic denervation of the parasympathetic pupillary innervation. Its cause is unknown, although it has been noted to occur following a viral infection. Those most often affected are women who are 20 to 30 years of age. To diagnose an Adie's pupil, 2.5% methacholine (Mecholyl) is instilled into both eyes. The affected pupil promptly contracts, but the normal pupil does not.

ARGYLL-ROBERTSON PUPIL

Pupils are bilaterally small and irregularly shaped, and react to accommodation but not to direct light. This condition is often seen with neurosyphilis (tabes dorsalis).

MIDBRAIN DAMAGE

Midposition, nonreactive pupils may be caused by a lesion in the dorsal portion of the midbrain or a nuclear midbrain lesion; in the former instance, the pupils are round and regular, whereas in the latter instance, they may be irregular and unequal. Potential causes of midposition pupils include midbrain damage from transtentorial herniation, tumors, infarction, and hemorrhage.

PONTINE DAMAGE

Small, bilateral, nonreactive pupils (*pinpoint pupils*) may result from the loss of sympathetic innervation. The cause is usually pontine hemorrhage, but this condition can also occur with the administration of opiate drugs.

(continued)

TABLE 7-6
Abnormal Pupillary Responses Continued

CONDITION/RESPONSE	CHARACTERISTICS
MIOTIC (SMALL) PUPILS	The most common causes of miosis are ophthalmic miotic drugs (acetylcholine chloride, carbachol, demecarium bromide, echothiophate iodide, isoflurophate, physostigmine, pilocarpine, and others), opiates (heroin, morphine sulfate, hydromorphone), and pontine hemorrhage. Miosis can occur with destruction of the sympathetic innervation and interruption of the inhibitory pathways to the oculomotor nuclei (Edinger-Westphal nucleus). Traumatic miosis is caused by direct injury to the eye and is often associated with orbital trauma. Miosis following trauma usually results from intraocular inflammation or injury.
MYDRIATIC (LARGE) PUPILS	Mydriatic pupils are most often caused by amphetamines, glutethimide (Doriden), ophthalmic mydriatics, and cycloplegic agents (atropine sulfate, cyclopentolate hydrochloride, homatropine hydrobromide, scopolamine hydrobromide, and tropicamide). Traumatic mydriasis is the result of direct injury to the eye, and is often associated with orbital injuries. Mydriasis is the usual result of local sphincter paralysis or tears in the sphincter muscle. In this instance, the pupil will have an irregular shape as a result of the tearing.

> A pupil may be abnormally large or small because of orbital trauma. When pupillary asymmetry is noted without other neurological deficits, such as consciousness, the possibility of orbital trauma should be explored.

CONDITION/RESPONSE	CHARACTERISTICS
SEVERE ANOXIA OR ISCHEMIA; DEATH	Bilateral, fixed, and dilated pupils are the clinical signs that are seen in the terminal state (they can also result from atropine-like drugs). An intact ciliospinal reflex may produce momentary bilateral dilation.

Acoustic (VIII) Nerve (Sensory)

The acoustic nerve is divided into two branches, the **cochlear (hearing)** and the **vestibular (balance).** Unless a history of vertigo, tinnitus, or disturbed balance is given, the vestibular branch is not tested. If evaluation is indicated, special testing methods and equipment will be required.

To test **hearing**, direct the patient to cover one ear. Standing on the opposite side, 1 to 2 feet away from the ear, whisper a few numbers or a word. The patient should be able to hear. Test the other ear. Hearing should be equal in both ears. The tympanic membrane can be examined with an otoscope.

Next, check for **lateralization** and compare **air** and **bone conduction.** The **Weber test** is used to evaluate lateralization, whereas the **Rinne test** evaluates air and bone conduction. Both tests require the use of a 512 Hz tuning fork (Fig. 7-6). For the **Weber test,** place a lightly vibrating tuning fork firmly on the top of the patient's head or in the middle of the forehead. Inquire whether the patient hears it more on the left side, the right side, or in the middle. Normally, the sound is heard in the middle or equally in both ears. In the **Rinne test,** place the base of a lightly vibrating tuning fork on the mastoid process until the patient can no longer hear the sound. Quickly place the vibrating fork near the ear canal with one side of the fork toward the ear. Ask whether it can be heard. Normally, the sound should be heard longer through air than through bone (AC > BC). In evaluating hearing acuity, it is important to differentiate between **conduction loss** and **sensorineural loss.** The findings for unilateral loss for each are as follows:

TYPE OF DEAFNESS	RINNE	WEBER
Conduction deafness	BC > AC (abnormal)	Lateralizes to deafer ear
Sensorineural deafness	AC > BC	Lateralizes **away from** deafer ear

Abnormal results from either test warrant further investigation with more sensitive testing procedures.

Glossopharyngeal (IX) and Vagus (X) Nerves (Both Mixed)

The glossopharyngeal and vagus nerves are usually tested together because their innervation overlaps in the pharynx.

The glossopharyngeal nerve supplies sensory components to the pharynx, tonsils, soft palate, tympanic membrane, posterior third of the tongue, and secretory fibers of the parotid gland. It also supplies motor fibers to the stylopharyngeal muscle of the pharynx, whose role is to elevate the pharynx. The patient is asked to open his or her mouth and say ''ah.'' The upward movement of the soft

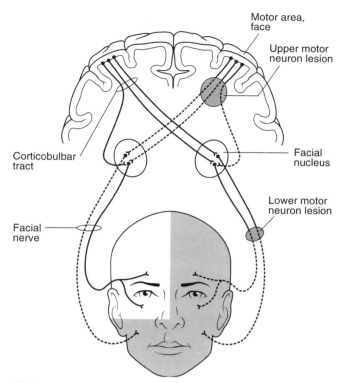

FIGURE 7-5
Sensory vectors of the face.

palate and uvula should be noted. The vagus nerve provides parasympathetic fibers to the viscera of the chest and abdomen. Sensory fibers innervate the external ear canal, pharynx, larynx, and viscera of the chest and abdomen. The vagus also provides motor control to the soft palate, larynx, and pharynx.

The soft palate is examined with the patient's mouth open. Normally, when the patient says "ah," the palate elevates and the uvula remains midline. Check to see whether the uvula deviates to one side or the other (Fig. 7-7). The gag reflex is innervated by cranial nerves IX and X. After warning the patient that you are going to check the gag reflex, touch the posterior pharyngeal wall with a tongue blade or applicator first on the left side and next on the right side. A gag response should be stimulated on each side.

The voice quality is evaluated by listening to the patient speak and noting hoarseness; a soft, whispery voice; or no voice. Difficulty in speaking, such as hoarseness or speaking in a whisper, is termed **dysphonia**. Both are due to paralysis of the soft palate (**palatal paralysis**) and can result in nasal-sounding speech. **Dysarthria** refers to defective articulation that may be caused by a motor deficit of the tongue or speech muscles. Slurred speech should be noted, as should difficulty in pronouncing the letters *m, b, p, t,* and *d* and the number *one*.

Spinal Accessory (XI) Nerve (Motor)

The accessory nerve, as it is sometimes called, is tested in two segments. First, the trapezius muscle is palpated and its strength evaluated while the patient shrugs the shoul-

ders against resistance provided by the examiner's hands. Second, the patient is asked to turn his or her head to one side and push the chin against the examiner's hand, thereby allowing the sternocleidomastoid muscle to be palpated and its strength evaluated. The same procedure is then repeated on the other side. The symmetry of the trapezius and sternocleidomastoid muscles is noted, along with any muscle wasting or spasm.

Hypoglossal (XII) Nerve (Motor)

The patient is asked to open his or her mouth. The tongue is first inspected as it lies on the floor of the mouth. Note any atrophy or fasciculation. Ask the patient to protrude the tongue. Note asymmetry, atrophy, or deviation from midline. Next, direct the patient to move the tongue from side to side. Note the symmetry of movement. Finally, ask the patient to push the tongue against

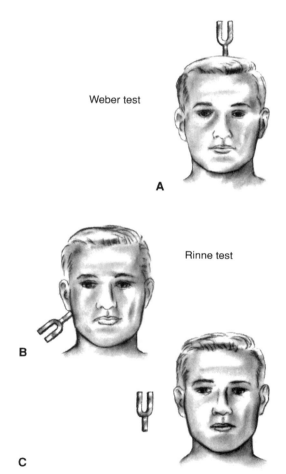

FIGURE 7-6
Weber test and Rinne test. Note the placement of a vibrating tuning fork (512 Hz) for each test. (*A*) Weber test for lateralization. Place the vibrating fork firmly on the top of the head or on the middle of the forehead. Normally the sound is perceived midline. Rinne test for comparing bone and air conduction: Place the base of the vibrating tuning fork on the mastoid process until the patient can no longer hear it (*B*); then, quickly place the fork near the external auditory canal, with one side toward the ear (*C*). Normally, the sound can be heard longer through air than through bone (AC > BC).

the inside of each cheek as the examiner palpates externally on the cheek for strength and equality.

MOTOR SYSTEM EXAMINATION

The third step in the neurological examination is the evaluation of motor function. The motor examination proceeds from the upper limbs to the neck and trunk and, finally, to the lower extremities. Limb evaluation proceeds from proximal to distal. It is impractical to test all muscles, but major groups are assessed; a more detailed examination can be conducted if deficits are noted in a particular area. The symmetry of each muscle or muscle group is noted. Consider five areas in the evaluation: (1) muscle size; (2) muscle tone; (3) muscle strength; (4) gait/posture; and (5) involuntary movements.

Muscle Size

Inspect symmetric muscles for both size and contour. When in doubt, a tape measure can be used to measure the same muscle on the opposite side of the body. Measurements must be taken from the same reference point for accuracy. Note muscle wasting, atrophy, or hypertrophy.

Muscle Tone

Tone is the normal state of muscle tension. The muscle is palpated while at rest and during passive stretching. With the patient relaxed, the joints are put through the normal range of motion (flexion and extension) by the examiner. The systematic evaluation proceeds from the shoulder, elbow, wrist, and fingers in the upper extremities and from the hip, knee, and ankle in the lower extremities. Findings from the left side and the right side are then compared. Abnormalities in muscle tone include spasticity, rigidity, and flaccidity.

Spasticity refers to increased resistance to passive movement, often more pronounced at the extremes of range of motion and usually followed by a sudden or gradual release of resistance. Spasticity is due to injury to the corticospinal system. **Clasp-knife spasticity** is increased resistance with a sudden release at the end of extension.

Rigidity is a state of increased resistance. **Cogwheel rigidity** is a series of ratchet-like, small, regular jerks that are felt on passive flexion or extension. **Lead-pipe rigidity** is resistance that persists throughout extension and flexion.

Flaccidity refers to decreased muscle tone or **hypotonia**. The muscle is weak, soft, flabby, and fatigues easily.

Special states of muscle tone in unconscious patients, decortication and decerebration, are discussed in Chapter 8.

Muscle Strength

In a conscious patient, the major muscles and muscle groups are evaluated by asking the patient to move actively against the resistance provided by the examiner. Muscle strength can be rated using a scale of 0 (no muscle contraction detected) to 5 (active movement against full resistance). Muscle strength is

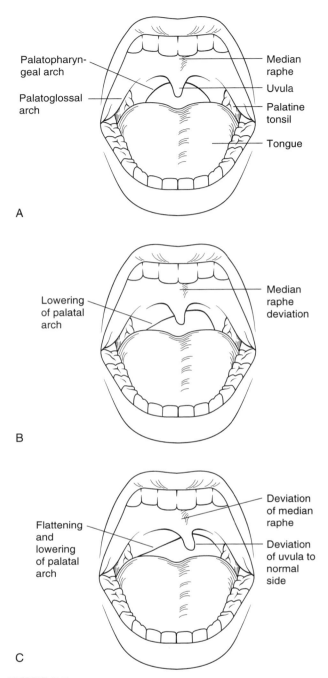

FIGURE 7-7
Observing the palate. (A) Normal palate with mouth open and at rest. (B) Right unilateral vagus paralysis with mouth at rest. (C) Right unilateral vagus paralysis when saying "ah."

recorded together with the maximum grade achievable on the scale (*e.g.*, 4/5) (Table 7-7). Another method of recording motor strength is drawing a stick figure and noting the numerical values of motor strength on the limbs. This recording system is shown in Fig. 7-8.

In the following section, the spinal nerve roots that innervate the muscles are shown in parentheses. If particular spinal nerves have a greater influence in the muscle or mus-

TABLE 7-7 *Grading of Muscle Strength*	
GRADE	**STRENGTH**
5	Active movement against gravity and full resistance; normal muscle strength
4	Active movement against gravity and some resistance; the examiner can overcome the muscle resistance
3	Active movement against gravity
2	Active movement of the body part when gravity is eliminated
1	A very weak muscle contraction is palpated; only a trace of a contraction is evident, but no active movement of the body part is noted
0	No muscle contraction is detectable

cle group, those roots are in bold. Note that there may be slight variations in texts in identifying spinal nerve roots. Examination of the unconscious patient is addressed in Chapter 8.

UPPER EXTREMITIES: CONSCIOUS PATIENT

To evaluate the upper extremities, ask the patient to close the eyes and stretch out the arms parallel to the floor with palms up for 20 to 30 seconds (Fig. 7-9). Downward drifting of an arm or pronation of the palm on one side, called **pronator drift**, suggests mild paresis of the involved extremity or weakness of the shoulder girdle. With the patient's arms outstretched and parallel to the floor, the examiner observes the scapula for increased prominence of the scapular tip (**winging**) accompanied by inward and upward displacement. Evaluating each scapula separately, the examiner tries to depress one outstretched arm against the resistance provided by the patient while observing for winging. Winging is suggestive of serratus anterior muscle (C5, C6, C7) weakness. Next, ask the patient to make "chicken wings" with the upper arms (flex forearms and extend upper arms to the sides). The examiner tries to push the arms down against resistance (C5, C6).

The arm is evaluated next. Ask the patient to "make a muscle" by flexing the upper arm. The examiner tries to pull the flexed forearm open; this is the biceps (C5–C6). Next, turn the lower arm so the hand faces a midsaggital line. Instruct the patient to pull toward himself or herself; this is the brachioradialis (C5–C6). Now tell the patient to push you away with the flexed lower arm; this is the triceps (C7–C8).

The wrist and hand are evaluated next. With the patient's hands flexed into fists, the examiner attempts to push the extended wrist downward against resistance (C6) and then to straighten the flexed wrist (C7). If successful, it is suggestive of wristdrop. The examiner extends his or her index and middle fingers to the patient with the instructions "Squeeze my fingers as hard as you can." Normally, the grips are firm and equal and the examiner should have some difficulty pulling the fingers out of the patient's grip (C8, T1). Next, instruct the patient to spread the fingers and

keep them spread as the examiner attempts to force the fingers together (T1). For thumb opposition, instruct the patient to place the index fingertip and thumb together into a circle (C8, T1). The examiner tries to pull them apart by pulling his or her finger through the circle. If this can easily be done, there is notable weakness.

LOWER EXTREMITIES: CONSCIOUS PATIENT

In examining the lower extremities, proceed from the hip to the feet. By positioning the hands appropriately, the examiner provides resistance to movement. The examiner compares the strength in the left and right muscle or muscle group and grades each side. While the patient is lying on the examining table or the bed, the following are tested:

- **Hip flexion (L1, L2,** L3; iliopsoas): the examiner places his or her hand on the upper leg. The patient is instructed to raise the leg against the examiner's hand.
- **Hip adductors (L2, L3,** L4; adductors): the patient is instructed to separate the extended legs about 6 inches. The examiner places the hands firmly on the bed between the patient's knees. The patient is instructed to bring the knees together against the examiner's hands.

(text continues on page 123)

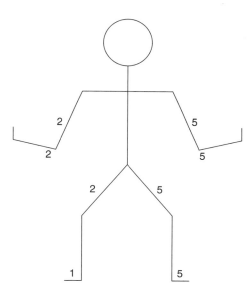

FIGURE 7-8
A stick figure can be used to record muscle strength using the following numbers to represent response: 5, active movement against gravity and full resistance (normal muscle strength); 4, active movement against gravity and some resistance; 3, active movement against gravity; 2, active movement of the body part when gravity is eliminated; 1, a very weak muscle contraction is palpated, but no active movement of the body part is noted; 0, no muscle contraction is detectable. *Note:* sometimes an examiner will use (+) or (−) in the "4" category to indicate how strong the patient's muscle was against the examiner's resistance. A "4+" indicates that a large amount of resistance by the examiner was necessary for the muscle to finally be overcome.

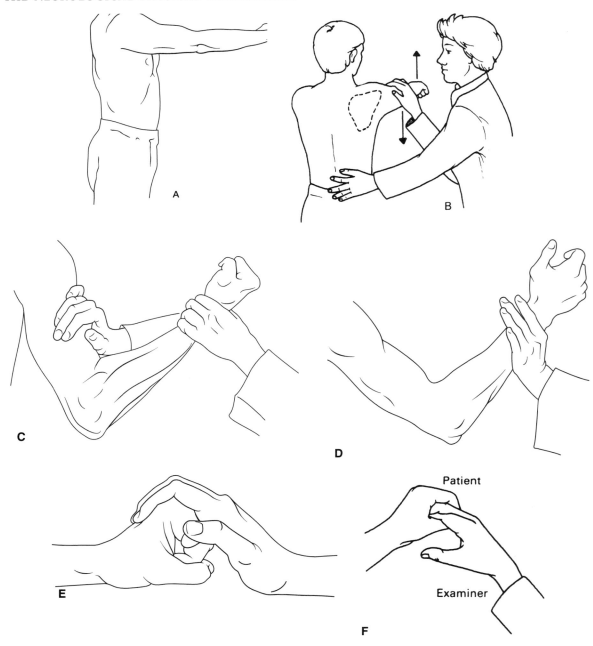

FIGURE 7-9

Testing muscle strength in the extremities. (*A*) Ask patients to hold their arms straight in front of them, with palms up, for 20 to 30 seconds. Watch how well they maintain this position. (Tendency to pronation suggests mild hemiparesis; downward drift of arm with flexion at the elbow may also occur.) (*B*) On each side, try to depress the patient's outstretched arms against his or her resistance. Note the patient's strength and watch the scapula on that side for winging or displacement. (Increased prominence of the scapular tip [winging] with displacement in and up suggests a weak serratus anterior muscle.) (*C*) Ask the patient to flex his or her upper arm. Try to pull the flexed forearm open; this will allow you to evaluate the biceps. (*D*) Ask the patient to push against your hand with the flexed lower arm to evaluate the triceps. (*E*) Test extension at the wrist by asking the patient to make a fist and resist your pulling it down. (There will be wristdrop in radial nerve disorders.) (*F*) Test the patient's grip by asking him or her to squeeze your fingers as hard as possible. You can avoid painful, hard gripping by offering the patient only your index and middle fingers, with the middle finger on top of the index. You should normally have difficulty removing your fingers from the patient's grip. (Grip may be affected by forearm muscle weakness and painful disorders of the hands.)

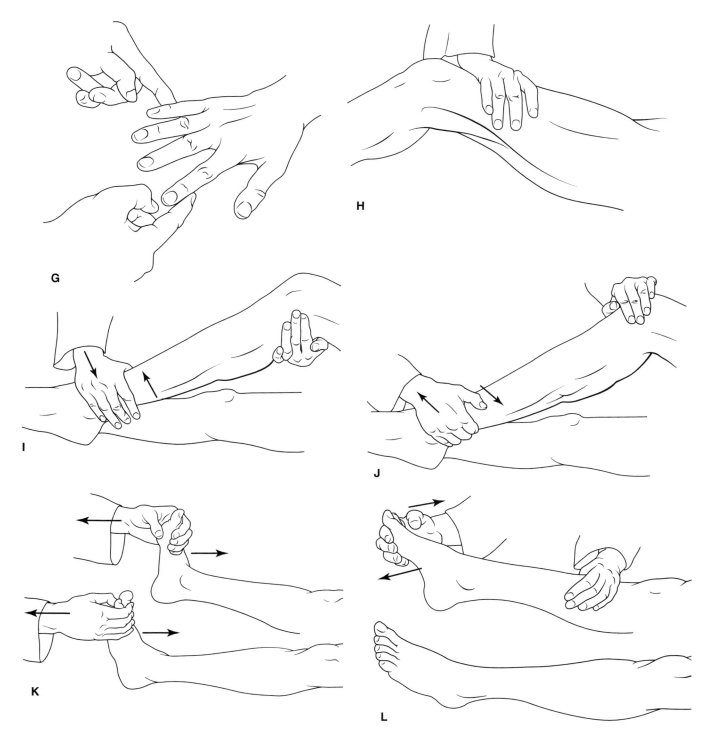

FIGURE 7-9

(Continued) (*G*) Ask the patient to spread his or her fingers. Check abduction by trying to force them together. (There will be weak abduction in ulnar nerve disorders.) (*H*) Test flexion at the hip by placing your hand on the patient's upper leg. Ask the patient to raise the leg against your resistance. (*I*) Test extension at the knee by supporting the patient's knee with one hand and placing the other on the lower leg about four inches above the ankle. Ask the patient to straighten the lower leg against your resistance. (*J*) Test flexion at the knee by placing one hand on the partially flexed knee and the other under the lower leg about four inches above the ankle. Ask the patient to flex his or her knee against your resistance. (*K*) Test dorsiflexion at the ankle by asking the patient to pull up against your hands. (*L*) Test plantar flexion by asking the patient to push down against your hands.

CHART 7-2
Gait Changes Associated With Anatomical Correlations

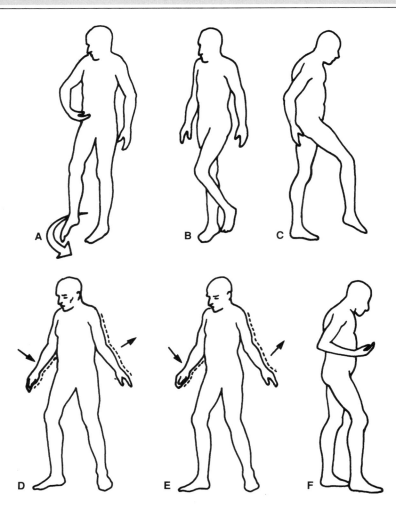

A   Spastic hemiparesis is associated with unilateral upper motor neuron disease. One arm is flexed, close to the side, and immobile; the leg is circled stiffly outward and forward (circumducted), often with dragging of the toe.

B   Scissors gait is associated with bilateral spastic paresis of the legs. Each leg is advanced slowly and the thighs tend to cross forward on each other at each step. The steps are short. Patients look as if they were walking through water.

C   Steppage gait is associated with foot-drop, usually secondary to lower motor neuron disease. The feet are lifted high, with knees flexed, and then brought down with a slap on the floor. Patients look as if they were walking up stairs.

D   Sensory ataxia is associated with loss of position sense in the legs. The gait is unsteady and wide-based (the feet are far apart). The feet are lifted high and brought down with a slap. Patients watch the ground to guide their steps. They cannot stand steadily with feet together when the eyes are closed (positive Romberg test).

E   Cerebellar ataxia is associated with disease of the cerebellum or associated tracts. The gait is staggering, unsteady, and wide-based, with exaggerated difficulty on the turns. The patient cannot stand steadily with feet together, whether eyes are open or closed.

F   Parkinsonian gait is associated with the basal ganglia of Parkinson's disease. The posture is stopped, the hips and knees slightly flexed. Steps are short and often shuffling. Arm swings are decreased and the patient turns around stiffly—"all in one piece."

(Adapted from Staab, A. S. and L. C. Hodges. [1996]. *Essentials of gerontological nursing: adaptation to the aging process.* Philadelphia: J.B. Lippincott.)

TABLE 7-8
Description of Gait Disturbances

NAME	DESCRIPTION	CAUSES
GENERAL GAIT DISTURBANCES		
• Steppage gait	Associated with footdrop and flaccidity of the leg. To compensate for footdrop, the patient lifts the upper leg high to clear the foot from floor; as a result, the foot slaps the floor.	Can be unilateral when caused by a lesion involving the external popliteal nerve. It is bilateral in cases of peroneal muscle atrophy (as in Charcot-Marie-Tooth disease) or bilateral L-5 and S-1 involvement (poliomyelitis or some polyneuropathies).
• Waddling gait	Broad base and lateral jerking movement of the hips and trunk	Weakness of the gluteal, psoas, and truncal muscles
• Hypotonic gait	Hyperextension of the knees, wide-based flail-like movements of the legs accompanied by a high step; the heel touches first, followed by the slap of the foot as the toes touch the floor.	Degeneration of the posterior columns (loss of proprioception)
SPECIAL GAIT DISTURBANCES CLASSIFIED ACCORDING TO ANATOMICAL AREAS		
• Cerebellar gait	Wide-based, staggering, lurching, and uncoordinated gait	Any disease involving the cerebellum (tumor, multiple sclerosis, Friedreich's ataxia)
• Corticospinal gaits		
Hemiplegic	Unilateral; the arm is semiflexed with the elbow held close to the waist; fingers are flexed and wristdrop is noted; the extended, spastic, stiff leg is swung in a semicircle when walking; the foot is inverted, and footdrop is evident.	Stroke
Spastic	Shuffling, with the legs stiff	Bilateral involvement of the corticospinal tract
Scissor	The legs cross, one in front of the other, with each step; the knees are brought inward; and the person often walks on toes because of the swaying motion. Bilateral condition	Severe spasticity of the adductor muscles of the legs
BASAL GANGLIA GAITS		
• Parkinsonian	Loss of automatic arm swinging is evident while walking; head and body are flexed forward; the arms are semiflexed and adducted; and the legs are rigid and flexed. A slow, shuffling gait is typical. Once walking begins, the person may propel forward with increased momentum.	Defect in the basal ganglia
• Athetoid	Sudden, wormlike movements of the arms, head, and legs which make forward progress difficult	Defect in the basal ganglia

- **Hip abductors** (**L4, L5**, S1; gluteus medius and minimus): the examiner places his or her hands on the bed on the outside of the patient's knees. The patient is instructed to spread both legs against the examiner's hands.
- **Hip extension** (L5, **S1**, S2; gluteus maximus): the patient is instructed to push the posterior thigh down against the examiner's hand, which is positioned on the posterior thigh.
- **Knee extension** (L2, **L3, L4**; quadriceps femoris): the examiner cradles the partially flexed knee and places his or her other hand on the top of the lower leg about 4 inches above the ankle. The patient is instructed to straighten the lower leg against resistance.
- **Knee flexion** (L5, **S1**, S2; hamstrings): the examiner cradles the partially flexed knee and places his or her other hand under the lower leg about 4 inches above the ankle. The patient is instructed to flex the knee against resistance.
- **Dorsiflexion of foot** (L4, **L5**; tibialis anterior): the examiner places both hands on the top of the feet with the thumbs on

the soles. The patient is instructed to pull the toes toward his or her nose.
- **Plantarflexion of foot** (**S1**, S2; gastrocnemius); the examiner places both of his or her hands on the soles of the patient's feet with the thumbs on top of the toes. The patient is instructed to "press on the gas pedal."

Gait and Posture

Gait may be evaluated with the motor examination or at the end of the cerebellar examination. **Gait** is the manner of walking, and **posture** is the position or orientation of the body in space. Any patient able to ambulate, even with assistive devices (cane, walker), should be observed walking, preferably without shoes or stockings. The examiner should be prepared to protect the patient from injury. Observe the patient walking back and forth naturally in the room. The points to note include gait (smooth or staggering); position of feet (broad based or normal); symmetry of arm and leg movement (do arms swing naturally?); presence of any un-

TABLE 7-9
Involuntary and Abnormal Movements

TYPE	DESCRIPTION	COMMENTS
Tremors	• Involuntary trembling movement of the body or limbs resulting from contraction of opposing muscles; tremors are characterized by rate, distribution, and relationship to movement.	• Seen with certain organic diseases; some forms of tremors are psychogenic in origin
• Physiologic	• The occasional tremors seen in healthy people and precipitated by extreme fatigue or stress.	
• Essential (familial, senile)	• Tremors occur when muscles are brought into action to support or move an extremity; they may also affect the jaw, lips, and head (head nods from side to side or to and fro). • Absent at rest • Tremor has characteristics similar to those of parkinsonian tremors.	• Improvement is usually noted with alcohol, sedatives, and propranolol.
• Toxic	• Tremors are caused by toxic states (*e.g.,* uremia) or ingestion of toxic substances (*e.g.,* drug withdrawal).	
• Cerebellar	• Tremors occur during movement and increase toward the end of the purposeful act.	• Caused by cerebellar lesions • May be seen in multiple sclerosis
• Parkinsonian	• These regular, rhythmic tremors are described as "pill-rolling tremors" (alternating flexion–extension of the fingers and adduction–abduction of the thumb). • Observed at rest • Associated with increased muscle tone	• Basal ganglia disorder seen in Parkinson's disease
• Resting tremors	• Tremor occurs when the patient is at rest and is diminished by purposeful activity.	
• Intentional tremors	• Tremor is increased or precipitated by purposeful activity.	
Choreiform movements	• Characterized by irregular, jerky, uncoordinated movements and abnormal posture • Represent a more generalized condition than tremors • May be evidenced by grimacing and difficulty in chewing, speaking, and swallowing • Increase with purposeful activity, making it difficult to complete the simplest of motor functions	
Clonus/myoclonus	• Sudden, brief, jerking contraction of a muscle or muscle group	
Athetosis	• Involuntary, repetitive, slow gross movements, particularly affecting posture • Arms tend to swing from a widely abducted base.	• Movements described as snakelike
Tics	• Involuntary, compulsive, stereotyped movements • Described as "nervous habits" • Repeated at irregular intervals • Often involve the face	• Often psychogenic in origin
Spasms	• Involuntary contraction of large muscle groups (arms, legs, neck)	• Oculogyric spasms, as seen in Parkinson's disease, are an example; these spasms are characterized by a fixed, upward gaze controlled by extraocular muscles.
Ballism	• More or less continuous, gross, abrupt contractions of the axial and proximal muscles of the extremities • Violent flail-like movements	• May involve one side of the body (hemiballismus) • Caused by a destructive lesion in or near the contralateral subthalamic nucleus

coordinated movements or tremors; height of step (shuffling, high, normal); and length of step (short, long, normal). Note how easily the patient can turn around and how many steps are required to turn.

Next, have the patient walk heel to toe (called **tandem walking**), walk on the toes only, and walk on the heels only.

An alternative is to ask the patient to hop on one foot and then the other. **Ataxia** is defined as incoordination of voluntary muscle action, particularly of the muscle groups used in activities such as walking or reaching for objects. Chart 7-2 and Table 7-8 list the most common gait disturbances seen with neurological conditions.

TABLE 7-10
Sensory System Assessment

SENSORY MODALITIES	DESCRIPTION/TECHNIQUE
Primary sensory modalities	
Superficial sensations	
Superficial tactile (light touch) sensation	A wisp of cotton is used as the stimulus. Patients are asked to close their eyes and signify with a word, such as "yes," when they feel a light touch. The examiner lightly touches the skin with the cotton wisp, beginning at the head and working downward. Each side of the body is assessed.
	Light touch sensation is often preserved when other sensory modalities are compromised in lesions of the spinal cord. This occurs because of an overlap of innvervation.
Superficial pain sensation	A pin or other sharp object is used as the stimulus. Care must be taken to prevent injury to the patient.
Within a few segments after entering the cord, fibers conveying pain and temperature synapse and cross the midline through the ventral commissure to the opposite lateral spinothalamic tract. This is important to note because there may be dissociation of pain and temperature loss with preservation of the ability to feel light touch.	The same systematic procedure is followed as for light touch.
Temperature sensation	Two test tubes, one filled with cold water and the other filled with warm water, are used for the stimuli. Alternate: use a cold tuning fork.
Note that the tracts conveying pain and temperature both cross to the opposite side of the spinal cord.	Following the same procedure as for light touch and pain, the patient is systematically touched and responses are noted.
Deep Sensations	
Sense of motion and position	Passive motion is tested in the upper extremities on the thumb and in the lower extremities on the big toe. The sides of the toe and thumb are lightly grasped by the examiner's index finger and thumb and moved up or down.
	Note that the thumb and toe should be touched lightly so that the pressure needed to move the appendage is not apparent to the patient.
	As the examiner moves the thumb and toe, the patient is asked to identify the direction of movement (up or down).
Deep pain	The Achilles tendon, calf, and forearm muscle are squeezed on each side of the body. Note the patient's sensitivity to the stimulus.
Vibration sensation	Using a vibrating tuning fork, place the instrument on the bony prominences (thumb and big toe).
	The patient is instructed to signal when the vibration is first felt and when it is no longer present.
	Compare the sensitivity of the two sides; compare proximal and distal portions of the same extremity. If abnormality is detected, more extensive testing is conducted.
Cortical discrimination (complex somatic sensations requiring cerebral cortex interpretation)	
Two-point discrimination	A small pair of calipers or other sharp instrument is used as the stimulus. Alternate: touch patient simultaneously or singularly.
Note: Body areas vary in sensitivity to discriminate simultaneous stimuli	The patient, with eyes closed, is simultaneously touched with two sharp objects and then asked whether he or she is being touched by one or two objects. This testing procedure continues over the surface of the body.
Point localization	The patient's skin is lightly touched at a particular point while his or her eyes are closed and is asked to identify where he or she was touched. Compare each side of the body for response.
Stereognosis	With the eyes closed, common objects, such as a pencil, comb, or coin, are placed in the patient's hand. The patient is then asked to identify the object.
Texture discrimination	With eyes closed, the patient is asked to differentiate between materials of varying textures. Each side of the body is tested and compared.

(continued)

TABLE 7-10 Sensory System Assessment Continued	
SENSORY MODALITIES	DESCRIPTION/TECHNIQUE
Traced-figure identification	The examiner traces a number or letter on the patient's palm, back, or other part of the body with his or her finger or an applicator stick; the patient is asked to identify the figure traced. Each side of the body is tested.
Double simultaneous stimulation (extinction)	Two corresponding body parts are touched simultaneously. The patient is asked to identify the area touched. The examiner notes whether the patient is aware of being touched on both sides.

Involuntary Movements

Any involuntary movements are noted. In observing for involuntary movement, consideration is given to rate (cycles per second), distribution (proximal muscles, distal muscles), and relationship to movement (increasing or decreasing with movement). Symmetrical weakness of the **proximal** muscles suggests a **myopathy**, a disorder of muscles; symmetrical weakness of **distal** muscles suggests a **polyneuropathy**, a disorder of peripheral nerves (Bates, 1995, p. 515). Common abnormalities of movement include tremors, choreiform movements, clonus, myoclonus, athetosis, tics, spasms, and ballism. Table 7-9 summarizes involuntary movements.

SENSORY SYSTEM EXAMINATION

In evaluating the sensory system, the examiner determines the patient's ability to perceive various types of sensations with the **eyes closed**. Each side of the body is compared with the other, as are sensory perceptions at the distal and proximal portions of each extremity. The testing proceeds in an orderly fashion. The body areas commonly evaluated include the face, neck, hands, forearms, upper arms, trunk, thighs, lower legs,

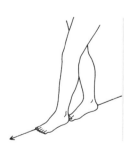

FIGURE 7-10
Assessment of cerebellar function. The integrity of the cerebellum can be tested by having the patient walk heel to toe along a line (tandem gait). With cerebellar hemispheric involvement, the patient often falls toward the side of the lesion, and there is ataxia. With midline cerebellar dysfunction, the gait is wide-based and tandem gait walking cannot be performed. (From Weber, J. [1992]. *Nurse's handbook of health assessment.* 2nd ed. Philadelphia: J. B. Lippincott.)

and feet. The perianal area is assessed only in special circumstances, such as when a sacral injury is suspected. Sensory function is rated according to the following scale:

2—normal
1—present, but diminished (abnormal)
0—absent

A detailed sensory examination is part of the **extended examination** and is undertaken when numbness, pain, trophic changes, or other sensory abnormalities are present. Although all sensory modalities are listed below, not all are tested even in an extended examination because some systems carry more than one modality. Assessing only one modality of each system is sufficient. The three main sensory systems entering the spinal cord are:

- Pain–temperature (spinothalamic tracts)
- Position and vibration (posterior columns)
- Light touch (involves both of the pathways)

Discrimination sensations involve some of the above sensory tracts, but also involve the cerebral cortex, especially the parietal lobe.

The following lists the sensory modalities with testing methods for evaluation (Table 7-10). A map of dermatomes should be used to guide the examination or to focus a detailed examination of a particular area. Usually, pain, vibration, and light touch are the modalities tested.

Superficial Sensation

- Light touch: A wisp of cotton is used to lightly touch various areas of the skin.
- Pain: An open safety pin or a broken wooden applicator is used to prick the skin. The skin is touched arbitrarily with the sharp or dull side. The bottom of the applicator or bottom of the pin is used for a "dull." (If pain sensation is intact, testing for temperature sensation is usually omitted.)
- Temperature: A tube of hot water and one of cold water are applied in succession to the same areas used in other tests. The patient is asked to identify "hot" or "cold." A cool tuning fork can also be used; it is placed on a particular part of the body and then moved to the opposite side of the body. The patient is asked if it feels the same on both sides of the body.

CHART 7-3
Major Muscle-Stretch Reflexes (Deep Tendon Reflexes)

In assessing deep tendon reflexes (DTRs), proper technique must be used to elicit an optimal response. The *briskness* of the response is noted. To remember the major DTRs, recall the ascending sequential order of $\frac{1}{2}-\frac{3}{4}-\frac{5}{8}-\frac{7}{8}$.

Achilles Reflex (S-1, S-2) (ankle jerk)

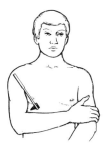

With the knee flexed, the Achilles tendon is struck; the foot should flex in a plantar direction.

Quadriceps Reflex (L-3, L-4) (knee jerk)

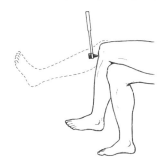

With the knee flexed, the patellar tendon is struck; the knee should extend.

Biceps Reflex (C-5, C-6)

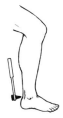

With the arm partially flexed at the elbow with palm down, the examiner's finger is placed on the biceps tendon; the examiner's finger is then struck and the stimulus is conveyed to the biceps; the elbow should flex.

Triceps Reflex (C-7, C-8)

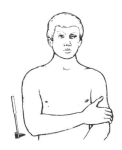

With the arm partially flexed at the elbow and the palm directed toward the body, the triceps tendon is struck above the elbow; the elbow should extend.

Deep Sensation

- Vibration: A tuning fork is placed on the bony prominence of the big toe and thumb; if the vibration is perceived, you can assume that this modality is normal in more proximal areas.
- Deep pressure pain: The Achilles tendon and gastrocnemius and forearm muscles are squeezed.
- Proprioception: The thumb and large toe are moved up or down. The patient should be able to identify "up" or "down."

Discriminative Sensation (usually, not all modalities are tested)

- Two-point discrimination: A part of the body is touched simultaneously with sharp objects to determine if one or two pricks can be felt. (The presence of receptors varies in different parts of the body.)
- Point discrimination: The patient is asked to name the location at which he or she was touched with the wooden end of an applicator or the examiner's hand.
- Recognition of shape and form: The patient is asked to identify common objects placed in his or her hand such as a key, pen, or coin. Inability to recognize objects by touch is called **astereognosis.**
- Texture discrimination: The patient is asked to differentiate among various textures (*e.g.*, silk, wool).
- Graphesthesia: A letter or number is written on the palm with a dull-pointed object; the patient is asked to identify the symbol.
- Extension phenomenon: If sensation is normal, being touched on the skin on both sides of the body simultaneously should result in both stimuli being felt.

TABLE 7-11
Major Superficial (Cutaneous) Reflexes

REFLEX	INNERVATION	TEST
Corneal	CNs V, VII	Touch cornea lightly with a wisp of cotton; lids should quickly close.
Gag	CNs IX, X	Stimulate the back of the pharynx with a tongue depressor; a retching or gagging response should be elicited.
Swallowing	CNs IX, X	Stimulate one side of the uvula with a cotton applicator; the uvula should elevate.
Upper abdominals	T8–T10	Stroke the outer abdomen toward the umbilicus using a tongue blade; the umbilicus should move up and toward the area being stroked (Fig. 7-11).
Lower abdominals	T10–T12	Stroke the lower abdomen toward the umbilicus using a tongue blade; the umbilicus should move down and toward the area being stroked (Fig. 7-11).
Cremasteric (male)	L1–L2	Lightly stroke the inner aspect of the thigh or lower abdomen; elevation of the ipsilateral testicle should occur (Fig. 7-12).
Bulbocavernous (male)	S3–S4	Apply direct pressure over the bulbocavernous muscle behind the scrotum, or pinch the glans penis; the muscle should contract, raising the scrotum toward the body.
Perianal	S3, S4, S5	Scratch the tissue at the side of the anus with a blunt instrument; there should be a puckering of the anus. Also, if a gloved finger is inserted into the rectum, a contraction should be felt.

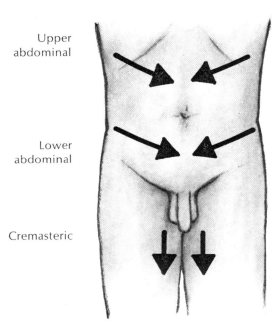

Upper abdominal

Lower abdominal

Cremasteric

FIGURE 7-11
The abdominal and cremasteric reflexes. Test the abdominal reflexes by lightly but briskly stroking each side of the abdomen and below the umbilicus in the direction illustrated. Use a key or a tongue blade to stroke the skin. Note the contraction of the abdominal muscles and the deviation of the umbilicus toward the stimulus. Obesity may mask an abdominal reflex. In this situation, use your finger to retract the patient's umbilicus away from the side to be stimulated. Feel with your retracting finger for the muscular contraction. Not routinely done. If tested the cremasteric reflex is assessed by lightly scratching the inner aspect of the upper thigh. Note the elevation of the testicle on that side. Abdominal and cremasteric reflexes may be absent in both upper and lower motor neuron disorders. (From Bates, B. 1983. *Guide to physical examination*, 3rd ed. Philadelphia: J.B. Lippincott.)

CEREBELLAR SYSTEM EXAMINATION

The following outlines the most common methods used to evaluate balance and coordination. (Gait, discussed with the motor examination, can be included at the end of the cerebellar examination). The patient is instructed to do *one* of the following in each category:

Upper Extremities

- The examiner raises his or her index finger about 2 feet and central–midface from the patient. The patient is given the instruction "With your left hand, touch my finger, then touch your nose; do this as fast as you can." Be sure that the upper arm is extended and parallel to the floor. This should be evaluated with the patient's eyes open and then closed. Repeat with other arm.
- Instruct the patient to rapidly pronate and supinate the hand in the other palm; repeat with other hand.
- Instruct the patient to rapidly tap his or her index finger on the thumb; then tap all four fingers, one at a time, against the thumb. Repeat with other hand.

If the finger-to-nose test is smooth and on the mark, further evaluation of the upper extremities is not necessary. **Dysmetria** is the inability to control accurately the range of movement in muscle action with resultant overshooting of the mark. Overshooting is also called **past-point**. The term *dysmetria* is used particularly with reference to hand movements.

Lower Extremities

- While lying on the back or sitting, the patient is instructed to move one heel down the shin of the opposite leg; repeat on the opposite side.

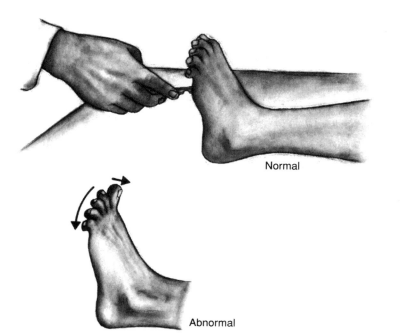

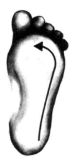

FIGURE 7-12
Babinski reflex. With a moderately sharp object, such as a key, stroke the lateral aspect of the sole from the heel to the ball of the foot, curving medially across the ball. Use the lightest stimulus that will provoke a response. Note any movement of the toes, normally flexion. Dorsiflexion of the great toe, with fanning of the other toes, indicates upper motor neuron disease.

Normal

Abnormal

• The patient is instructed to draw the number "8" with his or her foot in the air; repeat with the other foot.

Body Balance

The Romberg test assesses body balance. Ask the patient to stand erect with feet together, first with eyes open (cerebellar and visual input) then with eyes closed (cerebellar and dorsal column proprioception). To protect the patient from injury, stand beside him or her with your arms positioned to provide support should he or she begin to fall. If the patient loses balance with the eyes opened or can stand with the eyes opened but loses balance when the eyes are closed, it is a positive **Romberg's sign** and is indicative of cerebellar damage on the side to which he or she leans (Fig. 7-10).

REFLEXES

Testing the reflexes provides an important indication of the status of the central nervous system in both conscious and unconscious patients. A stimulus is mediated by a definite pathway through the receptor organ, afferent limb, spinal cord or brain stem, efferent limb, and effector organ. The reflex is modified by the simultaneous activity of other pathways, particularly the corticospinal tract. Alterations in reflexes may be the earliest signs of a pathological condition. Reflexes are classified into three categories: (1) muscle-stretch reflexes (also known as deep tendon reflexes or DTRs), (2) superficial or cutaneous reflexes, and (3) pathological reflexes.

Muscle-Stretch Reflexes

The muscle-stretch reflexes are evaluated first. These reflexes occur in response to a sudden stimulus, such as the percussion hammer that causes the muscle to stretch. Chart 7-3 lists the

major muscle-stretch reflexes tested. It is important to use the proper technique to elicit a reflex. With the muscle relaxed and the joint at midposition, the tendon is tapped directly using a percussion or reflex hammer. Normally, there is contraction of the muscle with a quick movement of the limb or structure innervated by the muscle. Both sides of the body are tested and the results are compared. The briskness of the response should also be noted. The muscle-stretch reflex ranges are graded on a scale from 0 to 4, as follows:

4+—Very brisk, hyperactive; muscle undergoes repeated contractions or clonus; often indicative of disease
3+—More brisk than average; may be normal for that person or indicative of disease
2+—Average or normal
1+—Minimal or diminished response
0—No response

Superficial Reflexes

Superficial reflexes are elicited by light, rapid stroking or scratching (depending on the tissue being tested) of a particular area of the skin, cornea, or mucous membrane. Table 7-11 lists the most common superficial reflexes tested. These reflexes are initiated by cutaneous receptors stimulated by stroking. The grading of superficial reflexes is different from the scale used with muscle-stretch reflexes. Superficial reflexes are graded as either present (+) or absent (0). If they are present but weak, they may be recorded as "weak."

Pathological Reflexes

Of the pathological reflexes, the **Babinski reflex** is the most important. The grading of pathological reflexes involves noting the presence or absence of the pathological sign. The presence of a pathological sign (+) is abnormal, whereas

CHART 7-4
Pathological (Primitive) Reflexes

Reflex	Associated Conditions
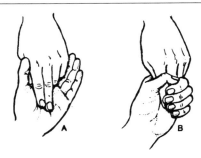 *Grasp reflex.* (A) Palmar stimulation. (B) Grasp response.	• Mostly frontal lobe disease • Sometimes occipital lobe disease • Bilateral cerebral atrophic disease (*e.g.,* Alzheimer's disease) • Bilateral thalamic degeneration • Advanced age and dementia *Note:* The reflex may be interpreted by family members and others as a voluntary act. It would be a voluntary act if the patient were able to release the grasp on command.
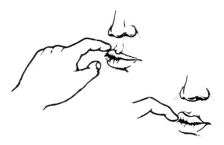 *Snout reflex.* Puckering of lips in response to gentle percussion in the oral region.	• Cerebral degenerative diseases (*e.g.,* Alzheimer's disease) *Note:* In late stages of dementia, some patients demonstrate continuous mouth and licking movements, along with pursing of the lips.
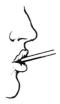 *Sucking reflex.* Sucking movement of the lips in response to tactile stimulation in the oral region	• Same as for snout reflex *Note:* The reflex may be noted when the patient is suctioned or when mouth care is administered.

absence of a pathological sign (−) is normal (Fig. 7-12). Other pathological reflexes are associated with damage to the cortical levels such as in dementia. These are termed *primitive reflexes* because they are seen in the early stages of development and subsequently disappear. If they do reappear, they are often associated with dementia. In addition to those reflexes discussed in Chart 7-4, the **palmomental reflex** can be added. This reflex, also referred to as the *palm-chin reflex*, consists of unilateral contraction of the mentalis muscle when the thenar eminence of the ipsilateral hand is stimulated briskly. When the palm at the thumb is scratched, the chin on the same side puckers toward the cheek. This reflex is more common in aging; it may or may not be associated with dementia.

A **flexion reflex**, a primitive central nervous system reflex, is a general term encompassing various polysynaptic reflexes.

Also known as the *withdrawal reflex*, it moves the limb away from the source of stimulation, thus resulting in flexion. Because the stimulus is polysynaptic, there is an after discharge in the interneuronal relays, and the motor response outlasts the stimulus. Activation of the flexor motor neurons in the leg is typically widespread, so that flexor muscles at the *ankle, knee, and hip* contract to withdraw the whole limb; this trigroup contraction is sometimes referred to as a **triple flexion** response.

References

1. Bates, B. (1995). *A guide to physical examination and history taking* (6th ed.). Philadelphia: J. B. Lippincott.
2. Evinger, L. C., Fuchs, A. F., & Baker, R. (1977). Bilateral lesions of the medial longitudinal fasciculus in monkeys: Effects on the hori-

zontal and vertical components of voluntary and vestibular induced eye movements. *Experimental Brain Research, 28,* 1–20.

Bibliography

Benton, A. L., Sivan, A. B., Hamsher, K., Varney, N. R., & Spreen, O. (1994). *Contributions to neuropsychological assessment* (2nd ed.). New York: Oxford University Press.

Fuller, G. (1993). *Neurological examination made easy.* New York: Churchill Livingstone.

Gilman, S., & Winmans, S. A. (1992). *Manter and Gatz's essentials of clinical neuroanatomy and neurophysiology* (8th ed.). Philadelphia: F. A. Davis.

Leigh, R. J. (1995). *Neuro-ophthalmology: Brainstem and cerebellar ocular motor control.* American Academy of Neurology, Annual Meeting, Seattle, WA, May 7.

Strub, R. L., & Black, F. W. (1993). *The mental status examination in neurology* (3nd ed.). Philadelphia: F. A. Davis.

Swartz, M. H. (1994). *Textbook of physical diagnosis: History and examination* (2nd ed.). Philadelphia: W. B. Saunders.

Westmoreland, B. F., Benarroch, E. E., Daube, J. R., Reason, T. J., & Sandok, B. A. (1994). *Medical neurosciences: An approach to anatomy, pathology, and physiology by systems and levels.* Boston: Little, Brown.

Willms, J. L., Schneiderman, H., & Algranati, R. S. (1994). *Physical diagnosis: Bedside evaluation of diagnosis and function.* Baltimore: Williams & Wilkins.

CHAPTER 8

Neurological Assessment

Joanne V. Hickey

The purposes of this chapter are (1) to provide an overview for establishing and updating a database for a hospitalized neuroscience patient; and (2) to provide a framework for understanding the purpose, organization, and interpretation of data from the systematic neurological assessment conducted at the bedside. Some content that appears in Chapter 7 has been also included in this chapter for the convenience of the reader.

ESTABLISHING A NURSING DATABASE

When admitting a patient, the nurse begins to collect a comprehensive database by completing a nursing admission history and general admission assessment prior to conducting a neurological assessment. Most nursing departments have adopted a special format for this purpose as part of their documentation system. The data may be entered in a written format or typed into a computerized documentation system. Regardless of how the data are entered or stored, the database is the foundation for ongoing assessment, planning, implementation, and evaluation of care and practice. The database is key to maintaining continuity of care as the patient moves through the various levels of care and to planning for discharge care and follow-up.

One section of the database includes demographics, route and circumstances of admission, vital signs, weight, and other general information (glasses, hearing aid, etc.). The largest section pertains to the comprehensive systematic assessment often based on body systems or functional patterns. The circumstances of admission affect data collection. Ideally, the nurse has an opportunity to interview the patient and family on admission. The interview is not only a mechanism for gathering data and dispensing information but also an opportunity to establish a good working relationship with both patient and family. If the patient is unable to provide information, a family member may be able to help.

Throughout the interview, the nurse should be alert for any misconceptions or misunderstandings held by the patient or family. Information should be corrected and clarified as necessary and appropriate referrals made. There often is a section that collects data for early identification of patients and families at high risk for problems that will have a negative effect on recovery, such as drug abuse or frequent readmissions in the past. By identifying high-risk indicators, they can be addressed early through appropriate referrals and interventions.

For a patient with altered consciousness or a personality change, it is helpful to talk with the family to learn about the patient's personality prior to the current illness. This baseline information detailing the patient's usual behavior and personality is very useful for future comparison throughout the course of hospitalization. In the event of an emergency admission, some of the data gathering will be postponed until the patient is stabilized or family can be reached. As soon as possible, the nurse should interview the patient and family to develop a written or computerized plan of care. If care maps are used, the appropriate care map should be reviewed and modified as necessary.

OVERVIEW OF NEUROLOGICAL ASSESSMENT

Purposes

Nursing management of the neurological patient is based upon highly developed nursing assessment and clinical reasoning skills. The nurse must know what parameters to assess, the proper technique for assessment, the appropriate method of documentation, and how to interpret the data to decide what action, if any, should be taken. Critical thinking skills are inherent in this process, both to detect subtle and obvious changes in the neurological examination and clinical condition, and to incorporate such information into the context of the overall patient profile. Well-developed critical thinking skills are the foundation for all patient management decision making.

The purposes of the care nurse's neurological assessment are different, in some respects, from those of neurological assessments conducted by the physician, the advanced practice nurse functioning in an expanded role, and other health professionals. The purposes of the neurological assessment conducted by the care nurse are to

- Identify the presence of nervous system dysfunction
- Determine the effects of nervous system dysfunction on activities of daily living and independent function
- Detect life-threatening situations
- Establish a neurological database for the patient
- Compare data to previous assessments to determine change, trends, and needed interventions
- Provide a database upon which nursing diagnoses will be based

A baseline assessment of neurological signs is made so that deviations and trends can be noted. A comparison is made between data derived from the current assessment and previously collected data in order to determine if neurological signs are stable, deteriorating, or improving. These data also provide the basis for denoting trends over time in making judgments about clinical progress. Changes in neurological signs may be rapid and dramatic or very subtle, developing over a period of hours, days, weeks, or even months.

There are a variety of sources from which information about the patient's neurological status can be derived, including the nursing admission history and comprehensive assessment, nurses' notes, neurological assessment sheets, and intershift nurses' reports. Other parts of the medical record are also a rich source of data that should be reviewed. In addition, the family can contribute a wealth of information about the patient's behavior and functional level before hospitalization.

Parameters of Neurological Assessment

The components to be included in a neurological assessment depend on the extent of assessment conducted (complete or focused), the patient's state of consciousness, and the frequency of the assessment. A **comprehensive neurological examination** has been discussed in Chapter 7 and includes level of consciousness including cognitive function; cranial nerve function; motor function; sensory function; cerebellar function; and reflexes.

If the patient's condition and circumstances of admission allow, the complete assessment may be conducted at the time of admission to establish a baseline. However, in practice it may be necessary to do a **problem-focused neurological examination** on a particular part or parts of the nervous system because of a functional change and the need for more in-depth data.

A **neurological assessment** is focused on selected critical components that are sensitive to change and that provide an overview of the patient's overall condition. The nurse must decide what other components, if any, should be added to best monitor the patient's condition. An assessment in the intensive care unit for an unconscious patient is quite different than the assessment in an intermediate care unit for a patient who is recovering from a stroke. This neurological assessment generally includes

- Level of consciousness (orientation and cognition)
- Pupillary signs
- Motor function (hand grasps, pronator drift, leg movement)

FREQUENCY OF ASSESSMENT AND DOCUMENTATION

The frequency and extent of the neurological assessment will depend on the stability of the patient and the underlying condition. For a stable patient who is doing well, an assessment may be ordered every 4 to 8 hours. However, a patient who is very unstable may warrant assessment every 5 to 15 minutes to monitor changes and the need for intervention. The nurse should use his or her independent clinical judgment to assess the patient more frequently or expand the assessment to include more parameters.

Most facilities use a standardized neurological assessment sheet or computerized assessment template to document neurological parameters. Sometimes, it is necessary to add a narrative description to expand upon the data recorded or to add other pertinent information to the data set. Most forms or computer documentation systems allow for these important entries.

The neurological assessment is the core nursing database for identifying nursing diagnoses and for planning nursing interventions. The accuracy of these assessment data and the nurse's critical thinking skills to identify change, interpret its significance, and take appropriate action form the foundation of neuroscience nursing practice.

ASSESSMENT OF CONSCIOUSNESS

Consciousness is a state of general awareness of oneself and the environment and includes the ability to orient toward new stimuli. It results from the integrated activities of numerous neural structures including the reticular formation. Difficulties in the assessment of consciousness arises as a result of the subjective evaluation of a person's appearance and behavior. Consciousness has traditionally been divided into two components:

- **Arousal** and **wakefulness**, which is concerned with the patient's appearance of wakefulness
- **Content** or **cognition**, which includes the sum of cerebral mental functions[1]

The content of consciousness is largely a cerebral cortical function, whereas arousal requires both the cerebral hemispheres and the upper brain stem.

Consciousness can be viewed as analogous to a double helix. The difficulties inherent in assessing altered consciousness and underlying pathological states, then, can be compared with the difficulty of trying to separate the strands of a double helix into distinct entities. As a result, consciousness terminology and concepts tend to be somewhat vague. For example, the level of arousal is described by terms such as *clouding of consciousness, drowsiness, obtundation, stupor,* or *coma,* and is assessed by evaluating the content of consciousness, especially as represented by the quality of the patient's perception of self and the environment. Because consciousness cannot be measured directly, it is estimated by observing behavioral indicators in response to stimuli. Consciousness is the most sensitive indicator of neurological change; as such, a change in the level of consciousness is usually the first to be noted in neurological signs. Consciousness is a dynamic state that is subject to change; it can occur rapidly (within minutes) or very slowly, over a period of hours, days, or weeks. When an assessment is conducted, the patient's arousability and behavior merely provide an estimate of consciousness at a given point in time.

Anatomical and Physiological Basis of Consciousness

The reticular formation (RF) is a complex network of nuclei and nerve fibers in the central tegmental portions of the brain stem, extending from the pyramidal decussation in the medulla to the basal forebrain area and thalamus. It was once believed that the central group of reticular nuclei composed the major part of the **ascending reticular activating system** (ARAS) which caused arousal when activated. The ARAS receives synaptic input from multiple sensory pathways and sends rostral impulses to the thalamus and then to the whole cerebral cortex. The nuclei that compose the system begin in the lower brain stem (medulla) and proceed through the pons, midbrain, and thalamus. From the reticular nucleus of the thalamus, fibers project to all parts of the cerebral cortex, and they can activate the cerebral cortex independent of specific sensory systems (Fig. 8-1). Thus, an increase in the level of sensory stimulation results in increased neuronal activity and heightened arousal and alertness.

It is now known that there are at least two more systems that contribute to arousal and consciousness in addition to the central thalamocortical fibers of the ARAS. The first tract ascends through the hypothalamus to influence basal forebrain structures including the limbic system. This pathway includes histamine secreting neurons which participate in arousal.[2] The second pathway is composed of axons of serotonergic neurons of the midbrain raphe nuclei and the norepinephrine neurons of the locus ceruleus, both of which provide a diffuse, widespread innervation of the neocortex. Raphe nuclei are active in deep sleep. The largest group of central noradrenergic neurons is the **locus ceruleus,** found in the pontomesencephalic junction rostral and lateral to the facial and trigeminal motor nuclei. The cells have long dendrites and receive afferent fibers from many parts of the central nervous system (CNS). The efferent fibers of the locus ceruleus travel rostrally in the central tegmental tract and medial forebrain terminating in the hypothalamus, forebrain, and basal ganglia. These three pathways are responsible for arousal and consciousness.

The reticular activating system (RAS) is a physiological entity rather than a localized anatomical system. Neurons of

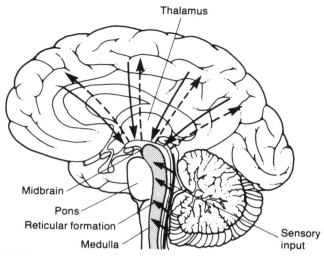

FIGURE 8-1
Reticular activating system.

the RF form a very diffuse interrelated system. Neurons of the RAS extend their dendrite fibers over large areas, providing for overlapping of fibers and an intermingling of dendrites with ascending and descending myelinated and unmyelinated bundles. This unique structure creates multiple opportunities for stimulation by collaterals coming from every major somatic and special sensory pathway, as well as from adjacent brain stem nuclei cranial nerves V through XII. The ARAS is essential for arousal from sleep, wakefulness, focusing of attention, perceptual association, and introspection.

Alterations in Consciousness
DEGREE OF DYSFUNCTION

Alteration of consciousness can vary in severity from slight to severe. An altered level of consciousness indicates brain dysfunction or brain failure. The longer the duration and the more severe the dysfunction, the less the chance of complete recovery. The change can occur rapidly, as is the case with an epidural hematoma, or very slowly over a period of weeks, as is the case with a chronic subdural hematoma in an elderly person.

MAJOR CAUSES

Alterations in the level of consciousness may occur because of

- Direct destruction of the anatomical structures of consciousness by a disease process
- Alterations in the energy substrates necessary for function of the anatomical structures involved in consciousness
- Toxic effects of endogenous or exogenous substances on the structures

COMA

Various states of altered consciousness will be discussed. However, a few points should be made about coma. Coma is the result of bilateral, diffuse cerebral hemispheric dysfunction or involvement of the brain stem (midbrain and pons, which includes the ARAS) or both. A focal hemispheric lesion (*e.g.*, small brain tumor) will not result in coma; only diffuse hemispheric conditions (*e.g.*, diffuse cerebral edema) result in coma. Coma is not a disease itself, but reflects some underlying disease processes involving either (1) primary CNS problems or (2) metabolic or systemic conditions. The following is a summary of the major causes of altered consciousness.[3]

Supratentorial Lesions. A lesion must affect the cerebral hemispheres **directly and widely** to cause diffuse bilateral cerebral hemispheric dysfunction and subsequent coma. Common lesions and associated secondary cerebral edema that can have diffuse effects on the brain include subcortical destructive lesions such as a thalamic lesion; hemorrhagic lesions (intracerebral, epidural, subdural hematomas); infarctions; tumors; abscesses; and head injuries.

Subtentorial (Infratentorial) Lesions. Subtentorial lesions **directly compress or destroy** the neurons of the RAS that lie in the central gray matter of the diencephalon, midbrain, and upper pons. Common compression lesions and associated secondary cerebral edema include basilar artery aneurysms; posterior fossa subdural or epidural hemorrhage; and cerebellar hemorrhage, abscess, tumor, or infarction. Common destructive lesions include pontine hemorrhage and brain stem infarction.

Metabolic Disorders. Altered consciousness may also be attributable to metabolic causes and systemic disease, such as deprivation of oxygen and other key metabolic requirements (hypoxia, ischemia hypoglycemia, or vitamin deficiency). It may also be caused by disease of organs excluding the brain, such as the following:

- Nonendocrine organs
  Kidney (uremic coma)
  Liver (hepatic coma)
  Lungs (carbon dioxide narcosis)
  Pancreas (exocrine pancreatic encephalopathy)
- Hypofunction or hyperfunction of endocrine organs
  Thyroid (myxedema and thyrotoxicosis)
  Parathyroid (hypoparathyroidism and hyperparathyroidism)

Adrenals (Addison's disease, Cushing's disease, pheochromocytoma)
Pancreas (diabetes mellitus and hypoglycemia)
- Electrolyte and acid–base imbalance
- Pharmacological agents
  Sedatives: barbiturates and nonbarbiturates, hypnotics, tranquilizers, ethanol, opiates, and bromides
  Acidic toxins: paraldehyde, methyl alcohol, ethylene glycol, and ammonium chloride
  Psychotropic drugs: amphetamines, lithium, tricyclic antidepressants, and others
  Other drugs: such as steroids, cimetidine, salicylates, anticonvulsants

The most common metabolic causes of altered consciousness seen in a hospitalized population are hypoxia, hypoglycemia, and sedative drug overdose. It is routine practice in most emergency departments to draw blood for glucose levels and toxicology screening, as necessary.

In assessing a comatose patient, the nurse should be aware that several problems outside the CNS can cause a decreased level of consciousness. A comparison of the changes that accompany coma caused by metabolic disorders and those occurring with nervous system structural lesions is summarized in Table 8-1.

Level of Consciousness

ASSESSMENT

The level of consciousness is assessed by applying stimuli and observing the response. The technique used depends on the type of stimuli applied. Auditory and tactile stimuli are the two used to assess consciousness and are considered on a continuum (Fig. 8-2).

Auditory Stimuli. Sound is the stimulus that is applied first. A normal speaking voice is used initially. If the patient responds, then the nurse can talk to the patient and ask questions to assess orientation and response to questions (discussed in the next section). If the patient does not respond to a normal voice volume, a louder voice or a loud noise, such as that produced by clapping the hands, is used. If a response is elicited, the nurse can then assess orientation by asking questions.

TABLE 8-1
Comparison of Coma Caused by Metabolic and Central Nervous System Structural Lesions

OBSERVATION	METABOLIC COMA	CNS STRUCTURAL COMA
Motor system deficits	**Diffuse** abnormal motor signs (tremors, myoclonus, and, especially, asterixis); symmetrical	**Focal** abnormal signs that are unilateral; asymmetrical
Motor abnormalities	Coma **precedes** motor abnormalities	Coma **follows** motor abnormalities
Pupils	Bilaterally **reactive**	Unilaterally nonreactive, or later, bilaterally **nonreactive**
Progression of neurological deterioration	**Partial** dysfunction affects many levels of the CNS while other functions are retained	**Orderly** rostral–caudal deterioration with supratentorial lesions
Electroencephalogram	**Diffusely** but not locally slow	May be slow, but will also show abnormal **focal** areas

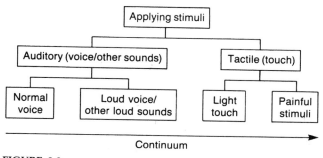

FIGURE 8-2
Assessment of consciousness: Applying stimulation.

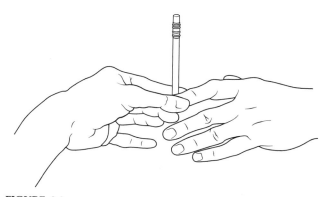

FIGURE 8-3
Applying pressure to the fingernails is one kind of stimulus used in assessing the patient's level of consciousness.

Tactile Stimuli. If there is no response to auditory stimulation, tactile stimulation is attempted. The patient's arm is gently shaken while calling his or her name. If no response is elicited by this means, painful (noxious) stimuli is applied.

The most common method of applying painful stimuli is to apply firm pressure to the nail beds (fingernails, toenails) then observe the motor response (Fig. 8-3). This is a peripheral stimuli; the response elicited could be a reflex response. A central stimuli such as pinching the trapezius muscle or grasping the pectoralis major are other methods for providing painful stimuli. The response elicited by a central stimulus is a more reliable and valid indicator of actual function in comatose patients. Some practitioners suggest using the "sternal rub" (vertically rubbing the tissue along the sternum). However, the soft tissue above the sternum bruises easily in most people. Applying supraorbital pressure is another form of stimulus. It is not recommended, especially if there is a possible facial fracture.

Motor response to painful stimuli is classified according to the following categories:

Purposeful: withdraws from the painful stimuli and crosses midline; may push the examiner's hand away (seen in light coma)
Nonpurposeful: the stimulated limb moves slightly, without any attempt to withdraw from the source of pain; painful stimuli to the pectoralis or trapezius may result in a contraction of a muscle or muscles, such as the quadriceps or biceps, but the arm does not cross midline
Unresponsive: patient shows no signs of reacting to painful stimuli (seen in deep coma)

IDENTIFYING THE LEVELS OF CONSCIOUSNESS

There is no internationally accepted taxonomy of definitions with which to label levels of consciousness, nor is there agreement on the definitive manifestations of the various stages of consciousness. Therefore, no precise terminology exists for conveying information about a patient from one clinician to another. This creates confusion in accurately assessing patients. As a result, the Glasgow Coma Scale is used universally to decrease the subjectivity and confusion associated with assessing level of consciousness.

Despite the problems with precise terminology, there are several commonly used terms in the literature to describe altered consciousness. These are included here to complete the discussion of this confusing problem, as an accurate description of the patient's behavior, motor response, pupillary signs, and vital signs is essential in monitoring neurological status.

For purposes of this discussion, consciousness can be viewed as a crude continuum, with full consciousness as the anchor on one end and deep coma as the anchor on the opposite end (Fig. 8-4). The following terms, although subject to a variety of definitions and interpretations, appear quite often in the literature and are frequently used in clinical discussion of patients:

Full consciousness: awake, alert, and oriented to time, place, and person; comprehends the spoken and written word and is able to express ideas verbally and/or in writing
Demonstrates reliable and responsible behavior
Confusion: disoriented in time, place, or person; initially becomes disoriented to time, then to place, and, finally, to person; shortened attention span; memory difficulty is common; becomes bewildered easily; has difficulty following commands; exhibits alterations in perception of stimuli; may have hallucinations; may be agitated, restless, irritable, and increasingly confused at night
High risk for injury (falls); requires special nursing management, including frequent observations

Full consciousness	Confusion	Lethargy	Obtundation	Stupor	Coma		
					Light coma	Coma	Deep coma

FIGURE 8-4
Continuum of consciousness. Arousal/wakefulness includes a wide range of levels that can be conceptualized as a crude continuum with "full consciousness" as the anchor on one end and "deep coma" as the anchor on the other end.

Side rails and perhaps a jacket restraint may be necessary to prevent injury

Lethargy: oriented to time, place, and person; very slow and sluggish in speech, mental processes, and motor activities

High risk for injury (falls, slips, spilling of hot liquids)

Needs increased supervision; cannot anticipate needs quickly; needs stimulation

May need a jacket restraint; side rails should be up

Obtundation: readily arousable with stimulation; responds verbally with a word or two; can follow simple commands appropriately when stimulated (*e.g.*, when asked to stick out tongue); otherwise appears very drowsy

High risk for injury; side rails and perhaps a jacket restraint are necessary

Needs frequent observation and supervision

Unable to assume any responsibility

Stupor: lies quietly with minimal spontaneous movement; generally unresponsive except to vigorous and repeated stimuli to which incomprehensible sounds and/or eye opening may be noted; responds appropriately to painful stimuli

High risk for injury; side rails and perhaps a jacket restraint may be necessary

Needs frequent observation and supervision

Unable to assume any responsibility for self

Coma: appears to be in a sleeplike state with eyes closed; does not respond appropriately to body or environmental stimuli; does not make any verbal sounds; differentiation of coma is based on motor responses (purposeful, nonpurposeful, or unresponsive)

High risk for injury and aspiration

Needs a standard of care appropriate for the comatose patient

A priority of care is maintaining a patent airway.

Confusion exists in describing the comatose state because of variations in the definition of coma and the inability to measure consciousness directly. Some authors classify coma according to depth by correlating motor responsiveness (purposeful, nonpurposeful, and unresponsive) to painful stimuli with deterioration in level of consciousness. As described previously, the RAS is a diffuse system within the brain stem and cerebral hemispheres with multiple connections among motor, sensory, and reticular systems. Most clinicians will attest that there are gradations of coma, based on motor responsiveness to painful stimuli, which are helpful in evaluating a patient's neurological condition in the clinical setting.

For the purposes of this discussion, **coma** is defined as a sustained pathological state of unconsciousness that results from dysfunction of the ARAS. Coma can be divided into three gradations: light coma (sometimes called semicoma), coma, and deep coma. The labels attached to each level are not universally accepted and thus are open to discussion. The critical element in each description is the response to painful stimuli:

Light coma (semicoma): unarousable; no spontaneous movement noted; withdraws purposefully to painful stimuli; usually, the brain stem reflexes, such as the gag, corneal, and pupillary reflexes, are intact.

Coma: unarousable; withdraws nonpurposefully to painful stimuli; brain stem reflexes may or may not be intact; decorticate or decerebrate rigidity may be present.

Deep coma: unarousable; unresponsive to painful stimuli; brain stem reflexes are generally absent; decerebrate rigidity is usually present.

THE GLASGOW COMA SCALE

The **Glasgow Coma Scale** (GCS), developed in Glasgow, Scotland in 1974, is widely used in the United States and internationally for assessment of comatose patients. The scale was developed to standardize observations for the objective and accurate assessment of level of consciousness. The GCS is especially useful for monitoring changes during the first few days after injury or in unstable comatose patients.

The scale is divided into three subscales: eye opening, best verbal response, and best motor response (Fig. 8-5). Within each subscale are a variety of categories. The information collected is plotted on a graph to provide a visual record of deterioration, improvement, or stabilization. In interpreting the GCS, the numerical values of each subscale are added for a total score. The range of possible scores is 3 to 15. A score of 15 indicates a fully alert, oriented person, whereas a score of 3, the lowest possible score, indicatives deep coma. Patients with a score of 7 or less are considered comatose, thus requiring a standard of nursing care appropriate for an unconscious patient.

CHANGES IN LEVEL OF CONSCIOUSNESS

Changes in the level of consciousness are, to some extent, predictable in that a patient who has been in a coma and now is arousable with repeated stimulation is described as displaying improvement in level of consciousness. Clinicians frequently say "The patient appears to be lighter." What they are actually implying is that the deteriorated level of consciousness appears to have improved since the last examination or the overall trend is one of improvement.

The various stages of consciousness are arranged on a crude continuum that aids the clinician in assessing changes in the patient's condition. It is possible, and indeed probable, that all of the levels of consciousness are not observable in particular patients as they recover from injury.

A few final points concerning the level of consciousness should be kept in mind:

1. A patient with a head injury who is evaluated during the posttraumatic period may arrive at an extended plateau of consciousness in the recovery process. For example, a patient can be comatose for a period of time and then become restless and agitated. This state may persist for days before it is followed by full consciousness. The pattern of recovery is based on the type, extent, and site of the injury and secondary injuries.

2. If the patient is sedated for agitation with very short-acting drugs such as propofol, turn off the drug 5 to 10 minutes before assessing the patient so that the drug response will not cloud the assessment.

3. It is important to record the time of observation of postoperative patients who have undergone intracranial sur-

Scoring of Eye Opening

- • 4 Opens eyes spontaneously when the nurse approaches
- • 3 Opens eyes in response to speech (normal or shout)
- • 2 Opens eyes only to painful stimuli (*e.g.,* squeezing of nail beds)
- • 1 Does not open eyes to painful stimuli

Scoring of Best Motor Response

- • 6 Can obey a simple command, such as "Lift your left hand off the bed"
- • 5 Localizes to painful stimuli and attempts to remove source
- • 4 Purposeless movement in response to pain
- • 3 Flexes elbows and wrists while extending lower legs to pain
- • 2 Extends upper and lower extremities to pain
- • 1 No motor response to pain on any limb

Scoring of Best Verbal Response

- • 5 Oriented to time, place, and person
- • 4 Converses, although confused
- • 3 Speaks only in words or phrases that make little or no sense
- • 2 Responds with incomprehensible sounds (*e.g.*, groans)
- • 1 No verbal response

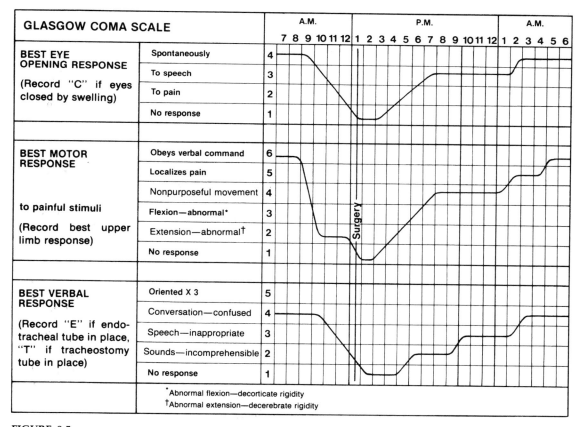

FIGURE 8-5
Glasgow coma scale.

gery. It makes a great difference whether there is a 1-hour or 4-hour interval between observations that indicate how rapidly the neurological status of the patient might be changing following surgery.

4. Recovery from an altered level of consciousness is influenced by age, type of injury, and premorbid health status. Younger patients (especially under 20 years) have a much better prognosis for recovery than do older patients.

5. The longer the coma, the worse the outcome. Absence of corneal, gag, pupillary, or oculocephalic responses initially or during the course of illness indicates a poor outcome. Decortication, decerebration, or flaccidity of the motor system also denotes a poor prognosis.

Special States of Altered Consciousness

According to Plum and Posner, nearly all comatose patients begin to awaken from their comatose state within 2 to 4 weeks after injury, regardless of the severity of brain damage, if they survive at all.[4] Once a sleep–wakefulness cycle has been reestablished, the patient is no longer comatose, even though there is no apparent awareness of or interaction with the environment. A few special states of altered consciousness are seen and discussed in the clinical setting and in the literature. These special states include persistent vegetative state, locked-in syndrome, brain death, and dementia. See Chart 8-1 for a description of the special states of altered consciousness.

Cognition

ASSESSMENT

Consciousness has been conceptualized as having two components: arousal and content. Arousal has already been discussed in the previous section. **Content** represents the sum of cognitive and affective function and is controlled by the cerebral cortex. As part of the assessment of level of consciousness, the nurse assesses orientation to time, place, and person. However, this provides limited information about the patient's overall cognitive function. Therefore, in the awake patient, the nurse conducts a cognitive assessment, or mental status examination, to determine the effect of neurological disease on the patient's ability to function in day-to-day living.

There are several areas to address in cognitive assessment (see Chap. 7). The following list includes the major areas covered in a mental status assessment, organized hierarchically:

- Orientation to time, place, and person
- Attention and vigilance (the ability to sustain attention over a period of time), as well as the ability to focus and concentrate on a task which requires self-regulation and screening out of distracting environmental stimuli
- Memory (short-term and long-term)
- Language—demonstrating an understanding of the written and spoken word, as well as the ability to use language appropriately (*e.g.*, identifying any difficulty with word finding or misuse of words)

- General fund of information
- Construction ability (ability to draw and copy on command)
- Sequencing activities
- Problem solving
- Abstraction
- Insight and judgment
- Special integrative skill deficits such as agnosias and apraxias

ASSESSMENT OF COGNITIVE FUNCTION AT THE BEDSIDE

In clinical practice and critical thinking, the question is how much of the cognitive (mental status) examination should be conducted and how frequently should particular parameters be assessed. The answer is, "it depends." It depends on the type of clinical setting and the need to monitor certain parameters. In the acute care hospital, especially in the intensive care environment, the level of consciousness is so depressed that assessing higher level function is impossible. As the patient begins to regain consciousness, an abbreviated bedside assessment will help the clinician to determine progress. For example, asking the patient to show you two fingers is a simple command that requires understanding of the spoken word and the motor ability to respond to the command. The following is a sample of questions that can be asked at the bedside to assess cognitive and motor function:

- What is the name of this place?
- What is the date?
- Show me two fingers.
- Stick out your tongue.
- Look toward me.
- Wiggle your thumb or toes.
- How much is a quarter, a dime, and a nickel?

Some cognitive functions are assessed within the context of providing care and observing the patient during activities of daily living (ADLs). Deficits may be obvious because of their impact on ADLs. Higher-level deficits may be more subtle because the patient may appear to be functional, having devised ways to compensate for deficits. Collaborative efforts with occupational therapy and possibly neuropsychology can be very beneficial in identifying the particular problems and developing interventions. The nurse documents findings and develops nursing diagnoses and interventions to assist the patient in relearning skills. The major nursing diagnosis for cognitive deficits is **altered thought processes**, a broad category that requires further delineation into specific nursing diagnoses. Chart 8-2 offers additional information on nursing management.

Standardized instruments such as the Mini-Mental Status Exam[5] may also be used to assess cognitive function. The Rancho Los Amigos Scale (Chap. 14) is another useful tool for determining behavioral patterns and includes interventions for various behavioral patterns.

RECOVERY AND REHABILITATION

Some improvement in cognitive function is often evident during the course of acute hospitalization owing to the natural recovery of the brain. The major amount of natural

CHART 8-1
Special States of Altered Consciousness

Persistent Vegetative State

Vegetative state is a term used to describe a subacute or chronic condition that usually occurs following severe cerebral injury. When the condition lasts for a month, it is called **persistent vegetative state (PVS).** Other terms formerly used to describe the vegetative state were *coma vigil* and *irreversible coma.*

Discussion about the definition and clinical course of PVS has been a topic of intense interest in the last few years and has raised many ethical questions about quality of life. In 1989, the American Academy of Neurology published guidelines on the vegetative state.* The Multi-Society Task Force on PVS has built on their work.

The Multi-Society Task Force on PVS defines the **vegetative state** as a clinical condition of complete unawareness of the self and the environment, accompanied by sleep–wake cycles, with either complete or partial preservation of hypothalamic and brain stem autonomic functions. In addition, patients in a vegetative state:†

- Show no evidence of sustained, reproducible, purposeful, or voluntary behavioral responses to visual, auditory, tactile, or noxious stimuli
- Show no evidence of language comprehension or expression
- Show no bowel or bladder control
- Cannot experience pain
- Demonstrate variable patterns of preserved cranial nerve and spinal reflexes (*e.g.,* pupillary light response, corneal, gag); primitive reflexes (*e.g.,* grasping, sucking)
- Maintain vital signs and spontaneous respirations
- Have open eyes and spontaneous eye movement. Sometimes the patient's eyes appear to follow people in the room; however, he or she is unable to follow a command to look in a particular direction.

Further, **PVS** is defined as a vegetative state present 1 month after acute traumatic or nontraumatic brain injury or lasting for at least 1 month in patients with degenerative or metabolic disorders or developmental malformations.

The clinical course and outcome of PVS depend on its cause. The Task Force identifies three categories of disorder that can cause PVS:‡

- Acute traumatic and nontraumatic brain injuries
- Degenerative and metabolic brain disorders
- Severe congenital malformations of the nervous system

Recovery of consciousness is unlikely or rare for both adults and children in the following situations:

- Posttraumatic PVS after 12 months
- Nontraumatic PVS after 3 months
- Degenerative metabolic disorders or congenital malformations after several months

The life expectancy of all PVS patients is substantially reduced; survival ranges from 2 to 5 years; survival beyond 10 years is very unusual.

PVS presents special ethical, moral, and legal issues that will be discussed in Chapter 4.

Locked-in Syndrome

The **locked-in syndrome** refers to a state in which full consciousness and cognition are intact but severe paralysis of the voluntary motor system makes movement and communications impossible.§† The usual cause is the interruption of the descending corticobulbar and corticospinal tracts at or below the pons; however, breathing is left intact. The locked-in syndrome can also be associated with peripheral motor neuron disease or paralysis produced with neuromuscular blocking drugs. Patients with this version of the locked-in syndrome can usually establish simple communications through eye blinking and vertical eye movement. The locked-in syndrome may be

(continued)

CHART 8-1 Special States of Altered Consciousness (Continued)

Locked-in-Syndrome (Continued)

seen in certain cerebrovascular diseases with ventral pontine infarction and such conditions as myasthenia gravis and poliomyelitis. The diagnosis is established by clinical examination.

Brain Death

Brain death is a state of irreversible loss of both cortical and brain stem activity.‖ It is characterized by irreversible coma and apnea; all brain stem reflexes and cranial nerve function is lost. The diagnosis of brain death is made based on requirements in three areas:¶

- Absence of brain stem reflexes
- Absence of cortical activity
- Demonstration that this state is irreversible

Criteria have been established for the diagnosis of brain death but are still controversial. These criteria and their implications for nurses in managing the patient and family are discussed in Chapter 14.

Dementia

Dementia is a progressive and permanent decline in global cognitive functions without a reduction in arousal. Advanced dementia may progress until the patient looses self-awareness and all evidence of learned behavior. Such a total decline results in a vegetative state.# The causes of dementia are many, including primary organic disorders of the cerebral cortex or hemispheres owing to diffuse injuries or degenerative disorders. Occasionally, the condition may be partially reversed, as in the case of normal pressure hydrocephalus or vitamin deficiency. However, dementia usually implies an irreversible disorder in which the person's ability to function independently and assume responsibility for self is seriously impaired or absent.

* American Academy of Neurology. (1989). Position of the American Academy of Neurology on certain aspects of the care and management of the persistent vegetative state patient. *Neurology, 39,* 125–126.
  † Multi-Society Task Force on PVS. (1994). Medical aspects of the persistent vegetative state (Part 2). *New England Journal of Medicine, 330*(22), 1572–1579.
  ‡ Multi-Society Task Force on PVS, p. 1573.
  § Plum & Posner, 1980; American Academy, 1989.
  ‖ Barnat, J. L., Culver, C. M., Nelson, J. R., et al. (1981). On the definition of death. *Annals of Internal Medicine, 94,* 389–395.
  ¶ Barnat et al.; President's Commission for the Study of Ethical Problems in Medicine and Biomedical and Behavioral Research. (1981). *Defining death: Medical, legal, and ethical issues in the determination of death.* Washington, DC: U.S. Government Printing Office.
  # Multi-Society Task Force on PVS. (1994). Medical aspects of the persistent vegetative state (Part 1). *New England Journal of Medicine, 330*(21), 1499–1509, p. 1503.

---

recovery occurs in the first 3 to 6 months after injury; recovery can still occur after this time, but at a much slower rate. Many patients will have persistent cognitive deficits that will require cognitive rehabilitation. Nurses identify cognitive deficits, document the findings, and develop appropriate interventions. In most hospitals, the occupational therapist can perform a short (approximately 30 minutes) cognitive assessment screening to determine areas affected by cognitive deficits. If necessary, a neuropsychologist can conduct a detailed cognitive assessment to pinpoint deficits and develop a treatment program. Often, a consultation with the neuropsychologist is postponed to allow for natural recovery. Specific patient management will depend on the overall assessment. Some patients will be referred for short-term cognitive rehabilitation in an in-house program, whereas others may be offered outpatient treatment.

NURSING IMPLICATIONS FOR ALTERED CONSCIOUSNESS

The nursing implications for accurate assessment can be derived from the previous discussion. There is no specific nursing diagnosis at present that captures the concept of altered arousal. Charts 8-3 and 8-4 list selected nursing diagnoses that are often associated with the patient with altered conscious-

CRANIAL NERVE ASSESSMENT

Occasionally, the nurse may be required to conduct a complete assessment of the 12 cranial nerves at the time of admission to establish a baseline (see Chap. 7 for the complete cranial

CHART 8-2
Nursing Management of the Patient With an Altered Level of Consciousness

The following are some basic management points for a patient with altered level of consciousness (LOC):

1. **Maintaining a patent airway is a top priority.** The patient should not be left lying on his or her back because of the increased possibility of aspiration. Position to facilitate drainage of oral secretions.

2. A change in the LOC is the **most sensitive indicator of neurological change** and, therefore, the first neurological sign to change when there is an alternation in neurological status. The LOC should be assessed periodically (as often as every 5 to 10 minutes in the acute, unstable patient and every 4 hours in the stable patient). Regardless of all the technological advances in healthcare, the observations of the nurse who knows the patient are still the most sensitive "sensors" of neurological changes. The nurse who is well acquainted with the personality and behavior pattern of the patient can best evaluate whether behavior changes are caused by pain, fatigue, or neurological deterioration. The nurse has the responsibility of advising the physician of changes in the LOC.

3. When the LOC has deteriorated, the nurse should talk to the patient in a calm, normal, reassuring voice, explaining in simple terms what is being done and orienting him or her to the environment. If the patient normally wears glasses or a hearing aid, they should be worn.

4. When talking to the patient, the nurse should try to screen out external environmental stimuli that might increase confusion. Also, a group of people entering the room and talking to the patient can be both overwhelming and confusing. In essence, it creates a sensory overload for the fragile recovering neurological circuits and can result in confusion and misinterpretation of stimuli.

5. Once patients begin to awaken and verbalize, they often recognize a void of time for which they cannot account. This can be very frightening. The nurse should fill the gaps of time by briefly recounting what has happened during the lapse. Also, when the patient begins to make incorrect statements, the nurse should matter-of-factly correct any misconceptions.

6. The nurse is responsible for **protecting the patient from injury.** As the LOC deteriorates, the nurse must assume total responsibility for the patient's safety. The methods employed depend on the availability of staff (usually fewer staff on evenings and nights), the patient's degree of agitation and impulsive behavior, the location of his or her room in relationship to the nurses' station, and the use of supportive equipment (ventilator, CVP and IV lines, ICP monitoring catheter, and others). Regardless of the circumstances, the standard of care for this patient requires much more nursing time and intervention than that required for an alert, oriented patient. The nurse should observe the patient frequently; talk in a calm manner; maintain the bed in low position, unless contraindicated; maintain all siderails in up position; and use restraints as necessary to protect the patient from injury, according to hospital policy.

7. Nighttime and darkness often lead the patient to misinterpretation of environmental and other stimuli. A night light and periodic visits by the nurse can help to control confusion, fear, and hallucinations.

8. The family and other visitors need instruction about how to visit a patient with altered LOC or cognitive functions. The specific guidelines will depend on the particular patient. The nurse should be available to intervene if problems occur during the visit, as well as to evaluate the effects of the visit on the patient and the visitors. If the patient is upset, the possible reasons for the reaction should be explored. Family members may need support after the visit to express their concerns and fears.

nerve assessment). Another complete cranial nerve assessment may be necessary at critical points during hospitalization when change is anticipated, such as postoperatively.

In the real world of clinical practice, the cranial assessment is, however, often abbreviated. There are two reasons for this. First, the patient may not be able to cooperate by following specific commands (*e.g.*, smile; stick out the tongue) or by reporting subjective changes in neurological function (*e.g.*, double vision). The inability to cooperate or to participate is often the result of altered consciousness (*e.g.*, coma) or cognitive/perceptual deficits. Second, after a comprehensive as-

sessment, it is often appropriate to tailor the assessment to the patient's specific condition.

Such tailoring implies an understanding of the pathophysiology of the specific condition and the need to monitor specific functions that are at high risk for dysfunction. For example, a patient who is admitted with a diagnosis of an acoustic neuroma (a tumor involving the eighth cranial nerve) requires assessment of cranial nerve VIII function to determine hearing loss and vertigo. Assessment of function would also be required for cranial nerve V (sensory loss to the face), cranial nerve VII (deficits in motor function of the

---

CHART 8-3
*Nursing Diagnoses Associated
With Altered Levels of Consciousness*

The following nursing diagnoses are often
identified for the patient who has an altered level
of consciousness caused by neurological
problems:

- Risk for injury
- Risk for aspiration
- Noncompliance
- Health maintenance, altered
- Elimination pattern, altered: bowel and bladder
- Physical mobility, impaired
- Self-care deficits, complete
- Home maintenance management, impaired
- Nutrition, altered, less than body requirement
- Communication, impaired, verbal
- Airway clearance, impaired
- Sleep pattern disturbance
- Thought processes, altered
- Sensory perception, altered
- Individual coping, impaired

---

face), and cranial nerves IX and X (loss of gag reflex or difficulty speaking). The reason for assessment of these cranial nerves is their anatomical proximity in the posterior fossa to cranial nerve VIII (the location of the acoustic neuroma). As the tumor grows, it may impinge on a number of adjacent cranial nerves, causing dysfunction. Because consciousness is usually not affected by an acoustic neuroma, the patient is able to cooperate with the assessment. By contrast, assessment of these cranial nerves is usually deferred in a patient with a frontal brain tumor.

Table 8-2 summarizes the components of cranial nerve assessment as conducted in actual clinical practice (see also Chap. 7). Pupillary signs are of particular importance in cranial nerve assessment and can be assessed in all patients regardless of level of consciousness or ability to cooperate. Other cranial nerves can be tested at the bedside for conscious, responsive patients. Still other cranial nerves can be tested in both conscious and unresponsive patients, using alternate techniques. The following sections describe these practical bedside techniques.

ASSESSMENT OF VISUAL FIELDS (OPTIC NERVE)

The visual field can be easily and quickly assessed for a conscious, cooperative patient at the bedside. This is done by asking the patient to focus on your nose and then introducing a varying number of fingers with both hands simultaneously into the bilateral upper quadrants; repeat in the bilateral lower quadrants (see Chart 7-1). You can quickly ascertain whether the patient has full visual fields or gaps in the visual fields

such as those that occur with neglect of one side. If a deficit is noted, further assessment may be necessary.

ASSESSMENT OF PUPILS (OCULOMOTOR NERVE)

Examination of pupil function is an extremely important part of patient assessment that can be carried out in either a conscious or unconscious patient. The general points to note when assessing the pupils include their size, shape, and reaction to light. Accommodation is **not** evaluated in every assessment. The findings in one pupil are always compared to the findings in the other pupil, and differences between the two are noted. Data are documented in the neurological database.

Size. Normally, the pupils are equal in size, measuring about 2 to 6 mm in diameter with an average diameter of 3.5 mm. Two methods are used to record pupillary size: the millimeter scale (most common) and descriptive terms.

If the millimeter scale is used, the examiner, using a diagrammatic gauge, estimates the size of each pupil by comparing the gauge with the patient's pupils (Fig. 8-6). This assessment is carried out for each pupil. The examiner then records a numerical value ranging from 2 to 9 mm to signify the size of each pupil.

If descriptive terms are used to evaluate the size of the pupils, the following terms are used: pinpoint, small, midposition, large, and dilated (Chart 8-5).

Shape. Normally, both pupils are round. Shape is assessed simply by looking at the contour of the pupils. Abnormal pu-

---

CHART 8-4
*Nursing Diagnoses Associated
With Altered Cognitive Function*

The following nursing diagnoses are often
identified for the patient who has alterations in
cognitive function caused by neurological
problems:

Major Nursing Diagnosis

- Thought processes, altered (including memory,
  planning, the perception of relationships,
  problem solving, abstraction, recognition of
  consequences of action, etc.)

Associated Nursing Diagnoses

- Sensory perception, altered
- Knowledge deficit
- Social interaction, impaired
- Personal identity disturbance
- Individual coping, impaired
- Adjustment, impaired
- Knowledge deficit
- Conflict, decisional

TABLE 8-2
Summary of Cranial Nerve Assessment at the Bedside

CRANIAL NERVE	ASSESSMENT	COMMENTS
I Olfactory	**Sense of smell** Usually deferred	Deficits noted in only a few cases, usually with lesion in the parasellar area
II Optic	**Vision** Monitor while working with patient; observe for difficulty with ADLs Ask patient to identify how many fingers are being held up or to read menu or newspaper Use Rosenbaum Pocket Vision Screener to assess vision in each eye Monitor for visual field cuts by checking upper and lower quadrants while patient focuses on your nose	Common deficits; deficits can cause blindness in one eye, bitemporal hemianopsia, or homonymous hemianopsia
III Oculomotor	**Pupil constriction; elevation of upper eyelid** Assess size, shape, and direct light reaction of pupils	Changes are common with a number of progressing neurological problems
III Oculomotor, IV Trochlear, & VI Abducens	**Extraocular movement** Tested together in conscious, cooperative patient; ask patient to follow a pencil tip through the six cardinal eye movement	Deficits are common; inability to move the eyes in one or more directions is called strabismus
V Trigeminal	**Sensation to face; mastication muscles** Often deferred If assessed, patient must be cooperative and able to accurately report facial sensation to stimulation **Afferent limb of corneal reflex**	Deficits found in trigeminal neuralgia and sometimes with acoustic neuroma Corneal reflex assessed in trigeminal neuralgia; can assess reflex in unconscious patient
VII Facial	**Muscles for facial expression; efferent limb of corneal reflex** In cooperative patient, ask him or her to smile, show teeth, puff cheeks, wrinkle brow; observe for symmetry of face In a comatose patient, tickle each nasal passage, one at a time, by inserting a cotton-tipped applicator; observe for facial movement	Total unilateral facial weakness called Bell's palsy Unilateral from below the eye and down, seen in stroke Note the difference between central and peripheral facial involvement
VIII Acoustic	**Hearing and balance** Usually deferred May note deficit while working with patient	Deficits with acoustic neuroma, cerebellar pontine angle tumors, Meniere's disease
IX Glossopharyngeal and X Vagus	**Palate, pharynx, vocal cords, and gag reflex;** tested together because of overlap In conscious patient, have patient open mouth and say "ah"; assess gag reflex Unconscious patient: assess gag reflex	Deficits common in posterior fossa lesions Gag reflex is a brain stem reflex and has prognostic value in unconscious patient
XI Spinal Accessory	**Shrug shoulders and move head side to side** Usually deferred	Deficits common in posterior fossa lesions
XII Hypoglossal	**Movement of tongue** In conscious patient, ask him or her to stick out the tongue	Deficits common in posterior fossa lesions

Note: *This table summarizes* **assessment at the bedside.** *Although a baseline assessment of all cranial nerves is recommended, this may not always be possible. In addition, whereas frequent assessment of particular cranial nerves is critical in certain conditions, it may be safely deferred in other conditions.*

pil shapes may be described as ovoid, keyhole, or irregular (Chart 8-6).

Reaction to Light. When light is shone into the eye, the pupil should immediately constrict. Withdrawal of the light should produce an immediate and brisk dilation of the pupil. This is called the **direct light reflex** (Fig. 8-7). Introducing the light into one pupil should cause similar constriction to occur simultaneously in the other pupil. When the light is withdrawn from one eye, the opposite pupil should dilate simultaneously. This response is called the **consensual light reaction.**

Pupillary reaction to light is recorded using descriptive terms or symbols (Chart 8-7). The descriptive terms that are used include brisk, sluggish, and nonreactive or fixed. Plus and minus signs are recorded if a symbol recording system is used. (Common abnormal pupillary responses and findings are found in Chart 8-8. Refer also to Chap. 7 for more information on pupillary assessment.)

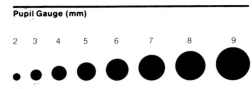

Pupil Gauge (mm)

2   3   4   5   6   7   8   9

FIGURE 8-6
Pupil gauge.

ABNORMALITIES

Nursing Assessment. Assessing the size and shape of the pupils and the direct light reaction are ways of gathering data about the condition of important selected intracranial structures that are known to respond in particular ways in the presence of brain dysfunction. The nurse must interpret what is observed to decide what action, if any, should be taken. As these signs are checked, the following questions should be asked:

- What do I see?
- What does it mean?
- How does it relate to previous assessments?
- How am I going to proceed?

The third question, "How does it relate to previous assessments?" is important because data are compared with the previous baseline assessments to denote change. The assessment can reveal no change, subtle change, or dramatic change from previous findings. Generally, a change of any kind is important to note because it is indicative of an intracranial change.

A change in any of the parameters included in the neurological assessment must be considered in conjunction with changes in other areas evaluated in the assessment. For instance, a rapidly developing hematoma or cerebral edema can affect other aspects of the assessment, such as the level of consciousness and motor function. If, however, the pupil appears to be dilated and fixed (a new finding from the last assessment) and the patient continues to be well oriented and maintains motor function, then the pupillary signs should be rechecked.

Assessment of Extraocular Movement (Oculomotor, Trochlear, and Abducens Nerves)

Extraocular movement and the position of the eyeballs are assessed; some modifications must be made in assessing an unconscious patient. The oculocephalic reflex is not usually assessed by the nurse. In the normal healthy person, one would expect the following:

- The eyes move conjugately in the orbital sockets.
- The eyes blink periodically.
- No nystagmus or abnormal eye movement is noted.
- The eyeball neither protrudes nor is sunken in the orbits.
- The upper eyelid does not droop and the palpebral fissures are equal bilaterally.

These are the established normal criteria that guide the assessment of ocular movement in the patient. Some of the data are collected simply through focused observation of the patient for 10 to 15 seconds. Appropriate technique is required to elicit other data.

ASSESSMENT OF THE CONSCIOUS, COOPERATIVE PATIENT

The Eyeballs. The position of the eyes within the sockets is assessed by observing the eyes frontally, in profile, and from above the patient's head. If no abnormality is noted, most clinicians will not comment about position in the documentation.

- Abnormal protrusion of one or both eyeballs is termed **proptosis or exophthalmos**.
- Abnormal recession of one or both eyelids is termed **enophthalmos**.

The Eyelids. The patient is asked to look straight ahead; observations of each eye are made and compared. The width of each palpebral fissure is observed. The palpebral fissure is the space between the upper and lower eyelid. Next, the position of the eyelid in relation to the pupil and iris is evaluated. Normally, the lid slightly covers the outer margin of the iris. A narrowed palpebral fissure usually indicates a droopy eyelid, also known as **ptosis**. Ptosis is seen in Horner's syndrome and conditions that affect the oculomotor nerve, such as transtentorial herniation syndromes and myasthenia gravis with ocular involvement.

Note the presence of edema of the eyelids. Edema can result from trauma to the orbit and may occur in the upper eyelid, the lower eyelid, or both.

Movement of the Eyes. Extraocular movement is assessed in conscious patients by asking them to follow a pencil or the examiner's finger through the six cardinal directions of gaze in an "H" sequencing (Fig. 8-8; see Fig. 7-3). Inability to move either eye in any one of the six cardinal directions should be noted. When both eyes move in the same direction at the same speed and maintain a constant alignment, the gaze is termed **conjugate gaze**. A lack of parallelism between the two visual axes or movement in opposite directions is called **dysconjugate gaze** or **strabismus**. If the dysfunction is limited to a specific movement or movements, an ophthalmoplegia is present. **Ophthalmoplegia** is defined as paralysis of one or more eye muscles (see Table 7-5 for a summary of ophthalmoplegias).

The patient is asked whether double vision, **diplopia**, is noticed when focusing in a particular direction. When a patient moves the eyes in a certain direction, visual images fall on the retina in different points, rather than on the same point on each retina. This lack of parallelism can cause double vision when the patient focuses in a particular direction.

Abnormal Movements. The patient is asked to focus straight ahead and then to follow the examiner's finger through the six cardinal directions. Any abnormal eye movements should be noted. **Nystagmus** is defined as involuntary movement of an eye, which may be horizontal, vertical, rotary, or mixed in direction. The tempo of the movements can be regular, rhyth-

CHART 8-5
Nursing Assessment of Pupillary Size

In assessing pupillary size using either descriptive terms or a gauge, each pupil is assessed individually and then the findings for each pupil are compared. This is very important because pupils are normally equal (see note on anisocoria).

Descriptive Term	Definition	Findings
Pinpoint	The pupil is so small that it is barely visible or appears as small as a pinpoint.	Seen with opiate overdose, pontine hemorrhage, ischemia.
Small	The pupil appears smaller than average but larger than pinpoint.	Seen normally if the person is in a bright room; also seen with miotic ophthalmic drops, opiates, pontine hemorrhage, Horner's syndrome, bilateral diencephalic lesions, and metabolic coma.
Midposition	When the pupil and iris are observed, about half of their diameter is iris and half is pupil.	Seen normally; if pupils are midposition and nonreactive, midbrain damage is the cause.
Large	The pupils are larger than average, but there is still an appreciable amount of iris visible.	Seen normally if room is dark; may be seen with some drugs, such as amphetamines; glutethimide (Doriden) overdose; mydriatics; cycloplegic agents; and some orbital injuries.
Dilated	When the pupil and iris are observed, one is struck by the largeness of the pupil with only the slightest ring of iris, which is barely visible.	Abnormal finding; bilateral, fixed, and dilated pupils are seen in the terminal stage of severe anoxia–ischemia or at death.

Note: **Anisocoria** is the term used to describe inequality in size between the pupils. About 17% of the population has slight anisocoria without any related pathological process. It is, therefore, important to make a baseline assessment of pupillary size and compare subsequent assessments with the baseline. If pupillary inequality is a new finding, it should be reported. If the patient is admitted with slight pupillary inequality and no other abnormalities are detected on the neurological assessment, the pupil inequality may not be significant.

mical, pendular, or jerky, with the movement having a fast and slow component. Nystagmus can result from several different problems. If nystagmus is present, the nurse should document the characteristics of the movement and include any information on circumstances that seem to cause the nystagmus (*e.g.*, focusing the eye in a certain direction). Specific types of nystagmus are discussed in Chapter 7. Periodic blinking is normal and expected. The nurse should assess blinking by observing the patient. In some conditions, such as Parkinson's disease, blinking is decreased.

ASSESSMENT OF THE COMATOSE PATIENT

General Observations. The comatose patient usually appears to be in a sleeplike state, with or without the eyes closed. If the eyes are closed, the eyelids can gently be raised to inspect the position and movement of the eyes. The eyes may assume a prolonged stare without any discernible movement, or they may move slowly from side to side. Absence of any movement usually indicates that the eye movement center in the brain stem is not functioning. This is a poor prognostic sign. Con-

CHART 8-6
Nursing Assessment of Pupillary Shape

Descriptive Term	Definition	Findings
Round	Like a circle	• Normal finding
Ovoid	Slightly oval "ovoid"	• Almost always indicates intracranial hypertension and represents an intermediate phase between a normal pupil (round) and a fully dilated fixed pupil; an early sign of transtentorial herniation
Keyhole	Like a keyhole	• Seen in patients who have had an iridectomy (excision of part of the iris). An iridectomy is often part of cataract surgery, a common procedure in the elderly population. (The reaction to light is very slight.)
Irregular	Jagged	• Seen in Argyll–Robertson pupils and with traumatic orbital injuries

versely, slow movement from side to side usually indicates an intact brain stem.

The Eyelids. After the eyes are inspected, the eyelids are released. It should be noted whether the lids slowly cover the eyes. This point is noteworthy when a differentiation between feigned coma and true coma is being made. In coma, the eyelids close slowly once they are released; in the hysterical patient, the eyes will close quickly.

Eye Movement. Because the patient is not conscious, eye movement cannot be assessed voluntarily. However, to determine whether the brain stem and the brain stem center for eye movement are intact, the **oculocephalic reflex (doll's eye phenomenon)** can be assessed by the physician (Fig. 8-9). If the oculocephalic response is inconclusive, the **oculovestibular reflex (cold caloric)** can be assessed, provided there are no contraindications (see Fig. 6-12). This is a more sensitive test of brain stem function. These are not routine reflexes that are assessed with neurological signs. The physician may choose to evaluate these reflexes in some patients to determine brain stem function for prognostic purposes or as part of brain death criteria.

FREQUENCY OF ASSESSING EYE MOVEMENT

Ocular movement parameters do not change as rapidly as other parameters of the neurological assessment. The nurse should assess eye movements once during a shift and more

often if indicated. Nursing diagnoses associated with eye movement deficits include:

• Sensory perception, altered, visual (major)
• Risk for injury

Assessment of Facial Movement (Facial Nerve)

If the examiner wishes to assess the facial nerve in the conscious, cooperative patient, the patient is asked to smile and show his or her teeth while the examiner observes for symmetrical bilateral facial movements. In the unconscious patient, the easiest and quickest way to assess the facial nerve is to tickle each nostril of the nose with a cotton-tipped applicator. The patient will wince in response to the stimulation and the facial muscles will contract; the examiner can determine whether there is symmetrical, bilateral facial movement.

Selected Reflexes

The corneal and gag reflexes, both brain stem reflexes, can be assessed in both the conscious and unconscious patient. These brain stem reflexes are helpful in determining the intactness of the brain stem. In the conscious patient or unconscious patient, touch each cornea with a wisp of cotton and observe for a blinking action. Another way to check the corneal reflex in an unconscious patient is to drop a small amount of water or

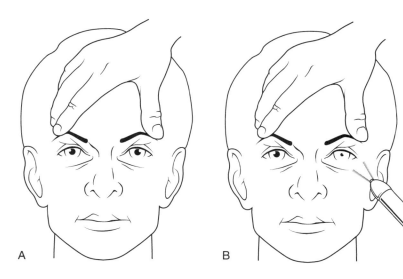

FIGURE 8-7
Evaluating pupillary reactions by checking pupil size (*A*) and reaction to light (*B*).

saline (from a plastic ampule used for instillation while suctioning) onto the cornea. If the reflex is intact, the eye will blink. Recall that the corneal reflex is mediated by cranial nerves V and VII.

To assess the gag reflex in the conscious patient, ask the patient to stick out his or her tongue so that a cotton-tipped applicator can be used to touch the posterior pharynx on each side. For an unconscious patient, a cotton-tipped applicator can be inserted into the mouth and the posterior pharynx touched on each side to illicit a gag response. Recall that the gag reflex is mediated by cranial nerves IX and X. Checking these reflexes provides excellent data about brain stem function.

MOTOR ASSESSMENT

Assessment

The motor assessment is conducted in an orderly fashion, beginning with the upper limbs and proceeding to the neck and trunk and, finally, to the lower extremities. Limb evaluation proceeds from proximal to distal.

The purposes of the neurological assessment are different from those of the neurological physical examination, which includes a detailed examination of the motor system. The neurological assessment provides a baseline from which to denote change. A sampling of a few key muscles or muscle groups provides a good indicator of function and change. Based on the patient's particular problem and deficits, other muscles can be monitored to determine change. In the neurological assessment, the motor assessment usually focuses on the arms and legs.

Noting changes in motor function helps the nurse to consider the patient's functional level and the effect on independence in ADLs. Deficits in motor function may indicate the need for adaptation of activities or assistive devices to meet the patient's individual needs.

The technique used to evaluate motor function depends on the patient's level of consciousness. In the conscious and alert patient, the assessment can be conducted by observing responses to directions such as "Squeeze my hands." The aphasic or apraxic patient may have difficulty following directions.

In an unconscious patient or one who is unable to participate, the nurse must rely on special testing techniques and observations for data. The basic approach to assessment of motor function is detailed in Chart 8-9. A few additional points will help to guide the assessment process. In assessing motor function, the following should be considered: (1) muscle size, (2) muscle tone, (3) muscle strength, (4) presence of involuntary movement, and (5) posture and gait, if appropriate for the patient's condition. When one muscle or muscle group is assessed, it is always compared with the same muscle or group on the opposite side of the body for symmetry.

Muscle Size and Tone

The muscle or muscles are observed for their size and palpated at rest and then during passive movement for tone. Abnormalities in muscle tone include spasticity, rigidity, and flaccidity.

Spasticity refers to increased resistance to passive movement, often more pronounced at the extremes of range of motion and usually followed by a sudden or gradual release of resistance. Spasticity is caused by injury to the corticospinal system. **Clasp-knife spasticity** is increased resistance with a sudden release at the end of extension.

Rigidity is a state of increased resistance. **Cogwheel rigidity** is a series of ratchet-like, small, regular jerks that are felt on passive flexion or extension. **Lead-pipe rigidity** is resistance that persists throughout extension and flexion.

Flaccidity refers to decreased muscle tone or **hypotonia**. The muscle is weak, soft, and flabby and fatigues easily.

Decortication and decerebration, special states of muscle tone seen in some unconscious patients, require more detailed explanation.

MUSCLE TONE IN THE UNCONSCIOUS PATIENT

In the unconscious patient, muscle tone can be assessed by guiding the extremities through passive range of motion. Rigidity, flaccidity, and spasticity can be noted by these simple maneuvers.

CHART 8-7
Nursing Assessment of Pupillary Light Responses

Descriptive Term	Symbol	Findings
Brisk	++	Normal finding
Sluggish	+	Found in conditions that cause some compression of the oculomotor (III) nerve; seen in early transtentorial herniation, cerebral edema, and Adie's pupil
Nonreactive or fixed	–	Found in conditions that include compression of the oculomotor nerve; seen with transtentorial herniation syndromes and in severe hypoxia and ischemia (terminal stage just before death)
Swollen closed	c	One or both eyes are tightly closed because of severe periorbital edema; the pupillary light reflex may be difficult to assess.

One other response—the Hippus phenomenon—is included; this does not usually appear on assessment sheets but may be observed in the clinical area and, therefore, needs to be recorded.

| Hippus phenomenon | None | With uniform illumination of the pupil, dilation and contraction are noted. This may be considered normal if pupils are observed under high magnification. The Hippus phenomenon is also observed in patients who are beginning to experience pressure on the third cranial nerve. This is often associated with early transtentorial herniation. |

Note: On some pupillary assessment sheets, other symbols are used in place of descriptive terms.

Unconscious patients can exhibit abnormal muscle tone or motor responses that appear as stereotyped postures and are initiated by noxious stimuli. The particular posture assumed varies according to the anatomical level of injury and motor tract interruption. This response results from rostral-to-caudal deterioration, which can occur when a hemispheric lesion extends into the midbrain or when a midbrain or upper pons lesion is present.

Decortication and Decerebration. Noxious stimuli can initiate rigidity and abnormal posture if the motor tracts are interrupted at specific levels. These abnormal postures are called *decortication* and *decerebration.* In some instances, either posture may be apparent without the application of noxious stimuli. Decortication and decerebration are indicative of cerebral damage at a certain level, as well as change in the patient's condition. The particular posture or stereotypic movement assumed by the patient differs depending on the anatomical level of injury.

Decortication, sometimes called *abnormal flexion response,* is characterized by flexion of the arms, wrists, and fingers, with adduction in the upper extremities and extension, internal rotation, and plantar flexion in the lower extremities (Fig. 8-10A). Simply stated, decortication is hyperflexion of the upper extremities and hyperextension of the lower extremities. Lesions of the cerebral hemispheres or internal capsule cause decorticate posturing by interrupting the corticospinal pathways.

Decerebration, sometimes called *abnormal extensor response,* includes adduction and hyperpronated arms, with stiffly extended legs and plantar flexion of the feet (see Fig. 8-10B). When fully developed, it may also include opisthotonus (tetanic spasms that arch the back with backward flexion of the head and feet). Stated simply, decerebration is hyperextension of both upper and lower extremities. This response results in rostral-to-caudal deterioration, which can occur when a diencephalic lesion of the hemisphere extends, thereby causing midbrain or upper pontine damage. (Both the midbrain and pons are brain stem structures.)

Intermittent Decortication and Decerebration. If there is a difference in an ischemic response or an injury between the deep cerebral hemispheric structures and upper brain stem, variations in adequate blood supply to these regions may cause intermittent decortication or decerebration. There may also be variations in adequate blood supply from the left to the right side on the structure. The patient can change from bilateral decerebration to bilateral decortication (or vice versa), from unilateral decerebration to unilateral decortication, or from one side of the body that is decorticate while the other side is decerebrate. Both decerebration and decortication are poor prognostic signs, although decerebration is a more ominous sign than decortication. Onset of either position or a change from decorticate to decerebrate posture must be reported immediately because this is an ominous sign of extension of the lesion into the upper brain stem.

CHART 8-8
Common Abnormal Pupillary Responses

Oculomotor Nerve Compression

Observation

One pupil (R) is larger than the other (L), which is of normal size. The dilated pupil (R) does not react to light, although the other pupil (L) reacts normally. A ptosis may be seen in the dilated pupil.

Interpretation

A dilated, nonreactive (fixed) pupil indicates that the controls for pupillary constriction are not functioning. The parasympathetic fibers of the oculomotor nerve control pupillary constriction. The most common cause of interruption of this function is compression of the oculomotor nerve, usually against the tentorium or posterior cerebral artery.

The compression of the oculomotor nerve is caused by a lesion, such as a hematoma, tumor, or cerebral edema, on the same side of the brain as the dilated pupil. This causes downward pressure so that the uncus of the temporal lobe herniates, trapping the oculomotor nerve between it and the tentorium.

Bilateral Diencephalic Damage

Observation

Upon examination, the pupils appear small but equal in size, and both react to direct light, contracting when light is introduced and dilating when light is withdrawn.

Interpretation

The sympathetic pathway that begins in the hypothalamus is affected. Because both pupils are equal in size and respond equally to light, the damage is bilateral. Therefore, it can be assumed that there is bilateral injury in the diencephalon (thalamus and hypothalamus).

Because metabolic coma can also result in bilaterally small pupils that react to light, this diagnostic possibility must be ruled out.

Horner's Syndrome

Observation

One pupil (L) is smaller than the other (R), although both pupils react to light. The eyelid on the same side as the small pupil droops (ptosis). There may be a sweating deficiency (anhidrosis) on the same side of the face as the ptosis. The collective symptoms of a small reactive pupil, ptosis, and anhidrosis are called *Horner's syndrome.*

Looking at the Patient

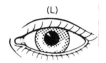

(R)   (L)

Ptosis

Action

Check assessments from previous data, compare. If the dilated pupil is a new finding, it should immediately be reported to the physician because the process of rostral-caudal downward pressure must be treated without delay. It would be expected that changes would also be apparent in the level of consciousness, motor function, and other parameters of the neurological assessment.

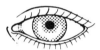

Action

These findings should be compared to previous assessments to determine whether this is a new development. The possibility of metabolic coma should be considered by reviewing blood electrolyte and blood glucose levels. For example, diabetic acidosis may result in a metabolic coma because of a high blood glucose level.

A review of blood chemistry values is particularly important if the patient is a recent emergency admission, for whom an adequate history may not have been collected. If the small, reactive pupils are a new finding, this information should be reported.

(R)   (L)

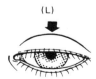

(continued)

CHART 8-8 Common Abnormal Pupillary Responses (Continued)

Oculomotor Nerve Compression

Interpretation

There is an interruption of the ipsilateral sympathetic innervation to the pupil that can be caused by hypothalamic damage (posterior or ventrolateral portion), a lesion involving the lateral medulla or the ventrolateral cervical spinal cord, and, sometimes, occlusion of the internal carotid artery.

Midbrain Damage

Observation

Both pupils are at midposition and are nonreactive to light.

Interpretation

When the pupils are midposition in size and nonreactive, neither sympathetic nor parasympathetic innervation is operational. This finding is often associated with midbrain infarction or transtentorial herniation.

Pontine Damage

Observation

Very small (pinpoint), nonreactive pupils are seen.

Interpretation

Most often, this finding indicates hemorrhage into the pons, a very grave occurrence as the pons controls many motor pathways and vital functions. Bilateral pinpoint pupils may also occur with opiate drug overdose, so this possibility should be ruled out.

Dilated Unreactive Pupils

Observation

Both pupils are dilated and nonreactive (fixed).

Interpretation

This finding is characteristic of the terminal stages of severe anoxia, ischemia, and death. Since atropine-like drugs will cause dilated pupils, this possibility must be ruled out. In addition, an intact ciliospinal reflex can produce momentary bilateral dilation.

Looking at the Patient

Action

If this is a new finding, it should be reported.

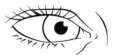
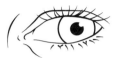

Action

The pupils should be evaluated in conjunction with other neurological assessments. The change in pupil size and reaction should be reported if this represents a new finding.

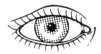
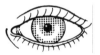

Action

Report this finding if it is new. The prognosis for patients with pontine damage is grave. Other changes in neurological status, such as a decreased level of consciousness and respiratory abnormalities, would also be expected.

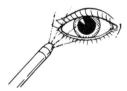

Action

Emergency action is necessary to reverse the anoxic state and prevent death. Oxygen therapy at high concentrations and a patent airway must be ensured to provide oxygen for the ischemic cerebral cells. Other signs and symptoms of neurological deterioration would be present.

- Hand grasps ("Squeeze my fingers hard.")
- Pronator drift ("Extend your arms in front of you.")

Lower Extremities

- Leg movement ("Wiggle your toes.")
- Dorsiflexion ("Pull your toes up.")
- Plantarflexion ("Step on the gas.")

The various techniques for assessing these functions in the upper and lower extremities of the conscious and comatose patient are included in Chart 8-9. Other muscles of interest can be added. For the patient who has some weakness in the arms, an alternative is to ask the patient to bend his or her arms at the elbows and position the forearms parallel to the floor. Rotate one forearm around the other. The weaker arm will have difficulty clearing the other arm and will hit the stronger arm. For weak lower legs, an alternative is to ask the patient to wiggle his or her toes.

In the **unconscious patient**, muscle strength is surmised through alternate techniques.

Upper Extremities. The unconscious patient is first observed for spontaneous movement as he or she lies in the bed. A noxious stimulus is then applied to elicit a motor response. *Note:* Apply a noxious stimulus centrally rather than peripherally. An example of a central stimulus is pinching the pectoralis major muscle. A peripheral stimulus, such as pressing on the nailbed, may result in a reflex response. Observe for withdrawal of the arm on the stimulated side. A purposeful response will be evident if the arm crosses the midline as it attempts to withdraw from the noxious stimulus. To assess each arm for paresis, place the patient in a neutral supine position. Position the forearms perpendicular to the bed, holding the patient's arms upright by the hands or wrists. The movement of both arms is then observed as the extremities are released simultaneously. A paralyzed or paretic arm will fall more quickly than an intact arm. The weaker arm may strike the patient's face as it falls.

Lower Extremities. Observe for spontaneous movements. Apply a noxious stimulus to observe for any movement. Although often impractical, the legs can be assessed for paralysis or paresis. The patient is positioned flat on the back with the knees flexed so both feet are flat on the bed. The knees are simultaneously released and the movement of the legs is observed. The paralyzed or paretic leg will fall to an extended position with the hip outwardly rotated. The normal leg will maintain the flexed position for a few moments and then gradually assume its previous position.

INVOLUNTARY MOVEMENT, POSTURE, AND GAIT

The presence of involuntary movements, such as tremors, choreiform movements, myoclonus, athetosis, tics, spasms, or ballism, is noted (see Table 7-9). **Posture** is the position or orientation of the body in space; **gait** is the manner of progression in walking. First, the patient's position while he or she is lying in bed is observed. Next, if weight bearing and ambulation are possible,

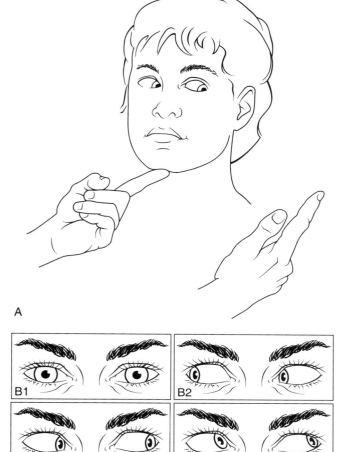

FIGURE 8-8
Extraocular movements.

MUSCLE STRENGTH

In the **conscious, cooperative patient**, muscle strength is assessed by active, passive, and active resistive movements. What muscle should be assessed as part of the abbreviated neurological assessment at the bedside? In the conscious patient, assess the following.

Upper Extremities

- Biceps ("Make a muscle.")
- Triceps ("Push me away.")

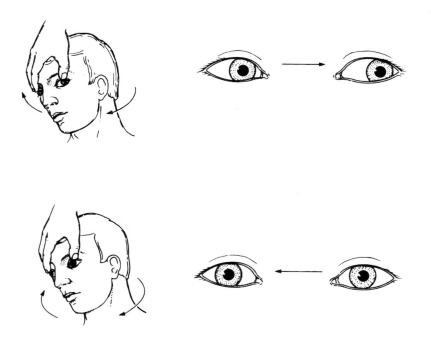

Assessment Technique for the Oculocephalic Reflex

1. Briskly rotate the head from side to side, or
2. Briskly flex and extend the neck.

Findings

1. When the head is rotated, the eyes should move in the direction opposite to the head movement. (If the head is rotated to the left, the eyes appear to move to the right.)
2. When the neck is flexed, the eyes appear to look upward; when the neck is extended, the eyes look downward.
3. When the doll's eye reflex is absent, the eyes do not move in the sockets and thus follow the direction of passive rotation.

   Loss of the oculocephalic reflex in the comatose patient indicates a severe lesion at the pontine–midbrain level of the brain stem.

FIGURE 8-9
Oculocephalic reflex. Eye movement in the unconscious patient can be assessed by the physician by means of the oculocephalic response (doll's eye phenomenon). In the presence or suspicion of a cervical fracture or dislocation, this test is contraindicated. (*Note:* If the presence of the oculocephalic reflex is questioned or the conduction of the test is contraindicated, the oculovestibular reflex is tested. In many hospital emergency departments, the oculovestibular reflex is tested more often than the oculocephalic reflex unless there are contraindications.)

observe the patient's posture while he or she is standing still. The patient is then observed while walking and the following characteristics are noted: erect, stooped, or leaning toward one side; position of the arms in relationship to the body; and quality and amount of movement in the lower extremities. A description of common gait abnormalities appears in Table 7-9 and Chart 7-2. See Chart 8-10 for nursing diagnoses associated with motor function deficits.

SENSORY ASSESSMENT

The sensory assessment is usually deferred unless the patient has spinal cord disease (secondary to trauma, neoplasm, infectious processes, or stenosis), intervertebral disk disease,

Guillain-Barré syndrome, or other conditions that affect the spinal cord or spinal nerves. The decision to include a sensory assessment is left to the judgment of the clinician. A sensory assessment is conducted in the patient who is conscious, cooperative, and able to respond appropriately. If a sensory assessment is conducted, the sensory modalities that can be assessed include:

- Superficial sensation
- Light touch (cotton-tipped applicator)
- Pain (pinprick)
- Deep sensation
- Proprioception (the big toe and fingers are moved in various positions)

CHART 8-9
Nursing Assessment of Motor Function at the Bedside

Conscious Patient Who Is Able to Follow Simple Commands

A sampling of the strength of key muscles in the extremities will provide an overview of motor function. Other muscle groups of interest can be added (see Chap. 7 and Fig. 7-9 for more information).

Upper Extremities:
A. Deltoids
B. Biceps
C. Triceps
D. Hand grasps
E. Pronator drift

Lower Extremities:
F. Hamstrings
G. Quadriceps
H. Dorsiflexion
I. Plantarflexion

Unconscious Patient

Unconscious patients can exhibit abnormal muscle tone or motor responses that appear as stereotyped postures and are initiated by noxious stimuli (see decortication and decerebration).

Upper Extremities: Unconscious Patient

- First observe for spontaneous movement as patient lies in the bed.
- Apply a noxious stimulus. *Note:* **Apply a noxious stimulus centrally rather than peripherally. An example of a central stimulus is pinching the pectoralis major muscle. A peripheral stimulus, such as pressing on the nailbed, may result in a reflex response and confuse findings.**

- Observe for withdrawal of the arm on the stimulated side. A purposeful response is present if the arm crossed the midline to noxious stimulus.

Sometimes added to the assessment:

- With the patient lying on his or her back, position the forearms perpendicular to the bed, holding the patient's arms upright by the hands or wrists.
- The movement of both arms is then observed as the extremities are released simultaneously.
- A paralyzed or paretic arm will fall more quickly than an intact arm. The weaker arm may strike the patient's face as it falls.

Lower Extremities: Unconscious Patient

- Observe for spontaneous movements.
- Apply noxious stimuli; observe for motor response.

Sometimes added to the assessment for paralysis or paresis, although often impractical because of abnormal posturing and increased tone:

- Position flat on the back with the knees flexed so both feet are flat on the bed.
- The knees are simultaneously released and the movement of the legs is observed.
- The paralyzed or paretic leg will fall to an extended position with the hip outwardly rotated. The normal leg will maintain the flexed position for a few moments and then gradually assume its previous position.

Pain and **light touch** are the most frequently assessed modalities. The technique for assessment follows these basic principles:

- With the patient's eyes closed, begin either at the face or feet and systematically assess and compare findings on both sides of the body. If you are assessing a patient with spinal cord or spinal nerve deficits, starting at the feet and working upward is helpful to determine the highest level of intact sensory function.
- Ask the patient to tell you when the sensory stimulation is felt.
- Record the highest level of function on each side of the body (there may be unilateral sensory functional loss).

Table 5-6 includes a list of dermatome levels. Chapter 7 discusses sensory assessment in greater detail. Chart 22-4 includes the sensory assessment for spinal cord injury.

FREQUENCY AND DOCUMENTATION OF SENSORY DATA

The frequency of assessment depends on the patient's acuity and stability. Patients with acute spinal cord trauma, acute transverse myelitis, or acute Guillain-Barré syndrome should be assessed for the highest level of function every 2 to 4 hours. In patients whose condition is stable, assessment once a shift is probably frequent enough to keep the nurse aware of functional level. Documentation of findings can be done in several ways. If a special Spinal Cord Assessment Sheet or dermatome territory map is used, data are entered using a checkmark format. The data may also be recorded in a narrative format, using dermatome landmarks to monitor function (*e.g.*, highest sensory level is one finger above the umbilicus). Chart 8-11 lists the nursing diagnoses associated with sensory deficits.

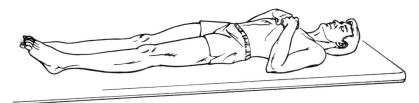

A *Flexor or decorticate posturing response*

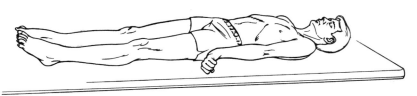

B *Extensor or decerebrate posturing*

FIGURE 8-10
Abnormal rigidity. (*A*) Decorticate rigidity. In decorticate rigidity, the upper arms are held tightly to the sides, with elbows, wrists, and fingers flexed. The legs are extended and internally rotated. The feet are plantar flexed. This posture implies a destructive lesion of the corticospinal tracts within or very near the cerebral hemispheres. (*B*) Decerebrate rigidity. In decerebrate rigidity, the jaws are clenched and the neck extended. The arms are adducted and stiffly extended at the elbows with forearms pronated, wrists and fingers flexed. The legs are stiffly extended at the knees, with the feet plantar flexed. Decerebration is caused by a lesion in the diencephalon, midbrain, or pons, although severe metabolic disorders, such as hypoxia or hypoglycemia, may also produce it. (From Fuller, J. and Schaller-Ayers, J. [1994]. *Health assessment: A nursing approach.* [2nd ed.]. Philadelphia: J. B. Lippincott)

CEREBELLAR ASSESSMENT

To assess cerebellar function at the bedside, a sample of upper extremity and lower extremity function is acceptable. See Chapter 7 for more details about assessment. For upper extremities assessment, ask the patient to touch your finger and then his or her nose. This movement should be done as fast as possible. Assess first with eyes open then with eyes closed. Note the smoothness of the movement and accuracy of touching the target. An alternative method is to ask the patient to rapidly pronate and supine the fingers of one hand onto the palm of the other several times.

For the lower extremities, ask the patient to run the heel of one foot down the shin of the other leg. Ataxia and dysmetria are abnormal findings. If the patient is ambulatory, the Romberg test can be used. However, be prepared to support the patient if he or she begins to sway or fall. In addition, observe the patient for any involuntary movements that may be associated with cerebellar dysfunction. Nystagmus is not uncommon with cerebellar dysfunction. Chart 8-12 lists the nursing diagnoses associated with cerebellar deficits.

VITAL SIGNS AND ASSESSMENT

Vital signs are taken on all patients, but in patients with neurological problems, there can be special considerations, particularly with increased intracranial pressure or brain stem pathophysiology. The relationship between vital signs and neurological function is based on hemodynamics. The brain requires a constant, large volume of oxygen-rich blood to support adequate cerebral perfusion pressure. Without adequate cerebral perfusion pressure, cerebral ischemia develops, cerebral metabolism is affected, and neurological dysfunction occurs.

The following are homeostatic mechanisms important to understanding cerebral hemodynamics.

CNS Ischemic Response. When cerebral blood flow to the brain stem vasomotor center is compromised sufficiently to cause ischemia, the neurons of the vasomotor center respond directly to the elevated carbon dioxide with excitation. This excitation causes a significant rise in systemic arterial pressure; it is called the CNS ischemic response.[6]

Cushing's Response (Reflex). A special type of CNS ischemic response that results from increased intracranial pressure is called Cushing's reflex. When cerebrospinal fluid (CSF) pressure approaches the pressure found within the intracranial cerebral arteries, the cerebral arteries become compressed and begin to collapse, compromising cerebral blood flow. To compensate, Cushing's response is activated, causing the arterial pressure to rise. When the arterial pressure has risen to a higher level than the CSF pressure, cerebral arterial flow is reestablished and the ischemia is relieved. Thus, the blood pressure is established and maintained at a new, higher level to provide adequate blood flow. Cushing's response is a com-

pensatory response that helps protect the brain from loss of
adequate blood flow.[7]

Cushing's Triad. *Cushing's triad* refers to three signs—bradycardia, hypertension, and bradypnea (often at an irregular
rate)—that are attributable to pressure on the medullary centers of the brain as a result of intracranial hypertension and
rostral–caudal herniation. It indicates rapid deterioration and
decompensation of protective reflexes.

Clinically, the nurse should realize that changes in vital
signs, such as Cushing's response and Cushing's triad, are late
findings, if they occur at all. Therefore, do not wait for these
responses before intervening, because it may be too late to
prevent irreversible neurological damage or even death.

In the discussion that follows, it is evident that the assessment of vital signs should be both quantitative and qual-
itative. The numerical value of each vital sign is important,
but the characteristic descriptive pattern and rhythm can provide diagnostic indicators of intracranial pathophysiology and
neurological progression.

General Anatomical and Physiological Considerations Related to Vital Signs

The "centers" for vital signs are located within the brain
stem. Complex networks of neurons in the brain stem RF
participate in the regulation of cardiovascular, respiratory,
and other visceral functions. Rather than being discrete anatomical centers for a particular function such as inspiration, neurons for autonomic functions are intermingled and
functionally related and have reciprocal connections. Observation of a physiological response, such as inspiration,
is seen after a particular pattern of the RF is stimulated. The
RF receives visceral sensory input polysynaptically through
collaterals from ascending spinal cord sensory pathways
and the nucleus tractus solitarius. (The **nucleus tractus so-**

litarius is the first brain stem structure for termination of
visceral afferent impulses; the site of initiation and integration of many autonomic reflexes; and the site for input to
the hypothalamus and other autonomic structures).[8] Other
afferent sensory impulses reach the RF through descending
fibers from the hypothalamus and from the limbic system
through the dorsal longitudinal fasciculus, medial forebrain
bundle, and mamillotegmental tracts.

Vasomotor Tone. The RF neurons that influence cardiovascular function are located primarily in the medulla. The
ventrolateral medulla contains a group of **vasomotor neurons** which control blood pressure. Some neurons project
directly to preganglionic parasympathetic cranial nerve nuclei (midbrain, CN III; pons, CN VII; and medulla, CN IX,
X). The preganglionic nuclei maintain arterial blood pressure, mediate sympathetic reflexes, and serve as relay sta-
tions for sympathetic pathways. The vagus (X) is very important because its efferent impulses have a major role in
control of respiratory, cardiovascular, and gastrointestinal
functions. Other neurons in the ventrolateral medulla, the
cardiovagal neurons, control heart rate. Finally, portions of
the medullary RF coordinate various respiratory and cardiovascular reflexes.

Respirations. Some centers in the RF control visceral motor
neurons and respiratory motor neurons. These neurons are
mostly located in the parabrachial area dorsal (pons), the
nucleus tractus solitarius (medulla), and several excitatory
neuron groups that sustain vasomotor tone and respirations
(ventral lateral medulla, respiratory groups). The several
respiratory groups include **inspiratory neurons** that project
to the spinal phrenic motor neurons and **expiratory neurons** that project to the intercostal respiratory motor neurons. Respiratory neurons found in the parabrachial area
(pons) are called pontine dorsal or the **pneumotaxic center**,
whereas the nucleus tractus solitarius (medulla) and ventrolateral medulla neurons together are called the **ventral**

respiratory groups. Some interneurons located proximal to
the ventral respiratory groups are key for the generation of
respiratory rhythm.

There is still much that is not known about the control of
respirations and central respiratory drive, although new understandings are reflected in recent literature. The respiratory
centers of the brain are located within the pons and medulla.
The pons contains a pneumotaxic area and the medulla contains the ventral respiratory groups (Fig. 8-11).

The **ventral respiratory groups** have a role in controlling inspiration and expiration. The **pneumotaxic center**
transmits impulses of varying magnitude for inspirations.
The primary function of the center is to limit inspiration;
however, by limiting respirations, it exerts a secondary effect on the rate of breathing. Strong pneumotaxic signals
can increase the rate of breathing (*e.g.*, 30 to 40 per min),
whereas weak signals will reduce the rate to only a few
breaths per minute. The Hering-Breuer reflex also has an
effect on turning off respirations.

The **Hering-Breuer reflex** is a protective reflex that prevents excessive lung expansion. Stretch receptors located in
the bronchi and bronchioles throughout the lungs transmit
signals through the vagus nerve to the dorsal respiratory
group when the lungs are overinflated and expiration is initiated. This reflex has a function similar to that of the pneumotaxic center in that it limits the duration of inspiration
through a feedback loop that "turns off" inspiratory effort and
reduces the time of inspiration so that the respiratory rate is
increased.

Body Temperature. The preoptic nucleus of the anterior hypothalamus is the center for the regulation of body heat and
acts by monitoring the temperature of blood. Regulation of
heat is accomplished by an integrated response of the sweat
glands, peripheral vessels, and skeletal muscles for shivering.
Through these structures, the body can conserve or divest itself of body heat.

Assessment of Vital Signs

RESPIRATIONS

The respiratory pattern can sometimes be correlated with dysfunction in a particular anatomical level. However, this is not
always possible because the patient may be on a ventilator
which is set for a particular rate and rhythm, thus overriding
an inadequate respiratory pattern. In some cases, respiratory
changes may not be seen until just before death.

Assessment. The rate, rhythm, and characteristics of the inspiratory and expiratory phases of respirations should be
noted. In addition to neurological causes of respiratory
changes, a number of other etiologies should also be considered, such as acidosis, alkalosis, electrolyte imbalance, congestive heart failure, anxiety, and various respiratory complications (*e.g.*, atelectasis, pneumonia, pulmonary edema).
Drugs, particularly narcotic analgesics, sedatives, and anesthetic agents, may have a depressant effect on the respiratory
system. Morphine sulfate depresses the respiratory rate in addition to causing constriction of the pupils. Because it causes
respiratory depression and masks the neurological signs of
pupillary response, use of morphine sulfate is limited in neurological patients. Small doses of morphine sulfate may be ordered to decrease rapid respirations when ongoing monitoring and respiratory support are available.

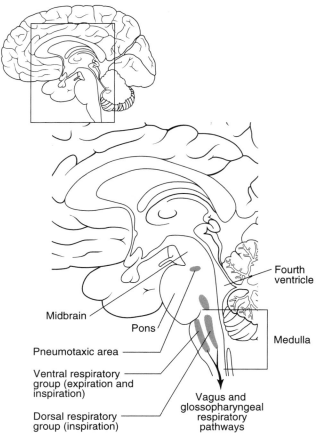

FIGURE 8-11
Major brain stem areas for respiratory control.

Changes in Respirations. Regulation of respirations is controlled by many neurological mechanisms. With cerebral injury, changes can occur in respiratory patterns; documentation by the nurse is important. Chart 8-13 describes types of abnormal respiratory patterns.

A few last points should be made with regard to respirations and intracranial pressure. Initially, an acute rise in intracranial pressure is reflected by a slowing of the respiratory rate. As the intracranial pressure continues to rise, the rate becomes rapid. These respirations are almost always noisy. The respiratory pattern will also change with a rising intracranial pressure. The nurse should consider the complete diagnostic data set when assessing respiratory function and planning interventions. Other metabolic, cardiac, and respiratory conditions mentioned previously can trigger changes in respiratory function. Trauma to the cervical spine may produce respiratory distress; if the injury is above the phrenic segment (C-4), total arrest may occur.

The major nursing diagnoses associated with respiratory dysfunction are:

- Impaired Breathing Pattern
- Impaired Gas Exchange
- Altered Cerebral Tissue Perfusion
- Risk of Aspiration
- Impaired Airway Clearance

The role of the nurse in relation to respiratory function is to (1) periodically assess and document rate, rhythm, and characteristics of respirations; (2) implement interventions to maintain a patent airway and promote respiratory function; (3) assess for secondary conditions that may cause respiratory complications; (4) assess for respiratory complications or insufficiency; and (5) notify the physician if respiratory problems occur. See Chapter 12 for a discussion of respiratory management.

PULSE

Assessment. The rate, rhythm, and quality of the pulse should be assessed, documented, and compared with previous data. Common changes that may occur in rate and rhythm are tachycardia, bradycardia, and cardiac arrhythmias. A bounding or thready pulse is a common change in pulse quality. A bounding pulse often accompanies rising intracranial pressure. A thready pulse is seen in the terminal stages or with accompanying intra-abdominal hemorrhage.

The major nursing diagnoses associated with pulse rate changes or arrhythmias are as follows:

- Tissue Perfusion, Altered, Cerebral
- Gas Exchange, Impaired
- Cardiac Output, Altered
- Activity Intolerance

Changes in Pulse. **Tachycardia** in a neurological patient can indicate that a patient is (1) hypoxic; (2) experiencing high intracranial pressure; or (3) bleeding internally in the abdominal, thoracic, or pelvic cavity.

Bradycardia can occur in the later stages of progressive increased intracranial pressure as part of Cushing's response. The blood is pumped to the edematous brain against great pressure so that the pulse is decreased to a rate of 40 to 60 per minute and bounding. Also, hypotension and bradycardia may be secondary to cervical spinal cord injury with interruption of descending sympathetic pathways.

Cardiac arrhythmias are rather common symptoms. Arrhythmias are seen more often in patients who have blood in the CSF (*e.g.*, subarachnoid hemorrhage, severe head injury); have undergone posterior fossa surgery; or have high intracranial pressure.

If there is evidence of abnormalities in rate or rhythm, a rhythm strip should be obtained immediately to document and identify the problem. Treatment should be instituted as necessary. Continuous cardiac monitoring and cardiac drugs are often necessary.

BLOOD PRESSURE

Assessment. In assessing blood pressure, the nurse monitors for hypotension, hypertension, and pulse pressure. A comparison is made with previous assessment data. The major nursing diagnoses associated with abnormal blood pressure are the following:

- Altered Cerebral Tissue Perfusion
- Impaired Gas Exchange
- Altered Cardiac Output
- Activity Intolerance

Changes in Blood Pressure. **Hypertension** in the neurological patient may be associated with sympathetic stimulation resulting from massive hypothalamic discharge or a rising intracranial pressure. An elevated systolic blood pressure, widening pulse pressure, and bradycardia are seen in the advanced stages of increased intracranial pressure and are known as **Cushing's response**.

Hypotension is rarely attributable to cerebral injury. When it is seen with severe neurological injury, it occurs only as a terminal event and is accompanied by tachycardia. Inadequate cerebral perfusion denies the cerebral tissue of an adequate oxygen supply, and the regulatory mechanisms no longer function. In this stage of decompensation, deterioration is rapid and death results. The suspicion of occult internal hemorrhage (thoracic, abdominal, pelvic, or long bone) should be raised when hypotension and **tachycardia** are seen together and hypovolemic shock is present. Hypotension and **bradycardia** may be seen in patients with cervical spinal injury as a result of interruption in the descending sympathetic pathways.

TEMPERATURE

Assessment. In the following situations, the temperature should be taken by the rectal route: a patient with a tracheostomy or nasogastric tube; a patient receiving oxygen; a combative, confused, or disoriented patient; and an unconscious patient. The nurse should stay with the patient while the thermometer is in place. The temperature and the route by which it was taken should be recorded on the flow sheets. If a continuous monitoring device has been used to monitor the temperature, this should

CHART 8-13
Abnormal Respiratory Patterns Associated with Intracranial Problems

The following abnormal respiratory patterns are seen in conditions that directly and indirectly affect the respiratory centers of the brain stem. *Primary* injury may occur as a result of ischemia, infarction, or invasion by a space-occupying lesion located in the brain stem respiratory centers. *Secondary* injury may be caused by (1) increased intracranial pressure (ICP) on the brain stem secondary to a supratentorial condition related to cerebral edema, hemorrhage, or infarction; or (2) CNS depression from such conditions as metabolic dysfunction and drug overdose. However, increased ICP is the major cause of respiratory complications.

Cheyne-Strokes respirations

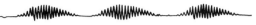

⊢ One Minute ⊣

Rhythmic waxing and waning in the depth and rate of the respiration followed by apnea. Pattern due to two factors: (1) increased sensitivity to carbon dioxide that results in the change in depth and rate; and (2) decreased stimulation from respiratory centers that results in apnea. Lesions are most often located *bilaterally deep* within the cerebral hemispheres, diencephalon (thalamus and/or hypothalamus), or basal ganglia.

Central neurogenic hyperventilation

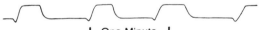

⊢ One Minute ⊣

Respirations increased in rate and depth; may lead to respiratory alkalosis. Pattern thought to be due to release of the reflex mechanisms for respiratory control in the lower brain stem and results in low arterial carbon dioxide tension and elevated pH; lesion location is unclear although midbrain and upper pontine lesions are usually considered the source.

Apneustic breathing

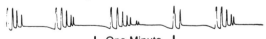

⊢ One Minute ⊣

A pause of 2 to 3 seconds noted after a full or prolonged inspiration; may alternate with an expiratory pause; lesion located in the lower pons area.

Cluster breathing

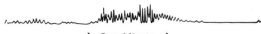

⊢ One Minute ⊣

Clusters of irregular breaths with periods of apnea at irregular intervals (gasping breathing occurs at a slow rate and has features similar to cluster breathing); lesion located in lower pons or upper medulla.

Biot's (ataxic) breathing

⊢ One Minute ⊣

Completely irregular, unpredictable pattern with deep and shallow random breaths and pauses; lesion located in the medulla.

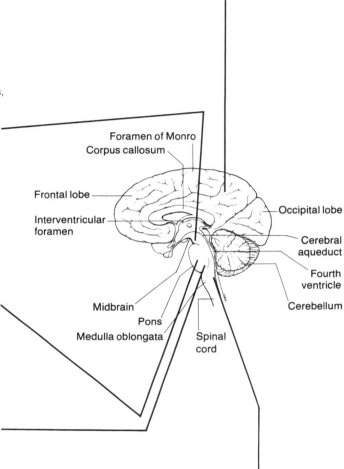

be noted on the flow sheets. If the temperature is elevated and the patient has been placed on a hypothermia blanket, the temperature should be monitored every half hour until it begins to drop to an acceptable level. Shivering increases intracranial pressure and should be avoided.

The major nursing diagnoses associated with abnormal body temperature are as follows:

- Hyperthermia
- Hypothermia

Changes in Temperature. **Hypothermia** is seen in certain conditions such as spinal shock when autonomic innervation is lost; metabolic or toxic coma of any origin; drug overdose, especially from depressant drugs (barbiturate overdose); and destructive brain stem or hypothalamic lesions. Specific treatment depends on the cause. Warm blankets and/or a warming blanket may be applied. Room temperature should also be adjusted.

Hyperthermia is much more common than hypothermia. Fever is a complex, coordinated autonomic, neuroendocrine, and behavioral response that is adaptive and is often part of the acute-phase reaction to immune challenge.[9] Fever can be caused by a wide range of infectious organisms, noninfectious inflammatory responses, and central fever. Regardless of the cause, the clinical presentation of fever is stereotypic and largely independent of the causative agent. Fever may be associated with any of the following conditions.

INFECTIOUS ORGANISMS. A variety of organisms such as *Staphylococcus aureus*, *Escherichia coli*, *Pseudomonas aeruginosa*, and others cause infections. Infections can result from open head wounds (meningitis), postoperative wounds or shunts, nosocomial pneumonia, and intravenous lines and tubes (central and peripheral lines, urinary catheters [urosepsis], ventriculostomies). In these cases, cultures will be positive in identifying the causative organism. Non-neurological causes of infection should also be considered such as septicemia, gram negative sepsis, and endocarditis.

Treatment is based on the selection of a sensitive antimicrobial drug. In addition, strict aseptic dressing technique and line- and tube-change protocols can significantly reduce infections. Prophylactic use of antimicrobials may be ordered in some instances to cover the patient. An example is ordering a course of an antimicrobial (*e.g.*, vancomycin hydrochloride) when a ventriculostomy is inserted.

NONINFECTIOUS INFLAMMATORY RESPONSES. Cultures from patients with the following conditions are negative.

- **Posterior fossa syndrome** mimics meningitis with a number of symptoms that include stiff neck, a low CSF glucose level, a possible elevated protein CSF level, and polymorphonuclear leukocytes. However, unlike meningitis, CSF cultures are negative. Posterior fossa syndrome is seen in patients who have had posterior fossa surgery or blood in the CSF and is often related to subarachnoid hemorrhage.
- **Drug induced fever** is caused by an immune response to a drug. Common causative drugs are anticonvulsants such as phenytoin (Dilantin) and carbamazepine (Tegretol); analgesics; phenothiazines; anticholinergic drugs; and antibiot-

ics. The diagnosis is established by withdrawal of the drug and subsequent rechallenge. Cultures of blood, urine, and sputum are negative and the patient looks better clinically than the temperature would suggest.

- **Neuroleptic malignant syndrome** is related to use of antipsychotic drugs and includes muscular rigidity, a catatonic-like state, altered consciousness, and a high fever of up to 41.5° C (107° F). Discontinuing the drug and supporting the patient are the components of a treatment plan.
- Other causes of an elevated temperature are pulmonary embolism and phlebitis; these should be considered in evaluating the patient.

CENTRAL FEVER. Central fever is caused by a central neurogenic etiology seen with space-occupying lesions, trauma or a lesion that involves the hypothalamus or base of the brain, or traction of the hypothalamus or brain stem. High fever up to 41.5° C is the cardinal finding and perspiration is absent.[10] This is a diagnosis of exclusion and is made only after all other causes of fever have been ruled out.

Effects of Steroids on Temperature. The neuroscience patient may be treated with large doses of steroids, often dexamethasone (Decadron). Steroids are anti-inflammatory agents that mask the classical clinical signs of infections, such as an elevated temperature and white blood count. Therefore, monitor the patient for signs of infection such as cloudy or foul-smelling urine; yellowish, foul-smelling sputum; or adventitious breath sounds. Cultures and blood counts should be monitored for evidence of infection.

How aggressively should an elevated temperature be treated? Most clinicians who manage neuroscience patients will treat an elevated temperature when it reaches a certain level (38° C or 39° C) because of the effect on the brain. An elevated temperature increases overall body metabolism and cell metabolism of all systems including the brain which, in turn, produces an increase in carbon dioxide and lactic acid by-products of cell metabolism. Carbon dioxide, a potent cerebral vasodilator, will cause an increase in intracranial pressure in a patient who may already have high intracranial pressure. If the oxygen supply to cerebral tissue is insufficient, cerebral ischemia develops. Therefore, treatment of hyperthermia to prevent neurological deterioration is a central concern in management. Usual treatment is aspirin or acetaminophen and possibly a cooling blanket for high temperatures.

The reason for the elevated temperature should be investigated carefully, as there may be a non-neurological cause. The nurse should listen to the chest for breath sounds and rales. The urine and the sputum should be considered for possible culture. Finally, all dressings and drainage, if present, should be assessed.

SUMMARY

The neurological assessment is the foundational database for the nurse to use in making nursing diagnoses, planning care, implementing interventions, and evaluating care for the patient. It is essential that the nurse develop the skills and knowledge to conduct this assessment competently and engage in the clinical reasoning for patient management.

References

1. Plum, F., & Posner, J. (1980). *The diagnosis of stupor and coma* (3rd ed.). Philadelphia: F. A. Davis, p. 2.
2. Barr, M. L., & Kiernan, J. A. (1993). *The human nervous system: An anatomical viewpoint.* Philadelphia: J. B. Lippincott, pp. 158–159.
3. Plum & Posner, 1980, pp. 178–180.
4. Ibid., pp. 178–179.
5. Folstein, M. F., Folstein, S. E., & McHugh, P. R. (1975). Mini-mental state: A practical method for grading the cognitive state of patients for the clinician. *Journal of Psychiatric Research, 12,* 189–198.
6. Guyton, A. C. (1986). *Textbook of medical physiology* (7th ed.). Philadelphia: W. B. Saunders, pp. 250–251.
7. Ibid., pp. 250-251.
8. Westmoreland, B. F., Benarroch, E. E., Danube, J. R., Reagan, T. J., & Sandok, B. A. (1994). *Medical neurosciences: An approach to anatomy, pathology, and physiology by systems and levels.* Boston: Little, Brown, p. 216.
9. Saper, C. B., & Breder, C. D. (1994). The neurological basis of fever. *New England Journal of Medicine, 330*(26), 1880.
10. Cunha, B. A., & Tu, R. P. (1988). Fever in the neurosurgical patient. *Heart and Lung, 17*(6, part 1), 611.

Bibliography

Books

Barr, M. L., & Kiernan, J. A. (1993). *The human nervous system: An anatomical viewpoint.* Philadelphia: J. B. Lippincott, pp. 364–376.

Bates, B. (1995). *A guide to physical examination and history taking* (6th ed.). Philadelphia: J. B. Lippincott.

Conn, P. M. (Ed.). (1995). *Neuroscience in medicine.* Philadelphia: J. B. Lippincott, pp. 227–235.

Westmoreland, B. F., Benarroch, E. E., Danube, J. R., Reagan, T. J., & Sandok, B. A. (1994). *Medical neurosciences: An approach to anatomy, pathology, and physiology by systems and levels.* Boston: Little, Brown, pp. 249–271.

Periodicals

Cunha, B. A., & Tu, R. P. (1988). Fever in the neurosurgical patient. *Heart and Lung, 17*(6, part 1), 608–611.

Saper, C. B., & Breder, C. D. (1994). The neurological basis of fever. *New England Journal of Medicine, 330*(26), 1880–1886.

Section 3

General Considerations in Neuroscience Nursing

CHAPTER 9

Nutritional Support for Neuroscience Patients

Joanne V. Hickey

Providing for the nutritional needs of neuroscience patients is a critical component in the healing and recovery process. Injury, physiological dysfunction, and stress often change the utilization of nutrients and water; adjustments in nutrition are then needed to meet basic requirements of energy and cellular function and to repair injured tissue. Reparative tissue consumes more protein, carbohydrate, lipid, water, and oxygen than does normal tissue. Dietary and nutritional modifications imposed by illness also have a direct effect on adequate nutrition and normal body function. The patient with neurological dysfunction may have deficits, such as an altered level of consciousness or paresis/paralysis of the muscles needed for chewing and swallowing, that further complicate ingestion of an adequate dietary intake. Consideration of these factors, plus the effect of illness on other body systems, suggests that there are special complexities that must be addressed in meeting the nutritional needs of the neuroscience patient. In managing the patient holistically, nutritional needs cannot be overlooked because no patient will recover from illness without adequate nutritional support.

BASIC NUTRITIONAL REQUIREMENTS

Caloric Intake

The caloric intake necessary for a person depends on the person's age, sex, body size, activity level, and body temperature, as well as the environment's ambient temperature. Women require 1,700 to 2,500 calories per day, whereas men need between 2,300 and 3,100 calories per day. The caloric intake needed increases in any stressful situation, such as physiological trauma, emotional stress, surgery, fever, seizure activity, decorticate or decerebrate rigidity, restlessness, agitation, hypermetabolic states, and sepsis. Caloric requirements can be increased two to three times for a patient with ongoing stress or serious injury, such as multitrauma or septic states. Patients with severe head injuries can require 4,000 to 5,000 calories per day. Metabolic rate studies can be helpful in assessing caloric needs of patients who are difficult to assess (*e.g.*, head injury, spinal cord injury, obese patients).

In the general population, a caloric intake of 25 to 35 kcal/kg of body weight is generally required. In determining the amount of calories required, the basal energy expenditure (BEE) is calculated using the Harris–Benedict formula. This formula considers weight, sex, height, and age in the calculations. A stress factor is generally added to the BEE based on the patient's condition.

Proteins

Proteins are organic substances composed of amino acids. Although carbohydrates, fat, and protein all contain carbon, hydrogen, and oxygen, only protein contains nitrogen. Nitrogen is a component of every cell in the body. When 6.25 g of protein are metabolized, 1 g of nitrogen results. By weight, 1 g of protein is 16% nitrogen. The primary function of protein is to build and repair body tissue. One gram of protein yields 4 calories when metabolized.

ESSENTIAL AND NONESSENTIAL AMINO ACIDS

Amino acids may be classified as either essential or nonessential. **Essential amino acids** are necessary for normal growth and development and cannot be manufactured by the body. **Nonessential amino acids** are defined as amino acids that are not necessary for normal growth and development and can be manufactured by the body. Table 9-1 lists both essential and nonessential amino acids.

TABLE 9-1
Essential and Nonessential Amino Acids

ESSENTIAL AMINO ACIDS	NONESSENTIAL AMINO ACIDS
Histidine*	Alanine
Isoleucine	Arginine*
Leucine	Asparagine
Lysine	Aspartic acid
Methionine	Cystine (Cysteine)
Phenylalanine	Glutamic acid
Threonine	Glutamine
Tryptophan	Glycine
Valine	Hydroxylysine
	Hydroxyproline
	Proline
	Serine
	Tyrosine

* Classified as semiessential because the need for these amino acids depends on the supply of the essential amino acids from which they are made.

COMPLETE AND INCOMPLETE PROTEINS

Protein can also be classified as either complete or incomplete. A **complete protein** is one that contains all of the essential amino acids in sufficient quantity and appropriate proportions to supply the body's needs. Proteins of animal origin, such as milk, meat, cheese, and eggs, are examples of complete proteins. An **incomplete protein** is defined as one that is deficient in one or more essential amino acids. Incomplete amino acids are of plant origin and include grains, legumes, and nuts.

DAILY PROTEIN REQUIREMENTS

The healthy adult requires 0.8 g/kg of protein per day. The protein requirement for the adult depends on age and sex. It is approximately 46 g/day for females and 56 g/day for males. Patients with major injuries or wounds will require a daily intake of protein that is two to four times the normal daily requirement.

NITROGEN BALANCE

Nitrogen is the major component of protein. Almost all of the nitrogen ingested comes from protein, and most of the nitrogen lost from the body is in the form of nitrogenous end products found in the urine as urea, creatinine, uric acid, and ammonium salts. A small amount of nitrogen loss occurs through the stool and skin. Nitrogen balance indicates whether the patient is anabolic (has a positive nitrogen balance) or catabolic (has a negative nitrogen balance). The normal healthy adult who is not growing, who consumes an adequate diet, and whose lean body mass remains the same is said to be in nitrogen balance. Nitrogen balance is calculated as follows:

- Nitrogen balance equals nitrogen intake/24 hours minus nitrogen output/24 hours.
- Nitrogen intake is calculated from the protein intake in 24 hours.
- Nitrogen output is calculated from a 24-hour urine urea nitrogen (UUN) excretion study.

Positive Nitrogen Balance. When the nitrogen intake is greater than the nitrogen output, the patient is said to be in positive nitrogen balance or an anabolic state. **Anabolism** is a constructive metabolic building process that is responsible for growth or repair of body tissues. A positive nitrogen balance indicates anabolism. Anabolism is the opposite of catabolism.

Negative Nitrogen Balance. When the nitrogenous output exceeds the nitrogen intake, a state of negative nitrogen balance exists. In this state, the lean body mass is being metabolized and decreases in quantity. Negative nitrogen balance occurs in states of inadequate essential amino acid intake and use, immobilization for any reason (*e.g.,* unconsciousness, paralysis, spinal cord injury), and exposure to stress (*e.g.,* trauma, surgery, disease processes). **Catabolism** is a destructive phase of metabolism in which complex substances are broken down and energy is released. The opposite of catabolism is anabolism. Anabolism is a building process in which nutrient material is converted into complex living matter. Any patient who is in a negative nitrogen balance will not recover from surgery, trauma, sepsis, or a disease process until an anabolic state (positive nitrogen balance) is created.

Carbohydrates

Carbohydrates are defined as starches and sugars that are used by the body for energy. One gram of carbohydrate yields 4 calories when metabolized. Carbohydrates are classified as monosaccharides, disaccharides, or polysaccharides. Table 9-2 describes the categories, types, and sources of carbohydrates. For carbohydrates to be used by the body, they must be broken down into glucose. Glucose is the simplest form of sugar that circulates in the blood; it is oxidized to release energy, and is the source of energy for cerebral cell metabolism. Glucose may be used in the body in any of three ways:

1. Glucose is oxidized in the body for energy.
2. Glucose is stored as a reserve in the liver (and in muscle tissue to a lesser degree) in the form of glycogen through a process called **glycogenesis.** Hydrolysis of glycogen to glucose is called **glycolysis** (the anabolic enzymatic conversion of glucose to lactate or pyruvate, resulting in energy stored in the form of ATP, as occurs in muscles).
3. Excess glucose can be converted into fat and stored in the body as adipose tissue.

Fats

Fats occurring as organic substances in the body are called lipids. **Fatty acids** are the basic units of structure in lipids; they can be divided into essential fatty acids and nonessential fatty acids. An **essential fatty acid** cannot be manufactured in the body and will cause a specific deficiency disorder if not ingested in an adequate amount. There is one essential fatty acid called linoleic acid that is important in the maintenance of the skin, hair, nerve linings, and cell membranes and is also a component of prostaglandins and other body chemicals. It is also necessary for forming other acids, such as arachidonic

TABLE 9-2
Types of Carbohydrates

CATEGORY	TYPE	SOURCES
Monosaccharides (simplest form of carbohydrates)	Glucose (dextrose)	Natural glucose found in food or formed in the body from starch digestion
	Fructose (levulose) (converts to glucose for energy)	Sugar found in fruits and honey
	Galactose (not found free in food); changed to glucose for energy	Produced from lactose (milk sugar)
	Alcohol derivatives	
	Mannitol	From mannose
	Sorbitol	From glucose
Disaccharides (more complex sugars made up of two monosaccharides)	Sucrose = glucose + fructose	Table sugar, brown sugar, molasses, maple sugar
	Lactose = glucose + galactose	Sugar in milk
	Maltose = glucose + glucose	Malt products and germinating cereals
Polysaccharides (very complex carbohydrates)	Starch	Potatoes; cereal grains, including rice; root vegetables; legumes
	Cellulose	Dietary fiber

acid. Nonessential fatty acids do not cause specific deficiency disorders if not ingested in sufficient amounts because they can be manufactured in the body.

The purpose of fat in the diet is primarily to produce energy, although it is also important in terms of fat-related compounds in the body, such as cholesterol, triglycerides, phospholipids, and lecithin. The major sources of fat in the normal diet are butter, margarine, oil, bacon, meat, fats, egg yolks, nuts, and legumes. When 1 g of fat is oxidized, 9 calories are generated.

Vitamins, Minerals, and Water

In addition to proteins, carbohydrates, and fats that are necessary for proper nutrition, vitamins, minerals, and water are requisites. Certain vitamins and minerals cannot be stored in the body, so the patient will quickly become deficient if an adequate diet is not consumed daily. Other vitamins can be stored in the body so that deficiencies will not be apparent until after a month or two of inadequate vitamin intake.

VITAMINS

Vitamins are classified as either water-soluble or fat-soluble. **Water-soluble vitamins** are vitamin C and the B-complex vitamins, which include thiamine, riboflavin, niacin (nicotinic acid), pyridoxine, pantothenic acid, biotin, folic acid, and cobalamin. The **fat-soluble vitamins** are A, D, E, and K. Vitamins and their functions are described in Table 9-3.

MINERALS

Minerals can be divided into major minerals and trace minerals. **Major minerals** include calcium, chloride, magnesium, phosphorus, potassium, and sodium. The **trace minerals** include cadmium, chromium, copper, fluoride, iodide, iron, manganese, molybdenum, nickel, selenium, silicon, tin, va-

nadium, and zinc. Minerals and their functions are described in Table 9-4.

WATER

The amount of water necessary for adequate nutrition depends on the temperature of the ambient environment, amount of perspiration, activity, endocrine function, urinary output, and other factors. Under normal conditions, the average person requires approximately 2,600 mL of water a day. A guideline for calculating water requirements is one mL/kcal energy expenditure. This can be subdivided into intake from three sources:

- In the form of liquids: 1,200 to 1,500 mL/day
- Within foods: 700 to 1,000 mL/day
- From oxidation of food: 200 to 300 mL/day

Hypermetabolic states, fever, profuse perspiration, significant drainage from wounds, and excessive urinary output are a few situations that warrant an increased fluid intake.

METABOLIC CHANGES FOLLOWING INJURY AND STARVATION

Significant differences accompany the body's response to injury (trauma, surgery, sepsis) and to fasting or starvation. The major differences are listed in Table 9-5.

Response to Stress and Injury

ACUTE PHASE

Any type of injury is a form of stress that triggers the stress response and arouses the central nervous system to activate the sympathetic nervous system. The body's response to stress or

TABLE 9-3
Vitamins and Their Functions

VITAMINS	FUNCTIONS
FAT-SOLUBLE VITAMINS	
Vitamin A	Growth and maintenance of epithelial tissue; bone development; visual acuity in dim light
Vitamin D	Facilitates absorption and utilization of calcium in bone and tooth development
Vitamin E	Cellular antioxidant
Vitamin K	Essential in prothrombin formation and blood clotting
WATER-SOLUBLE VITAMINS	
Thiamine	Key role in carbohydrate oxidation; participates in the Krebs' cycle; a component of enzymes
Riboflavin	Involved in amino acid and purine metabolism; necessary for generation of adenosine triphosphate (ATP)
Niacin	Essential in protein utilization and in the synthesis of fatty acids and cholesterol
Pyridoxine	Essential for protein metabolism
Pantothenic acid	Involved in the synthesis of acetylcholine, cholesterol, fatty acids, and steroids, as well as in oxidation of energy nutrients
Biotin	Important in the synthesis of fatty acids, utilization of glucose, and metabolism of protein
Folic acid	Essential in amino acid metabolism; important in the maturation of red blood cells
Cobalamin	Involved in the manufacture of enzymes necessary for the metabolism of nutrients and synthesis of deoxyribonucleic acid (DNA)
Vitamin C	Involved in production of collagen, hormonal synthesis, amino acid metabolism, integrity of capillary walls, and red blood formation; important in wound healing

TABLE 9-4
Mineral Requirements and Their Functions

NAME	FUNCTIONS
MAJOR MINERALS (RELATIVELY LARGE AMOUNTS NECESSARY FOR HEALTH)	
Calcium	Necessary for bone formation, teeth, blood clotting; involved in muscle contraction and relaxation, cardiac function, and transmission of nerve impulses; activates enzymes; affects the permeability of the cell membrane
Chloride	Regulates osmotic pressure and acid–base balance; activates the enzyme amylase in saliva
Magnesium	Important cation within the cell; involved in the function of B vitamins; necessary for the utilization of potassium, calcium, and protein; facilitates maintenance of electrical activity in muscles and nerves
Phosphorus	Involved in bone formation and nerve and muscle action, as well as in carbohydrate metabolism, fatty acid transport, and energy metabolism
Potassium	Involved in maintenance of intracellular osmotic pressure and acid–base balance, as well as in glycogen formation, contraction of muscle fibers, and transmission of electrical impulses within the heart
Sodium	Involved in maintenance of extracellular osmotic pressure and acid–base balance, as well as cell permeability, absorption of glucose, muscle irritability, and muscle contraction
TRACE MINERALS (SMALL AMOUNTS NECESSARY FOR HEALTH)	
Cadmium	Function not clear, but appears to be involved in basic biological systems
Chromium	Associated with glucose metabolism
Copper	Component of certain enzymes and elastin; involved in the formation of myelin and melanin pigment, in the synthesis of hemoglobin, and in the maintenance of bones and neurological function
Fluoride	Involved in the mineralization of bones and teeth and in the prevention of dental caries and osteoporosis
Iodine	Necessary for skin integrity, thyroid function, and neuromuscular function
Iron	Component of hemoglobin, myoglobin, and certain enzymes; involved in normal blood platelet production, oxygen transport and utilization, and in maintenance of the integrity of the mucous membranes
Manganese	Activates several enzymes; involved in formation of urea, in central nervous system function, in carbohydrate and fat metabolism, and in synthesis of cartilage
Molybdenum	Component of certain enzymes; involved in fatty acid utilization and bone formation
Nickel	Associated with thyroid hormone and ribonucleic acid (RNA)
Selenium	Associated with fat metabolism; component of the enzyme that protects red blood cells from damage
Silicon	Necessary in bone, cartilage, and connective tissue formation
Tin	Involved in protein synthesis and enzyme systems
Vanadium	Thought to be involved in bone and teeth formation
Zinc	Associated with skin integrity and wound healing; involved with normal sense of taste and smell, bone growth and strength, and sexual maturation; component of several enzymes

TABLE 9-5
Differences in Early Metabolic Responses to Fasting and Injury

METABOLIC ACTIVITY	FASTING	AFTER INJURY
Glucose levels	Low	High (hallmark of stress reponse)
Protein catabolism	Low	High
Fat catabolism	High	Low/none
Ketosis	Present	Absent
Ketosuria	Present	Absent
Basal metabolism rate	Low	High

injury is to **survive** by meeting increased metabolic needs to preserve vital functions. The sympathetic nervous system immediately stimulates the adrenal medulla to release catecholamines (epinephrine, norepinephrine), corticosteroids (glucocorticosteroids, mineralosteroids), glucagon, and insulin. Catecholamines act on the liver and muscles to convert stored glycogen into glucose by a process called *glycogenolysis* so that the glucose can be released into the bloodstream. At the same time, insulin secretion from the pancreas is suppressed so that hyperglycemia will meet the increased demand for energy. In addition, catecholamines increase lipolysis and gluconeogenesis. *Lipolysis* is a process by which fatty acids are released from fat stores and are then converted into glucose as another source of energy. *Gluconeogenesis* is the process of converting amino acids from skeletal muscles into glucose.

Glucocorticosteroids stimulate the pancreas to secrete glucagon. Cortisol acts by increasing the breakdown of lipids. At the same time, aldosterone, a mineralocorticoid, increases water and sodium retention. There is a decrease in serum potassium that may last for several days because, initially, the excretion of potassium through the urine is increased, whereas the excretion of sodium through the urine is decreased. The sodium retention phase is followed by diuresis. In the acute phase, fluid retention is also enhanced by the increased secretion of antidiuretic hormone (ADH) that is prompted by the hypothalamus.

Glucagon has a major effect on the liver—it causes the liver to convert amino acids into glucose (gluconeogenesis). It also suppresses the anabolic effect of insulin in protein synthesis (proteolysis). As mentioned previously, the initial response to stress is suppression of insulin secretion so that hyperglycemia and gluconeogenesis result, creating ready sources for increased energy demands. In the acute phase, the blood glucose level is elevated. There is rapid utilization of glycogen, amino acids, and fatty acids for energy. Within a few days or a week, the body then enters an adaptation phase.

LATER RESPONSE (ADAPTATION PHASE)

In the adaptation phase, there is a decrease in blood glucose and blood urea nitrogen (BUN) levels. At the same time, ketosis and ketosuria appear. In some instances of prolonged stress, such as that seen in neurosurgical patients, the body does not develop starvation ketosis of the adaptation phase but continues to break down body protein mass. There are

about 6 kg of protein in the average adult. Between 25 and 75 g will be metabolized daily, yielding 100 to 300 calories daily. In the catabolic phase, the patient can lose 10 to 30 g of nitrogen daily as the result of protein breakdown. The excessive amount of nitrogenous waste challenges the ability of the kidneys to excrete the urea. The increase in urea also has an effect on the osmotic pressure in the tubules, causing an increased amount of water to be excreted. Unless a high-protein diet is given, wound healing and recovery will be seriously hampered.

Response to Starvation
EARLY PHASE

After several hours without food intake, the body responds to frank starvation by **conservation.** Initially, the lowered glucose level causes a drop in the circulating insulin. The level of glucagon increases and activates glycogenolysis (glucose produced from glycogen liver stores for 24 to 36 hours). The liver then metabolizes amino acids for energy, which causes a gradual increase in the BUN level for 2 to 4 days. Protein catabolism provides energy for the glucose-dependent brain. The decreased level of insulin appears to be the major control in lipolysis. Lipolysis produces free fatty acids and glycerol. Utilization of body fat gradually increases over the next 20 to 40 days, so that the BUN level gradually decreases.

In brief starvation, the following characteristics are noted: increased urine nitrogen and urinary output; rapid weight loss; and decreased muscle mass, serum glucose level, and circulating insulin level.

LATER DEVELOPMENTS (KETO-ADAPTATION PHASE)

The body then enters the keto-adaptation phase as more body fat is metabolized. This period of prolonged starvation can last for several months. There is an increase in ketosis and ketosuria, both of which are related to the by-products of fat metabolism. Ketone bodies contribute to the conservation of muscle protein. Another important adaptive change noted at this time is that the brain utilizes ketone bodies as its major source of energy.

The characteristic changes noted in prolonged starvation can be summarized as follows:

- Increased fat catabolism
- Slow weight loss
- Slow loss of muscle mass
- Increased urinary ammonia levels
- Decreased UUN levels
- Metabolic acidosis that is usually compensated for by respiratory alkalosis
- Decreased basal metabolism rate and body temperature
- Increased extracellular fluid and peripheral edema (late finding)

PREMORBID STARVATION PHASE

When the fat stores of the body are exhausted, the patient enters a premorbid state of starvation. Protein muscle mass is utilized for energy so that decreased muscle mass and rapid weight loss ensue. Death will result unless aggressive nutritional support is given.

Effects of Malnutrition

A short period (less than 1 week) of catabolism can be tolerated by the well-nourished patient without negative effects. However, for patients who were poorly nourished before sustaining injury or who are unable to establish a normal eating pattern within a week of injury, serious problems will develop. The depletion of protein from the body produces a catabolic state of malnutrition with the following consequences:

- Compromised wound healing
- Predisposition to development of decubiti
- Decreased immunological response to infection
- Increased susceptibility to development of complications
- Increased mortality
- Failure to wean from a ventilator

Malnutrition Syndromes

Two types of malnutrition syndromes may be found in hospitalized patients:

1. In **marasmus**, the patient appears malnourished as a result of rapid loss of fat and muscle mass secondary to improper protein and caloric intake. The visceral protein is maintained until the muscle mass is severely depleted. Clinically, the patient appears grossly underweight, with loss of both muscle mass and subcutaneous fat. Diarrhea is common. Metabolic activity is decreased and prostration is seen.
2. A **protein deficiency state** may be found in normal or obese patients who undergo stress. These patients have an above-standard fat store and muscle mass, but the visceral protein store is depleted. This disorder is similar to kwashiorkor syndrome in children. Clinical evidence of protein deficiency includes edema, muscular wasting, depigmentation of hair and skin, scaly and flaky skin, hypoalbuminemia, moderate anemia, and diarrhea.

Other clinical signs and symptoms that are associated with malnutrition are hair loss, dull-looking hair, seborrhea, swelling of the tongue, and bleeding from the gums.

NUTRITIONAL ASSESSMENT

Various nutritional assessment profiles have been developed to determine the patient's nutritional status, identify specific nutritional deficits, and develop appropriate protocols of nutritional therapy to meet the patient's needs. In considering nutritional status and needs, age is an important component. For example, the potential for malnutrition among geriatric patients is high, and the usual parameters such an anthropometric measures are less dependable.

A collaborative team approach that includes the physician, nurse, and clinical dietitian is most effective. Other nutritional consultation available in a facility should be used as necessary. In some organizational structures, the physician and the nurse may be solely responsible for nutritional assessment. Patients should be screened for appropriate nutritional support soon after they have been hospitalized (within the first 24 hours).

Nutritional assessment can easily be forgotten when life-threatening events occur. However, without sufficient nutritional support, wound healing will be delayed, the patient will be increasingly susceptible to infections, and overall recovery will be seriously hampered.

The **goal** of the nutritional assessment is to

- Identify a daily nutritional goal for the patient based on his or her caloric, carbohydrate, and protein needs
- Select the particular type of feeding to be used (*e.g.*, Isocal HN for a goal of 80 cc/h)
- Determine if feeding will be given continuously or as a periodic bolus
- Advance, over a time schedule, the amount of feeding to be administered per hour or bolus feeding (*e.g.*, begin at 20 cc/h for 8 hours, then increase by 20 cc/h every 8 hours until goal is reached)
- Identify any specific criteria to determine tolerance (*e.g.*, aspirate gastric tube and hold feeding for > 100 cc)

In assessing the nutritional status of a patient, the following data are collected:

1. Physical inspection of the patient includes assessment of the following: skin for turgor, dryness, edema, or easy bruising; mucous membranes for dryness, color, bruising, or bleeding (especially gums for easy bleeding); tongue for swelling and papillary atrophy; eyes for pale or dry conjunctiva or sunken eyeballs; and muscles for atrophy or wasting.
2. Note the patient's weight and how that compares with recommended weight based on gender and height. Determine whether there has been unexplained weight loss or weight gain. An involuntary weight loss of 10% or more in 1 year is considered significant. Information on recent dietary changes and what constitutes normal daily dietary intake is noted.
3. Anthropometric measurements are considered, including weight, height, triceps skinfold (TSF) thickness, arm muscle circumference (AMC), and mid-upper arm circumference (MUAC). These data provide information about growth, development, and body composition (they measure body fat and lean body muscle). Abnormally low values indicate that protein stores have been depleted. Data can be distorted if the patient is obese or edematous.
   TSF thickness is calculated by lifting the skin of the posterior arm away from the triceps muscle and measuring the skinfold thickness with standard calipers. The measurement is made midway between the posterior aspect of the top of the shoulder and the bony projection of the elbow. If the patient can stand, the arm should hang freely. The bedridden patient should be positioned flat in bed with the arm raised upright. MUAC, which is measured at the same point as the TSF, indicates the fat and protein stores available. The AMC is a good indicator of protein nutrition and can be calculated from the other two arm measurements as follows:

$$\text{AMC (cm)} = \text{MUAC (cm)} - [3.14 \times \text{TSF (cm)}]$$

4. Laboratory studies (and normal ranges for each) include the following:
   - Serum creatinine (0.6 to 1.2 mg/dL): an end product of protein metabolism, indicates depletion of muscle mass
   - Serum albumin (3.3 to 4.25 g/dL): estimates visceral protein stores; a value of 2.1 to 3.0 g/dL indicates moderate malnutrition, whereas a value of less than 2.1 signifies severe malnutrition
   - Serum total protein (6.6 to 7.9 g/dL): estimates visceral protein stores
   - BUN (8 to 20 mg/dL): indicates the rate of protein metabolism
   - Blood glucose (70 to 100 mg/dL): indicator of a prime energy source
   - Serum transferrin (180 to 260 mg/dL): indicator of iron-transporting capacity and excess protein loss; a value of 100 to 150 mg signifies moderate malnutrition, whereas a value of less than 100 indicates severe malnutrition.
   - Total iron-binding capacity (300 to 400 mg/dL for men and 300 to 450 mg/dL for women): estimates visceral protein stores
   - Serum osmolality: estimates water balance
   - Serum free fatty acids: estimates fat breakdown
   - Liver function studies
   - Kidney function studies
   - 24-hour UUN (maximal clearance: 64 to 99 mL/min): measures nitrogen balance
   - 24-hour creatinine height index (84 to 90 mL/min): indicates the degree of muscle depletion
   - Serum sodium, chloride, potassium, calcium, phosphorus, magnesium, and cholesterol values: indicate electrolyte balance and nutritional status; recently, more emphasis has been give to monitoring and maintaining calcium, phosphorus, and magnesium at normal levels
   - Total white blood cell count, total lymphocyte count, hemoglobin, and hematocrit: indications of immune response, anemia, and fluid balance
5. Immune function is assessed by examining the total white blood cell count and the total lymphocyte count. When protein malnutrition exists, there is a decrease in peripheral lymphocytes (as well as a decreased ability to fight infection).
6. In the malnourished patient, the cellular immunity response shows a decrease in the synthesis of antibodies and the antibody response. Tests used to assess this response include purified protein derivative (PPD) skin test, mumps skin test, and others. In the malnourished patient, there is a delay (greater than 24 hours) in response. In the normal person, a response is noted within 24 hours.

Related Nursing Diagnoses

Based on a nutritional assessment, a number of nursing diagnoses can be made. The following nursing diagnoses are often identified for the patient with problems related to nutritional need:

Major Nursing Diagnoses

- Nutrition, Altered, More Than Body Requirements
- Nutrition, Altered, Less Than Body Requirement

- Fluid Volume Deficit
- Fluid Volume Deficit, Risk for
- Fluid Volume Excess

Associated Nursing Diagnoses

- Swallowing, Impaired
- Oral Mucous Membrane, Altered
- Hyperthermia
- Aspiration, Risk for
- Activity Intolerance

Ongoing Nursing Assessment

The nurse can monitor the patient's nutritional status by monitoring the following parameters:

- Weigh the patient twice a week, on designated days, and note trends in stability of weight.
- Observe skin turgor, the condition of the tongue and mucous membranes, muscle tone, and muscle bulk daily.
- Monitor intake and output and record measurements.
- Maintain a calorie count with the help of the diet therapist.
- If the patient is receiving continuous feeding via a food pump, monitor the equipment to ensure that it is working properly.
- Monitor tolerance of feeding by aspirating the feeding tube periodically (unless the tube is a jejunostomy tube).
- Monitor the patient's energy level and tolerance of activity, such as being up in a chair.
  In conscious patients, note verbal response to activity.
  In conscious patients and in those with an altered consciousness state, monitor vital signs and objective signs of fatigue.
- Monitor appropriate laboratory data.

The nurse should collaborate with the physician and diet therapist to meet the nutritional needs of the patient.

COMMON NEUROLOGICAL PROBLEMS THAT INTERFERE WITH NUTRITION

Common Neurological Deficits

For patients to consume a normal oral diet that will then be digested and supply the necessary nutrients for the body, several functions must be intact. Patients must be alert and oriented and have an attention span sufficient for concentrating on the task at hand; they must be able to feed themselves, chew, and swallow; and they must be able to digest and utilize the nutrients through a functional gastrointestinal (GI) tract. Many patients with neuroscience problems have deficits that interfere with adequate nutrition, such as the following:

- Altered levels of consciousness (*e.g.*, confusion, stupor, restlessness, coma)
- Alterations in mentation (*e.g.*, short attention span, distractibility, refusal to eat)
- Diminished or absent swallowing or gag reflex

- Paresis or paralysis of arms necessary for feeding self
- Paresis or paralysis of muscles of mastication and/or the tongue
- Anorexia, nausea, vomiting, and excessive weight loss secondary to irradiation or chemotherapy for nervous system neoplasms

Special protocols and alternative methods of providing nutrition are necessary to support the nutritional needs of these patients.

Special Neurological Disorders and Their Effects on Nutrition

A number of common neurological disorders affect the nutritional needs of the patient. Several of these disorders and the interventions used in addressing them are presented in Table 9-6.

Drugs can also affect adequate nutrition. For instance, dexamethasone (Decadron) is a drug frequently ordered for neuroscience problems. Several metabolic changes are associated with the use of the drug; these are particularly significant for the patient undergoing a stress response to injury or early starvation. If a steroid such as dexamethasone is ordered for the patient, it is usually ordered at the time of hospital admission, and the course of therapy lasts several days. This time period coincides with the early responses to stress. The specific points of steroid therapy that relate to the patient's nutritional status include the following:

- Increased salt and water retention and increased excretion of potassium
- Increased calcium excretion
- Decreased carbohydrate tolerance
- Development of negative nitrogen balance because of increased protein catabolism
- Possible development of hypercholesterolemia and hypertriglyceridemia
- Electrolyte imbalance
- Impaired wound healing
- Modification of the body's immune response

The nurse should keep these effects of glucocorticosteroid therapy in mind when considering the nutritional effects of illness on the patient.

METHODS OF PROVIDING NUTRITION FOR NEUROSCIENCE PATIENTS

Initially, hospitalized neuroscience patients may be given intravenous (IV) fluid if they are unable to consume a diet orally. For patients who are well nourished, a few days of IV therapy will probably not be harmful to their nutritional status. However, few calories can be administered by the peripheral IV route, and patients must rely on body stores to provide necessary nutrients and calories. A liter of 5% dextrose and water contains only 200 calories. If patients are unable to consume an adequate diet by the oral route within a few days, then a nasogastric tube or other enteral tube is used or, less frequently, total parenteral nutrition (TPN) is instituted. An individualized assessment is necessary to determine the patient's nutritional needs and the best method of delivery. Alternative methods for providing adequate nutrition (tube feeding, TPN), as well as special procedures for oral feeding, are discussed in the following sections.

Feeding Tubes

Feeding tubes can be employed to provide nutrition on a temporary basis to patients who are unable to ingest food by the normal oral route. The feeding tube is inserted through the nose and into the stomach or upper small bowel. The type and the size of feeding tube chosen vary, and each has certain advantages and disadvantages. Large-bore, rigid feeding tubes can cause erosion of the nasal passages, esophagus, and stomach, but the large bore of the tube ensures better delivery of the feeding without occlusion. Smaller, more pliable tubes are less likely to erode tissue, but the tube is more likely to become occluded by congealed tube feeding. Administering medications through a small bore tube can also clog the tube. It is best to give medications through a large-bore feeding tube or, if not possible, flush well with water before and after giving medication through a small-bore tube.

There is controversy about the merits of tube placement in the stomach or duodenum. Those who favor the duodenal placement cite a decreased probability of aspiration as compared with gastric placement. Others cite studies and their own clinical experience which supports no increase in aspiration with gastric placement. It is left to the preference of the physician to decide which placement site will be used.

In certain patients, the use of a feeding tube is undesirable or contraindicated. The following are some of the common situations in which a feeding tube may be avoided:

- When long-term nutritional support will be required
- In the presence of a basal skull fracture, facial fractures, or leakage of cerebrospinal fluid
- When injury has been sustained or there is a disease process affecting the oropharynx, esophagus, or other portions of the GI tract

In these situations, a gastrostomy or jejunostomy tube may be inserted.

BEGINNING FEEDINGS

Current research-based practice favors early use of the gut for feeding because of many advantages. Beginning a feeding at as little as 10 mL/h continuous rate will maintain the integrity of the endothelial lining of the gastrointestinal tract and decrease the incidence of sepsis. After the nasogastric, gastrostomy, or jejunostomy tube is inserted, feedings are not begun until an x-ray film of the abdomen confirms gut placement. Some will not begin feeding until bowel sounds have returned; others will start a feeding at 10 mL/h even if no bowel sounds are present. A small amount of water, 5% dextrose and water, or a low-residue feeding diluted with water is often the initial feeding. The following guidelines are observed in beginning feedings:

TABLE 9-6
Nutritional Implications in Specific Neurological Disorders

DISORDER	NUTRITIONAL EFFECTS	INTERVENTION
Epilepsy (drugs used in treating the various types of epilepsies may cause nutritional deficits)	Primidone, phenobarbitol, and phenytoin can cause decreased serum levels of several B-complex vitamins.	Supplement with B-complex vitamins.
	Phenytoin can cause Megaloblastic anemia	Provide supplemental folic acid.
	Carbohydrate intolerance (rarely) that can lead to hyperosmolar coma	Monitor serum glucose levels.
Parkinson's disease	Levodopa is not as effective if patient is on a high-protein diet and taking pyridoxine	Provide a protein redistribution diet. Avoid a high-protein diet. Avoid multivitamins that include pyridoxine.
Spinal cord injuries	Loss of calcium from bones occurs secondary to not bearing weight (increased possibility of urinary tract calculi)	Provide a fluid intake of at least 3,000 mL/day to "flush" the urinary tract, thereby preventing infection and calculi.
	Negative nitrogen balance (loss of protein from muscles)	Increase protein intake to about 125 g/day.
Head injuries and comatose state	Negative nitrogen balance as a result of nothing being taken by mouth and limited IV caloric intake	Administer supplemental vitamins. Provide high protein intake (1.5 to 2.0 g/kg/day)
	Dehydration from altered osmotic gradient caused by drugs that increase excretion of water (during catabolic phase)	Administer sufficient water. Give supplemental vitamins and minerals. Provide 2,000 to 5,000 calories/day.
	Loss of calcium from bones if not weight-bearing	
Infectious processes that increase body temperature (meningitis, encephalitis, abscess)	Increased metabolic rate secondary to elevated temperature	Increase caloric intake to 2,000 to 5,000 calories/day.
	Loss of fluid through perspiration with fever	Increase fluid intake to compensate for fluid loss.
Increased activity states as seen with decortication/decerebration, restlessness, agitation, seizure activity, delirium tremors, chorea	Additional calories needed to compensate for energy expanded	Increase caloric intake to 2,000 to 5,000 calories/day; a nutritional consultation should be conducted

- Begin with a small amount of feeding (10 to 50 mL) delivered by gavage feeding, and administer it slowly.
- If a food pump is to be used, begin at a slow rate of about 10 to 30 mL/h.
- If water is tolerated, begin a commercial tube feeding slowly. Some physicians order dilution of the feeding with half water initially to improve the patient's tolerance of the nutrients.
- Observe the patient for intolerance or any untoward effects (*e.g.,* abdominal distention, vomiting, diarrhea).
- Maintain an accurate intake and output record.

NURSING RESPONSIBILITIES IN ADMINISTERING NASOGASTRIC FEEDINGS

Nasogastric feedings may be administered in one of two ways: continuously with the use of a food pump or intermittently with the use of a gavage bag. Special nursing protocols are followed to prevent vomiting and aspiration of the feeding. The patient should be observed frequently and suction equipment should be handy should evidence of aspiration be noted. The nursing interventions and responsibilities for the patient receiving nasogastric feeding include the following:

1. Raise the head of the bed 45 degrees or higher.
2. Check the position of the tube to be sure that it is in the stomach. Aspirate gastric contents. Inject about 5 cc of air into the tube and listen with a stethoscope just below the xiphoid process for the sound of air entering the stomach. Place the end of the feeding tube into a cup of water; if there are periodic bubbles that synchronize with respirations, the tube is probably in the lung.
3. Aspirate the tube to determine if the previous feeding has been absorbed; if 100 mL or more of residual feeding is aspirated, the feeding should be withheld or the food pump turned off for 2 hours; this information should be reported. It may be necessary to reevaluate the patient's feeding schedule. In 2 hours, aspirate the tube again to reassess the amount of residual feeding present. If there is a minimal amount or no residual feeding remaining, begin the feeding again.
4. If the patient has a tracheostomy tube in place, inflate the cuff; keep it inflated for 1 hour after completion of the feeding. The purpose of this action is to prevent aspiration.
5. Intermittent feedings should be administered over a period of 30 to 60 minutes depending on the amount of the

feeding. On completion of the feeding, flush the tubing with 50 mL of water and clamp the tube.

6. Record the amount and type of feeding on the intake and output record.
7. Monitor the patient's weight; weighing the patient twice a week is usually adequate.
8. Monitor the following laboratory studies: BUN, serum electrolytes, and serum creatinine.
9. Observe the patient for signs and symptoms of dehydration from hyperosmolar feedings that can lead to hyperosmolar nonketotic coma. Be sure that adequate supplemental water is ordered for the patient, especially if hyperosmolar feedings are being administered.
10. Monitor the urine for specific gravity level and adequacy of output.
11. Observe the patient for signs and symptoms of abdominal distention, regurgitation, aspiration, nausea/vomiting, diarrhea, or intolerance to the feeding.

INDICATIONS FOR A GASTROSTOMY OR JEJUNOSTOMY

Many serious problems can develop from prolonged nasogastric intubation. Possible problems include erosion and/or necrosis of the nares or nasal septum, sinusitis, peptic esophagitis from gastric reflux along the tube, and gastric erosion or ulcers. The need for prolonged tube feeding is an indication for a simple surgical procedure whereby a gastrostomy or jejunostomy tube is sutured into position. After the tube is inserted, it is usually left to gravity drainage for the first 24 hours. When bowel sounds have returned, a small amount of water or a combination of glucose and water, as outlined earlier, is begun. The insertion site is treated like any other surgical wound:

- The incision and tissue around the tube are cleansed daily according to hospital protocols.
- A dry, sterile dressing is applied over the incision and around the tube; assess the incision the area around the tube for any signs or symptoms of infection.

Types of Tube Feedings

Tube feedings can be classified into three major categories: elemental, low-residue, and high-residue diets. An **elemental diet** provides nutrients in the simplest chemical form for easy absorption with no residue. Nitrogen and protein are given in the form of amino acids, and carbohydrate is supplied as simple sugar or glucose. Elemental formulas are prepared commercially and are fortified with vitamins and minerals.

A **low-residue diet**, a variation of the elemental diet, uses albumin as the protein source. It is more palatable than the elemental diet. Most commercial formulas are low residue. A **high-residue diet** is similar to the low-residue diet in composition except it contains fiber for bulk. For patients who are constipated, a high-residue diet is helpful. Examples of commonly used commercially prepared feedings are included in Table 9-7.

Feedings can be administered intermittently a few times a day, or a food pump may be used to provide nutrition on a continual basis.

Problems Associated With Tube Feedings

Several potential problems and complications are associated with tube feedings. These potential problems and the appropriate nursing interventions are presented in Table 9-8.

One important consideration with the use of continuous enteral tube feeding concerns those patients who are receiving oral phenytoin (Dilantin). Patients receiving continuous feedings require increased doses of phenytoin to maintain therapeutic levels because phenytoin binds to protein. These patients also tend to develop signs and symptoms of phenytoin toxicity when tube feedings are discontinued if the same dosage is maintained. As many patients receive both continuous enteral feedings and phenytoin therapy simultaneously, increased doses of phenytoin will be required in these patients. The dosage will need to be evaluated and probably decreased when the tube feeding is discontinued. Patients should have phenytoin levels monitored more frequently when receiving

TABLE 9-7
Composition of Selected Commercially Prepared Tube Feedings

PRODUCT	kcal/mL	PROTEIN (g/L)	CARBOHYDRATES (g/L)	FAT (g/L)	mOsm/kg*	COMMENT
Ensure	1.06	37	143	37	450	Lactose free; may be used as a full liquid diet, liquid supplement, or tube feeding
Ensure Plus	1.5	54	197	52.5	600	High-calorie liquid diet intended for tube or supplemental oral feeding
Isocal (reg)	1.06	34	138	44	270	Isotonic, moderate protein
Isocal HN	1.06	44	123	46	270	Isotonic, high protein
Sustocal	1.01	61	140	23	670	High protein, oral or tube feeding
Sustocal Plus	1.50	61	190	57	650	High calorie, high protein, oral or tube feeding (comes in flavors)
Traumocal	1.50	82	145	69	560	High calorie, high protein for acute stress
Deliver 2.0	2.00	75	200	45	640	High calorie, high protein, concentrated for fluid restriction

Formulas of higher osmolarity (>450 mOsm) increase the risk of diarrhea; most formulas are lactose free.

TABLE 9-8
Potential Problems Encountered With Tube Feedings

PROBLEM	POSSIBLE CAUSES	NURSING ACTIONS
Diarrhea	Hyperosmolarity of feeding (usually 450 mOsm/L or more)	Begin very slowly and allow patient to adapt to formula. Dilute feeding or give free water. If ordered by the physician, a few drops of deodorized tincture of opium (DTO) may be added. Try a fiber-containing formula.
	Rapid rate of infusion	Administer very slowly until GI tract adapts to the feeding. Feeding may have to be discontinued and started again slowly in a diluted form. If diarrhea is not extensive, paregoric or diphenoxylate (Lomotil) may be given temporarily.
	Lactose intolerance	Avoid feeding with lactose unless patient normally drinks milk daily without ill effects.
Constipation	Diet high in milk content	Change type of feeding to a fiber-containing formula.
	Inadequate fluid intake	Give sufficient free water in diet.
	No bulk in diet	Record frequency of bowel movements. Administer stool softeners and mild laxatives if necessary.
Vomiting	Feeding too soon after intubation or suctioning	Allow patient a rest period before beginning feeding.
	Too rapid a rate of infusion	Run infusion slowly.
Dumping syndrome	Too rapid an infusion of hyperosmolar solutions	Run infusion slowly. Administer free water after intermittent feeding to dilute intake.
Dehydration	Rapid infusion of hyperosmolar carbohydrates that cause hyperglycemia → osmotic diuresis → dehydration	Administer slowly. Check sugar and acetone periodically (usually every 6 hours). May need to administer regular insulin to cover glycosuria.
	Excessive protein and electrolytes (have an osmotic effect)	Adjust formula. Administer free water. Monitor serum electrolytes and balance as necessary.
Edema	Excessive sodium in formula	Change feeding as necessary. Monitor serum electrolytes. Balance electrolytes with drug therapy as ordered.
Aspiration	Feeding tube not in stomach/jejunum	Check position of tube *before* beginning feeding.
	Vomiting (see vomiting for description)	Position with head of bed elevated 30 to 45 degrees.
	Note: Aspiration can cause pneumonia; every precaution should be taken to prevent aspiration.	Have suction equipment handy.
Plugged feeding tube	Coagulation of feeding solution in tube owing to spoilage of feeding	Place container with feeding solution into a basin of ice. Rock salt may be added to ice to keep it from melting quickly in hot weather.
	Low pH of gastric secretions causing plugging at the end of the feeding tube	Flush tubing with water after each feeding. Change connecting tube daily if it is disposable or washable.
Excessive feeding solution in stomach upon aspiration	Malabsorption of feeding	Give feeding at a slower rate. Aspirate feeding tube periodically (every 4 to 6 hours; if more than 75 to 100 mL is obtained, report it and postpone feeding; check again in 2 hours to see if contents have been absorbed (if the patient receives feedings through a food pump, turn off the machine for 2 hours and then recheck). May need to change type of feeding.
Other intolerance to feeding	Renal or hepatic disease (patient may not tolerate even normal levels of amino acids)	Change feeding. Monitor kidney and liver blood studies before and during administration of feedings.
Malnutrition	Inadequate diet (protein, carbohydrate, fats, minerals, or vitamins)	Check type of feeding; supplement with vitamins, minerals, and other requirements as necessary.
Negative nitrogen balance	Inadequate intake of nitrogen (protein is chief source of nitrogen)	Monitor blood urea nitrogen and creatinine levels. Weigh the patient periodically.
	Catabolic state	Increase nitrogen intake.

enteral nutrition therapy, and they should be assessed for signs and symptoms of toxicity. Because intravenous phenytoin is not metabolized in the gastrointestinal tract, drug levels are unaffected by concurrent enteral feeding.

Total Parenteral Nutrition

TPN, also known as parenteral hyperalimentation, is a method of administering a highly concentrated hypertonic solution of essential nutrients intravenously to provide the total nutritional needs of the patient over an extended period. This method of providing nutrition can be initiated early in the acute stage of illness or trauma (within 24 to 48 hours) to maintain the nutritional needs of the patient. Some patients may be able to convert to enteral feedings, while others will need to continue TPN for an extended period of time. The usual criteria used in the selection of patients for TPN are as follows:

- Inability to eat or use the GI tract for digestion and absorption of food
- Involuntary loss of 10% of body weight
- A state of malnutrition
- A hypermetabolic or catabolic state

Neuroscience patients who are good candidates for TPN include the following:

- Multitrauma patients with GI injuries that interfere with digestion and absorption of nutrients
- Patients with severe sepsis
- Malnourished patients who are in a severe catabolic state (negative nitrogen balance) associated with such conditions as prolonged coma, spinal cord trauma, and other major injuries

A large-bore catheter is inserted into the subclavian vein or vena cava for administration of the TPN solution. The solution administered is usually prepared in the pharmacy under strict aseptic conditions. The solution provides the following:

- Carbohydrates: 20% to 25% glucose
- Protein: amino acids as a nitrogen source to counteract the negative nitrogen balance
- Vitamins, minerals, electrolytes, and water

TPN provides sufficient amounts of nutrients to allow for tissue repair and building and normal physiological activity. Each liter of solution can provide 1,000 calories. The usual precautions for administering a hyperosmolar solution should be followed. The patient should be monitored according to the following parameters:

- Stable rate of fluid infusion that is checked at least every hour
- Blood glucose monitored every 6 hours
- Urine specific gravity checked every 6 hours
- Intake and output record maintained
- Weight determined and recorded at least twice a week
- Complete nutritional profile of laboratory studies recorded, as discussed earlier

Patients receiving TPN usually also receive fat emulsions, such as 500 mL of Intralipid, to prevent essential fatty acid deficiency. The administration schedule can vary from 1 to 2 times a week to daily. It is given slowly over a period of 12 hours.

The use of TPN is less popular than it was in the past. Current thinking is that there are important advantages to feeding via the gut, as discussed previously.

Oral Feedings

The goal of enteral or parenteral nutritional management is to allow the patient to be rehabilitated so that an adequate diet can be consumed by the oral route. Before beginning to feed the patient by the oral route, several nursing actions should be initiated:

- Assess the gag and swallowing reflexes. Do not initiate oral feedings if the gag or swallowing reflexes are not intact, because aspiration is possible.
- Note the presence of any facial weakness. The paresis or paralysis may be confined to only one side of the face.
- Auscultate the abdomen for the presence of bowel sounds. Oral feedings are *not* begun or resumed if bowel sounds are absent.
- Elevate the head of the bed to 45 degrees.
- Be certain that suction equipment is readily available, should it be needed.
- If the patient has a tracheostomy tube in place, inflate the cuff before beginning to offer oral intake. The cuff is kept inflated for 45 to 60 minutes after the feeding is completed.

Consider consulting speech therapy to conduct a swallow study if dysphagia or silent aspiration is suspected. The speech therapist can determine problems with the muscles of swallowing or the mechanics of swallowing as well as the degree of difficulty. As a result, a dysphagia diet and/or the need for thickened liquids can be ordered.

Once the preliminary assessment and necessary precautions have been taken to prevent aspiration, the nurse can initiate oral nutrition. The following guidelines should be observed:

- Begin with clear liquids. Patients should be encouraged to take a small sip through a straw, hold it in the mouth, and then swallow it.
- If they cannot manage a straw, offer a gelatin dessert from a spoon. (If the patient has any facial weakness, offer the food on the nonaffected side.)
- Give small feedings; frequently assess the response to and tolerance of the feeding.
- If clear liquids are well tolerated, the patient can progress to pureed foods and then to a soft diet. Continue to assess tolerance of the diet and progress slowly.
- Progress to a regular diet, as tolerated. Encourage a well-balanced diet.
- Assess the patient's ability to self feed. Cognitive, motor, and coordination deficits may interfere with this activity. Several problems that interfere with eating may be identified. These problems and appropriate nursing actions are described in Table 9-9.

TABLE 9-9
Potential Problems Associated With Oral Feedings

PROBLEM	DESCRIPTION	NURSING ACTIONS
Distractibility/short attention span	Patients become interested in the activity around them and stop eating; patients forget what to do with their food once they get it on their eating utensil	Screen patient from the distraction. Take excess dishes off the meal tray. Redirect patient's attention to eating; cue as necessary. Screen patient from excessive environmental stimuli. Break activity of eating into steps and direct the patient in the steps of eating (*e.g.*, pick up the potatoes with your spoon; lift the spoon to your mouth; open your mouth).
Disorientation	Not always aware of time, place, person. May think that the food belongs to someone else or that it is poisoned	Provide reality orientation and assist patients in feeding themselves. Give many verbal cues for eating. Correct any misconceptions. Reassure the patient in a calm voice. Be sure the patient is wearing eyeglasses if appropriate
Visual deficits		
Diplopia	Double vision	Apply an eye patch to one eye or cover one lens if double vision is present.
Hemianopia	Loss of vision in half of the visual field	If patient eats food from only one side of the dish, turn the dish; remind the patient to turn his or her head to scan the dish.
Dimness of vision	Visual images may be dim or fuzzy	Provision of a good light may be of some help in dimness.
Motor deficits (plegia or paresis) Muscles of chewing or of the face or tongue Arm or hand	May involve deficits of cranial nerves V, VII, or XII Associated with hemiparesis or hemiplegia; monoplegia of one extremity may be present	Encourage patient to chew food on the unaffected side. Have the patient try to eat with the other hand. Use built-up eating utensils. Use special equipment, such as a guard around the plate to prevent food from spilling off the dish. Consult the occupational therapist for suggestions. Prepare the patient's tray (*e.g.*, cut up meat, pour milk).

Although it can be time-consuming to supervise a patient while eating, it is an important consideration in the rehabilitation process and achievement of independence. Every effort should be made to assist the patient in achieving this goal.

Fluid Restriction

One component of the overall approach to management of increased intracranial pressure and cerebral edema is a fluid-restricted diet. The purpose of the diet is to limit fluid intake so that the patient is kept slightly underhydrated. The resultant hemoconcentration draws fluid across an osmotic gradient and decreases cerebral edema and intracranial pressure. Overhydration of a patient will contribute to increasing intracranial pressure and cerebral edema.

Fluid restriction is ordered according to the number of milliliters of fluid allowed in a 24-hour period. The patient must stay within the fluid restriction. All intake, regardless of the route—oral, enteral, or IV—is calculated in the total. For example, a patient may be placed on a 1,500-mL fluid-restricted diet. The nurse must assess the patient's dietary intake, IV fluid intake, and need for other fluid intake. Let's assume that the patient is receiving a tray from the dietary

department three times a day. An IV infusion is maintained as a "keep open" because the patient is receiving an IV antibiotic every 8 hours. The drug must be given in 50 mL of fluid, and a 10-mL flush is necessary after each administration of the drug. The patient also receives oral medication (tablets) four times a day. The nurse must plan how to allocate the overall fluid allotment. The following calculations are made:

"Keep open" infusion	400 mL/24 hours
Fluid for intravenous medication	180 mL/24 hours
Fluid for oral medications (60 mL × 4)	240 mL/24 hours
Total fluids for three meals	680 mL/24 hours
	1500 mL/24 hours

The nurse must carefully check the patient's trays to be sure that no more than 680 mL was consumed as the combined fluid intake for all three meals. For a patient who chooses to have only coffee and orange juice for breakfast (for a total of 200 mL), the remaining 480 mL is the total allocation for lunch and dinner. Patients and their families need to understand the purpose of a fluid-restricted diet. An accurate intake and output record must be maintained, and good communication between nurses on all shifts is needed.

Let us further assume that this same patient completes the course of antibiotic therapy and the IV infusion is discontinued. The only sources of intake then are the diet and the fluid needed to swallow the medication; thus, the nurse must redistribute the fluid intake. The nurse and the patient may decide to allocate some of the intake to an afternoon and a bedtime beverage. The distribution of fluid intake for the day is based on the patient's needs and the nurse's judgment, but the overall intake must be within the limits of the fluid restriction.

SUMMARY

The nutritional needs of a patient must be addressed early during hospitalization to prevent states of malnutrition and negative nitrogen balance. The patient with a severe head injury or other serious neurological dysfunction will often have increased caloric needs that may exceed 4,000 or 5,000 calories per day. Unless nutritional requirements for energy and tissue repair are met, a patient will not recover to the fullest extent possible.

Bibliography

Bell, S. J., Borlase, B. C., Swails, W., Dascoulias, K., Ainsley, B., & Forse, R. A. (1994). *Journal of the American Dietetic Association, 94*(4), 414–419.

Buckley, S., & Kudsk, K. A. (1994). Metabolic response to critical illness and injury. *AACN Clinical Issues in Critical Care Nursing, 5*(4), 443–449.

Clifton, G. L, Robertson, C. S., & Choi, S. C. (1986). Assessment of nutritional requirements of head-injured patients. *Journal of Neurosurgery, 64*, 895–901.

Clifton, G. L., Robertson, C. S., & Constant, C. F. (1985). Enteral hyperalimentation in head injury. *Journal of Neurosurgery, 62*, 186–193.

Clifton, G. L, Robertson, C. S., Grossman, R. G., et al. (1984). The metabolic response to severe head injury. *Journal of Neurosurgery, 60*, 687–696.

Dupuis, R. E, & Maranda-Massari, J. (1991). Anticonvulsants: Pharmacotherapeutic issues in the critically ill patient. *AACN Clinical Issues in Critical Care Nursing, 2*(4), 639–656.

Evans, N. J. (1994). The role of total parenteral nutrition in critical illness: Guidelines and recommendations. *AACN Clinical Issues in Critical Care Nursing, 5*(4), 476–484.

Galindo-Ciocon, D. J. (1993). Tube feeding: Complications among the elderly. *Journal of Gerontological Nursing, 19*(6), 17–22.

Goins, W. A., Wiles, C. E., & Cerra, F. B. (1993). Pharmacology, monitoring, and nutritional support. *Critical Care Clinics, 9*(4), 689–713.

Gora, M. L., Tschampel, M. M., & Visconti, J. A. (1990). Considerations of drug therapy in patients receiving enteral nutrition. *Nutrition in Clinical Practice, 4*, 105–110.

Grant, J. P. (1994). Nutritional support in critically ill patients. *Annals of Surgery, 220*(5), 610–616.

Jacob, R. A, & Milne, D. B. (1993). Biochemical assessment of vitamins and trace metals. *Clinics in Laboratory Medicine, 13*(2), 371–385.

Karstaedt, P. J, & Pincus, J. (1992). Protein redistribution diet remains effective in patients with fluctuating Parkinsonism. *Archives of Neurology, 49*, 149–151.

Koehler, K. N, & Garry, P. J. (1993). Nutrition and aging. *Clinics in Laboratory Medicine, 13*(2), 433–454.

Lipkin, E. W, & Bell, S. (1993). Assessment of nutritional status: The clinician's perspective. *Clinics in Laboratory Medicine, 13*(2), 329–352.

Lord, L. M, & Sax, H. C. (1994). The role of the gut in critical illness. *AACN Clinical Issues in Critical Care Nursing, 5*(4), 450–458.

Medley, F., Stechmiller, J., & Field, A. (1993). Complications of enteral nutrition in hospitalized patients with artificial airways. *Clinical Nursing Research, 2*(2), 212–213.

Metheny, N. (1993). Minimizing respiratory complication of nasoenteric tube feedings: State of the science. *Heart and Lung: Journal of Critical Care, 22*(2), 213–223.

Ouellette, F. (1995). Pulmonary aspiration of enteral feedings: A model for prevention. *Journal of Home Health Care Practice, 7*(2), 45–55.

Romito, R. A. (1995). Early administration of enteral nutrients in critically ill patients. *AACN Clinical Issues, 6*(2), 242–256.

Sax, H. C. (1993). Can early enteral feeding reduce postoperative sepsis and multiple organ failure? A review of recent studies. *Journal of Critical Care Nutrition, 1*(1), 5–14.

Shuster, M. H. (1994). Enteral feeding of the critically ill. *AACN Clinical Issues in Critical Care Nursing, 5*(4), 459–475.

Stanford, G. G. (1994). The stress response to trauma and critical illness. *Critical Care Nursing Clinics of North America, 6*(4), 693–702.

Toto, K. H., & Yucha, C. B. (1994). Magnesium: Homeostasis, imbalances, and therapeutic uses. *Critical Care Nursing Clinics of North America, 6*(4), 767–783.

CHAPTER 10

Fluid and Electrolyte Management in Neuroscience Patients

Joanne V. Hickey

INTERRELATEDNESS OF FLUID AND ELECTROLYTE BALANCE

Fluid and electrolyte balance is controlled by several interrelated mechanisms in the body. Metabolic derangement is common in neuroscience patients and can be related to neurological problems or a complication of therapeutics. The conditions that are discussed in this chapter include diabetes insipidus (DI), syndrome of inappropriate secretion of antidiuretic hormone (SIADH), cerebral salt wasting, hyperosmolar nonketotic hyperglycemia (HNKH), and major electrolyte imbalances.

Distribution of Water in the Body

The major compound in the body is water, which is distributed between the intracellular and extracellular spaces. Sodium is the major ion in the extracellular space, whereas potassium is the major intracellular ion. Overall fluid balance is maintained through a process called **osmosis**. Electrolytes, mainly potassium and sodium, are involved in osmosis.

Osmolality refers to the concentration of solute (ion particles) in a solvent (water) per unit of total volume of solution; it is the ability of fluid to hold water or draw it through a semipermeable cell membrane. Hyperosmolality occurs when there is a depletion of body water or an excess of salt. Hypoosmolality occurs when there is an excess of water or a depletion of salt. This relationship can be remembered by the following: high and dry; low and wet. The high and low refer to osmolality, whereas the dry and wet refer to fluid volume. Normal values for osmolality are as follows:

- Serum: 280 to 295 mOsm/L
- Urine: 50 to 400 mOsm/L (The normal ratio of urine to serum osmolality is 4:1.)

PHYSIOLOGICAL CONTROL OF WATER BALANCE

Several neurohumoral and renal physiological mechanisms control water balance within a very narrow range by controlling volume, concentration, and composition of body fluids. These mechanisms are controlled by the neurohypophysial system, the thirst center, and the renin-angiotensin-aldosterone system.

The Neurohypophysial System

The production, storage, and secretion of **antidiuretic hormone** (ADH) affect the reabsorption of water by acting on the collecting tubules of the kidney. Within the hypothalamus are two pairs of nuclei cell groupings called the **supraoptic nuclei** and **paraventricular nuclei**, so named for their anatomical locations (Fig. 10-1). Most ADH is synthesized within magnocellular neurons of the supraoptic and paraventricular nuclei. ADH is then loosely bonded with a carrier protein called **neurophysin**. From the supraoptic and paraventricular nuclei, the combined ADH and neurophysin are transported down the **pituitary stalk** or **infundibulum** through terminal nerve fibers and terminal nerve endings. ADH is then stored in large secretory granules in the nerve endings of the posterior pituitary gland (also called the **neurohypophysis**). Secretion of ADH is controlled by electrical impulses generated by the supraoptic and paraventricular nuclei. The impulses travel down the nerve fibers and nerve ending tracts, and ADH is released from the nerve endings. Because of the loose bonding of neurophysin to ADH, the neurophysin immediately separates from ADH. ADH is then absorbed into adjacent capillaries and circulation.

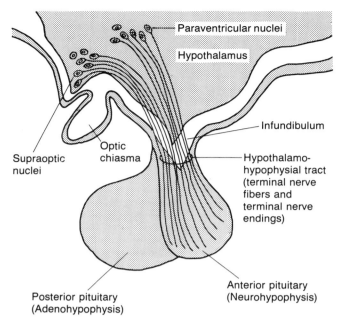

FIGURE 10-1
Within the hypothalamus are the supraoptic nuclei and paraventricular nuclei, which produce antidiuretic hormone (ADH). This hormone combines with neurophysin and travels down the terminal nerve fibers and terminal nerve endings to be stored in large secretory granules in the nerve endings of the posterior pituitary gland (neurohypophysis). (The lateral hypothalamic area, where the thirst center is located, is not shown.) (From De Graaff, K. M., & Fox, S. I. [1988]. *Concepts of human anatomy and physiology*, [2nd ed.]. Dubuque, IO: Wm. C. Brown.)

ADH is very potent, and even minute amounts (as little as 2 μg) have an appreciable effect on water balance. The half-life of ADH is 15 to 20 minutes, with metabolic degradation occurring in the liver and kidney. The immediate release and rapid breakdown of ADH account for the quick response time for even minute changes in volume, concentration, and composition of body fluids. The target organ of ADH is the kidney. With ADH, the collecting ducts and tubules become very permeable to water so that fluid is reabsorbed and conserved within the body. Conversely, without ADH, the renal collecting ducts and tubules are almost totally impermeable to water so that fluid is not reabsorbed; therefore, it is excreted in the urine.

REGULATION OF ADH PRODUCTION

Three type of receptors provide negative feedback loops to control the secretion of ADH. **Osmoreceptors** are located in the hypothalamus near the cells that produce ADH; they respond to changes in concentration of **extracellular fluid** (ECF). These receptors are affected by the degree of concentration of the ECF. Concentrated ECF stimulates the supraoptic nuclei to send impulses to release ADH, which will cause reabsorption of water in the kidney. Conversely, dilute ECF around the hypothalamic osmoreceptors inhibits the generation of impulses for the release of ADH. ADH has a potent influence on sodium ion concentration. Because about 95% of the total osmotic pressure of the ECF is determined by the sodium ion

concentration, in effect, ADH also controls the concentration of sodium ions.

Stretch receptors located in the atria of the heart have a potent constricting effect on the arterioles, thus increasing arterial blood pressure. The relaxation of atrial stretch receptors increases ADH secretion. **Baroreceptors**, located in the carotid sinus and aortic arch, respond to pressure changes; hypotension will increase ADH secretion.

CONTROL OF ANTIDIURETIC HORMONE SECRETION

Factors That Increase Release of Antidiuretic Hormone. Certain conditions or circumstances increase ADH secretion, thereby conserving water in the body. They include the upright position; hyperthermia; hypotension; hypovolemia, especially that caused by severe blood loss; pain; stress; anxiety; nausea; emesis; hypoxia; and trauma. Drugs that increase ADH release also have been identified: morphine sulfate, chlorpromazine hydrochloride (Thorazine), chlorpropamide (Diabinese), chlorothiazide (Diuril), carbamazepine (Tegretol), barbiturates, angiotensin II, beta-adrenergic agents, cholinergic drugs, clofibrate (Atromid S), cyclophosphamide (Cytoxan), vincristine sulfate (Oncovin), acetaminophen (Tylenol), meperidine hydrochloride (Demerol), and nicotine.

Factors That Decrease Release of Antidiuretic Hormone. Some conditions and circumstances decrease the release of ADH. They include the recumbent position, hypothermia, hypertension, hypo-osmolarity, and an increase in blood volume. Drugs that decrease ADH secretion include adrenergic agents, anticholinergic agents, ethanol, phenytoin (Dilantin), glucocorticosteroids (*e.g.*, dexamethasone), lithium carbonate, and demeclocycline (Declomycin).

The Thirst Center

Within the lateral hypothalamus is the **ventromedian nucleus**, also known as the **thirst center**. The osmoreceptors that stimulate the supraoptic and paraventricular nuclei also stimulate the thirst center. The thirst center, in turn, stimulates the cerebral cortex, signaling the need to drink fluids. As long as the person is able to respond to this impulse, fluid and electrolyte balance can be maintained. However, motor deficits, dysphagia, or a decreased level of consciousness may interfere with the person's ability to respond appropriately to the thirst stimuli.

The ADH feedback system and the thirst center are the major mechanisms for maintaining normal fluid balance in the body. In addition, aldosterone contributes to water balance.

The Renin-Angiotensin-Aldosterone System

Renin, which is released into the blood by the kidney's juxtaglomerular cells, acts on **angiotensinogen**, which has been produced by the liver, to form **angiotensin I**. When angiotensin I circulates through the lungs, two amino acids are removed. This reaction results in the formation of **angiotensin II**, a substance that stimulates the adrenal cortex (adrenal zona glomerulosa) to produce aldosterone. **Aldosterone** acts on the distal tubule of the nephron to promote readsorption of sodium while increasing excretion of potassium and hydrogen ions. Secretion of aldosterone from the adrenal cortex is activated by stimulation of volume receptors in the juxtaglomerular apparatus in response to a low renal perfusion pressure.

Antinatriuretic Factor

The **antinatriuretic factor** (ANF) promotes sodium excretion and vasodilation. ANF is released from the cardiac atria into the systemic circulation in response to increased atrial pressure. This may be a counteraction to the previously mentioned sodium-retaining mechanisms.

DIABETES INSIPIDUS

Diabetes insipidus is a condition of decreased secretion of ADH. Affected patients void large amounts of dilute urine daily and are at high risk for fluid and electrolyte imbalance and dehydration. The signs and symptoms include the following:

- Polyuria (urine volumes ranging from 4–10 L daily; hourly output exceeding 200 mL)
- Low urine-specific gravity (1.001–1.005)
- Extreme thirst (polydipsia) if the patient is conscious and the thirst center is intact
- High serum osmolality

Pathophysiology

The pathophysiology of DI is related to decreased production or release of ADH, increased breakdown of ADH, and less commonly, a defect in the kidney tubule's response to ADH. Dehydration, electrolyte imbalance, and hypovolemia can occur if fluid replacement is not provided.

Classification

DI has been classified by location and etiology (central neurogenic, nephrogenic), pattern of development, and permanency (transient, permanent).

LOCATION AND ETIOLOGY

Central neurogenic DI is defined as cessation of the pituitary gland's secretion of ADH because of a disease process or injury to the hypothalamus, the supraoptic-hypophysial tract, or the posterior lobe of the pituitary gland (neurohypophysis). Central neurogenic DI can be subdivided into the following four types:

- **Classical severe DI**, in which there is failure to synthesize or release ADH
- **Defective osmoreceptor DI**, in which very high osmolarity fails to trigger secretion of ADH, although the hormone is released in response to hypovolemia

- **Reset osmoreceptor DI**, in which secretion of ADH is not triggered until the plasma osmolarity is higher than the usual threshold
- **Partial DI**, in which ADH is released at the usual threshold, but the amount of hormone secreted is decreased

The most common cause of central DI is neurosurgery or head trauma, especially around the sella tursica; it is common in brain death. Less commonly, DI develops as a result of certain infections, neoplasms, vascular lesions, granulomatous disease, or severe head injury. Postsurgical central DI can occur any time within 14 days of neurosurgery, although it usually occurs within the first few postoperative days (see section entitled Patterns of Development).

Nephrogenic DI is a rare form of the disorder caused by an inability of the kidneys to respond to ADH.

PATTERN OF DEVELOPMENT

Central DI can develop in three distinct patterns following surgery:

- **Initial DI**. Significant polyuria lasts a few days and then gradually subsides during the next 1 to 7 days; it is associated with edema secondary to surgery.
- **Delayed DI** (may be permanent). The hypothalamus is damaged with some destruction of the ADH secretory cells; there is persistent polyuria of varying degree. The polyuria does not begin for about 3 to 4 days after injury because previously synthesized ADH has been released.
- **Triphasic DI**. Polyuria begins 1 to 2 days after surgery and lasts for 1 to 7 days. This is followed by 1 to 5 days of normal urinary output and then recurrence of polyuria. The period of normal urinary output is probably attributable to ADH being released until retrograde degeneration of damaged ADH production cells is complete.

PERMANENCY

The classification of DI can also be made according to permanency of the condition. Transient DI can develop secondary to surgery around the supraoptic hypophysial or head trauma. Normal secretion of ADH will usually be reestablished within a few days or a few weeks. Patients may or may not require treatment, depending on the severity of the condition and their ability to balance intake and output. A condition of permanent DI will develop only if 80% or more of the ADH-producing nuclei of the hypothalamus and the proximal end of the pituitary stalk are destroyed. This situation requires lifelong treatment with replacement hormonal therapy.

Diagnosis

The diagnosis of DI is based on the clinical finding of polyuria coupled with low urinary-specific gravity levels and high serum osmolality. A dehydration test may be ordered to determine which type of DI is present when the cause is unclear.

Treatment

The treatment of DI initially includes the replacement of fluids if the patient is unable to take an adequate amount of fluid orally. Administration of ADH (vasopressin) also is possible if a fluid deficit develops. The various types of drug preparations that are available and frequently ordered are listed in Table 10-1. For patients with mild DI, other drugs known to stimulate the hypothalamus to produce more ADH or to enhance the kidney's response to the hormone may be ordered. These drugs also are included in Table 10-1.

If the DI is a permanent condition, the patient will require a teaching program and ongoing medical management.

Nursing Management

ASSESSMENT

The nurse caring for a neurosurgical patient should be aware of the possible development of DI and should monitor the patient accordingly. The following parameters should be assessed:

- Urinary output every 1 to 2 hours
- Urinary-specific gravity every 1 to 2 hours
- Intake and output balance
- Serum osmolarity and electrolytes
- Signs and symptoms of dehydration
- Daily weight, if possible

When assessing the fractional urinary output for a patient with an altered level of consciousness, an indwelling catheter is usually used to measure urinary output on a specific time schedule. The amount of urinary output in just 1 hour can be extraordinary. If the urinary output is 200 mL/h or more for 2 consecutive hours, this should be reported to the physician.

In most instances, neurosurgical patients and those subject to increased intracranial pressure are maintained in a slightly dehydrated state to control intracranial pressure. An output of 200 mL/h or more for 2 consecutive hours can quickly lead to dehydration in these patients. The nurse will notice that the urine is very pale (straw colored) and dilute. The specific gravity will be 1.005 or less. These two concurrent findings are usual signs of DI. Other findings include a rising serum osmolality, extreme thirst, and dehydration.

NURSING DIAGNOSES

Following are the major nursing diagnoses associated with a patient with DI:

- Fluid Volume Deficit (R/T dehydration)
- Altered Cerebral Tissue Perfusion (R/T hypovolemia, dehydration)

INTERVENTIONS

The nursing responsibilities for the patient with DI include hourly monitoring of urine output and specific gravity. Serum osmolarity, electrolytes, and blood urea nitrogen levels should also be monitored carefully. The patient should be weighed daily, and intake and output records should be maintained. The nurse should also observe the patient for signs and symptoms of dehydration, electrolyte imbalance, and hypovolemia.

A major nursing responsibility is managing fluid replacement. The oral route may be used if the patient is conscious

TABLE 10-1
Drugs Used in the Treatment of Diabetes Insipidus

NAME	USUAL ADULT DOSE	DURATION	COMMENTS
Aqueous vasopressin	5–10 U SC	3–6 h	Short duration; used for patients who have immediate postoperative diabetes insipidus or who cannot be monitored frequently
Vasopressin tannate in oil	5 U IM	24–72 h	Painful injection; preparation must be warmed and shaken to mix properly; injection site must be rotated; used if diabetes insipidus is expected to last for a period of time
Lypressin nasal spray	Spray intranasally three to four times a day	4–6 h	Nasal mucosa must be intact; useful for mild diabetes insipidus; patient may develop nasal congestion, which will interfere with absorption
Desmopressin acetate (DDAVP)	0.1–0.4 mL intranasally	12–24 h	Causes minimal nasoconstriction; administered once or twice a day; used for severe permanent, or transient complete, central diabetes insipidus

In milder forms of diabetes insipidus (when ADH is secreted in small amounts), the following drugs may be used to enhance the secretion of ADH or to increase the response of the kidney to ADH:

NAME	USUAL ADULT DOSE	DURATION	COMMENTS
Fludrocortisone (Florinef)	0.1–0.2 b.i.d. PO (only)	6–12 h	Mineralocorticoid that favors reabsorption of potassium and sodium
Chloropropamide (Diabinese)	250–500 mg/d PO	24 h	Stimulates release of ADH from the posterior pituitary and enhances its action on renal tubules
Clofibrate (Atromid S)	500 mg q.i.d. PO	24 h	Same as above
Carbamazepine (Tegretol)	400–600 mg/d	24 h	Same as above
Hydrochlorothiazide (Hydrodiuril)	50 mg/d (or b.i.d.) PO	12–24 h	Used for nephrogenic diabetes insipidus

and able to swallow adequate amounts of fluid. If this is not possible, the intravenous route should be used. The rate of infusion should be monitored frequently and the amount of intake compared with the amount of output. In the patient who has triphasic DI, care should be taken to prevent water intoxication during the period of normovolemia of urine.

For the patient with permanent DI, a patient teaching plan should be developed and implemented. The following information should be included in the teaching plan:

- Information about DI
- Suggestions as to how to adjust one's daily schedule to accommodate the care needs associated with DI
- Information about the drug protocol (frequency, side effects, overdose)
- Information about follow-up care
- Recommendations regarding a medical alert bracelet

See the sections entitled Risk for Knowledge Deficit and Risk for Noncompliance in the nursing care plan for the patient undergoing transsphenoidal surgery in Chapter 18.

SYNDROME OF INAPPROPRIATE SECRETION OF ANTIDIURETIC HORMONE

Syndrome of inappropriate secretion of antidiuretic hormone is characterized by an abnormally high level or continuous secretion of ADH so that water is continually reabsorbed from the kidney tubules, resulting in water intoxication.

Clinically, SIADH is seen in three disease groups: carcinomas, pulmonary disorders, or central nervous system (CNS) disorders (Diringer, 1992). SIADH may occur in the following common conditions:

- Almost any CNS disorder, including head trauma, infections (meningitis, encephalitis, abscesses), tumors, cerebrovascular disease, subarachnoid hemorrhage, and Guillain-Barré syndrome
- Carcinoma, especially bronchogenic carcinoma (oat cell carcinoma)
- Pulmonary disorders, such as pneumonia, lung abscess, or tuberculosis

In addition, other conditions may cause temporary SIADH:

- Pain, fear, or major temperature change
- Positive pressure breathing on a respirator
- Increased secretion of ADH secondary to certain drugs (oral hypoglycemics, general anesthetics, chemotherapeutic agents, sedatives, opiates, and carbamazepine [Kinzie, 1987])

The criteria for the diagnosis of SIADH include the following:

- Low serum osmolality (usually <275 mOsm/L)
- Low serum sodium, which is a dilutional hyponatremia (<130 mEq/L)

- High urine sodium (25 mEq/L)
- High urine osmolality (higher than serum)
- Decreased urinary output (400–500 mL/24 hours)
- Generalized weight gain
- Absence of renal or endocrine disease (hypothyroidism or hypoadrenalism)

Pathophysiology

The negative feedback mechanisms that normally control the release of ADH fail to function in SIADH, and there is continuous release of ADH. The ADH causes excessive water retention by the kidney, resulting in *dilutional hyponatremia* and expansion of ECF. The syndrome can be temporary or permanent; the severity of signs and symptoms depends on the amount of salt depleted and the amount of water retained. SIADH is a major cause of hyponatremia in patients with CNS disease; it is usually temporary in CNS problems. The fluid retention involves the total body rather than a particular area or compartment of the body, such as the lower extremities.

Diagnosis

The possibility of an underlying renal or adrenal disease must first be ruled out before the diagnosis of SIADH is considered. Diagnosis of SIADH is based on the clinical and laboratory findings associated with the disorder. Associated CNS or respiratory system pathophysiology or drug therapy known to increase ADH secretion can usually be identified as the cause.

Treatment

The treatment of SIADH depends on its severity and the underlying cause of the problem. The underlying cause should be identified and managed. Often SIADH is self-limited in neurological patients. The principles of treatment include the following:

- Fluid restriction (<1,000 mL/24 hours). This may be the definitive treatment.
- Judicious replacement of sodium with a hypertonic solution (3%) of sodium chloride administered slowly. Hyponatremia is not corrected aggressively because of the risk of pontine myelinolysis (Chedid & Flannery, 1995). Correction usually occurs in 3 to 6 days.

Drug therapy for SIADH includes the following:

- Furosemide (Lasix) for diuresis
- In some instances, demeclocycline hydrochloride, 300 mg q.i.d., to suppress ADH activity
- Lithium carbonate, 900 to 1,200 mg, to inhibit the renal response to ADH

Nursing Management
ASSESSMENT

The patient with SIADH should undergo assessment of the following parameters:

- Intake and output
- Daily weight for gain, if possible
- Urine and serum sodium and osmolalities
- Urine-specific gravity
- Blood urea nitrogen
- Signs and symptoms of fluid and electrolyte imbalance (sodium depletion), lethargy, confusion, muscle weakness and cramping, headache, seizures, coma)
- History of kidney or adrenal disease

NURSING DIAGNOSES

The following nursing diagnoses may be appropriate for the patient with SIADH:

- Fluid Volume Excess
- Altered Oral Mucous Membrane
- Risk for Impaired Skin Integrity

INTERVENTIONS

The nurse caring for the patient with SIADH must monitor the laboratory values for serum and urine sodium and osmolalities. Intake and output must be carefully recorded and monitored. If an intravenous infusion is ordered, it should be administered slowly.

Most patients with SIADH are placed on a fluid restriction. The reason for this restriction should be explained to the patient and family. A strict intake and output record is maintained to keep the patient within the prescribed fluid restriction. Frequent mouth care is provided for comfort, because fluid restriction will cause the patient to have a dry mouth.

Because weight gain is common with SIADH, the patient is weighed daily. The accumulation of fluid also predisposes the bed-ridden patient to skin breakdown. Frequent skin care, turning, and repositioning should be included in the plan of care.

The hyponatremia associated with SIADH can lead to neurological changes in the sensorium, muscle cramping, headache, seizures, and even coma. The nurse must be aware of the signs and symptoms of sodium depletion and must notify the physician of any such changes so that definitive action can be taken before serious deficits develop.

SPECIAL METABOLIC AND ELECTROLYTE IMBALANCES

Cerebral Salt Wasting

Cerebral salt wasting, a condition characterized by true hyponatremia, primary loss of sodium and concurrent loss of ECF, decreased plasma volume, decreased body weight, increased blood urea nitrogen values, and a negative salt balance, has been discussed in the literature. It challenges the previously held belief that most hyponatremia is caused by SIADH. Table 10-2 presents a comparison of cerebral salt wasting and SIADH. Wijdicks and associates (1985) measured plasma volume, fluid, sodium balance, and vasopressin levels in patients with ruptured saccular aneurysms. They found that vasopressin (ADH) values were elevated at the time of hospitalization and then subsequently declined in the first week, regardless of the presence of hyponatremia. (By definition, SIADH is associated with an increased level of vasopressin.) Thus, they concluded that the natriuresis and hyponatremia were attributable to primary salt wasting rather than SIADH. Further, they recommended that the natriuresis and hyponatremia should be corrected with fluid replacement rather than by fluid restriction, the usual treatment for SIADH.

The role of ANF has been considered in cerebral salt wasting. Cells located in the two atria, but especially in the right atrium, produce ANF, a hormone-like substance. It is thought to be secreted in response to stimulation of the stretch receptors in the atrial wall. ANF is a potent hormone that increases renal excretion of sodium. Concomitantly, ECF volume and blood volume decrease slightly. ANF has a role in blood volume regulation, but the specifics of the mechanism are unclear.

Hyponatremia and decreased fluid volume are recognized as high risk factors for the development of vasospasm. The result of vasospasm is decreased cerebral blood flow to the affected arterial territory, causing ischemia and extension of cerebral deficits. Treatment of symptomatic vasospasm is directed at the primary goal of increasing cerebral perfusion pressure with hypervolemic-hypertensive therapy. Chapter 28 discusses hypervolemic-hypertensive therapy. Because the treatment of SIADH is fluid restriction, compared with fluid

---

TABLE 10-2
A Comparison of the Signs and Symptoms of the Syndrome of Inappropriate Secretion of Antidiuretic Hormone (SIADH) and Cerebral Salt Wasting

SIADH	SALT WASTING
Hyponatremia (dilutional)	Hyponatremia (primary)
Increased extracellular fluid	Decreased extracellular fluid
Serum hypo-osmolality (<280 mOsm/L)	Serum hypo-osmolality
Increased plasma volume	Decreased plasma volume
Increased body weight	Decreased body weight
Low blood urea nitrogen (BUN)	High BUN
Not necessarily a negative salt balance	Excessive natriuresis
Urine osmolality inappropriately concentrated compared with serum osmolality	Negative salt balance (primary loss of sodium)

volume replacement in cerebral salt wasting, the physician must make the distinction between the two conditions. Fluid restriction in a patient with cerebral salt wasting places that patient at high risk for the development of vasospasm and cerebral ischemia.

HYPEROSMOLAR NONKETOTIC HYPERGLYCEMIA

Hyperosmolar nonketotic hyperglycemia, a serious metabolic complication seen in some neurological patients, is characterized by high levels of hyperglycemia (600–1,400 mg/dL) without concurrent ketoacidosis. The syndrome can develop slowly and is usually seen in older patients (50–70 years of age) with a history of non–insulin-dependent diabetes mellitus. However, some patients without a history of diabetes mellitus have developed HNKH.

Some conditions appear to place patients at risk for the development of HNKH. The most common associated conditions seen in neurological patients are infections (especially those caused by gram-negative organisms, such as certain pneumonias and acute pyelonephritis), enteritis, acute trauma, severe physiological stress, hyperalimentation, and drugs known to interfere with diabetic control (*e.g.,* thiazide diuretics, mannitol, steroids, phenytoin). Most patients who develop HNKH have concurrent renal or cardiovascular disease.

Clinically, the patient develops polyuria, which leads to dehydration, hemoconcentration, hypovolemia, high serum osmolality (about 350 mOsm/L), and elevation of serum blood urea nitrogen. The serum ketone level is negative, and the acetone breath and Kussmaul respiration seen in diabetic coma are usually not present. The skin and mucous membranes are dry, with decreased skin turgor. Neurologically, the level of consciousness deteriorates from confusion to stupor and finally, to coma. Other neurological findings may include seizures, hemisensory deficits, and visual field cuts.

The treatment of HNKN is directed at cautious replacement of fluids, correction of the electrolyte imbalance and hyperglycemia, and treatment of the underlying cause. Half saline (0.45) with potassium replacement is given slowly. High doses of insulin are not necessary, because the patient does not have a problem with insulin use. The major problem in HNKN is dehydration. The major nursing diagnosis related to the care of the patient with HNKN is **Fluid Volume Deficit.** Clinically, the patient will be very dehydrated, and as a result of the severe dehydration, he or she may be comatose. The nurse monitors vital signs and hemodynamics and provides supportive care to these seriously ill, unconscious patients. (See Chap. 16 for more information on the care of the unconscious patient.)

MAJOR ELECTROLYTE IMBALANCES

When considering fluid and electrolyte balance, the nurse should be attuned to the various signs and symptoms of imbalance. As part of the assessment of patients, a review of the blood chemistry values should be included and correlated with the clinical presentation. Some patients can tolerate a wide deviation from the normal range of values, while others are sensitive to even slight changes. Note that there may be slight differences in normal values between laboratories.

The following information summarizes the major electrolytes and the various states of imbalance that can develop.

POTASSIUM

Potassium (3.5–5.0 mEq/L) is important in cell metabolism, such as protein and glycogen synthesis, and in cellular membrane potential; it is the chief intracellular ion.

Signs and symptoms of **hyperkalemia** (mild symptoms if the potassium level is 5–7 mEq/L; severe if the level is >7.0 mEq/L) include the following:

- Electrocardiographic changes or cardiac arrhythmias
  Tall peaked T waves
  Widening of the QRS complex or shortening of the QT interval
- Ventricular fibrillations leading to cardiac arrest
- Muscle weakness with decreased reflexes
- Bradycardia and hypotension
- Paresthesia
- Respiratory paralysis

Signs and symptoms of **hypokalemia** (potassium levels <3.5 mEq/L) include the following:

- Electrocardiographic changes or cardiac arrhythmias
  U waves
  Prolonged QT interval
  Depressed ST segment
  Low, flat T waves

SODIUM

Sodium (135–145 mEq/L) is the chief extracellular ion; it is important in osmolality and water balance.

Signs and symptoms of **hypernatremia** (sodium levels >145 mEq/L) include the following:

- Dehydration (poor skin turgor, dry skin and mucous membranes, sunken eyeballs)
- Stupor
- Thirst
- Oliguria

Signs and symptoms (not severe until the sodium level is 125 mEq/L or less) of **hyponatremia** (sodium levels <135 mEq/L) include the following:

- Confusion, lethargy, coma
- Seizures
- Hypotension, tachycardia (thready pulse), cold, clammy skin

CALCIUM AND MAGNESIUM

About one-half of the total calcium (4.5–5.5 mEg/L) and magnesium (1.3–2.1 mEq/L) is found as free ions in the plasma. The free form is physiologically active; the other half is bound to albumin and is inactive. When calcium and magnesium fall, they usually fall together because both are bound to albumin. Calcium is involved in blood coagulation, skeletal and cardiac muscle contractility, and several membrane and cellular functions. Calcium and magnesium are important in neuromuscular conduction and activation. Deficiency of magnesium has been associated with failure to wean from a ventilator.

Signs and symptoms of **hypercalcemia** (calcium levels >5.5 mEq/L) include the following:

- Deep bone pain
- Flank pain from renal calculi
- Muscle hypotonicity
- Nausea and vomiting
- Dehydration
- Progression from stupor to coma

Signs and symptoms of **hypocalcemia** (calcium levels <4.5 mEq/L) include the following:

- Tingling of fingertips
- Tetany
- Abdominal cramps
- Muscle cramps
- Carpopedal spasms
- Seizures
- Prolonged QT interval

Hypomagnesemia (magnesium levels <1.3 mEq/L) is a common clinical disorder, especially in the intensive care unit. It is a deficiency usually related to gastrointestinal or kidney problems. It is also common with long-term diuretic therapy.

Signs and symptoms include the following:

- Neuromuscular: twitching and tremors, muscle weakness, paresthesias, hyperreflexia
- Mentation and consciousness: depression, delirium, agitation, confusion
- Cardiac: premature ventricular contractions (PVCs), ventricular fibrillations or tachycardia; Torsades de pointes; electrocardiographic changes

Signs and symptoms of **hypermagnesemia** (>3 mEq/L; symptoms related to degree of elevation) include the following:

- Cardiovascular: hypotension progressing to prolonged QRS and PR intervals and finally to heart block
- Neuromuscular: sedation, hyporeflexia, muscle paralysis, respiratory weakness
- Other: nausea, vomiting, and skin warmth

Phosphorus is a form of phosphate ion (1.8–2.6 mEq/L). It is a key component of ribonucleic acid and deoxyribonucleic acid and is essential for intracellular storage and conversion of energy (adenosine triphosphate, creatine phosphate), carbohydrate metabolism, and regulatory compounds, and dissociation of oxygen.

Signs and symptoms of **hyperphosphatemia** (phosphorus levels >2.6 mEq/L) are usually not present. When high phosphorus levels are maintained for an extended time, phosphate deposits may develop in the body. Elevated phosphorus levels are often associated with renal failure.

Signs and symptoms of **hypophosphatemia** (phosphorus levels <1.8 mEq/L) are not present in patients with acute deficits. In those with prolonged deficiencies, bone pain, dizziness, anorexia, and muscle weakness may be noted. This condition is usually associated with hyperparathyroidism.

Although management and correction of electrolyte imbalances are collaborative problems, the effects of specific imbalances require nursing assessment and monitoring of specific parameters, such as apical pulse and level of consciousness.

Bibliography

Chedid, M. K., & Flannery, A. M. (1995). Head trauma. In J. E. Parrillo & R. C. Bone (Eds.), *Critical care medicine: Principles of diagnosis and management* (p. 1252). St Louis: C.V. Mosby.

Diringer, M. N. (1992). Management of sodium abnormalities in patients with CNS disease. *Clinical Neuropharmacology, 15*(6), 427–447.

Kinzie, B. J. (1987). Management of the syndrome of inappropriate secretion of antidiuretic hormone. *Clinical Pharmacology, 6*, 625–633.

Schultz, N. J. (1993). Body electrolyte homeostasis. In J. T. DiPiro, R. L. Talbert, P. E. Hayes, G. C. Yee, G. R. Matzke, & L. M. Posey (Eds.), *Pharmacotherapy: A pathophysiologic approach* (2nd ed.) (pp. 764–796). Norwalk, CT: Appleton & Lange.

Wijdicks, E. F. M., Vermeulen, M., ten Haaf, J. A., Hijdra, A., Bakker, W. H., & van Gijn, J. (1985). Volume depletion and natriuresis in patients with a ruptured intracranial aneurysm. *Annals of Neurology, 18*(2), 211–216.

CHAPTER 11

Pharmacological Management of Neuroscience Patients

Stephen W. Janning
Timothy F. Lassiter

OVERVIEW

Role of the Pharmacist in Patient Management

Traditionally, the profession of pharmacy has been devoted exclusively to dispensing a high-quality drug product. With advancement in technology, pharmacists have been safely able to devote less time to drug distribution services while assuming new roles in multidisciplinary patient management. At the same time, as medical science has advanced, pharmacological management of patients has become increasingly complex. Pharmacists are drug therapy experts whose primary responsibility is preventing and solving drug-related problems and providing drug information to all health care providers and patients. These circumstances have empowered pharmacists to become proactively involved in patient care as part of the multidisciplinary health care team. Pharmacists also develop and implement drug therapy monitoring plans, such as scheduling and reviewing serum drug concentrations, to achieve therapeutic endpoints and avoid toxicity.

Impact of Pharmacotherapy on the Nervous System

Pharmacotherapy has a tremendous impact on the assessment and care of the neuroscience patient. For example, many drugs commonly prescribed in the acute care setting can alter the level of consciousness (LOC). This is an obvious desired endpoint for narcotic analgesics, benzodiazepines, and other sedatives. However, many other drugs can also alter the LOC, either as a side effect (clonidine, H_2 receptor antagonists) or as a symptom of toxicity (relative overdose of imipenem in a patient with renal failure). Toxicity is of particular concern in

the elderly and any patient in the intensive care unit (ICU). In both cases, patients may be more sensitive to the pharmacological effects or toxicities of a medication. This sensitivity is frequently compounded by an impaired ability to eliminate the offending agent due to renal or hepatic insufficiency.

Despite the risks involved, properly managed adjuvant pharmacotherapy can indeed be life saving. In addition, drug therapies are being developed that may directly prevent neurological damage or improve recovery. For example, high-dose corticosteroids improve neurological recovery following acute spinal cord trauma. Several distinctly different approaches to pharmacologically limiting secondary brain injury following trauma are under investigation. Neuronal growth factor has been identified and reproduced in the laboratory.

Therapeutic Decision Making

Determining optimal pharmacological management of the neuroscience patient depends on numerous factors. Ultimately, a risk-benefit assessment must be made for each therapeutic decision. Occasionally, this process results in a drug being prescribed that carries with it a high risk of producing a deleterious effect but is also potentially life saving. This is frequently the case when amphotericin B or an aminoglycoside is prescribed. Another example includes a patient given sedatives and neuromuscular blockers for ventilator compliance at the expense of a reliable neurological examination.

Once a careful risk-benefit assessment has been made, one comparable therapy can be selected over another based on cost. Such decisions become more difficult when a more expensive drug can potentially shorten a hospitalization or avoid an expensive adverse effect. Unfortunately, studies that comprehensively examine health care costs from a pharmacoeconomic perspective are only beginning to emerge.

COMMONLY USED DRUGS ALONG THE CONTINUUM OF CARE

The discussion of drug therapy in this chapter is focused on practical information necessary to manage the neuroscience patient. Tables are included for a quick reference. Drugs are addressed by body systems. For those who wish more detailed information, pharmacology texts should be consulted.

Hemodynamic Support and Associated Drugs

In addition to proper fluid management, neuroscience patients in the ICU often require therapy with vasoconstrictors, vasodilators, or inotropes. Proper monitoring is essential and typically includes frequent measurement of mean arterial pressure, heart rate, central venous pressure, urine output, and cardiac output as determined by a pulmonary artery catheter. The goal is to meet the oxygen requirements of the body. More definite therapeutic endpoints, such as specifically targeted oxygen delivery values or a minimum acceptable blood pressure, are controversial. Therapy must be individualized for each patient. Hemodynamic regimens often involve multiple drugs, making physical and chemical compatibility an issue with respect to concomitant fluids and intravenous (IV) access. The pharmacist can help solve these complex problems. Never assume compatibility when appropriate data are lacking.

In the neuroscience patient, recent research has focused on cerebral oxygen delivery and consumption optimization, rather than cerebral perfusion pressure, as a therapeutic endpoint for hemodynamic manipulation. This is particularly useful when vasodilators and other antihypertensives are prescribed due to the complex interrelationships between vascular tone and cerebral perfusion in the setting of an acute neurological insult (see Chap. 17).

VASOCONSTRICTORS

Vasoconstrictors are helpful when hypotension is the result of a loss of vascular tone. This is commonly due to either sepsis or spinal shock. They are relatively contraindicated in untreated hypovolemic or cardiogenic shock. A high-dose requirement of vasoconstrictors for a prolonged period is an ominous sign because these drugs preserve blood pressure at the expense of organ perfusion. Extended periods of vital organ hypoperfusion contribute to multiple organ dysfunction syndrome, which carries with it a high mortality rate.

Dopamine is notable in that its pharmacological effects are dose dependent. At low doses ("renal-dose dopamine"), it is thought to increase blood flow to the kidneys and mesentery by selective vasodilatation. As the dose is increased, inotropic (increased cardiac contractility) and chronotropic (increased heart rate) effects predominate. At high doses, it is a potent vasoconstrictor, effectively overriding any selective vasodilatation activity. **Phenylephrine** is a potent vasoconstrictor devoid of direct inotropic or chronotropic activity. Some clinicians consider it the drug of choice for spinal shock, and it is being used more frequently for septic shock. Reflex bradycardia develops occasionally with its use. **Norepinephrine** is a potent vasoconstrictor with concomitant inotropic and chronotropic activity. **Epinephrine** acts as a positive inotropic or chronotropic agent at low doses and a vasoconstrictor with higher infusion rates (Table 11-1).

Regardless of the dose prescribed, great care must be taken to avoid extravasation of these vasoactive substances. This complication can produce extensive skin necrosis due to intense local vasoconstriction. Local instillation of phentolamine is indicated when this occurs.

INOTROPES

The inotropes are useful when cardiac contractility needs to be increased to optimize cardiac output. Careful titration is necessary because these agents can increase heart rate. Exces-

---

TABLE 11-1
Vasoconstrictor Agents

DRUG	DOSE	ADVERSE EFFECTS	COMMENTS
Dopamine	2–4 μg/kg/min	Polyuria, tachycardia, skin necrosis with extravasation	"Renal dose" dopamine may protect kidneys when giving other vasopressors.
	4–8 μg/kg/min	Tachycardia compared with equipotent dose of dobutamine, skin necrosis with extravasation	With inotropic dose may begin to see vasoconstrictor effects.
	8–20 μg/kg/min	Tachycardia, hypertension, skin necrosis with extravasation	Prolonged high doses produce organ hypoperfusion and renal dysfunction.
Phenylephrine	30 μg/min; titrate to effect (usually <300 μg/min required)	Reflex bradycardia, skin necrosis with extravasation	May be drug of choice for spinal shock; may be useful when other vasoconstrictors cause excessive tachycardia.
Norepinephrine	2 μg/min; titrate to effect (typically <30 μg/min)	Tachycardia, skin necrosis with extravasation	Useful for patients not responding to dopamine, organ hypoperfusion, and renal dysfunction with prolonged high doses.
Epinephrine	2–10 μg/min	Tachycardia	Primarily has an inotropic effect.
	10–20 μg/min	See above	Vasoconstricting dose preserves coronary and cerebral flow.

sive tachycardia can be deleterious due to decreased cardiac output as a result of shortened filling time and diminished stroke volume or from prolonged excessive myocardial oxygen demand in the setting of ischemic heart disease. The inotropes can also cause vasodilatation, which is usually tolerated poorly in this setting (Table 11-2).

Dobutamine is the most frequently prescribed positive inotrope. It is usually well tolerated and infrequently causes tachycardia. **Amrinone** is a newer inotrope that does not have direct chronotropic activity. It is also a vasodilator, however, so blood pressure must be monitored closely. Amrinone is associated with a high incidence of thrombocytopenia. **Milrinone** is similar to amrinone but is probably a more potent inotrope. It is also the most expensive drug in this class. Patients with severely impaired cardiac contractility are sometimes prescribed both milrinone and dobutamine. **Isoproterenol** is used infrequently as an inotrope due to its strong concomitant chronotropic activity. It is useful, however, for treating symptomatic bradycardia unresponsive to atropine.

VASODILATORS

Vasodilators are routinely prescribed in the neuroscience patient. They can be used in patients with impaired cardiac output to decrease the workload of the heart (afterload) and improve cardiac performance. More typically, they are used to control blood pressure in hypertensive patients with neurological sequelae. Blood pressure goals must be individualized to prevent further damage related to elevated pressures without also worsening cerebral ischemia. As mentioned previously, the most common side effects are hypotension and tachycardia (Table 11-3).

The calcium channel blockers are frequently used. **Nicardipine** is available in IV form and is a smooth-acting vasodilator when given as a continuous infusion. **Nifedipine** given orally or sublingually has been used extensively to treat hypertensive urgencies. It is more potent than nicardipine. Careful monitoring of vital signs and neurological status is required because nifedipine has rarely been associated with worsened ischemic stroke. **Nimodipine**, although an effective antihypertensive, is exclusively used to prevent cerebral va-

sospasm. In addition to having antihypertensive properties, any calcium channel blocker may help interrupt the development of secondary brain injury after trauma. **Verapamil** and **diltiazem** are effective when given as an IV bolus or infusion for supraventricular arrhythmias. They also lower blood pressure but are not routinely used in acute situations. Verapamil and diltiazem are often prescribed chronically to treat hypertension. Sustained-release oral dosage forms are available. They should not be crushed and given through any kind of enteral tube, because this will place the patient at risk for hypotension from the relative overdose. Similarly, non–sustained-release calcium channel blockers given once a day are likely to be ineffective unless they have a long half-life like amlodipine.

Nitroglycerin is a vasodilator but is often ineffective in managing severe hypertension. **Sodium nitroprusside** is a potent arterial and venous vasodilator that has been used for many years for hypertensive urgencies and emergencies. It should be avoided in patients with acute neurological injury because it tends to override any remaining vascular protection and expose the brain to excessively high pressures. High doses given for a prolonged period can lead to thiocyanate toxicity, particularly if the risk of renal failure is high. Unexplained acidosis is usually the first sign. Concomitant **sodium thiosulfate** has been advocated to prevent thiocyanate toxicity.

Beta blockers are also useful vasodilators. **Esmolol** is an ultra-short-acting beta blocker that can be given as escalating IV boluses or by a continuous infusion. It is also effective for supraventricular tachycardia. **Labetalol** is a more potent direct vasodilator. Many consider it to be the drug of choice for acutely managing hypertension in the neuroscience population because of its safety record and because it does not cause as much tachycardia as other potent vasodilators. All beta blockers have negative inotropic effects that can limit their use in patients with congestive heart failure. They can also worsen glucose control in diabetics, worsen pulmonary function in asthmatics, and (rarely) cause hyperkalemia.

Prior to the arrival of labetalol and other newer antihypertensives, **alpha-methyldopa** was frequently used for blood pressure management in the neuroscience ICU. Sedation is a common side effect. Other nonsedating vasodilators are now

---

TABLE 11-2
Inotropic Agents

DRUG	DOSE	ADVERSE EFFECTS	COMMENTS
Dobutamine	2.5 μg/kg/min; titrate up to 20 μg/kg/min	Hypotension, ischemia tachycardia	Wean slowly (1 μg/kg/min per hour); useful for low cardiac output unresponsive to fluids.
Dopamine, epinephrine, norepinephrine			See Table 11-1 for details.
Amrinone	0.75 mg/kg once for 3 min, then 5 μg/kg/min; titrate up to 15 μg/kg/min	Hypotension, ischemia, thrombocytopenia, tachycardia	Primarily a vasodilator; typically used with dobutamine.
Milrinone	50 μg/kg once over 10 min, then 0.375–0.75 μg/kg/min	Hypotension, ischemia, tachycardia	More potent than amrinone, typically used with dobutamine.
Isoproterenol	2–10 μg/min	Tachycardia, hypotension, ischemia	Excessive tachycardia limits use to severe bradycardia only.

TABLE 11-3
Vasodilators

DRUG	DOSE	ADVERSE EFFECTS	COMMENTS
CALCIUM CHANNEL BLOCKERS			
Nicardipine	5 mg/h IV; titrate q15min up to 15 mg/h; onset: 1–5 min	Hypotension, tachycardia	Doses > 15 mg/h not effective; fluid load can be substantial; max. concentration = 0.2 mg/mL.
Nifedipine	PO/SL: 10–30 mg q4–8h; max daily dose = 180 mg; onset: 5–15 min	Hypotension, tachycardia, headache, flushing	SL has been associated with worsened ischemic stroke.
Nimodipine	60 mg PO/SL (sublinguil) q4h × 21 d	Hypotension, tachycardia	For preventing vasospasm after aneurysm repair only; 30 mg q2h has been used in hypotensive patients.
Verapamil	PO: 80 mg q8h up to 480 mg/d	Heart block, worsened congestive heart failure, constipation	IV is useful for supraventricular arrhythmias, not for acutely elevated blood pressure.
Diltiazem	PO: 30 mg q6h up to 360 mg/d	Similar to verapamil but less pronounced	See verapamil.
Nitroglycerin	20–300 µg/min; onset: 1–2 min	Hypotension, headache, methemoglobinemia	Tachyphylaxis can occur; oral and topical forms are available. Provide "nitrate free" interval qd to lessen tachyphylaxis.
Sodium nitroprusside	0.5–10 µg/kg/min; onset: seconds	Hypotension, cyanide toxicity, especially with concurrent renal failure	Avoid in setting of increased intracranial pressure; some advocate concurrent sodium thiosulfate to minimize risk of cyanide toxicity.
BETA BLOCKERS			
Labetalol	IV: 10–20 mg over 2 min; may increase to 40–80 mg and repeat q10min up to total of 300 mg; onset: 5 min	Bradycardia, bronchospasm, worsened glucose control in diabetes	May be the drug of choice for many neuroscience patients; may use continuous infusion starting at 2 mg/min and titrate to effect.
Esmolol	500 µg/kg once, then 25–50 µg/kg/min up to 400 µg/kg/min; onset: 1–3 min	See labetalol; worsened congestive heart failure	Also useful for supraventricular tachycardia; it is very short acting.
Enalaprilat	IV: 0.625–5 mg over 5 min q6h; onset: 15 min PO: 2.5–40 mg/d	Hypotension, hyperkalemia, rash, cough, laryngeal edema	Intensity of response depends on fluid status of patient; IV form is at least twice as potent as oral form.

preferred because they do not affect neurological assessment. The angiotensin-converting enzyme inhibitor, **enalaprilat,** is now available for IV use in the acute care setting. The relative efficacy of this drug fluctuates depending on the volume status of the patient. Hypovolemic patients tend to have an exaggerated response, while fluid overloaded patients tend to respond poorly. Enalaprilat also can cause hyperkalemia.

Anticonvulsants

Anticonvulsants are a mainstay of therapy for patients with seizure disorders. These agents are effective for control of seizures from a variety of etiologies. Most patients with seizure disorders can be managed with pharmacotherapy alone. More than 20 different drugs are used to control convulsive episodes, but most patients are effectively managed with four to five agents used alone or in combination. A review of commonly used anticonvulsants is presented in Table 11-4. A more complete discussion of selected agents and nursing implications is offered below.

PHENYTOIN (DILANTIN)

Phenytoin is a member of the hydantoin class of anticonvulsants. It blocks synaptic post-tetanic potentiation and subsequent propagation of electrical discharge in the motor cortex. The drug blocks sodium transport and thereby stabilizes membrane sensitivity to hyperexcitable states. Phenytoin is used for management of tonic-clonic and psychomotor seizures. It may be used alone or in combination with other drugs. When used in combination, it is often possible to reduce the adverse effects of the respective agents and achieve a synergistic effect on controlling seizures. Phenytoin is also used prophylactically in neurosurgical patients to prevent seizures in the postoperative period.

Drug Level Monitoring. The accepted therapeutic range for phenytoin is 10 to 20 mg/L. Above this, side effects, such as nystagmus, ataxia, and altered cognition, are more apparent. The half-life of phenytoin varies considerably among patients and increases with dosage and plasma level. Steady state levels are normally reached in 7 to 14 days but may take up to

TABLE 11-4
*Drugs Used to Treat Seizure Disorders**

DRUG	INDICATION	ADULT DOSE	PEDIATRIC DOSE	THERAPEUTIC SERUM LEVEL	SIDE EFFECTS, TOXICITIES	COMMENTS
BARBITURATES						
Phenobarbital (Luminal)	Generalized and partial tonic-clonic seizures, cortical focal seizures, status epilepticus	60–240 mg/d†	3–5 mg/kg/d	15–40 mg/L	Sedation, rash, hyperactivity, ataxia, respiratory depression, hypotension (IV)	Induces hepatic enzymes—may increase elimination of drugs
Primidone (Mysoline)	Tonic-clonic, focal, or psychomotor seizures	750–2,000 mg/d	10–25 mg/kg/d	5–20 mg/L	Sedation, ataxia, nausea, dizziness, rash (similar to phenobarbital)	Active metabolites: PEMA and phenobarbital
HYDANTOINS						
Phenytoin (Dilantin)	Tonic-clonic and psychomotor seizures, status epilepticus	300–600 mg/d (15–20 mg/kg as IV load)	4–8 mg/kg/d	10–20 mg/L	Nystagmus, rash, sedation, fever, gingival hyperplasia, ataxia hypotension, and bradycardia (IV)	IV administration: limit 50 mg/min, as direct push into running IV line
Mephenytoin (Mesantoin)	Tonic-clonic, focal, psychomotor, and Jacksonian seizures	200–800 mg/d	100–400 mg/d		Nystagmus, rash, dizziness, ataxia	
SUCCINIMIDES						
Ethosuximide (Zarontin)	Absence seizures	500–1,500 mg/d	20–40 mg/kg/d	40–100 mg/L	Drowsiness, rash, headache, nausea, vomiting	Protein binding minimal, low potential for long-term toxicity
Methsuximide (Celontin)	Absence seizures	300–1,200 mg/d	5–20 mg/kg/d	40–100 mg/L	Drowsiness, rash, headache, nausea, vomiting	
OTHER AGENTS						
Carbamazepine (Tegretol)	Tonic-clonic, mixed, and psychomotor seizures	400–1,200 mg/d	10–40 mg/kg/d	4–12 mg/L	Dizziness, ataxia, nystagmus, rash, diplopia	Induces own metabolism and metabolism of other drugs
Valproic acid (Depakene, Depakote)	Simple and complex absence seizures	500–4,000 mg/d	15–60 mg/kg/d	50–100 mg/L	Nausea, vomiting, drowsiness, liver toxicity, diarrhea	Hepatic enzyme inhibitor
Felbamate (Felbatol)	Partial seizures, partial/generalized associated with Lennox-Gastaut syndrome	1,200–3,600 mg/d	15–45 mg/kg/d		Nausea, vomiting, diarrhea, anxiety, insomnia, rash, headache, hypophosphatemia	Risk of fatal aplastic anemia or liver failure; use recommended only if benefits exceed risks
Gabapentin (Neurontin)	Partial seizures with and without secondary generalization	900–3,600 mg/d	Safety not established in children younger than 12 y		Drowsiness, ataxia, dizziness, fatigue, nystagmus	Not expected to interfere with metabolism of other anticonvulsants
Lamotrigine (Lamictal)	Simple and complex partial seizures	100–500 mg/d	0.5–15 mg/kg/d		Dizziness, diplopia, headache, ataxia, nausea, vomiting, drowsiness, rash	Not expected to interfere with metabolism of other anticonvulsants
Clonazepam (Klonopin)	Absence seizures, Lennox-Gastaut syndrome	1.5–20 mg/d	0.01–0.2 mg/kg/d	20–80 ng/mL	Drowsiness, ataxia	Tolerance to anticonvulsant effect may occur in up to 30% of patients

* The agents in this table represent therapies commonly used in the treatment of seizure disorders. Dosing guidelines are ranges and may vary considerably among patients. For a more complete review of these agents or others not listed here, the reader should consult other standard references on pharmacotherapy or the management of epilepsy.
† d = day.

28 days in some patients. Except when patients are loaded on phenytoin, obtaining levels more frequently than every 3 to 4 days is rarely necessary.

Phenytoin is highly protein bound, with about 90% of drug in serum bound to albumin. Only the unbound (free) drug is available to exert a pharmacological effect. Serum phenytoin levels are normally reported as total drug concentrations. Thus, the free concentration is approximately 10% of the total phenytoin concentration, or 1 to 2 mg/L. In patients with hypoalbuminemia, total serum phenytoin levels may appear low, when the active free phenytoin component may actually be normal or high. In such patients, measurement of free levels are a better indicator of clinical response. When free phenytoin concentrations are not readily available, adjusted total phenytoin levels may be estimated by the following equation:

$$\text{Adjusted phenytoin level} = \frac{\text{measured phenytoin}}{(\text{serum albumin}) \, (0.2) + 0.1}$$

Drug interactions with agents that displace phenytoin from albumin will also increase the free concentration and lead to increased therapeutic effect or toxicity.

Administration. Phenytoin is available as an IV preparation, chewable tablets, oral suspension, and extended-release capsules. The IV and capsule formulations contain phenytoin sodium, whereas the chewable tablets and suspension contain phenytoin acid. Phenytoin sodium is 92% phenytoin. In some patients, changing formulations may result in altered serum concentrations due to the different percentages of phenytoin. The extended capsule formulation is the only oral form approved for once-a-day dosing.

In patients with feeding tubes, administration of phenytoin can present problems. The suspension tends to settle out in the bottle, making it difficult to deliver a specific dose consistently. Vigorous shaking is required to resuspend the drug. When administered concurrently with tube feedings, phenytoin may bind to the feedings, reducing absorption of the drug. While theoretically possible with all oral forms, this is most frequently reported with the suspension formulation. If serum levels begin declining in patients previously maintained on a fixed dosing regimen, administration may need to be staggered with feedings to allow time for complete absorption. Chewable tablets may be crushed and put down feeding tubes, and the capsules may be emptied and instilled through the tube. The extended phenytoin sodium contained in the capsule formulation retains its delayed release properties even when removed from the capsule shell.

Parenteral formulations of phenytoin are insoluble in water and contain solvents (propylene glycol and alcohol) to produce a solution. These solvents contribute to the problems associated with parenteral administration. The manufacturer recommends direct push into a running IV line at no more than 50 mg/min. Rates exceeding this lead to cardiac toxicity and hypotension. When administering large loading doses, however, this can be inconvenient. Dilution in various fluids can cause precipitation of the drug. Though not recommended by the manufacturer, various researchers have studied administration of phenytoin in 0.45% or 0.9% sodium chloride or lactated Ringer's with good results. Most studies mixed the drug in 100 to 500 mL of these fluids and used an in-line filter to prevent transmission of microcrystals to the patient. This technique may offer an alternative to IV push when large doses of phenytoin are given. Intramuscular administration is not advisable because absorption is highly erratic, and the extreme alkaline pH of the injection causes tissue damage.

Drug Interactions. Phenytoin is subject to many drug interactions. As mentioned previously, any agents that displace phenytoin from binding sites will potentiate its effect. Warfarin, tricyclic antidepressants, and aspirin are examples of agents causing displacement interactions. Because phenytoin is metabolized in the liver, drugs inhibiting (*e.g.*, cimetidine, valproic acid) or inducing (*e.g.*, phenobarbital, carbamazepine) hepatic metabolism will alter serum phenytoin concentrations. Additionally, phenytoin can alter effects of other anticonvulsants by unpredictable, complex mechanisms. Phenytoin may increase or decrease the action of phenobarbital and valproic acid and decrease the effect of carbamazepine. Patients should be carefully monitored when adding or discontinuing any medications to their regimen when taking phenytoin. Drug–food interactions may be clinically relevant. Chronic phenytoin administration can lower folic acid levels in patients, while folate replacement therapy may decrease its anticonvulsant effects.

Side Effects and Toxicities. With increasing plasma levels, common side effects include nystagmus, drowsiness, ataxia, fatigue, and cognitive impairment. Gastrointestinal (GI) symptoms of nausea, vomiting, or diarrhea are seen frequently. Administering phenytoin with meals can reduce the occurrence of these effects. Some patients will exhibit a fever while on phenytoin. An erythematous morbilliform rash may occur requiring discontinuation of the drug. Gingival hyperplasia is a frequent side effect with chronic phenytoin use. Patients should be counseled on the importance of good oral hygiene to minimize this problem. Rare complications include hepatotoxicity and blood dyscrasias.

VALPROIC ACID (DEPAKENE, DEPAKOTE)

Valproic acid is a carboxylic acid compound that exerts its anticonvulsant activity through increased brain levels of gamma-aminobutyric acid. There may also be some effect on potassium channels or direct membrane-stabilizing effects. The drug is usually used for treatment of absence seizures or in combination with other agents for control of various convulsive disorders. The enteric-coated formulation, divalproex sodium (Depakote) is metabolized to valproic acid in the gut.

Drug Level Monitoring. Accepted therapeutic levels for valproate are 50 to 100 mg/L. However, more recent studies have shown that higher levels may be necessary for effective seizure control. The toxicities associated with valproic acid do not seem to be correlated with serum concentration as much as with total dose administered. Steady state plasma levels are normally achieved in 2 to 4 days.

Drug Interactions. Valproic acid is a potent inhibitor of hepatic microsomal enzymes. As such, drugs that are metabolized in the liver will be eliminated more slowly from the body. Phenobarbital clearance is decreased considerably when combined with valproic acid. Valproate is also 90% bound to plasma proteins, creating the potential for displacement interactions. These effects may occur simultaneously, leading to unpredictable results when valproic acid is combined with other anticonvulsants. Combinations with phenytoin or carbamazepine are representative of this phenomenon, leading to increased toxicities or loss of seizure control when adding or removing agents from a patient's regimen.

Side Effects and Toxicities. GI complaints are the most frequently reported problem with valproic acid therapy and include nausea, vomiting, indigestion, diarrhea, and anorexia. These can be reduced by administering the dose with food or by changing to an enteric-coated formulation. Central nervous system (CNS) symptoms of drowsiness, ataxia, and tremor are also reported. Hepatotoxicity may occur, usually within the first 6 months of therapy. This has been most commonly reported in children younger than 2 years on multiple anticonvulsants. Minor elevations in liver function tests are often seen and appear to be dose related. Some physicians recommend l-carnitine treatment to protect against hepatotoxicity, but this has not been clearly proven to be effective. Valproic acid also affects platelet aggregation and may cause thrombocytopenia and other blood dyscrasias. Reduction in dose usually results in an increase in the platelet count.

CARBAMAZEPINE (TEGRETOL)

Carbamazepine is an iminostilbene derivative chemically related to the tricyclic antidepressants. It is is believed to reduce polysynaptic responses and block post-tetanic potentiation. The drug is useful in the treatment of tonic-clonic, mixed, and psychomotor seizures.

Drug Level Monitoring. Serum levels from 4 to 12 mg/L are considered therapeutic for carbamazepine. Steady state levels are initially reached in 3 to 5 days. Carbamazepine, however, has the unique property of inducing its own metabolism. Initial drug half-life ranges from 25 to 65 hours but decreases to 12 to 17 hours with chronic dosing. This effect is first seen in the first few days of therapy and is normally complete in 3 to 4 weeks. Thus, patients stabilized on a given dose early in the course of therapy may experience decreased levels and loss of seizure control with time. Frequent monitoring and dosage adjustments are necessary in the first few months of treatment to optimize drug therapy.

Drug Interactions. In addition to inducing its own metabolism, carbamazepine can induce the metabolism of other drugs. Interactions have been documented with valproic acid, warfarin, and ethosuximide, resulting in decreased blood levels of these agents. Carbamazepine is 76% bound to plasma proteins; thus, displacement reactions are less of a problem compared with other anticonvulsants. Other drugs induce (phenobarbital, phenytoin, primidone) or inhibit (valproic acid, cimetidine, erythromycin) the metabolism of carbamazepine and require careful monitoring with concomitant use.

Side Effects and Toxicities. The most common side effects of carbamazepine therapy are drowsiness, dizziness, headache, diplopia, nausea, and vomiting. These may be minimized by slow titration of dose and tend to decrease with time. Serious bone marrow toxicities have been reported, including aplastic anemia, agranulocytosis, and thrombocytopenia. Fortunately, these are rare. Leukopenia is the most common blood abnormality seen in about 10% of patients but is usually transient. Skin rashes may occur, ranging from a mildly eczematous form to a Stevens-Johnson type syndrome. Carbamazepine may also induce a hyponatremic hypo-osmolar condition similar to the syndrome of inappropriate antidiuretic hormone (SIADH).

PHENOBARBITAL (LUMINAL)

Phenobarbital is a barbiturate that exerts its anticonvulsant effect by depression of post-synaptic excitatory discharge. Therapeutic levels are between 15 and 40 mg/L. The half-life is extremely long (100 hours); thus, steady state levels will not be reached for 3 to 4 weeks after initiating therapy. However, this does allow for convenient once daily dosing in most patients.

Drug Interactions. Phenobarbital is a potent inducer of hepatic microsomal enzymes. Thus, it may reduce blood concentrations of any drug cleared by the liver, including phenytoin, carbamazepine, and valproic acid. Phenobarbital metabolism may be inhibited by valproic acid and alcohol (ethanol).

Side Effects and Toxicities. Sedation, fatigue, and depression are the primary side effects of phenobarbital, but tolerance does develop with chronic use. In children and the elderly, the drug may produce the opposite effect, causing insomnia and hyperactivity. Hypotension can occur with IV administration. Intramuscular injections are painful and can produce tissue necrosis. Respiratory depression can be profound after IV injections, especially when combined with benzodiazepines.

OTHER AGENTS

Newer anticonvulsants have been marketed recently for the management of seizure disorders. These include **felbamate (Felbatol), gabapentin (Neurontin),** and **lamotrigine (Lamictal).** These agents are indicated for adjunct use in a variety of convulsive disorders. Gabapentin and lamotrigine are unique among the anticonvulsants because they have not been found to interfere with the metabolism of other seizure medications. This is a desirable property when adding these agents to complex medication regimens. Lamotrigine may affect one metabolite of carbamazepine by a pharmacodynamic mechanism, but this has not been confirmed by controlled data. In these cases, patients can be managed by reducing the carbamazepine dose or by separating the administration of both medications by 1 hour. Felbamate, first introduced in 1993, was noted to cause aplastic anemia and liver failure in some patients. Given this, the Food and Drug Administration issued a warning in 1994 that patients should be withdrawn from felbamate treatment when possible. Patients should not discontinue treatment without medical supervision. When the risk of uncontrolled seizures outweighs the potential risk of hematological or hepatic problems, physicians are encouraged to obtain informed consent and should perform frequent monitoring for associated symptoms.

CHRONIC MANAGEMENT OF ANTICONVULSANTS

Patients with epilepsy or other secondary seizure disorders will often require long-term therapy with anticonvulsants to keep symptoms under control. Compliance with their medication regimen is crucial, because the most frequent cause of seizures in this population is abrupt withdrawal from anticonvulsants. Patients will need to be counseled on the importance of maintaining dosing schedules, potential side effects and their management, and the possibility for other drugs to interact with their antiepileptic medications. Frequent blood level monitoring may be necessary, especially when titrating doses of newly added agents. Establishing a relationship with a community pharmacist is essential to ensure safe management of this disease. Pharmacists can help the patient understand the side effects they encounter and provide close monitoring for drug interactions with prescription and nonprescription medications.

Sedation and Neuromuscular Blockade

The decision to give neuroscience patients sedatives is complex. On one hand, untreated agitation can contribute to ventilator noncompliance, self-extubation, and decannulation; worsen hypertension; and elevate intracranial pressure. However, agitation can also be an important symptom of hypoxemia, evolving sepsis, worsening neurological injury, or pain. Potentially reversible causes of agitation must be identified and treated prior to giving sedatives because the patient's neurological assessment will be compromised once therapy is started.

Once the decision to implement sedation is made, careful monitoring is important. Aspiration precautions should be instituted when appropriate. Respiratory depression and hypotension are common side effects of sedative regimens, so excessive sedation should be avoided. Prolonged sedation from overzealous administration of these drugs can delay extubation and complicate brain-death protocols. Sedation can also mislead clinicians into suspecting acute neurological deterioration and prompt otherwise unnecessary computed tomography scans. For these reasons, it is preferable to titrate sedative administration according to a sedation scale, such as the Ramsay, rather than giving an arbitrary amount. Continuous infusions of sedatives are probably more likely to result in excessive sedation than intermittent administration. Either way, the patient must be allowed to recover at regular intervals to allow neurological assessment. Recent research has focused on developing shorter acting sedatives to minimize these concerns and make them easier to use. Specific details regarding the use of individual sedatives and neuromuscular blockers can be found in Table 11-5.

BENZODIAZEPINES

Benzodiazepines remain the mainstay for sedation of the neuroscience patient. They can be given as an intermittent IV bolus or a continuous infusion. Benzodiazepines are relatively insoluble in water. This can be an important consideration when fluid limitation is necessary and dose requirements are high. This situation commonly occurs in neuroscience patients with benzodiazepine tolerance for whatever reason (tachyphylaxis) or a history of significant ethanol abuse (accelerated metabolism). The pharmacist should be consulted prior to dilution when concentrated continuous infusions are required.

Diazepam is the oldest injectable benzodiazepine. It is still frequently used for initial control of seizures. **Lorazepam** has also been available for several years and is particularly useful in patients with liver or hepatic dysfunction because its safe elimination tends to be preserved under these conditions compared with other benzodiazepines. **Midazolam** is the newest parenteral benzodiazepine, and some clinicians consider it the drug of choice due to its short half-life. However, more recent data have shown that the duration of sedation of all of the injectable benzodiazepines is roughly equal. In fact, numerous case reports describe long recovery times (*i.e.,* days) after midazolam infusions are stopped in critically ill patients.

Flumazenil is a specific benzodiazepine antagonist that can quickly reverse excessive sedation from these drugs. However, using flumazenil this way is specifically discouraged because it can cause severe withdrawal symptoms and seizures in benzodiazepine-tolerant patients. Patients who receive flumazenil should be monitored closely because it is very short acting. Resedation once it wears off is common.

OTHER SEDATIVES

Propofol is a very short-acting sedative that is being used in some ICUs. It is particularly useful when the anticipated duration of sedation is short, because recovery is rapid. Patients with long-term sedation requirements should receive a different agent because the short sedation duration is no longer advantageous. It is the most expensive sedative in routine use. Attempts at using propofol to lower intracranial pressure have been unsuccessful. Individual propofol preparations should not hang for longer than 12 hours because it is provided as a lipid emulsion, and is therefore an excellent medium for microbial growth. **Haloperidol** is a useful sedative and is particularly effective for patients experiencing delirium. Low doses tend to be prescribed, often with disappointing results. However, a properly titrated dose can be safe and effective. Extremely high doses (in excess of 100 mg per dose) and continuous infusions have been used safely. Haloperidol can lower seizure threshold and is usually not used in patients with known epilepsy. It can also cause hypotension if administered too quickly. The barbiturate **pentobarbital** is usually reserved for inducing pharmacological coma in the setting of status epilepticus or elevated intracranial pressure unresponsive to other treatment. High doses can suppress cardiac function. Serum pentobarbital concentrations are monitored, but the correlation with efficacy or toxicity is poor. Low concentrations need to be documented prior to declaring brain death in patients who have received high doses of pentobarbital.

CHRONIC MANAGEMENT OF SEDATIVES

Chronic sedative use should be reserved for patients in whom agitation secondary to a residual neurological deficit places them or others at risk for harm. Sedatives should be carefully

TABLE 11-5
Sedation and Neuromuscular Blockade

DRUG	DOSE*	ADVERSE EFFECTS	COMMENTS
BENZODIAZEPINES			
Diazepam	0.1–0.2 mg/kg q1–2h; onset: 1–3 min	Excessive sedation, respiratory depression, hypotension	Commonly used for initial control of seizures; active metabolite, vein irritant; considerably higher doses in patients tolerant to benzodiazepines (see text)
Lorazepam	0.04 mg/kg q2–4h; onset: 5–15 min	See diazepam	See diazepam; inactive metabolites; predictable response in critically ill
Midazolam	0.025–0.035 mg/kg q1–2h; onset: 1–3 min Infusion: 0.05–5 µg/kg/min	See diazepam; prolonged sedation, especially with continuous infusions	Unpredictable elimination in critically ill patients
Propofol	Bolus: 1–2 mg/kg Infusion: 5–50 µg/kg/min	Cardiovascular depression, infection risk with long hang times, hypotension	No withdrawal syndrome; quick recovery; expensive; does not directly lower intracranial pressure
Haloperidol	Initial: 2–10 mg; may double q30min until symptoms improve; onset: 3–5 min Maintenance: 5–40 mg q4h	Extrapyramidal side effects, lowers seizure threshold, hypotension (uncommon)	Works particularly well for delirium; up to 100-mg doses and continuous infusions tolerated well
Pentobarbital	3–5 mg/kg over 30 min, then 1 mg/kg/h, onset: <1 min	Cardiac depression	Serum concentration of 30–50 µg/mL may produce coma with low risk of cardiac side effects; must have level <10 µg/mL to determine brain death
NEUROMUSCULAR BLOCKERS			
Pancuronium	0.01–0.015 mg/kg; q1–2h	Tachycardia	Active metabolite accumulates in renal failure; "train of four" monitoring with nerve stimulator best for monitoring efficacy
Vecuronium	0.01–0.015 mg/kg; repeat q1h or start 1 µg/kg/min infusion	Prolonged paralysis increasingly reported	Partially active metabolite may accumulate in renal failure; expensive; use "train of four" monitoring
Atracurium	0.08–0.1 mg/kg, then 5–10 µg/kg/min	Histamine release	Does not accumulate in renal or hepatic failure; expensive; monitor "train of four"

* Sedative doses provided are for parenteral management of acute agitation only. Considerably higher doses are occasionally required with long-term use (see text). Chronic oral dosing (when appropriate) will differ and is highly patient specific.

withdrawn at intervals to make sure they are still indicated because excessive or unnecessary sedation can mask or impede neurological recovery. Fall precautions should be observed, even in patients taking these drugs chronically. Aspiration is also a long-term risk. Sudden discontinuation of long-term benzodiazepine therapy can precipitate a withdrawal reaction. Depending on the benzodiazepine, the onset can be delayed for as long as 7 days after cessation of therapy. Extreme agitation with hyperdynamic vital signs is a routine symptom. Seizures are not uncommon. The shorter acting benzodiazepines alprazolam and lorazepam may have a higher risk of seizure with sudden withdrawal.

NEUROMUSCULAR BLOCKADE

Occasionally, a patient may be so combative that neuromuscular blockade (NMB) is warranted. Other indications include short-term paralysis for a bedside procedure, elevated intracranial pressure unresponsive to other treatments, decrease work of breathing in patients with the adult respiratory distress syndrome, and increased ventilator compliance, particularly when nonphysiological modes, such as inverted inspiratory-expiratory ratio, are used. **Pancuronium, vecuronium**, and **atracurium** are the most frequently prescribed neuromuscular blockers. Vecuronium is probably used the most, but they all have advantages and disadvantages, so selection should be individualized. Specific details are listed in Table 11-5.

Careful monitoring is important when continuous NMB is prescribed. All the neuromuscular blockers are associated with tachyphylaxis. Therefore, as the patient becomes "tolerant" to a drug, higher doses are required. Patients requiring amounts that greatly exceed maximum recommended doses will usually respond to a different agent. Doses should be titrated so one or two twitches are maintained when a "train of four" is assessed by a nerve stimulator. Failure to do so increases the risk of excessively prolonged NMB after the drug is stopped. Complete blockade lasting several days after drug discontinuation has been reported, with abnormal neuromuscular weakness lasting several weeks after initial recovery. In addition, excessive doses waste health care dollars, because NMB regimens are very expensive.

NMB should be stopped regularly to allow a full neurological evaluation, because many of the signs and symptoms of acute deterioration will be masked while the patient is paralyzed. Furthermore, the patient must be adequately sedated (and when appropriate, receive adequate analgesia) at all times while the blockade is in effect. These drugs do *not* have sedative or analgesic properties. Hyperdynamic vital signs may be the only clue that sedation or analgesia is ineffective.

Antibiotics

INDICATIONS

Many neuroscience patients require antibiotic therapy at some point during their hospitalization. Antibiotics are often prescribed as prophylaxis in conjunction with neurosurgical procedures. The initial dose should be infused as close to the time of initial incision as possible (within 2 hours is optimal) for maximal efficacy. Therefore, they are best given in preoperative holding, as opposed to "on call to OR," to avoid ineffective prophylaxis due to unanticipated delays. The value of postoperative doses is controversial.

Occasionally, patients may have an unrelated preexisting infection, such as a urinary tract infection or community-acquired pneumonia, that requires treatment. In contrast, meningitis and ventricular shunt infections are examples of established CNS infections that require hospitalization for aggressive therapy with antibiotics.

Some patients come with an evolving infection as a result of prehospital events. For example, aspiration of gastric contents during an episode of status epilepticus often causes bacterial pneumonia in addition to a chemical pneumonitis. Presumptive antibiotics are often prescribed under these circumstances. Trauma victims may present with an open skull fracture or other systemic injuries, such as penetrating abdominal trauma, that require presumptive antibiotics for proper management.

Despite strict adherence to aseptic technique and optimal overall management, neuroscience patients are at high risk for developing nosocomial infections. Neurological impairment increases the risk of pneumonia, either as a result of continued aspiration, atelectasis, or prolonged mechanical ventilation. Indwelling devices, such as external ventricular drains, all methods of vascular access, and bladder catheters, are associated with infectious complications. Corticosteroid therapy and inadequate nutritional support also increase risk of nosocomial infection in the neuroscience patient.

GENERAL PRINCIPLES

Proper selection of antibiotics depends on numerous factors. These include the presumed site of infection, local antibiotic sensitivity trends, and patient-specific considerations. For example, preexisting conditions, such as drug allergies, a seizure disorder, or renal dysfunction, may preclude the use of one antibiotic over another in applicable patients. The selection of an antibiotic regimen for meningitis must take into account the penetration of that drug across the blood–brain barrier.

Once therapy is selected, the patient is monitored for response and adverse effects. Response is usually determined based on trends in core body temperature, white blood cell count and differential, and results of culture and sensitivity testing. Other tests specific to the infectious source, such as chest radiographs in patients with pneumonia, are also important when grading response. Generally, at least 72 hours is required to gauge the clinical response to a new regimen of antibiotics. Neuroscience patients can be particularly difficult to assess in this capacity. For example, depending on the primary neurological insult, certain patients may remain febrile due to a centrally mediated "resetting" of their core temperature, despite proper treatment of their infection. Corticosteroids can confuse the clinician either by masking an ongoing fever due to their antipyretic action or causing a sustained leukocytosis. Neuroscience patients may become "colonized" with nosocomial bacteria during a long hospitalization. This results in consistently positive cultures, despite the absence of a clinical infection. Thus, the whole patient must be assessed when determining response to antibiotic therapy.

Compared with other classes of pharmaceuticals, antibiotics (with important exceptions, see Table 11-6) are remarkably safe to administer. In general, few adverse reactions are related to IV administration. Drug incompatibilities, as always, should be checked prior to coadministering an antibiotic with another IV fluid or drug infusion. Most IV antibiotics, with the exception of trimethoprim-sulfamethoxazole and amphotericin B, can be given in reasonable volumes of 0.9% Normal Saline (NS). See Table 11-6 and the discussion of specific antibiotics below for details. Known allergies to antibiotics are common because they are so widely prescribed. Therefore, it is necessary to screen each patient for drug allergies before giving the first dose of any antibiotic. The assistance of a pharmacist can be invaluable in assessing the risk of cross-sensitivity in patients with allergies to certain antibiotics who require treatment for infection.

All antibiotics can disrupt the normal bacterial flora due to their antimicrobial action. Often, this does not cause a detectable problem or may result only in mild diarrhea. Unfortunately, this can also lead to superinfection by allowing other endogenous microorganisms resistant to the antibiotics to multiply unchecked. One possible outcome, pseudomembranous colitis, is characterized by high output diarrhea (which is occasionally bloody) and can be life threatening. The diagnosis is usually confirmed by the detection of *Clostridium difficile* toxin in a stool sample. Treatment consists of discontinuing the offending antibiotic(s) and starting enterally administered antibiotics, such as metronidazole, to treat the *C. difficile*. Antidiarrheals and antimotility agents are contraindicated until the cause of the diarrhea is identified. Another common example of superinfection is a serious nosocomial infection caused by "selected" multiply-resistant microorganisms that typically develops after a lengthy regimen of broad-spectrum antibiotics. The selection of resistant microorganisms (such as *Pseudomonas*) through the prolonged use and misuse of antibiotics ultimately affects the ecology of the entire health care facility. The recent emergence of vancomycin-resistant *Enterococcus faecium* as a serious nosocomial pathogen is an example. This unfortunate development in particular impacts the neuroscience patient, because the propagation of this new pathogen seems to be related to excessive use of vancomycin, which is commonly prescribed as prophylaxis in neurosurgical patients.

TABLE 11-6
*Antibiotics**

DRUG	DOSE†	ADVERSE EFFECTS‡	COMMENTS‡
Beta-lactams		Adverse effects common to all beta-lactams and related antibiotics: phlebitis, nausea, diarrhea, pseudomembranous colitis, hypersensitivity reactions (see text), rare disturbances in blood counts	All beta-lactams can cause neurotoxicity, including seizures with prolonged excessive doses
PENICILLINS			
Penicillin G	5–30 M.U./d	See above	Particularly useful for *Streptococcus* infections, including *Enterococcus,* weak activity against *Staphylococcus aureus*
Ampicillin	4–12 g/d		
Antistaphylococcal penicillins			
Nafcillin	4–12 g/d	Interstitial nephritis not rare, especially with methicillin; see above	Little activity against anything but *S. aureus;* strains resistant to methicillin are resistant to all three
Methicillin	4–12 g/d		
Oxacillin	4–12 g/d		
Extended Spectrum			
Piperacillin	8–18 g/d	See above; ticarcillin in particular inhibits platelet function	Useful for hospital-acquired gram-negative bacteria; can inactivate aminoglycosides in serum samples, resulting in falsely low values
Ticarcillin	4–24 g/d		
Mezlocillin	6–18 g/d		
Cephalosporins		See above; general adverse effect statement for beta-lactams	Most cephalosporins can falsely elevate creatinine
First generation			
Cefazolin	2–6 g/d	See above	Most often used for surgical prophylaxis
Second generation			
Cefuroxime	2.25–4.5 g/d	See above; hypoprothrombinemia	Cefuroxime is particularly useful for community-acquired pneumonia
Cefamandole	2–12 g/d		
Cephamycins			
Cefoxitin	3–8 g/d	See above; can cause hypoprothrombinemia	Expanded spectrum against enterics and anaerobes is good for intra-abdominal infection
Cefotetan	1–2 g q12h		
Third generation			
Ceftriaxone	1–4 g/d	See above	All are useful for hospital-acquired pneumonia; ceftizoxime and ceftazidime in particular are effective for meningitis
Ceftazidime	1.5–6 g/d		
Ceftizoxime	2–12 g/d		
Cefoperazone	2–4 g/d		
Cefotaxime	2–12 g/d		
Beta-Lactamase Inhibitor Combinations			
Ampicillin/Sulbactam	6–12 g/d	See above	See information on individual drugs; all have expanded spectrum against enterics, *S. aureus,* and anaerobes
Ticarcillin/Clavulanate	12.4–18.6 g/d		
Piperacillin/Tazobactam	13.5 g/d		
Aztreonam	3–8 g/d	See above	Similar spectrum as ceftazidime; does not cross-react in penicillin-allergic patients.
Imipenem/Cilastatin	1.5–4 g/d	See above; highest incidence of neurological toxicity, including seizures	Very broad spectrum; usually reserved for patients with known resistant bacteria.
Aminoglycosides			
Gentamicin	3–5 mg/kg/d	Nephrotoxicity, ototoxicity (?), neuromuscular blockade	Serum concentration monitoring is required to ensure efficacy, minimize toxicity (see text); therapeutic amikacin: peak = 25–35, trough = 5–10 μg/mL.
Tobramycin	3–5 mg/kg/d		
Amikacin	15 mg/kg/d		

(continued)

TABLE 11-6
Antibiotics Continued

DRUG	DOSE†	ADVERSE EFFECTS‡	COMMENTS‡
Vancomycin	IV: 2 g/d PO: 125 mg q6h Intrathecal: 5–10 mg q48–72h	Red man's syndrome, ? nephrotoxicity, ? ototoxicity	Role of concentration monitoring is controversial: peak = 20–40 µg/mL, trough at least 5 µg/mL typical therapeutic goals if measured; oral form only useful against *Clostridium difficile*
Antifungals Amphotericin B	0.25–1.0 mg/kg/d	Nephrotoxicity, electrolyte depletion, fever, chills, hypotension, anaphylaxis	Drug of choice for most serious systemic fungal infections; infuse over 4–8 h; not compatible in saline; 250–500 mL dilution is required
Fluconazole	100–800 mg/d	Rash, elevated liver function tests	Excellent enteral absorption; limited antifungal spectrum; drug interactions (see text)
Chloramphenicol	50 mg/kg/d	Aplastic anemia, grey syndrome, fever	Excellent penetration across blood–brain barrier

Fluoroquinolones
  Ciprofloxacin
  Ofloxacin
	400–1,200 mg/d
	400–800 mg/d
		Headache, restlessness, agitation	Significant drug interactions (see text); do not give with antacids or sucralfate

Acyclovir	15–30 mg/kg/d	Crystalluria, tremors, seizures	Effective for viral meningitis; infuse over at least 1 h
Trimethoprim/sulfamethoxazole	8–20 mg/kg/d (trimethoprim)	Allergic reactions, nausea, renal failure	Requires dilution in high volumes of dextrose; interacts with warfarin (see text)
Clindamycin	900–2,700 mg/d	Highest risk of pseudomembranous colitis, neuromuscular blockade (rare)	Effective against anaerobes and *S. aureus*; useful for aspiration pneumonia and intra-abdominal infection
Metronidazole	1–2 g/d	Diarrhea, metallic taste, disulfiram reaction	Active against gram-negative anaerobes only; useful in intra-abdominal infections; oral form is drug of choice for treatment of *C. difficile*

* Antimicrobials listed are restricted to those most frequently encountered in neuroscience patients.
† All dosing information refers to intravenous administration except where indicated.
‡ Adverse effects and comments listed for groups of antimicrobials apply to all antimicrobials in group unless otherwise specified.
d = day; M.U. = million units.

SPECIFIC ANTIMICROBIALS

The following is a discussion of specific classes of antibiotics, with special emphasis on nursing implications and application to the neuroscience patient. Specific details regarding dose ranges, clinical use, and adverse effects are listed in Table 11-6.

Beta-Lactam Antibiotics. Beta-lactam antibiotics are the most frequently prescribed class of antimicrobials. This category includes various *penicillins* and *cephalosporins, beta-lactamase inhibitor combinations, monobactams,* and *carbapenems.* They are effective for a wide variety of clinical infections and prophylaxis. Of particular note in the neuroscience patient are the third-generation cephalosporins, which, unlike most antibiotics, penetrate the blood–brain barrier well. **Ceftazidime** in particular is useful for gram-negative meningitis and has largely replaced the intrathecal instillation of aminoglycosides. Most beta-lactams are eliminated by the kidneys. When high doses of these antibiotics are given to patients with renal failure, subsequent accumulation of the drug can cause neurological side effects, including generalized seizures. The incidence of this adverse drug reaction is probably highest with the carbapenem antibiotic imipenem. A pharmacist can assist with questions regarding the proper dosing of these drugs in patients with renal insufficiency.

A common dilemma encountered in patients prescribed beta-lactam antibiotics is cross sensitivity. When a beta-lactam is ordered for a patient with a history of hypersensitivity to a similar antibiotic, the allergy must first be ascertained. A history of a severe reaction, such as anaphylaxis, to any beta-lactam precludes the use of any related antibiotic, with the possible exception of the monobactam aztreonam. Patients with a history of less severe reactions, such as a rash or hives, to a penicillin, for example, should probably not receive another penicillin but will probably tolerate a cephalosporin without incident. Careful monitoring is required, however. The reported incidence of cross-sensitivity of penicillin-allergic patients to a cephalosporin is probably about 5%. Cross-sensitivity with imipenem is rare but has been reported. Aztreonam does not cross-react in penicillin-allergic patients.

Because cephalosporin allergies are relatively uncommon, the incidence of cross-sensitivity with other beta-lactam antibiotics is unknown. Chemically distinct antibiotics should probably be used. It is worth noting that allergic-type adverse drug reactions can occur at any time during a course of antibiotics.

Aminoglycosides. The aminoglycosides are powerful antibiotics that are commonly prescribed for *nosocomial pneumonia, intra-abdominal infections,* and *urinary tract infections.* They need to be dosed carefully to maximize efficacy and minimize toxicity. Critically ill neuroscience patients often fail to attain therapeutic peak concentrations with typical doses. Furthermore, impaired renal function can lead to excessive aminoglycoside accumulation and may result in nephrotoxicity. Therefore, *peak and trough serum concentration* monitoring is necessary to ensure that the dose selected is safe and effective. These serum samples are usually obtained when the patient has reached a steady state, typically after three to four consecutive, properly timed doses. The recommended time these drug concentrations ("levels") are measured relative to the dose infused varies somewhat. Whatever the strategy, accurate documentation of *actual* infusion times and serum sampling times is critical to allow proper interpretation of aminoglycoside concentrations and prevent inappropriate adjustments. Pharmacists can be of great assistance when questions regarding serum drug concentration sampling arise. Peak concentrations of **gentamicin** or **tobramycin** need to be 6 to 12 μg/mL to treat most infections adequately, while trough concentrations should be less than 2 μg/mL to reduce the risk of kidney damage.

Recently, an alternative dosing strategy for the aminoglycosides called single daily dosing (SDD) has gained acceptance in many institutions. With SDD, patients with normal renal function receive their entire daily dose as a single 5 to 7 mg/kg infusion. This dosing strategy is supposed to increase efficacy and reduce toxicity, but definitive data are still evolving. Therapeutic peaks for SDD are 12 to 20 μg/mL, which needs to be considered if an aminoglycoside concentration is reported by the laboratory as toxic. Previously, peaks this high were thought to cause ototoxicity, but this is probably not true. Trough concentrations with SDD are usually undetectable. Therefore, instead of measuring a trough, the second serum level is usually obtained 8 hours after the peak is drawn. Aminoglycosides should be avoided in patients with myasthenia gravis because they have been shown (rarely) to potentiate neuromuscular junction blockade.

Vancomycin. **Vancomycin** is a chemically distinct antibiotic that is prescribed for many infections, such as catheter-related sepsis and meningitis caused by gram-positive bacteria (staphylococci, streptococci). It is particularly useful in patients with documented allergies to beta-lactam antibiotics. Vancomycin is the drug of choice for the treatment of documented infections with methicillin-resistant *Staphylococcus aureus* (MRSA). Empiric vancomycin prescribing in patients at low risk for MRSA is discouraged by the Centers for Disease Control and Prevention due to the emergence of *vancomycin-resistant microorganisms.*

An unusual acute flushing or erythematous reaction involving the upper torso and neck, dubbed "red man's syndrome," has been associated with the rapid infusion of van-

comycin. It resolves spontaneously by slowing down the infusion rate. Hypotension has also been associated with brisk vancomycin administration. To minimize infusion-related adverse effects, each gram of vancomycin should be given over at least 1 hour. Longstanding concerns about the association of excessive vancomycin accumulation with adverse effects, such as ototoxicity and nephrotoxicity, have not been supported in well-designed studies.

Patient-specific vancomycin regimens are calculated based on weight and kidney function. In addition, empiric vancomycin regimens are routinely monitored with peak and trough serum drug concentrations (see the section "aminoglycosides"). This practice has recently been challenged because the relationship between vancomycin concentrations and efficacy or adverse effects is unclear. The need for vancomycin serum concentration monitoring is less controversial in patients with meningitis, in whom high serum concentrations are needed due to poor penetration of the drug through the blood–brain barrier. In severe cases of meningitis when aggressive vancomycin therapy is indicated, the drug may be given intrathecally to overcome this problem. Patients receiving strictly prophylactic regimens certainly do not benefit from vancomycin concentration monitoring.

Antifungal Therapy. Antifungals are occasionally prescribed in neuroscience patients, usually for meningitis or urinary tract infections. **Amphotericin B** is the drug of choice for most serious systemic fungal infections. It is associated with numerous side effects, including hypotension, fever, nephrotoxicity, hypomagnesemia, and hypokalemia. These adverse drug reactions occur to a greater or lesser extent in virtually every patient who receives amphotericin B. Close monitoring is essential. *Potassium supplementation* requirements in excess of 200 mEq/d are not uncommon. Each dose of amphotericin B should be infused over at least 4 hours in an attempt to minimize these side effects. In addition, some clinicians advocate giving a 1-mg test dose prior to the first dose because anaphylaxis has been reported rarely. There is some evidence that sodium chloride repletion may decrease the risk of nephrotoxicity. Patients with fungal urinary tract infections may benefit from local treatment with amphotericin B, using either intermittent instillations or a continuous bladder irrigation. Systemic absorption is nil, thus avoiding the many side effects mentioned previously.

Fluconazole is a newer antifungal that is usually well tolerated, but resistance has been reported, and its efficacy for many indications is still under investigation. Its excellent blood–brain barrier penetration makes it particularly useful for cryptococcal meningitis in patients with the acquired immunodeficiency syndrome. Oral absorption is excellent. Fluconazole interacts with several drugs, including warfarin and phenytoin. Reducing the dose of warfarin or phenytoin is usually required to prevent bleeding complications or phenytoin toxicity.

Other Antimicrobials. Information about specific antimicrobials not discussed previously is listed in Table 11-6. Specific issues regarding these antimicrobials in neuroscience patients are discussed below.

Chloramphenicol is a broad-spectrum antibiotic that for years was the drug of choice for meningitis due to its excellent penetration into the CNS. Serious hematological toxicities and the availability of equally effective alternatives limit its use today.

The *fluoroquinolones* (**ciprofloxacin**, others) are useful for many nosocomial and community-acquired infections. Patients with concomitant renal failure require reduced doses to avoid neurological toxicity (see beta-lactams). Fluoroquinolones can interact with several drugs, including warfarin and theophylline. Patients receiving these drugs will have an increased risk of toxicity due to an amplification of their pharmacological effect when the fluoroquinolone is added. Doses of antacids, oral calcium or magnesium supplements, or sucralfate should not be given within 2 hours of an enterally administered dose of a fluoroquinolone, because absorption of the antibiotic will be impaired.

Acyclovir is an antiviral drug that is indicated for patients with serious viral meningitis. IV doses should be infused over at least 1 hour to avoid kidney damage from crystallization in the nephrons.

Trimethoprim-sulfamethoxazole is routinely prescribed for urinary tract infections. Occasionally, larger IV doses are prescribed for serious systemic infections with resistant microorganisms, such as *Xanthomonas maltophilia* or *Pneumocystis carinii*. Large volumes of 5% dextrose are required for proper administration. Check with a pharmacist prior to dilution when fluid restriction or isotonic fluids are important. A history of sulfa allergy, which is common, should always be ruled out before giving trimethoprim-sulfamethoxazole. Dermatological allergic reactions can be severe (Stevens-Johnson syndrome). Concomitant trimethoprim-sulfamethoxazole can also interact with warfarin and increase the risk of bleeding complications.

Metronidazole and **clindamycin** are two antibiotics with strong activity against anaerobic bacteria. Clindamycin is particularly useful for treating aspiration pneumonia because it also has activity against *S. aureus*. Diarrhea and, uncommonly, pseudomembranous colitis (see previous discussion) are associated with clindamycin. Metronidazole, in addition to being commonly used for intra-abdominal infections, is the drug of choice for pseudomembranous colitis (see previous discussion). The beta-lactamase inhibitor combinations (see Table 11-6) also have excellent antianaerobic activity, thus negating the need for concomitant metronidazole or clindamycin.

CHRONIC MANAGEMENT OF ANTIMICROBIALS

Neuroscience patients usually finish antibiotic therapy for serious infections while still hospitalized. However, home-based IV antimicrobials may rarely be encountered in patients finishing long regimens for difficult to treat infections, such as fungal meningitis. Proper education of the patient and family is crucial for the safety and efficacy of these comparatively complicated therapies.

Unfortunately, patients with incomplete neurological recovery requiring long-term care are still at an increased risk of developing new infections (see indications). Prophylactic antibiotics have been prescribed under these circumstances. However, this is generally discouraged because prophylactic antibiotics have not been shown to decrease

reliably the risk of clinically significant infections. In addition, when infections occur, they tend to be more difficult to treat due to selection of resistant organisms (see general principles). Furthermore, avoidable drug interactions, adverse drug effects, and increased health care expenditures are associated with these unnecessary antibiotics. When antibiotics become necessary, proper education of the patient and other caregivers is important, because noncompliance contributes directly to therapeutic failure. Having all prescriptions filled at the same pharmacy can decrease the risk of undetected drug interactions.

Stress Ulcer Prophylaxis

Neuroscience patients in the ICU are at high risk for developing what is now called stress-related mucosal damage (SRMD). SRMD can result in hemodynamically significant and occasionally life threatening upper GI hemorrhage. In addition to being "stressed" like other critically ill populations, neuroscience patients tend to secrete abnormally large amounts of stomach acid. This risk is further compounded when corticosteroids are concomitantly prescribed. Thus, pharmacological prophylaxis is necessary. Whether adequately tolerated upper GI feedings provide acceptable protection against SRMD is controversial. Agents prescribed strictly for SRMD prophylaxis are not typically required as part of the chronic management of neuroscience patients because the risk is only temporary.

HISTAMINE TYPE 2 ANTAGONISTS

Histamine type 2 antagonists (H_2 blockers) are effective in preventing SRMD. They act by decreasing stomach acid production. Attempts have been made to correlate a specific targeted gastric aspirate pH with efficacy, but there is no consensus about what that target value should be. A gastric pH that is consistently 3 or less may need higher doses of H_2 antagonists. A continuous infusion that can be titrated according to gastric pH may be indicated. H_2 antagonists can also be given enterally in patients with functional GI tracts. Refer to Table 11-7 for specific details.

H_2 antagonists are usually well tolerated. They have been associated with acute mental status changes (delirium, sedation), particularly in elderly patients in the ICU. There is also a potential for drug interactions involving these agents. In the neuroscience patient, **cimetidine** can decrease clearance of phenytoin, resulting in potentially toxic phenytoin concentrations. This is particularly significant when cimetidine is started or stopped in a patient already stabilized on a phenytoin regimen. **Rantidine** and **famotidine** do not appreciably interact with phenytoin. H_2 antagonists may also predispose patients to nosocomial pneumonia. The stomach is usually sterile because it is strongly acidic under normal circumstances. Acid suppression allows bacterial overgrowth, which is then available for aspiration and subsequent infection. However, studies to date comparing acid-reducing SRMD prophylaxis regimens with cytoprotective regimens (see following discussion) have not consistently shown a difference in infectious complications.

TABLE 11-7
Stress Ulcer Prophylaxis

DRUG	DOSE	ADVERSE EFFECTS	COMMENTS
H$_2$ antagonists			
Ranitidine	IV: 50 mg q8h Infusion: 6.25 mg/h PO: 150 mg q12h	Altered mental status, elevated liver enzymes, thrombocytopenia	Continuous infusions can be titrated based on gastric pH—see text.
Cimetidine	IV: 300 mg q8h Infusion: 37.5 mg/h PO: 300 mg q6h	See above	See above; interacts with phenytoin, warfarin, theophylline
Famotidine	IV: 20 mg q12h Infusion: 1.67 mg/h PO: 20 mg q12h	See above	See above; continuous infusion is not as well studied as ranitidine and cimetidine
Sucralfate	1 g PO/NG q6h (dissolve in 10–30 mL H$_2$O for NG use)	Constipation, hypophosphatemia	Does not affect gastric pH; do not give through any tube that empties anywhere but the stomach
Antacids	PO/NG (nasogastric): 30 mL q2h	Magnesium containing: diarrhea, hypermagnesemia in renal failure Aluminum containing: constipation, hypophosphatemia	Adverse effects depend on antacid used; dose can be titrated if gastric pH remains low; ? aspiration risk with higher volumes
Omeprazole	PO: 20 mg q24h	Diarrhea, abdominal pain	Not well studied for stress ulcer prophylaxis; do not empty capsule contents for administration by tube

SUCRALFATE

Sucralfate has been extensively studied for SRMD prophylaxis. It is as effective as H$_2$ antagonists in preventing SRMD. Sucralfate acts by covering the stomach with a protective coating. It is not systemically absorbed. Therefore, it is ineffective if given through an enteral access tube that empties anywhere but in the stomach. Likewise, suspensions or slurries should not be administered orally, because most of the dose will coat the upper pharynx and esophagus. Because gastric pH is unaffected, it may cause fewer infectious complications. These factors, coupled with sucralfate being the cheapest SRMD prophylaxis regimen, make it the drug of choice. Sucralfate should not be given at the same time as a fluoroquinolone, because absorption of the antibiotic will be impaired. Separating the administration of these drugs by 2 hours will minimize this effect.

OTHER PROPHYLAXIS REGIMENS FOR STRESS-RELATED MUCOSAL DAMAGE

The first SRMD prophylaxis regimen identified was antacids. Large doses have to be given every 1 to 2 hours. This requires considerable nursing time and may predispose to aspiration and subsequent infection (see previous discussion). **Omeprazole** is a strong inhibitor of gastric acid secretion. It has not been well studied for SRMD prophylaxis. It is only available in capsule form. The contents of the capsule should not be removed and given through a tube because this impairs the bioavailability of the drug.

Steroids

Steroids have several potential indications in the neuroscience patient. However, they can also cause significant side effects. Steroids can have either mineralocorticoid activity, glucocorticoid activity, or both. The mineralocorticoid effect causes sodium and water retention, along with potassium wasting. The anti-inflammatory effect of steroids is due to the glucocorticoid activity, which causes most of the therapeutic and adverse effects of these drugs. The following discussion is limited to systemic applications of these drugs in neuroscience patients.

DEXAMETHASONE

Dexamethasone is a potent steroid that has only glucocorticoid activity. This is advantageous in patients who require limited fluid intake to prevent edema or minimize swelling. It is usually prescribed for patients with vasogenic edema secondary to tumor. Currently available glucocorticoids are ineffective for the cytotoxic edema that commonly accompanies acute head injury, but research on newly discovered steroid derivatives (tirilazad, for example) continues. Dexamethasone is also commonly used to minimize inflammation after spinal cord surgery.

OTHER STEROIDS

Methylprednisolone has mineralocorticoid and glucocorticoid activity. Extremely high doses have recently been shown to improve recovery after spinal cord injury if started within

8 hours of the initial insult. It has also been used for certain neuromuscular disorders. Steroids should be avoided in myasthenia gravis, however. Fluid and sodium retention limit the usefulness of methylprednisolone in many neuroscience patients.

Hydrocortisone also possesses mineralocorticoid and glucocorticoid activity and closely resembles the cortisol normally produced by the body. It is routinely used in "stress doses" (200–400 mg/d) after trauma or major surgery in patients who take chronic steroids. **Corticotropin** or its synthetic form, **cosyntropin**, triggers cortisol secretion by the adrenal glands. Intermittent therapy has helped some patients with multiple sclerosis. It can also be used as a one-time dose to assess adrenal function.

Fludrocortisone is a pure mineralocorticoid. It is used to reverse the temporary sodium wasting that can occur in neuroscience patients It may also be required chronically after pituitary resection. It usually takes 2 to 3 days to assess the maximum effect of fludrocortisone. In patients with diabetes insipidus, desmopressin or vasopressin are preferred due to their rapid onset of action.

ADVERSE EFFECTS

Most of the serious adverse effects of steroids are due to glucocorticoid activity. Steroids lower glucose tolerance, leading to hyperglycemia and its complications. White blood cell counts rise, but the result is immunosupression because the cells do not function properly, predisposing the patient to infection. Steroids further confuse the evaluation for infection because they are antipyretics. They also can prevent or delay wound healing, contribute to muscle atrophy, and cause osteoporosis. While profound steroid deficiency can make a patient unresponsive to vasopressors, quick IV administration of large doses can cause cardiovascular collapse. Glucocorticoids can also cause significant GI bleeding. Antacids or H₂ antagonists are routinely prescribed concomitantly but have not been effective in preventing this complication. Steroids are appetite stimulants. They can also induce a profound psychological dependence and other neuropsychological changes. Excessive sodium and fluid retention and hypokalemia are common when agents with mineralocorticoid activity are administered. This can be particularly deleterious in patients with underlying heart disease or hypertension.

CHRONIC MANAGEMENT OF STEROIDS

While many neuroscience patients who receive steroids acutely tolerate them fairly well, the incidence of significant adverse effects rises with long-term therapy. Therefore, the risk-to-benefit ratio needs to be carefully weighed before patients are committed to chronic steroids. Once the decision is made, the minimally effective dose should be used. Drug-free holidays or intermittent ("pulse") therapy should be considered when feasible. However, patients receiving long-term steroids should be instructed never to stop taking them unless instructed to do so by the health care provider. Eventually, the body stops making its own cortisol when high doses of steroids are given for prolonged periods. Abrupt withdrawal can lead to cardiovascular collapse and other complications due to the sudden acute deficiency of this vital hormone. A slow

tapering of the dose can minimize these complications. Patients should also be instructed to watch for and report signs of infection (fever, thrush) or GI bleeding (melena, sharp abdominal pain).

Diuretics

Diuretics are used in neuroscience patients either as part of the hemodynamic management in general or to lower intracranial pressure. The osmotic diuretic **mannitol** is preferred for managing intracranial hypertension because it relieves intracellular edema in addition to prompting a diuresis. Patients with preexisting congestive heart failure should be monitored carefully, because the osmotic load of the drug may shift enough fluid into the intravascular space to cause vascular congestion and pulmonary edema. Serum osmolality should be monitored, especially in patients with renal failure, because the mannitol will accumulate. The drug is ineffective when the serum osmolality exceeds 320 mOsm/kg H₂O. Mannitol is also used to prompt diuresis in an attempt to minimize renal complications after angiography.

Loop diuretics decrease chloride and water reabsorption in the nephron. Therefore, a loop diuretic, such as **furosemide**, may assist in the fluid management of patients with elevated intracranial pressures; however, unlike mannitol, it does nothing to reverse intracellular edema directly. Furosemide is also a vasodilator and can lower blood pressure and relieve pulmonary congestion prior to the onset of diuresis. For this reason, IV doses should be given no faster than 10 mg/min. Patients with acute renal failure may receive very large doses in an effort to maintain an adequate urine output. Continuous infusions of furosemide have also been used in this setting. Other more expensive diuretics, such as bumetenide, have been tried, but they provide no advantage over furosemide when given in equipotent doses.

Hypokalemia and hypomagnesemia occur in virtually 100% of patients who receive a loop diuretic. Monitoring serum values and supplementing when necessary are important to minimize the cardiac sequelae associated with these deficiencies. Some clinicians feel that high doses of loop diuretics may be nephrotoxic, but the effects are probably mostly due to excessive diuresis and kidney hypoperfusion from hypovolemia. IV doses need to be doubled when switching to enteral therapy, because absorption is only about 50%. Likewise, patients maintained on oral therapy need to have their dose reduced by 50% when converted to a parenteral regimen unless a more vigorous diuresis is desired.

Gastrointestinal Agents

Neurology and neurosurgical patients often experience problems related to the GI tract. Many situations contribute to hypoactive bowel function, including surgery, paralysis, inability to ambulate, and medications, such as sedatives and narcotic analgesics. In patients receiving enteral feeds, delayed gastric emptying can lead to increased residuals and possible aspiration. The drugs commonly used for treating these conditions are GI prokinetics and stool softeners or laxatives. *GI prokinetics* stimulate the stomach and intestinal tract to improve gastric emptying and intestinal transit time. Two primary agents are available, metoclopramide and cisapride.

METOCLOPRAMIDE (REGLAN)

Metoclopramide was first introduced to treat diabetic gastroparesis but is often used in various hypoactive GI conditions. It is also used for gastroesophageal reflux disease and as an antiemetic for cancer chemotherapy. Metoclopramide sensitizes GI receptors to acetylcholine. It primarily affects the upper GI and intestinal tracts, with little effect on colon or gall bladder motility. Doses range from 10 to 20 mg given four times daily, 30 minutes before meals or every 6 hours in patients on continuous feeds. Available formulations include tablets, oral liquid, and injection.

Side effects from metoclopramide are related to its dopaminergic actions. The drug antagonizes central and peripheral dopamine receptors. Extrapyramidal and Parkinson-like symptoms may occur in 1% to 9% of patients, but in nonchemotherapy regimens, the incidence of these side effects is lower. CNS complaints occur in 12% to 24% of patients and consist of drowsiness, restlessness, fatigue, akathisia, and dizziness. GI symptoms reported include nausea and diarrhea. In patients requiring neurological assessments, metoclopramide's CNS actions may affect the examination findings.

CISAPRIDE (PROPULSID)

Cisapride is the second prokinetic agent marketed. It promotes the release of acetylcholine from the myenteric plexus in GI smooth muscle. It has stimulant effects on gastric, intestinal, and colonic function. Unlike metoclopramide, cisapride has no direct cholinergic effects or significant blocking action on dopaminergic receptors. Thus, it produces a more benign effect on the neurological examination compared with metoclopramide. The dose of cisapride is also 10 to 20 mg four times a daily. The drug is only available as an oral tablet. *Side effects* are primarily limited to the GI tract and consist of abdominal cramping and diarrhea. CNS side effects reported include headache and dizziness.

STOOL SOFTENERS AND LAXATIVES

These agents are used to promote passage of feces in patients with decreased bowel function. The many available products can be grouped in five primary classes. Bulk-forming laxatives (*e.g.*, psyllium, Metamucil) add fiber to facilitate normal passage of intestinal contents. However, if not given with sufficient fluid, bulk laxatives can have a constipating effect. In fact, these are sometimes given in minimal volume to treat diarrhea. Lubricants (*e.g.*, mineral oil) coat the stool in the intestinal tract to facilitate passage through the colon. Stool softeners (*e.g.*, docusate, Colace) are surfactants that increase the wetting efficiency of intestinal fluid, thus softening fecal mass. Saline laxatives (*e.g.*, milk of magnesia, sodium phosphate) draw water into the bowel through an osmotic process. Finally, stimulant laxatives (*e.g.*, bisacodyl) directly irritate the intestinal wall to promote peristalsis. Overuse of stimulant laxatives can lead to cathartic colon, in which the luminal wall loses tone and functions poorly. Any agent that increases intestinal transit and emptying have the potential to reduce absorption of medications from the gut.

Anticoagulants and Antiplatelet Agents

Drugs that affect coagulation are often encountered in neurology and neurosurgical patients. These may be used to treat primary disease, such as embolic stroke, or for prophylaxis of embolic complications in immobilized patients. The major anticoagulants used are heparin and warfarin. Antiplatelet agents include dypyridamole, sulfinpyrazone, aspirin, and ticlopidine, but the latter two are most commonly used for neurological conditions (Table 11-8).

HEPARIN

Heparin is used for the treatment and prevention of venous thromboembolism. It acts by combining with antithrombin III, which inhibits the intrinsic clotting cascade (activated factors XII, XI, IX, X, and thrombin). Thus, by inhibiting coagulation, heparin stops formation and growth of a thrombus and allows endogenous thrombolytics to eliminate the clot.

Dosing. Traditionally heparin is dosed by giving a 5,000-U bolus intravenously followed by a 1,000 U/h continuous infusion. The rate of infusion is titrated to achieve an activated

---

TABLE 11-8
Anticoagulant and Antiplatelet Agents

DRUG	ADULT DOSE	SIDE EFFECTS, TOXICITIES	MONITORING
Warfarin (Coumadin)	2–10 mg/day	Bleeding, skin necrosis	PT 1.3–1.5 × control or INR 2–3 (DVT, PE, stroke); PT 1.5–2.0 or INR 3.0–4.5 (cardiac origin)
Heparin	50–100 U/kg bolus, followed by 15–25 U/kg/h infusion	Bleeding, thrombocytopenia	aPTT 1.5–2.0 × control or 40–80 sec
Enoxaparin (Lovenox)	30 mg twice daily	Bleeding, thrombocytopenia	INR, PT, aPTT not routinely needed; CBC periodically
Aspirin	325–1,500 mg/day	GI upset, bleeding	
Ticlopidine (Ticlid)	250 mg twice daily	GI upset, bleeding, neutropenia	Routine complete blood counts

partial thromboplastin time (aPTT) of 1.5 to 2.0 times control. This normally equates to 40 to 80 seconds in most patients. Recent studies have shown reduced bleeding complications by using a weight-based dosing formula. Patients receive a bolus of 50 to 100 U/kg, followed by an infusion of 15 to 25 U/kg per hour. The half-life of heparin ranges from 30 to 150 minutes. Accordingly, serum aPTT measurements should be made 4 to 6 hours after initiation of therapy or any dosage changes. For prophylaxis, heparin may also be administered subcutaneously. Common regimens call for 5,000 U given every 8 to 12 hours.

Side Effects. The primary complication of heparin therapy is bleeding. The risk of bleeding is greater when the aPTT is above two times the control value. Given its short half-life, reduction or cessation of the infusion will rapidly reverse the effects. Heparin is a combination of different size polymers, of which only a small portion is believed to cause its anticoagulant effect. Low molecular weight heparin is thought to provide effective anticoagulation while reducing bleeding complications. One such product, **enoxaparin** (Lovenox) is dosed at 30 mg subcutaneously twice daily. Heparin may be reversed by administration of protamine sulfate. A dose of 1 mg of protamine will neutralize approximately 100 U of heparin.

Thrombocytopenia is also a complication of heparin therapy. Two primary effects on platelets are seen. One type presents as a slight fall in the platelet count soon after initiation of therapy. This effect is usually transient, with platelet counts tending to stabilize or return to baseline with continued therapy. The second type is normally seen after 3 to 5 days on heparin and is characterized by a continual decline in the platelet count. This form of thrombocytopenia is serious and requires cessation of heparin therapy if counts do not stabilize.

WARFARIN (COUMADIN)

Warfarin (Coumadin) is an anticoagulant that prevents synthesis of vitamin K-dependent clotting factors in the liver (factors II, VII, IX, and X). It is used to treat or prevent complications from venous thrombosis, atrial fibrillation with embolization, or pulmonary embolism. While the anticoagulant effect occurs within 24 hours of initial treatment, the antithrombotic effect is not present for 4 to 7 days. Because warfarin inhibits the *synthesis* of clotting factors, those in circulation are not affected. For this reason, patients should be maintained on heparin and warfarin for 5 days to allow for the full antithrombotic effect of warfarin to occur.

Dosing and Therapeutic Monitoring. Normal dosing ranges for warfarin are 2 to 10 mg/day. Doses are titrated to achieve a prothrombin time (PT) of 1.3 to 1.5 times control for deep venous thrombosis or 1.5 to 2.0 times control for prophylaxis in patients with prosthetic heart valves. The World Health Organization now advocates the use of the international normalized ratio (INR) for monitoring warfarin therapy. This method eliminates the variability seen between controls when using the PT. The target INR for most thrombotic conditions is 2.0 to 3.0; for prosthetic heart valves, it is 3.0 to 4.5.

Side Effects and Drug Interactions. Bleeding is the major concern with warfarin therapy. Warfarin overdoses may be treated by administration of vitamin K, but this will adversely affect continuation of warfarin therapy due to the synthesis of new clotting factors. Mild bleeding may often be resolved by holding one or more doses. Severe bleeding that is life threatening should be treated with IV fresh frozen plasma. A rare complication of warfarin involves skin necrosis. This occurs within the first 10 days and is due to a hypercoagulable state induced prior to achieving the full antithrombotic effect of the drug. Overlapping heparin administration for the first 5 days of warfarin use helps to minimize this complication. Warfarin is more than 98% bound to albumin, presenting a major bleeding risk from interactions with other highly bound drugs. Because warfarin is eliminated by the liver, enzyme inhibitors can also lead to increased anticoagulant effects.

ANTIPLATELET DRUGS

These drugs prevent platelet aggregation and subsequently reduce formation of arterial thrombi, which could lead to stroke or myocardial infarction. **Aspirin** is the most frequently prescribed antiplatelet agent. It irreversibly acetylates platelet cyclooxygenase, affecting function for the lifespan of the platelet (5–7 days). A number of studies have shown benefits in neurological conditions, including symptomatic relief of transient ischemic attacks and reduction in incidence of stroke. Doses ranged in these studies from 1.0 to 1.5 g/day. Newer studies are looking at the benefits of low-dose aspirin therapy for stroke. In myocardial infarction trials, benefits were seen with doses of 81 to 325 mg/day. Side effects from these doses are minimal and primarily consist of GI complaints.

Ticlopidine (Ticlid) is another irreversible inhibitor of platelet aggregation and is indicated for patients with cerebral ischemic symptoms or for poststroke patients. It blocks the adenosine diphosphate pathway and has no effect on cyclooxygenase. The recommended dose is 250 mg twice daily, taken with food. Because aspirin and ticlopidine act on platelets through different mechanisms, there may be some beneficial effects to using both together. However, this combination potentiates the effects of aspirin and may lead to toxicities. Ticlopidine is associated with severe neutropenia; thus, routine blood counts are necessary to monitor for this complication. Given this, it is often reserved for patients intolerant of aspirin therapy. Other ticlopidine side effects include diarrhea, rash, and minor bleeding.

CHRONIC MANAGEMENT OF ANTICOAGULANTS

Patients with thromboembolic disease often require long-term anticoagulation to prevent further complications. Some conditions in which this may be indicated include deep vein thrombosis, pulmonary embolism, and embolic stroke. The patient must understand the nature of the disease and the need for strict compliance with the medication regimen. Patients should be counseled to watch for any signs or symptoms of bleeding. They should also understand the need for frequent PT monitoring. Dietary counseling is also necessary, because foods rich in vitamin K can blunt the effect of warfarin. Those taking warfarin should be able to identify such foods and maintain consistency in their diet. Patients should be educated about the potential for drug interactions with warfarin.

The pharmacist can play a vital role in monitoring the patient's medication regimen for potential problems and offering advice on over-the-counter drugs that may adversely interact with warfarin.

Volume Expanders and Intravenous Fluids

In patients with cerebral ischemic injury from stroke or vasospasm, one cornerstone of treatment involves hypervolemic or hemodilution therapy. This is accomplished by administration of IV fluids (**crystalloids**) or plasma volume expanders (**colloids**). The goal is to increase systemic blood pressure to a level adequate to maintain cerebral perfusion. There is considerable debate among practitioners as to whether colloids or crystalloids are better, so a brief discussion of their respective use follows.

CRYSTALLOIDS

Crystalloids consist of solutions containing sodium chloride as their osmotic component. When fluids such as 5% dextrose and water (D5W) are infused, the dextrose is rapidly metabolized, leaving free water. This will rapidly equilibrate with extravascular tissues and fluid compartments and can contribute to fluid overload and edema. For this reason, isotonic fluids (0.9% sodium chloride, NS) are preferable for hypervolemic therapy. Because the solution is osmotically consistent with body fluids, the solution remains in the vasculature longer. NS will ultimately equilibrate with other body compartments, so the effect is short lived and requires continuous infusion of large volumes to maintain desired pressures. Alternatively, some clinicians choose to use hypertonic saline solutions (1.8% or 3% sodium chloride) for hypervolemic therapy. These solutions draw fluid from other compartments into the intravascular space, allowing for longer effects on blood pressure with lower administered volumes. Caution should be used when infusing hypertonic solutions through peripheral veins due to the potential for irritation and hemolysis. Using central venous catheters for administration avoids this problem. Frequent electrolyte monitoring is also necessary to avoid hypernatremic complications.

COLLOID

Colloid solutions contain osmotically active protein or starch molecules that increase plasma oncotic pressure. As with hypertonic solutions, colloids draw fluid from extravascular spaces and provide more sustained hemodynamic effects. Colloid solutions are normally isotonic, minimizing the potential for hemolysis. The effects from colloid administration usually persist for hours, allowing for intermittent dosing and reduction in total fluid given to the patient relative to crystalloids. **Albumin** is the major contributor to plasma oncotic pressure in the body. Commercially, it is available as a 5% or 25% solution. The 5% solution is isotonic and used when the patient is hypovolemic or fluid status is not an issue. More concentrated 25% solutions are hypertonic, which is beneficial in fluid-restricted patients or those with cerebral edema. **Plasma protein fraction (Plasmanate, PPF)** comes as a 5% solution of plasma proteins, of which 83% to 90% is albumin. Adverse effects from albumin and PPF are rare and usually are from hypersensitivity reactions to the proteins. Reactions are more common with PPF than albumin and more prevalent when PPF is infused at greater than 10 mL/min. **Hetastarch (Hespan)** is a synthetic colloid used to expand plasma volume. It produces hemodynamic effects much longer than albumin and PPF, ranging from 3 to 12 hours. Recommended doses should not exceed 1,500 mL/day; some patients have tolerated larger doses. The large starch molecule in hetastarch adversely affects coagulation and may precipitate bleeding in various patient populations. Case reports of bleeding and neurological deterioration have been noted in neurosurgical patients treated with hetastarch. In fact, the manufacturer recommends against its use in patients with subarachnoid hemorrhage and resultant vasospasm or in any neurosurgical patient in whom the possibility of intracranial bleeding exists.

Electrolyte Management

Patients hospitalized with neurological conditions often experience electrolyte abnormalities, especially in the intensive care setting. Surgery, fluid balance, medications, and the patient's own pathophysiology may contribute to imbalances in electrolytes. Without correction, such imbalances may worsen the patient's clinical condition. A discussion of key electrolyte disturbances and treatment follows.

SODIUM

This is the main extracellular cation in the body. Sodium performs two principal roles: regulating osmotic pressure and water balance between intracellular and extracellular compartments and maintaining acid–base balance. The normal serum level is 135 to 145 mEq/L. Hypernatremia is normally due to some form of dehydration and is treated by fluid replenishment. Hyponatremia can be due to a number of causes. Some reasons include fluid overload, cerebral salt-wasting syndrome, SIADH, and medications, such as diuretics. Treatment may include fluid restriction for SIADH or sodium replacement. Replacement may be accomplished with hypertonic saline (1.8% or 3% sodium chloride) or by increasing dietary salt intake. Dietary sodium replacements may be added to enteral feeds or taken by mouth in the form of salt tablets. **Fludrocortisone (Florinef)** is a mineralocorticoid that produces significant sodium retention and increases urinary potassium excretion. Fludrocortisone is useful in patients who remain hyponatremic despite aggressive sodium repletion. Doses range from 0.1 to 0.2 mg twice daily.

POTASSIUM

This is the primary intracellular cation and is important in the regulation of acid–base balance, balance of intracellular volume, and maintenance of electrical conduction in cardiac and skeletal muscle. The normal serum range is 3.5 to 5.0 mEq/L.

Hypokalemia is normally due to net body losses (nasogastric suctioning, vomiting, diarrhea, diuretics) or redistribution into cells (alkalosis). Symptoms include confusion, muscle weakness, diminished reflexes, arrhythmias, hypotension, and electrocardiogram (ECG) changes. Treatment consists of potassium replacement through the oral or parenteral route. Many available oral products may be used interchangeably according to patient acceptance. Enteric-coated potassium tablets should be avoided due to lesions resulting from dose dumping in the intestines. IV potassium replacement must be performed cautiously to avoid hyperkalemia secondary to a lag in redistribution into cells. Potassium may be administered safely at a rate of 10 mEq/h in most patients. Rates of 20 to 40 mEq/h have been used but should be accompanied by close ECG and serum potassium monitoring, which may not be possible in a non-ICU setting. Peripheral infusions of more than 10 mEq/100 mL are associated with burning during administration. Thus, central venous lines or larger veins should be used whenever possible.

Hyperkalemia is usually the result of excessive potassium repletion, shifts out of cells as with acidosis, and renal failure. Patients experience irritability, nausea, muscle weakness, and ECG changes. Therapeutic interventions for hyperkalemia include calcium chloride (cardioprotective), sodium bicarbonate or glucose plus insulin (shift potassium intracellularly), or exchange resins like sodium polystyrene sulfonate (Kayexelate, increase potassium elimination). Severe hyperkalemia may require hemodialysis.

CALCIUM

The role of calcium in the body is complex and involves a number of mechanisms, including coagulation, propagation of nerve impulses, insulin release, and cardiac contractility. The accepted normal serum (total) calcium concentration is 8.5 to 10.5 mg/dL. Most laboratories measure total calcium concentrations, but the free or ionized fraction is the active component. Thus, physiological changes can alter ionized calcium levels and make the total level seem abnormally low or high. Acidosis can raise free levels, whereas alkalosis increases calcium binding to albumin. This can cause a clinically relevant hypocalcemia while total calcium levels appear normal. Hypoalbuminemia can also result in lowered calcium levels. Total serum calcium values will decrease 0.8 mg/dL for each 1.0 g/dL deviation of albumin below 4.0 g/dL. When the patient's clinical condition complicates interpretation of total serum levels, ionized calcium concentrations may be necessary.

Hypercalcemia is most commonly due to malignancy or hyperparathyroidism. Symptoms include nausea, vomiting, bone pain, renal stones, muscle weakness, coma, and cardiac arrhythmias. Treatment modalities include loop diuretics, calcitonin, gallium nitrate, plicamycin, pamidronate, and oral phosphorus supplementation.

Hypocalcemia may result from a number of causes, including poor nutritional status, low serum albumin, pancreatitis, vitamin D deficiency, and hypoparathyroidism. Symptoms consist of tetany, abdominal and skeletal muscle cramping, convulsions, irritability, confusion, and cardiac changes. Correction of symptomatic hypocalcemia requires replacement through the IV route. Calcium chloride or calcium gluconate injection are the most common agents used. Most patients receive 1 to 2 g as a single dose repeated as needed based on blood chemistries. Administration of a 10% solution (1 g/10 mL) at a rate of 1 mL/min. is considered safe in most patients. The dose may also be added to maintenance IV fluids. Calcium chloride contains more elemental calcium per gram (13.5 mEq) than calcium gluconate (4.5 mEq).

MAGNESIUM

This is the second major intracellular cation and plays a role in nerve conduction, muscular contractility, and activation of multiple enzyme systems. Normal serum values range from 1.6 to 2.4 mEq/L. Hypermagnesemia almost always is due to renal insufficiency and is treated by dialysis or aggressive diuresis. Hypomagnesemia is characterized by paresthesias, muscle weakness, tremor, hyperreflexia, nystagmus, ataxia, seizures, and cardiac arrhythmias. Causes include inadequate intake, reduced GI absorption, primary renal diseases, and iatrogenic renal wasting secondary to medications (e.g., amphotericin, diuretics). Magnesium replacement may be accomplished orally or intravenously; however, oral magnesium absorption is variable, and large doses can induce diarrhea. Examples of oral regimens include milk of magnesia 5 mL or magnesium oxide 400 mg four times daily. Parenteral magnesium sulfate in doses of 1 to 4 g is commonly used to replete magnesium stores. Solutions more concentrated than 2 g/100 mL are associated with pain during infusion. A 10% solution may be administered as a bolus at a rate of 1.5 mL/min.

PHOSPHORUS

Primarily an intracellular anion, phosphorus is involved in bone formation and is the energy source of adenosine triphosphate to drive numerous physiological processes. The accepted range for serum phosphorus is 2.5 to 5.0 mg/dL. Hyperphosphatemia is normally a condition accompanying renal failure. Treatments involve administration of phosphate binders, such as aluminum hydroxide or calcium acetate. Hypophosphatemia occurs most commonly from insufficient nutritional intake, acid–base disturbances, or phosphate binding drugs (e.g., antacids, sucralfate, calcium salts). Symptoms include malaise, paresthesias, weakness, confusion, seizures, and coma. Phosphate salts can be given by the oral or parenteral routes. Oral intake for moderately low phosphorus levels should start at 50 to 60 mmol/d in three to four divided doses. Doses for IV administration range from 0.08 to 0.25 mmol/kg of lean body weight, depending on the degree of hypophosphatemia and whether the patient is symptomatic. Infusions should be run slowly over 4 to 6 hours to avoid phosphate intoxication.

Respiratory Drugs

Occasionally, neurology and neurosurgical patients will require medications to improve respiratory function. Conditions such as asthma, chronic obstructive pulmonary disease (COPD), or pneumonia can increase the work of breathing and complicate the patient's recovery. Bronchodilators are often used in this setting to reverse airway obstruction and help mobilize secretions. A brief review of agents used in the hospital setting is presented below. For a more complete coverage of therapeutic management of asthma and COPD, the reader should consult standard references on the subject.

ALBUTEROL (VENTOLIN, PROVENTIL)

Albuterol is a sympathomimetic that acts on β_2 receptors in the lung to stimulate bronchodilation. The resultant dilation of the airways is often beneficial to help the patient expectorate pulmonary secretions. Albuterol is available as a metered-dose inhaler, solution for nebulization, and a variety of oral dosage forms. In the ICU patient, dosing usually consists of treatments every 4 hours administered by a respiratory therapist. The nebulizer solution is used most frequently in mechanically ventilated patients, but metered-dose inhalers may be administered as well. In this scenario, the normal dose (two puffs) may be exceeded to account for drug loss in the ventilator tubing. Side effects of albuterol include tremor, headache, anxiety, tachycardia, nausea, and hypokalemia. These effects are minimized when the drug is given as an inhalation but may be encountered more frequently at higher doses. Other sympathomimetics seen in the hospital setting include *metaproterenol (Alupent)*, *isoetharine (Bronkosol)*, and *isoproterenol (Isuprel)*. These agents are less β_2 specific compared with albuterol and may cause more cardiac effects. In the neurosurgical ICU, these effects may translate to increased intracranial pressure in some patients and thus would make such agents less attractive bronchodilators.

IPRATROPIUM (ATROVENT)

Ipratropium is a quaternary amine anticholinergic bronchodilator. Its mechanism of action consists of blocking the effect of acetylcholine to maintain bronchial tone. Concomitant use with sympathomimetics provides an additive bronchodilating effect. The drug comes as a metered-dose inhaler and nebulizer solution. Standard doses are two puffs or one nebulizer treatment every 6 hours. Adverse effects from ipratropium are minimal due to its quaternary structure and consist primarily of dry mouth and cough.

Bibliography

Books

AHFS Drug information 95. (1995). Bethesda, MD: American Society of Health-System Pharmacists.

Boucher, B. A., & Phelps, S. J. (1993). Acute management of the head injury patient. In J. T. DiPiro, R. L. Talbert, P. E. Hayes, et al. (Eds.), *Pharmacotherapy: A pathophysiologic approach* (pp. 904–912). Norwalk, CT: Appleton and Lange.

Bradberry, J. C. (1993). Stroke. In J. T. DiPiro, R. L. Talbert, P. E. Hayes, et al. (Eds.), *Pharmacotherapy: A pathophysiologic approach* (pp. 336–356). Norwalk, CT: Appleton and Lange.

Chernow B. (Ed.) (1995). *Pocket book of critical care pharmacotherapy.* Baltimore: Williams and Wilkins.

Erdman, S. M., Rodvold, K. A.., & Friedenburg, W. R. (1993). Thromboembolic disorders. In J. T. DiPiro, R. L. Talbert, P. E. Hayes, et al. (Eds.), *Pharmacotherapy: A pathophysiologic approach* (pp. 312–335). Norwalk, CT: Appleton and Lange.

Gahart, B. L. (1995). *Intravenous medications* (11th ed.). St. Louis: Mosby-Year Book.

Garnett, W. R. (1993). Epilepsy. In J. T. DiPiro, R. L. Talbert, P. E. Hayes, et al. (Eds.), *Pharmacotherapy: A pathophysiologic approach* (pp. 879–903). Norwalk, CT: Appleton & Lange.

Knoben, J. E., & Anderson, P. O. (Eds.) (1993). *Handbook of clinical drug data* (7th ed.). Hamilton, IL: Drug Intelligence Publications.

Lott, R. S. (1992). Seizure disorders. In M. A. Koda-Kimble & L. Y. Young (Eds.), *Applied therapeutics: The clinical use of drugs* (pp. 1–22). Vancouver, WA: Applied Therapeutics.

Olin, B. R. (Ed.) (1995). *Drug facts and comparisons*. St. Louis, MO: Facts and Comparisons.

Samuels, M. A. (Ed.) (1995). *Manual of neurologic therapeutics* (5th ed.). Boston: Little, Brown, and Company.

Schultz, N. J. (1993). Body electrolyte homeostasis. In J. T. DiPiro, R. L. Talbert, P. E. Hayes, et al. (Eds.), *Pharmacotherapy: A pathophysiologic approach* (pp. 764–769). Norwalk, CT: Appleton & Lange.

Susla, G. M., Masur, H., Cunnion, R. E., et al. (Eds.) (1994). *Handbook of critical care drug therapy*. New York: Churchill Livingstone.

Wilson, R. F., & Janning, S. W. (Eds.) (1995). *Handbook of antibiotic therapy for surgery-related infections* (3rd ed.). Springfield, NJ: Scientific Therapeutics Information.

Young, L. Y., & Smith, G. H. (1992). Interpretation of clinical laboratory tests. In M. A. Koda-Kimble & L. Y. Young (Eds.), *Applied therapeutics: The clinical use of drugs* (pp. 1–17). Vancouver, WA: Applied Therapeutics.

Periodicals

Bracken, M. B., Shepard, M. J., Collins, W. F., et al. (1995). A randomized, controlled trial of methylprednisolone or naloxone in the treatment of acute spinal cord injury. *New England Journal of Medicine, 322,* 1405–1411.

Cully, M. D., Larson, C. P., & Silverberg, G. D. (1987). Hetastarch coagulopathy in a neurosurgical patient (letter). *Anesthesiology, 66,* 706–707.

Davidson, J. E. (1994). Neuromuscular blockade: Implications, peripheral nerve stimulation, and other concurrent interventions. *New Horizons, 2,* 75–84.

Durbin, C. G. (1994). Sedation in the critically ill patient. *New Horizons, 2,* 64–74.

Fabian, T. C., Boucher, B. A. , Croce, M. A., et al. (1993). Pneumonia and stress ulceration in severely injured patients: A prospective evaluation of the effects of stress ulcer prophylaxis. *Archives of Surgery, 128,* 185–192.

Gilman, J. T. (1995). Lamotrigine: An antiepileptic agent for treatment of partial seizures. *Annals of Pharmacotherapy, 29,* 144–151.

Janning, S. W., Stevenson, J. G., & Smolarek, R. T. (1996). Implementing comprehensive pharmaceutical services at an academic tertiary care hospital. *American Journal of Health-Systems Pharmacy, 53,* 542–547.

Lollgen, H., & Drexler, H. (1990). Use of inotropes in the critical care setting. *Critical Care Medicine, 18,* S56–S60.

Pohlman, A. S., Simpson, K. P., & Hall, J. B. (1994). Continuous intravenous infusions of lorazepam versus midazolam for sedation during mechanical ventilatory support: A prospective, randomized study. *Critical Care Medicine, 22,* 1241–1247.

Toole, J. G. (1987). Use of hetastarch for volume expansion-response. *Journal of Neurosurgery, 66,* 636 (letter).

Wagner, B. K. J., & D'Amelio, L. F. (1993). Pharmacologic and clinical considerations in selecting crystalloid, colloidal, and oxygen-carrying resuscitation fluids, part 1. *Clinical Pharmacy, 12,* 335–346.

Wagner, B. K. J., & D'Amelio, L. F. (1993). Pharmacologic and clinical considerations in selecting crystalloid, colloidal, and oxygen-carrying resuscitation fluids, part 2. *Clinical Pharmacy, 12,* 415–428.

Wallace Laboratories. (1994). *Felbatol package insert*. Cranbury, NJ.

CHAPTER 12

Respiratory Management of Neuroscience Patients

Christine L. Willis

Care of the pulmonary system has become increasingly complicated as sophisticated technology and knowledge continue to develop. Many advances, such as computerized ventilators with enhanced capabilities, are now available. There are more precise mechanisms for evaluating respiratory function and response and the overall effectiveness of therapy. These and other advances offer many additional options for patient care but also challenge the care provider to stay current and well informed about the respiratory information that is generated. As data are gathered during the course of patient care, physiological principles must be applied to clinical problems that arise. New therapies, devices, and approaches to treatment require constant appraisal of the treatment interventions that are most appropriate for each patient's conditions and situations, based on identified, specific outcomes.

Each member of the health care team has an integral function in providing comprehensive care, and nurses play a crucial role in this continuous monitoring process and in the clinical decision making that takes place. While the physician determines the diagnosis and course of treatment, the nurse's role is to be a patient advocate, providing ongoing assessment and intervention. The overall plan of care should be the product of the entire team's efforts, with the nurse overseeing the process and keeping all details aligned.

The respiratory therapist is one of the nurse's most valuable allies and resources. Therapists can provide invaluable information, including technical assessment and determination of the most appropriate mode of treatment based on individualized patient needs. Their expertise with the mechanical and technical aspects of care can do much to achieve optimal outcomes in patient care. Their role includes assistance in determining the most effective delivery technique and how to modify treatment as the patient's condition or needs change. Using arterial blood gases (ABGs), pulse oximetry,

capnometry, and determination of rates, volumes, pressures, and inspired oxygen levels, they can assist and be a supplemental source of information for the nurse, especially in the areas of physical assessment and response to therapy.

A well-integrated team approach, incorporating all members within the system, provides an optimal approach to care delivery. Each discipline must supply input based on their expertise. The patient can then achieve the maximal benefit possible.

THE CRITICALLY ILL NEUROSCIENCE PATIENT

Neuroscience patients offer a unique challenge to the care provider, especially when they experience respiratory compromise in addition to their primary neurological diagnosis. The interrelationships between the two systems must be kept in mind and monitored throughout the course of treatment.

While oxygenation is essential to the normal maintenance of overall body function, the critically ill neuroscience patient offers a unique challenge when pulmonary complications are also involved. In normal circumstances, respiratory function requires both an intact nervous system and a fully functioning pulmonary circuit. Without adequate oxygenation, cerebral metabolism is quickly compromised, and decreased levels of consciousness, coma, and brain death can occur.

Central control mechanisms are located in the medulla and the pons and regulate the autonomic functions of respiration. These centers provide feedback to regulate inspiration and expiration based on input from chemoreceptors and proprioceptive receptors throughout the body. The chemoreceptors are located in the bifurcation of the common carotid arteries and are sensitive to changes in $PaCO_2$. In normal conditions, an increase in $PaCO_2$ will stimulate ventilatory drive and increase the rate and depth of respiration. The proprioceptive receptors are stimulated by changes in the lung tissue and airways and transmit information through the vagus nerve back to the brain. The spinal cord is another active participant; it carries impulses to the brain from peripheral motor nerves originating in cervical and thoracic cord areas over myoneural junctions to respiratory muscles, the most important of which is the diaphragm. As the diaphragm moves downward, it creates space within the chest, increasing the intrathoracic pressure and allowing atmospheric air to enter (inspiration). Expiration occurs as the diaphragm relaxes, and the air is allowed to exit the thoracic cavity. Any interruption in these pathways or functions will affect respiration and ventilation.

Spinal cord injury and neuromuscular dysfunction may interrupt the pathway of impulses and interfere with respiration. In this situation, the muscles responsible for respiration are no longer stimulated to function effectively. Loss of normal protective functions of the airway or loss of appropriate muscle stimulation or function are the two most common problems faced when patients present with respiratory dysfunction as a result of neurological insult to the spinal cord or malfunction of neuromuscular circuits.

Central nervous system disease is another clinical situation that can interrupt the control of breathing. Increased intracranial pressure (ICP; tumor, injury, abscess, hydrocephalus, or vascular disruption), direct injury to the brain stem (infarction or tumor), or cerebral depression from drugs or metabolic disturbance can all lead to the need for intervention. Any of these processes will impact on the central chemoreceptors, affecting how they respond to normal respiratory stimulation.

Normal cerebral metabolism includes aerobic and anaerobic functions that provide the energy essential for functional demands. The brain must be continuously supplied with adequate blood flow because it has no intrinsic capacity for glucose storage. The brain requires approximately 20% of the body's total oxygen supply; it is dependent on the competency of the heart as a pump and on the lungs as a site for adequate gas exchange. Without sufficient mean systemic arterial pressure, cerebral autoregulatory mechanisms will not protect the brain from hyperemia (engorgement of the cerebral blood vessels) or cerebral ischemia. The balance of blood flow is reported as cerebral perfusion pressure. It is a measure of the blood entering versus the blood leaving the brain. ICP is a key factor when considering some of the interventions required in the care of the patient with pulmonary and neurological compromise. Changes in $PaCO_2$ will cause vasoconstriction or vasodilation, markedly altering the cerebral blood flow and ICP.

NORMAL PHYSIOLOGY

The lungs can be viewed as a bellows system that exchanges carbon dioxide for oxygen on a controlled basis. However, on closer examination, the process includes many other aspects associated with the overall integrity of the body. Several disparate functions occur simultaneously, including acid–base regulation, endocrine function, local and systemic immune function, and excretion. The pulmonary vascular bed also coordinates the flow of blood from the right side of the heart to the left and can affect cardiac output positively or negatively. One method to evaluate respiratory function is in terms of how effectively *ventilation, diffusion,* and *transport* of oxygen occur.

Ventilation is the process through which gas moves through the airways to the lung tissue and alveoli. Many factors can affect this movement of oxygen. These include function of the muscles that allow chest wall expansion (intercostals, diaphragm, accessory), the patency of the airways themselves, and the neural regulation that controls both of these actions. Neural output dysfunction can affect central respiratory centers (medulla and pons) and can be an obstacle to the conduction of impulses to the muscles responsible for ventilation. In addition, pain and "guarding" can alter breathing patterns and decrease the amount of gas that reaches the alveoli and is subsequently available for exchange.

Diffusion of oxygen from the alveoli to the arterial circulation depends on the physiological pressure gradients present between the arterial and venous blood that surrounds the alveoli in the pulmonary capillary vascular bed. This can be affected by the amount of tissue available for exchange (parenchyma) and by the amount of blood circulated through the pulmonary vascular bed from the heart. Loss of viable alveoli (emphysema), scarred lung tissue (pneumonitis, fibrosis), consolidation (pneumonia, atelectasis), and pneumothorax can interfere with the transfer of oxygen and carbon dioxide.

Transport of adequate amounts of gas is determined not only by the oxygen available, but also by the number of red blood cells and the amount of hemoglobin that carries the oxygen to the cells of the body. The heart and blood vessels must be functioning and patent to ensure that the pathways are used effectively. pH, $PaCO_2$ levels, amounts of **2,3-diphosphoglycerate,** and hypothermia or hyperthermia can also be factors and can hamper or facilitate transfer of oxygen and carbon dioxide at the cellular level. The **oxyhemoglobin dissociation curve** represents this graphically (Fig. 12-1). As the

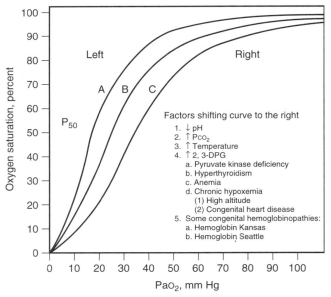

FIGURE 12-1
Oxyhemoglobin dissociation curve.

curve shifts to the right, hemoglobin loses its affinity for oxygen and readily unloads in the tissues. Conversely, a shift to the left causes hemoglobin to retain its oxygen, and it will not release it to the tissues as readily. Loss of red blood cells or hemoglobin (anemia, hypovolemia), loss of vascular pressure (shock, septicemia, hypovolemia), or blockage of a pathway (deep vein thrombosis, pulmonary embolus) are all examples of problems that can affect the transport process.

PATIENT ASSESSMENT

Developing standards of care for respiratory management is essential and is facilitated by identifying specific outcomes for therapy. When faced with respiratory dysfunction, several generic outcomes are common to all patients whether or not they also have neurological problems. These include (1) maintenance of adequate oxygenation and acid–base status, (2) provision for and maintenance of a patent airway, (3) prevention of complications associated with respiratory therapies (*e.g.*, necrosis of airway mucosa from prolonged intubation, aspiration, loss of hypoxic drive to breathe, barotrauma), (4) removal of secretions, and (5) resolution or stabilization of the respiratory dysfunction.

The need and degree of pulmonary support will vary according to the patient's clinical picture. In some instances, this need for support will increase or decrease on a dynamic basis. While the basic assessments include respiratory rate, level or degree of dyspnea, and other vital signs, additional specific tools can supplement diagnostic decision making. The assessment process to determine whether or not a patient will benefit from the initiation of respiratory therapy may be complex. The vital connection between the organ systems should be kept in mind to guide clinical decision making.

One of the best methods to ascertain concurrent or past pathology is to obtain an accurate health history from the patient or a reliable family member. The presence of chronic respiratory disease cues the caregiver that any additional insult to a major organ system will only complicate the clinical picture. Patients with known respiratory compromise will need oxygen supplementation and may need additional pharmacological intervention. Careful assessment of breathing patterns, the shape of the chest (normal thoracic configuration versus barrel shaped), and extremities will also yield valuable information. Further attention to inspection, percussion, and auscultation of the chest is helpful in determining specific problem areas that can be monitored.

Lung volumes and flow rates are additional indices of respiratory efficiency (Fig. 12-2). Pulmonary function studies can be completed in special laboratories, while less complicated assessments can be accomplished at the bedside. The information obtained will help pinpoint the current physiological problem and monitor the response to therapy. The respiratory therapist often must perform this task. The patient's results are then compared with standards based on age, sex, weight, and height. The information gathered can provide evidence of obstructive or restrictive processes within the lung. Changes from the patient's baseline can then be treated and evaluated on a continuing basis. As an example, patients with obstructive disease may increase the volume and flow rate of air following treatment with a bronchodilator. This response

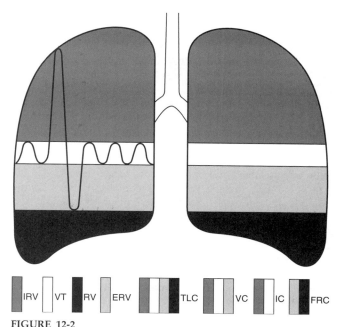

FIGURE 12-2
Normal lung volumes and capacities. (IRV = inspiratory reserve volume; V_T = tidal volume; RV = residual volume; ERV = expiratory reserve volume; TLC = total lung capacity; VC = vital capacity; IC = inspiratory capacity; FRC = functional residual capacity.)

can be detected by using previous and current pulmonary function studies.

Specifics of Assessment

The initial step is to determine whether or not the patient has a patent airway. If not, an artificial airway must be considered, such as an endotracheal tube or tracheostomy. Gas exchange must be evaluated, keeping in mind that increased $PaCO_2$ levels are a potent vasodilator. This is an important consideration when evaluating patients with neurological problems. Patients with increased $PaCO_2$s may need to be iatrogenically hyperventilated to reduce the CO_2 levels, thus lowering the ICP. In severe cases, the $PaCO_2$ should be maintained in the 25 to 30 mm Hg range, somewhat below the normal of 35 to 45 mm Hg.

Hypoxemia can also cause increased cerebral blood flow, and procedures such as suctioning can cause rapid and dangerous increases in ICP by temporarily decreasing levels of oxygen. When repeated suctioning is needed, it may be necessary to sedate the patient and hyperventilate using 100% oxygen before, during, and after the procedure. New "in-line" suction catheters that do not require the patient to be separated from the ventilator are now in use. In addition, some of the more modern ventilators have built-in mechanisms for delivering 100% at the touch of a button just before, during, and after the suctioning procedure.

The Assessment Process

The most definitive picture of oxygenation can be obtained through the analysis of ABGs. These values are a reflection of (1) arterial oxygenation (PaO_2), (2) alveolar oxygenation

($PaCO_2$), (3) acid–base status (pH), and (4) oxygen delivery to the tissues (PvO_2 determined by cardiac output, hemoglobin, and O_2 saturation).

Arterial oxygenation (PaO_2) is the portion of oxygen that is dissolved in the plasma of the blood. It is what remains once the hemoglobin molecules have been saturated completely with oxygen. Normal values are 80 to 100 mm Hg.

Alveolar oxygenation is evaluated by analyzing the level of CO_2. Like oxygen, it is carried by the red blood cells. Only 5% of it is dissolved in the plasma. It is also carried in the circulation as bicarbonate once it has entered the red blood cells and dissolved into hydrogen and bicarbonate ions. If the CO_2 is too high, the patient is hypoventilated, not eliminating enough CO_2 through adequate ventilation and the gas exchange process. Conversely, if below normal, it is a reflection of hyperventilation or too rapid elimination of CO_2. Normal values are 35 to 45 mm Hg.

The pH is the relationship between the amount of acid (carbonic acid, H_2CO_3) in the blood in relation to the amount of base (bicarbonate HCO_3^-) in the blood. The normal ratio is 20:1 which yields a pH of 7.40. If the pH is below 7.35, acidemia occurs and is caused by an increase in $PaCO_2$ (respiratory control) or a decrease in bicarbonate (renal or metabolic control). When the pH is above 7.45, alkalosis occurs and is the result of decreased $PaCO_2$ (respiratory control) or increased bicarbonate (metabolic control).

The body strives to maintain the pH within the narrow margins of 7.35 and 7.45. The lungs are the most rapid regulator, able to shift the rate and depth of ventilation within minutes to coordinate the amount of CO_2 retained or eliminated. Other metabolic exchanges regulated in the kidney control bicarbonate release or conservation. These metabolic processes take longer to act but will eventually aid in the compensation process when imbalance occurs for a prolonged period.

Actual calculation of tissue level O_2 consumption requires invasive monitoring devices (Swan-Ganz catheters). It is obtained using the Fick equation, calculating consumption based on cardiac output times the difference between arterial and venous O_2 levels. The product of the equation is the amount of oxygen used at the cellular level.

$$V\,O_2 = Q \times (Ca\,O_2 - Cv\,O_2)$$

Pulse oximetry is noninvasive; however, the data generated provide only saturated hemoglobin values (SaO_2). It is used as an adjunct to ABGs. The technique uses spectrophotometry emitting light from a probe that is directed through a capillary bed. It is read by measuring the amount of oxygen bound to hemoglobin. The monitor provides a percentage of saturation. Probes can be positioned at several body sites, such as the finger, ear lobe, or bridge of the nose. Several factors can cause inaccurate readings: reduced blood flow, severe anemia, hypotension, hypothermia, darkly pigmented skin, nail polish, an increase in ambient environmental light, or any distortion of the arterial pulse. A normal reading is between 92% and 100%. The presence of hemoglobinopathies can also effect the reading.

Alternatively, *capnometry* can be used to determine approximate levels of PCO_2. This technique analyzes exhaled carbon dioxide. It is a noninvasive method using mass spectrometry. Two types are currently used: mainstream and sidestream analyzers. Mainstream units analyze for CO_2 content directly from the endotracheal tube. Sidestream devices analyze for CO_2 away from the airway itself and carry the sample to a separate chamber for analysis. The uses of capnometry are limited; although there is correlation between arterial $PaCO_2$ and PCO_2, during crucial times, such as ventilator weaning, it is usually best to rely on serial blood gas measurements to assess the effect of therapy and guide further treatment.

CAUSES OF INCREASED PCO_2	CAUSES OF DECREASED PCO_2
Increased CO_2 production	Decreased CO_2 production
Decreased alveolar ventilation	Increased alveolar ventilation
Machine failure (*e.g.*, leak in circuit)	Machine failure (*e.g.*, esophageal intubation, disconnection, cuff leak)

WHEN TO INITIATE OXYGEN THERAPY

Once it has been determined that a patient requires supplemental oxygen therapy, it is necessary to determine how much to administer and the most effective route. The goals for therapy are based on information gained using the oxyhemoglobin dissociation curve. It is essential to deliver enough oxygen to maintain the PaO_2 at or greater than 70 mm Hg. At this level, the hemoglobin is saturated to ensure adequate delivery of oxygen to the tissues. One general rule of therapy is not to use more oxygen than is necessary because of the risk of toxic damage by FiO_2 levels above 50%. It is important to remember that the patient with chronic obstructive pulmonary disease (COPD) is a special case and may be injured by even minimal levels of supplemental oxygen. This phenomenon occurs because of compensatory mechanisms. With time, the chronically high level of CO_2 is no longer the stimulus to breathe, making the patient dependent on low levels of oxygen rather than on high levels of CO_2. Supplemental therapy for this patient population must be gauged carefully to avoid reducing this hypoxic drive.

A specific guideline to use in the initiation of supplemental oxygen is a PaO_2 of 50 mm Hg or more. Below this level, the oxyhemoglobin dissociation curve drops off sharply, and the saturation of the hemoglobin molecule is in jeopardy. It is wise to begin therapy cautiously and to adjust the level according to serial blood gas measurements. Pulse oximetry is not appropriate in this situation because it will not monitor pH and CO_2 levels adequately. Avoid nitrogen washout atelectasis and oxygen toxicity caused by using too high levels of inspired oxygen.

Two categories of oxygen therapy are available for adults who are able to breathe spontaneously. Low-flow (or variable performance equipment) and high-flow (or fixed performance) equipment. Low-flow systems will entrain certain amounts of room air so that the absolute delivery depends on (1) the liter flow, (2) the size of the reservoir (size of the face mask), (3) the amount of the physiological reservoir in the naso-oropharynx, (4) the capacity of the reservoir to refill during the various phases of inspiration and expiration, and (5) the ventilatory pattern of the patient. High-flow systems provide a consistent FiO$_2$, essentially providing an excess of flow well beyond the calculated needs of minute volumes or inspiratory flow rates. Examples are Venturi masks and high-volume aerosol systems. These are not always the most efficient and precise alternative and may be difficult to quantify especially in precarious clinical situations.

The most commonly used systems are those that use low-flow methods. These include the nasal cannula, the simple face mask (without the reservoir), the partial rebreather mask, and the nonrebreather mask.

The nasal cannula is the most frequently used device and is usually considered the most comfortable. It has its drawbacks because it can be a source of breakdown of tissue, which can occur from drying of the nasal mucosa or pressure around the ears and nares. The actual amount of inspired oxygen can vary based on the patient's rate and depth of respiration. It also requires the patient to breathe through the nose and not the mouth. In most instances, though, the delivered FiO$_2$ can be estimated roughly using the increments in the following table:

L/min	FiO$_2$
1	0.24
2	0.28
3	0.32
4	0.36
5	0.40
6	0.44

The simple face mask is another alternative. Its efficiency depends on the patient's ventilatory pattern and depth of respiration. It is generally available in only one size. The fit of the mask impacts the amount of oxygen delivered. If the fit is not optimal, more room air will be entrained with a dilution of the FiO$_2$ as a result. The high flow of gas that must be used with this type of device washes out the residual CO$_2$ of exhalation so that there is very little CO$_2$ rebreathing. The drawbacks of the mask include the same type of pressure sores associated with the nasal cannula, an increased risk of aspiration, and drying of the eyes from the high flow of gas through the system. Use of the mask may also increase a dyspneic patient's feelings of claustrophobia. Because of the associated discomfort, patients will often remove the mask, making the issue of compliance a concern as well. The following table illustrates the comparison of the types of masks:

MASK	L/min	FiO$_2$
Simple	>5	0.40–0.60
Partial rebreather	>8	>0.60
Nonrebreather	>10	>0.80

Ideally the use of the nonrebreather should prevent the entrainment of gas from the outside atmosphere. In practice, because of fit, this is not always the case. The nonrebreather usually supplies an FiO$_2$ of about 80%.

High-flow O$_2$ systems provide a patient's entire inspired minute volume. These devices include (1) air entrainment masks (Venturi masks), (2) large-volume aerosol systems, and (3) large-volume humidifier systems. All of these operate using a specific volume of room air with every liter of O$_2$ flow through the mask. The amount of air entrained depends on the size of the nozzle entering the mask. The FiO$_2$ delivered can range from 50% with the air entrainment methods to 100% with the high-volume aerosol systems.

Several assessments must be made when choosing a particular route of therapy: (1) What is the exact FiO$_2$ needed? (2) Are consistency and accuracy of FiO$_2$ needed on a controlled basis? (3) Is humidity needed, or will it hinder comfort or compliance? (4) Is there an adequate airway in place through which the FiO$_2$ can be delivered? Not only must the method of delivery be determined, but also whether or not the patient will wear the device. If the level of consciousness is decreased, this is not an issue, but for those who are conscious, anxious, or dyspneic, the best route may be the one that the patient will use consistently.

There are several goals of therapy when oxygen is initiated. The reduction of hypoxemia is the most important, but other factors will also be influenced. The myocardium will be at lower risk for insult. In addition, the work of breathing is significantly reduced. Specifically, the patient's ABGs pulse oximetry, respiratory rate, use of accessory muscles, pulse, blood pressure, and subjective evaluation of well-being can be monitored.

INDICATIONS FOR INTUBATION

When the patient is unable to breathe spontaneously, has an obstructed airway, or loses a patent airway, a decision to intubate must be made. The four primary reasons to intubate include (1) to provide positive pressure ventilation, (2) to bypass or prevent airway obstruction, (3) to prevent aspiration, and (4) to facilitate secretion clearance. Intubation is a means to ensure a precise and consistent delivery of inspired oxygen (FiO$_2$). The exact nature of the situation will help to determine whether or not to intubate, but several factors may be evaluated when making the decision. These include the severity of the problem that threatens the airway, the underlying respiratory status, the expected duration of the threat, and whether or not alternatives for reversal of the problem are available (*e.g.*, drugs to reverse oversedation or the depressant effects of other agents).

Endotracheal intubation may be accomplished using the nose or the mouth. Tubes come in various designs and may be manufactured for the nose, mouth, or both. The shaft of the tube is curved, and the tip is beveled to ease insertion into the nasal passageway and through the vocal cords. Tube length varies from 12 to 38 cm. The shaft of the tube is marked in centimeters to help to estimate and maintain tube position while inserting or repositioning the tube. A radiopaque line runs along the shaft of the tube to help locate its position on x-ray. Sizes range from an inner diameter (ID) of 2.0 mm for a newborn to 11 mm for a large adult. Adult tubes have a 2-to 4-cm long cuff bonded to the distal end of the tube that, when inflated, allows stabilization of the tube so that no air escapes when positive pressure ventilation is applied. Neonatal and pediatric tubes do not have cuffs to avoid doing damage to the narrow portion of the child's upper airway. During the intubation procedure, a variety of sizes of tubes should be available. On average, an average female requires a 7.5 to 8.0 mm ID and an average male, 8.5 to 9.0 mm ID.

When properly positioned, the tube should be approximately 2 to 7 cm above the carina, and its position should be verified by x-ray immediately. Potential complications of intubation with an endotracheal tube include insertion trauma, hypoxia and ischemia, cardiac arrhythmias, gastric aspiration, esophageal intubation, laryngospasm, bronchospasm from stimulation of airway irritant receptors, and right bronchial intubation. Careful attention during the procedure and vigilant observation following will help to prevent complications. It is important to inspect the chest for bilateral symmetric expansion and to auscultate for equal breath sounds throughout all lung fields. The stomach should be auscultated as well, and if the sounds over the stomach are louder than those heard over the anterior chest wall, the tube should be withdrawn right away. Once the tube has been evaluated for correct position, it needs to be secured. It is wise not to retape the tube too often because of the danger of dislodgment. Some sources recommend doing this only once every 3 days.

Once the tube is in place, it requires meticulous care to prevent the many complications that may arise. Nasal tubes can lead to accumulation of fluid in the sinuses because they obstruct normal sinus drainage. Oral tubes can lead to stomatitis or tooth damage. Mouth care needs to be given thoroughly and frequently. The artificial airway also provides a port of entry for contamination by the patient's own organisms and those that may be introduced through nosocomial transmission. Colonization with microorganisms occurs rapidly in patients who are intubated. Laryngeal damage begins shortly after the intubation occurs. Erosion of the laryngeal mucosa can occur in as little as 1 day. Usually these lesions will heal soon after extubation. However, in some patients, it may take several weeks for the healing process to be completed; during this time, swallowing and speech may be affected.

Normally when there is no longer a need for an endotracheal tube, an order is written for extubation. The evaluation process of when to remove the tube may require several days, especially if the patient has recently been weaned from mechanical ventilation. The patient needs to be well rested and alert to cooperate during and after the procedure. Once the patient no longer needs artificial ventilation, has a patent natural airway, and has recovered enough to protect his or her airway with the gag and cough reflex, the tube may be removed.

Equipment for immediate reintubation should be kept at the bedside for at least 12 hours following tube removal should the need to reintubate occur. Special care to keep the patient well informed during the procedure is vital to reduce anxiety. The patient is positioned at a 90-degree angle and suctioned through the tube and orally to remove secretions. The cuff is deflated, and the patient is given several breaths to hyperoxygenate the lungs and to assess for a slight leak around the cuff. If this leak is not detected, the physician needs to be notified because this may be a sign of laryngeal edema and can result in total airway obstruction if the tube is removed at this point. Once it has been determined to be safe, the tube should be removed in one smooth movement, applying suction as it is removed. This helps to reduce any secretions that may be retained at the end of the tube. Following the removal, supplemental oxygen is given with high humidity to help decrease airway irritation. The patient is reminded that the hoarseness and sore throat are to be expected and will decrease during the next few days.

Following the procedure, ABGs and careful monitoring of the patient are essential. Breath sounds should be evaluated frequently and any evidence of respiratory distress reported at once. Laryngeal spasm, tracheal edema, or ventilatory failure are some of the complications that can occur.

TRACHEOTOMY AND TRACHEOSTOMY

In several instances, endotracheal intubation is not desirable or can no longer be tolerated by the patient. At this time, it is necessary to decide whether or not a tracheotomy should be done. The *tracheotomy* is the surgical incision that provides an opening into the tracheal wall. The *tracheostomy* is the stoma or opening through which the tracheostomy tube is inserted to maintain patency of the opening.

Certain criteria dictate when and if to do this procedure, but they are not always rigidly followed within the clinical setting. Each situation must be evaluated in light of the patient's needs, prognosis, and goals. As a general rule, it is best to consider this procedure when prolonged intubation is anticipated or when other contraindications to nasal or oral intubation exist. These may include obstruction of the upper airway or predisposition for aspiration (glottic incompetence) or when airway management may be a problem, such as in certain neurosurgical operations, flail chest, or head or neck trauma.

In general, the care of the tracheostomy tube and stoma is much simpler than that of the endotracheal tube. Once the stoma has begun to heal (about 4–7 days), drainage and the possibility of infection dramatically decrease. At this point, it is also much easier to replace the tube should it be dislodged. The presence of a tracheostomy also allows more meticulous mouth care and oral suctioning. In some instances, it may also allow the patient to eat, thus lessening the need for more invasive means of nutrition. While aspiration is still a concern, the need for central venous catheters for total parenteral nutrition is minimized. For patients who are unstable, the tracheostomy also allows for quick reinstitution of mechanical ventilation when needed.

The tracheostomy tube is similar to the endotracheal tube but is shorter (2–6 in long). Adult tubes may be made of plastic, nylon, or metal and may or may not have a cuff. All tubes have the basic component parts, consisting of an outer cannula, an inner cannula, and an obturator, which is a guide for insertion of the outer cannula. Sizes are determined by ID, inner diameter, or a size between the two called a Jackson size. The distal end of the tracheostomy tube is squared off and not

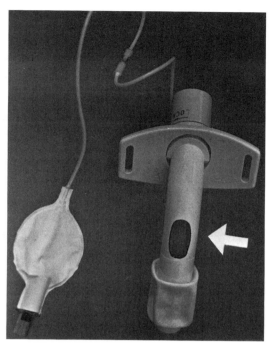

FIGURE 12-3
Fenestrated tracheostomy tube.

beveled as an endotracheal tube is. This prevents the tube from adhering to the wall of the trachea and causing occlusion.

Specially designed tubes are available for almost all patient needs. For those who require only maintenance of an airway, a cuffless tube (Jackson) may be appropriate. If a patient requires mechanical ventilation, a cuffed tube must be placed. When inflated, the cuff allows the ventilator to provide positive pressure into the lungs. Without an inflated cuff, the delivered volume would escape back through the trachea. Once decannulation (removal of the tracheostomy tube) is anticipated, a fenestrated tube may be placed initially (Fig. 12-3), allowing for progressive trials; this allows the patient periods of time that simulate total closing off of the stoma. During this process, the cuff is deflated, the inner cannula is removed, and a small cap is placed over the stoma opening.

Some patients may require long-term management of their airway, such as in the case of permanent spinal cord injury or irreversible damage to a vital structure or function. If the patient does not require mechanical ventilation, a Jackson or metal tracheostomy tube may be more comfortable and more durable for long-term needs. The patient or caregiver is then taught how to accomplish total tube removal and cleaning. Removing the tube daily allows for complete cleaning and inspection of the stoma and the outer cannula.

SUCTIONING

Critical care patients often require frequent suctioning of the airway. This procedure is not benign and has great potential for complications. Indications for suctioning should be evaluated carefully to determine whether or not the procedure is absolutely necessary. The local complications that can occur

include microatelectasis around the tip of the catheter, erosion of the tracheal mucosa, and stripping of the ciliated epithelium, impairing the mucociliary clearing escalator, which protects the tracheobronchial tree.

The most important physiological hazard that can occur as a result of suctioning is hypoxemia. This can have serious consequences on the cardiac system and can lead to bradycardia, tachyarrhythmias, premature ventricular contractions, and even cardiac arrest. Other side effects include hypotension, hypertension, increased ICP, atelectasis, trauma to the airway, nosocomial infection, tachypnea, cyanosis, and dyspnea. Endotracheal suctioning has special implications for the neurological patient because of the effects on ICP. PO_2 and PCO_2 are both affected, as is mean arterial pressure. In patients with known increased ICP, it is vitally important to include some method of hyperoxygenating the patient prior to suctioning. This helps to prevent excessive hypoxemia and hypercapnia during the procedure. The time spent suctioning should not exceed 10 to 15 seconds. If possible, the head of the bed may also be raised 20 to 30 degrees. This helps to reduce ICP, but it may also lower cerebral perfusion pressure (CPP). Each patient situation must be considered individually.

It is not unusual for the patient to panic during suctioning as air is removed from the lungs. the patient must be well informed as to why and how the procedure will be performed. Repeated attempts to suction can also promote bacterial colonization of the respiratory tree, which can lead to pneumonia, especially in patients who are already compromised by age, comorbid conditions, or drugs.

To avoid the complications associated with suctioning, some basic safeguards can be used to help to ensure that the least amount of compromise occurs. It is helpful to keep one hand clean and maintain sterility with the other. Hyperventilate the patient with 100% oxygen for at least 60 seconds before introducing the catheter to reduce the effects of hypoxemia. When a patient is being mechanically ventilated, it may be easier to have a second person assist with removing the patient from the ventilator and with using the Ambu bag for hyperventilation. Pass the catheter without applying suction. Advance the catheter until resistance is felt, and then draw back approximately 1 to 2 cm and apply suction, carefully rotating the catheter as it is withdrawn. Circular rotational movement of the catheter will prevent it from adhering to the tracheal wall for any extended period. This helps prevent damage to the wall. The length of time spent in the airway should never exceed 10 to 15 seconds. Once the catheter is withdrawn, hyperventilate the patient again using 100% oxygen. Repeat the procedure as needed, allowing the patient recovery time between passes with the catheter. The oral airway may be suctioned with the catheter at this point, but once the catheter is contaminated with nasal or oral secretions, it cannot be used to suction the lower airway again. New gloves and catheter must be used if the procedure must be repeated.

Every time the procedure is required, the potential for complications exists, so the least amount of suctioning needed is always best. Some sources suggest that specific guidelines for when to suction should be outlined so that the decision is not based entirely on subjective assessment. Once completed, document the type of procedure done, the time involved, the number of passes, the character of the secretions (color, consistency, amount, and odor), the response of the patient, and any adverse reactions.

In recent years, new devices have been introduced to ease the suctioning procedure. Closed tracheal suction systems, which consist of a catheter within a sleeve, require using only clean gloves. Because the patient does not have to be removed from the ventilator circuit, the risk of contamination is minimized. Ventilator technology has also been developed to allow the hyperventilation with 100% oxygen at the touch of a button, thus eliminating the need for separating the patient from the system and eliminating use of the Ambu bag.

VENTILATORY SUPPORT

To meet ventilatory demands, the patient must have an intact medullary control system, adequate neuromuscular function, adequate volumes, and pulmonary compliance within reasonable limits. When the patient is unable to maintain spontaneous adequate ventilation or when hypoxemia is present, mechanical ventilation is indicated. Neuroscience patients may require mechanical ventilation to induce hypocapnia, lowering the PCO_2 to 25 to 35 mm Hg and creating an alkalosis that reduces cerebral edema and ICP. In general, inadequate ventilation or hypoxemia is caused by inadequate lung expansion, respiratory muscle dysfunction, excessive work of breathing, unstable respiratory drive, or the use of potent pharmacological agents that can severely affect these functions.

The primary symptom of acute respiratory failure is usually dyspnea. Patients may describe shortness of breath, air hunger, or breathlessness. The severity and time during which dyspnea occurs may provide cues as to how rapidly the process is progressing. Other more subtle signs may be an increased agitation, change in the level of consciousness, or a general feeling of discomfort and foreboding.

In contrast, when a patient experiences chronic ventilatory failure, such as with neuromuscular diseases (amyotrophic lateral sclerosis or Duchenne muscular dystrophy), the sensation of dyspnea is usually absent. When it does occur, it may be precipitated be the onset of pneumonia or pulmonary embolism.

In addition to evaluating ABGs to determine the appropriateness of mechanical ventilation, other laboratory data are also of benefit. Blood levels need to evaluated for polycythemia (hemoglobin >15 g) and high venous bicarbonate levels, which reflect a chronic compensatory process. The presence of imbalances in electrolytes, especially potassium, magnesium, calcium, phosphate, and the amount of hemoglobin, can also affect ventilatory capability. Certain tests will also yield information regarding potential reversible causes for the respiratory failure, such as a nutritional deficit that will further complicate the weaning process when the time is appropriate. Total lymphocyte count, serum albumin, and transferrin levels indicate protein stores vital to muscle function. Chest radiographs are helpful to rule out pneumothorax, pulmonary edema, and other possible diagnoses. Sputum examination for culture and sensitivity will give valuable information to determine the most effective antibiotic when infection is present.

Two common clinical situations require immediate attention. The first is when the patient is unable to regulate rising PCO_2 levels, which then causes a decrease in serum pH or acidosis. While not absolute, this is a fairly consistent indicator that mechanical ventilation is needed. The second instance is when hypoxemia worsens, and an increased FiO_2 is required. When more conservative methods, such as the use of a rebreather, partial rebreather, or other type of mask, are ineffective, mechanical ventilation may be the safest and most reliable means to ensure a precise level of delivered oxygen. While a high FiO_2 may initially be required to correct hypoxemia, the initiation of mechanical ventilation may lessen the work of breathing and improve breathing patterns to the point that the high levels may be gradually decreased to safer ones below 50%.

The chief goals of mechanical ventilation are to (1) adjust the alveolar ventilation to a level optimal for each patient; (2) improve the ventilation or perfusion ratios, thus improving overall oxygenation; (3) decrease the work of breathing and reverse respiratory muscle fatigue; (4) relieve acute respiratory acidosis; and (5) provide prophylaxsis in certain high-risk situations, such as immediate postoperative periods when the use of anesthetics may compromise ventilation.

Types of Ventilators

Many types of mechanical ventilators are available on the market. In the acute care setting, positive pressure is the method most often used. This type of device allows the power source (ventilator) to force gas into the patient's lungs and expand the chest wall. When the process is complete, the chest relaxes, and the patient exhales passively as the airway pressures return to normal.

While highly sophisticated devices are available, the basic types are pressure-cycled ventilators and volume-cycled ventilators. Pressure-cycled machines offer a distinct disadvantage in that a desired tidal volume (Vt) is not always delivered secondary to the differences in airway pressures within individual patients. If lung compliance or resistance changes, gas delivery can be adversely affected. As an example, in COPD patients, the presence of retained secretions or bronchospasm can cause hypoventilation because the preset airway pressures are met before adequate oxygen is delivered.

In addition, the FiO_2 cannot be controlled because the air source is attached to an oxygen blender, preventing a precisely delivered oxygen level. Examples of this type of ventilator are the Bird Mark 7, 8, 10, or 14.

Volume-cycled ventilators allow gas to flow into the lungs until a preset volume of air has been delivered to the patient or expelled from the ventilator. This capability allows a wide variety of lung conditions to be treated. These devices can generate pressures up to 120 cm of H_2O, which may be necessary to deliver the desired volume.

In critical situations in which lung function and mechanics are profoundly affected, this capability allows the ventilator to deliver a constant Vt despite changing airway conditions or the degree of lung compliance. *Adult respiratory distress syndrome* (ARDS) is an example and is commonly seen in patients with head injury or subarachnoid hemorrhage. This particular clinical diagnosis often requires the use of these high-technology ventilators. Their capabilities allow for the application of subtle and precise means of delivering preset volumes and pressures within the lungs. Examples of this type of ventilator are the Bear 1 and Bear 2, the MA 1 and the MA 2, and the Monaghan 225/SIMV.

The newest ventilators have computers, microprocessors, or both built into a volume- or time-cycled device. These allow the control of breath-to-breath ventilation with electronic memory and digital displays to assist the management of the patient's changing condition. These also allow the addition of pressure support, which is a feature that maintains a preset amount of positive pressure to the airway during inspiration. It is triggered by the patient's spontaneous breaths and helps to reduce the patient's work of breathing and the demands on the muscles responsible for ventilation. It is a feature often used during the weaning process because it allows a gradual decrease in the work done by the machine, allowing the patient to assume more and more of the work as his or her strength and endurance return.

In chronic care settings, other types of ventilators may be used for patient care. Negative-pressure ventilation has been available for many years, and its popularity and application have waxed and waned. In certain populations, this type of ventilator may be much less invasive because it works on a mechanical basis, pulling the chest wall outward, creating negative pressure within the thoracic cavity, and causing air to enter the lungs passively. As the outward pressure is released, the chest wall collapses back to its resting state, and passive expiration occurs. This mode is useful in patients who have anatomical deformities or who suffer from disorders where the mechanics of respiration are jeopardized.

Ventilator Settings

As ventilators become more and more sophisticated, the nurse must understand the settings and the implications they have for patient care. While the respiratory therapist is one of the best resources for the information regarding the technical aspects of the ventilator, the nurse is in a key position to assemble the entire picture for comprehensive evaluation and modification of the treatment plan.

Once again, team work cannot be emphasized enough, as the nurse, therapist, and physician collaborate to arrive at the best alternative for the patient.

There are many working parts to a modern ventilator. The circuit usually consists of the same type of tubing that is found on other respiratory equipment. In addition, it also has a spirometer device that detects flow and is able to display the volume of each breath. Humidifiers are placed to warm and humidify the inspired air as the patient's natural mechanisms for this are being bypassed. There may also be thermometers and indicators for sampling the gas delivered and probes for measuring the airway pressures.

The particular *mode* of ventilation is usually determined by the patient's individual condition. These various modes include assist, assist-control, controlled, intermittent mandatory ventilation, and synchronized intermittent mandatory ventilation. The assist-control mode allows the patient to trigger the machine spontaneously while still providing backup ventilation should the rate or volume decrease. The advantages of the assist-control mode are several: The tendency to hyperventilate the patient is decreased because fewer mechanical breaths are delivered and the patient is allowed to control PCO_2 levels. Also the need for sedation and muscle relaxants

to control the ventilatory rate is decreased. The use of lower mean airway pressures are possible, which decreases the potential for complications. The uniform ventilation assists in the even distribution of muscle use and air flow throughout all lung regions. Assist-control also lessens the possibility of increased intrathoracic pressures. When increased, these higher pressures can lead to cardiac decompensation, causing decreased cardiac output and a compromise in circulation.

Positive end expiratory pressure (PEEP) is another setting frequently used in patients who need ventilatory support. The mechanisms of PEEP are not well understood, but the benefits are believed to be derived from the back pressure created within the lungs, which prevents atelectasis and airway collapse. By stenting the airways open and creating additional functional residual capacity, better oxygenation is usually achieved, reducing the need for high levels of inspired oxygen and the toxic damage it can cause. It also helps in the recruitment of previously collapsed airways, thus enhancing the ventilation perfusion ratios and increasing the number of alveoli available for gas exchange. Optimal PEEP is defined as that which allows the maintenance of a PO_2 of 60 mm Hg or greater with an FiO_2 of less than or equal to 50% while still maintaining an adequate cardiac output. The range used is normally between 10 and 20 cm H_2O but may go as high as 45 cm H_2O in patients with ARDS who have severely decreased compliance or increased consolidation. For neurological patients, ICP may be elevated with the addition of PEEP to the ventilatory system. Its application should be limited to situations in which it is specifically necessary, and levels of greater than 15 cm should be avoided.

Pressure support ventilation is the delivery of a preset amount of positive pressure to the airway during inspiration. It is applied to augment spontaneous breaths, reducing the patient's work of breathing and the effort that must be expended. This allows some respite for the muscles used for breathing; the aim is to increase these muscles' endurance and strength. This setting is particularly helpful when patients are being weaned from mechanical ventilation. It allows the patient to control the rate and frequency of ventilation and therefore promotes greater patient comfort.

The other principle settings of which the nurse should be aware are the *inspired levels of oxygen* (FiO_2), *the tidal volume,* the *sigh volume,* the *I:E ratio,* and the *inspiratory flow rate.*

The FiO_2 may be set as high as 100% initially during an acute episode. The goal of therapy is to remedy the clinical problem with the hope of being able to reduce the FiO_2 to a level that maintains the PO_2 at or above 60 mm Hg without having the FiO_2 above 50%. Each time a change is made in this setting, an oxygen analyzer should be used to determine the precise level of O_2 being delivered.

Vt is calculated using the patient's weight in kilograms. It is set at 10 to 15 mL/kg of ideal body weight, normally between 500 and 1,000 mL. The rate of ventilation is normally set between 10 and 16 breaths per minute. These may need to be recalculated periodically to be sure that adequate minute ventilation is occurring.

The sigh volume is set at approximately $1\frac{1}{2}$ times the patient's Vt. In the past, this maneuver was considered routine in the care of a patient being mechanically ventilated, but this practice is not as common as it once was.

The sensitivity setting determines the patient effort required to initiate assisted breathing. It is normally not used while the patient is in the control mode. It is manipulated until the patient generates -0.5 to -1.5 cm H_2O of pressure. If the sensitivity is set too high, the ventilator will trigger too quickly; if it is too low, the patient may not be able to trigger the breaths needed, and hypoventilation will result.

Inspiratory and expiratory times may be set in the range of 1.5 to 2.0 seconds. If set higher, it may result in patient discomfort and have adverse effects on the cardiopulmonary circulation. In patients with obstructive lung disease, the ratio may be set at 1:3 to 1:5 to facilitate complete alveolar emptying during expiration. This setting may also be uncomfortable, and the patient may require sedation to control this parameter.

The *inspiratory flow rate* is the volume of gas that travels through the airways during the period of respiration. It is controlled by a calibrated knob that can be set at values of 20 to 120 L/min. An average rate of flow is between 40 and 60 L/min. Higher flow rates of up to 100 L/min may be required for patients with significant lung disease or who need a higher minute ventilation. With COPD patients, high flow rates will increase the distribution of the gas available for exchange, opening under ventilated alveoli. A too high flow rate may create additional airway turbulence and offset any advantage that is created. Flow rate will directly affect the inspiratory time, so this must be kept in mind when considering the total picture.

Peak inspiratory pressure is measured by observing the needle on the pressure manometer, which swings upward during inspiration. The highest observed level is defined as the peak pressure. The optimal place to take this measurement is at the closest point to the patient rather than close to the ventilator. It is an indication of airway mechanics and the compliance within the lung tissue. With time, serial measurements will yield trends reflecting worsening or improving conditions within the lungs. Too high levels (above 30 cm H_2O) may indicate decreased lung function and the need to be aware of the potential for barotrauma, hypotension, and other complications associated with increased pressures within the airways. This can at times lead to an increase in arterial carbon dioxide tension (PCO_2). This is termed permissive hypercapnia and needs to be monitored carefully. Alarms are usually set to indicate when the patient is repeatedly exceeding the preset safe pressure limits. This can alert the caregiver to investigate the cause of worsening compliance or increased airway pressure.

In summary, all of the ventilator settings should be monitored regularly, but the following components should be assessed routinely: (1) ventilator mode, (2) FiO_2, (3) respiratory rate per minute, (4) Vt, (5) peak inspiratory pressure, (6) PEEP levels, and (7) whether or not the alarm system is on and functioning appropriately.

Monitoring the Patient on Ventilatory Support

The patient who is being maintained on mechanical ventilatory support needs to monitored on a continuous basis. In addition to the complications of intubation, adding another set of invasive manipulations may endanger the patient further if not assessed frequently and consistently. The process of mechanical ventilation can adversely affect all of the major organ systems. These effects include the following:

Pulmonary

Pulmonary emboli
Barotrauma (from alveolar overdistention)
Pulmonary fibrosis (from oxygen toxicity of FiO_2 >50%)

Gastrointestinal

Pneumoperitoneum
Alterations in gastric motility (ileus)
Gastrointestinal hemorrhage

Cardiovascular

Arrhythmia
Myocardial ischemia
Alterations in hemodynamics (fall in cardiac output)

Infectious complications

Nosocomial pneumonia
Bacteremia or sepsis

Nutritional complications

Malnutrition
Complications of invasive nutritional support (central lines for parental nutrition)

Associated problems

Complications of pulmonary artery catheters
Tracheal intubation
Ventilator-induced injury

Most of the complications that occur are the result of other major organ failures but should be kept in mind as part of the comprehensive picture. In the neuroscience patient, the addition of positive pressure ventilation may have profound effects on the ICP through changes in the cerebral perfusion pressure produced when changes occur in the systemic blood pressure. Central venous pressure always increases when positive pressure is added, depending on the patient's lung compliance and chest wall distensibility. The effect of positive pressure ventilation is normally mediated through the pleural space to the central venous pressure. As the CVP increases, this rise is communicated to the cerebral circulation, resulting in concomitant increases in the cerebral perfusion pressure. The biggest risk occurs with patients who have increased lung compliance and decreased chest wall compliance because this translates into the greatest increase in CPP. If the patient also has decreased intracranial compliance, the ICP is likely to increase as a result of positive airway pressure. In summary, both the ventilatory parameters and the ICP must be monitored carefully in conjunction with each other. It is best to avoid removing the patient repeatedly from the ventilator because this causes swings in the pressures, which may affect overall stability of the CPP.

Infectious Complications Associated With Mechanical Ventilation

Although many organ systems have the potential for infection, the pulmonary tree is perhaps the most vulnerable while the patient is intubated and consequently compromised. Placement of an artificial airway beyond the vocal cords always involves some degree of contamination, especially with gram-positive organisms that may inhabit the oropharynx normally. Hospitalized patients experience the additional threat of exposure to even more resistant and virulent organisms found within the hospital environment. Nosocomial pneumonia occurs in 0.5% to 5% of all hospital admissions, but the incidence increases with severity of illness and when patients must be artificially ventilated. When the patient is compromised by additional insults or drugs that may limit the immunological response, infection may be unavoidable.

The caregiver needs to be alert for changes in the amount, color, consistency, and odor of sputum that is produced. The presence of crackles and wheezes may signal the development of infiltrates as a result of a bacterial overgrowth. Fever, an increased number of white blood cells and the presence of immature white blood cells, and a change in the baseline chest x-ray are other indicators. A change in the oxygenation status (ABGs) can be another measure of infectious involvement as pneumonia develops and causes consolidation and limited gas exchange.

Many infections are caused by more than one organism and may require more than one antimicrobial. These pathogens include gram-negative bacilli, gram-positive cocci, and other organisms, such as fungi, viruses, *Pneumocystis*, and *Legionella*. Sources of infection include multiple and invasive monitoring devices, respiratory therapy equipment, medical personnel, and environmental reservoirs (*e.g.,* sinks, counter tops, telephones). Usually the host's response determines the course and outcomes of these infections.

During recent years, more attention has been focused on the role of the gastrointestinal tract as a source of oropharyngeal colonization by gram-negative bacilli and subsequent development of nosocomial pneumonia.

Often mechanically ventilated patients may exhibit these symptoms of infection that can be associated with other clinical problems. A new appearance of an infiltrate on chest x-ray may be from an infectious cause, but it may also be the result of atelectasis, hemorrhage, contusion, congestive heart failure or pulmonary edema, or subclinical aspiration. With the myriad symptoms present, accurate diagnosis of nosocomial pneumonia is often difficult to determine. Taken a step further, it is even more difficult to treat the specific organisms present. Some data suggest that use of empiric antibiotics may not only be ineffective, but may even decrease the drug's efficacy for future use when needed. Newer and more refined methods of detection and qualification of organisms are needed. Procedures using bronchoscopy and bronchoalveolar lavage are under investigation for future use, which will make precise isolation and identification of microorganisms easier.

Prevention of nosocomial infection in ventilated patients may be one key to the solution of the problem. Simple common sense measures can help, such as (1) resolving the patient's underlying disease, (2) keeping the patient's head elevated when the airway is at risk, (3) maintaining adequate nutritional status to keep patient reserves at their optimum, (4) extubating as soon as possible, and (5) limiting the use of inappropriate antibiotics as much as possible. Meticulous care of the ventilator circuitry, appropriate change of equipment and proper disinfection, and consistent handwashing by staff all help to limit the rate, growth, and spread of infection. Constant reinforcement of these principles with staff also may encourage more consistent adherence to good practices.

Weaning From the Ventilator

The process of weaning the patient from mechanical ventilation is usually begun when the patient has made sufficient improvement and can be expected to support his or her respiratory function spontaneously again. This occurs when the underlying disease process that necessitated the mechanical ventilation has been resolved. When there is significant lung disease, the process may be more difficult, but overall, the steps used in the process are consistent with a few modifications. The major determinant is whether or not the patient has the mechanical and neurological capability to sustain independent ventilation.

By definition, the process of weaning is the gradual shift of the work of breathing from the ventilator to the patient. The American College of Chest Physicians Consensus Conference on Mechanical Ventilation defines weaning as the gradual reduction of ventilatory support and its replacement with spontaneous ventilation. Most clinicians use a much broader definition than this, and in clinical practice, there may be wide diversity in how physicians and the remainder of the care team accomplish weaning within a particular setting.

For most patients, weaning and extubation take place within a limited time frame, which may be only several hours. For others, it can be a long and arduous process that involves slow and steady progress interspersed with setbacks.

When considering when to begin, it is important to correct as many of the patient's medical problems as possible before attempting the weaning process.

Factors to Correct Before Weaning

Acid–base abnormalities	Altered levels of consciousness
Anemia	Arrhythmias
Decreased cardiac output	Electrolyte abnormalities
Fever	Fluid imbalance
Hyperglycemia	Infection
Pain	Malnutrition
Renal failure	Shock

CLINICAL INDICATORS OF WHEN TO WEAN

The patient's readiness to be weaned includes assessment of inspiratory muscle endurance, work of breathing (WOB), oxygenation and ventilation, and left ventricular function.

A patient's normal response to the withdrawal of mechanical ventilatory support includes (1) a decreased Vt and respiratory rate, (2) a slight drop in PaO$_2$ sometimes due to a degree of atelectasis, (3) a slight drop in cardiac output, and (4) a decrease in alveolar ventilation and ventilation-perfusion, which may cause a rise in $PaCO_2$ with a subsequent drop in pH. If the patient is an appropriate candidate for weaning or extubation, these responses should not present any major problems. However, if they become marked, they may result in failure to wean.

Over the years, several specific parameters have been proposed to help to determine when patients may be ready to begin the weaning process.

Respiratory mechanics measure respiratory muscle endurance, efficiency, and WOB. They include spontaneous respiratory frequency, spontaneous Vt, resting minute ventilation, maximum voluntary ventilation, vital capacity, and negative inspiratory force (NIF). These values are helpful in predicting whether or not a patient is ready to breathe without mechanical support. Obtaining these values requires the cooperation and effort of the patient. It also necessitates the patient's understanding of the process and the goal to be achieved. A good therapist and nurse are essential in helping the patient achieve the maximal results when these values are being assessed.

The patient's *respiratory rate* is an important factor to assess. If greater than 25/min, the WOB required may be too high to wean successfully. It may indicate that there is an increase in dead space ventilation (VD/VT) and an overall decreased alveolar ventilation. Paradoxical respiratory effort can also be detected when the abdomen and the thorax work in opposition, moving inward during inspiration and outward during expiration. These patterns represent an inefficient mechanism and will lead to failure in weaning because of the huge amounts of energy required to sustain the effort.

Vt is the amount of exhaled air measured in milliliters. A spontaneous Vt of 4 to 5 mL/kg is recommended prior to beginning the weaning process. Normal minute ventilation is the product of the respiratory rate and the Vt and should be between 5 and 10 L/min. If greater than this, the WOB and the resultant fatigue may impair weaning.

Maximum voluntary ventilation is the maximum amount of air that can be inhaled and exhaled as rapidly as possible for 1 minute. It is determined be measuring the patient's maximum exhaled volume for 15 seconds and multiplying by 4. This measurement is an indication of respiratory muscle endurance, thoracic compliance, and airway resistance. It is a good indicator of the patient's reserve and ability to maintain effective ventilation. Normal values are 50 to 250 L/min. Lower values may be found in older patients.

Vital capacity and NIF will indicate whether or not the patient is able to take a deep breath. Without adequate respiratory excursion, the patient may not be able to clear secretions and prevent atelectasis. A normal vital capacity is 10 to 15 mL/kg. The negative inspiratory force (sometimes also called the maximum inspiratory pressure) is measured using the inspiratory force manometer and should be 20 cm H_2O or greater if weaning is to be successful. The greater the NIF, the easier it is for the patient to take a deep breath.

ABGs are also an essential part of the assessment picture. The values are not absolute but help to identify trends for the patient: (1) the presence of acidosis or alkalosis or other metabolic imbalances that must be corrected to ensure

success with weaning, and 2) the PaO_2, which should be greater than 60 mm Hg on an inspired fraction of oxygen of 50% or less.

The level of PEEP required is also an important indicator. PEEP improves oxygenation by stenting open the small airways, improving the distribution and ventilation, and thus improving the diffusion of gas from alveoli to blood. Levels of 5 cm H_2O are considered physiological and may be used on all patients who require mechanical ventilation. When a patient requires an FiO_2 of greater than 50% and levels of PEEP greater than 5 cm H_2O, the FiO_2 is usually decreased first before attempting to decrease the PEEP. Once a PaO_2 of 60 mm Hg is achieved at <50% FiO_2, the PEEP can gradually be reduced by 2 to 3 cm increments until 5 cm is reached. Lowering of the FiO_2 can be guided with the use of pulse oximetry and ABGs, attempting to keep the saturation at a level greater than 90%.

An additional calculation is necessary to determine the efficiency of the lungs' gas exchange. The intrapulmonary shunt is the portion of the pulmonary blood flow not exposed to functioning alveoli. It is determined by calculating the arterial-alveolar ratio. This gradient is measured by dividing the arterial partial pressure of O_2 by the alveolar oxygen.

$$\text{A-a gradient} = FiO_2 \times [(760 \text{ mm Hg} - 47 \text{ mm Hg})] - (PaCO_2/0.8)$$

A normal A-a gradient should be greater than .75; if less than this, it indicates an increased intrapulmonary shunt that may interfere with weaning attempts.

Left ventricular function indicates the patient's cardiac status and is assessed by measuring the cardiac index. Normal cardiac index is 2.4 to 4 L/min/m². Without sufficient blood flow, the increased demands placed on the system during weaning may outstrip the patient's capacity to compensate. If not available, heart rate and blood pressure can also be used to assess the cardiac response and the delivery of oxygen to the tissues. A change in systolic pressure correlates with increased WOB and increased left ventricular work, which will also hamper weaning success.

Ongoing evaluation of the weaning process is important in the course of pulmonary care, but equally important is knowing when the weaning attempt is not progressing. It is just as important to know when to stop the attempt so that the patient is not totally defeated by the frustration and futility of the situation. Many factors will influence the process, including the physical factors (oxygenation, workload, ventilation requirements, ventilatory drive, muscle strength, and hemodynamic status), but other parameters must also be considered. These include environmental factors (sensory overload, sleep deprivation, decreased mobility) and personal variables (anxiety, fear or panic, pain, disorientation, previous success with coping). Psychological factors will also affect the weaning attempt (*e.g.*, hopelessness, depression, perceived ability to succeed). It is important to analyze the cause of weaning failure to determine whether the patient may be a candidate for future trials.

When the patient repeatedly fails weaning attempts, long-term mechanical ventilation must be considered. Most acute care hospitals do not have the resources to care for these types of patients for prolonged periods. Because of this, there are usually a limited number of alternatives for patients who are faced with this situation.

Chronic long-term ventilator facilities have grown in number throughout this country in the last several decades. Many of these facilities offer not only pulmonary care, but also extensive rehabilitation. In many instances with their specialized focus on the restorative aspects of care, patients who were not immediately able to wean and recover in an acute care setting may do so over an extended period in these institutions.

RESPIRATORY MANAGEMENT IN THE HOME

With the increased interest in cost containment and decreased length of stay, greater numbers of ventilator-dependent patients and their families are choosing to be discharged to their homes instead of long-term facilities. Modern technology has met this demand, and now specialized ventilators are available that are less sophisticated and complicated than the ones used in hospitals. Although these devices do not have all of the "high tech" capabilities, they are exceptionally "user friendly" and easily adapted to the home setting.

In the home, mechanical ventilation may involve positive or negative pressure devices. Negative pressure is used most often in patients who have neuromuscular disease and mild respiratory failure. These include the tank (iron lung), cuirass (external shell), or wrap, which surrounds the chest wall. These devices are cumbersome, large, and difficult to maneuver. In addition, they do not allow the delivery of precise amounts of air flow or oxygen levels. Despite their drawbacks, many patients are able to live for extended periods with them.

Positive pressure ventilators are usually chosen for home mechanical ventilation. These require placement of a tra-

cheostomy for long-term management. Many different models are available using either volume-cycled or pressure-cycled modes for delivery of oxygen.

The process of discharge planning and training of family members is an extensive and detailed process. Careful assessment must take place to determine whether or not this alternative is feasible and safe. There must be total commitment of the patient and the family to the decision. Financial and environmental factors must be evaluated carefully, especially when the duration of therapy is uncertain. Over months and sometimes years, the psychological and emotional drain of the situation may take a toll on even the most resourceful and healthy family. Community resources must also be capable of responding to the needs of a patient who is "chronically critically ill." The home care companies that provide the equipment and the respiratory therapists must be available at a moment's notice, helping the patient's family to troubleshoot problems as they arise.

The process of teaching the family before discharge involves many areas, including the following:

Tracheostomy care

1. Stoma care
2. Tie changes
3. Suctioning, use of an Ambu device, hyperoxygenation
4. Instructions on reinserting the tracheostomy tube if coughed out
5. Cuff monitoring
6. Inner cannula removal and cleaning

Use and maintenance of the mechanical ventilator

1. Alarms, emergency situations (*e.g.,* power failure)
2. Circuitry cleaning
3. Addition of supplemental oxygen to the system

General nursing care

1. Hygiene
2. Administration of medications
3. Restorative care (physical therapy, occupational therapy)
4. Monitoring of vital signs and functions, when to access the medical system
5. Psychological care
6. Aspects of nutrition and hydration

A collaborative approach with all team members (Fig. 12-4) is the optimal method in developing a teaching plan for the family. Very few patients qualify for prolonged private duty nursing support in the home. For this reason, one family member should be identified as the one responsible for the delivery of care. Additional family members should also learn the skills required to serve as backup.

PHARMACOLOGY OF THE RESPIRATORY SYSTEM

Many families of pharmacological agents are available to enhance respiratory function. These range from bronchodilators, methylxanthines, mucolytics, corticosteroids, stimulants, de-

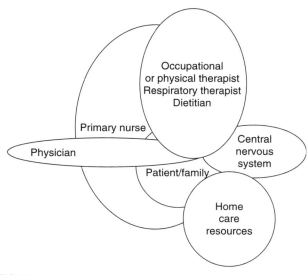

FIGURE 12-4
Model of collaboration.

pressants, and antitussives to a wide category of antibiotics and anti-infectives that are used to treat acute and chronic infections. In general, the four goals of respiratory drug therapy to consider are (1) maintenance of the airway (bronchodilation and reduction of spasm), (2) promotion of secretion clearance, (3) improved alveolar function, and (4) restoration of a normal breathing pattern. The discussion in this chapter is limited to the drugs that are most likely to be encountered within the hospital setting versus the drugs that may be used for more chronic problems.

Beta-2 agonists and anticholinergics are the most often used drugs used for bronchodilation. They work by relaxing the smooth muscles of the large airways, thus promoting dilation. Some examples include albuterol (Ventolin, Proventil) and ipatropium bromide (Atrovent). They are usually delivered via an aerosol system or a metered-dose inhaler and are effective on a long- or short-term basis, depending on the agent used.

Methylxanthines are controversial because of the potential for toxicity and the other organs that may be affected. They have some influence on respiratory muscles (diaphragm), renal function, and the myocardium. The therapeutic range for this family of drugs varies with each individual patient, and the side effects can be more of problem than the beneficial effects achieved. Examples of these drugs are theophylline or aminophylline preparations. The blood levels of these drugs need to be monitored routinely.

The corticosteroids may be used to reduce inflammatory changes within the airways. These can be given systemically or by direct inhalation. The potential detrimental effects of steroid use must be considered whenever they are given (*e.g.,* gastrointestinal irritation, Cushingoid effects, psychosis). Examples are prednisone, methylprednisolone, and beclomethasone. The negative side effects of systemic steroids can be minimized using direct inhalation, but in acute situations, the levels achieved may not be sufficient to achieve the desired result.

Mucolytics and expectorants can be of great benefit when airway clearance must be considered. These too can be delivered systemically or by direct inhalation, depending on the drug. Examples include acetylcysteine, potassium iodide, and guaifenesin.

Respiratory stimulants will directly affect the medullary center and need to be used cautiously because they may also cause excessive central nervous system stimulation. Examples are doxapram and progesterone. Doxapram is an analeptic and is often used to stimulate patients following anesthesia. It must be given intravenously and monitored carefully. Progesterone is a hormone that acts centrally in the respiratory center. It is helpful in patients with chronic CO_2 retention and in the morbidly obese with Pickwickian syndrome. The effect is not immediate, and its use is primarily for long-term benefit.

Any drug that sedates or calms a patient will also diminish the drive to breathe. This may include narcotics, benzodiazepines, and other agents used to reduce pain, provide sedation, or reduce anxiety. They must be used cautiously.

The elderly population, which is a large number of the patients seen in acute care settings, may need special consideration when determining drug dosing and frequency. This group is often compromised by age-related changes, such as absorption, metabolism, distribution, and elimination. The levels achieved may vary significantly in the elderly and are affected by the amount of lean body mass and fat, decreased hydration, and diminished blood flow to the kidneys and liver.

THE ROLE OF NUTRITION IN THE NEURORESPIRATORY PATIENT

The vital connection between respiratory capability and nutrition may be overshadowed by more overt clinical concerns. Many patients suffer the effects of starvation while more obvious and urgent physiological issues are being addressed. The respiratory system suffers several effects when this starvation process occurs: (1) catabolism of muscle protein, resulting in weakened respiratory muscles and leading to fatigue or difficulty in weaning from mechanical ventilation; (2) decreased surfactant production, resulting in decreased lung compliance and increased work of breathing; (3) impairment of the immune system; (4) decreased circulating albumin over time, decreasing the colloid osmotic pressure; (5) decreased tissue integrity; and (6) a decreased respiratory response to hypoxic drive.

All of these factors will influence the outcomes of care and should be considered and treated aggressively from the outset of treatment. Technology and advanced knowledge have helped in this area. Many routes for nutrition delivery are available, such as total parental nutrition, gastrostomy and jejunostomy tubes, and nasogastric tubes. In addition, there are multiple formulas to treat even the most complicated metabolic problems.

Bibliography

Ackerman, M. H. (1993). The effect of saline lavage prior to suctioning. *American Journal of Critical Care, 2*(4), 326–330.

Aloi, A., & Burns, S. A. (1995). Continuous airway pressure monitoring in the critical care setting. *Critical Care Nurse, 15* (4), 66–74.

Barker, E. (1994). *Neuroscience nursing.* St. Louis: C.V. Mosby.

Bolton, P. J., & Kline, K. A. (1994). Understanding modes of mechanical ventilation. *American Journal of Nursing, 94*(6), 36–42.

Briones, T. L. (1992). Pressure support ventilation: New ventilatory technique. *Critical Care Nurse, 12*(4), 51–58.

Burns, S. M., Fahey, S. A., Barton, D. M., & Slack, D. (1991). Weaning from mechanical ventilation: A method for assessment and planning. *AACN Clinical Issues in Critical Care Nursing, 2*(3), 372–387.

Burton, G. G., Hodgkin, J. E., & Ward, J. J. (1991). *Respiratory care* (3rd ed.). Philadelphia: J.B. Lippincott.

Campbell, B., & Ferguson, D. (1995). Endotracheal suctioning: Time worn ritual or timely intervention? *American Journal of Critical Care, 4*(2), 100–105.

Chipps, E. M., Clanin, N. J., & Campbell, V. G. (1992). *Neurologic disorders.* St. Louis: C.V. Mosby.

Christensen, M. A., Bloom, J., & Sutton, K. R. (1995). Comparing arterial and end tidal carbon dioxide values in hyperventilated neurosurgical patients. *American Journal of Critical Care, 4*(2), 116–121.

Colchesy, J. M., Daly, B. J., & Montenegro, H. D. (1995). Weaning chronically critically ill adults from mechanical ventilatory support: A descriptive study. *American Journal of Critical Care, 4*(2), 93–99.

Colice, G. (1993). How to ventilate patients when ICP elevation is a risk. *Journal of Critical Illness, 8*(9), 1003–1020.

Dantzker, D. R., Mac Intyre, N. R., & Bakow, E. D. (1995). *Comprehensive respiratory care.* Philadelphia: W.B. Saunders.

DesJardins, T., & Burton G. G. (1995). *Clinical manifestations and assessment of respiratory disease.* St. Louis: C.V. Mosby.

Elpern, E. H. (1991). Prolonged ventilator dependence: Economic and ethical considerations. *Critical Care Nursing Clinics of North America, 3*(4), 601–607.

Findeis, A., Larson, J. L., Gallo, A., & Shekleton, M. (1994). Caring for individuals using home ventilators: An appraisal by family caregivers. *Rehabilitation Nursing, 19*(1), 6–11.

CHAPTER 13

Behavioral and Psychological Responses to Neurological Illness

Joanne V. Hickey

The purpose of this chapter is to address the psychosocial aspects of neuroscience nursing practice and to present nursing interventions for the major emotional and behavioral responses to neurological illness. The emotional needs of the family are considered, as are the stresses and responses precipitated in the nursing staff who work with neuroscience patients.

Injury or disease involving the nervous system often has far-reaching effects, not only on the neurological-physiological body system, but also on the cognitive and affective functions, personality, and individual characteristics that give a person uniqueness, individuality, and identity. These compounded deficits and devastating losses create stresses for the patient and family that tax coping and adaptive skills. Because many neurological conditions can alter a person's cognitive abilities, patients often lack an awareness of the change in their behavior and cognitive functions. If these changes in higher level functions are recognized, patients may not have an insight into the cause, amount or degree, significance, or implications of the behavioral changes in relationship to their lifestyle.

Family members and significant others are better able to accept physiological changes in their loved ones than behavioral, cognitive, or personality changes. Changes in a patient's behavior affect group dynamics and interpersonal relationships as well. The normal patterns of family interactions are altered, and family structure changes accordingly. Changes in patterns of interaction and family structure also alter methods of problem solving and the use of effective coping mechanisms. These factors contribute additional stresses to the already stressful experience of neurological illness.

STRESS AND THE STRESS RESPONSE

The writings of Selye provide a basic foundation for understanding physiological and psychological responses to stress. According to Selye, stress is defined as "the nonspecific response of the body to any type of increased demands upon it."[1] The increased demands on an organism, termed *stressors*, cause stress. Regardless of whether the stressor is associated with a desirable effect *(eustress)* or an undesirable effect *(distress)*, the same physiological responses are precipitated.[2] The interaction and integration of physiological and psychological responses to stress were documented by Selye and other writers who preceded him, such as Cannon and Jacobson. Cannon is credited with recognizing that the physiological reactions of the sympathetic system that occur in response to various emotional states are similar to those that occur in response to biological precipitators.[3] Jacobson noted similar reactions in the sympathetic nervous system and skeletal muscles in response to emotional states.[4]

Selye is credited with the introduction of the term *general adaptation syndrome* into the literature. This syndrome refers to the nonspecific reactions of the hypothalamic–pituitary–adrenocortical system to any type of stress. The general endocrine changes associated with the response are enlargement of the adrenal cortex, shrinkage of the thymus gland, and ulceration of the stomach (stress ulcers). These responses are mediated by the pituitary–adrenocortical axis of the neuroendocrine system and cause a multisystem response. Much interest and numerous research studies have been devoted to understanding the neuroendocrine influence during stress.

When considering the general adaptation syndrome, three phases can be identified: (1) the alarm reaction, in which the sympathetic system is activated and subsequently activates the neuroendocrine system; (2) resistance to stress, a period of adaptation to the stress; and (3) exhaustion from stress, a time when the coping mechanisms are insufficient or ineffective for continuing to deal with the stress. The degree to which the general adaptation syndrome is implemented and the amount of time during which it is operational depend on the intensity and type of stress experienced. Selye suggested that continued intense stimulation from stress would deplete the organism's ability to respond at all, or to respond effectively, to stress.

The concept of stress as a psychological phenomenon has evolved from the work of various theorists. The conceptualization of stress has taken on many diverse models. The critical components that contribute to the understanding of stress have been identified as follows: The stimulus (stressor) must be viewed as a threat by the individual; the stimulus, regardless of whether it is positive or negative, must be viewed as being significant or relevant to the individual's welfare; and the organism's capacity for adaptation must have been exceeded. These critical components address the type and intensity of a stimulus, the individual's perception of the stimulus, and the duration of the stimulus that depletes the capacity to cope.

What kinds of stimuli activate the stress response in the neurological patient? Any intense physical or psychological stimuli, such as forced immobilization, trauma, pain, fear, threat of loss, lack of control, or anxiety, can cause a multisystem stress response. There are degrees of intensity of stimuli that cause a proportional stress response. For example, one would expect a much less intense stress response in a patient who has been admitted for an elective cranioplasty for cosmetic purposes long after an injury occurred than in a patient who has been admitted for a craniotomy for removal of a brain tumor of unidentified histological origin.

HUMAN ADAPTATION AND COPING

Adaptation is the process of change undertaken by an organism in response to a change in the internal or external environment for the purpose of maintaining equilibrium. Physiological adaptation supports survival and homeostasis within the organism. Psychological adaptation is directed toward maintaining a psychological homeostasis and supporting the self-concept and the self-esteem of the individual. Adaptation may be positive or negative in that the process either supports or is detrimental to the well-being of the individual. Behaviors that are detrimental to the individual are termed maladaptive behaviors, whereas those that support the well-being of the individual are called adaptive behaviors.

Much has been written about how individuals adapt to changes in their internal and external environment. The conceptualization of adaptation is central to the practice of nursing because much of the nurse's time and energy are directed at supporting healthy adaptation.

The word *coping* refers to the methods, skills, or processes used by an individual in adapting to stresses in the internal or external environment. Coping has been defined in the literature in many different ways to fit the needs of particular models. However, the definition just presented is broad enough to provide a basic conceptual structure. Coping mechanisms are normal—everyone uses them—but some may be effective in dealing with a stressor (problem), whereas others may be ineffective. The choice of coping mechanisms and the manner in which they are applied affect the promotion of health in the health care setting. The roles of the nurse are to help patients identify previously used effective coping mechanisms and assist and support patients so that they can use effective coping skills and mechanisms to deal with the stresses precipitated by illness. Coping is viewed as the individual's attempt to remove stress and restore physical and emotional equilibrium.

NEUROLOGICAL CONDITIONS AND THEIR PSYCHOLOGICAL EFFECTS

Illness is a stressor that creates physiological and psychological stress for the person involved. Stress responses may be viewed on a scale that varies according to the amount of noxious stimuli, the patient's perception of the significance of the stimuli, and the length of time the stimuli remain. So far, this discussion of stress, adaptation, and coping could be applied to either physiological or psychological stress. The discussion now focuses on psychological stresses and psychological responses to neurological illness.

In the case of neurological illness, the psychological stressors and stress response can be particularly taxing in terms of the person's ability to cope and adapt to the illness. Common situations, concerns, and losses precipitated by neurological illness may include the following:

- Threat to survival
- Threat to the quality of life as it was known before the illness—lifestyle, occupation, social and recreational activities, freedom to make changes, and control over one's being and destiny
- Development of neurological deficits:
  Paresis or paralysis (interferes with mobility, swallowing, self-control, speech)
  Bowel or bladder dysfunction
  Communication deficits
  Sexual dysfunction
  Emotional deficits and responses (emotional lability, aggression, depression, anxiety)
  Cognitive deficits (difficulty in reasoning, making judgments, memory)
  Sensory deficits (hearing loss, loss of visual acuity, diplopia, paresthesias, anesthesia)
  Autonomic deficits (orthostatic hypotension, loss of ability to perspire, difficulty controlling body temperature)
- Important and significant losses, such as loss of the following:
  Independence in the activities of daily living
  Control over decisions that affect one's destiny

The ability to perceive the environment accurately through the senses (stimuli may be perceived as meaningless, confusing, or absent)

The ability to understand language and to express oneself verbally and in writing

The ability to be responsible for oneself

When assessing the patient's ability to cope and adapt to the emotional and behavioral responses necessitated by the impact of neurological illness, the nurse seeks feedback from the patient to validate perceptions, clarify information, and ascertain whether the patient understands the information provided. The feedback collected is verbal and nonverbal, or it may be only nonverbal in some patients, depending on the type and degree of neurological deficits sustained. For the patient with neurological illness, these interactions may be severely compromised or impossible (*e.g.*, those who are comatose or aphasic).

Many patients' neurological deficits compromise normal interpersonal relationships and the ability to express themselves and comprehend information. Such situations create additional stress. Stress will cause various emotional and psychological responses that may require the intervention of the nurse.

GENERAL PRINCIPLES FOR CONSIDERING THE PATIENT'S EMOTIONAL AND PSYCHOLOGICAL RESPONSES TO NEUROLOGICAL CONDITIONS

Certain emotional and psychological responses can be expected in patients with any illness. Although the nurse can anticipate responses, patients must be assessed carefully to determine how they have responded to their circumstances. The nurse would expect the person who is alert and well oriented to be fearful of anticipated surgery. However, the specific reasons for or perceptions of the planned events that contribute to the fear can vary from patient to patient. For example, for some patients (particularly adolescents), the most terrifying aspect of undergoing a craniotomy may be having their head shaved. If the nurse recognizes that this issue is the source of greatest fear or stress to these patients, discussing their concerns may help to alleviate some of their fear, especially if they are provided with information and encouraged to participate in problem solving to deal with the temporary loss of hair. Although the shaving of the head will still cause a certain amount of fear, much can be done to dispel some of the underlying concerns, thus modifying the emotional and behavioral response of the patient.

Nursing Assessment and Ongoing Assessment

In assessing the psychological responses of the patient, the nurse should do the following:

1. Observe the patient's behavior when alone and while interacting with others (family members, significant others,

staff, other patients); note facial expressions, body language, tone of voice, and reactions to particular individuals.
2. Establish rapport with the patient; provide opportunities for communication in whatever way possible, depending on which communication skills are intact.
3. Focus communication on the patient by using open-ended questions, provided the patient has adequate neurological function to respond.
4. Listen to what the patient has to say and how it is said (*e.g.*, how things are described, use of analogies).
5. Collect information from the patient and family or significant others on the following:
   Previous adjustment patterns and use of coping mechanisms
   Personality before illness
   Previous emotional and behavioral responses to stress
   Means for dealing with stress (*e.g.*, jogging, withdrawal)
   Support systems
   Family interactions
6. Validate the information collected with the appropriate person(s) (*e.g.*, family, other health professionals), as necessary.
7. Consult with others to broaden the base of information about the patient.
8. Validate perceptions.

Assessment is an ongoing process involving data collection, analysis, and formulation of nursing diagnoses. Once the nursing diagnoses have been made, the nurse must then plan appropriate nursing interventions.

Nursing Diagnoses

The catastrophic and disabling nature of many neurological conditions precipitates many emotional and psychological responses in patients and their families. A number of nursing diagnoses, listed in Chart 13-1, may be appropriate.

Nursing Interventions

The nursing interventions necessary for dealing with the many emotional and behavioral responses to the stress of neurological illness are directed at helping patients maintain their identity, a positive self-concept, and self-esteem. General principles that can guide the nurse to help the patient deal with the many emotional and behavioral responses to the stress of neurological illness include the following:

1. Provide an open, nonjudgmental environment.
2. Be supportive.
3. Develop alternate ways of communication if communication deficits exist.
4. Accept the patient's perceptions and behavior.
5. Matter-of-factly correct any inaccurate factual information.
6. Encourage the patient to express feelings in whatever way is possible.
7. Listen empathetically and attentively; reflect the pa-

CHART 13-1
Nursing Diagnoses Related to Emotional and Psychological Responses of Patients or Family to Neurological Conditions

The following nursing diagnoses are often identified for the patient or family with an altered emotional or psychological response to neurological conditions:

Major Nursing Diagnoses	Associated Nursing Diagnoses
• Fear	• Chronic Low Self Esteem
• Personal Identity Disturbance	• Situational Low Self Esteem
• Anxiety	• Anticipatory Grieving
• Hopelessness	• Dysfunctional Grieving
• Powerlessness	• Social Isolation
• Body Image Disturbance	• Risk for Altered: Parenting
• Altered Role Performance	• Altered Parenting
• Impaired Social Interaction	• Parental Role Conflict
• Altered Family Processes	• Risk for Violence: Self-directed or directed at others
• Impaired Verbal Communication	• Sleep Pattern Disturbance
• Ineffective Individual Coping	• Decisional Conflict
• Impaired Adjustment	• Post-Trauma Response
• Ineffective Family Coping: Compromised	• Ineffective Family Coping: Disabling
	• Defensive Coping
	• Ineffective Denial
	• Spiritual Distress

tient's thoughts and perceptions for clarification and validation.
8. Help the patient use positive adaptive coping mechanisms.
9. Allow the patient to make decisions and maintain control to the degree that he or she is able.
10. Allow the patient to be involved in problem solving as much as possible.
11. Provide information and reinforcement as necessary.
12. Make referrals to other health professionals when appropriate.
13. Help the patient set realistic goals.
14. Support a positive self-concept and self-esteem.
15. Stay calm and relaxed; nurses are role models for the patient and family.

COMMON EMOTIONAL AND PSYCHOLOGICAL RESPONSES TO THE STRESS ASSOCIATED WITH NEUROLOGICAL CONDITIONS

The general management principles of assessment and nursing intervention discussed in the previous section can be applied to the management of the common emotional and psychological responses seen in many patients as they face the prospect of acute or chronic neurological disease. The emo-

tional and psychological responses discussed include anxiety, frustration, anger, hostility, fear, regression, denial, guilt, depression, powerlessness, and stigma. Although these common responses are discussed as separate entities, several responses can occur concurrently in the patient.

Anxiety

Anxiety is a feeling of uneasiness, apprehension, or dread that is associated with an unrecognized, subjective source of anticipated danger. It results from the real or perceived conflicts and frustrations of living. For patients who are unable to speak because of neurological disability or a tracheostomy, their ability to ventilate feelings of frustration, anger, and hostility is negated. This causes anxiety for the patient and perhaps for the nurse. Anxiety is often classified as mild, moderate, or severe to convey the notion that the feeling can range from the mild awareness of fear or anticipatory danger to outright panic. Physiological alterations in the autonomic system, such as an elevated pulse rate and blood pressure, perspiration, tightness in the stomach, or diarrhea, may accompany this mood state. The patient who is anxious will demonstrate various recognizable behaviors associated with the degree of anxiety, including irritability, uneasiness, apprehension, demanding or unreasonable behavior, and often verbal abusiveness. Such a patient is often described as "very difficult." Occasionally, a patient may be charming and agreeable but noncompliant with established treatment protocols. This, too, is a way of dealing with anxiety.

NURSING INTERVENTIONS

Because anxiety is associated with an unrecognized, subjective source of anticipated danger, time should be spent trying to discover what is generating the anxiety. Often, several concerns are responsible for anxiety, some of which cannot be identified on the conscious level. For the patient who cannot communicate, the nurse must try to anticipate potential sources of anxiety and provide information. Alternate methods of communication should be developed, and the nurse must become very good at reading body language.

Recognizing potential sources of anxiety must be a major concern when caring for the patient. To alleviate anxiety, nurses should explain to the patient what is going to be done before beginning and then keep the patient apprised of what is being done while care is administered. Care should also be explained to the "unresponsive" or "unconscious" patient because there is no way to determine whether sensory stimuli are getting through to the brain and being processed. The caregiver must assume that some verbal stimuli will penetrate the barriers of neurological illness, providing information and comfort to the patient.

For patients who are able to follow directions and cooperate, relaxation therapy may reduce anxiety. This is a systematic approach to tightening and relaxing muscle groups to relieve muscle tension. Another relaxation technique is the use of imagery. Patients are encouraged to select an image that is particularly relaxing and pleasing. They are taught to close their eyes, relax, and focus on experiencing all of the pleasing sensations of being in this chosen setting. Any type of relaxation technique takes time to learn and must be practiced to achieve optimal results. Appropriate patients must be selected for this therapy.

Frustration

Frustration is the feeling that occurs when a course of action or activity cannot be carried out or brought to a desirable conclusion. Irritability, anxiety, and verbal outbursts often accompany frustration. The amount of frustration experienced will be proportional to the value and desirability the patient places on the thwarted action.

NURSING INTERVENTIONS

The nurse can help patients identify the basis for their frustration. Once identified, problem solving should be used to determine why the desired result was not achieved. It may be that the patient had set unrealistic goals. In this instance, realistic goals should be identified. Another possibility may be that an alternate approach is necessary to achieve the desired goal. The patient must be encouraged to examine the situation realistically and to select appropriate strategies or alter the goals. Expressing frustration is helpful in dissipating feelings of frustration.

Anger

Anger is an intense feeling of displeasure and antagonism in response to mounting frustration, conflict, or anxiety. It connotes strong feelings in response to the actual prevention or threat of prevention of achievement or maintenance of a desired goal or state. Anger that is turned inward is called **depression.** The behavioral manifestations of anger may include aggressive or destructive acts, verbal attacks, silence, or depression.

NURSING INTERVENTIONS

Patients who are angry need the same kind of help and support that anxious or frustrated patients need. If an angry patient is apt to lose self-control and cause injury to another or to self or if the patient is prone to cause property damage, he or she must be controlled. A quiet environment, drug therapy, or other forms of therapy directed at preventing self-harm may be necessary. The patient must be provided with an appropriate outlet for feelings of anger. If the source of the anger can be identified, it may be possible to alleviate the situation.

Hostility

Hostility is usually seen in association with anger. It is a feeling of antagonism directed toward another and is associated with a wish to hurt, humiliate, or discredit that person. Hostility is generally thought to be the result of frustrated or unfulfilled needs or wishes. According to Horney, repressed hostility is one of the major sources of anxiety.[5] Kiening describes the development of hostility in the following way:[6]

- A person experiences frustration, loss of self-esteem, or unmet needs for status, prestige, or love.
- Within a given situation, the person has certain expectations for self and for others.
- The expectations are not met.
- The person feels inadequate, hurt, or humiliated.
- The person experiences anxiety, which becomes hostility, causing one of three reactions:
  The hostility is repressed and the person withdraws.
  The feeling is disowned and the person behaves in an extremely polite and compliant manner.
  The person behaves in an overtly hostile manner. This may be manifested verbally or nonverbally.

NURSING INTERVENTIONS

Patients who are hostile need help in understanding the origin of their feelings. They also need to be able to express their feelings in a safe, nonjudgmental environment. The nurse caring for a hostile patient can use a similar approach as would be appropriate for the anxious patient.

Fear

Fear is a feeling of extreme apprehension or dread associated with a potential or real threat to the well-being of the individual. Fear may be associated with the unknown, mutilation, loss of control, pain, disability, or other factors. Behavioral manifestations of fear often include excitability, irrational behavior, and irrational and inaccurate beliefs about the feared object. Physiological signs and symptoms of the activated sympathetic nervous system (fight or flight response) include pallor, tachycardia, pupillary dilation, dry mouth, and cold, clammy hands.

NURSING INTERVENTIONS

The nurse should try to identify the basis of the patient's fear. Identifying the source of fear will require exploring concerns with the patient. Once the source of the fear is identified, the nurse may be able to correct any misinformation. The need to verify the patient's understanding and perceptions and to clarify and amplify information is an ongoing, necessary aspect of communication. The nurse may also need to make appropriate referrals to assist the patient in alleviating the fears.

Regression

The person who is subjected to extreme and continued stress may retreat to the use of behavioral patterns that were appropriate during an earlier developmental stage. This response is called **regression.** On a temporary basis, regression can be a protective mechanism that preserves the person's limited ego strength. A certain amount of regression occurs with all serious illness as part of the response to the illness. The behavioral manifestations vary and may include helplessness, crying, temper tantrums, withdrawal from responsibilities, preoccupation with self, dependency, giddiness, and stubbornness.

NURSING INTERVENTIONS

The patient who demonstrates evidence of regression needs a supportive, safe environment. The regression indicates that the patient is overwhelmed by the current stressors and cannot cope effectively. The nurse needs to implement methods for stress reduction and support effective coping mechanisms.

Denial

Denial is a defense mechanism, sometimes called a temporary protective mechanism, whereby the person refuses to acknowledge the existence or significance of a known fact. The known fact is too painful for the person to deal with, so its existence is denied. The degree of denial varies from person to person. Denial can be an effective, temporary method of dealing with a stress-producing situation until the person is able to muster the ego strength to deal with the problem. Continued denial, however, becomes a negative mechanism, in that the person does not incorporate the known information into reality for problem solving and realistic planning. Rather, the patient behaves as if the situation does not exist or refuses to discuss the topic in relation to himself or herself. Denial is likely to be carried out in fantasy, daydreaming, or games so that reality is temporarily pushed aside.

NURSING INTERVENTIONS

At some point, denial becomes an ineffective coping mechanism for dealing with stress. The seriousness of the illness or the probable outcome can no longer be denied. An enormous amount of stress is associated with this realization. Patients gradually begin to acknowledge some of the more obvious aspects of their illness. They need the support of the nursing staff to make this adaptation. Questions should be answered honestly and as completely as possible based on the known facts so that patients can gradually face most of the realities of their illness. Depression and grieving are characteristic of this period. Once the painful information is incorporated into reality, the patient is able to make realistic decisions based on an altered and realistic self-concept.

Guilt

The feeling that one has done something wrong and is directly responsible for negative outcomes, pain, or frustration of goals is called **guilt.** The behavioral manifestations of guilt include a feeling of regretful responsibility for negative consequences, self-deprecation, lowered self-esteem, and possibly self-hate.

NURSING INTERVENTIONS

The nurse should help the patient identify the source of the guilt and deal with the situation realistically and honestly.

Depression

Depression is a feeling of sadness and self-depreciation accompanied by difficulty in thinking and conducting usual activities and responsibilities, a lowered energy level, and self-preoccupation. The depressed person is unable to express feelings and instead internalizes them. Depression has also been defined as anger turned inward. The characteristic behaviors associated with depression are a sad, expressionless face; flat affect; listlessness; lack of interest in others or the environment; possible crying spells; and a sense of hopelessness. Some people who are depressed see no possible resolution to their situation and may contemplate suicide. Allusions to suicide may be made either directly or indirectly and should be taken seriously.

NURSING INTERVENTIONS

There are varying degrees of depression. The person who is severely depressed may need psychiatric consultation and help. Drug therapy may be helpful in treating temporary depression. However, the reason(s) for the depression must be sought, identified, addressed, and treated. Suicide precautions may need to be instituted.

Powerlessness

Powerlessness is defined as a perceived or real lack of control over one's body, mind, environment, or life. The typical behavioral characteristics of powerlessness include a feeling of frustration, anger, hopelessness, depression, and apathy.

NURSING INTERVENTIONS

Patients who perceive themselves as powerless, in the psychological sense, may need to be reminded that they have more power than they believe they do. Because of illness, power is often altered, but it is not lost. Patients need to recognize the power that they have and should be encouraged to use it appropriately.

Neurological illness may have deprived the patient of power over certain physiological functions. Participating in a rehabilitation program may help the patient reclaim his or her altered control and power over body functions. If complete rehabilitation is not possible, the patient may benefit from adaptive devices or altered methods of accomplishing tasks.

Stigma

When a person feels devalued or unable to meet minimum societal norms, this is termed a **stigma.** The feeling of stigmatization can result from physical or emotional deficits, behavioral abnormalities, or violation of societal laws or codes. The person who feels stigmatized demonstrates characteristic behaviors that include feelings of shame, alienation, or being devalued; a decreased feeling of self-esteem or social worth; isolation from normal relationships; rejection of attempts by others to reach out to him or her; suspiciousness; paranoid behavior; loneliness; hostility; and anger.

NURSING INTERVENTIONS

Dealing with patients who feel stigmatized can be difficult. Their feelings are usually based on deep-seated beliefs and values. These patients need assistance in exploring their feelings so that they can better understand them. The nurse needs to present reality and correct any erroneous information that the patient expresses. It is also important to support and build the patient's self-esteem.

EMOTIONAL AND PSYCHOLOGICAL RESPONSES TO SPECIFIC ASPECTS OF ILLNESS: NURSING IMPLICATIONS

Some emotional and psychological responses associated with certain aspects of neurological illness and hospitalization call for specific nursing interventions in addition to the general nursing approaches discussed previously in this chapter. The following experiences are discussed: loss, grief and bereavement, immobility, dehumanization, change in body image, sensory deprivation, isolation, sensory overload, intensive care unit (ICU) response, and transfer anxiety.

Loss

Loss is defined as a state in which a person experiences deprivation or the complete lack of something that was previously present and available to him or her. The person who has sustained a significant loss will demonstrate behaviors consistent with grieving and bereavement. (See the section that follows on grief and bereavement for specific behavioral manifestations.)

Loss can be sudden or gradual, predictable or unexpected, and temporary or permanent. Paralysis can be used to illustrate sudden and gradual loss. Patients who sustain a spinal cord injury in a motor vehicle accident may experience sudden loss of motor function below the level of injury. By contrast, patients with progressive multiple sclerosis often experience a gradual decline in motor function until they are completely paraplegic. In the first instance, paralysis occurs in a split second; in the second example, it develops gradually over years.

Some losses are predictable, whereas others are unexpected. The patient diagnosed as having amyotrophic lateral sclerosis will probably develop severe difficulty with speech and swallowing as the illness progresses. On the other hand, the patient with a right hemispheric stroke is not expected to develop aphasia.

Some losses are temporary, whereas others are permanent. For example, the patient who has had surgery on the left parietal lobe of the brain may be temporarily aphasic postoperatively because of cerebral edema. Given a few days of treatment of the cerebral edema, speech ability would be expected to return gradually over the next several days. An example of a permanent loss may be seen in the patient who has undergone removal of a large acoustic neuroma that involved the trigeminal (V) and facial (VII) cranial nerve. Unilateral loss of sensation to the face and drooping of the side of the mouth may remain despite the surgery.

Significant losses may include loss of spouse, family members, or significant others; body parts; life; possessions; and physical, psychological, or cognitive functions. The individual's response to the loss will depend on the value that is placed on the lost object or body function, the societal and cultural value placed on the loss, and the cultural, economic, and support groups available to assist the individual in dealing with the loss. Each person has a unique value system. How the person values an object, person, or function influences the response to loss. For example, a person who loses the use of the right arm may be devastated if he or she is right-handed and enjoys activities that require fine motor control of the hands, such as painting. Another patient who is left-handed, retired, and spends his or her leisure time reading or watching television would be inconvenienced by the loss, but it would not alter the basic lifestyle or self-concept to the same degree as the other patient.

Certain body functions, such as continence of the bladder and bowel and sexual function, are highly valued functions. Loss of these functions may be viewed as major, even catastrophic, losses by the person and society and have a great impact on lifestyle.

Cultural values also dictate an individual's response to loss. If the culture places a high value on the ability or body part lost, then the impact on the individual as a respected member of the culture is significant. When a person sustains a loss, the response and the adjustment to the loss will depend on the cultural, economic, and support groups available. All societies, regardless of whether they are primitive or highly sophisticated, have customs and rituals that are followed when someone dies. However, no such customs exist when there is loss of body function. Often, the loss of body function (disability) renders the person socially unacceptable because other people feel uncomfortable being around that person. For example, the person who has dysphagia may not be a welcome guest at the dinner table. Even if other people were able to accept the patient's difficulty in managing food, the patient may feel humiliated by uncontrolled drooling or food falling from the mouth.

The economic impact resulting from some losses is significant. Life insurance is helpful when a family member dies. Various health insurance policies assist with the cost of health care, and some people elect to purchase policies that provide payments if disability occurs. However, disability often results in an inability to participate in one's occupation, resulting in loss of salary. If the person is able to benefit from a rehabilitation program, he or she may be able to return to work at some job, but it may be at a much lower salary than previously. The resultant decreased financial income lowers the patient's economic status and lifestyle. The spouse or other family member may have to seek employment or in some cases, may need to leave a job to care for the patient. This decrease in income at a time when extra expenses from loss are incurred has a dramatic effect on the patient's lifestyle and self-concept.

Support groups are available for some patients with particular problems, such as head injuries or multiple sclerosis. The purpose of these support groups is to assist the patient and family members with the loss of health and the disabilities incurred from the illness. The particular services offered vary from organization to organization but may include practical information on how to live with the particular illness, psychological and emotional support, and identification of resources to assist the patient and family.

NURSING INTERVENTIONS

The nurse must explore with the person the significance of the loss. What does the loss mean to the patient within the context of lifestyle and self-concept? Until the nurse can appreciate the significance of the loss from the patient's point of view, it will be difficult to be supportive. Once the nurse understands the significance of the loss, information and assistance can be provided to the patient and family. Referrals to other professionals or organizations may be appropriate.

Grief and Bereavement

According to Engel,[7] the loss of any valued object or function is followed by three stages that lead to healthy resolution: (1) shock and disbelief, (2) development of an awareness (recognition) of the loss, and (3) restitution (reconciliation).

The shock phase immediately follows the loss. Patients are stunned, appear to be out of contact with the environment, and are in a state of disbelief. They may be able to intellectualize the loss but cannot accept it emotionally. They do not believe that this is happening to them and may verbalize that this cannot be true.

During the recognition phase, patients begin to realize that the loss is real. Characteristic behaviors include anger, blaming themselves, depression, and asking, "why me?" These individuals are often preoccupied with the loss and what it means to them. The loss is internalized.

The final stage, restitution, is consistent with a realistic acceptance of what has happened. Gradually, interest in others and the environment returns. Patients begin to see themselves realistically and to integrate the change in body image into a positive self-concept. They are able to make decisions about themselves and the future and to see a realistic future for themselves.

NURSING INTERVENTIONS

During the shock phase, accept the patient's behavior. Denial may be a protective coping mechanism. Allow patients to deny the loss if they must. Listen to them in an accepting, nonjudgmental manner, and refrain from telling them that you understand how they feel unless you have experienced the same loss.

During the recognition phase, accept the patient's anger. Allow for opportunities to express his or her feelings, and correct any misinformation. Support the patient through depression. Explain the patient's response to the loss to the family. Be supportive of the family. As the period of restitution emerges, encourage the patient to express his or her views and to plan realistically. Help the patient collect necessary information, either personally or by making appropriate referrals. Be supportive, and help the patient adapt and integrate the altered body image into his or her self-concept. Allow the patient to be as independent as possible and to assume responsibility for self.

Immobility

The prescribed, enforced, or unavoidable limitation of movement that occurs over a prolonged period is called **immobility**. Immobility can occur in the physical, psychological, intellectual, or social domains. The person who is physically immobilized may develop psychological immobility. Immobility reduces the quality and quantity of sensory input available to the person. This leads to a reduction in the individual's ability to interact with the environment. The behavioral manifestations of immobility include (1) a sense of confinement and limitation of space, resulting in frustration and anxiety; (2) a lack of control, which can lead to anger and depression; and (3) a forced change in body image and self-concept.

The neurological patient may suffer immobility in all domains. Paresis or paralysis can impose involuntary confinement and immobilization. The patient is not able to move freely; movement is a means of control that is highly cherished as a requisite for independence. Certain types of equipment, such as ventilators, food pumps, urinary catheters, intravenous lines, and orthopedic traction, enforce varying degrees of immobility on the patient. Cognitive and psychological deficits precipitated by neurological disease block or severely compromise psychosocial and intellectual input, making the patient feel confined or immobilized. The patient with an altered level of consciousness may be completely isolated from input in all domains. Social immobility may result from the manner in which other people treat the patient because of physical condition and disabilities.

NURSING INTERVENTIONS

The goal of the nurse caring for immobile patients is to draw them into the mainstream of life, involving them to the extent that the therapeutic plan allows. Provide reality orientation (by using clock, calendar, or radio or telling patients what is happening in their immediate vicinity) so that they will be drawn into the environment. Extend the environment of these patients, if possible, by taking them out of their room, moving them near a window, or providing them with a wheelchair. Encourage social interaction and expression of feelings.

Dehumanization

Viewing patients as disease entities and divesting them of human capacities, qualities, and functions so that they are considered merely objects is called **dehumanization**. When dehumanization exists, the focus of attention is not on the person or unique individual who is experiencing illness, but rather on signs, symptoms, diagnostic data, and equipment. When patients are thus divested of their humanity, they are not consulted on decisions concerning themselves, provided with information, or treated with the respect and consideration normally extended to a person. Instead, the caregivers take over the day-to-day decisions affecting the patient.

It is not necessarily the uncaring nurse who treats the patient as less than human. When caring for an unresponsive patient, it is easy to lose sight of the patient as a person. Human relationships are built on interactions between individuals. If this interchange is not ongoing, it is easy to lose sight of the humanity of the other individual.

NURSING INTERVENTIONS

Address patients by name; think of them by name and as unique individuals rather than as a room number or diagnosis. Treat patients as the unique individuals that they are. Speak to them, and involve them in the environment and in decisions about their care as much as possible. Allow them to assume as much control and responsibility for themselves as possible.

Change in Body Image

A concept basic to one's sense of identity, security, self-esteem, and self-concept is body image. **Body Image** is defined as the conscious and unconscious perceptions (feelings and attitudes) that one has about his or her body as a separate and distinct entity. It is a developmental and social creation that is subject to very slow change in adult life. Illness, disability, and loss of function force a change in body image on the patient. If the change can be integrated realistically within the patient's self-concept without altering self-esteem, then the adaptation and adjustment are positive.

The behavioral manifestations associated with a change in body image often include those that accompany loss, grief, and bereavement. The change is viewed as a threat or significant loss, and the patient passes through the characteristic stages of shock, recognition, and reconciliation.

NURSING INTERVENTIONS

If the nurse views the patient's change in body image within the conceptual framework of loss, grief, and bereavement, the nursing intervention will follow a similar approach. Accept the patient's perception of self. Recognize that changing one's body image is a slow process. Support patients as they begin to recognize the impact of illness on their concept of body image. Help patients to accept and adapt to the change with positive reinforcement.

Sensory Deprivation

Sensory deprivation is defined as a lack of or decreased sensory input from the external or internal environment. There is a lack of or decreased perception of multisensory input of various intensities and meanings to the person. The behavioral manifestations of sensory deprivation vary, depending on the degree of deprivation. They may include abnormalities in feeling states, disorientation, impairment of the ability to think, distortion of perception, and illusions and hallucinations. The patient with neurological illness may experience any number of neurological deficits that contribute to sensory deprivation, such as an altered level of consciousness, paresis or paralysis, paresthesias, visual deficits, hearing loss, taste or smell deficits, and cognitive or emotional deficits. Head injury, spinal cord injury, cerebrovascular accident, multiple sclerosis, and any number of other neurological conditions can precipitate sensory deprivation. Therapeutic protocols, such as instituting aneurysm precautions, may also cause sensory deprivation.

NURSING INTERVENTIONS

The nurse should be aware of the frequency with which sensory deprivation occurs, especially in neurological patients, and should assess patients for its presence. The nurse must identify the causes and the specific types of sensory deficits present. Once these questions are answered, the nurse can develop an approach to provide multisensory stimuli to the patient as a means of compensation. Sensory input can be provided by talking to the patient; playing the radio, television, or tape recordings of family members' voices; providing reality orientation and touch; and positioning. Reality orientation is a process of actively making patients aware of their environment (*e.g.,* describing ongoing activities, weather, date, time, place, people, objects). Sensory deprivation, rather than physiological deficits of the reticular activating system, may be the cause of a patient's disorientation.

Sleep Deprivation

Sleep deprivation is defined as a lack of adequate sleep or dream time in relation to prior or usual sleep patterns. People who are deprived of sleep for prolonged periods experience behavioral, psychological, and physiological alterations. Behavioral manifestations are similar to those seen in psychosis (alterations in perceptions, cognition, mood, affect). Patients admitted to ICUs, requiring constant care and monitoring, receiving certain medication, and experiencing extreme stress are prime candidates for sleep deprivation. The strange environment and constant activity of the hospital predispose patients to this common phenomenon. Because of injuries to the brain and their need for attention, neurological patients often experience sleep deprivation.

NURSING INTERVENTIONS

The nurse should assess the patient's 24-hour sleep–wakefulness cycle to determine how much sleep time is actually provided. Nursing care should be planned to provide uninterrupted sleep time. Drug therapy can also have an effect on the quality of sleep and dream time. Certain drugs may alter the depth of sleep and the sleep pattern. Deprivation of the various levels of sleep, such as the rapid eye movement stage, is thought to have a negative effect on the patient. The nurse should be aware of the various factors that influence that patient's ability to sleep and control the environment as much as possible to facilitate sleep.

Sensory Overload

Sudden, excessive, sustained, multisensory experiences that are perceived as confusing, bothersome, meaningless, and extremely stressful to the patient are defined collectively as **sensory overload.** The behavioral manifestations of sensory overload are confusion, disorientation, irritability, restlessness, agitation, anger, panic, and auditory or visual hallucinations.

Neurological patients may experience sensory overload from equipment (*e.g.*, respirator, cardiac monitor), conditions that intensify sensory input (meningitis, encephalitis), or the constant stimuli of nursing care, particularly if they are critically ill.

NURSING INTERVENTIONS

The nurse should identify the various sensory levels and sources of input in the patient's environment. Every effort should be made to control and moderate the intensity of stimuli. Special situations sometimes exist, such as when subarachnoid precautions are instituted. The purpose of these precautions is to decrease all stimuli so that the patient will not rebleed. In patients with meningitis or encephalitis, tactile stimuli should be minimized, and all other environmental stimuli should be controlled.

Intensive Care Unit Response

Admission to the alien environment of the ICU is very stressful for the patient and family for many reasons. The ICU environment is characterized by strange noises, smells, and bright lights, and the open floor plan characteristic of most ICUs offers little privacy. The pervasive atmosphere is one of urgency, danger, and death being held in abeyance by technology and heroic measures of the staff. Ironically, the patient and family can feel profound isolation within this charged environment. Fear, anxiety, depression, and delirium are common responses to the situation, and the patient or family may panic. According to Cassem and Hackett,[8] nothing else distorts personality quite like panic.

Disorientation is common in patients. Sleep deprivation or an altered sleep–wakefulness cycle contributes to disorientation and misinterpretation of reality. Patients may exhibit agitation, hallucinations, delusions, and psychosis. This phenomenon is called **ICU psychosis.** The changes in behavior can be difficult to interpret. When neurological patients exhibit a change in behavior, one often attributes the change to a neurological cause. However, psychological responses and drug side effects should also be considered as possible etiologies.

NURSING INTERVENTIONS

Institute strategies to provide emotional support, reassurance, and information to the conscious patient, and plan activities to allow for periods of uninterrupted sleep. Provide for the safety needs of agitated patients. In an unconscious patient, provide for "soft stimuli," such as light touch, soft voices, and family visits whereby family members talk quietly to the patient about pleasant topics.

Transfer Anxiety

The increased anxiety and feelings of insecurity experienced by patients when they are moved from one unit or facility to another are called **transfer anxiety.** Patients may be transferred from the ICU to a regular acute care unit. Neurological patients may also be transferred to a rehabilitation facility, chronic care facility, or nursing home. Patients and their families may be concerned that the quality of care and the commitment of the nursing and medical staff will not be as good in the new setting. There may be the underlying feeling that the quality of care will deteriorate and that the person will not be recognized as a unique individual. The unit to which a patient is currently assigned may be perceived as one that offers a higher level of nursing, medical, and technological support than the unit to which the patient is being transferred. Patients may experience fear of the unknown and may view the transfer as a threat to their security and well-being.

The major behavioral manifestation is anxiety that may develop into a panic-like state as the day of transfer approaches. The patient may also experience physiological responses (psychosomatic responses) to the stress of an impending transfer. Common signs and symptoms may include elevation of blood pressure, shortness of breath, tightness in the chest, palpitations, or elevation in body temperature.

NURSING INTERVENTIONS

Comprehensive discharge planning should include the psychological preparation of the patient and family to ensure a smooth transition from the acute care setting to another facility or home. The liaison nurse from the new facility may need to visit the patient to help facilitate the transition and provide information about the new facility. Questions should be encouraged and complete information provided to dispel the patient's fear of the unknown facility. A visit to the new unit or facility is desirable so that the patient (if possible) or family members can tour the facilities and meet members of the staff.

If the neurological patient is going home, the physical environment should be evaluated, and the delivery of any necessary equipment should be arranged before the day of discharge. Patient and family teaching should be conducted in plenty of time so that they will feel comfortable. If possible, a weekend home visit by the patient should be arranged. In this way, problems can be addressed and resolved before the actual discharge is made. Every attempt should be made to anticipate potential problems so that a smooth transition can occur.

Regardless of the plans after discharge, the patient and family should be given an opportunity to terminate (*i.e.*, say good bye) with the staff.

PSYCHOLOGICAL, EMOTIONAL, AND BEHAVIORAL RESPONSES OF THE FAMILY OR SIGNIFICANT OTHERS

Neurological illness has serious consequences, not only for the patient, but also for family members and significant others. The family structure, relationships, and methods of dealing with stress and crisis become important considerations for the nurse. Family members will react to illness individually within the entire gamut of responses, including anxiety, anger, depression, denial, grieving, and fear. Neurological illness often takes the form of a chronic condition with permanent or progressive disabilities that compel the patient to depend on family or significant others to meet basic needs. The stresses incurred by neurological illness are significant and require the support and assistance of health professionals for the family to make a realistic adjustment. The ability of the family to accept the situation and adapt will directly influence the emotional well-being of every member of the family unit, including the patient. See Chart 13-1 for nursing diagnoses related to the family.

NURSING INTERVENTIONS

The role of the nurse in supporting the family includes the following:

- Talk to the family to determine their understanding and perception of the patient's illness.
- Determine the schemata of family interactions and support systems.
- Allow the family members to express their feelings.
- Correct misinformation, and provide data as necessary.
- Make referrals as necessary.
- Allow the family to become involved in the care of the patient, if they so wish.
- Promote normalcy.
- Support the family in their decision about patient's care or plans for posthospital care.
- Be prepared to repeat information.

EMOTIONAL AND PSYCHOLOGICAL RESPONSES OF THE NURSE CARING FOR NEUROLOGICAL PATIENTS

Care of the Caretakers: Secondary Traumatic Stress

Traumatic events affect the lives of many people besides the immediate victims. Working with patients who have suffered neurological illness is challenging and difficult. The literature to date has focused on the patient and family. Some attention should be focused on the nurse and what she or he brings to the therapeutic relationship and how she or he is affected by these relationships. The conscious and the unconscious responses of the nurse need to be examined. These responses include affective, cognitive, and somatic components. Nurses need ongoing and regularly scheduled supportive relationships with their supervisors in which they are able to talk about their feelings and are urged to attend to their own self-care and spiritual renewal.

Common job-related stressors include caring for patients who have the following:

- Neurological injury as a result of trauma (*e.g.*, motor vehicle accidents, assaults, self-inflicted injuries)
- Terminal diagnoses, especially if they are young
- Cognitive and emotional disabilities
- Neurological deficits that render them completely dependent on the nurse
- Tracheostomy tubes, ventilators, and support equipment
- Significant pain that does not respond to the normal modalities of pain control
- Multiple trauma or a critical illness
- Agreed to a donor organ transplant
- Been designated as brain dead
- Been discharged to another facility after a long stay on the unit

Other factors in the work environment that are sources of stress include the following:

- Experiencing interpersonal conflict with coworkers or administrative personnel
- Dealing with the family of a dying patient
- Dealing with a disoriented, demanding, noisy, or "difficult" patient or family
- Having to assume responsibilities that the nurse is not prepared to manage
- Dealing with physicians, residents, nursing students, and faculty
- Rotating shifts and working double shifts
- Working with insufficient staff
- Working with inadequate supplies or auxilliary staff (*e.g.*, transport services, laboratory services)
- Working without effective leadership
- Observing curtailment of programs due to lack of adequate funding
- Seeing patients who will receive inadequate rehabilitation due to lack of funds
- Receiving no recognition
- Having to channel communications through the bureaucracy to get results
- Downsizing of hospitals resulting in rapid turnover of staff
- Being unable to organize staff as a cohesive group due to rapid changes in staffing patterns
- Feeling devalued with acknowledgment of the shift in care from hospitals to outpatient settings

Unless nurses take the time to protect themselves from the acute and chronic stresses of their job, their mental and physical health are at risk. Burnout is the result of chronic stress, and it affects the quality of the care administered to the patient and the professional and personal life of the nurse. Nurses must learn to recognize the signs and symptoms of stress and do something positive to deal with them before serious problems result. Nurses are encouraged to choose appropriate coping mechanisms to deal with stress and to practice good health habits themselves (*e.g.*, eating well, avoiding drugs and alcohol abuse, participating in an exercise program or other recreation).

Many articles and continuing education offerings have addressed the needs of the nurse as a person and professional who is subject to significant stress. The concept of burnout is well documented and discussed in the literature. Nurses as caregivers are very vulnerable to stress, and measures should be taken to protect and support them. Each nurse must assume responsibility for his or her own mental health and practice appropriate methods of stress control.

References

1. Selye, H. (1956). *The stress of life.* New York: McGraw-Hill.
2. Selye, H. (1974). *Stress without distress.* Philadelphia: J.B. Lippincott.
3. Cannon, W. B. (1936). *The wisdom of the body.* New York: W.W. Norton.
4. Jacobson, E. (1965). *Anxiety and tension control.* Philadelphia: J.B. Lippincott.
5. Horney, K. (1937). *Collected works of Karen Horney* (Vol. 1) (p. 63). New York: W.W. Norton.
6. Kiening, M. M., Sr. (1978). Hostility. In C. E. Carlson & B. Blackwell (Eds.), *Behavioral concepts and nursing interventions* (2nd ed.) (p. 131). Philadelphia: J.B. Lippincott.
7. Engel, G. L. (1964). Grief and grieving. *American Journal of Nursing, 64,* 93.
8. Cassem, N., & Hackett, T. (1978). The setting of intensive care. In T. Hackett & N. Cassem (Eds.), *Massachusetts General Hospital handbook of general hospital psychiatry.* St. Louis: C.V. Mosby.

Bibliography

Books

Aguilera, D. C., & Messick, J. M. (1990). *Crisis intervention: Theory and methodology* (6th ed.). St. Louis: C.V. Mosby.

American Psychiatric Association (1994). *Diagnostic and statistical manual of mental disorders* (4th ed.). Washington, DC: Author.

Brooks, N. (Ed.) (1984). *Closed head injury: Psychological, social, and family consequences.* Oxford: Oxford University Press.

Carpenito, L. J. (1989). *Nursing diagnosis: Application to clinical practice* (3rd ed.). Philadelphia: J.B. Lippincott.

Coehlo, G. V., Hamburg, D. A., & Adams, J. E. (1974). *Coping and adaptation.* New York: Basic Books.

Derogatis, L. R. (1982). Self-report measures of stress. In L. Goldberger & S. Breznitz (Eds.), *Handbook of stress: Theoretical and clinical aspects.* New York: Free Press.

Dimond, M., & Jones, S. L. (1983). *Chronic illness across the life span.* Norwalk: Appleton-Century-Croft.

Henderson, G., & Bryan, W. V. (1984). *Psychosocial aspects of disability.* Springfield: Charles C. Thomas.

Lazarus, R. S. (1984). *Stress appraisal and coping.* New York: Springer.

Lewis, S., Granger, R. D. K., McDowell, W. A. et al. (Eds.) (1989). *Manual of psychosocial nursing interventions: Promoting mental health in medical-surgical settings.* Philadelphia: W.B. Saunders.

Miller, J. F. (1983). *Coping with chronic illness: Overcoming powerlessness.* Philadelphia: F.A. Davis.

Rosenthal, M., Griffith, E. R., Bond, M. R., & Miller, J. D. (1990). *Rehabilitation of the head-injured adult* (2nd ed.). Philadelphia: F.A. Davis.

Wood, R. L. (1987). *Brain injury rehabilitation: A neurobehavioral approach.* Rockville: Aspen Publishing.

Periodicals

Bell, T. (1986). Nurses' attitudes in caring for the comatose head-injured patient. *Journal of Neuroscience Nursing, 18,* 279–283.

Bernstein, L. P. (1990). Family-centered care of the critically ill neurologic patient. *Critical Care Nursing Clinics of North America, 2*(1), 41–50.

Braulin, J. L. D., Rook, J., & Sills, G. M. (1982). Families in crisis: The impact of trauma. *Critical Care Quarterly, 5*(3), 38–46.

Burckhardt, C. S. (1987). Coping strategies of the chronically ill. *Nursing Clinics of North America, 22*(3), 543–550.

Caine, R. M. (1989). Families in crisis: Making the critical difference. *Focus on Critical Care, 16*(3), 184–189.

Campbell, C. H. (1988). Needs of relatives and helpfulness of support groups in severe head injury. *Rehabilitation Medicine, 13,* 320–325.

Clum, M. N., & Ryan, M. (1981). Brain injury and the family. *Journal of Neurosurgical Nursing, 13,* 165–169.

Craig, M. C., Copes, W. S., & Champion, H. R. (1988). Psychosocial considerations in trauma. *Critical Care Quarterly, 11,* 51–58.

Evans, R. L., & Bishop, D. S. (1987). Predicting post-stroke family function: A continuing dilemma. *Psychology Report, 60,* 691–695.

Frye, B. (1987). Head injury and the family: Related literature. *Rehabilitation Nursing, 12,* 135–136.

Grinspun, D. (1987). Teaching families of traumatic brain-injured adults. *Critical Care Quarterly, 10,* 61.

Gull, H. J. (1987). The chronically ill patient's adaptation to hospitalization. *Nursing Clinics of North America, 22*(3), 593–601.

Hegeman, K. M. (1988). A care plan for the family of a brain-trauma client. *Rehabilitation Nursing, 13,* 254–262.

Lambert, C. E., & Lambert, V. A. (1987). Psychological impacts created by chronic illness. *Nursing Clinics of North America, 22*(3), 527–533.

Leske, J. S. (1986). Needs of relatives of critically ill patients: A follow-up. *Heart & Lung, 15,* 189–193.

Lust, B. L. (1984). The patient in the ICU: A family experience. *Critical Care Quarterly, 6*(4), 49–57.

Martin, K. M. (1987). Predicting short-term outcome in comatose head-injured children. *Journal of Neuroscience Nursing, 19*(1), 9–13.

Mathis, M. (1984). Personal needs of the family members of critically ill patients with and without acute brain injury. *Journal of Neurosurgical Nursing, 16*(1), 36–44.

Mauss-Clum, N., & Ryan, M. (1981). Brain injury and the family. *Journal of Neurosurgical Nursing, 13*(4), 165–169.

McCann, I. L., & Pearlman, L. A. (1990). Vicarious traumatization: A contextual model for understanding the effects of trauma on helpers. *Journal of Traumatic Stress, 3*(1), 131–149.

Podrasky, D. L., & Sexton, D. L. (1988). Nurses' reactions to difficult patients. *Image, 20*(1), 16–21.

Pollock, S. E. (1987). Adaptation to chronic illness: Analysis of nursing research. *Nursing Clinics of North America, 22*(3), 631–644.

Pollock, S. E. (1984). The stress response. *Critical Care Quarterly, 6*(4), 1–13.

Printz-Feddersen, V. (1990). Group process effect on caregiver burden. *Journal of Neuroscience Nursing, 22*(3), 164–168.

Soderstrom, S., Fogelsjoo, A., Fugl-Meyer, K. S., & Stensson, S. (1988). I. Head injury. A program for crisis-intervention after traumatic brain injury. *Scandanavian Journal of Rehabilitation Medicine, 17*(Suppl.), 47–49.

Tilden, V. P., & Weinert, C. (1987). Social support and the chronically ill individual. *Nursing Clinics of North America, 22*(3), 613–620.

CHAPTER 14

Rehabilitation of Neuroscience Patients

Joanne V. Hickey

This chapter provides nurses caring for neuroscience patients with basic information about the principles and concepts of rehabilitation as they apply to neuroscience patient populations. There is a specialty area of rehabilitation practice in nursing; however, rehabilitation principles and concepts are a fundamental component of nursing practice and cut across all practice areas.

FRAMEWORKS FOR DISABILITY

For a number of years, there were two widely used conceptual frameworks regarding disability and rehabilitation: the International Classification of Impairments, Disabilities, and Handicaps (ICIDH)[1] and the functional limitations model or Nagi framework[2]. Using these two frameworks as a foundation, the Institute of Medicine proposed a new model in 1991.

The International Classification of Impairments, Disabilities, and Handicaps

The ICIDH was developed by the World Health Organization to organize information about the consequences of disease. In addition to defining disease, it includes three distinct classifications, impairment, disability, and handicap, each relating to a different level of response or consequence to disease. Because each level is distinct and independent of the other, a person can be impaired without being disabled and disabled without being handicapped.

- **Disease** is the underlying diagnosis and pathological process.

- An **impairment** is an abnormality of a psychological, physiological, or anatomical structure and function; it represents disturbance on the *organ* level.
- A **disability** is the consequences of impairment as it relates to individual functional performance and activity; it represents disturbance on the *person* level.
- A **handicap** refers to the disadvantages experienced by an individual that limit or prevent fulfillment of roles that are normal for the individual as a result of impairment or disability; it represents disturbance on the *societal* level.

Functional Limitations Model

The functional limitations framework consists of four concepts:[3]

- **Pathology** refers to the cellular and tissue alterations occurring from disease, trauma, infection, or congenital problems.
- **Impairment** is the specific abnormalities of physical, mental, and biochemical functioning.
- **Functional limitations** occur when there is a decrease in an individual's actual or potential performance.
- **Disability** occurs when conditions interfere with the performance of personal, social, and culturally expected roles.

Institute of Medicine Model

In 1991, a new model of disability was proposed by the Institute of Medicine that combined the ICIDH and Nagi framework. The term *handicap* was deleted, and to the Nagi framework was added *risk factors* and *quality of life* to create a new model of the disabling process.[4] The addition of these two dimensions are in line with current thinking about disability.

CONCEPTS OF REHABILITATION

Rehabilitation is a dynamic process through which a person is assisted to achieve optimal physical, emotional, psychological, social, and vocational potential and to maintain dignity, self-respect, and a quality of life that is as self-fulfilling and satisfying as possible. According to Brummel-Smith, the major goals of rehabilitation are improving function, promoting independence and life satisfaction, and preserving self-esteem.[5] To be effective, rehabilitation must be a philosophy of care and an integral part of health care delivery.

Rehabilitation refers to a continuum of functional restoration. In some situations, complete functional restoration is possible, as in the case of a patient who sustains a mild concussion. In this instance, complete recovery is the rule. However, when complete recovery of function is not possible and a permanent disability is likely, the patient must be helped to accept, adjust to, and compensate for the existing deficit and to establish an optimal level of function. For example, a paraplegic patient who sustained a severed spinal cord is expected to be permanently paralyzed. Present medical technology cannot restore the severed cord to its premorbid condition, although this may be possible sometime in the future. However, a comprehensive rehabilitation program helps the person live a useful, relatively independent life from a wheelchair.

Another aspect of rehabilitation addresses chronic health problems and degenerative diseases, such as multiple sclerosis. Although currently no cure exists for multiple sclerosis, a rehabilitation program can optimize quality of life through health promotion, symptom management, prevention of complications, and patient education to promote independence for the longest possible time. As the disease progresses, rehabilitation offers alternate ways of carrying out activities of daily living (ADLs) with adaptive devices and alternate methods of performing skilled acts.

A PHILOSOPHY OF REHABILITATION

A **philosophy** is a set of broad statements about fundamental beliefs and values. A philosophy of rehabilitation offers a framework to shape the overall rehabilitation process and often includes the following premises:

1. *A person with a disability has intrinsic worth that transcends the disability; each person is a unique holistic being who has the right and the responsibility to make informed personal choices regarding health and lifestyle.*[6] Restoring an individual's capacity to a level sufficient to resume roles such as homemaking, parenting, and gainful employment offer many social, emotional, psychological, and financial returns to society.

2. *Rehabilitation is an integral component of all care administered by all health care providers.* Rehabilitation begins the moment a person seeks health care so that prevention is incorporated into the rehabilitation process. A major goal in educating all health care providers is to prepare them to "think rehab" from the moment of initial contact with the patient.

3. *Comprehensive rehabilitation requires the active participation and collaboration of all health care providers through ongoing communication and management.* Scheduled team conferences, informal discussion, written plans of care, and progress notes provide a means of communication. Multidisciplinary collaboration and management mean that all health team members collaborate to achieve specific, identified, mutual goals.

4. *Rehabilitation requires the active participation of the patient to achieve optimal rehabilitative potential.* The patient must be motivated to be actively involved in the rehabilitation process.

5. *Rehabilitation actively involves the patient's family or significant others; they are the patient's potential support systems and assist with the transition back to the home and community.* Family members must be reached at their individual levels of understanding, considering their educational, socioeconomic, and cultural backgrounds to understand the rehabilitative goals and methods selected to meet these goals. The nurse usually interprets this information for the family, helping them to understand how they can best participate. In addition, the family is a rich source of information about the patient's personality and lifestyle that will be helpful in the transition back to the community.

6. *An individual patient and family evaluation is necessary to determine their ability to contribute to the rehabilitation process.* All families cannot contribute in the same way or to the same degree. Because each family and patient present different problems, individual evaluation is necessary.

7. *The patient experiences illness and disability within the context of her or his previous adjustment patterns.* The strengths and weaknesses of the patient's personality are essentially the same during illness. The team members must recognize the social and cultural influences that affect the patient's adjustment patterns and acceptance of care.

8. *Rehabilitation takes place within the context of the patient's whole life: the sociocultural aspects of life, his or her job or vocation, family, home, place in the community, religion, and relationship to self.* When illness strikes, family life is abruptly interrupted and altered. Illness affects not only the patient, but also the family. Therefore, rehabilitation should also include the needs of the family.

9. *Rehabilitation is a dynamic process with progress, plateaus, and setbacks.* Only through ongoing assessment and problem solving is achievement of patient goals possible.

10. *Transitions in care include plans for continued rehabilitation services. Options include acute or subacute inpatient rehabilitation, community re-entry, outpatient rehabilitation, or home health therapies.* The patient and family should be presented with various care alternatives and helped to evaluate the implications of each choice, including cost and health insurance issues. The patient and family should actively participate in the decision-making process of discharge planning to the degree that they are able and willing to participate for a relatively smooth transition and adjustment.

Terminology of Rehabilitation

The following terms are used consistently in rehabilitative health care:

- **Rehabilitative potential**—dormant power for rehabilitation within a person that exists as a possibility that can eventually become actualized
- **Short-term goals**—goals to be achieved in the immediate future (usually set for 1 week); discrete units or steps involved in the learning of a skill that must be achieved before more complex skilled acts can be accomplished; the steps through which long-term goals are achieved
- **Long-term goals**—goals projected for completion in the distant future; can be considered the ultimate objectives of a rehabilitation program
- **Optimal goals**—optimal rehabilitation goals that may be expected barring significant setbacks or complications
- **Realistic goals**—goals that reflect a realistic appraisal of the person and achievable outcome
- **Acute disability**—a disability that has a finite duration and is completely resolved in a short period of time; reversible; temporary
- **Chronic disability**—an ongoing disability that limits the person in some way; permanent; irreversible
- **Collaborative model of practice**—multidisciplines working collaboratively together to achieve measurable functional outcomes for people with disabilities
- **Multidisciplinary team rounds**—activity in which the various health team professionals visit the patient as a group to assess the person's current functional level, problems, and concerns; usually daily or weekly; provide data for further discussion at a team meeting or conference
- **Family meetings**—planned meetings with one or more health professionals and family members to discuss patient or family education; recognizes the importance of the family in the rehabilitation of the patient and helps to maintain open communication

Framework for Rehabilitation Decisions

Decisions related to rehabilitation are based primarily on information gathered during a screening examination. The goal is to determine the best possible match between the needs of the patient and capabilities of the rehabilitation programs in the community. In this complex health care environment, decisions regarding health care and expenditure of dollars are scrutinized. One of the key initial decisions regarding rehabilitation is if the person is a candidate who can benefit from rehabilitation. Figure 14-1 summarizes the process of reaching a rehabilitation decision. This information and figure are taken from the Agency for Health Care Policy and Research (AHCPR) clinical practice guidelines, *Post-Stroke Rehabilitation* (1995), but they are applicable to all initial and subsequent transitional rehabilitation decisions.[7]

Multidisciplinary Team

Several health care disciplines may participate in a multidisciplinary collaborative model of practice to provide a comprehensive rehabilitation program. The central focus of care is the patient and family, and each multidisciplinary team member works with the patient and family to achieve functional outcomes. Although all patients will not require the services of every discipline, they are available for consultation as necessary.

The rehabilitation process begins with a comprehensive functional assessment. The functional independence measure (FIM) is the most widely used standardized instrument to measure severity of disability based on a functional assessment.[8] The FIM assesses self-care, sphincter control, transfers, locomotion, communication, and social cognition. In addition, each health team member can further assess the patient using other instruments specific to the particular discipline.

Once a database has been collected, a comprehensive rehabilitation plan is developed with functional outcome measurements identified. Team conferences are one example of a formal communication mode. Informal communications between and among team members are ongoing. These reinforce collaboration among team members, promoting continuity of care and moving the plan forward. Because of the complexity of care and the numbers of people involved, it is easy for communication to break down. Therefore, planned, formal, patient-centered conferences are essential for the vitality of the process.

ASSESSMENT OF ACTIVITIES OF DAILY LIVING

ADLs are activities that must be accomplished independently for patients to assume responsibility for their own needs and to participate actively in society. Independence can be measured by the degree of responsibility assumed by the patient for these ADLs that are necessary for successful functioning at home, at work, and in social situations.

A variety of ADLs focus on different aspects of function:

- **Personal ADLs**: bathing, toileting, grooming, eating, performing oral hygiene, dressing, ambulating within the home, and communicating. The ability to perform these activities makes the person independent in self-care.
- **Instrumental ADLs**: using the telephone, shopping, using transportation to get around in the community, and walking distances outside the home. Independence in these activities makes the person independent in basic activities outside the home.
- **Occupational and role activities**: roles in the home, such as homemaking, parenting, and spousal roles and jobs outside the home. The skills necessary to assume any role or job are identified; the occupational therapist, family counselor, or vocational counselor can assist in assessing critical skills.

Helping the patient relearn ADLs begins with an assessment of the skills that are intact, those that are lost, and those that cannot be accomplished without some help. The major barriers to relearning ADL skills in the neurological patient are deficits affecting perception, motor activity, communication, vision, and cognitive functions.

The teaching plan is based on the individual needs of the patient and the principles of learning and teaching. For example, the occupational therapist can be helpful in making

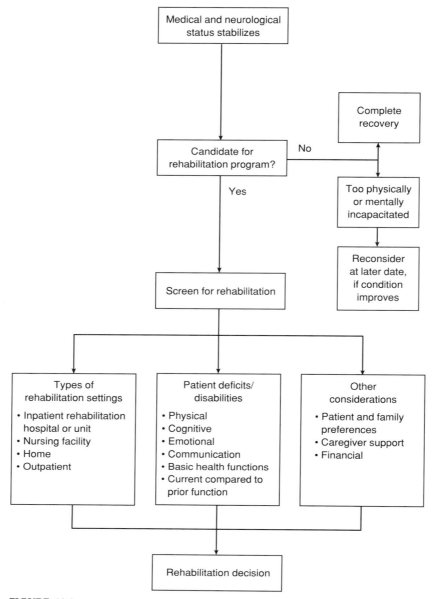

FIGURE 14-1
Framework for rehabilitation decisions. (Gresham, G. E., Duncan, P. W., Stason, W. B., et al. [1995] *Post-stroke rehabilitation*. Clinical practice guideline, No. 16. Rockville, MD: U.S. Department of Health and Human Services. Public Health Service, Agency for Health Care Policy and Research. AHCPR Publication No. 95-0662. May.)

suggestions for teaching the patient ADLs. If the patient is being seen by the occupational therapist on a regular basis, the nurse should coordinate nursing activities with those of the therapist so that the patient will not become confused.

Each activity to be relearned must be analyzed to identify the critical components involved in the overall task. Use of adaptive devices may be necessary to compensate for neurological deficits and to allow the patient to perform ADLs independently. For example, a spoon with a bulky stem may allow the patient with contractures of the hand to grasp the spoon, an act that could not be accomplished if the spoon were

of regular size or shape. Chart 14-1 details the principles of learning and teaching. The information in Chart 14-2 applies specifically to patients with cerebral injury.

PRINCIPLES OF REHABILITATION NURSING

The principles of rehabilitation are an integral component of independent nursing practice and include the major elements of **prevention, maintenance,** and **restoration**. Many nursing

CHART 14-1
Principles of Learning and Teaching

Patient and family education are important components of the rehabilitation process. Effective teaching rests on an understanding of the principles of learning and teaching as applied to the clinical setting.

The following basic principles can serve as a guide in teaching the patient:

- The objectives of the teaching session should be defined clearly; it is wise to write down behavioral objectives to identify the knowledge and skills the patient is expected to learn.
- The skills involved in the activity should be limited to small, critical units to facilitate learning.
- People learn best when they are able to perceive a need or value in the learning.
- Readiness to learn is important if patients are to benefit from the material presented; they must have sufficient physical and mental function to learn successfully.
- The patient should be rested and comfortable before the teaching session begins to enhance concentration.
- The nurse should demonstrate the skill and then have the patient perform the skill under supervision; if the skill is not performed correctly, it should be demonstrated again. The patient may need extensive supervision and opportunity for repetition to master the skill.
- The more senses involved in learning, the more apt the patient is to learn. (For example, the nurse can demonstrate the skill while telling the patient what is being done; gestures may also be used.)
- Reinforcement of learning should be followed through with consistency by all staff members working with the patient. Such reinforcement should be based on a written teaching plan.
- The patient's age, neurological deficits, educational background, fluency, and intelligence should be considered when individualizing a teaching plan that is appropriate for his or her needs.
- The patient should be given positive verbal feedback for accomplishments.
- The patient should be motivated to participate actively in the learning process.
- The patient and family should be encouraged to ask questions.

protocols and procedures contain elements of all three components. Preventive measures include special skin care, proper positioning and realignment, frequent turning, and range of motion exercises. The maintenance of intact skills and functions is supported by such activities as getting the patient out of bed to a chair and encouraging the patient to be as independent as possible in ADLs. Instituting exercise programs designed to increase range of motion, teaching ADLs to a patient with a paralyzed limb, and helping a patient relearn names of common objects are examples of restorative nursing activities. This framework can be kept in mind when planning and administering nursing care to address particular deficits.

A fundamental concept of rehabilitation is to do **with** the patient and not do **for** or **to** the patient. According to the American Nurses Association and the Association of Rehabilitation Nurses, the goal of rehabilitation nursing is to assist people with disability and chronic illness to attain maximum functional ability, maintain optimal health, and adapt to an altered lifestyle.[9] Rehabilitation nurses assist patients to identify goals that are realistic and attainable and consider the patient's continuing accountability for optimal wellness.[10] Once a skill has been mastered, a patient is expected to maintain it and build on that skill when possible. A patient is guided to do any part of a task even if he or she is unable to perform the complete activity. For example, the nurse may soap and squeeze a face cloth, but the patient may be able to wash one side of the face. This is a beginning, and it helps to develop the complete skill in the future. Unlike other aspects of nursing, rehabilitation is often a very slow process requiring continued dedication and effort. The long-lasting reward is that a human being has been helped to achieve maximal potential.

Rehabilitation is a collaborative process involving health professionals from various disciplines working together to achieve mutual goals. As the member of the rehabilitation team who spends the most time with the patient on a daily basis, the nurse provides continuity of care through coordination. The nurse can help coordinate and manipulate the patient's daily schedule so that optimal benefit will be derived from therapy. For example, the patient should be at a high energy level for the strenuous activity of mat work or ambulating in physical therapy. Scheduling these activities when the patient is tired is counterproductive to the goals of physical therapy. The nurse also assesses and address the patient's physical, emotional, and psychological responses to various therapeutic regimens.

The family often approaches the nurse with questions and concerns about the overall plan of care. In some instances, information and clarification is provided. In other instances, it may be necessary to refer questions to other team members or to initiate a family team meeting. Keeping the lines of communication open is a tedious and difficult job that is compounded by the large number of people involved in the patient's care. The nurse often becomes the clearinghouse for information, concerns, and confrontations.

Patient and family education is key to optimal recovery. Excellent community resources are available through a variety of agencies, such as the American Heart Association for stroke information. The patient and family need to be aware of these resources and need assistance in making contact.

CHART 14-2
Teaching the Patient With Cerebral Injury

Patients with cerebral injury present special problems in learning because of certain cognitive deficits, such as easy distractibility, short attention span, inability to think abstractly, memory deficits, poor judgment, and inability to transfer learning from one situation to another. An assessment to identify deficits and to develop an individualized teaching plan that reflects modifications designed to compensate for deficits is necessary. A few principles should be remembered when teaching such a patient:

- Be realistic in your expectations.
- Assume a calm and positive attitude toward the patient's ability to learn.
- Develop a written teaching plan for use by all nursing staff; be consistent.
- Plan short teaching sessions with specific goals.
- Choose a time when the patient is not tired.
- Use simple, specific instructions.
- Proceed systematically, in a step-by-step fashion.
- Motivate the patient.
- Facilitate learning by repetition and reinforcement.
- For the patient who is easily distracted, structure the environment to minimize distractions.
- Praise any accomplishment.
- Incorporate behavior modifiction principles.
- Tailor teaching methods to the patient's functional level (*e.g.*, may need visual aids and demonstration rather than explanation).

Nursing Management of Patients With Impaired Physical Mobility

ASSESSMENT

The nurse assesses mobility by conducting a motor function examination and reviewing the data from the FIM. Independence is closely correlated to a person's ability to move individual body parts or the body as a whole. Loss of mobility imposes severe constraints on the individual's freedom and independence.

Nursing management will depend on the nursing diagnosis. The following are possible nursing diagnoses:

- Impaired Physical Mobility
- Fatigue
- Risk for Injury (from falls)
- Risk for Altered Skin Integrity
- Activity Intolerance

The following are possible collaborative problems:

- Pathological fractures
- Joint dislocation

The major nursing diagnosis of **Impaired Physical Mobility** is applied to a patient experiencing limited physical movement in the environment, including bed mobility, transfers, and ambulating. When considering altered mobility, the nurse develops interventions directed at preventing edema of the extremities, skin breakdown, contractures, subluxation, deconditioning of muscles, pneumonia, and deep vein thrombosis.

Patients with concurrent cerebral injury and impaired physical mobility may not have sufficient cognitive ability to comprehend fully the extent and implications of their disability or the relationship of prescribed treatment to the maintenance, prevention, and restoration of functional loss. They will need direct supervision. They are at high risk for injury due to falls.

The nursing diagnoses of **Fatigue** and **Activity Intolerance** are related to bed rest reconditioning. Endurance for activity must be developed. As a rule, one day for every day in bed is necessary to build endurance; in elderly patients, it is longer. The nurse deals with these barriers to help the patient achieve an optimal level of independence.

Finally, the nurse has a role in the prevention of the possible collaborative problems listed previously.

INTERVENTIONS

As a member of the multidisciplinary team, the nurse works collaboratively with other team members to assist the patient to regain function. The philosophy of rehabilitation nursing is an integral part of care provided. The specifics of care depend on the patient's functional deficits and needs.

THE BASIS OF MOVEMENT AND TREATMENT OF MOVEMENT DISORDERS

Normal movement patterns originate in genetically programmed configurations of neurons. The maturation of the central nervous system follows a predetermined pattern of elaboration and refinement of movement. Reflex and voluntary control proceed in cephalic to caudal and proximal to distal directions. For example, voluntary head movement is learned before voluntary trunk movement. Most motor systems are modifiable within limits, thus providing the basis for developing acquired motor skills.

The maturation and concurrent development of movement and posture follow a deliberate pattern for learning of skilled acts. Mobility develops from synchronized coactivated flexor and extensor muscles that provide the stabilizing forces for posture. Hand and finger control develops from visually directed grasping and releasing of objects.[11] Understanding the development of movement patterns is the basis of treatment.

Neurophysiological and Developmental Treatment Approaches

There are five recognized rehabilitation treatment programs for people with motor control deficits related to cerebral injury: the Root approach; the Bobath neurodevelopmental approach; the Brunnstrom approach; the proprioceptive neuromuscular facilitation; and the Carr and Shepard approach of motor relearning. Because the Bobath neurodevelopmental approach is used by many nurses, it is discussed in more detail.

BOBATH NEURODEVELOPMENTAL TREATMENT APPROACH

The Bobath approach is used primarily for patients with hemiplegia caused by stroke, brain injury, and cerebral palsy. The major goal is normalization of muscle tone, posture, movement, and function. Underlying premises include the following[12-14]:

- The sensation of movement is learned and not the movement itself.
- Every skilled activity takes place against a backdrop of basic patterns of postural control, righting, equilibrium, and other protective reactions.
- When cerebral injury occurs, abnormal patterns of posture and movement develop that interfere with the performance of ADLs.
- The abnormal patterns develop because sensation is diverted into the abnormal patterns; this diversion must be stopped to reinstitute control over the motor output in developmental sequence.
- Eliciting the basic patterns of postural control, righting, and equilibrium is necessary, thus providing the normal stimuli while inhibiting abnormal patterns.
- People are allowed to feel, and thus relearn, normal movement patterns and postures.

Nurses can incorporate major principles of treatment into positioning, turning, transferring, and ADLs. These principles include the following[15]:

- Reintegration of function of the two sides of the body is emphasized during movement, ADLs, and bed or chair positioning so that bilateral segmental movement will occur.
- Proximal to distal positioning is recommended (tone in the limbs can be reduced from proximal points, such as the head, shoulder, or pelvic girdle).
- Weight bearing is provided on the affected side to normalize tone. This includes in sitting, lying, or rising.
- Tasks should begin from a symmetrical midline position with equal weight bearing on the affected and unaffected sides.
- Movement toward the affected side is encouraged.
- Straightening of the trunk and neck is encouraged to promote symmetry and normalization of tone and posture.

- Hemiplegic patients should be positioned in opposition to the spastic patterns of flexion and adduction in the upper extremity and extension in the lower extremity.

Positioning

Positioning the patient in proper body alignment is necessary to prevent the development of musculoskeletal deformities, such as contracture and ankylosis; skin breakdown and pressure ulcers; and decreased vascular supply, thrombosis, and edema.

Positioning of the neuroscience patient may be complicated by nuchal rigidity, spasticity, abnormal posturing (*e.g.,* decerebration), presence of a cast, position restriction secondary to surgery, and lacerations or abrasions associated with multiple trauma. These specific problems encountered in positioning change as the muscles undergo the various phases of recovery (Table 14-1).

A few basic principles are guides for positioning the patient in bed:

- The unconscious patient should be repositioned every 1 to 2 hours around the clock. As consciousness is regained, independent movement in bed and participation in self-care activities are encouraged to maintain muscle strength and tone. Proper positioning should be taught to the patient if he or she has the cognitive ability to participate.
- If spasticity is present, frequent repositioning will be necessary. Splinting and casting to inhibit tone may be applied by a physical therapist.
- Any restriction of position should be posted conspicuously at the head of the bed and included in the nursing care plan.
- A sufficient number of pillows should be available to maintain body alignment.
- Trochanter rolls, sand bags, and other positioning devices may be used.
- If an arm is weak or paralyzed, it should be positioned to approximate the joint space in the glenoid cavity. The affected arm should not be pulled. A pillow or small wedge in the axillary region will help prevent adduction of the shoulder.
- Special resting hand splints may be ordered to prevent contracture; they should be removed periodically to assess the skin for pressure areas.
- Edema of the extremities, particularly the hands, can be controlled by positioning and elevating the hand higher than the elbow.
- An elastic glove may be ordered to control hand edema.
- Prevention of footdrop is a concern in the lower extremities. Foot positioning devices, such as high-top sneakers or special splints, may be ordered.
- Heels should be kept off the bed to prevent pressure ulcers from developing. A pillow placed crosswise to elevate the lower legs may be helpful, or heel guards may be applied. (In many instances, the patient will be wearing elastic stockings and air boots.)

SIDE-LYING POSITION

An unconscious patient, or one with a diminished or absent swallowing or gag reflex, should not be positioned supine because the possible aspiration of secretions or occlusion of the

TABLE 14-1
Patterns of Muscle Recovery in Hemiplegia

STAGE	NAME	ONSET	DESCRIPTION
I	Flaccidity	From the time of injury to 2 or 3 d after	No tendon reflexes or resistance to passive movement
II	Spasticity (late onset of spasticity indicates a poor prognosis)	2 d to 5 wk	Hyperactive tendon reflexes and exaggerated response to minimal stimuli
III	Synergy (flexion, then extension)	2–3 wk	Simultaneous flexion of muscle groups in response to flexion of a single muscle (*e.g.,* an attempt to flex the elbow results in contraction of the fingers, elbow, and shoulder)
IV	Near normal, possible weakness or slight incoordination may still be present (late return of tendon reflexes indicates a poor prognosis)	1 wk to 6 mo	Control of voluntary movement; recovery occurs predictably from the proximal muscles of the extremity to the distal muscles (*i.e.,* voluntary movement of the hand and foot is last to recover and tends to be weaker)

airway by the tongue. Therefore, positioning in the true supine position is reserved only for the conscious patient. The side-lying position with the head of the bed elevated 10 to 30 degrees facilitates drainage of secretions from the mouth. The head should positioned in a neutral position. A soft collar or towel rolls can be used to maintain the neutral position and prevent hyperflexion, which would partially obstruct the airway and impede venous drainage from the brain. Proper body alignment is maintained through the use of pillows (Fig. 14-2).

With a patient for whom long-term bed rest is ordered, a modified position halfway between the supine and side-lying position may be necessary to relieve pressure on body surfaces. This patient can be positioned in good body alignment with the head turned slightly to facilitate drainage of oral secretions and to maintain a patent airway.

Exercise Programs

Voluntary muscles will lose tone and strength if they are not used. Patients with neurological deficits involving paresis and paralysis and those confined to prolonged bed rest are subject to these deleterious muscle effects of immobility (Table 14-2).

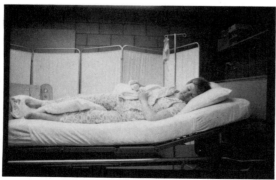

FIGURE 14-2
Positioning of the patient in side-lying position.

Because the flexor and adductor muscles are stronger than the extensors and abductors, contractures of the flexor and adductor muscles will develop quickly if preventive measures are not instituted. An exercise program must be followed aggressively to maintain muscle tone and function, prevent additional disability, and aid in the restoration of motor function.

Range-of-motion exercises include the full range of movement that each joint of the body can *normally* perform. A patient who cannot carry out independent range-of-motion exercises should be assisted in this activity by the nurse. Once radiographical studies have ruled out fractures and no other medical problems or medical treatments contraindicate movement of a particular body part, range-of-motion exercises should begin.

Exercises can be classified into the following categories:

- **Passive**—motion provided to a body joint by another person or outside force
- **Active**—voluntary motion to a body joint that is independently executed by the individual
- **Active assistive**—motion to a body joint accomplished by the patient with the assistance of another person
- **Active resistive**—motion voluntarily provided to a body joint against resistance
- **Isometric** or **muscle-setting**—exercises accomplished by alternately tightening and relaxing the muscle without joint movement

The exercise program prescribed will depend on the stage of illness and the particular disabilities. In the acute stages of illness, a physical therapist may come to the patient's bedside once or twice daily to administer specific exercises. If only range-of-motion exercises are prescribed, nurses will be the care provider administering these exercises. Once the patient's condition improves, he or she will be taken to the physical medicine department where equipment is available for a more sophisticated, aggressive rehabilitation program. The nurse can reinforce and integrate the skills into other aspects of care.

TABLE 14-2
The Effects of Prolonged Immobilization on the Musculoskeletal System

STRUCTURE	INITIAL CHANGES	ADVANCED CHANGES
Bones	Skeletal malalignment; calcium loss	Skeletal deformities Generalized osteoporosis
Joints	Joint stiffness; mobility limitation; shortening or stretching of ligaments	Ankylosis
Muscles	Muscle weakening; shortening or stretching of tendons	Muscle atrophy Fibrotic changes and muscle contractures

In addition, the patient's family can be taught how to carry out the prescribed exercises.

PASSIVE RANGE-OF-MOTION EXERCISES

When passive range-of-motion exercises are administered, two factors must be considered: the joint being exercised and the placement of the caregiver's hands when carrying out the exercise properly. One hand is placed above the joint to provide support against gravity and any unwanted movement. The other hand gently moves the joint through its normal range of motion.

Passive range-of-motion exercises are usually administered at least four times daily and may be incorporated, in part, with other procedures, such as bathing or repositioning.

- Choose a time when the patient is rested, comfortable, and pain-free to gain cooperation.
- Explain what is being done, even if the patient is apparently unconscious.
- Position in proper body alignment, and drape, as necessary, to avoid undue exposure. Drawing the curtains offers privacy and excludes environmental stimuli in the instance of an easily distracted patient.
- Provide a comfortable room temperature to prevent chilling, shivering, and unwanted muscle contractions.
- Maintain good posture to ensure efficient body movement; face the patient to observe facial reaction to the exercises.
- The movements of the exercise should be slow, smooth, and rhythmical.
  Move the body part to the point of resistance and stop.
  Move the body part to the point of pain and stop.
  If the patient becomes excessively fatigued, discontinue the exercises.

Although the physiotherapist may move a body part beyond the point of pain or resistance for selected patients, this is not within the scope of nursing practice and should be avoided unless specifically prescribed. As the patient's condition improves, self-care should be encouraged for as many activities as possible. Because return of motor function is a slow process, the patient should be encouraged to carry out the exercises and be reminded of the need to continue with these activities as part of the rehabilitation program.

OTHER EXERCISES

Specific exercises, such as lifting hand weights, may be ordered to strengthen a weakened arm. Encourage the patient to engage in these activities. Be sure that the necessary equipment is at hand. Adapt activities to provide movement for specific muscle groups. For example, providing a ball of yarn for a female patient who enjoys knitting can improve motor function of a weakened hand while providing sensory stimulation.

BALANCING AND SITTING ACTIVITIES

Once the patient's condition has stabilized and range-of-motion exercises have begun, the next skill is balancing and sitting. For patients who have been confined to bed for a long time, it will be necessary to progress slowly. The head of the bed must be raised gradually over days to overcome orthostatic hypotension. Monitor the physiological response by assessing the blood pressure and pulse, skin color and dryness, and asking the patient if he or she is experiencing dizziness or lightheadedness. Record baseline signs and symptoms. After the head of the bed is raised the prescribed number of degrees, again assess for a drop in blood pressure; a thready, rapid pulse; paleness; diaphoresis; dizziness; or lightheadedness. If these signs quickly reverse, no action may be necessary. Sustained symptoms require lowering the head of the bed slightly until symptoms subside. Because many neurological patients are placed at a 30-degree angle while confined to bed, much adjustment may not be necessary for them to tolerate the change to a vertical position. For those maintained in a flat position or at a 10-degree angle, the adjustment will take longer.

For paraplegic or quadriplegic patients, orthostatic hypotension can be a stubborn problem to manage, as extensive vasomotor paralysis results in a subsequent drop in blood pressure when the vertical position is assumed. An abdominal binder and thigh-high elastic stockings and elevating the leg rests of the wheelchair are helpful to combat hypotension. These patients, particularly quadriplegics, may require a special program in the physical therapy department in which a tilt table is used to raise the patient gradually over several days.

Balancing. **Balancing**, the ability to sit or stand erect, can be achieved through consciously using both sides of the body, focusing on the symmetrical midline point, and using support devices that help to steady the patient's center of gravity. The use of a back or neck brace for a cord injury patient can make the difference between success and failure. The hemiplegic patient should be helped to the sitting position and instructed to support himself or herself with the unaffected arm and hand. The hand should be placed flat on the bed slightly behind or at the side as a means of support. Because there is a tendency to slouch to the affected side, the patient should be reminded to sit straight and erect, focused on a balanced midline. Some conscious patients who have difficulty balancing while sitting in bed do well when they are helped to sit at the side of the bed or in a chair with their feet flat on the floor.

In unconscious patients, the same process for overcoming orthostatic hypotension can be used; however, information regarding the adjustment of these patients must be derived from objective signs. Ability to balance will not be possible until the level of consciousness improves; however, the patient can be propped to the required position.

Once balancing in the sitting position has been mastered, the patient is ready to begin balancing in the standing position at the bedside.

Sitting. Both the conscious and unconscious patient can sit in a chair, although the unconscious patient is not positioned in the sitting position on the side of the bed for obvious safety concerns. The conscious patient may sit on the side of the bed, using the overbed table and pillows for support. The chair selected should provide firm support and have a high back and arms, especially if the patient has motor weakness or paralysis. For the weak, debilitated patient who cannot hold up the head or neck, a high-back chair that extends to the top of the head is most effective. This patient often has a neck brace, which should be applied for sitting.

A lapboard, pillows, and the overbed table, rolled down to a comfortable height, are helpful for providing added support while positioning a patient in a chair. Pillows or rolls are used to support the arms in the desired position. The feet are positioned flat on the floor. The pressure on the bottom of the feet assists in stretching the heel cord. Footdrop may develop if stretching of the cord is not provided. The head must be positioned carefully so that the airway or tracheostomy is not obstructed. Any equipment that is in place, such as a urinary catheter or feeding tube, should be checked to ensure patency and freedom from traction.

If the patient has some independent motor function, necessary equipment is placed nearby, possibly on an overbed table that has been lowered and placed in front of the patient's chair. The call bell is placed close or attached to the patient's clothing if there are neurological deficits that could interfere with the ability to find the cord easily.

The patient is observed often and tolerance to being out of bed evaluated. The patient should not be allowed to become overtired. It is best to plan a schedule that allows for periods of bed rest and out-of-bed activity based on an individual assessment of the patient's tolerance and fatigue.

Mobility: Transfer and Ambulation

When considering a patient's mobility, the type(s) of transfer used reflect a continuum from complete dependency to complete independence:

- Two-person lift—physical transfer by at least two nursing staff members; no active patient participation
- Hoyer lift—transfer using a lifting device that is operated by nursing staff members; no active patient participation

Once the patient is able to balance and sit, he or she is ready for transfer activities:

- The patient stands and pivots with assistance from one or more nursing staff members and stands and pivots on the

unaffected leg; moderate patient participation is required. A leather belt worn around the patient's waist will allow the nurse to grasp the belt and support the patient.
- With the assistance of a slide board, the patient is able to transfer from the bed to the chair with or without assistance.
- Independent transfer is the patient's ability to transfer independently.

The degree of assistance necessary for transfer and ambulating can be classified as follows:

- Dependent—maximal, moderate, or minimal
- Contact guard—provision of verbal cues and minimal physical support during the activity, such as holding the arm or waist during ambulation
- Supervision—provision of verbal cues only, as necessary

TRANSFER ACTIVITIES

A few basic principles for assisting patients should be kept in mind:

- As a rule, transfer toward the unaffected side.
- Patients should wear well-fitting, sensible shoes rather than slippers, because most slippers offer little support and tend to slide on the floor.
- If a paretic arm is in need of support, it should be supported by gently holding the forearm. The nurse should never tug on the paretic arm by pulling on the upper arm or shoulder.
- If balance is unsteady, the nurse should stand on the affected side, ready to grasp a belt around the patient's waist (can grasp the top of pants of pajama bottoms, but not as secure). A belt is strongly recommended.
- If the patient's knees buckle and additional assistance is required, the nurse stands in front of the patient and pushes with his or her knee against the patient's unaffected knee to lock the knee in position and prevent it from buckling. This action enables the patient to bear some of his or her body weight.
- A walker or four-point cane may be used for support.
- The patient must learn to stand erect before ambulation training can begin. If difficulty is encountered in raising the affected foot, a special shoe with a plastic foot brace may be helpful.
- Other transfer activities that the patient may need to learn, depending on the permanence of the disability, include transferring from the wheelchair to the toilet, bathtub, or automobile.

TRANSFER ACTIVITY: FROM LYING IN BED TO A SITTING POSITION

Hemiplegic Patients. For the hemiplegic patient who wants to assume a sitting position from a position lying in bed on the back (Fig. 14-3), these steps are followed:

- Move toward or roll onto the side of the bed on which you intend to sit.
- Slip the unaffected leg under the affected leg at an angle so that the unaffected leg becomes a transfer cradle for the affected limb.

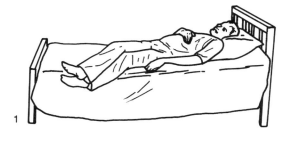

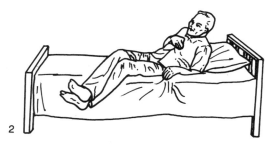

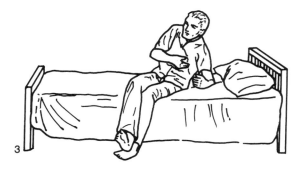

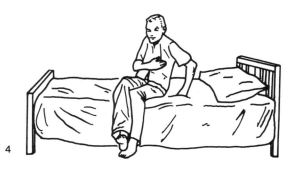

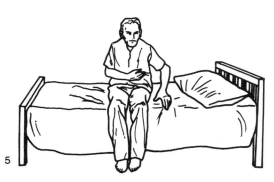

FIGURE 14-3
Getting up and sitting on side of the bed. *Clockwise:* (*1*) Use strong hand to place weak arm across abdomen. Slide strong foot under weak ankle; move both legs to side of the bed on strong side and over side. (*2*) Grasp edge of mattress as illustrated and push with elbow and forearm against the bed. (*3*) Come to a half-sitting position, supporting body weight on strong forearm. (*4*) Move hand to the rear, pushing up to a full sitting position. (*5*) Move around until sitting securely on side of bed; uncross legs. (*Up and Around.* Reprinted with permission of the American Heart Association.)

- Place the affected arm on the abdomen or lap.
- Push off the mattress with the unaffected elbow, raising your upper body, while turning your hips toward the side of the bed on which you intend to sit.
- Swing the unaffected leg (on which the affected leg rests) over the side of the bed, and use the unaffected hand to push up.
- Once in the sitting position, lean on the unaffected hand to maintain an erect position.

Paraplegic or Incomplete Quadriplegic Patients. Most transfer activities need to be done for quadriplegic and some incomplete quadriplegic patients. A trapeze over the bed and a sliding board can be used to assist paraplegic patients and some quadriparetic patients.

TRANSFER ACTIVITY: FROM SITTING ON THE SIDE OF THE BED TO A BACK-LYING POSITION

Returning to the back-lying position from a sitting position on the side of the bed involves the following steps (Fig. 14-4):

- Sit slightly above the center on the side of the bed so that you will be in the proper position on the mattress once the back-lying position is assumed.
- Place the affected arm on your lap.
- Slip the unaffected foot under the affected ankle.
- Place the unaffected hand on the edge of the mattress near the unaffected hip.
- Press the hand into the mattress, lowering your body onto the bed while the elbow bends.

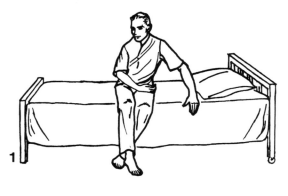

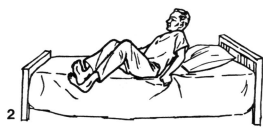

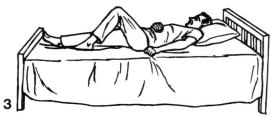

FIGURE 14-4
Moving from a sitting position on edge of bed to a back-lying position. (*1*) Place weak arm across the lap. Slide strong foot under weak ankle. (*2*) With strong hand, grasp edge of mattress near the hips and press against bed, lowering body to the bed as the elbow bends. At the same time, swing legs onto bed. (Note: Patient should be seated in the proper spot so that head will be on pillow after lying down.) (*3*) Uncross legs. Bend the strong hip and knee and push against bed with heel to move body up or down in bed to proper position. (*Up and Around.* Reprinted with permission of the American Heart Association)

- Simultaneously swing the unaffected leg onto the bed as your body is lowered.
- Uncross the ankle and bend the unaffected knee; push up or pull down on the bed, as necessary, with the bending and pulling action of the knee to position yourself comfortably.

TRANSFER ACTIVITY: FROM A SITTING POSITION ON THE BED TO A CHAIR

Transferring from the bed into a chair requires planning. If a chair is used, it should provide firm support and have arms. In the case of a wheelchair, the wheels of the chair should be locked with the footrests up.

Hemiplegic Patients. Hemiplegic patients may complete this type of transfer by following these steps (Fig. 14-5):

- Free any catheter or tubes secured to the bed.
- Place the chair at a slight angle as close as possible to the bed on the unaffected side.
- With feet close together, lean forward slightly, put the unaffected hand on the mattress edge, and push off to a standing position, bearing weight on the unaffected side.
- Once balance has been maintained and is steady enough for momentary release of support, move the strong hand to the farthest armrest of the chair.
- Keep the body weight well forward; pivot on the unaffected foot, and slowly lower to a sitting position.

Paraplegic or Incomplete Quadriplegic Patients. The paraplegic or quadriplegic patient will need a dependent slide board transfer, which is less strain on the back than a lift into the chair; the aid of two or three people will be needed, depending on the patient's height and weight. Some paraplegic patients can learn to transfer themselves from the bed to a chair with the use of a slide board.

TRANSFER ACTIVITY: FROM CHAIR TO BED

When transferring from a chair to a sitting position on the bed, the following technique is used (Fig. 14-6):

- The chair should be at a slight angle, as close to the bed as possible; the unaffected side should be closest to the bed.
- Place feet firmly on the floor close to the chair, with the unaffected heel slightly in back and directly under the edge of the seat.
- Move forward in the chair, placing the unaffected hand on the front portion of the arm of the chair.
- Leaning forward over the unaffected leg; push off to a standing position so that the feet are slightly apart with most of the weight being borne by the unaffected leg.
- After regaining balance with the support of the armrest, lean slightly forward, reach for the edge of the mattress with the unaffected hand, and pivot on the unaffected foot, slowly lowering to a sitting position.

AMBULATION

Hemiplegic Patients. Before hemiplegic patients can ambulate, they must first learn to stand and balance themselves in an upright position. Standing exercises can begin at the bedside and proceed to the parallel bars in the physical therapy department. Standing helps to reinforce a positive body image and a feeling of wholeness and improves overall physical fitness.

Once standing has been mastered, an evaluation is conducted to determine if any special bracing or support equipment is necessary. If the patient is developing footdrop or has a tendency to drag the foot, a short leg plastic brace or a brace with a spring in it can be helpful. These types of braces are designed to prevent extreme plantar flexion. If the patient is weak, a crutch, four-point cane, or walker may be necessary (Fig. 14-7). A sling may be applied to the affected arm for balance only while walking. The sling should be adjusted to approximate the glenoid (shoulder) joint space. The affected arm should not be pulled.

Ambulation or gait training often begins at the parallel bars, where the patient learns to bend a knee and then extend it again.

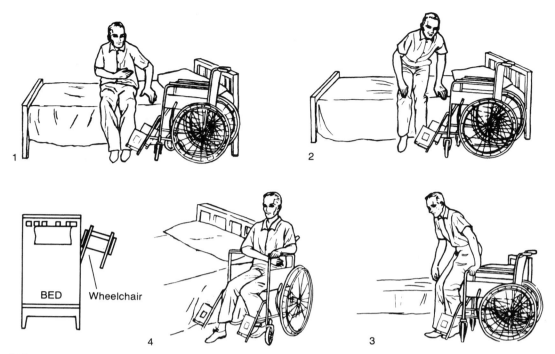

FIGURE 14-5
Doing a standing transfer from bed to wheelchair. *Clockwise:* (*1*) Place wheelchair at 45° angle to bed on patient's stronger side; lock brakes and raise footrest; move to the edge of bed. (*2*) Push down on bed with stronger arm; push off bed and stand, keeping weight on the stronger leg. (*3*) Move stronger arm and leg to opposite side of wheelchair. (*4*) Lean forward and sit down while holding on to wheelchair arm. (*Up and Around.* Reprinted with permission of the American Heart Association.)

This exercise is alternated from one knee to the other. If the affected knee continues to be weak and tends to buckle, a longer leg brace can be designed to compensate for this disability.

When helping the patient to ambulate, the nurse should walk on the patient's affected side. Added support may be given by grasping the patient's belt or the top of the patient's pants or by applying a safety belt. The patient may feel more secure walking near the wall with the unaffected side nearest the wall. A handrail in the corridor or room is another source of support and security. In the physical therapy department, climbing and descending stairs are taught.

For the patient who is unable to master ambulation, wheelchair mobility may be achieved using the unaffected hand to propel the wheelchair on a level surface. This provides a degree of independence. An electric (battery-operated) wheelchair is another alternative for providing mobility.

It is impossible to state the exact intervals when balancing, sitting, standing, and walking should be introduced and mastered. Age, severity of illness, other neurological deficits, chronic conditions, endurance, and complications are all factors. Attitude and motivation are important factors in the rehabilitation process. Frequent assessment allows systematic evaluation of the patient's needs so that rehabilitation can progress steadily toward the greatest level of independence.

Paraplegic or Incomplete Quadriplegic Patients. The physiological and psychological benefits of ambulation need to be considered. Research has contributed greatly to ambulation options for spinal injured people. Some paraplegic and a few quadriparetic patients can walk with the help of braces and canes. For others, ambulation is possible using functional electrical stimulation and a walker.

For a person who needs a wheelchair, many different types are available that need to be matched to the needs of the particular patient. Battery-operated wheelchairs that are activated by a breath sensor located near the mouth of the quadriplegic patient provide a degree of independence. Even a quadriplegic patient with an injury at C-5 can use this type of wheelchair. Incomplete quadriplegics with a C-2 to C-5 injury can use chin, eye, or tongue control systems. The paraplegic patient does well in a standard wheelchair or an electric wheelchair operated by hand controls.

Computer-operated equipment programmed to execute many mundane activities, such as closing draperies or turning out lights, has afforded a greater degree of independence to the disabled person. Computer technology for adaptive living is developing rapidly. As the technology improves, the cost decreases, making the equipment more accessible for the patient.

MANAGEMENT OF THE SKIN

The neuroscience patient is at high risk for the development of pressure ulcers because of motor, sensory, and vasomotor deficits related to neurological disease and immobility. According to the AHCPR clinical practice guideline, *Pressure Ulcers in Adults: Prediction and Prevention* (1992), a **pressure ulcer**

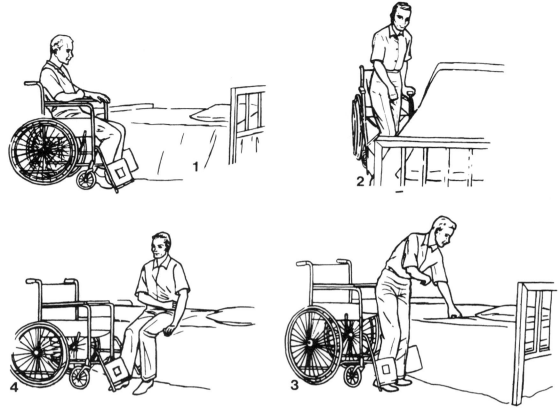

FIGURE 14-6
Moving from wheelchair to bed. *Clockwise:* (*1*) Place wheelchair at 45° angle to the bed on the patient's stronger side; lock brakes and raise footrest; move to edge of chair. (*2*) Grasp chair arm with stronger arm and push off the chair to a standing position bearing weight on stronger leg. (*3*) Move strong hand to edge of bed for support. (*4*) Lean forward, pivot on stronger foot, and slowly sit down. (*Up and Around.* Reprinted with permission of the American Heart Association).

is any lesion caused by unrelieved pressure resulting in damage of underlying tissue.[16]

Nursing Management of the Patient With Altered Skin Integrity

ASSESSMENT

Pressure ulcers are usually over bony prominences and are graded or staged to classify the degree of tissue damage observed. **Impaired Skin Integrity** related to immobility or the effects of pressure, friction, shearing, or maceration is the nursing diagnosis.

The AHCPR Pressure Ulcers Guideline (1992) is the standard of practice for prediction, prevention, and early treatment of pressure ulcers in adults. It also cites supporting research evidence for each recommendation. This publication sets the standard of practice to which all nurses are held, and this is the standard of care for neuroscience patients.

INTERVENTIONS

Follow the AHCPR guidelines mentioned previously.

SENSORY-PERCEPTUAL DEFICITS

Perception is a complex intellectual process of recognizing, interpreting, and integrating sensory stimuli into meaningful information from the internal and external environments. Whereas the left side of the brain is dominant for language, the right side of the brain is dominant for perception of two- and three-dimensional shapes, faces, color, spatial positions, and orientation in space. The parietal lobe is particularly important in perception. Perceptual deficits are often seen in patients with head injury and stroke and may take many forms, including deficits in perception of self, body image, illness, spatial relationships, agnosia, and apraxia.

Nursing Management of Patients With Perceptual Deficits

ASSESSMENT

The major perceptual deficits are summarized in Table 14-3. A number of nursing diagnoses are applicable; the following are possible nursing diagnoses:

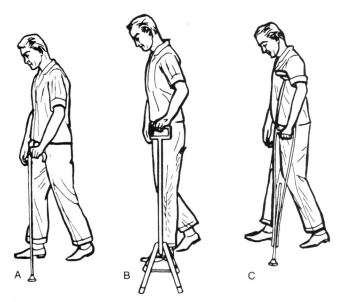

FIGURE 14-7
Assistive devices, such as a cane (*A*), a wide-base cane (*B*), or crutches (*C*), may be necessary for ambulation. (*Up and Around.* Reprinted with permission of the American Heart Association.)

- Sensory/Perceptual Alterations
- Body Image Disturbance
- Impaired Environmental Interpretation Syndrome
- Impaired Memory
- Self Esteem Disturbance
- Risk for Injury
- Confusion
- Personal Identity Disturbance

A possible collaborative problem may be neglect syndrome.

Interventions. Nursing interventions are directed at helping the patient to compensate for any deficits. Patients with perceptual deficits are impulsive and often lack of awareness of their deficits. This behavior also places a patient at high risk for injury.

COMMUNICATION DEFICITS

Aphasia is the loss of ability to use language and to communicate thoughts verbally or in writing. It is the result of injury to the cortex of the left hemisphere in the posterior frontal or anterior temporal lobes. Aphasia can be subdivided into non-fluent and fluent aphasia. The nursing diagnosis for a patient with aphasia is Impaired Verbal Communication. Chart 14-3 summarizes aphasia and the nursing guidelines for working with affected patients. See Chapter 7 for further discussion of aphasia.

Generally, the greatest degree of spontaneous functional return occurs in the first 3 to 6 months following injury, although substantial deficits may persist. Additional improvement can occur for 2 or 3 more years. Each patient must be

viewed as an individual in the rehabilitative process. Age, area of injury, presence of other health problems, and motivation are a few factors having a direct bearing on recovery.

Nursing Management of Patients With Altered Communication
ASSESSMENT

The nurse will need to assess the patient's communication system to determine which skills are intact or deficient. Assess the following abilities:

- Speak in response to an open-ended question, such as "Tell me about your hobbies"
- Use vocabulary, grammar, and syntax correctly; spontaneity, hesitancy in pronunciation, and speed of speech
- Respond appropriately to verbal instructions that are one to three steps in complexity
- Respond appropriately to written instructions that are one to three steps in complexity
- Express ideas in writing; write a response to such requests as "Write your name" or "Describe this room"

Note difficulty in expressing thoughts verbally, finding the correct word (word finding), forming words or sentences, following written instructions, and expressing ideas in writing. Other abnormal findings include slurring of speech. As a result of stroke, some patients may be unable to speak the primary language that they had been using and revert to language spoken in the past.

Several factors associated with neurological illness can mask an accurate assessment of communication skills, such as the following:

- Altered level of consciousness
- Decreased visual acuity
- Hearing loss
- Dysarthria
- Cognitive deficits (decreased attention or concentration) or short-term memory deficits
- Visual field cuts (hemianopsia)
- Absence of prescribed lenses
- Absence of hearing aid normally worn
- Unfamiliarity with the language

A short attention span or inability to concentrate influences the ability to follow verbal or nonverbal cues. Because concentration and attention seem to vary from day to day or even minute to minute, there can be great differences in the patient's ability to communicate at any time.

The following are possible nursing diagnoses (no particular collaborative problem is noted):

- Sensory/Perceptual Alterations
- Impaired Verbal Communication
- Impaired Memory

TABLE 14-3
Summary of Major Perceptual Deficits and Nursing Management

DEFICIT	ASSESSMENT	INTERVENTION
PERCEPTION OF ILLNESS • Denial of hemiplegia or other motor or sensory deficits • *Anosognosia*—the inability to recognize, denial of, or unawareness of a loss of or defect in physical function	• Fails to use the involved side of the body without being reminded to do so • Shows a lack of concern about the disability and fails to understand how the paralysis and other deficits will affect lifestyle • Lacks awareness or denies outright the presence of paralysis or other deficits on the involved side • May deny all sensory input on the affected side	• Accept the patient's perception of self, and provide for the safety and cleanliness of the area. • Provide tactile stimuli to the affected side by touching or stroking the affected side by itself, rather than stimulating both sides simultaneously. • Teach the patient to position the affected extremity carefully and to check its position by looking at it; if the patient completely ignores the area, use positioning to improve his or her perception (*e.g.,* position the patient facing the affected side so that the area is in view).
BODY IMAGE • *Body image*—the concept one has of the sum of one's body parts in relationship to the whole —Nursing diagnosis: Body Image Disturbance • *Unilateral neglect*—a condition in which the patient ignores the hemiplegic side —Nursing diagnosis: Unilateral Neglect	• If asked to draw a clock, will not draw the side of the clock on which neglect is present	• Encourage the patient to handle the affected side. * Teach visual scanning of the environment to overcome one-sided neglect. * Approach the patient from the unaffected side until ready to learn compensatory scanning techniques. * Place the food tray toward the unaffected side. * Use verbal cues to guide the patient toward the affected side. * Provide a mirror, if possible. * Position the call light and other equipment on the patient's unaffected side.
SPATIAL RELATIONSHIPS • *Hemianopia*—the loss of vision in half of the visual field. —Nursing diagnosis: Sensory/Perceptual Alterations	• Neglects input from the affected side	• See last six interventions listed above (asterisks). • *Note* visual changes commonly present and change about every 6 months. No ophthalmological check-up is necessary until 6 months have transpired.
• Defects in: —Localized objects in space —Estimating size —Judging distances —Remembering arrangement of objects in the environment —Finding way to places or back to room —Telling time —Right–left discrimination	• Has difficulty walking through a doorway • Exhibits impaired recall of the placement of objects in a familiar environment, such as the locations of windows and doors in the room • Has difficulty learning the way around the hospital unit (such as how to go from the hospital room to the kitchen and back) • Experiences difficulty reading and computing figures because of an inability to move eyes from left to right on a page or to line up numbers accurately to compute figures • Is unable to identify left or right	• Provide verbal cues. • Do not allow the patient to wander around the unit alone. • Use descriptive terms to identify areas, rather than "left" or "right" directions (*e.g.,* "Lift the unaffected leg" but not "good/bad"). • Use a mirror to help patients adjust position if they have difficulty maintaining their position.

(continued)

TABLE 14-3
Summary of Major Perceptual Deficits and Nursing Management Continued

DEFICIT	ASSESSMENT	INTERVENTION
AGNOSIA		
• Inability to recognize familiar environmental objects through the senses —Visual agnosia: inability to recognize familiar objects by sight (Nursing diagnosis: Sensory/Perceptual Alterations) —Auditory agnosia: inability to recognize familiar objects through sound (Nursing diagnosis: Sensory/Perceptual Alterations) —Tactile agnosia (astereognosis): inability to recognize familiar objects through the sense of touch (Nursing diagnosis: Sensory/Perceptual Alterations)	• Ask patient to identify common objects by sight. • Observe the patient's response to common sounds, such as a ringing telephone. • With the patient's eye closed, place a common object in his or her hand, and ask the patient to identify the object.	• Use other, intact senses to identify environmental stimuli (*e.g.,* if the patient has visual agnosia, have him or her use voices and sounds to identify familiar objects). • Use the drill method of teaching to help the patient relearn objects that cannot be identified. • Protect the patient from injury • Interpret the patient's behavior for the family.
APRAXIA		
• Inability to carry out a learned, voluntary act in the absence of paralysis —Constructional apraxia (Nursing diagnosis: Self-Care Deficit) —Dressing apraxia (Nursing diagnosis: Dressing Self-Care Deficit)	• May exhibit clumsiness or an inability to carry out activities of daily living (ADLs) correctly; may be unable to sequence components of a skilled act • May have difficulty completing the task of drawing a clock and placing the hands at a given time • May have difficulty dressing self (*e.g.,* may put both arms in the same sleeve)	• Encourage the patient to participate in ADLs. • Correct any misuse of equipment or incorrect actions; guide the patient's hand, if necessary. • Reteach any forgotten skills. • Protect the patient from injury. • Interpret the patient's behavior for the family.

Interventions. To work effectively with the patient, the nurse should assume a calm, reassuring, and supportive manner that conveys acceptance of the patient's behavior. Spending time and assuming an unhurried approach reinforce this message. Guidelines for working with the aphasic patient are included in Chart 14-3. Deficits in the ability to communicate are devastating and frustrating to the patient and may result in fear and depression.

SWALLOWING DEFICITS

Swallowing is a complex process of ingesting food of a solid or liquid consistency while protecting the airway (Fig. 14-8). Glenn cites four phases of swallowing[17]:

• **Oral preparatory phase:** Food is taken into the mouth and chewed, forming a bolus.
• **Oral phase:** The bolus of food is centered and moved to the posterior oropharynx.
• **Pharyngeal phase:** The swallowing reflex carries the bolus through the pharynx.
• **Esophageal phase:** Peristalsis carries the bolus to the stomach

A number of cranial nerves are involved in functions related to swallowing:

CRANIAL NERVE	MOTOR INNERVATION	SENSORY INNERVATION
Trigeminal (V)	Mandibular muscles for chewing and mastication	Two sensory areas of face (maxillary, mandibular)
Facial (VII)	Facial expression, including movement of lips; submandibular and sublingual salivary glands	Taste to anterior two-thirds of tongue
Glossopharyngeal (IX)	Stylopharyngeus muscle to pull up pharynx	Pharynx, tongue, and taste receptors of posterior one-third of tongue
Vagus (X)	Muscles of soft palate, pharynx, and larynx	Pharynx and larynx
Spinal accessory (XI)	Sternocleidomastoid and trapezius to hold head up and rotate head	None
Hypoglossal (XII)	Intrinsic muscle of tongue to move tongue	None

Regardless of whether the food is liquid or solid, protection of the airway is imperative to prevent the most serious of complications—aspiration. Aspiration is serious

CHART 14-3
Deficits In Communications: Descriptions and Nursing Guidelines

Nonfluent Aphasia (Broca's Aphasia)

- The patient will have difficulty expressing thoughts verbally or in writing.
- The degree of difficulty can range from mild word finding difficulty to limitation of expression to "yes" and "no."
- The ability to understand the written and spoken word remains intact.
- The site of injury is Broca's area (in the frontal lobe close to the area of the motor cortex and controls the movement of the lips, jaw, tongue, soft palate, and vocal cords).
- Broca's area contains the memory for motor patterns of speech.

Fluent Aphasia (Wernicke's Aphasia)

- Wernicke's area (in the temporal lobe flanked by Heschl's gyrus on one side and the angular gyrus on the other) is the site of injury.
- Heschl's gyrus is the primary receptor area for auditory and visual fields.
- Wernicke's area provides the connective pathways that bridge the primary auditory cortex and the angular gyrus.
- The patient hears the sounds of speech, but the parts of the brain that give meaning to the sounds of speech are not activated, so that comprehension of speech is impaired.
- Because the control of the musculature for speech is not impaired, the patient can speak but makes many errors when using words.
- Because patients are unaware of their imperfect messages, they may talk at great length.
- The patient's ability to express words in writing may also be compromised.

Mild Nonfluent Aphasia

- Stimulate conversation and ask open-ended questions.
- Allow patients time to search for the words to express themselves.
- Disregard choice of incorrect words.
- Be supportive and accepting of the patient's behavior as he or she deals with the frustration of finding the right words of expression.
- Assure patients that their speech will gradually improve with time.

Severe Nonfluent Aphasia

- Accept self-expression by whatever means possible (e.g., pantomime, pointing).
- Do not pressure the patient into self-expression.
- Be supportive of patients, and accept their behavior if they show frustration (by crying or some other means) because of difficulty encountered in expressing themselves.
- Provide a loose-leaf book with pictures of common objects so that the patient can point to the picture when unable to say the word.
- Tell the patient that speech skills can be relearned, given time.
- Anticipate the patient's needs.

Mild Fluent Aphasia

- Stand close to patients (within their line of vision) so that they can also observe lip movements as an added cue to communication.
- Speak slowly and distinctly, using simple sentences and a common vocabulary.
- Use simple gestures as an added cue in speaking.
- Repeat or rephrase any instructions if they are not understood.
- Speak in a normal speaking voice.

Severe Fluent Aphasia

- Use whatever vocabulary the patient can still understand.
- Use very simple sentences or phrases that express only the critical essence of a thought.
- Divide any tasks into small units, working with the individual units to accomplish the task.
- Use pantomime, pointing, touch, and so forth to express ideas.
- Anticipate the patient's needs.

(continued)

CHART 14-3 Deficits In Communications: Descriptions and Nursing Guidelines (Continued)

Global Aphasia

- Results from a massive stroke or lesion involving Broca's and Wernicke's areas of the brain.
- Global aphasia is a combination of expressive and receptive aphasia whereby the patient is left with little, if any, intact communication system.
- Affected patients can neither understand what they hear or read nor convey their thoughts in speech or writing.
- The prognosis is poor.

---

because it causes a chemical pneumonia. When thinking about aspiration, a picture of someone coughing vigorously comes to mind. This is the case if the gag and cough reflex are intact. However, there is much discussion about "silent aspiration." A person with a diminished or absent gag and cough reflex can aspirate material without the usual evidence of coughing. In a conscious patient, a moist, wet voice may be noted. Usual symptoms of aspiration are absent. Silent aspiration may first be evident by an elevated temperature or adventitious lung sounds followed by a diagnosis of pneumonia by chest film.

With neurological disease, there can be deficits in the mechanisms controlling swallowing, and aspiration can result. The nursing diagnoses associated with swallowing deficits are Impaired Swallowing and Risk for Aspiration.

Nursing Management of the Patient With Impaired Swallowing

ASSESSMENT

Swallowing is a complex process (see Fig. 14-8 for normal swallowing). The defining characteristics for impaired swallowing, according to the North American Nursing Diagnosis Association,[18] are also related to the specific phases of swallowing listed previously:

PHASES OF SWALLOWING	CHARACTERISTIC OBSERVATIONS; ALSO OBSERVE FOR EVIDENCE OF ASPIRATION
Oral phase	Drooling or food particles on affected or side of chin
	Pocketing of food
	Excessive chewing
	Facial asymmetry or weakness
	Tongue weakness or limitation of movement
	Inability to close lips tightly or move lips
	Weakness or absence of gag reflex
	Weakness or absence of swallowing reflex
	Nasal drainage due to nasal regurgitation
	Loss of internal or external sensation of the oral cavity or face
Pharyngeal phase	Noted delayed or absence of swallowing
	Coughing while drinking fluids or eating liquids (*e.g.,* soup)
	History of aspiration pneumonia
	Wet, gurgling, moist, or nasal voice, particularly during eating
	Frequent clearing of throat
	Complaints of burning (from drugs or other irritating material sticking and irritating tissue) or something sticking in back of throat
Esophageal phase	Burping or substernal distress due to esophageal reflux
	Coughing or wheezing

Before offering any food or drink orally, the gag and swallowing reflexes are assessed. The gag reflex on each side should be assessed, because an asymmetrical response is possible. The swallowing reflex can be assessed by placing the examiner's index finger on the top of the larynx and asking the patient to swallow. If the reflex is intact, the larynx will elevate (the epiglottis closes over the trachea), displacing the examiner's finger. If the gag or swallowing reflex is not intact, *nothing should be given orally* because the patient cannot protect the airway and will aspirate. Diagnostic tests may be ordered to identify the specific etiology of the dysphasia. Common diagnostic tests include the bedside swallow examination, modified barium swallow with video-fluoroscopy, and video-endoscopy. A review of the video film will help to identify the specific portion of the sequence of swallowing that is problematic.

The following are major nursing diagnoses:

- Impaired Swallowing
- Risk for Aspiration

A possible collaborative problem is aspiration pneumonia.

Interventions. Supervise the patient during mealtime and snack time. There are some general interventions to facilitate swallowing. Specific suggestions, based on specific patient needs, may also be made. Consider these general points:

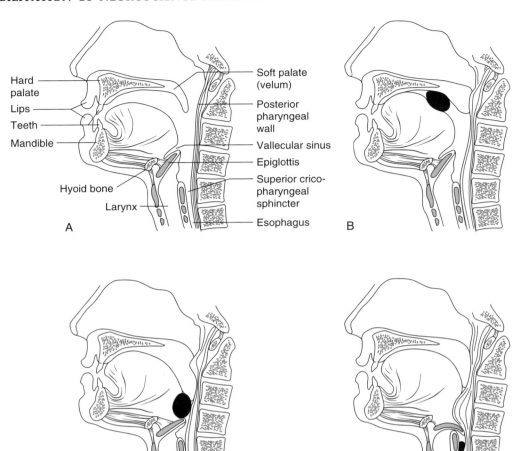

FIGURE 14-8
Swallowing process.

- Feed or eat in the upright, sitting position at a 90-degree angle; avoid slumping.
- The head should be tilted forward and the chin tucked in to prevent food moving to the posterior oropharynx before it has been chewed; if the patient is unable to maintain the head position, the nurse can support the head with the palm of the hand against the forehead.
- Encourage small bites and thorough chewing.
- For patients with hemiplegia or hemiparesis, place food on the unaffected side.
- The nurse should note consistency of food that is troublesome. (Some people have more difficulty with solid foods and others will have more difficulty with liquids.)
- If "pocketing" of food is a problem, have the patient sweep the mouth with his or her finger after each bite to clear the food.
- The speech therapist can be helpful by suggesting an adaptive cup and special techniques to ensure swallowing.
- Discuss with the physician any persistent problems. If oral feeding is contraindicated, a feeding tube or gastrostomy tube can be considered (see Chap. 9).

- If cognitive deficits are present, the patient may have poor impulse control and may stuff the mouth hurriedly with food. If this occurs, the basis of the swallowing problem may be behavioral rather than neurological, and nursing interventions should be directed at managing the behavior and controlling distractions from the focus of eating. This patient requires mealtime supervision and verbal and nonverbal cues.

BLADDER DYSFUNCTION AND RETRAINING

Normal Bladder Function

Bladder control is an integrated function of the brain stem, spinal, and cerebral levels[19] (see Chap. 5).

- **Brain stem pontine level**. The true micturition centers are located the dorsal pons. During micturition, the medial pontine region is activated, and the lateral pontine region is inhibited. This activity produces coordinated bladder contraction and sphincter relaxation, resulting in bladder emptying. Disruption in the central nervous system *above* the sacral reflex center usually causes a hyperreflexic bladder and is classified as an upper motor neuron injury.

- **Spinal level.** The *sacral reflex control center* of the bladder is located in spinal segments S-2 to S-4. The parasympathetic innervation of the pelvic nerve is responsible for bladder emptying, while the sympathetic (hypogastric nerve) and somatic (pudendal nerve) innervations promote retention of urine. Micturition involves a supraspinal-spinopontospinal reflex triggered by stimulation of tension receptors, which result in coordination of the contracted detrusor muscle and relaxation of the sphincter. Interruption of the descending suprasegmental pathways results in micturition through segmental spinospinal sacral reflexes that are triggered by perineal or nociceptive stimulation. The sphincter contractions are not well coordinated. Disruption at the sacral reflex center or in the peripheral nervous system causes an areflexic bladder, which is classified as a lower motor neuron injury.
- **Cerebral level.** The micturition centers are controlled by input from the hypothalamus and the medial frontal cortex. Cortical input is responsible for voluntary control of the initiation and cessation of micturition. Lesions of the medial frontal lobes or hypothalamus can interrupt these pathways, resulting in involuntary micturition sometimes called **uninhibited bladder**.

SUMMARY OF EFFECTS OF NEUROLOGICAL LESIONS ON MICTURITION

People with neurological disease or injury may be unable to maintain normal urinary elimination patterns because of dysfunction at the brain stem, spinal, or cerebral levels. Any disruption of the sensory or motor pathways in the central or peripheral nervous systems that have input to the bladder will cause a disruption in urinary elimination patterns.

Types of Bladder Dysfunction: Alterations in Urinary Elimination Patterns

There are many conceptual frameworks regarding altered urinary elimination, including upper motor neuron and lower motor neuron injury and a classification of neurogenic bladder types. (A **neurogenic bladder** is defined as any bladder disturbance that is attributable to motor or sensory pathways in the central or peripheral nervous systems that have input to the bladder. See Table 14-4 for a listing of neurogenic bladder types.) From a nursing perspective, nurses focus on assisting people to improve function through a functional health pattern framework; this is the approach taken in this chapter.

Alterations in urinary elimination patterns can be classified generally into urinary incontinence (UI) and urinary retention. Each of these two major classifications can be further subdivided into categories based on cause, characteristics, and pathophysiology. It is important to be able to categorize accurately the type of altered urinary elimination pattern present to treat the problem effectively. The following sections discuss UI and urinary retention with emphasis on altered function in neurological patients.

Urinary Incontinence

UI can be associated with various problems, such as a diminished level of consciousness; cerebral injury, especially to the frontal lobe; or spinal cord injury. The Clinical Practice Guidelines for *Urinary Incontinence in Adults*, published in 1992, is the definitive resource for health professionals in the management of adult UI in ambulatory and nonambulatory patients in outpatient, inpatient, home care, and long-term care settings.[20]

CLASSIFICATION OF URINARY INCONTINENCE

The Clinical Practice Guidelines for *Urinary Incontinence in Adults* have classified UI into four major categories: urge incontinence, stress incontinence, overflow incontinence, and other types of functional incontinence.

- **Urge incontinence** is the involuntary loss of urine associated with an abrupt and strong desire to void (urgency).
- **Stress incontinence** is the involuntary loss of urine during coughing, sneezing, laughing, or other physical activities that increase abdominal pressure.
- **Overflow incontinence** is the involuntary loss of urine associated with overdistension of the bladder.
- **Functional incontinence** is urine loss caused by factors outside the lower urinary tract; this category includes UI not classifiable into the three categories listed previously.

See Table 14-5 for descriptions, related findings, and patient populations associated with each type of UI.

CAUSES OF URINARY INCONTINENCE

The nurse should consider the many common causes of transient UI when assessing the patient for risk factors and related contributing factors for UI. Common cause of UI include altered states of consciousness (*e.g.*, confusion, coma); urinary tract infections; atrophic urethritis or vaginitis; depression; excessive urine production related to excess intake, diuresis from drugs, or endocrine conditions, such as diabetes mellitus; restricted mobility related to bed rest, poor eye sight, Parkinson's disease, and restriction to getting out of bed; deconditioning, such as orthostatic hypotension, weakness, and fatigue; and stool impaction.

In addition, a number of drugs may contribute to UI secondarily by clouding the sensorium or by directly affecting the organs of micturition. They include sedative hypnotics; diuretics that may overwhelm bladder capacity and lead to polyuria, frequency, and urgency; anticholinergics with related urinary retention and associated urinary frequency and overflow UI; alpha-adrenergic agents, in which sphincter tone in the proximal urethra can be decreased with alpha antagonists and increased with alpha agonists; and calcium channel blockers, which can reduce smooth muscle contractility in the bladder, resulting in urinary retention and overflow UI.

TABLE 14-4
Classification of Neurogenic Bladder Types*†‡*

NEUROGENIC BLADDER TYPES	ANATOMICAL LEVEL OF DISRUPTION	CHARACTERISTICS AND DESCRIPTION	ASSOCIATED CLINICAL PROBLEM	MANAGEMENT
Uninhibited neurogenic	Lesion in the frontal brain or pontine micturition centers	• Cortical control of initiation and inhibition to suppress voiding urge diminished • Reduced bladder capacity with little or no residual urine • Urgency, frequency, nocturia, urge incontinence	Stroke, traumatic brain injury, multiple sclerosis (MS), and brain tumor	• Timed voiding • Condom type catheter for male, and "padding" of bed with absorbent pads for female
Reflex neurogenic	Spinal cord lesion above T12–L1	• Upper motor neuron (UMN) lesion with disruption of sensory and motor innervation *above* segments S2–S4 • Control lost from higher brain centers, resulting in uninhibited, involuntary detrusor contractions and uncontrolled voiding; spinal reflex arc takes over • Inability of distal sphincter to relax in coordination with detrusor contraction; results in ↑ bladder pressure with emptying and large amounts of residual urine	Lower spinal cord lesion or patient with blood supply interruption to cord secondary to trauma, tumor, vascular lesion, or MS	• Reflex triggering techniques • Intermittent catheterization • Drugs
Autonomous or areflexic neurogenic	Spinal cord lesion *at or below* T12–L1	• Disruption of sensory and motor innervation of sacral spinal reflex arc (S2–S4), a lower motor neuron (LMN) injury • ↓ sensation of bladder fullness, weak or absent detrusor contractions, and ↑ bladder capacity with high residual urine.† • Loss of voluntary voiding except with straining; overflow incontinence is common	Spina bifida, meningocele, or herniated intervertebral disc with LMN injury	• Intermittent catheterization • Straining using Valsalva's maneuver • Crede's method
Motor paralytic neurogenic	Anterior horn cells of S2–S4 ventral roots	• Partial or complete motor loss of bladder function with intact sensation • Difficulty with starting stream • ↑ bladder capacity; high residual urine; overflow incontinence common	Herniated intervertebral disc, spinal trauma, spinal tumor, and poliomyelitis	• Intermittent catheterization • Straining using Valsalva's maneuver • Crede method
Sensory paralytic neurogenic	Dorsal roots of sacral reflex center (S2–S4) or in sensory pathways to cerebral cortex	• ↓ or absent sensation of pain or fullness in bladder • Infrequent voiding with large output; ↑ bladder capacity with overflow incontinence common	Diabetic neuropathy, tabes dorsalis, syringomyelia, and MS	• Timed voiding • Intermittent catheterization

* McCourt, A. E. (Ed.) (1993). Specialty practice of rehabilitation nursing: A core curriculum (3rd ed.) (pp. 101–102). Skokie, IL: Rehabilitation Nursing Foundation.

† Hoeman, S. P. (1996). Rehabilitation nursing: Process and application (pp. 427–432). St. Louis: C.V. Mosby.

‡ Lapides, J., & Diokno, A. C. (1976). Urine transport, storage, and micturition. In J. Lapides (Ed.), Fundamentals of urology. Philadelphia: W.B. Saunders.

Urinary Retention

Urinary retention is often associated with spinal cord injured patients. In the acute phase of spinal cord injury, the abrupt interruption of the spinal innervation is lost, resulting in spinal shock and an areflexic bladder. The bladder becomes distended, causing overflow UI (see Tables 14-4 and 14-5). The bladder gradually converts to a hypersensitive bladder as the spinal shock diminishes over days or weeks. If the spasticity and hypersensitivity of the bladder are severe, any slight stimulus, such as a minimal amount of urine in the bladder (20–50 mL) or stroking of the abdomen, thigh, or genitals, will cause the bladder to empty by reflex.

Nursing Management of Patients With Altered Urinary Elimination Patterns

ASSESSMENT

The nurse assesses the patient to determine the altered urinary elimination pattern present (Table 14-6). The parameters considered in the assessment include confirming voiding pattern by monitoring the voiding pattern and characteristics over 24 hours, intake and output record, recent urinalysis and culture, and functional level. Factors that may be contributing to or

TABLE 14-5
*Types, Descriptions, Related Findings, and Patient Populations Associated With Urinary Incontinence**

TYPES	DIAGNOSIS/ DESCRIPTION	RELATED FINDINGS	PATIENTS AFFECTED AND COMMENTS
Urge	• Diagnosed by urodynamics • Usually associated with urodynamic findings of involuntary detrusor contractions • Urodynamic finding of detrusor hyperactivity with impaired bladder contractility (DHIC) • DHIC can mimic other types of urinary incontinence (UI) and result in wrong treatment.	• If associated with neurological disorder, called detrusor hyperreflexia • If no neurological disorder, called detrusor instability • Patients with DHIC have involuntary detrusor contractions, yet must strain to empty bladder either completely or incompletely; in addition to urge UI with ↑ post-void residual volumes, patients with DHIC may also have obstruction, stress UI, or overflow UI.	• Stroke; in suprasacral spinal cord lesions or multiple sclerosis, detrusor hyperreflexia often accompanied by external sphincter dyssynergia; can cause urinary retention, vesicoureteric reflux, and renal damage† • Frail elderly often have DHIC.
Stress	Diagnosed by observed urine loss with an ↑ in abdominal pressure, absence of detrusor contraction, or an overdistended bladder‡	Two possible causes: • Hypermobility or significant displacement of urethra and bladder neck during exertion. • Intrinsic urethral sphincter deficiency (ISD); may be related to congenital sphincter weakness	• Patients with myelomeningocele, post-trauma, radiation, or sacral cord lesions; in women may be associated with many surgeries for incontinence • May leak continuously or leak with minimal exertion
Overflow	• Many presentations: constant dribbling, urge UI, or stress UI symptoms	• May be due to: (1) an underactive or acontractile detrusor; or (2) a bladder outlet or urethral obstruction, resulting in overdistention and overflow; and (3) weak detrusor from idiopathic causes	• Underactive detrusor related to certain drugs, fecal impaction, diabetic neuropathy, or low spinal cord injury • Outlet obstruction common in men with prostatic hypertrophy, pelvic prolapse in women, and suprasacral spinal cord injured and multiple sclerosis patients, detrusor external sphincter dyssynergia
Other types of Functional UI	• A diagnosis of exclusion • Caused by factors outside the urinary tract, such as chronic impairments of physical or cognitive functioning • May be caused by ↓ bladder compliance	• May be improved or cured by improving functional level, treating other medical conditions, discontinuing certain drugs, adjusting hydration status, or reducing environmental barriers • May have a combined urge UI and stress UI, which is called **mixed UI** • Severe urgency associated with bladder hypersensitivity without detrusor overactivity called **sensory urgency**	• Immobilized and cognitively impaired may also have other types and causes of UI • Patients with ↓ bladder compliance resulting from inflammatory bladder conditions (chemical or interstitial cystitis) and some patients with myelomeningocele often have *sensory urgency.*

* *U.S. Department of Health and Human Services, Agency for Health Care Policy and Research (1992). Urinary incontinence in adults, No. 92-0038. Washington, DC: U.S. Department of Health and Human Services, Agency for Health Care Policy and Research.*
† *McGuire, E. J., Woodside, J. R., Borden, T. A., & Weiss, R. M. (1981). Prognostic value of urodynamic testing in myelodysplastic patents. Journal of Urology, 132(2), 205–209.*
‡ *International Continence Society for the Standardization of Terminology of the Lower Urinary Tract Function (1990). British Journal of Obstetrics and Gynaecology, 6(Suppl.), 1–16.*

resulting from the altered elimination pattern must be identified, as should the areas in need of further evaluation before therapeutic interventions are begun. The pathophysiology should be considered in relation to normal function. The nurse should discuss with the physician and other team members the need for further evaluation and the best approach to the management of the urinary elimination pattern (Chart 14-4).

Nursing management will depend on the nursing diagnoses. The following are possible nursing diagnoses:

• Altered Urinary Elimination
• Stress Incontinence
• Reflex Incontinence
• Urinary Retention
• Risk for Altered Skin Integrity
• Urge Incontinence
• Functional Incontinence
• Total Incontinence
• Risk for Urinary Tract Infection

TABLE 14-6
Nursing Assessment for Altered Patterns of Urinary Elimination

CHARACTERISTICS OF VOIDING PATTERN

- Frequency of voiding and time during day and night
- Amount of voiding each time
- Evidence of dribbling (frequency, amount)
- Urgency
- Ability to delay voiding until in appropriate place
- Awareness of full bladder
- Distended bladder
- Sensation of incomplete bladder emptying
- Difficulty starting stream
- Dysuria
- Foul-smelling urine
- Residual urine greater than 150 mL

RELATED FACTORS

- Neurological disease or injury
- Cognitive deficits
- Sensory deficits with vision or hearing
- Altered sensorium or consciousness (confusion, coma)
- Neuropathies
- Comorbidity
- Urinary tract infection
- Vaginitis or atrophic urethritis
- Drug therapy that influences urinary output or bladder function
- Depression
- Large amounts of oral or intravenous intake; evaluation intake and output record
- Environmental barriers to getting to bathroom
- Restricted mobility
- Stool impaction

The following are possible collaborative problems:

- Acute urinary retention
- Renal insufficiency
- Renal calculi

Interventions. Various methods of managing altered urinary elimination patterns are discussed in the next section. Within a collaborative interdisciplinary model of practice, input regarding management of urinary function is provided by the multidisciplinary team. However, the nurse is primarily responsible for managing the complex multifactorial problem of an altered urinary elimination pattern, integrating all the components of the treatment plan, and preventing complications, such as urinary tract infection and skin breakdown.

To prevent urinary tract infection, remove the indwelling catheter as soon as possible and use alternate methods of emptying and stimulating the bladder on a regular schedule. Follow all the research-based guidelines for maintaining aseptic technique related to catheters, catheterization, and skin care. For example, meatal care is controversial and not recommended.

Maintain an intake and output record, and review it periodically. Fluid intake is an important factor to adjust when trying to establish continence and regular emptying of the bladder. UI is a risk factor for skin breakdown. Provide for meticulous skin care, and keep the patient dry.

TREATMENT OPTIONS FOR MANAGEMENT OF ALTERED URINARY ELIMINATION PATTERNS

The three major categories of treatment outlined for UI are behavioral, pharmacological, and surgical.[21] This can be used as a framework for nursing management and is summarized in Table 14-7.

"Acute urinary retention" is a collaborative problem to be addressed with the physician. Management of acute urinary retention is always directed at using some method of evacuating the bladder to prevent reflux and infection. Chronic urinary retention is usually treated with intermittent catheterization.

Whenever possible, the patient should be involved in selecting treatment options from established methods. As a rule, the least invasive and least dangerous procedure should be the first choice. According to the AHCPR guidelines for UI in adults, behavioral techniques are low-risk interventions that decrease the frequency of UI in most in-

CHART 14-4
Possible Diagnostic and Evaluative Procedures for Patients With Urinary Elimination Problems

Patient Data

- Medical history
- Physical examination
  - Abdominal, genital, pelvic, rectal, neurological

Addition Tests Related to Voiding

- Estimated postvoid residual volume
- Provocation stress test
- Data related to urinary elimination
  - Voiding diary, voiding pattern, and so forth

Laboratory Tests

- Urinalysis
- Blood urea nitrogen, creatinine, protein, complete blood count
- Urine culture

Specialized Tests

- Urodynamic tests
- Endoscopic tests
- Imaging tests
  - Upper tract
  - Lower tract with and without voiding

TABLE 14-7
Management of Altered Urinary Elimination Patterns

URINARY PATTERNS	PATIENT TYPES	TREATMENT
Urge urinary incontinence	Strokes	Timed voiding; bladder training and every 2 hour prompt
Reflex urinary incontinence	Spinal cord injured upper motor neuron (UMN) and lower motor neuron lesions	Anticholinergic drugs and intermittent catheterization Condom catheter for men and "padding" for women
Overflow urinary incontinence	Spinal cord injuries with UMN lesion	Intermittent cauterization
Functional urinary incontinence	Various types of patients with functional deficits	Assistance for toileting and timed voiding • May use condom type catheter for men and "padding" for women
Urinary retention	Spinal cord injuries; some stroke patients	• Intermittent cauterization for life with a goal of 400 mL per catheterization (no voiding on own) • Trigger voiding philosophy for some practitioners

dividuals when provided by knowledgeable health professionals. All behavioral techniques involve educating the patient and providing positive reinforcement for effort and progress.[22] Behavioral techniques include bladder training (retraining), habit training (timed voiding), prompted voiding, and pelvic muscle exercises. These are discussed further. Additional techniques that may be used in conjunction with behavioral methods are biofeedback, vaginal cone retention, and electrical stimulation. These are not discussed further. In addition, the many drugs that can be used to treat urinary elimination problems are not discussed. For those interested in the additional techniques and drug therapy, other references should be consulted.

Once the particular type of altered urinary elimination pattern has been identified, treatment options are considered.

BEHAVIORAL TECHNIQUES

The following behavioral techniques have been effective and are recommended by AHCPR in the adult patient with incontinence.[23]

Bladder Training. **Bladder training**, also called bladder retraining, includes a number of variations. The time at which a bladder training program is initiated is critical to the success or failure of the program. Patients must be conscious, alert, and oriented. A bedpan, bedside commode, or access to the bathroom is necessary. The patient should be stable and preferably free from urinary tract infection.

Bladder training includes the three primary components of education, scheduled voiding, and positive reinforcement. The patient needs to be educated to understand the physiology, pathophysiology, technique, and desired outcome. The method of education depends on the patient with consideration for any cognitive or perceptual deficits that may interfere with learning.

A bladder retraining program assists the patient to learn to resist or inhibit the sensation of urgency, postpone voiding, and urinate according to a timetable rather than the urge to void.[24] The strategies of a bladder retraining program vary and may include adjusting the fluid loads and postponing voiding so that progressively larger volumes of urine distend the blad-

der, and longer intervals between voiding are achieved.[25] Motivating the patient is an important component of bladder training. The initial goal interval may be 2 to 3 hours, although it is not followed during sleep. Bladder retraining may continue for several months, during which time setting realistic goals, reinforcing patient education, and overall health monitoring and supervision are necessary.

Habit Training. **Habit training**, also called *timed voiding*, is scheduled toileting on a planned basis with the goal of keeping the person dry by asking him or her to void at regular intervals. Unlike bladder training, there is no systematic effort to motivate the patient to delay voiding and resist the urge. An attempt is made to match the timed voiding with the person's usual voiding schedule. The time interval may be from 2 to 4 hours.

Prompted Voiding. **Prompted voiding** is a technique used primarily with dependent or cognitively impaired people. Prompted voiding attempts to teach the incontinent person awareness of his or her incontinence so that toileting assistance is requested either independently or after being prompted by a caregiver. There are three major elements to prompted voiding:

• Monitoring: The person is checked by caregivers on a regular basis and asked to report verbally if he or she is wet or dry.
• Prompting: The person is asked (prompted) to try to used the bathroom and void.
• Praising: The person is praised for maintaining continence and attempting to use the toilet.

Pelvic Muscle Exercises. **Pelvic muscle exercises**, also called Kegel exercises, are a behavioral technique that require repetitive active exercises of the pubococcygeus muscle to improve urethral resistance and urinary control by strengthening the periurethral and pelvic muscles in women. The woman must gain awareness of her pelvic muscles and be taught the correct exercise method of "drawing in" the perivaginal muscles and anal sphincter as if to control urination or defecation without contracting abdominal, buttock, or inner thigh muscles.[26] Muscles are contracted to a count of 10 and then relaxed to a count of 10. About 50 to 100 of these exercises must be done daily to be effective. It takes about 4 to 6 weeks to notice improvement.

BLADDER-TRIGGERING TECHNIQUES

A few bladder-triggering techniques facilitate bladder emptying. They include suprapubic stimulation, the Valsalva's maneuver, and the Credé's maneuver.

Suprapubic Stimulation. **Suprapubic stimulation** is stimulation of the sacral-lumbar dermatomes by manually tapping the suprapubic area, pulling pubic hairs, or stroking the medial thighs. This is used for patients with upper motor neuron (UMN) lesions.

Valsalva's Maneuver. The **Valsalva's maneuver** is straining against a closed epiglottis while contracting the abdominal muscles and bearing down on the bladder. The straining is sustained or the breath held until the urine flow ceases. This maneuver is used for patients with lower motor neuron (LMN) lesions.

Credé's Maneuver. The **Credé's maneuver** is placing the hands flat just below the umbilical area and pressing firmly down and inward toward the pelvic arch. The purpose of this maneuver is to express urine from the bladder. It may be repeated as many times as necessary to express all of the urine in the bladder. This method is used only with LMN lesions (sacral reflex arc is not intact). Generally, Credé's maneuver is not used in patients with UMN bladder because it triggers sphincter closure and can cause reflux.

CATHETERS AND CATHETERIZATIONS

In the acute phase of spinal injury or other acute conditions, an indwelling catheter for continuous urinary drainage may be necessary. However, it should be removed as soon as possible and an intermittent catheterization schedule established.

Intermittent Catheterization. Intermittent catheterization means that the patient is straight catheterized at regular intervals of 2 to 4 hours or more to empty the bladder at regular intervals. Bladder-triggering techniques should be incorporated as a means of emptying the bladder before straight catheterization. Once the patient begins to void by reflex, the interval between catheterizations can be extended using postvoid residual urine amount as a guide. Indications to stop intermittent catheterization include an adequate amount of urine voided, residual urine volume of 100 to 150 mL or less, or genitourinary tract free of pathological changes or infection.[27]

Self-Catheterization. If intermittent catheterization is needed long term or in the home, many patients can be taught intermittent catheterization using a "clean technique" rather than the "sterile technique" used in care facilities. With the clean technique, the patient starts with a clean catheter rather than sterilized equipment. Warm tap water and soap are used to wash the perineal area. Hands are meticulously washed with soap and water, but sterile gloves are not worn. If the patient is not able to self-catheterize, use of an external condom type catheter connected to a leg bag may be used by male patients. This method can also be used for continuous drainage during sleep.

"Padding." **Padding** is the placement of absorbent pads in the bed or chair to adsorb the urine of incontinence. Use of padding is preferred to maintaining an indwelling catheter long term for patients who do not respond well to behavioral techniques or are not candidates for behavioral or other techniques.

BOWEL ELIMINATION AND DYSFUNCTION

Normal Function

The act of bowel evacuation is called **defecation**. The anus, the terminal end of the large bowel, is controlled by two sphincters: the involuntary proximal anal sphincter (smooth muscle) and the voluntary distal anal sphincter (striated muscle).

Defecation is a coordinated reflex of sacral segments S-3, S-4, and S-5, which is initiated by stimulated stretch receptors located in the anus that initiate peristaltic waves. These waves propel fecal matter toward the anus and open the proximal sphincter. If the distal sphincter is also open, bowel evacuation will occur.

The sacral reflex for bowel evacuation is weak and is aided by parasympathetic responses (peristalsis caused by ingestion of food and increased pressure within the lower bowel, which opens the proximal sphincter). Also, contraction of the abdominal wall aids bowel evacuation by increasing pressure on the bowel. See Chapter 5 for further discussion of defecation.

Types of Altered Bowel Function Patterns

A variety of neurological conditions and treatment protocols can cause alterations in bowel elimination patterns (constipation, diarrhea, or incontinence). Several risk factors have been identified for these abnormal patterns:

- **Constipation**: fluid restriction, prolonged immobility, nothing by mouth status as a result of swallowing deficits or unconsciousness, decreased bulk in diet, drugs known to decrease peristalsis (*e.g.,* codeine), spinal nerve compression, paralytic ileus, lack of sensation, lack of privacy, interruption of usual bowel routine, failure to respond to defecation stimuli
- **Diarrhea**: intolerance to tube feeding, antibiotic therapy, and fecal impaction
- **Incontinence**: Altered consciousness, cognitive deficits (*e.g.,* social disinhibition, lack of impulse control, inability to recognize and respond to defecation impulses), impaired communication, and neurogenic bowel without sensation or control (related to spinal cord injury above T11 or involving sacral reflex arc S2 to S4)

Nursing Management of Patients With Altered Bowel Elimination Pattern

ASSESSMENT

The nurse assesses the patient to identify the functional bowel elimination problem present. Parameters to be considered include bowel elimination pattern (frequency, characteristics of stool, presence of discomfort), presence of bowel sounds and abdominal distention, previous elimination pattern, and presence of risk factors (see previous list). Nursing management will depend on the nursing diagnosis. The following are possible nursing diagnoses:

- Diarrhea
- Colonic Constipation
- Bowel Incontinence

The following are possible collaborative problems:

- Paralytic ileus
- Gastrointestinal bleeding

Interventions. The nursing management for altered bowel elimination patterns will depend on the particular problem identified. However, the goal is for the patient to eliminate a soft, formed stool every 1 to 3 days. An individualized bowel program is developed for each patient following established standards of care and is included in the patient's care plan. See Chart 14-5 for a sample bowel program. Daily documentation should be included in the record.

If the patient is constipated, the following points may need to be considered:

- Determine which risk factors can be controlled or altered.
- Increase fluid intake if not contraindicated.
- Administer any drugs ordered by the physician as part of the bowel program.
  Bulk former (*e.g.,* Metamucil, 15 mL daily)
  Stool softeners (*e.g.,* docusate sodium, 100 mg three times daily)
  Mild laxatives (*e.g.,* Milk of Magnesia, 30 mL daily)
  Suppositories (glycerin or Dulcolax as needed)
- Enemas may be ordered.

The nurse should keep in mind the following guidelines when instituting any bowel program:

- Start with an empty lower bowel and then individualize a bowel program to meet needs.
- Get the patient onto the commode if at all possible.
- Try to establish an evacuation pattern at the same time of day that mimics the patient's preadmission pattern.

In addition to the treatment plan outlined, digital stimulation of the rectum can be used in patients with spinal cord injuries to stimulate defecation. Initiation of the Valsalva's maneuver or a push-up on the commode may also aid defecation. (Both hands are placed on the commode seat, and the patient raises himself or herself slightly off the seat.) Autonomic hy-

CHART 14-5
Sample Bowel Program to Establish Normal Elimination

The following protocol includes the basic components of a bowel program, although different physicians may prefer slight variations. Once a normal bowel elimination pattern has been established, an individualized protocol should be followed.

- Make sure the lower bowel is empty; an enema may be necessary before beginning the training program.
- Establish a time of day for a bowel movement based on the patient's previous pattern; adhere to this designated time of day rigidly.
- Encourage a diet high in roughage (whole-grain bread and cereal, fresh fruits, and vegetables); in addition, offer prune juice.
- Unless contraindicated by a fluid restriction, increase fluid intake to 2,000 to 2,500 mL/d.
- Insert a suppository on the first day. If it does not work, you may wait until the next day
- On the following day, repeat the insertion of the suppository. If it is effective, continue with the protocol every other day; but every day may be necessary for some patients.
- If at all possible, the patient should be seated on the commode or taken into the bathroom for defecation.
- Administer medications and collaborate with patient and health team members to adjust regimen individualized to the patient.

perreflexia may be triggered by impaction in patients with high spinal cord injuries (see Chap. 22).

COGNITIVE REHABILITATION

Cognitive deficits are one of the most disabling categories of deficits resulting from brain injury because they impact on every aspect of life. Deficits in higher level cognitive functions can be overlooked without careful assessment of the patient. If they are overlooked, the patient is often set up for failure and will not achieve the highest level of independence and quality of life possible.

Nursing Management of Patients With Cognitive Deficits

ASSESSMENT

The patient's cognitive function can be assessed by observing the patient's behavior, interactions, and function in the care setting or by using various assessment techniques and instruments to evaluate cognitive function.

TABLE 14-8
Rancho Los Amigos Scale: Levels of Cognitive Function

COGNITIVE LEVEL	DESCRIPTION	NURSING MANAGEMENT
	For levels I–III, the key approach is to *provide stimulation*.	
I: No response	Completely unresponsive to all stimuli, including painful stimuli	Multiple modalities of sensory input should be used. Examples are listed below, but should be individualized and expanded based on available materials and patient preferences (determined by obtaining information from the family).
II: Generalized response	Nonpurposeful response; responds to pain, but in a nonpurposeful manner	*Olfactory:* perfumes, flowers, shaving lotion *Visual:* family pictures, card, personal items
III: Localized response	Responses more focused: withdraws to pain; turns toward sound; follows moving objects that pass within visual field; pulls on sources of discomfort (*e.g.,* tubes, restraints); may follow simple commands but inconsistently and in a delayed manner	*Auditory:* radio, television, tapes of family voices or favorite recordings, talking to patient (nurse, family members). The nurse should tell patient what is going to be done, discuss the environment, provide encouragement. *Tactile:* touching of skin, rubbing various textures on skin *Movement:* range of motion exercises, turning, repositioning, use of water mattress
	For levels IV–VI, the key approach is to *provide structure*.	
IV: Confused, agitated response	Alert, hyperactive state in which patient responds to internal confusion/agitation; behavior nonpurposeful in relation to the environment; aggressive, bizarre behavior common	For level IV, which lasts 2–4 wk, interventions are directed at decreasing agitation, increasing environmental awareness, and promoting safety. • Approach patient in a calm manner, and use a soft voice. • Screen patient from environmental stimuli (*e.g.,* sounds, sights); provide a quiet, controlled environment. Remove devices that contribute to agitation (*e.g.,* tubes), if possible. • Functional goals cannot be set, because the patient is unable to cooperate.
V: Confused, inappropriate response	When agitation occurs, it is the result of external rather than internal stimuli; focused attention is difficult; memory is severely impaired; responses are fragmented and inappropriate to the situation; there is no carryover of learning from one situation to the other.	For Levels V and VI, interventions are directed at decreasing confusion, improving cognitive function, and improving independence in performing ADLs. • Provide supervision. • Use drill method and cues to teach ADLs. Focus the patient's attention and help to increase his or her concentration.
VI: Confused, appropriate response	Follows simple directions consistently but is inconsistently oriented to time and place; short-term memory worse than long-term memory; can perform some ADLs	• Help the patient organize activity. • Clarify misinformation and reorient when confused. Provide a consistent, predictable schedule (*e.g.,* post daily schedule on large poster board).
	For levels VII and VIII, the key approach is *integration into the community*.	
VII: Automatic, appropriate response	Appropriately responsive and oriented within the hospital setting; needs little supervision in ADLs; some carryover of learning; patient has superficial insight into disabilities; has decreased judgment and problem-solving abilities; lacks realistic planning for future	For Levels VII and VIII, interventions are directed at increasing the patient's ability to function with minimal or no supervision in the community. • Reduce environmental structure. • Help the patient plan for adapting ADLs for self into the home environment. • Discuss and adapt home living skills (*e.g.,* cleaning, cooking) to patient's ability.
VIII: Purposeful, appropriate response	Alert, oriented, intact memory; has realistic goals for future; judgment and problem solving skills intact; has realistic plans for community integration	• Discuss integration into the community setting (outside home, church, social activities, possibly the work environment). • Help the patient plan, anticipate concerns, and problem solve.

The nurse should observe the patient's reaction to stimuli, ability to perform ADLs, memory, way of dealing with minor stresses, problem-solving abilities, and judgment. The nurse should also identify cognitive deficits that impact on patient safety and implement interventions to protect the patient from injury.

Various instruments may be used to assess specific cognitive functions, such as memory, attention span, affect and general behavior, sequencing skills, problem solving, insight, judgment, and abstract thinking. The Mini-Mental State Examination, Neurobehavioral Cognitive Status Examination, and the Rancho Los Amigos Scale[28] are commonly used in the clinical setting. The Rancho Los Amigos Scale is very helpful in clinical practice, because it provides a practical framework for assessment and nursing interventions (Table 14-8). Mitchell provides an excellent discussion of this scale in her text.[7]

In many facilities, a short (half-hour) cognitive screening assessment may be conducted by the occupational therapy department. The information derived from this evaluation is helpful to the nurse in planning care if cognitive deficits can be identified. Many physicians prefer this approach rather than a full neuropsychological assessment, which takes many hours, because some recovery is expected during the early weeks after cerebral insult. If problems persist, a complete neuropsychological assessment is reserved for 3 to 6 months after injury.

INTERVENTIONS

Nurses can provide interventions for many cognitive problems in the acute care setting (see Table 14-8). With a knowledge of the patient's cognitive deficits, the nurse can identify realistic goals and expectations for the patient. An important role for the nurse is to explain the patient's behavior to the family and be supportive of their concerns. Family members should be told what kind of behavior to expect and how to interact with the patient.

The patient with severe cognitive deficits will require ongoing treatment following discharge from the acute care setting to a rehabilitation facility or to the patient's home. If a home discharge is planned, referrals for follow-up care should be arranged.

DISCHARGE PLANNING

Some patients will require long-term rehabilitation, which will necessitate the use of community resources if they are living at home or admission to a rehabilitation center or extended care facility. The nurse should evaluate the patient's level of independence in terms of ADLs to assess how much help the patient will need. This information, along with evaluations by other health team members, will provide a database for designing a comprehensive rehabilitation plan.

Family members must also be assessed to determine their ability to participate in the rehabilitation program. Some families are willing and able to care for the patient at home with the help of various community agencies. Other families do not want to care for the patient or are unable to do so because of other family responsibilities. **Caregiver stress** needs to be considered. The decision of how and where to provide for the

long-term rehabilitative needs of the patient must be a collaborative one that includes input from the physician, nurse, other health team members, family, and patient, if possible.

Regardless of whether the patient is going home to be cared for by family or to an extended care facility, the nurse will need to compile a summary assessment of the patient's needs and abilities in performing ADLs. Referral forms must be completed and sent to appropriate resources. (See Chap. 15 for information about discharge planning.)

Rehabilitation Legislation and Entitlement Programs

The value of rehabilitation for the individual and society is well appreciated and has been supported through many legislative programs. Information about entitlement programs and rehabilitation can be obtained from a variety of sources, such as the following:

- The social worker
- Local and state health departments through their departments of social service, rehabilitation, or vocational rehabilitation
- Special focus groups, such as the Multiple Sclerosis Society and National Head Injury Foundation

References

1. World Health Organization (1980). *Rehabilitation International classification of impairment, disabilities, and handicaps* (pp. 7–43). Geneva: World Health Organization.
2. Nagi, S. Z. (1965). Some conceptual issues in disability and rehabilitation. In M. B. Sussman (Ed.), *Sociology and rehabilitation* (pp. 100–113). Washington, DC: American Sociological Association.
3. Ibid, pp. 100–113.
4. Ibid, pp. 5–7.
5. Brummel-Smith, K. (1990). In B. Kemp, K. Brummel-Smith, & J. W. Ramsdell (Eds.), *Geriatric rehabilitation* (pp. 3–12). Austin, TX: PRO-ED.
6. American Nurses Association and the Association of Rehabilitation Nurses (1988). *Rehabilitation nursing: Scope of practice; process and outcome criteria for selected diagnoses.* Kansas City, MO: American Nurses Association.
7. U.S. Department of Health and Human Services, Agency for Health Care Policy and Research (1995). *Post-stroke rehabilitation*, No. 95-0662. Washington, DC: Author.
8. State University of New York at Buffalo, The Center for Functional Assessment Research (1993). *Guide for the uniform data set for medical rehabilitation (adult FIM)*, version 4.0. Buffalo, NY: Uniform Data System for Medical Rehabilitation.
9. McCourt, A. E. (Eds.) (1993). *The specialty practice of rehabilitation nursing: A core curriculum* (3rd ed.) (p. 13). Skokie, IL: The Rehabilitation Nursing Foundation.
10. Ibid.
11. Borgman-Gainer, M. F. (1996). Independent function: Movement and mobility. In S. P. Hoeman (Ed.), *Rehabilitation nursing: Process and application* (2nd ed.) (pp. 232–233). St. Louis: C.V. Mosby.
12. McCourt, A. E. (Eds.) (1993). *The specialty practice of rehabilitation nursing: A core curriculum* (3rd ed.) (p. 32). Skokie, IL: The Rehabilitation Nursing Foundation.
13. Borgman-Gainer, M. F. (1996). Independent function: Movement and mobility. In S. P. Hoeman (Ed.), *Rehabilitation nursing: Process and application* (2nd ed.) (pp. 232–233). St. Louis: C.V. Mosby.

14. Bobath, B. (1990). *Adult hemiplegia: Evaluation and treatment* (3rd ed.). Oxford, England: Butterworth-Heinemann.
15. McCourt, A. E. (Eds.) (1993). *The specialty practice of rehabilitation nursing: A core curriculum* (3rd ed.) (p. 32). Skokie, IL: The Rehabilitation Nursing Foundation.
16. U.S. Department of Health and Human Services, Agency for Health Care Policy and Research (1992). *Pressure ulcers in adults: Prediction and prevention*, No. 92-0047. Washington, DC: Author.
17. Glenn, N. H. (1996). Eating and swallowing. In S. P. Hoeman (Ed.), *Rehabilitation nursing: Process and application* (2nd ed.) (pp. 347–360). St. Louis: C.V. Mosby.
18. North American Nursing Diagnosis Association (1992). *NANDA nursing diagnosis: Definitions and classification 1992*. St. Louis: Author.
19. Westmoreland, B. F., Benarroch, R. R., Daube, J. R., Reagan, T. J., & Sandok, B. A. (1994). *Medical neurosciences: An approach to anatomy, pathology, and physiology by systems and levels* (pp. 237–240). Boston: Little, Brown.
20. U.S. Department of Health and Human Services, Agency for Health Care Policy and Research (1992). *Urinary incontinence in adults*, No. 92-0038. Washington, DC: Author.
21. Ibid, pp. 27–65.
22. Ibid, pp. 27–28.
23. Ibid, pp. 29–35.
24. McCormick, K. A., & Burgio, K. L. (1984). Incontinence: An update on nursing care measures. *Journal of Gerontological Nursing*, 10(10), 22–23.
25. Keating, J. C., Schulte, E. A., & Miller, E. (1988). Conservative care of urinary incontinence in the elderly. *Journal of Manipulative and Physiological Therapeutics*, 11(4), 463–464.
26. Rose, M. A., Baigis-Smith, J., Smith, D., & Newman, D. (1990). Behavioral management of urinary incontinence in homebound older adults. *Home Healthcare Nurse*, 8(5), 10–15.
27. McCourt, p. 103.
28. Rancho Los Amigos Hospital (1980). *Rehabilitation of the head-injured adult*. Downey, CA: Author.

Bibliography

Books

Bobath, B. (1990). *Adult hemiplegia: Evaluation and treatment* (3rd ed.). Oxford, England: Butterworth-Heineman.

Dobkin, B. H. (1996). *Neurologic rehabilitation*. Philadelphia: F. A. Davis.

Kottke, F. J., & Lehman, J. F. (1990). *Krusen's handbook of physical medicine and rehabilitation* (4th ed.). Philadelphia: W.B. Saunders.

Hoeman, S. P. (1996). *Rehabilitation nursing: Process and application*. St. Louis: C.V. Mosby.

Lezak, M. (1995). *Neuropsychological assessment* (3rd ed.). New York: Oxford University Press.

McCourt, A. E. (Eds.) (1993). *The specialty practice of rehabilitation nursing: A core curriculum* (3rd ed.). Skokie, IL: The Rehabilitation Nursing Foundation.

Storck, I. F., & Thompson-Hoffman, S. (1991). Disability in the United States: A portrait from national data (pp. 1–12). New York: Springer Publishing.

Periodicals

American Heart Association (1986). *Recovering from a stroke*. Author.

Davis, A. E., & White, J. J. (1995). Innovative sensory input for the comatose brain-injured patient. *Critical Care Nursing Clinics of North America*, 7(2), 351–361.

Davis, L. L., & Grant, J. S. (1994). Constructing the reality of recovery: Family home care management strategies. *Advanced Nursing Science*, 17(2), 66–76.

Harper, C. M., & Lyles, Y. M. (1988). Physiology and complications of bed rest. *Journal of the American Geriatric Society*, 36(11); 1047–1054.

Lugger, K. E. (1994). Dysphagia in the elderly stroke patient. *Journal of Neuroscience Nursing*, 26(2), 78–84.

Palmer, J. B., & DuChane, A. S. (1991). Rehabilitation of swallowing disorders due to stroke. *Physical Medicine and Rehabilitation Clinics of North America*, 3(3), 529–546.

Price, M. E., & DiIorio, C. (1990). Swallowing: A practical guide. *American Journal of Nursing*, 90(7), 42–46.

CHAPTER 15

Transitions in Care and Discharge Planning

Joanne V. Hickey

In Chapter 2, the continuum of care is discussed from the perspective of levels of care within the health care delivery system. In this chapter, the focus is on the processes necessary to facilitate the transition from one care environment to another to meet patient-centered health care needs. This chapter also focuses on the process of a special transition, discharge planning to the home. For many neurological patients, recovery does not mean a return to preillness or preinjury state of health. Cognitive or communications deficits may make it impossible for the patient to participate in decision making related to health care needs. Many neurological patients have new, complex needs to support optimal health. Transitions and associated planning are reviewed within the context of neuroscience patients.

Transitions can move a patient through acuity-based levels of care within a hospital, to transitional care units, to community-based care, or to home discharge. The term "discharge planning" is used to denote the process of planning patient health care needs when patients move from one place to another. Viewed from a broader context, patients have ongoing health care needs that do not end at discharge from the hospital. Patient-centered care recognizes that hospitalization is a single "incident" along a continuum of health care, and health care needs continue after hospitalization.[1]

TRANSITIONS IN CARE

Transition is a passage from one state, stage, or place to another; it is a change. Passage suggests movement from one place to another, and the movement is along some path or trajectory. Whenever movement occurs, the goal is that the movement is smooth with bridges in place to facilitate the process. A smooth transition is facilitated through **coordination of care** that anticipates potential problems, removes obstacles, addresses unmet needs, and prevents fragmentation. The coordinated care that prevents fragmentation is called **continuity of care.** Although a transition may represent some recovery, it is also frightening to the patient and family to move into an unknown environment and culture. Transitions in care can be within an institution, between institutions, between an institution and community-based care, and between an institution and home. All require a coordinated approach to promote continuity.

Depending on the services available in a facility, a neuroscience patient may move from a high-acuity unit, such as an intensive care unit (ICU), to one of lesser acuity, such as an intermediate unit. The patient and family need to be prepared for the transition through education and counseling that includes a brief description about the new unit, such as the kind of patients in the unit, visiting hours, what physicians will be taking care of them, and the ratio of nurses to patients. The 1:1 or 1:2 ratio of nurse to patient common in ICUs is much lower in intermediate units, and patients and families need to be prepared for decreased nursing intensity. They need to be reassured that the transfer is a positive sign of recovery and that their needs for care will continue to be met by health team members. A visit to the new unit to meet with a staff representative can alleviate anxiety.

If the patient is going to a special unit in the hospital, such as a rehabilitation unit or transitional care unit, education about the unit, its philosophy, and the focus of care offered should be shared. In particular, they need to know what patient and family involvement is expected. For example, in a comprehensive rehabilitation program, the focus is on functional recovery and self-care to promote independence. There is greater emphasis on the patient for self-care. Family members are prepared to assist the patient with care after discharge. These skills must be taught and practiced in a supportive environment.

Transitional units, such as Cooperative Care at New York Hospital, focus on enhancing patient and family participation through creation of a homelike environment that mimics the "real world." Patients are prepared to take their own medications and select their own meals from a cafeteria-style dining center. Although there are nurses, pharmacists, and nutritionists to provide education and support, the responsibility for care belongs to the patient. Another example of transitional care is the trend for large centers that have a national and international referral base to place patients and family members into a hospital-affiliated motel or hotel where they can assume responsibility for their own care. They have the option for education, consultation, and direct care if necessary. This model is useful for patients and family to adjust and feel confident about their recovery and ability to manage their own care. Another example is the trend for hospitals to extend care into the community by offering a home care program. One advantage of this arrangement is that the patient stays within the same health care organization and receives better continuity of care. In addition, if the patient needs readmission, that transition is simplified.

Continuity of care for a transition within an institution is usually easier to coordinate because the system is the same, and there are usually procedures for transferring a patient. However, the need for person-to-person communication between the present and new health provider must take place to provide for continuity of care. When the transition is between the institution and another institution, community-based care, or home, more complex discharge planning is needed.

DISCHARGE PLANNING FOR TRANSITIONS IN HEALTH CARE NEEDS

The standards of the Joint Commission on Accreditation of Healthcare Organizations (JCAHO) require discharge planning to be part of the care provided to patients, and that planning must involve the patient and family. Discharge planning is addressed in many different areas of the JCAHO Manual of Accreditation as a necessary part of service to the patient and a responsibility of health care providers. Patients with neurological dysfunction often have extensive and complex health needs that must be met beyond the acute care setting. Discharge planning is the vehicle through which the patient's health care needs can be met within the continuum of health care services.

Discharge planning is a logical, coordinated, multilevel process of decision making and other activities involving the patient, the family or significant other, and a team of multidisciplinary health professionals working together to facilitate a smooth, coordinated transition from one environment to another. The transitional environment may be an acute care facility, a chronic care or rehabilitation hospital, a nursing home, or the patient's home. The purpose of discharge planning is to assist the patient to make a smooth transition from one environment or level of care to another without sacrificing the progress that has already been achieved and to provide for other health care needs that are still unmet. Numerous studies have shown that hospitals and patients benefit from facilitating the transition out of the hospital. Benefits cited include improved patient outcomes, increased patient and family satisfaction, decreased length of stay, decreased hospital readmissions, enhanced cost effectiveness, decreased complications, and decreased mortality.

According to Shine,[2] discharge planning includes a systematic, multilevel process of the following activities:

- Assesses patients' resources and limitations early in hospitalization to determine needs
- Provides patient and family with the education necessary to care for themselves at home
- Counsels patients and families to facilitate the stressful transition between hospital and home, dependence and independence
- Plans for continuity in health care needs at discharge from the hospital
- Coordinates individual, family, hospital, and community resources needed to implement the plan for transition
- Follows-up at home to determine the effectiveness of the discharge plan and to assess changes in needs

Because hospitalizations are shorter, planning for transitions occurs in a compressed period with cost containment and continuity of care as goals.

Cost containment is a major force driving health care delivery. The current political climate regarding health financing is volatile.[3] Medicare and Medicaid, major federal and state programs that finance health care for large numbers of people, have serious financial problems that will only become worse in the future. Even with diagnosis-related groupings and prospective payment for hospital services, health care costs are out of control. There will certainly be changes in Medicare, Medicaid, and other government-supported programs.

More health care is provided in managed care environments. Managed care contracts emphasize early and aggressive discharge planning for cost containment and continuity of care (see Chaps. 1 and 2).

Continuity of care is a concept of coordinated delivery of health care on a continuum. The continuum of health care services includes various facilities, such as acute care hospitals, long-term and rehabilitation hospitals, nursing homes, intermediate care facilities, and day care centers. It also includes various types of services within and outside the hospital setting (*e.g.*, ICUs, specialty units, rehabilitation units, self-care units, ambulatory care services) and community resources, such as neighborhood health centers, Meals on Wheels, and specialty organization programs. For some patients, help is needed to prepare for death, and a hospice program may be the best support for these patients. As the patient's health care status changes, health care needs change, and the kind of services necessary to support these needs also change. The appropriate resource or facility that can best support and administer the necessary care most economically should be used. Current health care policy does not necessarily encourage or support the *most economical provision of care*. For example, Medicare pays for only he highest level of postacute care, skilled nursing, but will not pay for sitters or adult day care, which is less expensive, favored by patients and family, and can help avoid or delay institutional care, especially in patients with dementia.[4]

Meeting health care needs is predicated on selection of the appropriate resources and effective communications between health care providers. Therefore, continuity of care means quality care, because it involves matching the needs of the patient with the appropriate resources. Continuity of care and quality of care are maintained through the process of discharge planning.

ORGANIZATIONAL STRUCTURE FOR DISCHARGE PLANNING

Mechanisms and structures for discharge planning must be incorporated into the organizational or operational structure. Discharge planning must be placed in a department that assumes responsibility and accountability for it. Staff assigned to this department include continuing care nurses, case managers, and clinical social workers who have primary responsibility for discharge planning in that facility. Discharge planning begins during admission to a facility, and mechanisms for early identification of "high risk" patients are needed. Data collection on admission should include an assessment of projected discharge planning needs so that high risk patients can be identified and planning can begin immediately. This information should be communicated to the nurse caring for the patient and the clinical social worker assigned to the unit.

On the unit level, weekly collaborative multidisciplinary discharge planning rounds are the mechanism for discharge planning. Members of the team include nurses (*e.g.,* primary care nurse, utilization review nurse), physicians, clinical social worker, physical therapist, occupational therapist, and speech therapist. A vocational counselor, neuropsychologist, or representative from other disciplines is involved as necessary. All disciplines work collaboratively in the discharge planning process. Each patient's record is reviewed to determine needs for discharge planning. Team members provide input, and the clinical social worker or discharge planner and primary nurse work to together to develop a plan.

The nurse and clinical social worker strive to function as "co-discharge planners." The primary nurse has expertise in subacute and home nursing care needs and medical equipment. The primary nurse may want to involve a clinical nurse specialist in preparing the patient and family for discharge. The clinical nurse specialist has knowledge and skills in educating the patient, family, and team about the specific impact of the disease or injury on the patient and family. Because patients leave acute care "sicker and quicker," the clinical nurse specialist plays a vital role in training the patient and family to assume care (*e.g.,* tube feedings, injections). The clinical social worker has expertise in available resources for providing care, mechanisms for accessing needed care, and financing issues. The clinical social worker identifies barriers to a smooth discharge plan and collaborates with the team to seek solutions. The clinical social worker provides counseling, support, and education regarding advanced directives and coping with illness. The responsibilities of the nurses and the clinical social worker are shared and sometimes overlap. This can lead to role strain if roles and responsibilities are not clearly discussed and negotiated in each situation.[5]

The effectiveness of discharge planning depends on the conceptualization of discharge planning within the institution, the discharge planning program developed, the resources committed to the program, and the quality control and evaluative mechanisms incorporated in the process. How discharge planning is viewed by the health professionals and administration of the facility will shape the type of discharge planning program developed. The program includes the philosophy, objectives, and specific protocols developed to implement the steps of the discharge planning process. Whatever the program may be, it must be workable and realistic for that facility, and it must be supported by the commitment of the individuals and administration involved to make it a viable and effective process.

THE STEPS OF DISCHARGE PLANNING

The steps of discharge planning follow the usual flow of steps in any schemata of logical problem solving. The steps include (1) assessment of the patient and family; (2) analysis of data to identify specific patient and family needs; (3) planning to meet patient and family needs (*e.g.,* exploration of appropriate resources, development of a patient teaching plan); (4) implementation of the plan, including actual transfer; and (5) evaluation of the discharge planning process and the results.[6] Even though the steps in the process have been identified as distinct, there is much overlap, with simultaneous activity occurring in the process (Fig. 15-1). In the last few years, these phases have been collapsed as managed care has shortened acute care stays.

Assessment of the Patient and Family

Discharge planning begins the moment the patient enters the health care system; the initial patient assessment begins the process. Assessment is an ongoing process in which the database is constantly being refined, clarified, validated, and updated. Data are analyzed frequently to determine their significance. They may point out the need for the collection of other data, or they may be of sufficient magnitude to merit immediate planning and implementation of action because the patient has been identified as a high-risk patient with complex needs to be addressed.[7]

The significance of some data may be impossible to determine in some instances, particularly for the unstable or acutely ill patient. It is impossible to predict long-term needs when the impact of illness on the physical, cognitive, emotional, psychosocial, financial, and vocational status of a person are uncertain. However, the knowledge and experience of the health care professional will help in anticipating patient needs and projecting implications. Although in some instances, a "wait and see" attitude is assumed, the involvement of health professionals from other disciplines is helpful when monitoring potential patient and family needs. Once the patient is well stabilized, discharge planning can proceed in a more certain and organized manner.

Analysis of Data to Identify Specific Patient and Family Needs

Data analysis is an ongoing process because the practitioner must determine the significance and priority of that information. Some information does require immediate action, but

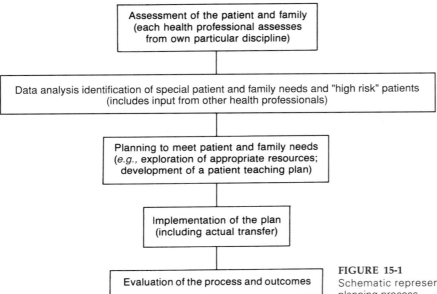

FIGURE 15-1
Schematic representation of the steps involved in the discharge planning process.

most data contribute to a body of information that should be analyzed systematically. Each professional health care discipline collects and analyzes its data and is responsible for sharing its expertise with professionals from other disciplines to work collaboratively in developing a comprehensive discharge plan.

The systematic analysis and sharing of information may be done in several ways, such as through consultation, multidisciplinary rounds, weekly unit or interdisciplinary conferences, and written and computerized patient records. The records include progress notes, referral forms (interagency referral forms), consultations, and checklist evaluation tools. It is important to develop an effective mechanism for written documentation of the discharge planning process to keep everyone involved updated and to facilitate reimbursement and quality assurance review.

Planning to Meet Patient and Family Needs

Once the specific patient and family needs have been identified, possible alternatives and resources in the community and health care system can be considered. It is most important for the patient and family to be an integral part of the process. Often, various alternatives must be explored to determine what best meets the needs identified and which approach is most acceptable to the patient and family. To be effective, the discharge plan must be individualized, realistic, and acceptable to the patient and family.

If the patient needs placement in an extended care facility, nursing home, or rehabilitation center, a member of the discharge planning department can suggest appropriate facilities in the area that can meet the patient's needs. A site visit can be arranged for the patient or family to assess the facility and talk with staff members. Cost, types of programs offered, distance of the facility from home, and other considerations need to be weighed when making a decision about placement. Pa-

tients may require referral to community resources for particular needs. Referral forms or telephone contacts are usually necessary to make these arrangements.

For patients and families who need patient teaching, a detailed written teaching plan is developed (see Chap. 14).

Implementation of the Plan (Including Actual Transfer)

Once a discharge plan has been developed, many activities need to be set in motion and coordinated to ensure a smooth transition to another facility or home. One person must assume the responsibility for the coordination of the plan and for keeping all involved people informed, including the patient and family. Team conferences and conferences that include the patient and family are very helpful.

The day of discharge is a culmination of the efforts and cooperation of many people. The patient has been prepared emotionally and psychologically for the transition, but most patients will nevertheless demonstrate some degree of transfer anxiety. By reassuring patients that they are ready and able to make the transition, the nurse can provide support for a smooth transition. The day of discharge can be a bittersweet experience for the staff who have worked with the patient, especially if the patient has been hospitalized for a long time. The caregivers must deal with their own feelings about the closure of the relationship.

Evaluation of the Discharge Planning Process and the Results

It is important to evaluate what is of value in the discharge planning program and process at a facility and what needs to be changed or fine tuned. Such an evaluation focuses on the opinions of the health professional involved in the process. It is also important to evaluate the process as perceived by the patient, family, and transfer agency. This is accomplished by follow-up telephone calls, conversations, visits from patients, visits by staff to the other facility, and evaluation forms. Evaluation is important for providing quality and continuity of care in the most cost-effective means possible. The feedback collected provides the data to make necessary changes in the process and helps to evaluate the quality of the extended care facility to which the patient has been transferred.

Necessary Conditions for Effective Discharge Planning—A Summary

A few basic principles can help to guide the process of discharge planning:

- Incorporation of discharge planning as an integral part of delivery of care within the objectives of the institution
- Incorporation of the responsibility for anticipating a patient's posthospital needs within all professional roles; should be written into job descriptions and fulfillment demonstrated
- Delegation of responsibility to the staff nurse or primary nurse to initiate the formal discharge planning process in enough time to allow for effective discharge planning
- Use of a multidisciplinary, collaborative approach to discharge planning
- Development of effective mechanisms and tools for communication among the patient, the family, health professionals, and others to implement the discharge planning process
- Written documentation of the steps involved in the discharge planning process and the various communications involved

APPLICATION OF THE PROCESS TO NEUROLOGICALLY IMPAIRED PATIENTS

The process of discharge planning often increases in complexity when it is applied to neurologically impaired patients because they have many complex and multifaceted needs. The discharge planning process may involve multitrauma patients who have sustained injury, not only to the nervous system, but also to other body systems: patients with head injury or spinal cord injuries; with neurological degenerative diseases, such as multiple sclerosis and amyotrophic lateral sclerosis; with neurological deficits from infectious processes; with central nervous system neoplasms; and others. The specific needs of each patient must be assessed separately and the discharge planning process individualized.

The process of discharge planning may need to be organized differently for neurological patients than for patients with other problems, although the steps in discharge planning are the same. As with any process, the steps involved are not compartmentalized, and there is simultaneous activity in multiple steps, even though the major focus may be on one particular step. Shorter hospital stays require acceleration of all processes, including discharge planning.

Assessment

It is often necessary for the neuroscience patient to be managed by a multidisciplinary team. The nursing staff collects an admission history and conducts ongoing assessments. For patients with neurological motor impairment, an assessment and treatment plan are developed by the physical therapist. The clinical social worker completes a comprehensive psychosocial assessment usually within 24 to 48 hours of admission. A pool of information exists to begin to predict special needs, rehabilitative potential, and expected outcomes for the patient.

Once the patient is medically stabilized, the extent and degree of deficits and needs can be validated with greater certainty. Consultation and evaluation by other health professionals (*e.g.*, the occupational therapist) can be requested to provide a complete database for discharge planning.

Data Analysis

The database is analyzed first by a practitioner from each discipline to consider the implications for that discipline. The information then needs to be analyzed by the team members collaboratively to consider interdisciplinary implications and how the information will be used in the overall discharge planning process. Data analysis is undertaken in conferences within the discipline and is considered during discharge planning rounds. Written documentation and plans should be available. Once data are analyzed and problems are identified, the next logical step is planning to deal with the problem.

Early Identification of Difficult Placement Problems

Certain socioeconomic and health issues render some patients difficult to place for extended care in facilities or in the community. These patients include those who are uninsured, the homeless, drug abusers, patients with acquired immunodeficiency syndrome, and those with dysfunctional families or without families. A patient admitted with a head injury may also have a concurrent cocaine abuse problem. Aftercare must include provisions for special needs, such as drug abuse rehabilitation, and consideration of the primary problem and deficits associated with the health injury.

Early identification of patients who are high risk and are difficult placement problems is important so that the multiple issues related to their care can be addressed early. This may require application for a Medicare or Medicaid number or other complicated processes that take time.

Planning

Planning, like other steps in the discharge process, is ongoing and collaborative. Planning is based on identification of short- and long-range realistic goals. The short-term goals become the steps for achieving long-range goals. The plan must be flexible to accommodate the changes that are apt to occur in the patient. It is impossible to predict with certainty the degree of recovery that can occur when a nervous system is injured. At times, the amount of improvement is a pleasant surprise, whereas with other patients, hopes for improvement are not realized. Therefore, the health team members must be able to readjust the discharge plan based on changes in the patient's condition and a realistic appraisal of potential outcomes.

Conferences with team members or with the patient and family are the usual methods for planning. It must be emphasized that inclusion of the patient and family is an absolute necessity for effective discharge planning. The plan for discharge should be documented in writing and updated as necessary. A reasonable time frame should be developed so that there is adequate time to complete activities, such as patient and family teaching.

Implementation

Implementation of the discharge plan involves the collaborative effort of many individuals working together to actualize the plan. A team member, often the social worker, will contact a potential transfer facility if the patient needs to be placed in a long-term or rehabilitative hospital or nursing home. Many times, a clinician from the transfer facility will visit patients to assess the feasibility of their transfer. Rehabilitation beds are scarce, and the patient must be able to benefit from the rehabilitation program offered by the facility to make transfer worthwhile. The clinician assessing the patient may decide if (1) the patient is a good candidate for the facility and is ready for transfer; (2) the patient is a good candidate but is not ready for transfer and another assessment of the patient should be scheduled in a few weeks; or (3) the patient is not a good candidate for transfer to the facility. In the case of aggressive rehabilitation programs, the patient must be alert, oriented, and able to retain information; follow simple instructions; and cooperate with caregivers to benefit from the rehabilitation program. After acceptance for transfer, it is helpful for the patient or a family member to visit the facility and talk with staff members before transfer plans are formalized, if this is feasible.

Once the transfer is formalized, information about the patient must be shared by the nursing staffs to promote continuity of care. This may be accomplished through meetings, telephone calls, or written referral forms. Most often, all three methods of communication are used. The physician will communicate with the accepting physician to provide necessary information relating to the medical management. For the patient who is going home, arrangements should be made well in advance for any necessary equipment. If community agencies will provide services, these arrangements should also be made.

The patient and family must be prepared emotionally and psychologically for the transfer. Transfer can be very frightening to the patient who has been hospitalized for an extended period. Therefore, much reassurance must be provided as the day approaches. Support groups in the community may be helpful to the patient or family. One such group is the National Head Injury Foundation, which has chapters throughout the country. Information about the purposes of such an organization and how to contact it should be provided. Printed materials, visuals, and small group conferences with other patients and families may be helpful. A discharge handbook or other form of printed material is especially useful because the patient or family member can read it at leisure and then ask questions as necessary.

As caregivers, health professionals often experience mixed emotions about the discharge of a patient for whom they have cared. Many patients with neurological dysfunction are hospitalized for extended periods, with the result that strong bonds are forged between patients and caregivers. Health professionals should recognize and deal with their feelings about the transfer of the patient.

Evaluation

Evaluation is a critical component in quality assurance. Health team members should evaluate the discharge planning process to identify any areas that need to be changed or improved. This can be done during team conferences or through periodic written review. Another focus of evaluation is patient and family satisfaction and benefit from treatment. This information can be collected in a follow-up contact. The quality of the discharge planning system should be monitored through a hospital-wide quality assurance program.

Summary

Discharge planning is a complex process of problem solving and ongoing independent and collaborative activities and communication directed at helping the patient make a smooth transition from one environment to another without negating any progress already made. The new environment may be home or an extended care facility that will provide continued care based on unmet needs of the patient. Throughout the discharge planning process, health professionals work with the patient and family to achieve mutually accepted and specific goals. Unless the health team, patient, and family share mutual and congruent goals, there will be confusion, frustration, discouragement, and fragmentation of effort. If this happens, the patient will not reach his or her optimal rehabilitation potential.

References

1. Ellers, B., & Walker, J. D. (1993). Facilitating the transition out of the hospital. In M. Gerteis, S. Edgman-Levitan, J. Daily, & T. L. Delbanco (Eds.), *Through the patient's eyes: Understanding and promoting patient-centered care.* (pp. 204–223). San Francisco: Jossey-Bass Publishers.
2. Shine, M. S. (1983). Discharge planning for the elderly patient in the acute care setting. *Nursing Clinics of North America, 18*(3), 403–410.
3. Keigher, S. M. (1995). Managed care's silent seduction of America and the new politics of choice. *Health and Social Work, 20*(2), 53–59.
4. Wallace, R. M. (1995). Personal communication. May 31.
5. Egan, M., & Kadushin, G. (1995). Competitive allies: Rural nurses' and social workers' perception of the social work role in the hospital setting. *Social Work in Health Care, 20*(3), 1–24.
6. McKeehan, K. M. (Ed.) (1981). *Continuing care: A multidisciplinary approach to discharge planning.* St. Louis: C.V. Mosby.
7. Rock, B. D., Beckerman, A., Auerback, C., Cohen, C., Goldstein, M., & Quitkin, E. (1995). Management of alternative level of care patient

using a computerized database. *Health and Social Work, 20*(2), 133–139.

Bibliography

Books

Cohen, E. L., & Cesta, T. G. (1993). *Nursing case management: From concept to evaluation.* St. Louis: C.V. Mosby.

Rorden, J. W. (1990). *Discharge planning guide for nurses.* Philadelphia: W.B. Saunders.

Periodicals

Gilmartin, M. (1994). Transition from the intensive care unit to home: Patient selection and discharge planning. *Respiratory Care, 39*(5), 456–480.

Houghton, B. A. (1994). Discharge planners and cost containment. *Nursing Management, 25*(4), 78–80.

Pray, D., & Hoff, J. (1992). Implementing a multidisciplinary approach to discharge planning. *Nursing Management, 23*(10), 52–52, 56.

Weinstein, R. (1991). Hospital case management: The path to empowering nurses. *Pediatric Nursing, 17*(3), 289–293.

Section 4

Special Considerations in Neuroscience Nursing

CHAPTER 16

Management of the Unconscious Patient

Joanne V. Hickey

Unconsciousness is a physiological and psychological state in which the patient is unresponsive to sensory stimuli and lacks awareness of self and the environment. Primary lesions of the central nervous system or dysfunction of other body organs can result in unconsciousness. The depth and duration of unconsciousness span a broad spectrum of presentations from fainting, with momentary loss of consciousness, to prolonged coma lasting weeks or months. The term coma is reserved for a clinical presentation in which the state of unconsciousness is maintained for a prolonged period, from hours to months. The pathophysiological basis for coma is damage in both cerebral hemispheres or damage to the brain stem or both. (See Chap. 8 for discussion of coma.) In addition, metabolic disorders can lead to coma by interfering with the normal cellular metabolic environment of neurons.

In neuroscience nursing practice, the nurse often cares for patients who are unconscious for prolonged periods. Unconscious patients are immobilized and in the supine position most of the time. The physiological consequences of short- and long-term immobilization predispose that person to functional decline and reduced quality of life. Not only does patient survival directly depend on the quality of care provided, but the realization of optimal rehabilitation potential hinges on the quality of nursing care. In addition to managing the primary neurological problem, the nurse must also incorporate a rehabilitation framework to maintain intact function, prevent complications and disabilities, and restore function to the degree possible.

The purpose of this chapter is to provide a basic nursing care framework for the unconscious, immobilized patient to achieve optimal patient outcomes and to include specific points of care relative to the management of the neuroscience patient. Not all that is discussed will be found on clinical pathways because it is assumed that meticulous detailed care will be provided. However, unless a standard is set, outcomes cannot be measured. Key points of the standard of care for the unconscious patient are outlined in this chapter. (See Chart 16-1 for a sample nursing care plan.)

MOBILITY AND IMMOBILITY

Kinesis, a word of Greek origin, means motion, or to move. The human body is designed for physical activity and movement. Moderate activity contributes to health, whereas lack of activity, regardless of reason, leads to multisystem deconditioning and physiological changes along a continuum. Bed rest was first recognized in the 1860s as a therapeutic modality. The therapeutic value of bed rest includes decreased oxygen consumption, prevention or reduction of trauma to a body part, and redirection of allocation of energy resources toward healing.[1] Immobility has also been described as the most potentially dangerous treatment prescribed today.[2]

Immobility is a disuse phenomenon that results in interrelated physiological and psychosocial effects. The morbidity of immobility is directly associated with the length of time of immobilization and other patient risk factors. Some physiological effects occur immediately on institution of bed rest, whereas other physiological and pathophysiological changes occur over a longer time. Therefore, although there are physiological changes with short periods (*e.g.,* 1–3 days) of immobility, they are less severe and may be reversible. Prolonged periods of immobility, which often occur with coma, spinal cord injury, or Guillain-Barreé syndrome, result in pathophysiological changes associated with serious morbidity and permanent disabilities. Risk factors that increase the probability of serious complications from immobility include length and degree of immobility, incontinence, poor nutrition, hypotension, infection, altered motor or sensory function, multiorgan failure, obesity, advanced age, and comorbidity. The elderly are particularly vulnerable to the deleterious effects of immobility.

(text continues on page 284)

CHART 16-1
Nursing Care Plan for the Unconscious Patient

Nursing Diagnosis	Nursing Intervention(s)	Outcome Criteria
Self-Care Deficit: R/T immobility and unconsciousness* Self-care deficit syndrome: —Bathing/Hygiene —Dressing/Grooming —Feeding —Toileting	• Provide basic hygienic care. • Dress and groom patient. • Provide nutritional support by alternate means (total parenteral nutrition; tube feeding), as ordered by the physician. • Provide for the elimination needs of the patient.	• Basic self-care needs will be provided for by the nursing staff.
Risk for Disuse Syndrome: R/T immobility/unconsciousness	See specific system, problem, and interventions.	• The multisystem effects of immobility will be recognized and minimized with appropriate interventions.
Respiratory Function		
Risk for Altered Respiratory Function: R/T immobility	• Apply preventive strategies to maintain respiratory function and prevent deconditioning and complications. • Conduct a risk assessment of respiratory function.	• Respiratory function will be maintained.
Risk for Aspiration	• Conduct a risk assessment. • Maintain a patent airway by suctioning prn. • Do not feed if patient has problems with swallowing. • Position to facilitate oral drainage. • Follow precautions to prevent enteral feeding aspiration.	• Patient will not aspirate.
• Ineffective Airway Clearance: R/T immobility and ineffective cough reflex	• Keep the patient's neck in a neutral position. • In the neurological patient, limit suctioning to 15 seconds or less. • If the patient has a tracheostomy tube in place, administer trachoestomy care every 4 h. • Position the patient in the lateral recumbent position on one side; reposition every 1 to 2 h. • Elevate the head of the bed, if possible.	• A patent airway will be maintained. • Drainage of secretions from the oropharynx will be facilitated.
• Ineffective Breathing Pattern: R/T immobility and underlying neurological problem(s)	• Monitor the rate, depth, and pattern of respirations frequently. • Monitor tidal volume and blood gas levels. • Observe the patient frequently for signs and symptoms of respiratory distress.	• The patient will establish and maintain an effective breathing pattern.

(continued)

CHART 16-1 Nursing Care Plan for the Unconscious Patient (Continued)

Nursing Diagnosis	Nursing Intervention(s)	Outcome Criteria
	• Auscultate the patient's chest frequently. • Elevate the head of the bed if possible. • Position the patient properly to facilitate respirations. For patients maintained on a ventilator: • Monitor the patient's synchrony or asynchrony on the respirator; report asynchrony to the physician.	
• Impaired Gas Exchange: R/T immobility	• Turn the patient at least every 2 h. • Provide for periodic chest physiotherapy. • Monitor the patient for cyanosis and respiratory distress. • Hyperinflate the patient's lungs with 100% oxygen before and after suctioning (with approval of the physician). • Administer oxygen as ordered. • Use an Ambu bag on the patient every 1 to 2 h. • Auscultate the patient's chest every 2 h.	• The patient will be free of signs of cyanosis and respiratory distress.
Cardiovascular Function		
• Cardiac output, altered: R/T immobility	• Monitor vital signs frequently. • Monitor the rate, rhythm, and quality of the patient's radial and apical pulses. • Document any arrhythmias. • If a cardiac monitor is being used, observe the monitor every $\frac{1}{2}$ to 1 h. • Note any correlations between pulse and blood pressure, and make appropriate observations.	• Cardiac output will be maintained within safe limits.
• Altered Peripheral Tissue Perfusion: R/T immobility	• Apply thigh-high elastic stockings and sequential compression air boots. • When placing the patient in a lateral recumbent position, position the upper leg so that it will not cause extreme pressure on the lower leg. • Do not use the foot gatch under the patient's knees. • Do not apply pillows or constricting objects to the backs of the patient's knees.	• Adequate peripheral perfusion will be maintained. • Dependent edema will not develop in the arms.

(continued)

CHART 16-1 Nursing Care Plan for the Unconscious Patient (Continued)

Nursing Diagnosis	Nursing Intervention(s)	Outcome Criteria
• Altered Cerebral Tissue Perfusion: R/T immobility	• Position the patient so the distal end of the extremity will be elevated. • Monitor the patient for signs of deep vein thrombosis. • Maintain the patient's head and neck in a neutral position. • Elevate the head of the bed 30–45 degrees. • Avoid positions that are known to cause a rise in intracranial pressure (*e.g.,* hip flexion, prone). • If an intracranial pressure monitor is being used, observe the monitor periodically for a rise in pressure. • Do not cluster nursing activities; let the pressure fall before beginning another procedure. • Maintain normothermia. • Provide "soft" stimuli (*e.g.,* soft music, family voices).	• Adequate cerebral perfusion pressure will be maintained.
Integumentary System		
• Risk for Impaired Skin Integrity: R/T immobility	• Provide skin care frequently (daily baths; mouth, back, and perineal care every 4 h). • Lubricate dry skin with cream or lanolin. • Lubricate the patient's lips. • Use nonallergenic or burn linen on the bed if the patient develops a rash or irritation from the bed linen. • Observe every square inch of skin at least every shift, some areas more frequently. • Do not position the patient on reddened areas of skin. • Check the patient's ears, elbows, and heels carefully for signs of skin breakdown. • If patient has a nasogastric or endotracheal tube taped to the mouth, remove the tape daily, wash the skin, and protect it with tincture of benzoin. Do not apply new tape in the same place. • Keep the patient's heels off the bed at all times.	

(continued)

CHART 16-1 Nursing Care Plan for the Unconscious Patient (Continued)

Nursing Diagnosis	Nursing Intervention(s)	Outcome Criteria
• Risk for Impaired Tissue Integrity (corneal): R/T immobility	• Cut and file fingernails and toenails. • Turn and reposition the patient at least every 2 h. • Inspect the eyes every 4 h for signs of irritation. • Position the patient on his or her side so that there is no possibility of eye or corneal irritation. • Cleanse the eyes frequently with normal saline and cotton balls. • Instill lubricating drops every 3 h. • Apply an eye shield over the eye, as necessary.	• Skin will remain intact. • The tissue of the eye will be maintained; corneal ulceration will not develop.
• Altered Oral Mucous Membrane: R/T dryness, decreased saliva	• Provide oral hygiene every 2–4 h. • Brush the patient's teeth once every shift. • Monitor the patient's mouth for lesions, dryness, or bleeding.	• The oral mucosa will remain intact and free of dryness, lesions, and white coating (tongue).

Musculoskeletal Function

Nursing Diagnosis	Nursing Intervention(s)	Outcome Criteria
• Impaired Physical Mobility: R/T immobility and underlying neurological problem(s) causing paresis, paralysis, or rigidity	• Administer passive range-of-motion exercises at least four times a day. • Position the patient in proper body alignment; reposition every 2 h. Use rolls, pillows, and the like as needed. Apply splints, if ordered. • Reposition decorticate or decerebrate patients every hour; control noxious stimuli that may increase the tendency for abnormal positioning. • Collaborate with the physical therapist. • Use splints, slings, a trochanter roll, or pillows to support affected extremities. • Apply sneakers or other supportive shoes as necessary.	• Movement of the joints will be maintained, and contracture will be prevented.
• Risk for Trauma; Stress fracture and joint dislocation	• Administer passive range-of-motion exercises at least four times a day. • Position in proper body alignment. • Provide rolls and pillow to maintain position. • Do not pull or tug on joints.	• No stress fractures or joint dislocations will occur.

(continued)

CHART 16-1 Nursing Care Plan for the Unconscious Patient (Continued)

Nursing Diagnosis	Nursing Intervention(s)	Outcome Criteria
Genitourinary Function		
• Altered Urinary Elimination: R/T immobility: —Incontinence —Retention —Large amounts of residual urine	• Monitor intake and output. • If an indwelling catheter is in place, maintain a closed system, and follow protocol for catheter care. • Remove the catheter as soon as possible. • Assess the intermittent catheterization program. • Provide perineal care. • Palpate the bladder to check for distention.	• The bladder will be emptied.
• Risk for Infection: R/T immobility —Urinary tract infection —Urinary stasis —Urinary calculi	• Follow strict aseptic technique in the care of the patient's catheter. • Remove the catheter as soon as possible. • Keep the patient's urine acidic. • Monitor urine pH. • Turn the patient from side to side. • Monitor urinalysis and urine culture and sensitivity results. • Monitor the patient and urinary output for signs and symptoms of infection.	• Factors contributing to infection will be considered and controlled when providing care.
Gastrointestinal Function		
• Altered Bowel Elimination: R/T immobility	• Monitor and record the frequency of bowel movements. • Monitor the characteristics of the stool. • Auscultate the patient's abdomen for bowel sounds. • Initiate a bowel program.	• Stools will be soft and formed. • Bowels will be evacuated every 1–3 d.
Neurological Function		
• Hyperthermia: R/T underlying neurological problem(s) or infection	• Monitor the patient's temperature periodically. • Remove excess clothing and top linen. • Provide sponge baths. • Use order for hyperthermia blanket. • Consider the underlying reasons for hyperthermia; implement appropriate interventions.	• Normothermia will be achieved and maintained.

(continued)

CHART 16-1 Nursing Care Plan for the Unconscious Patient (Continued)

Nursing Diagnosis	Nursing Intervention(s)	Outcome Criteria
• Sensory/Perceptual Alterations: R/T unconsciousness —Auditory —Gustatory —Kinesthetic —Olfactory —Tactile —Visual	• Provide sensory stimuli while caring for the patient by providing tactile stimulation, talking to the patient and telling him or her what is being done, and addressing the patient by name. • Structure sensory input by telling the patient in a clear, concise manner about surroundings, treatments, procedures, and policies. • Turn on the radio, TV, or tape recorder when no one is with the patient. • Use reality orientation techniques. • Use orientation instruments, such as a clock, calendar, window, favorite objects, or family pictures. • Encourage the family to touch and talk to the patient. • Promote social interactions. • Stimulate as many of the patient's senses as possible.	• Multisensory stimuli will be provided throughout the day.
Nutrition and Hydration		
• Altered Nutrition: Less than body requirements: R/T unconsciousness	• Monitor the patient's weight at least twice a week and record. • Maintain a daily calorie count. • Request a nutritional consultation. • Collaborate with the physician regarding a nutritional consult and nutrition orders as soon as the patient is stabilized. • Maintain an accurate intake and output record.	• Adequate nutrition will be provided. • An appropriate weight level will be maintained.
• Fluid Volume Deficit: R/T unconsciousness	• Maintain an accurate intake and output record. • Monitor skin turgor and mucous membranes for dryness. • Monitor vital signs, urine specific gravity, and serum osmolarity values.	• Adequate fluid volume will be maintained.

* R/T, related to

Minimal Physiological Mobility Requirement

Mobility is a topic of extensive study. The normal healthy adult changes position on average every 11.6 minutes during sleep; this physiological requirement for movement is termed the **minimal physiological mobility requirement**. Immobilized, bed-ridden patients can no longer move because of their disability, and the multiple complications of immobility begin to develop within hours, progressing along a continuum of early to late problems. The complications of immobility that affect the skin and respiratory, cardiovascular, gastrointestinal (GI), musculoskeletal, genitourinary, and nervous systems are well known. However, efforts to prevent the ravages of immobility have resulted in varying degrees of success despite the best efforts of many nurses and physicians.

SPECIAL BEDS FOR THE IMMOBILIZED PATIENT

Special beds have been designed to reduce the complications of immobility. These beds are especially helpful for the patient who is at high risk for skin breakdown and pressure ulcers from the constant pressure on the body caused by bed rest. A number of beds, marketed under the trade names of Kin-Air, BioDyne, Effica, Restcue, and others, are available. Each manufacturer offers special features that may be of particular value to patients depending on their individual needs. The cost effectiveness of ordering a special bed must be considered. Managed care plans and hospitals have established criteria for identifying high-risk patients for whom special beds will be helpful and cost effective. Institutional guidelines should be followed in the selection and use of such beds.

THE BASIS FOR NURSING MANAGEMENT OF THE UNCONSCIOUS PATIENT

Clinical reasoning is based on a systematic assessment of the unconscious patient to identify nursing diagnoses and collaborative problems and develop interventions. Because the patient is immobilized and multiple body systems are threatened, the *nursing diagnosis* of **Risk for Disuse Syndrome** and **Self-Care Deficit Syndrome** can be used to encompass all systems. The specific nursing diagnoses applicable for self-care deficits include **Feeding, Bathing/Hygiene, Dressing/Grooming, Toileting,** and **Instrumental Self Care Deficits**. In addition to nursing diagnoses, a number of *collaborative problems* are applicable.

Respiratory Function

Assuming the supine position causes physiological changes in the mechanics of breathing and in some lung volumes. Mechanical restriction occurs as a result of decreased overall respiratory muscle strength and a reduction of intercostal, diaphragmatic, and abdominal muscle excursion in supine breathing with a consequent decrease in thoracic volume. In normal people, tidal breathing in the upright position is pre-dominantly due to rib cage movement, while in the supine position, abdominal muscles predominate. Maximal inspiration capacity is decreased, resulting in a decrease in vital and functional respiratory capacities.[3]

All lung volumes decrease except for tidal volume. The decrease in thoracic size and increase in intrathoracic blood volume associated with the supine position cause a decrease in residual volume and functional residual capacity (FRC).[4] Normally, FRC is greater than closing volume to maintain an open airway. When the FRC is exceeded by the closing volume, the partial or complete closure of lung units causes atelectasis and regional differences in ventilation-perfusion ratio (V/Q mismatch), poorly ventilated and overly perfused areas, and arteriovenous shunts. If increased metabolic demands occur, hypoxia results.[5]

In addition, impaired mucociliary function causes mucous secretions to accumulate in the dependent respiratory bronchioli, which contributes to the development of atelectasis and hypostatic pneumonia.

ASSESSMENT

Respiratory function is assessed by a number of parameters: airway patency; rate, quality, and pattern of respirations; chest auscultation; and objective signs of oxygenation. The highest priority in managing a patient is assigned to airway patency. **Airway patency**, openness of the upper airway (nose, mouth, pharynx, and trachea), provides the route for air exchange. Obstruction of the airway may be caused by tissue injury, edema, mucus, or other drainage. The patient's ability to maintain a patent airway is assessed frequently.

Clinical evidence of an ineffective breathing pattern includes apnea, dyspnea, shortness of breath, stridor, rapid or shallow respirations, a prolonged expiration or inspiration phase, nasal flaring, pursed lips, intercostal or substernal retraction, abdominal breathing, and altered chest expansion.

Assess and monitor the following:

- Airway patency
- Rate, quality, and pattern of respirations
- Adventitious breath sounds by chest auscultation
- Correlation of findings of recent chest x-ray with clinical findings
- Amount and characteristics of airway secretions (for infection)
- Capillary refill and subtle cyanosis or dustiness in periorbital area, ear lobes, and fingernails
- Oxygen saturation with an oximeter
- Periodic blood gases
- Lung volumes and respiratory mechanics

RESPIRATORY PROBLEMS

The unconscious patient is at high risk for developing respiratory problems. The secondary effect of compromised respiratory function is cerebral hypoxia, which leads to further neurological deterioration unless the early signs and symptoms of respiratory insufficiency are recognized and interventions initiated expeditiously. The respiratory problems to be considered include airway obstruction, aspiration, atelectasis, and pneumonia. Other conditions seen in relation to trauma and intracranial hemorrhage are neurogenic pulmonary edema, adult respiratory distress syndrome, and disseminated intravascular coagulation; these conditions are discussed in Chapters 12 and 20.

Airway Obstruction. In the unconscious patient, a partially or completely obstructed airway can occur because of mucus or plugging of other foreign materials or posterior displacement of oropharyngeal soft-tissue structures, particularly the tongue, as a result of improper positioning of the head and neck.[6] The comatose patient is unable to reposition the head and neck to maintain airway patency. Other mechanical deficits affecting respiratory structures include postanesthesia recovery phase insufficiency, airway edema following extubation, and diaphragmatic or intercostal muscle paralysis related to spinal cord injury or neuromuscular diseases. The possible results of airway obstruction include alveolar hypoventilation, hypoxia, hypercarbia, increased respiratory rate, and atelectasis. The early signs and symptoms observed are shallow and noisy respirations, increased secretions from the mouth, and restlessness.

Aspiration. The unconscious patient is unable to protect the airway and therefore is at high risk for aspiration of foreign materials, such as pharyngeal secretions or regurgitated gastric contents. In the unconscious patient, passive regurgitation and microaspiration, rather than actual vomiting of gastric contents, is likely to occur, resulting in a chemical pneumonitis. Aspiration of tube feedings from a dislodged feeding tube or vomiting from a distended stomach can also lead to aspiration pneumonia.

Atelectasis and Pneumonia. Atelectasis, a state of alveolar collapse in a segment of pulmonary tissue, has long been known to be a consequence of prolonged bed rest and immobility. The concurrent stasis and pooling of secretions collect in the depended position, leading to hypostatic pneumonia and creating a medium ripe for bacterial growth. If the patient is dehydrated or receiving drugs that effect the tenacity of the secretions, bacteria can rapidly develop. In addition, patients are at high risk for nosocomial infections as a result compromised immunological state and colonization of the endotracheal tube.

The following are common related nursing diagnoses:

- Ineffective Airway Clearance
- Ineffective Breathing Pattern
- Impaired Gas Exchange
- Dysfunctional Ventilatory Weaning Response
- Risk for Aspiration
- Risk for Altered Respiratory Function
- Risk for Infection
- Risk for Impaired Swallowing Response

The following are common related collaborative problems:

- Hypoxemia
- Atelectasis, pneumonia

NURSING INTERVENTIONS

Nursing interventions are aimed at maintaining a patent airway and facilitating adequate respirations.

Airway Patency. A patent airway is the highest priority. The unconscious patient is defenseless against threats to a patent airway, particularly if the cough reflex is absent. In these patients and in conscious patients who do not have an intact cough reflex and are therefore at high risk for aspiration, suctioning will be necessary. If there is evidence of inability to protect the airway, then an endotracheal tube is urgently needed to prevent aspiration and the risk of infection due to aspiration. If unconsciousness is prolonged and the patient continues to need an artificial airway, a tracheostomy tube will be needed.

Oxygenation of the Lungs. Because an unconscious patient cannot respond to instructions to take deep breaths, alternative methods are used to improve total lung expansion and prevent pooling or stasis of secretions in the lungs. If allowed to develop, these conditions can lead to atelectasis or hypostatic and bacterial pneumonia. An Ambu bag can be used for a few minutes every hour to expand and oxygenate the patient's lungs, thus eliminating dead air space that could lead to pneumonia or atelectasis.

Positioning. Placing the unconscious, immobile, or weak patient in a lateral recumbent position promotes drainage of secretions, facilitates respirations, prevents pooling of secretions, and prevents the tongue from obstructing the airway. The patient should be turned from side to side at least every 2 hours to prevent pooling of secretions (Fig. 16-1). Unconscious patients are never positioned on their backs because of the risk of soft-tissue obstruction of the airway and the threat of aspiration.

Unless contraindicated, the patient's head should be elevated and turned to the side to facilitate drainage of secretions when lying in bed. If hemiplegia is present, the patient may be positioned on the paralyzed side, but special care and careful observations must be instituted to prevent injury (to soft tissue and nerves), edema, or any compromise of the vascular supply, particularly in the limbs. Because vasomotor tone is decreased in the affected area, adverse effects from improper positioning can develop rapidly. In this case, the patient may need to be turned more frequently than every 2 hours.

Suctioning. Periodic oropharyngeal or tracheal suctioning may be necessary to clear the airway of mucus, blood, or other drainage. When suctioning, the patient's head is turned from side to side (unless contraindicated) so that each bronchus can be suctioned. A patient should not be suctioned nasally if there is any possibility of a basal skull fracture or cerebrospinal fluid drainage from the nose or ear. In a patient with increased intracranial pressure, suctioning must be limited to 15 seconds or less. This is important to prevent hypercapnia, a known potent cerebrovascular vasodilating condition that increases intracranial pressure. The lungs are oxygenated (using an Ambu bag) with 100% oxygen with a few breaths before and after suctioning to control hypoxia and hypercapnia. (A patient with chronic obstructive lung disease should not receive

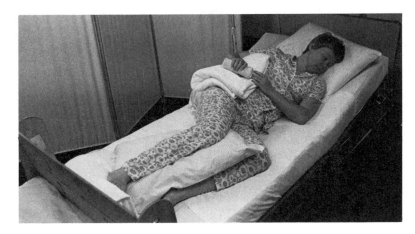

FIGURE 16-1
Positioning the unconscious patient.

100% oxygen; a lower concentration is used.) Suction equipment should be checked at the beginning of every shift and maintained in a ready state for immediate use.

Meticulous Aseptic Technique. Strict aseptic technique should be followed to prevent nosocomial infections. Patients may be immunocompromised from drug therapy and severe illness.

Other. Managing a patient on a ventilator and ventilator weaning are discussed in Chapter 12.

Cardiovascular Function

Physiological changes in cardiovascular function associated with immobility include increased cardiac workload and heart rate, decreased cardiac output, decreased stroke volume, increased peripheral vascular resistance, and decreased blood pressure.

Interestingly, cardiac workload increases in the resting supine position, rather than in the resting erect position. The pathophysiological basis for this involves changes in the vascular resistance and hydrostatic pressure associated with the recumbent position because blood distribution within the body is altered. When the vertical position is abandoned in favor of the horizontal position, about 11% of the blood volume leaves the legs to be distributed to other parts of the body. This increases the total volume of circulating blood that must be handled by the heart. The cardiac output and stroke volume are also increased when the patient is lying down.

Cardiac workload is also effected by the Valsalva's maneuver. The **Valsalva's maneuver** is defined as a forced expiration against a closed epiglottis. The physiological alterations include a period of thoracic fixation without expiration, which elevates intrathoracic pressure, thereby impeding venous blood from entering the large veins. When the patient exhales, there is a significant decrease in intrathoracic pressure, and a surge of blood is injected into the heart, thus increasing the workload of the heart.

Neuroscience nurses are well aware of the effect of intracranial pressure spikes that result from the Valsalva's maneuver. Spikes are potentially dangerous to patients with already elevated intracranial pressure. Pulling the patient up in bed and improper positioning are some common instances that can initiate the Valsalva's maneuver. The nurse should appreciate this and understand the effects on the patient.

ASSESSMENT

Assessment of cardiovascular function in the unconscious patient includes the following: rate, rhythm, and quality of the apical pulse and radial pulses.

- Chest auscultation of heart sounds
- Blood pressure, including ranges of systolic and diastolic over time
- Evidence of orthostatic hypotension with head elevation
- Periodic electrolytes
- Complete blood count, including hematocrit and hemoglobin
- Other hemodynamic parameters, such as cardiac output, peripheral vascular resistance, pulmonary artery wedge pressure, if centrally monitored

All vital signs should be considered collectively to assess relationships and trends over time for clinical reasoning and decision making. For intensive care unit patients who are being monitored by central lines, vital signs and hemodynamic variables are displayed on a monitor; data are usually stored for review and trend data.

CARDIOVASCULAR PROBLEMS

A number of cardiovascular changes and problems result from immobility, including alterations in vital signs related to cardiac deconditioning, deep vein thrombosis or pulmonary embolus, and orthostatic hypotension.

Alterations in Vital Signs. Alterations in blood pressure and pulse may be the result of immobility or may be related to the primary neurological problem. A brief discussion is included here for the reader to consider when evaluating the patient. Hypotension or hypertension should be viewed in relation to the patient's pulse rate, pulse quality, and pulse pressure.

- **Hypotension and pulse variations.** Hypotension is rarely attributable to brain injury. In these rare instances, hypotension is associated with severe cerebral injury and occurs only as a terminal event. The concurrent findings of hypotension and tachycardia should raise suspicion of occult internal hemorrhage (intra-abdominal, intrathoracic, pelvic, or long bone injury) and hypovolemic shock. Other signs of hypovolemic shock include restlessness, ashen skin color, cold and clammy skin, and a rapid, thready pulse. The combination of hypotension and bradycardia may be secondary to cervical spinal cord injury, in which descending sympathetic pathways have been interrupted. Hypotension and tachycardia can also be a hemodynamic response to prolonged bed rest.

- **Hypertension and pulse variations.** Hypertension may occur with increases in intracranial pressure related to a number of problems, such as hypertensive stroke or subarachnoid hemorrhage. The combination of an elevated blood pressure, widening pulse pressure, and bradycardia is called Cushing's response (see Chap. 8). Hypertension may also be attributable to preexisting hypertension or pain. The patient should be assessed carefully to determine the underlying cause of the hypertension. Drug therapy is instituted to control and maintain the blood pressure within specified systolic and diastolic parameters. These parameters may be set in a hypertensive range to maintain cerebral perfusion if increased intracranial pressure is present.

Deep Vein Thrombosis or Pulmonary Emboli. The patient who is immobilized is at high risk for the formation of deep venous thrombus with the potential for pulmonary emboli. Thrombus formation is caused by venous stasis, decreased vasomotor tone, pressure on the blood vessels, and hypercoagulable state. A number of factors make the patient high risk for the development of thrombi:

- Muscle contraction of the legs ordinarily promotes venous return to the heart, but in the case of the immobilized unconscious patient, the blood pools and venous stasis results.
- Hypercoagulability is a common finding. Immobility is often associated with dehydration and resulting hemoconcentration. In addition, dehydration and a state of hypercoagulability, common in these patients, contribute to venous thrombosis.[7] In addition, increased serum calcium contributes to hypercoagulation. (Calcium is liberated from the bones of any person who is not bearing weight.)
- Prolonged external pressure leads to intimal layer injury of blood vessels. Platelets collect at the injured intimal site, forming a layer that can become the foundation for clot formation. External pressure can result from pillow placement under the knees, with the upper leg resting on the lower leg in the lateral recumbent position and the continual resting of the heels on the bed.

Orthostatic Hypotension. The third major effect of immobility on cardiovascular function is **orthostatic hypotension**, which is the inability of the autonomic nervous system to maintain an adequate blood supply to the upper regions of the body when the patient is place erect or upright in bed. In the immobilized patient, orthostatic hypotension is attributable to a loss of general motor tone and decreased efficiency of the orthostatic neurovascular reflexes (which normally cause contraction of the blood vessels so that blood can flow upward against gravity).

The following are common related nursing diagnoses:

- Decreased Cardiac Output
- Peripheral Neurovascular Dysfunction
- Altered Peripheral Tissue Perfusion
- Altered Cerebral Tissue Perfusion
- Activity Intolerance

The following are common related collaborative problems:

- Decreased cardiac output
- Dysrhythmias
- Deep vein thrombosis
- Hypovolemia
- Pulmonary embolism

INTERVENTIONS

Appropriate nursing interventions and nursing management designed to support cardiovascular function in the unconscious immobilized patient include the following:

- Elevate the head of the bed, if possible; this will alter the intravascular pressure and stimulate the orthostatic neurovascular reflexes.
- Turn and position the patient carefully at frequent intervals, usually every 2 hours.
- When positioning in the lateral recumbent position, position the upper leg to prevent pressure on the lower leg.
- Do not use a foot gatch or place pillows under the knees (causes pressure and venous stasis).
- Administer range-of-motion exercises at least four times daily to improve blood return to the heart and prevent venous stasis.
- Apply thigh-high elastic stockings and sequential compression air boots to improve blood return to the heart and minimize venous stasis.
- Sit the patient in a chair, if at all possible; this alters intravascular pressure and stimulates the orthostatic neurovascular reflexes.
- Try to synchronize moving the patient with exhalation to prevent initiating the Valsalva's maneuver.
- Consider the relationship among hemodynamic variables and trends in specific variables.
- Monitor the patient for signs and symptoms of deep vein thrombosis or thrombophlebitis.

Once consciousness is regained, a period of reconditioning is needed before the erect position can be assumed. Because of prolonged bed rest, orthostatic hypotension must be managed before proceeding out of bed. Toward this end, the bed is elevated gradually each day, and the blood pressure, pulse, and objective signs and symptoms are monitored to determine successful adaptation to the change in position. Once the vertical position is tolerated, progress to sitting in a chair and ambulation can proceed, unless neurological deficits make it unfeasible. A physical therapy evaluation is conducted to determine the feasibility of ambulation and the short-term goals to accomplish that end. Need for special devices, such as braces, a walker, or crutches, is addressed. A beginning step toward ambulation is relearning balance and coordination of body parts in the vertical position.

The Skin and Related Structures

The skin is an important barrier to infection; it assists in heat regulation through sweating and piloerection in the cold and cushions bony prominence. Sustained pressure from immobilization is the most important cause of skin breakdown. Pressure transmitted to the skin, subcutaneous tissue, and muscles, particularly over bony prominences, can result in ischemia and necrosis. Shearing forces and friction related to moving patients can cause direct injury to the skin that results in pressure ulcers. In addition, incontinence, profuse perspiration, poor nutrition, and obesity are factors related to pressure ulcer development. Immobilized unconscious patients are at high risk for developing pressure ulcers.

ASSESSMENT

The skin and related structures (hair, fingernails, toenails, scalp, hair, eyes, and oral cavity) should be assessed according to the following guidelines:

Skin

- Identify all risk factors present for skin breakdown. Use the *Clinical Practice Guideline, Pressure Ulcers in Adults: Prediction and Prevention for Assessment and Management of Patients.*[8]
- Assess the skin using the Braden or Norton scale.
- Assess the skin for color, temperature, dryness, redness, abrasions, and pressure ulcers.
- Every square inch of skin should be observed and assessed in an 8-hour period (many areas are observed more frequently).
- Bony prominences, such as the elbows, iliac crest, or outer aspect of the ankle, can become irritated and red; assess all bony prominences for redness, irritated, or broken tissue.
- Do not position on a reddened or broken skin area.
- Assess fingernails and toenails for length and cleanliness.

Other

- Assess the mucous membranes of the oral cavity for dryness, irritation, signs of oral infections (yeast and others), and broken areas; the tongue may be coated with a whitish material.
- Assess eyes for redness and drainage.
- Assess scalp and hair for reddened areas (especially at occiput), abrasions, and pediculosis.

SKIN AND OTHER INTEGUMENTAL PROBLEMS

Abnormal findings may include redness of the skin, broken skin, pressure ulcer, dry lips and oral cavity, cracked lips, oral infection, eye infection, dryness of the eye, inability to close the eye, matted hair, pediculosis, long fingernails that cut into the palms of hand, and long toenails that scratch the skin. The following are common related nursing diagnoses:

- Risk for Impaired Skin Integrity
- Impaired Skin Integrity
- Altered Oral Mucous Membrane
- Risk for Infection
- Risk for Impaired Tissue Integrity (corneal)

NURSING INTERVENTIONS

An abundance of good research guides the nurse in providing research-based care to predict and prevent pressure ulcers. This is all outlined in the *Clinical Practice Guideline, Pressure Ulcers in Adults: Prediction and Prevention.* This is an outstanding resource and the standard to which all nurses are held when providing care. Every nurse must be well versed on the Guideline and incorporate it into practice. Nurses should refer to this resource for the specifics of care.

The following lists additional points for the nurse to consider when providing care.

Skin Care. When providing skin care, the nurse should do the following:

- Keep the skin clean and dry; provide frequent skin care.
- Male patients should be shaved daily. If the patient is receiving anticoagulation therapy, an electric razor should be used.
- Trophic skin changes, such as dryness, can occur with some neurological conditions; lubricate the skin with lotion to prevent skin breakdown.
- Provide frequent skin care.
- Turn and reposition every 2 hours; be sure the heels are off the bed and other vulnerable areas are positioned to prevent pressure.
- When moving the patient, turn and lift rather than causing shearing and friction on skin.
- Consider using a special bed to prevent skin breakdown in high-risk patients.

Mouth Care. When administering mouth care, the nurse should do the following:

- Cleanse and lubricate the mouth and tongue every 3 hours to prevent dryness, oral infections, and gum disease.
- Brush the teeth three to four times daily with the aid of a toothbrush and suction catheter.
- Lubricate the lips to prevent dryness and cracking.

Eye Care. When caring for the eyes and periocular area, the nurse should do the following:

- Inspect for signs of edema, ecchymosis, eye drainage, irritation, or abrasions.
- Periocular edema and ecchymosis are common after trauma or cranial surgery. Apply cold compresses or an ice bag for the first 24 hours, or alternate cold and warm compresses to reduce edema; follow hospital protocol.
- Cleanse the corners of the eyes with cotton balls and saline; the eyes should be irrigated four times daily with normal saline, or a commercially prepared solution (*e.g.,* Tearisol ophthalmic solution) should be instilled. The unconscious patient cannot blink periodically to cleanse and lubricate the

eyes. Corneal drying or injury to the eye can lead to corneal ulcerations and blindness.

- Apply an eye patch or eye shield, as necessary, to protect the eye from injury, especially if the eyes do not close completely (cranial nerve VII).

Scalp and Hair Care. The scalp and hair require attention:

- Examine the scalp for abrasions, pressure ulcers (especially in the occiput region), and edema. Treat any bruised or broken area.
- Patients with head trauma may have hair that is matted with blood, dirt, or glass; remove by combing and washing the hair, if not contraindicated, according to hospital procedure.
- Comb the hair; long hair can be braided or pulled to the side with an elastic band.

Fingernails and Toenails. An unconscious patient may clench the fists, digging the nails into the hands and causing injury. File and clip fingernails and toenails to protect the patient from injury.

Musculoskeletal Function

Immobility has a profound effect of the musculoskeletal system, including decreased muscle strength, muscle atrophy, contractures, and osteoporosis.

- **Decreased muscle strength**. Loss of muscle strength occurs with immobilization. The degree of loss of strength varies with muscle groups and the degree of immobility. The antigravitational muscles of the legs lose strength twice as fast as the arm muscles.[9] Recovery of strength occurs much slower than loss of strength, taking about 4 weeks to regain strength that was lost in 1 week even when a strengthening exercise program was offered.[10]
- **Muscle atrophy**. In addition to decreased muscle strength, muscles atrophy and shorten with immobilization. Muscle fiber length and total muscle length decrease during immobilization. Muscle atrophy means loss of muscle weight and bulk. When a muscle is immobilized in the shortened length, it atrophies about twice as fast as those held in a stretched position.[11] Because increased muscle tone prevents complete atrophy, patients with upper motor neuron disease, spastic paralysis, or immobilization lose only about 30% to 35% of muscle bulk. In the case of lower motor neuron disease and flaccid paralysis, muscle bulk is lost by about 90% to 95%. Muscle fibers are replaced by connective tissue if recovery does not occur.[12]
- **Contractures**. A contracture is a loss of full range of motion of a joint usually due to mechanical factors in the immobilized patient. When a muscle is maintained in a shortened position for even a 5 to 7 days, the muscle belly shortens. If the position is maintained for about 1 month, loose connective tissue in muscles and around joints changes to dense connective tissue of a contracture.
- **Osteoporosis**. Weight-bearing forces on joints and muscle activity are critical to maintaining the balance of bone formation and reabsorption. Immobilization results in significant bone loss. In a study of bone density of the lumbar vertebrae, healthy men with disc disease were placed on bed rest. Bone loss was calculated as 0.9% per week, about 50 times greater than predicted involutional bone loss.[13] Hypercalcemia and hypercalciuria, which reflect loss of total body calcium, occur with bed rest. The high level of calcium in the urinary tract contributes to urinary calculi formation. Osteoporosis predisposes the patient to vertebral compression fractures and long bone and hip fractures from minor trauma.

ASSESSMENT

The muscles of the upper and lower extremities, neck, and shoulders should be assessed for tone, bulk, and range of motion, and both sides of the body should be compared.

MUSCULOSKELETAL PROBLEMS

Abnormal musculoskeletal findings include decreased muscle tone (flaccidity, paresis, paralysis), increased muscle tone (rigidity, decortication, decerebration, tremors), muscle atrophy, contractures, ankylosis, and joint dislocation.

The following are common related nursing diagnoses:

- Impaired Physical Mobility
- Risk for Trauma (stress fractures, joint dislocation)

The following are common related collaborative problems:

- Pathological fractures
- Joint dislocation

NURSING INTERVENTIONS

The following nursing interventions are useful for preserving musculoskeletal function in the unconscious patient:

- Administer passive range-of-motion exercises every 4 hours.
- Reposition in proper body alignment every 2 hours; pillows, rolls, and special accessories, such as positioning boots or splints, can be used. An unconscious patient, unlike a conscious patient, is unable to change a malaligned position spontaneously in response to pain or discomfort.
- Reposition weak or paralyzed body parts to prevent deformity. For example, external hip rotation can develop if the leg is not properly positioned. The external hip rotation substantially prolongs the rehabilitation process and limits reaching optimal function.
- Position limbs to prevent dependent edema. For example, the hands should be slightly elevated. Edema limits range of motion, and lack of movement contributes to the development of ankylosis and contractures. Therefore, once any deficit impeding normal range of motion develops, the problem is compounded by additional impairments.

Genitourinary Function

Assuming the supine position with immobility results in urinary stasis in the renal pelvis and urinary bladder, a medium for bacterial growth. In addition, urinary retention and bladder distention are common. An unconscious patient will be incontinent due to an altered level of consciousness and the effects of the supine position.

The unconscious patient is at risk for two major problems: urinary tract infections and kidney and bladder stones (calculi). The causes of infection are the catheter and the stasis of urine. The stasis of urine in the bladder promotes bladder infections and ascending infections, which can involve the kidneys. The stasis of urine in the renal pelvis and bladder encourages the formation of calculi. The increased levels of calcium being excreted from demineralized bones, another effect of immobilization, results in hypercalciuria and contributes to the formation of urinary calculi.

ASSESSMENT

- Monitor intake and output.
- Determine the voiding pattern.
- Identify the characteristics of the urine.
- Be aware of the results of recent urinalysis and urine cultures.

The following are common related nursing diagnoses:

- Altered Urinary Elimination
- Total Incontinence
- Functional Incontinence
- Risk for Infection

The following are common related collaborative problems:

- Acute urinary retention
- Renal insufficiency
- Renal calculi

NURSING INTERVENTIONS

In an unconscious patient, methods of managing urine must be considered. On admission, an indwelling catheter is usually inserted. This may be necessary to monitor fractional urinary output for patients receiving diuretic therapy (*e.g.,* mannitol), those with diabetes insipidus, or other patients in whom careful and frequent monitoring of output is necessary. Another reason for inserting an indwelling catheter is to keep the patient dry, because urinary incontinence can quickly lead to skin breakdown. The catheter itself is a foreign body and an irritant to the urinary tract. The literature supports a direct relationship between urinary catheters and urinary tract infection. There are some special considerations when weighing the benefits and risks of inserting an indwelling catheter in an unconscious patient.

- If an indwelling catheter is necessary temporarily, remove it as soon as possible.
- For the male patient, a condom catheter is a possible choice.
- An alternate to continuous urinary drainage is an intermittent catheterization program useful in both genders.
- For some patients, absorbent incontinence pads that are changed frequently may be chosen to avoid the risk of infection from a catheter.

- Consider the condition of the skin. If areas of skin breakdown already exist, being wet for even a short time could increase that breakdown. (See Chap. 14 for further discussion, which includes *Urinary Incontinence in Adults, Clinical Practice Guideline.*[14])

Gastrointestinal Function

Constipation and fecal impaction are common in immobilized and unconscious patients. Normal stimulants to peristalsis, such as physical activity and a high-fiber diet, are absent. Nutrition is commonly provided by enteral tube feeding, which does not generally stimulate peristalsis. Components of the therapeutic plan, such as fluid restriction and drugs, contribute to constipation. Loose stools or diarrhea are also common in the unconscious immobilized patient, most often in response to poorly tolerated enteral feeding or drugs, especially antibiotics.

ASSESSMENT

- Auscultate the abdomen for bowel sounds.
- Note and record the consistency, color, size, and frequency of stools.
- Review the intake and output record and 24-hour balance for the last several days to determine the hydration status of the patient.
- Review the patient's medication sheet to determine drugs that can affect peristalsis and bowel evacuation.
- Ascertain the amount of fiber in the tube feeding.
- Test each stool for occult blood, and record the results.
- If possible, monitor gastric aspiration for occult blood.

GASTROINTESTINAL PROBLEMS

Abnormal findings may include a distended abdomen with decreased or absent bowel sounds, paralytic ileus, hyperactive bowel sounds, or positive hemo-occult gastric aspirant or stools.

The following are common related nursing diagnoses:

- Bowel Incontinence
- Diarrhea (related to intolerance of tube feeding or effects of drugs)
- Colonic Constipation

The following are common related collaborative problems:

- Paralytic ileus
- GI Bleeding

NURSING INTERVENTIONS

A hospital-approved bowel program (stool softeners, bulk former, mild laxatives) should be instituted and followed. These drugs can be given through a feeding tube, gastrostomy, or jejunostomy tube. (See Chap. 14 for a sample protocol.) If constipation is a problem, a few points should be kept in mind.

- Constipation increases intra-abdominal pressure which, in turn, increases intracranial pressure.
- In patients with increased intracranial pressure, enemas using 750 to 1,000 mL of fluid are often contraindicated because of the potential to initiate the Valsalva's maneuver, which can lead to further elevation of intracranial pressure.
- If not contraindicated, an unconscious patient can be positioned on a bedpan while lying in bed and given a limited fluid (about 300 mL) enema. The nurse will need to wear a glove and hold the rectal tube in position.
- A drug to stimulate peristalsis may be added, such as metoclopramide (Reglan).

In the case of diarrhea, the following should be kept in mind:

- Review the type and rate of enteral feeding ordered; feeding intolerance, especially to lactose, may be present. Change the feeding to one of increased bulk, or slow the rate of administration.
- Concurrent drug therapy, especially antibiotics, can cause diarrhea. Discuss discontinuing a high-suspect drug or changing it to another drug.
- Consider adjusting the dosage and frequency of the drug.
- Add drug therapy to decrease peristalsis and control diarrhea.

Gastric aspirations through an enteral tube and stools should be monitored for occult blood. This is necessary because GI bleeding in the neurological patient is common, especially if a head injury or intracranial insult has occurred. A gastric ulcer associated with neurological problems is called Cushing's ulcer. Another risk factor for GI bleeding is concurrent drug therapy, such as dexamethasone, which is irritating to the GI tract.

Metabolic Effects and Nutrition and Hydration Needs

A number of metabolic changes occur in response to immobility. Increased calcium excretion from bones is due to the elimination of weight-bearing forces on the long bones rather than inactivity.[15] These changes, seen in all age groups, are noted after only a few days of bed rest and continue for a number of weeks. See previously discussed musculoskeletal changes. Hypercalcemia and hypercalciuria result.

Glucose-insulin intolerance is altered with inactivity, and it correlates positively with the length of bed rest. To maintain a normal glucose level, increasing levels of serum insulin are necessary. The underlying mechanism is unclear, but reversal is noted after activity is resumed.[16]

While unconsciousness may last for days, months, or even years, the metabolic and nutritional needs of the patient must continuously be met to maintain body function, support tissue repair, and combat infections. (See Chap. 9 for physiological and pathophysiological responses.)

ASSESSMENT AND INTERVENTIONS

A nutritional consultation should be ordered as soon as the patient is stabilized (within 24–48 hours). At that time, the patient's nutritional and metabolic needs are assessed, and nutritional support is prescribed to meet the total needs based on consideration of the diagnosis, comorbidity, specific energy demands (*e.g.,* hyperthermia or agitation) for increased metabolic activity and tissue repair, loss of fluid (*e.g.,* from perspiration, diarrhea, or drainage), and basic life functions. Selected laboratory studies, such as albumin, are helpful to determine patient needs.

Methods of administering nutritional support to the unconscious patient include total parenteral nutrition and complete enteral nutritional feedings administered by way of a nasogastric, gastrostomy, duodenal, or jejunostomy tube. Chapter 9 provides a thorough discussion of nutritional support and nursing process related to nutrition. Although hydration is considered a part of nutrition, a special point should be made about hydration and the neurological patient. Fluid restriction may be ordered to control cerebral edema and increased intracranial pressure by keeping the patient slightly underhydrated. The intake is correlated with the output; therefore, an accurate intake and output record must be maintained.

Serum glucose, complete blood count with differential, electrolytes, and trace elements, such as magnesium, calcium, and phosphorus, should be monitored. Replacement therapy to achieve normal levels and determine the need for insulin administration needs to be considered.

The following are common related nursing diagnoses:

- Altered Nutrition: Less than body requirements
- Altered Nutrition: Potential for more than body requirements
- Fluid Volume Deficit
- Fluid Volume Excess

The following are common related collaborative problems:

- Hypoglycemia or hyperglycemia
- Electrolyte imbalance
- Acidosis (metabolic, respiratory)
- Alkalosis (metabolic, respiratory)
- Negative nitrogen balance
- Adrenocorticosteroid therapy, adverse effects

Infections in High-Risk Patients

Patients who are unconscious for prolonged periods are at high risk for infection for several reasons. Serious illnesses, often involving multiple body systems, challenge the body's immune system. Invasive procedures (*e.g.,* surgery) and invasive equipment (*e.g.,* central lines and urinary catheters) can lead to infection. Moreover, the use of antibiotics may result in opportunistic infections (Table 16-1). Immunosuppression related to steroid therapy (*e.g.,* dexamethasone), which is often prescribed for neuroscience patients, is common. All of these factors cause immunosuppression, so serious infection can be present with none or minimal clinical signs and symptoms of infection. Knowing that a patient is immunocompromised

TABLE 16-1
Causes and Prevention of Infections

TYPE OF INFECTION	PREDISPOSING FACTORS	COMMON CAUSATIVE ORGANISMS	PREVENTIVE MEASURES
Urinary tract (most common type of hospital-acquired infection)	Indwelling catheters Straight catheterization Traction on meatus (in males)	*Escherichia coli* (most common cause in nonhospitalized patients); *Proteus, Klebsiella, Enterobacter, Pseudomonas, Serratia* organisms (hospital-acquired infections)	• Maintain a sterile closed urinary drainage system. • Administer meatal and perineal care. • Maintain dependent drainage. • Maintain strict aseptic technique. • Prevent cross-contamination by strict adherence to handwashing protocol.
Respiratory	Respiratory assistance equipment Dehydration Presence of tracheostomy or endotracheal tube	*Staphylococcus aureus* and *Streptococcus;* about half of nosocomial pneumonias are caused by *Klebsiella, Enterobacter,* and *Pseudomonas* organisms	• Change ventilation equipment every 24 h. • Change the water in respiratory reservoirs every 8–12 h. • Maintain aseptic suctioning procedure. • Administer tracheostomy care every 4 h. • Adhere to strict handwashing technique. • Adhere to principles of aseptic technique.
Wound	Contamination of surgical incision (*e.g.,* as a result of a confused or disoriented patient pulling on the dressing)	*S. aureus, E. coli*	• Adhere to strict aseptic technique for dressing changes. • Change the dressing immediately if contamination occurs.
Vascular	IV and arterial catheters Swan-Ganz catheters Hyperalimentation	*S. aureus; E. coli; Streptococcus, Klebsiella, Serratia, Enterobacter,* and *Pseudomonas* organisms	• Change tubing every 24 h. • Apply iodophor ointment to the site with each dressing change. • Change dressings frequently, using strict aseptic technique.
Cerebrospinal fluid (CSF)	Intracranial pressure monitors Contamination of craniotomy or spinal surgery incisions Leakage of CSF, as may occur in basal skull fractures	*Streptococcus, Neisseria meningitidis, Haemophilus influenzae, E. coli*	• Maintain a closed system. • Use strict aseptic dressing technique. • Treat patients with CSF leakage aggressively with antibiotic therapy.

alerts the nurse to use meticulous aseptic technique. The nursing diagnosis frequently made is Risk for Infection.

Sensory Deprivation

Although unconscious patients appear to be completely unaware of their environment, it is impossible to determine if they are aware of any stimulus in the immediate environment. Many patients have regained consciousness and given accurate accounts of what happened and what was said to them when they were supposedly unconscious; therefore, it is important to maintain a positive attitude in the presence of these patients and assume that some stimuli will penetrate the complexities of unconsciousness. Stimuli can be provided by playing the radio, touching the patient, and talking. Patients should be told what will be done and should be oriented to time, place, person, and reality by describing the surroundings (weather and so forth).

Because visual impairment is generally another form of sensory deprivation in the unconscious patient, as the patient slowly begins to regain consciousness, there may be some continued visual deficits. (Visual deficits are common with head injuries because the visual system is a complex network that traverses several areas of the brain.)

REGAINING CONSCIOUSNESS

Awakening from unconsciousness is usually a gradual process that tends to vary from patient to patient. The amount of reconditioning and retraining needed to achieve optimal rehabilitation potential will depend on the length of unconsciousness, concurrent illness and complications, comorbidity, and age. See Chapter 14 for rehabilitation of patients.

References

1. Szaflarski, N. L. (1993). Immobility phenomena in critically ill adults. In J. M. Clochesy, C. Breu, S. Cardin, E. B. Rudy, & A. A. Whittaker (Eds.), *Critical care nursing.* Philadelphia: W.B. Saunders.
2. Brouse, N. L. (1965). *The physiology and pathology of bedrest.* Springfield, IL: Charles C. Thomas.
3. Sharp, J. T., Goldberg, N. B., & Druz, W. S. (1975). Relative contributions of rib cage and abdomen to breathing in normal subjects. *Journal of Applied Physiology, 39,* 608.
4. Ibid, Szaflarski, p. 34.
5. Harper, C. M., & Lyles, Y. M. (1988). Physiology and complications of bed rest. *Journal of the American Geriatric Society, 36,* 1047–1054.
6. Kennedy, S. K. (1993). Airway management and respiratory support. In A. H. Ropper (Ed.), *Neurological and neurosurgical intensive care* (3rd ed.) (pp. 69–95). New York: Raven Press.
7. Saleem, S., & Vallbona, C. (1995). Immobilization. In S. J. Garrison (Ed.), *Handbook of medicine and rehabilitation basics* (pp. 185–196). Philadelphia: J.B. Lippincott.
8. Panel for the Prediction and Prevention of Pressure Ulcers in Adults (1992). *Pressure ulcers in adults: Prediction and prevention,* Clinical Practice guideline, Number 3. AHCPR Publication No. 92-0047. Rockville, MD: Agency for Health Care Policy and Research, Public Health Service, U.S. Department of Health and Human Services.
9. Greenleaf, J. E., Van Beaumont, W., Convertino, V. A., et al. (1983). Handgrip and general muscular strength and endurance during prolonged bedrest with isometric and isotonic leg exercise training. *Aviation Space Environmental Medicine, 54,* 696.
10. Ibid, Saleem & Vallbona, p. 186.
11. Harper, C. M., & Lyles, Y. M. (1988). Physiology and complications of bed rest. *Journal of the American Geriatric Society, 36,* 1047–1054.
12. Ibid, Saleem & Vallbona, p. 188.
13. Krolner, B., & Toft, B. (1983). Vertebral bone loss: An unheaded side effect of therapeutic bed rest. *Clinical Science, 64,* 537.
14. Urinary Incontinence Guideline Panel (1992). *Urinary Incontinence in Adults: Clinical Practice Guideline.* AHCPR Publication No. 92-0038. Rockville, MD: Agency for Health Care Policy and Research, Public Health Service, U.S. Department of Health and Human Services.
15. Issekutz, B., Blizzard, J J., Birkhead, N. C., et al. (1966). Effect of prolonged bedrest on urinary calcium output. *Journal of Applied Physiology, 21,* 1013–1020.
16. Szaflarski; p. 38.

Bibliography

Books

Haler, E. M., & Bell, K. R. (1988). Contractures and other deleterious effects of immobility. In J. A. DeLisa (Ed.), *Rehabilitation medicine: Principles and practice* (pp. 448–462). Philadelphia: J.B. Lippincott.

Steinberg, F. U. (1980). The immobilized patient. In *Functional pathology and management.* New York: Plenum.

Periodicals

Bohachick, P. A. (1987). Pulmonary embolism in neurological and neurosurgical patients. *Journal of Neuroscience Nursing, 19*(4), 191–197.

Creditor, M. C. (1993). Hazards of hospitalization of the elderly. *Annals of Internal Medicine, 118*(3), 219–223.

Dittmer, D. K., & Teasell, R. (1993). Complications of immobilization and bed rest. Part 1: Musculoskeletal and cardiovascular complications. *Canadian family Physician, 39,* 1428–1432, 1435–1437.

Gradon, J. (1995). Immobility and infection: A practical review for the neurologist. *The Neurologist, 1,* 115–124.

Miller, M. (1981). Emergency management of the unconscious patient. *Nursing Clinics of North America, 16*(1), 59–73.

Olson, E. V. (1990). The hazards of immobility. *American Journal of Nursing, 90*(3), 43–48.

Puma, J. L., Schiedermayer, D. L., Gulyas, A. E., & Siegler, M. (1988). Talking to comatose patients. *Archives of Neurology, 45,* 20–22.

Rousseau, P. (1993). Immobility in the aged. *Archives of Family Medicine, 2*(2), 169–177.

Teasell, R., & Dittmer, D. K. (1993). Complications of immobilization and bed rest. Part 2: Other complications. *Canadian family Physician, 39,* 1440–1442, 1445–1446.

Von Rueden, K. T., & Harris, J. R. (1995). pulmonary dysfunction related to immobility in the trauma patient. *AACN Clinical Issues, 6*(2), 212–228.

Whitney, J. D., Stotts, N. A., Goodson, W. H., & Janson-Bjerklie, S. (1993). The effects of activity and bed rest on tissue oxygen tension, perfusion, and plasma volume. *Nursing Research, 42*(6), 349–355.

CHAPTER 17

Intracranial Pressure: Theory and Management of Increased Intracranial Pressure

Joanne V. Hickey

Clinically significant increased intracranial pressure (ICP) is a common pathophysiological problem addressed daily by nurses and physicians who care for neuroscience patients. However, the specific sequence of pathophysiological events leading to a sustained or unstable ICP is still poorly understood. This chapter reviews the underlying physiological cerebral hemodynamics and ICP concepts and applies this knowledge to the assessment and interventions for patient management.

CONCEPT OF INTRACRANIAL PRESSURE

ICP is the pressure normally exerted by cerebrospinal fluid (CSF) that circulates around the brain and spinal cord and within the cerebral ventricles referenced to the atmosphere on which cardiac and respiratory components are superimposed. The normal range of ICP is 0 to 10 mm Hg; many consider less than 15 mm Hg as normal. Homeostatic mechanisms maintain a mean pressure below 15 mm Hg (range 0–14 mm Hg). The monitoring of ICP in the clinical setting thus provides an average or mean CSF pressure. If the ICP is observed for an extended period and remains unchanged, the homeostatic mechanisms controlling the ICP are in a state of equilibrium or a *steady state*. However, abrupt changes in ICP from a stable level in response to activity or a sudden change in volume is called *transient increased ICP*. It may be that different physio-

logical mechanisms control steady and transient states of ICP.[1] With cerebral trauma or neurological disease, the normal homeostatic mechanisms controlling ICP may be disrupted, resulting in a sustained high ICP and eventual neurological and clinical death.

The implication of ICP is that only one ICP pressure exists within the intracranial space. This is a misconception; with cerebral trauma or disease, the pressure can vary widely within different areas of the brain. For example, the pressure in the tissue adjacent to an expanding, space-occupying lesion can be elevated, while the intraventricular pressure remains within a normal range. Also, elevated ICP is not always conveyed to the lumbar subarachnoid space where it would be reflected during a lumbar puncture. It is, therefore, more accurate to think in terms of ICPs, rather than a single, uniform ICP pressure.

Physiological Considerations
MONRO-KELLIE HYPOTHESIS

The average intracranial volume in the adult is approximately 1,700 mL, composed of the brain (1,400 mL), CSF (150 mL), and blood (150 mL). Basic to an understanding of the pathophysiological changes related to ICP is the **Monro-Kellie hypothesis**. It states that the skull, a rigid compartment, is filled to capacity with essentially noncompressible contents—brain matter (80%), intravascular blood (10%), and CSF (10%). The volume of these three components remains nearly constant in a state of *dynamic equilibrium*. If any one component increases in volume, another component must decrease reciprocally for the overall volume and dynamic equilibrium to remain constant; otherwise, ICP will rise. This hypothesis applies *only* when the skull is fused. Infants or very young children who have skulls with nonfused suture lines have some space for expansion of the intracranial space in response to increased volume, at least initially.

THE VOLUME–PRESSURE RELATIONSHIP WITHIN THE INTRACRANIAL CAVITY

According to the Monro-Kellie hypothesis, reciprocal compensation occurs among the three intracranial components—brain tissue, blood, and CFS—to accommodate any alterations within the intracranial contents. The compensatory mechanisms that maintain the intracranial volume in a steady state include the following:

- Displacement of some CSF from the ventricles and cerebral subarachnoid space through the foramen magnum to the spinal subarachnoid space and through the optic foramen to the perioptic subarachnoid space (basal subarachnoid cisterns)
- Compression of the low pressure venous system, especially the dural sinuses
- Decreased production of CSF
- Vasoconstriction of the cerebral vasculature

However, the amount of displacement of the brain, CSF, or blood is limited. Once compensatory mechanisms are exceeded, ICP rises and intracranial hypertension results.

Compliance. **Compliance** is a measure of the adaptive capacity of the brain to maintain intracranial equilibrium in response to physiological and external challenges to that system. It has been described as a measure of brain "stiffness." Compliance represents the ratio of change in volume to the resulting change in pressure. It is represented by the following formula, in which δ represents the symbol for change, V = volume, and P = pressure:

$$C = \delta V / \delta P$$

Applying this concept to intracranial dynamics, compliance is the ratio of change in ICP as a result of change in intracranial volume.

The intracranial dynamics are shown in Figure 17-1. The vertical axis represents pressure or ICP (measured in mm Hg). The horizontal axis represents intracranial volume. The shape of the curve demonstrates the effects on ICP when volume is added to the intracranial space. The ICP remains constant from point A to just before point B with the addition of volume. The compensatory mechanisms are adequate, and the compliance is high. Point B is a threshold; even though the ICP is still within normal limits, compliance is decreased. From points B to C, the slope begins to increase, reflecting a decrease in compensatory mechanisms and low compliance. With even a small increment in volume (points C to D), the compensatory mechanisms are exceeded, compliance is lost, and a disproportionate elevation in ICP is noted.

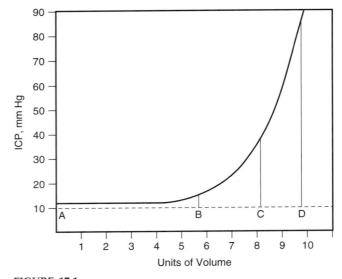

FIGURE 17-1
Pressure-volume curve. From point A to just before B, the ICP remains constant although there is addition of volume (compliance is high). At point B, even though the ICP is within normal limits, compliance begins to change, as evidenced by the slight rise in ICP. From points B to C, the ICP rises with an increase in volume (low compliance). From points C to D, ICP rises significantly with each minute increase in volume (compliance is lost).

Factors that influence compliance include the amount of volume increase, the time frame for accommodation of the volume, and the size of the intracranial compartments. Small-volume increments can usually be accommodated more readily than large-volume increments. Volume increases made over long periods can be accommodated much more easily than a comparable quantity introduced within a much shorter interval. The size of the intracranial compartments can vary because of cerebral atrophy, craniectomy, or immaturity of the cranium (suture lines not fused). For example, an adult with an acute epidural hematoma, a rapidly enlarging lesion, will develop increased ICP much more rapidly than a patient with a large, slowly growing brain tumor, such as a meningioma. In addition, some cerebral atrophy occurs with normal aging, thus creating a little more space in the cranial vault. Because of this extra intracranial space, a subdural hematoma may go unnoticed for weeks or months before there is a rise in ICP. However, a critical point is eventually reached beyond which compensation is exhausted, and there is a dramatic rise in ICP, regardless of how slowly minute-volume increments are added.

Estimating Compliance by Morphological Changes in Intracranial Pressure Waveform. Cerebral compliance can be estimated clinically by examining morphological changes in ICP waveforms in patients with an ICP monitor in place. The ICP wave is observed on a continuous real time display monitor. The pulse wave arises primarily from arterial pulsations and to a lesser degree from the respiratory cycle. Arterial influence comes from arterial sources that pump 10 to 15 mL of blood into the brain per cardiac cycle. In addition, effects from retrovenous pulsation and choroid plexus pulsations also influence the waveform.[2] Observing any variations in waveform

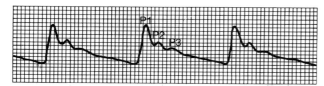

FIGURE 17-2
Normal ICP wave form (ICP = 8 mm Hg).

during activities, treatments, or environmental changes allows one to determine the effects of these activities on patients and to protect them from risk if necessary.

The ICP waveform has three peaks that are of clinical importance. Other lesser peaks sometimes occur after P3, but their significance is unknown.[3] The principal wave forms, in order of appearance, follow:

- P_1, the percussion wave, which originates from pulsations of the arteries and choroid plexus, is sharply peaked and fairly consistent in amplitude.
- P_2, the tidal wave, is more variable, and it terminates in the dicrotic notch.
- P_3, the dicrotic wave, immediately follows the dicrotic notch.

The pressure tapers down to the diastolic position after P_3 unless retrograde venous pulsation creates additional waves. At low ICP pressure, the pulse wave formation appears as a descending sawtooth pattern (Fig. 17-2). The P_2 wave is a reflection of intracerebral compliance. A rise in ICP is reflected as a progressive rise in P_2. The P_1 and P_3 waves rise to a much lesser degree so that the overall pulse wave has a rounded appearance (Fig. 17-3).

Clinical application of ICP waveform analysis is used to identify patients who exhibit low compliance as evidenced by an elevated P_2 wave. It is unclear whether the height of individual wave components indicates a continuum of compliance compromise from slight to severe. Because it is possible to observe responses to patient activities, treatments, and environmental factors immediately, it may be possible to use this information to develop an individual plan of care based on avoidance of individual risk factors. ICP waveform analysis should be a focus of more clinical research to explore its ramifications for integration into clinical practice.

CEREBRAL HEMODYNAMICS

Several concepts related to cerebral hemodynamics are important to an understanding of the pathophysiology of increased ICP.

Cerebral Blood Volume. **Cerebral blood volume** (CBV) refers to the amount of blood in the brain at a given time. Normally, blood occupies about 10% of the intracranial space. Most blood is contained in the low-pressure venous system. CBV is affected by the autoregulatory mechanisms that control cerebral blood flow (CBF). A limited compensatory mechanism is operational when ICP begins to rise. The mechanism responds by decreasing CBV. However, as the compensatory reserve is

exhausted, pressure in the venous system rises, CBV increases, and ICP rises.[4] Depending on the rate of decline in CBF and the duration of ischemia, cerebral infarction can occur.

Cerebral Blood Flow. Adequate blood flow and oxygenation are required to maintain normal neural function. The approximate blood flow through the brain is 750 mL/min. Although the brain is only 2% of body weight, it receives 15% of cardiac output and 20% of oxygen consumed in the basal state. In normal conditions, the total oxygen consumed by the brain and CBF are almost constant. Local demand for blood can vary depending on different metabolic needs. Cortical gray matter receives about six times the amount of blood as white matter, and changes in blood flow respond to demands of varying neural activity.[5] CBF is represented by the following equation, in which MAP = mean arterial pressure, CVP = central venous pressure, CPP = cerebral perfusion pressure, and CVR = cerebrovascular resistance:

$$CBF = (MAP - CVP)/CVR \quad \text{or}$$
$$CPP/CVR \quad \text{Note: } (MAP - CVP = CPP)$$

If the CBF exceeds the required amount of blood for metabolism, a state of hyperemia is said to exist. **Hyperemia**, also called "luxury perfusion," is an excess of blood to a part of the body.

Factors That Modify Cerebral Blood Flow. CBF can be increased or decreased by a number of extracerebral and intracerebral factors.[6]

EXTRACEREBRAL FACTORS. These factors are primarily related to the cardiovascular system and include systemic blood pressure, cardiac function, and blood viscosity.

- **Blood pressure.** *The main force that maintains cerebral circulation is the pressure difference between the arteries and the veins.* In the brain, cerebral venous pressure is low (approximately 5 mm Hg) so that arterial blood pressure is the most important factor in maintaining CBF. Under normal circumstances, intrinsic regulatory mechanisms maintain CBF at a constant level even with systemic arterial blood pressure changes unless the MAP dips to less than 50 to 70 mm Hg.
- **Cardiac function.** Systemic arterial blood pressure is dependent on the cardiac output and the peripheral vasomotor tone (resistance), which are primarily under autonomic control from the vasomotor center of the medulla. Cardiac arrhythmias, altered myocardial function, and cardiac disease can affect cardiac output, thus influencing CBF. In addition, a number of carotid sinus and aortic arch reflexes

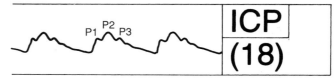

FIGURE 17-3
Abnormal ICP wave form (ICP = 18 mm Hg).

assist in maintaining a constant blood pressure. Advanced age, atherosclerosis, and certain drugs can alter these reflexes, thus affecting arterial blood pressure and CBF secondarily.

- **Blood viscosity.** Anemia may increase blood flow up to 30%, while polycythemia may decrease flow by more than 50%.

INTRACEREBRAL FACTORS. The primary intracerebral factors that influence CBF are widespread cerebrovascular artery disease and increased ICP.

Widespread cerebrovascular artery disease can increase cerebrovascular resistance, resulting in reduced CBF. Processes that rapidly shunt blood from arteries to veins (as in an arteriovenous malformation) can produce an increase in total CBF and a reduction in local tissue perfusion.

When **increased ICP** is present, it is transmitted to the low-pressure venous system, thus increasing cerebral venous pressure and decreasing CBF.

Regulation of Cerebral Blood Flow. Several other intracerebral regulator mechanisms can modify CBF and include autoregulation, chemical-metabolic regulation, and neurogenic regulation.[7]

AUTOREGULATION. The ability of an organ (such as the brain) to maintain a constant blood flow within a broad range despite marked changes in arterial perfusion pressure is called **autoregulation.** Autoregulation operates within limited parameters in healthy people—a mean arterial blood pressure of 60 to 150 mm Hg; below 60 mm Hg, CBF decreases, and above 150 mm Hg, CBF increases. Also, autoregulation generally operates with an ICP of less than 40 mm Hg.

Autoregulation is a major homeostatic and protective mechanism occurring in large and small arterioles and is sometimes called myogenic autoregulation. Arterioles contain smooth muscles that respond to stretch receptors and intraluminal pressure causing vasoconstriction to increase intraluminal pressure and vasodilation to decreased intraluminal pressure. Specifically, *autoregulation is primarily a pressure-controlled myogenic mechanism that operates independently, yet synergistically, with other chemical-metabolic and neurogenic autoregulatory mechanisms.* Autoregulation provides a constant CBF, maintained within the normal range by adjusting the diameter of blood vessels.

As with most compensatory mechanisms, a critical point is reached when other forces overcome autoregulation, thereby causing it to be impaired or lost locally or globally in an unpredictable pattern due to an ICP exceeding 40 to 50 mm Hg; local or diffuse injury, ischemia, or inflammation in cerebral tissue; or mean blood pressure in excess of 60 to 150 mm Hg. In patients with chronic hypertension, both the upper and lower limits of autoregulation are elevated.[8]

Without autoregulation, there is reduced cerebrovascular tone, known as **vasomotor paralysis,** and the CBF and CBV become passively dependent on changes in blood pressure.

CHEMICAL-METABOLIC REGULATION. Chemical and metabolic regulation exert a strong influence on CBF. Carbon dioxide, oxygen, and pH are important chemical regulators.

- **Carbon dioxide** (CO_2), found in the blood and locally in cerebral tissue as a end-products of cell metabolism, is the most potent agent that influences CBF. Cerebral blood vessels respond to changes in local carbon dioxide ($PaCO_2$) by vasodilating when $PaCO_2$ is high, thus increasing blood flow, and constricting when $PaCO_2$ is low, causing a decrease in blood flow.
- **Oxygen** (O_2) has the opposite effect: Reduction in local oxygen (PaO_2) produces vasodilation, and an increase in local PaO_2 produces vasoconstriction. The mechanism by which this is achieved is unclear.
- **H+** ions are also powerful agents that influence CBF. In body fluids, CO_2 combines with water to form carbonic acid, with subsequent dissociation of hydrogen ions. Hydrogen ion concentration can also be increased by lactic acid, pyruvic acid, and other acids that result from cell metabolism.
- **pH** changes also have an effect on cerebral arterioles; a low pH (acidosis) results in vasodilation and increased CBF, and a high pH (alkalosis) results in vasoconstriction and a decreased CBF. A buildup of the metabolic end-products of cell metabolism (lactic acid, pyruvic acid, carbonic acid) causes a localized acidosis. An increase in the concentration of these acids will also increase CBF.

Neurogenic Regulation. Neurogenic factors play a lesser role in regulation of CBF than the chemical-metabolic regulators. Neurogenic regulation includes a rich neural network that is extrinsic and intrinsic to the brain.[9]

- **Extrinsic neurogenic control.** Sympathetic innervation comes from postganglionic fibers of the superior cervical sympathetic ganglion that innervate the carotid and vertebral arteries and major intracranial branches. Norepinephrine, a vasoconstrictor, is released from the sympathetic fibers. Parasympathetic fibers come from the facial and superficial pertrosal nerves to innervate large- and small-diameter cerebral blood vessels. They use acetylcholine as a neurotransmitter, which causes vasodilation.
- **Intrinsic neurogenic control.** The intrinsic pathways originate in the brain stem and interneurons in the cerebral cortex. Brain stem pathways are from the locus ceruleus (neurons use norepinephrine to produce microcirculatory vasodilation), raphe nuclei (neurons use serotonin, a vasoconstrictor), and fastigial nuclei of the cerebellum. Cortical interneurons contain both vasoconstrictor and vasodilator substances.

Other Factors. An increase in CBF and CBV can also result from pharmacological agents, such as volatile anesthetic agents and some antihypertensives, and from rapid eye movement (REM) sleep, arousal, pain, seizures, elevations in body temperature (about 6% per degree centigrade), and cerebral trauma.

Cerebral Perfusion Pressure. **Cerebral perfusion pressure** is defined as the blood pressure gradient across the brain. The CPP found in a *normal* adult is in the range of 70 to 100 mm Hg. In the laboratory, ischemia is not seen until the CPP falls below 40 mm Hg.[10] However, in head-injured people, the observations regarding global blood flow and ICP changes may not accurately reflect areas of severe regional ischemia. Therefore, in cerebral trauma, the lower limits of CPP are probably 70 to 50 mm Hg.[11] Rosner recommends a CPP of 70 to 80 mm Hg for patients with cerebral injury and intracranial hypertension.[12] If CPP is inadequate, ischemia develops; if ischemia is not reversed, infarction results.

CPP is calculated as the difference between the incoming MAP and the opposing ICP. It is represented by the following formula:

$$CPP = MAP - ICP$$

CPP is an estimate of the adequacy of cerebral circulation. To calculate CPP, it is first necessary to compute the MAP. This is calculated as follows:

$$MAP = (systolic - diastolic)/3 + diastolic$$
Example: systolic = 130; diastolic = 82; ICP = 15
$$MAP = (130 - 82)/3 + 82 = 98$$
$$MAP - ICP = CPP$$
$$98 - 15 = 83$$

Cerebrovascular Resistance. **Cerebrovascular resistance** (CVR) is the pressure across the cerebrovascular bed from the arteries to the jugular veins, which is influenced by inflow pressure, outflow pressure, the diameter of the vessels, and ICP. (The cerebral venous system does not have valves as do other veins in the body. Thus, any condition that obstructs or compromises venous outflow may also increase CBV because blood is backed up into the intracranial cavity.) CVR is the amount of resistance created by the cerebral vessels, and it is controlled by the autoregulatory mechanisms of the brain. The CVR increases with vasoconstriction, decreases with vasodilation, and varies inversely with CBV.

Cerebral Metabolism. Under normal circumstances, the brain depends almost exclusively on glucose to obtain its energy needs. The energy needed is supplied from adenosine triphosphate (ATP), which is synthesized through the glycolytic pathway, Krebs' cycle, and respiratory chain. This accounts for the brain's high and critical dependence on oxygen.

Aerobic metabolism is the usual pathway for glucose metabolism. Glucose is metabolized through the previously mentioned pathways to yield 38 moles of ATP per mole of glucose. However, if anaerobic metabolism occurs, Krebs' cycle and the respiratory chain cannot be activated due to lack of oxygen. In these circumstances, pyruvate derived from glycolysis is metabolized to lactate, yielding only 2 moles of ATP per mole of glucose. Therefore, much less ATP is available to fuel the ATP-dependent sodium-potassium pump of cell membranes.

Pathophysiology

CEREBRAL ISCHEMIA AND CEREBRAL INFARCTION: THE ISCHEMIC CASCADE

Ischemia is a state reversible alteration in cell function due to a decreased oxygen supply. **Infarction** is irreversible alteration in function due to a lack of oxygen. Ischemia becomes infarction if no reversal action is taken. When the brain is deprived of an adequate blood supply, a chain of events occurs

called the ischemic cascade. The ultimate end-point of this process, unless reversed, is neuronal dysfunction and neuronal death. The ischemic cascade, as outlined by Westmoreland, Benarroch, Daube, Reagan, and Sandok, includes the following:[13]

- In the center of the ischemic area is a core of dead or dying cells surrounded by an ischemic area of minimally surviving cells called the **penumbra (halo)**. The cells of the penumbra receive marginal blood flow, but their metabolic activities are altered.
- Local autoregulation, responsiveness to chemical-metabolic factors, and perfusion pressure are impaired or lost.
- The lack of oxygen and glucose causes a switch to anaerobic metabolism.
- The absence of oxygen and glucose results in failure of ATP production; this, in turn, leads to ineffective cellular function and dysfunction of ATP-dependent neurotransmitter reuptake.
- The release of the excitatory neurotransmitter, glutamate, is increased; this results in increased neuronal necrosis. (Glutamate's neurotoxic effect occurs through activation of N-methyl-d-asparate receptors, which cause increased cell permeability to sodium ions, cellular swelling and lysis, and massive entry of calcium ions into the postsynaptic neuron.)
- The increase in intracellular calcium activates phospholipases and proteases, which generate oxygen-free radicals and nitric oxide. This leads to membrane, mitochondrial, and microtubular cellular damage and eventual death.

The survival of the penumbral cells depends on the successful re-establishment of an adequate circulation, the amount of end-products present, cerebral edema, and the alterations in local blood flow. If the cells of the penumbra die, the core of dead tissue enlarges, and the volume of surrounding tissue at risk increases.

With the breakdown in the blood–brain barrier, water content of the tissue increases, resulting in cerebral edema.

CEREBRAL EDEMA

Cerebral edema is an abnormal accumulation of water in the intracellular space, extracellular space, or both that is associated with an increase in brain tissue volume.[14] The edema can be a local or generalized problem, and it is usually associated with increased ICP. Cerebral edema can be serious and life-threatening because the increase in brain bulk produces pressure on the tissue, resulting in neurological deficit and exacerbation of the increased ICP. Severe cerebral edema can produce transtentorial herniation with progressive brain stem compression, herniation, and death.

Three types of cerebral edema are recognized: vasogenic, cytotoxic, and interstitial edema.

Vasogenic Edema. **Vasogenic edema** is an extracellular edema due to an increase in capillary permeability of the arterial walls to large molecules caused by a breakdown of the blood–brain barrier. As a result, a plasma-like filtrate, including large molecules of protein, leaks into the extracellular space. Vasogenic edema is seen locally around brain tumors, although it can develop around a cerebral infarct or a cerebral abscess.

Generalized vasogenic edema may occur with cerebral trauma or meningitis. Use of corticosteroids (dexamethasone) is effective especially with brain tumors. An osmotic diuretic (mannitol) may be helpful in the acute phase.

Cytotoxic Edema. **Cytotoxic edema** is increase in fluid in the intracellular space as a result of ATP-dependent sodium-potassium pump failure so that fluid and sodium accumulate within the cells, leading to diffuse brain swelling. The development of cytotoxic edema is associated with a hypoxic or anoxic episode, such as a cardiac arrest or asphyxiation. It is also seen with hypo-osmolarity conditions, such as water intoxication, hyponatremia, and the syndrome of inappropriate secretion of antidiuretic hormone.

Corticosteroids (dexamethasone) are not effective in treating cytotoxic edema. It is questionable whether furosemide is helpful. Osmotic diuretics may be beneficial in the acute stage when hypo-osmolarity is present.

Interstitial Edema. **Interstitial edema** occurs in the periventricular tissue when the intraventricular pressure is greater than the ability of the ependymal cells to contain the CSF within the ventricle. This forces the CSF across the ependymal tissue into the periventricular white matter. It is associated with acute and subacute hydrocephalus and possibly with benign intracranial hypertension (pseudotumor cerebri).

Corticosteroids or osmotic diuretics are ineffective, although acetazolamide (Diamox) may be administered to decrease CSF production. Treatment options include the temporary drainage of CSF until the condition corrects itself or surgical placement of a shunt.

Summary. Vasogenic and cytotoxic edema may be seen concurrently. Cerebral edema is considered to be proportional to the severity of injury or insult and reaches its maximum level in approximately 72 hours. It then gradually begins to subside, although it can persist to some degree for several months, depending on the degree of injury and other circumstances.

INTRACRANIAL HYPERTENSION

Intracranial hypertension, more commonly called increased ICP, is a symptom rather than a distinct disease entity. **Intracranial hypertension** is a sustained elevated ICP of 15 mm Hg or higher. The term **malignant hypertension** has been used by some authors to describe a sustained ICP of 20 mm Hg or higher. The underlying cause of increased ICP must be identified and treated to manage the problem effectively (Table 17-1).

Conditions that can cause intracranial hypertension can be classified as follows:

- Conditions that increase brain volume
  Space-occupying masses (*e.g.*, hematomas, abscesses, tumors, aneurysms)
  Cerebral edema (*e.g.*, head injuries, Reye's syndrome)
- Conditions that increase blood volume
  Obstruction of venous outflow
  Hyperemia
  Hypercapnia
- Conditions that increase CSF

TABLE 17-1
Correlation of Values of Intracranial Pressure Measurements (mm Hg and mm H₂O)

DESCRIPTION	mm HG*	mm H₂O‡
Normal	4–15	50–200
Slightly elevated	16–20	201–272
Moderately elevated†	21–39	286–530
Severely elevated	40 or greater	530 or greater
Correlation between mm Hg and mm H₂O data	10	136
	20	270
	30	410
	40	540
	50	670
	60	800
	70	900
	80	1050
	100	1360

* Also recorded in torr.
† Intracranial pressure ≥ 20 mm Hg is termed malignant hypertension.
‡ Approximate/mm Hg = 13.597 mm Hg.

Increased production of CSF (*e.g.*, choroid plexus papilloma)
Decreased absorption of CSF (*e.g.*, communicating hydrocephalus, subarachnoid hemorrhage)
Obstruction to flow of CSF (*e.g.*, communicating hydrocephalus)

The rate of development and extent of involvement of increased ICP and intracranial hypertension is related to cellular dysfunction and its consequences. Several factors influence the process. Once cerebral edema and increased ICP become established, a sequence of physiological events contributes to the perpetuation of dysfunction at the cellular level. The sequence of events is as follows:

↓ regional CBF → ↓ CPP in areas →↑ CO_2 (hypercapnia) ↓O_2 (hypoxia) → ↑ acidosis from end-products of cell metabolism → vasodilation → ↑CBF → ↑CBV → ↑ ICP → possible impairment of local autoregulation.

Moreover, decreased regional CBF and increased ICP activate the vasopressor ischemic response, resulting in increased MAP and increased CBF. This, in turn, leads to increased edema and ICP.

This circular sequence continues until the autoregulatory mechanisms are inactivated. The CBF passively responds to arterial blood pressure. The CBF and CPP cannot be maintained in relation to the rising ICP. The CPP approaches zero, and the CBF ceases. Blood vessels and brain tissue are compressed, and herniation and death follow.

SUMMARY OF FACTORS KNOWN TO INCREASE INTRACRANIAL PRESSURE

A number of factors known to increase ICP are included in Table 17-2. Many of these factors have been identified as a result of nursing research and are discussed further in the section on nursing management.

TABLE 17-2
Factors Known to Increase Intracranial Pressure

FACTORS AND DESCRIPTION	MECHANISMS
HYPERCAPNIA $Pco_2 \geq 45$ mm Hg Excessive levels of CO_2 in the blood Potent cerebral vasodilator	Elevated CO_2 results in increased CBF, which leads to increased CBV and ICP Hypercapnia results from underventilation of a patient in such circumstances as the following: • Sleep • Pulmonary diseases/conditions (*e.g.,* atelectasis, pneumonia, COPD, neurogenic pulmonary edema, ARDS) • Sedation from drugs • Shallow respirations, as seen with anxiety reactions, severe pain, or asynchrony with a respirator • Pressure on brain stem respiratory centers • Improperly calibrated respirator (*e.g.,* rate, sensitivity)
HYPOXEMIA $Po_2 < 50$ mm Hg Decreased O_2 in the blood Has a much lesser effect as a vasodilator compared to CO_2	Decreased O_2 does not increase cerebral vasodilation until it is 50 mm Hg or less. Hypoxemia results from the following: • Insufficient concentration of O_2 administered during O_2 therapy • Insufficient ventilation during and after suctioning • Inadequate ventilation during intubation • Partial or complete airway obstruction
RESPIRATORY PROCEDURES • Suctioning • PEEP • Asynchrony of respiratory rate when Ambu bag is used • Intubation • Increased airway pressure	Suctioning causes a decrease in O_2 and an increase in CO_2 and partially obstructs the airway with a catheter. PEEP causes increased intrathoracic pressure, which leads to increased central venous pressure, cerebral venous pressure, and ICP. Asynchronous use of the Ambu bag causes a response that is similar to the PEEP response. Same as suctioning
VASODILATING DRUGS Anesthetic agents (halothane, enflurane, isoflurane, nitrous oxide) Some antihypertensives Some histamines	Vasodilation causes increased CBF, resulting in increased ICP.
SOME BODY POSITIONS Trendelenburg position (always contraindicated in neuroscience patients) Prone position (increased intra-abdominal and intrathoracic pressures; also, neck flexion impedes venous drainage) Extreme hip flexion (increased intra-abdominal pressure) Hip flexion on a pendulous abdomen (increased intra-abdominal pressure) Angulation of the neck; neck flexion, even from a small, improperly positioned pillow, or improper lateral positioning when turned (which impedes venous return from the brain) Turning the patient laterally if the head of the bed is up and the knees are flexed on the abdomen (increased intra-abdominal pressure)	Obstruction of venous return from the brain increases CBV, which results in increased ICP. The venous cerebrovascular system has no valves; thus, an increase in intra-abdominal, intrathoracic, or neck pressure is communicated as increased pressure throughout the open venous system, thus impeding drainage from the brain and increasing ICP. It has been an accepted practice to elevate the head of the bed 30 degrees to facilitate drainage from the brain; current research is inconclusive as to what is the best degree of head elevation for promoting venous drainage from the brain.
PRESSURE ON NECK Snug "track tape," soft collar, or other constricting material	These impede venous drainage from the brain.

(continued)

TABLE 17-2

Factors Known to Increase Intracranial Pressure Continued

FACTORS AND DESCRIPTION	MECHANISMS
ISOMETRIC MUSCLE CONTRACTIONS	
Increased muscle tension without lengthening of the muscle	Isometric muscle contractions raise systemic blood pressure and contribute to further elevation of increased ICP in the patient who is on the borderline of brain compliance or who already has increased ICP.
Examples: pushing against the bed with one's feet, as in pushing oneself up in bed; pulling on an extremity restraint; shivering; decortication; decerebration; other rigidity	Passive range of motion (PROM) exercises do not involve isometric contractions because the length of the muscle does change during contraction. Therefore, PROM exercises should be included in the plan of care.
	Chlorpromazine (Thorazine) has been used to control shivering; pancuronium bromide (Pavulon) and baclofen (Lioresal) have been used for decerebration in the patient at risk for ICP spikes.
VALSALVA'S MANEUVER	
Exhalation against a closed epiglottis	Increased intra-abdominal or increased intrathoracic pressure impede venous return from the brain, thereby increasing ICP.
Examples: straining at stool, moving in bed, sneezing	If the patient's ICP is already elevated or brain compliance is borderline, spikes in ICP may occur.
COUGHING	
Increases intra-abdominal and intrathoracic pressure as a result of muscle visceral contractions	The increased intra-abdominal and intrathoracic pressure impede venous drainage from the brain.
	Also, the increased pressure is transmitted through the spinal subarachnoid space to the intracranial subarachnoid space and through the veins that communicate with the dural venous sinuses and intracranial subarachnoid space. The venous return from the cranial vault is impeded, resulting in increased ICP.
EMOTIONAL UPSET AND NOXIOUS STIMULI	
Upsetting conversations (*e.g.*, about prognosis, legal matters)	Activation of the sympathetic nervous system is probably the major cause of increased blood pressure, increased CBF, and increased ICP, particularly in the patient who already has increased ICP.
Noxious stimuli (*e.g.*, invasive procedures, such as lumbar puncture, or painful nursing procedures, such as removal of tape from skin)	
ACTIVITIES THAT INCREASE CEREBRAL METABOLISM	
Arousal from sleep	A focal or generalized increase in cerebral metabolism results from these activities. There is regional or generalized increased CBF, which is reflected in increased CBV, which causes an increase in ICP.
REM phase of sleep	
Seizure activity	
Hyperthermia	
CLUSTERING OF ACTIVITIES	
In a patient with already increased ICP, clustering of patient care activities (*e.g.*, bathing, turning) and other activities known to increase ICP can cause dangerous elevations in ICP and plateau waves in the patient at risk. The impact of nursing activities may be compounded after having blood drawn or undergoing an invasive procedure.	The compounding effect of activities causes an increase in blood pressure, CBF, and ICP; elevations of ICP can be high enough to cause plateau waves and cerebral ischemia.
Note that suctioning is notorious for increasing ICP in the patient at risk.	Spacing of procedures allows the patient's ICP to return to a safe baseline level. Observing the effects and the return to baseline on an ICP monitor provides a guide for delivering safe care to the patient at risk.

CBF, cerebral blood flow; CBV, cerebral blood volume; ICP, intracranial pressure; COPD, chronic obstructive pulmonary disease; ARDS, adult respiratory distress syndrome; PEEP, positive end expiratory pressure; PROM, passive range of motion; REM, rapid eye movement.

SIGNS AND SYMPTOMS OF INCREASED INTRACRANIAL PRESSURE

A Perspective

Increased ICP is a syndrome. A large percentage of neuroscience patients are at risk for developing ICP. Nursing assessment of neurological signs is directed at detecting *early* signs and symptoms of increased ICP when nursing and medical interventions are still effective. The baseline neurological assessment and ongoing assessments by knowledgeable practitioners are the most sensitive indicators of neurological change. When *late* signs appear (brain stem signs or changes in vital signs and alterations in respiratory pattern), it may be too late for effective interventions to reverse cerebral deterioration, herniation, or even death.

As discussed previously, several cerebral compensatory

mechanisms provide adequate CBF, CPP, and substrates for cerebral metabolism. These compensatory mechanisms act even when there is evidence of increased ICP. **Cushing's response** is a compensatory response that attempts to provide adequate CPP in the presence of rising ICP. The signs include the following:

- A rising systolic pressure
- A widening pulse pressure
- Bradycardia

These signs profile late brain stem dysfunction resulting from rising ICP and correlate with decreasing brain compliance.

Cushing's triad includes the following:

- Hypertension, usually with a wide pulse pressure
- Bradycardia
- Abnormal respiratory patterns

Cushing's triad is a very late presentation of brain stem dysfunction and correlates with low or loss of brain compliance. In such cases, cerebral herniation has probably already occurred, and the patient is critically ill. Interventions are directed at life-saving measures; cerebral dysfunctions may be irreversible at this point. Therefore, neurological assessment is directed toward *early* identification of neurological alterations so that interventions can be instituted when the chances of control and reversal are good.

Before discussing the traditional signs and symptoms associated with increased ICP, it may be helpful to consider a few points about ICP and how it can be masked or misinterpreted.

Clinical Variations in Increased Intracranial Pressure

Practitioners rely on clinical assessment for detection of the signs and symptoms of increased ICP and compromised CPP, but these are not necessarily apparent on clinical assessment of neurological signs. The overriding principle in explaining these dynamics is the *degree of compliance in the brain,* as explained by the pressure-volume curve (see Fig. 17-1). One cannot determine by clinical inspection where the patient is in relation to the pressure-volume curve. The patient's brain may be at the high compliance end of the curve or at the *low compliance* end when the slightest increase in ICP will result in decompensation and a significant elevation in ICP.

Direct Brain Stem Injury. Many of the signs and symptoms of increased ICP often cited (*e.g.,* decerebration, loss of the corneal reflex, changes in vital signs) relate to brain stem dysfunction. Direct primary brain stem injury can also produce similar signs and symptoms in the absence of increased ICP.

Transient Pressure Signs. The ICP is a dynamic rather than a constant pressure. Certain activities, such as straining and coughing, can elevate ICP. In a patient at risk who already has an elevated ICP, initiating an activity known to increase ICP

can precipitate *transient signs of increased ICP,* also known *as transient pressure signs* or *transient ischemic signs* (Chart 17-1). At the time of such a transient episode, the nurse may observe confusion or difficulty in arousal; a sluggish, slightly dilated pupil; or monoplegia or hemiparesis in a patient whose previous neurological assessment was normal. Reassessment within 5 to 20 minutes may reveal reversal of all symptoms. A transient elevation in ICP caused by a temporary interference with CPP resulting in transient ischemia is responsible for the clinical deterioration noted. This may explain why one nurse's observations of change may not be noted by another nurse who assesses the patient later.

Special Syndromes Associated With Increased ICP and CSF

Two special syndromes associated with increased ICP and CSF flow are benign intracranial hypertension and hydrocephalus.

BENIGN INTRACRANIAL HYPERTENSION (PSEUDOTUMOR CEREBRI)

Adams and Victor discuss pseudotumor cerebri, now called benign intracranial hypertension, in some detail.[15] This syndrome is seen most often in obese adolescent girls and young women. The chief complaint is headache, and in some instances, the patient experiences blurred vision, diplopia, slight numbness in the face, or dizziness. On physical examination,

---

CHART 17-1
Transient "Pressure Signs"

The following signs and symptoms are associated with transient elevations in ICP and cerebral hypoxia whereby there is temporary interference with CPP, resulting in transient ischemia. The signs and symptoms last a few minutes, occurring most often at the peak of plateau waves and then disappearing as the pressure decreases and CPP is once again reestablished. The signs and symptoms of transient "pressure signs" include the following:

- Decreased level of consciousness (*e.g.,* confusion, lethargy)
- Pupillary abnormalities
- Visual disturbances
- Motor dysfunction (hemiparesis or hemiplegia)
- Headache
- Aphasia
- Changes in respiratory pattern (*e.g.,* Cheyne-Stokes)
- Changes in vital signs

ICP, intracranial pressure; CPP, cerebral perfusion pressure

the patient is alert, aware, conversant, and seems otherwise well. The only abnormal finding is papilledema. On lumbar puncture, CSF pressure is usually about 250 to 450 mm H$_2$O. On computed tomography scan or magnetic resonance imaging, ventricles are of normal size, and there is no evidence of an intracranial mass or obstruction of CSF. Visual testing may find slight peripheral deficits. The immediate management concern is to reduce the papilledema to prevent visual impairment.

Treatment options include the following:

1. Repeated lumbar puncture to remove CSF until normal pressure is maintained (performed daily and then at increasing intervals)
2. Drug therapy if CSF pressure continues to be elevated and papilledema persists
   Prednisone (40–60 mg/d)
   Acetazolamide (Diamox; 750 to 1.0 g/d in two to four divided doses; carbonic anhydrase inhibitor that decrease CSF production)

In patients (approximately 10%) who do not respond to these treatments, trial of lumbar drainage, followed by placement of a lumbar peritoneal shunt may be necessary.

HYDROCEPHALUS

Hydrocephalus refers to a progressive dilatation of the cerebroventricular system because the production of CSF exceeds the absorption rate. Hydrocephalus is a clinical syndrome rather than a disease entity. Abnormalities in overproduction, circulation, or reabsorption of CSF can result in hydrocephalus. (See Chap. 5 for a review of CSF and circulation.)

Classification. Hydrocephalus can be subdivided into noncommunicating and communicating hydrocephalus:

- **Noncommunicating hydrocephalus** is a condition in which CSF in the ventricular system does not communicate properly within the subarachnoid space. Obstruction can be caused by a mass, such as a tumor within or adjacent to the ventricular system, a congenital obstruction, or an obliteration from an inflammatory process.
- **Communicating hydrocephalus** is a condition in which too few or nonfunctional arachnoid villi are unable to reabsorb CSF sufficiently. Subarachnoid hemorrhage secondary to aneurysmal rupture or a head injury can produce transient or lasting communicating hydrocephalus. The arachnoid villi become plugged and cannot reabsorb CSF. Plugging can occur from the end-products of blood cell breakdown or the exudate from meningitis.

The signs and symptoms of hydrocephalus depend on the type of hydrocephalus and the age of the patient. For noncommunicating hydrocephalus, treatment of the primary problem is necessary, usually with surgery. In communicating hydrocephalus, CSF drainage may be attempted to clear the arachnoid villi of exudate so that normal function will be resumed in the future. If this is ineffective, a surgical shunting procedure will be necessary. Selection of the particular procedure

will depend on the age of the patient and any preexisting health problems.

Because the scope of this text is limited to adult problems, no discussion of hydrocephalus in the infant or child is included. The reader is directed to a pediatric text for discussion of this topic.

Normal-Pressure Hydrocephalus. An important type of communicating hydrocephalus seen in older adults is called **normal-pressure hydrocephalus**; it is usually reversible. (This syndrome is also called occult hydrocephalus, low-pressure hydrocephalus, and normotensive hydrocephalus.)

In **normal-pressure hydrocephalus**, there is ventricular enlargement with compression of the cerebral tissue, but normal CSF pressure is noted on lumbar puncture. Various circumstances have been associated with the development of normal-pressure hydrocephalus:

- Plugging of the arachnoid villi secondary to subarachnoid hemorrhage
- Thrombosis of the superior sagittal sinus
- Head trauma, either accidental or following surgery, in which scarring of the basal cistern is thought to occur
- Bacterial meningitis, in which there is plugging and possible fibrotic changes of the arachnoid villi

After careful evaluation of some patients, particularly those 60 to 70 years old, if no associated precipitated condition has been found, the diagnosis is **idiopathic normal pressure hydrocephalus.**

Signs and Symptoms. The onset of normal-pressure hydrocephalus is insidious and slow to develop (over weeks or months). Changes occur so slowly that they can easily be overlooked by the patient and family, or they may be attributed to the aging process when an older patient is involved.

The cardinal symptoms include mental changes, urinary incontinence, and disturbances in gait. Mental changes may begin as mild forgetfulness along with a diminished level of generalized cognitive function and progress to severe impairment. In advanced cases, mutism and hypokinesia may be apparent. Gait disturbances begin with a slowed pace that includes wide-based, zigzag steps; subsequently, gait is unsteady, and falling is common. Upper extremity movement may be unaffected or slowed. With progression, independent ambulation is lost.

Urinary incontinence is not an early sign but appears later. Lost social inhibition and forgetfulness caused by cerebral atrophy are the probable causes. No headache or papilledema is noted, although unexplained nystagmus is apparent in many patients. Tendon reflexes, particularly in the lower extremities, are increased. In advanced cases, the Babinski, grasping, and sucking reflexes may be present.

Diagnostic Studies. The most common diagnostic studies are computed tomography and magnetic resonance imaging. Atrophy and enlarged ventricles are noted. A history of a slowly developing progression of symptoms is essential in establishing the diagnosis. Normal CSF pressure is noted on lumbar puncture.

Treatment. The accepted treatment for normal-pressure hydrocephalus is a ventricular shunt. When cerebral atrophy has occurred, reversal of symptoms is minimal. The following describes optimal outcomes from successful ventricular shunting:

- The most dramatic improvement that may be apparent almost immediately is in mental status. The patient will be much more alert, oriented, and manageable. Others will show gradual improvement.
- Incontinence may be quickly reversed.
- Reversal of gait disturbance takes longer; a permanent residual deficit may result.

Specific Signs and Symptoms of Increased Intracranial Pressure

The presenting signs and symptoms of increased ICP observed will depend on the following:

- The compartmental location of the lesion (supratentorial or infratentorial)
- The specific location of the mass (cerebral hemispheres, brain stem, or cerebellum)
- The degree of intracranial compensation (compliance)

The signs and symptoms of increased ICP may include the following:

Early Findings

- Deterioration in the level of consciousness (LOC; *e.g.,* confusion, restlessness, lethargy)
- Pupillary dysfunction
- Motor weakness, such as monoparesis or hemiparesis
- Sensory deficits
- Cranial nerve palsies (especially the oculomotor; slight ptosis); dysfunction of extraocular movement (EOM)
- Headache
- Possible seizures

Later Findings

- Continued deterioration in the LOC (coma)
- Possible vomiting
- Possible papilledema
- Headache
- Hemiplegia, decortication, or decerebration
- Changes in vital signs
- Impaired brain stem reflexes (corneal, gag reflexes)

The following signs and symptoms associated with increased ICP are discussed to clarify their relationship to the cluster of clinical observations found in increased ICP. Guidelines for assessment are found in Chapter 8.

DETERIORATION IN LEVEL OF CONSCIOUSNESS

Although deterioration in the LOC can be considered a generalized sign of neurological deficit, it is a reliable and sensitive *early* indicator of neurological deterioration. The LOC may be the first sign of deterioration for two reasons. First, the most highly specialized cells of the cerebral cortex are the most sensitive to the decreased oxygen supply that occurs with increased ICP. The patient responds to the oxygen deficit by becoming confused, restless, or drowsy or by having difficulty with cognition (memory and orientation to time, place, or person). Second, the LOC is altered with increased ICP because the cerebral cortex is supplied by the terminal arteries, which are most apt to be compromised, thereby decreasing the oxygen supply to the sensitive cells of the cerebral cortex.

The earliest changes in a deteriorating LOC are confusion, restlessness, and lethargy. Generally, disorientation is noted, first to time, then to place, and finally to person. As the ICP continues to rise, the patient becomes lethargic, stuporous, and finally comatose. In the terminal stages, there is no response to painful stimuli, and the patient is deeply comatose.

PUPILLARY DYSFUNCTION

With increased ICP caused by supratentorial masses or edema, changes in pupillary size, shape, and reaction to light are noted. In the early stages, the pupil begins to gradually dilate. In addition, it may become slightly ovoid, and its response to light may be sluggish. The hippus response (see Chap. 8) to light or an ovoid pupillary shape may be observed with the beginning of pressure on the oculomotor nerve. Because the source of the rising ICP (edema, space-occupying lesion) tends to be compartmentalized in the early stages, the pupillary dysfunction is ipsilateral to the lesion. In the later stages of increased ICP, the ipsilateral pupil becomes dilated and nonreactive (fixed) to light. Finally, in the terminal stages when a rising ICP has led to herniation, both pupils become bilaterally dilated and fixed. Compression on the oculomotor nerve from mass effect accounts for the pupillary dysfunction.

Pupillary reaction to light is an upper brain stem function (cranial nerve III) and provides data about brain stem function that are especially helpful when assessing the unconscious patient.

VISUAL AND EXTRAOCULAR MOVEMENT ABNORMALITIES

Visual deficits that can develop in the early stages of increasing ICP include decreased visual acuity, blurred vision, diplopia, and field cuts, all of which are subjective signs. These subjective symptoms require a conscious, conversant patient to provide this information to the examiner. EOM assessment can be conducted with a conscious, cooperative patient or by using the oculocephalic response in the unconscious patient.

Decreased acuity and blurring are probably associated with early hemispheric pressure because the visual pathways transect all of the lobes of the cerebral hemisphere. Diplopia is associated with paresis or paralysis of one or more of the extraocul muscles. With an attempt to focus in one direction, the images from both eyes will not fall on the same point on each retina, resulting in double vision. Visual fields and field cuts can be assessed by confrontation testing, again, requiring a cooperative, conscious patient.

Assessment of EOM is conducted to determine full EOM or EOM paralysis restricted to a particular plane. EOM can be tested by directing the patient to follow the examiner's finger through the full range of movement, or in an unconscious patient, the oculocephalic reflex can be assessed. The oculocephalic reflex provides data on the reflex ability of the eyes to cross midline. Dysfunction may be due to pressure from intracranial bulk that affects any EOM. EOM is innervated by cranial nerve III, IV, and VI in the brain stem and provides data about brain stem function that is especially helpful when assessing the unconscious patient.

DETERIORATION OF MOTOR FUNCTION

In the early stages, monoparesis or hemiparesis develops contralateral to the intracranial lesion due to pressure on the pyramidal tracts. In the later stages, hemiplegia, decortication, or decerebration develops because of increasing pressure on the brain stem. Decortication or decerebation may be unilateral or bilateral. In the terminal stages, the patient becomes bilaterally flaccid.

Clinically, there may be confusion about one of the most primitive flexion reflexes, sometimes called **triple flexion**, seen in the late stages. Flexor motor neuron activation is widespread, and the reflex results in flexor muscle contraction away from the source of the stimuli. This means that the flexor muscles at the ankle, knee, and hip contract to withdraw the whole limb. The clinical significance of this sign is that it is a primitive spinal reflex.

HEADACHE

In the early stages of rising ICP, some patients complain of a slight or vague headache. Headaches are not as common as one might expect. The following hypothesis of headaches and intracranial pathophysiology may be helpful.

The intracranial structures that are sensitive to pain are the middle meningeal arteries and branches, the large arteries at the base of the brain, venous sinuses, bridging veins, and the dura at the base of the skull. The brain is normally cushioned by CSF. When the volume of CSF is reduced, the cushion is decreased or eliminated. When the head is in the erect position, the brain sinks. In the horizontal position, the brain shifts to one side. To compensate for the decrease in CSF and to provide an adequate cerebral blood supply, the cerebral vessels dilate, particularly in the venous components. Dilation of the vessels, traction on the bridging veins, and stretching of the arteries at the base of the brain cause a headache.

Headache associated with increased ICP is worse on arising in the morning. This can be explained by noting that ICP rises to very high levels during the REM phase of sleep, which increases metabolism and produces carbon dioxide as an end-product. The associated hypercapnia causes vasodilation; this results in traction on proximal venous vessels and arterial stretching at the base of the skull. The result is headache.

VOMITING

Vomiting caused by increasing ICP is associated with infratentorial lesions or direct pressure on the vomiting center, the vagal motor centers located in the floor of the fourth ventricle in the medulla. The vagal motor center also mediates the motility of the gastrointestinal tract. An increase in ventricular pressure transmitted to these centers probably accounts for

vomiting. When the vomiting mechanism is directly affected by a neurological lesion, the afferent limb is short-circuited to produce vomiting without nausea. Without the warning of nausea, vomitus is ejected with unadulterated force because of the suddenness with which the thoracic and abdominal muscles contract.[16] The term projectile vomiting is used to describe the character of the vomiting.

CHANGES IN VITAL SIGNS

Blood Pressure. Blood pressure and pulse remain relatively stable in the early stages of rising ICP. In the later stages, when there is pressure on the brain stem, changes in blood pressure occur. An *ischemic reflex* is triggered by ischemia in the medullary vasomotor center, and systemic arterial pressure is increased. The intraluminal arterial pressure must be greater than the ICP for continued blood flow. As ICP rises, the blood pressure rises reflexively to compensate. Cushing's response is activated. The resultant elevation in blood pressure increases cardiac output so that the heart pumps with greater force, thus widening the pulse pressure. Increasing systemic blood pressure with a widening pulse pressure is the compensatory phase of increasing ICP. With deterioration the decompensation phase begins and blood pressure decreases.

Pulse. In the early stage of increasing ICP, the pulse is relatively stable. Bradycardia is probably due to pressure on the vagal control mechanism in the medulla. With a continued rise in pressure, the pulse drops to 60 bpm or less and becomes full and bounding. The decreased rate and bounding quality are compensatory to pump blood upward into vessels on which pressure is being exerted from expanding intracranial bulk. In the decompensatory stage, the pulse becomes irregular, rapid, and thready and then ceases.

Respirations. Alterations in the respiratory pattern are associated with direct pressure on the brain stem respiratory centers of the pons and medulla. The various patterns and associated anatomical levels are discussed in Chapter 8.

An acute increase in ICP can trigger development of acute neurogenic pulmonary edema in the absence of cardiac disease. Other possible acute respiratory complications include adult respiratory distress syndrome and disseminated intravascular coagulopathy. These conditions are discussed in Chapter 12.

Temperature. Variations in temperature are usually associated with hypothalamic dysfunction either by direct injury or due to traction on connecting tracts. During the compensatory phase of increasing ICP, temperature will probably be within normal limits. During the decompensatory phase, high temperatures are frequently observed (39°–41°C). Elevations in either phase need to be evaluated and differentiated between neurogenic hyperthermia and a temperature elevation due to an infection such as pneumonia.

LOSS OF BRAIN STEM REFLEXES

In the late stages of rising ICP, pressure on the brain stem causes loss or dysfunction of reflexes mediated by the brain stem. These reflexes include the pupillary, corneal, gag, swallowing, oculocephalic, and oculovestibular reflexes. The prognosis is poor for patients who have lost their brain stem reflexes.

PAPILLEDEMA

Papilledema, discussed in Chapter 8, is a blurring of the optic disc margin as noted in an ophthalmoscopic examination. Because the subdural and subarachnoid spaces continue along the optic nerve, increased pressure within the intracranial cavity is transmitted along the nerve. The result is edema of the head of the optic nerve viewed as the optic disc.

Depending on the circumstances, papilledema may be a late finding with increased ICP. It does not occur until the ICP has reached markedly elevated levels. Papilledema is not a universal observation made in all patients with increased ICP. In some patients, this may be the first sign observed if an elevated ICP has developed gradually.

Relationship of Increased Intracranial Pressure to Herniation Syndromes. Increased ICP that continues to develop will result in herniation. **Herniation** is defined as the abnormal protrusion of an organ or other body structure through a defect or natural opening in a covering membrane, muscle, or bone. When considering cerebral herniation, the tentorium cerebelli and the foramen magnum need consideration. The tentorium cerebelli is a double fold of dura mater that forms a partition between the cerebrum and cerebellum. The foramen magnum is the hole at the base of the skull (occipital bone) through which the spinal cord passes. If an elevated ICP continues to rise unchecked, a portion of the cerebrum will be herniated through the tentorium, with resulting exertion of pressure on the brain stem. This will eventually result in cerebellar tonsil herniation through the foramen magnum, the only opening in the closed cranial vault. Cerebellar tonsillar herniation is a sure cause of death because of pressure on the vital structures in the medulla.

The most common type of transtentorial herniation is uncal or lateral transtentorial herniation. Central herniation is less common because fewer masses are located on the midline axis.

In summary, there is an important relationship between increasing ICP and herniation syndromes. Increased ICP will lead to a herniation syndrome with serious consequences or death if not treated aggressively (Table 17-3).

HERNIATION SYNDROMES OF THE BRAIN

To understand the pathophysiology of cerebral mass lesions, it is most important to understand the principles that govern herniation of the brain caused by cerebral edema or a space-occupying lesion, such as a tumor or hematoma. The intracranial cavity is divided into several smaller compartments by folds of the fibrous, relatively rigid dura mater. The most important dural folds follow:

- **Falx cerebri** drops into the longitudinal fissure and partially divides the supratentorial space into a left and right side.

- **Tentorium cerebelli** separates the occipital lobes from the cerebellum and much of the brain stem; it creates a partition between the area above the tentorium, the supratentorial space, and the area below the tentorium, the infratentorial space. The tentorium is a tentlike structure higher in the center than on the sides of the skull. To allow the brain stem, blood vessels, and accompanying nerves to pass through the tentorium, there is an oval opening in the tentorium called the **tentorial notch** or **incisura**.

When cerebral edema or a mass occurs within a compartment, the pressure exerted by the lesion is not evenly distributed, resulting in shifting or herniation of the brain from a compartment of high pressure to one of lesser pressure. The shifting of cerebral structures due to pressure is called the **mass effect**. In the wake of this shifting, there is pressure or traction on some structures, which is evidenced by malfunction of the particular cerebral tissue.

Supratentorial Herniation

Three major patterns of herniation, described by Plum and Posner in their classic work, identify syndromes caused by expanding supratentorial lesions[17]: (1) cingulate herniation, (2) central or transtentorial herniation, and (3) uncal or lateral transtentorial herniation (Fig. 17-4).

CINGULATE HERNIATION

An expanding lesion in one cerebral hemisphere can cause pressure medially so that the cingulate gyrus is forced under the falx cerebri, displacing it toward the opposite side. The displacement of the falx can create compression of the local blood supply and cerebral tissue, causing edema and ischemia, which further increase the degree of ICP elevation. Cingulate herniation is common, but little is known about its clinical signs and symptoms.

CENTRAL OR TRANSTENTORIAL HERNIATION

The usual causes of rostral-caudal downward displacement of central transtentorial herniation follow:

- A lesion located on the central neural axis
- An extracerebral lesion located around the central apex of the cranium
- Bilaterally positioned lesions in each hemisphere
- Unilateral cingulate herniation

The lesion produces a downward displacement of the cerebral hemispheres, basal ganglia, diencephalon, and midbrain through the tentorial incisura. The diencephalon can be compressed tightly against the midbrain with such force that edema and hemorrhage result. Often, anterior choroidal artery depression is noted on the cerebral arteriogram. Central transtentorial herniation may or may not be accompanied by uncal herniation.

The early symptoms of central transtentorial herniation include the following:

TABLE 17-3
Progressive Signs and Symptoms of Uncal and Central Herniation*

LATERAL TRANSTENTORIAL HERNIATION (UNCAL SYNDROME)

Parameter	Local Early Signs	Diencephalon-Midbrain	Midbrain-Upper Pons	Lower Pons-Upper Medulla	Medulla
Pupils	Unilateral, dilated pupil; sluggish, nonreactive	Unilateral, dilated, and fixed	Bilateral, dilated, and fixed	→	→
Extraocular signs	May have ptosis Slight weakness → of oculomotor innervated muscles	Slight weakness becomes paralysis	→ →	→ →	→ →
Level of consciousness	Little effect on consciousness; restlessness Once deterioration begins, quick progression to a deep coma	Stupor; coma	Deep coma	→	→
Motor	Slight weakness (pronator drift)	With Kernohan's notch, hemiparesis on side of lesion Contralateral monoparesis; hemiparesis to hemiplegia; decerebration	Bilateral decerebration	Flaccidity with occasional decerebration	→
Sensory	Progressive deterioration	→	→	→	→
Babinski's sign	Negative	Bilateral positive	→	No reflexes	→
Respirations		Cheyne-Stokes	Central neurogenic hyperventilation	Shallow	Ataxia; then respirations cease
Other			Bradycardia Elevated systolic blood pressure Widening pulse pressure Wide variations in temperature; may be grossly elevated	Deterioration of vital signs Elevated temperature	No vital signs and temperature of 104°F or higher Temperature of 104°F or higher

TRANSTENTORIAL HERNIATION (CENTRAL SYNDROME)

Parameter	Local Early Signs	Diencephalon-Midbrain	Midbrain-Upper Pons	Lower Pons-Upper Medulla	Medulla
Pupils	Bilaterally small and reactive	→	Not equal in size, but each about midpoint and nonreactive	→	Dilated and fixed
Extraocular signs	May be normal or slightly roving; eventually, difficulty with upward gaze may be noted	Difficulty with → upward gaze	Dyconjugate gaze	→	→
Level of consciousness	Difficulty with concentration; becomes agitated or drowsy, then stuporous	Stuporous; coma	Deep coma	→	→
Motor	Contralateral hemiparesis to hemiplegia	Rigidity on ipsilateral side, which becomes decorticate	Bilateral decerebration	Flaccidity with occasional decerebration	→

(continued)

TABLE 17-3
Progressive Signs and Symptoms of Uncal and Central Herniation*
Continued

		TRANSTENTORIAL HERNIATION (CENTRAL SYNDROME)			
Parameter	*Local Early Signs*	*Diencephalon-Midbrain*	*Midbrain-Upper Pons*	*Lower Pons-Upper Medulla*	*Medulla*
Sensory	Progressive deterioration	→	→	→	→
Babinski's sign	Negative	Bilaterally positive Babinski's sign	→	→	→
Respirations	Cheyne-Stokes	→	Central neurogenic hyperventilation	Shallow	Ataxia; then respirations cease
Other			Wide variations in temperature (often very high)	Elevated temperature	Temperature of 104°F and higher
			Many develop diabetes insipidus		
			Bradycardia	Erratic pulse (fast and then slow)	No vital signs
			Elevated systolic blood pressure	Decreased blood pressure	
			Widening of pulse pressure		

* *An important point to keep in mind when observing a patient with a possible herniation syndrome is that there is predictable order to the development of signs and symptoms. The neurological deterioration in both central and uncal herniation proceeds in an orderly rostral-caudal scheme; the diencephalon, midbrain, pons, and finally, the medulla are affected from the increasing pressure. Signs and symptoms characteristic of each area can be identified. Notice that the last stages of central and uncal herniation are the same.*

- Stupor to coma
- Cheyne-Stokes respirations
- Small, reactive pupils (in early diencephalic stage)
- Gradual loss of vertical gaze
- Contralateral hemiplegia
- Ipsilateral rigidity that develops into decorticate and decerebrate posturing

The progression of symptoms with continued pressure is detailed in Table 17-3.

UNCAL OR LATERAL TRANSTENTORIAL HERNIATION

The most common cerebral herniation syndrome is uncal herniation. An expanding lesion of the lateral middle fossa, most often of the temporal lobe, causes shifting of the inner basal medial edge of the temporal lobe. This area contains the uncus and hippocampal gyrus; the uncus is forced through the tentorial incisura. The diencephalon and midbrain are compressed and displaced to the opposite side by the uncal herniation. With this lateral displacement, the cerebral peduncle (contralateral to the unilateral uncal herniation) may be compressed against the firm, unyielding edge of the tentorium incisura, producing **Kernohan's notch**. This is important because it results in an oculomotor localizing sign of hemiparesis on the same side as a cranial nerve deficit, rather than on the opposite side as would be expected (Fig. 17-5).

The oculomotor nerve (III) and the posterior cerebral artery on the same side of the expanding temporal lobe lesion are frequently caught between the overhanging edematous uncus and the free edge of the tentorium or another resistive structure. The entrapment of the oculomotor nerve results in ipsilateral pupillary dilation, which is usually an early sign of uncal herniation.

The signs of uncal herniation include the following:

- Ipsilateral pupillary dilation
- Ptosis
- Paralysis of the extraocular muscles
- Restlessness, then a deteriorating LOC
- Decrease or loss of sensory function
- Contralateral hemiparesis or hemiplegia
- Bilateral Babinski's signs
- Respiratory changes (*e.g.*, Cheyne-Stokes, ataxic patterns)
- Decorticate and decerebrate posturing
- Finally, dilated, fixed pupils; flaccidity; and respiratory arrest

The progression of symptoms with continued pressure is described in Table 17-3.

Any of the supratentorial herniation syndromes can initiate vascular and obstructive complications that can further exaggerate the seriousness of the neurological deterioration. Compression of the aqueducts of the ventricular system can cause CSF circulation to be interrupted. As a result, major spikes in ICP and hydrocephalus can develop. Cingulate herniation can compress both arterial and venous vessels (portions of the anterior cerebral artery and the great cerebral

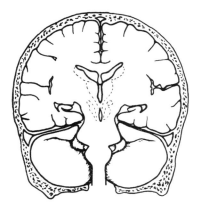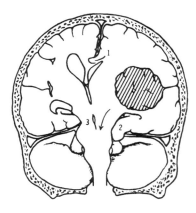

FIGURE 17-4

Cross section of a normal brain (*left*) and a brain with intracranial shifts from supratentorial lesions (*right*). (*1*) Herniation of the cingulate gyrus under the falx. (*2*) Herniation of the temporal lobe into the tentorial notch. (*3*) Downward displacement of the brain stem through the notch. (From Plum, F., & Posner, J. [1972]. *Diagnosis of stupor and coma.* [2nd ed.]. Contemporary neurology series. Philadelphia: F.A. Davis.)

vein), causing exacerbation of already present ischemia and edema.

When there is uncal herniation, the herniated tissue through the tentorial incisura compresses the posterior cerebral artery, resulting in partial occipital lobe infarction and edema. Brain stem edema, ischemia, and hemorrhage can develop from the diencephalon to the pons-medulla area secondary to the downward displacement from central herniation.

The result of progressive downward displacement from any of the supratentorial herniation syndromes is brain stem herniation, in which the medulla herniates into the foramen magnum. Death is immediate and is attributable to medullary compression. The medulla controls vital functions, such as respiration, blood pressure, cardiac function, and vasomotor tone, all of which are absolutely necessary for life.

Infratentorial Herniation

Lesions of the infratentorial compartment contributing to herniation are much less frequent than those involving the supratentorial region. The three possible effects of an expanding lesion of the infratentorial compartment follow:

• Direct compression of the brain stem, cerebellum, attached cranial nerves, and vascular supply
• Upward transtentorial herniation of the brain stem and cerebellum through the tentorial incisura, resulting in maximal pressure on the midbrain
• Downward herniation of both or one cerebellar tonsil through the foramen magnum with compression of the medulla (Fig. 17-6)

An expanding lesion causes direct pressure on selected structures. The increased pressure interferes with the normal function of the involved tissue and causes edema, ischemia, infarction, and necrosis if the process is not reversed. As the lesion continues to expand, the only sources of egress from the infratentorial compartment are the tentorial incisura or the larger orifice, the foramen magnum.

The brain stem structures, particularly the medulla, contain centers for vital functions. If medullary compression develops, death from respiratory and cardiac arrest is possible. Infratentorial expanding lesions can also encroach on a portion of the ventricular system so that hydrocephalus develops. The signs and symptoms noted with the various types of in-

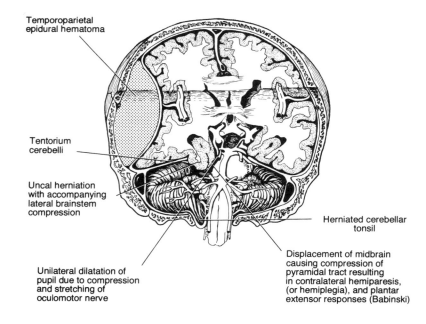

Temporoparietal epidural hematoma

Tentorium cerebelli

Uncal herniation with accompanying lateral brainstem compression

Unilateral dilatation of pupil due to compression and stretching of oculomotor nerve

Displacement of midbrain causing compression of pyramidal tract resulting in contralateral hemiparesis, (or hemiplegia), and plantar extensor responses (Babinski)

Herniated cerebellar tonsil

FIGURE 17-5

Crosssection of the brain showing herniation of part of the temporal lobe through the tentorium as a result of a temporoparietal epidural hematoma. (Kentzel, K. C. [1997]. *Advanced concepts in clinical nursing* [2nd ed.]. Philadelphia: J. B. Lippincott.)

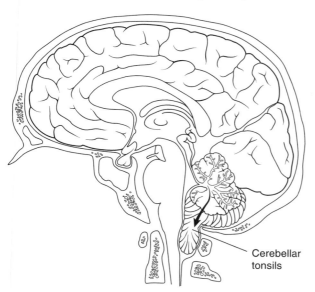

FIGURE 17-6
Herniation of the cerebellar tonsils into the foramen magnum is the final outcome of increased intracranial pressure. Respiratory centers within the medulla oblongata are compressed, and apnea leads to cardiac arrest and death.

fratentorial herniation syndromes vary depending on the brain stem area most involved.

The reader is cautioned to recognize the wide range of possible signs and symptoms with brain stem lesions. Clear-cut clinical syndromes are not present in the infratentorial compartment.

The most prominent signs associated with lesions compressing the brain stem include the following:

- Coma
- Abnormal respiratory patterns (Cheyne-Stokes, central neurogenic hyperventilation)
- Pupillary changes
- Ophthalmoplegias (*e.g.*, loss of upward gaze)
- Hemiparesis and hemiplegia
- Decortication or decerebration, which can progress to flaccidity
- Cranial nerve dysfunction (cranial nerves III through XII)
- Vital sign abnormalities

In summary, herniation syndromes are life-threatening occurrences that can progress rapidly. Early recognition of signs and symptoms is important for prompt intervention to prevent neurological demise. Signs and symptoms of impending herniation are summarized in Chart 17-2.

MANAGEMENT OF PATIENTS WITH ACUTE INCREASED ICP: MANAGING A COLLABORATIVE PROBLEM

Management of patients with acute increased ICP (intracranial hypertension) is a collaborative problem in which the nurse and physician share responsibilities for patient outcomes.

Medical and nursing management is directed toward early diagnosis and treatment of the underlying cause(s), control and management of intracranial hypertension, support of all body systems with particular attention to adequate cardiopulmonary function, and prevention of complications.

Technology and the Intensive Care Unit

The use of computers and computerized, integrated, databases and documentation systems, such as the CareVue (Hewlett-Packard) system, are changing how health professionals practice. In addition, an integrated database allows development of more sophisticated data-driven alerting, quality assurance, and decision-making programs that reduce errors and improve care. Databases also facilitate research, manage prognostication and scoring systems, enhance administrative record keeping and procedures, and facilitate some tasks that would otherwise be difficult or impossible to accomplish.

Patients with acute increased ICP will most likely receive care from a highly skilled critical care team within an intensive care unit (ICU) setting that has technological capabilities for bedside diagnostics, treatment, and invasive and noninvasive continuous monitoring. In addition to highly skilled professional care, most patients require continuous physiological monitoring to determine the need for interventions, adjust interventional strategies to meet desired end-points or physiological target parameters, and determine the response to therapy.

Arterial and central lines, such as Swan-Ganz and central venous pressure lines, are common in ICU settings. Arterial blood pressure, pulmonary artery pressure, central venous pressure, mixed venous oxygen saturation (SVO_2), and ICP are the most common physiological parameters monitored. (ICP monitoring is discussed later in this chapter.) Both continuous waveforms and continuous digital values are available. Other physiological values, such as cerebral perfusion pressures, are computer calculated and are available as continuous digital values.

Because of the critical reliance of the brain on oxygen, there is great interest, especially in neurocritical care, on monitoring oxygen delivery and consumption. Total body oxygen delivery and consumption are measured by a fiberoptic cath-

---

CHART 17-2
Signs and Symptoms of Impending Herniation

- Decreased level of consciousness (coma)
- Pupillary abnormalities
- Motor dysfunction (hemiplegia, decortication, or decerebration)
- Impaired brain stem reflexes (corneal, gag, swallowing)
- Alterations in vital signs, including respiratory irregularities

eter located in the pulmonary artery. Jugular bulb catheterization through retrograde internal jugular cannulation for cerebral venous blood access provides information about the adequacy of CBF and a global composite measure of whole-brain oxygen extraction by measuring mixed venous oxygen saturation (SVO$_2$).[18] The noninvasive pulse oximeter is easy to use and provides continuous data about oxygen saturation (SaO$_2$) from a sensor placed peripherally on a finger or an earlobe. In addition, continuous intra-arterial determination of blood gas analysis is now available. Monitoring of target organ oxygenation is critical to preserving neuronal tissues.

Monitoring of ventilatory function is vital. This can be accomplished from continuous data provided by sophisticated ventilators. Data provided include minute ventilation, ventilatory drive, and ventilatory distribution. Other data that can be collected include respiratory system mechanics and muscle function. Physiological data, along with data from ongoing clinical assessment, provide the foundation for clinical reasoning and decision making for patient care and the achievement of desired outcomes.

Strategies and Interventions for Increased Intracranial Pressure

Strategies and interventions used to manage patients with increased ICP include respiratory and airway support, oxygen therapy, hyperventilation, cardiac support, pharmacological agents, temperature control, seizure control, fluid restriction, CSF drainage, barbiturate coma, and surgery. These are discussed in the following sections. When considering the efficacy of any intervention, the effect on an increased ICP must be considered.

RESPIRATORY SUPPORT

In a previous section, the effects of CO$_2$ and O$_2$ on ICP are discussed. Adequate oxygen, a patent airway, and possibly ventilation support are necessary. If use of a ventilator is indicated, pressure support mode and positive end expiratory pressure may be used within limitations.

Positive airway pressure from mechanical ventilation is transmitted to the intracranial cavity through the mediastinal structures. The mean airway pressure is the key factor that indirectly affects the intracranial compartment. One of the factors alleged to raise ICP is **positive end expiratory pressure** (PEEP). It elevates the mean airway pressure and thus decreases mean arterial and cerebral perfusion pressure. Any event, such as pneumonia or neurogenic pulmonary edema, that decreases pulmonary compliance also attenuates the transmission of positive airway pressure through the lungs to the mediastinal cavity. As a result, PEEP has less of an effect on ICP. PEEP of 5 to 15 cm H$_2$O is well tolerated in patients with increased ICP.[19] Concurrent ICP monitoring is the best way to determine the actual effect.

Hyperventilation. Use of **hyperventilation** to reduce increased ICP is controversial. However, hyperventilation is a rapid and effective method of reducing ICP by inducing hypocarbia that results in vasoconstriction of the cerebral arteries, reduced CBF, and increased venous return from the brain.

Serum and CSF alkalosis causes cerebral vasoconstriction; this results in reduced intracranial volume and decreased ICP.

The response time for reduction of ICP by hyperventilation is almost immediate. The usual method to induce hyperventilation in a ventilated patient is to increase the ventilatory rate while maintaining a tidal volume of 12 to 15 mL/kg. The target level of PCO$_2$ is two-tiered and adjusted to target physiological values. Tier one of target PCO$_2$ is 30–35 mm Hg; tier two is a PCO$_2$ of 27–30 mm Hg. If the ICP and other physiological parameters improve with the first tier of PCO$_2$, it is not necessary to reduce PCO$_2$ further. However, if no improvement is noted, the provider may choose to lower the PCO$_2$ to the 27–30 range. Adjustments are made based on ICP, CPP, and arterial blood gas monitoring. The PCO$_2$ should be lowered gradually to prevent a "rebound effect" from overcorrecting. When hyperventilation is discontinued, it should also be withdrawn gradually over 12 to 24 hours.

Hyperventilation using an Ambu bag is sometimes necessary to decrease ICP in a patient who is demonstrating "pressure signs" and needs rapid reduction of ICP when a ventilator is not present. Ambu hyperventilation is done only until a ventilator can be obtained.

The effectiveness of hyperventilation appears to be time limited and thus transient. It is unclear how long hyperventilation should be maintained. Clinicians vary from 1 to 3 days to up to 1 week for appropriate use of the intervention.

What is controversial about hyperventilation? First, hyperventilation can increase mean airway pressure that is transmitted to the intracranial cavity, especially in compliant lungs, as seen in young, otherwise healthy patients. This will lead to an increase in ICP, the opposite desired effect. Second, PEEP can result in decreased cardiac filling pressures, which will be further aggravated by hyperventilation. Hypotension and compromised cerebral perfusion would then occur. The proactive approach to this potential problem is to maintain adequate intravascular volume and monitor the patient with a central line to assess hemodynamic stability. Third, severe vasoconstriction may result in ischemia. Fourth, barotrauma caused by high pressure of ventilation is possible. Fifth, it is unclear if hyperventilation improves patient outcome or functional level.

CARDIAC SUPPORT AND BLOOD PRESSURE CONTROL

Managing blood pressure is an important concern because of the serious consequences related to extremes in blood pressure. **Hypotension** can cause cerebral ischemia, whereas **severe hypertension** may aggravate edema in injured cerebral tissue in which the blood–brain barrier has been disrupted. Much is still unknown about the *best* level of blood pressure to maintain in terms of the "big picture" of dynamic intracranial equilibrium in a brain-injured patient with increased ICP. Certainly, maintaining adequate CPP is critical in preventing ischemia, but the optimal CPP for a particular patient can vary, depending on the circumstances.

The decision to treat systemic hypertension is difficult. If the systemic blood pressure is elevated because of the compensatory mechanism of Cushing's response, it should not be treated. Cushing's response is a compensatory ischemic response that reflexively raises the blood pressure in response to a rising ICP. If the blood pressure did not rise, the ICP would be equal to the blood pressure, and CBF would cease. Therefore, blood pressure is not lowered until an elevated ICP is controlled. Maintenance of adequate CPP is the best guide for the control of systemic hypertension. The goal should be to maintain a CPP of approximately 70 mm Hg.

Clinical judgment and experience guide selection of appropriate antihypertensive drugs. Some antihypertensives cause vasodilation, thus increasing CBF and ICP. The following can raise ICP:

- Vasodilators, such as nitroprusside, hydralzaine, and nitroglycerin
- Some calcium channel blockers (Nimodipine, however, does not affect ICP.)

If antihypertensive drugs are indicated, those most often used are intravenous beta blockers or the combined alpha and beta blocker, labetalol. These drugs be may given in combination with diuretics. If a hypotensive event occurs, a fluid bolus and a vasoactive drug are indicated. The drug of choice is phenylephrine hydrochloride (Neo-Synephrine).

PHARMACOLOGICAL INTERVENTIONS SPECIFIC FOR INCREASED INTRACRANIAL PRESSURE

Osmotic Diuretics. Osmotic diuretics work on the principle of establishing a high osmotic gradient to draw water from the extracellular space of the edematous cerebral tissue into the plasma. The extracellular fluid is hypotonic in relation to the hypertonicity of the serum. Water is drawn from the brain, thus reducing the bulk (volume) of the brain. Although glucose, urea, glycerol, and mannitol have been used as osmotic diuretics to treat increased ICP, only mannitol is discussed because it is the mainstay of hyperosmolar therapy.

Mannitol. Mannitol (Osmitrol) does not cross the blood–brain barrier. Its osmotic effect causes water to be drawn from the extracellular space of the edematous brain into the plasma, thereby reducing brain volume and decreasing ICP. Mannitol (20%–25%) is considered relatively safe and is administered intravenously through a filter. The filter is necessary because of the risk of crystallization of the drug. The current practice is to give small, frequent doses of mannitol to maintain the patient. Ropper and Rockoff suggest 0.75 to 1 g/kg initially, then 0.25 to 0.5 g/kg every 3 to 5 hours, infused rapidly.[20] The dose and frequency are correlated with ICP, CPP, and serum osmolality. Therapy is directed at keeping the serum osmolality at approximately 310 to 315 mOsm/L, depending on multiple variables. The maximal effect of mannitol should be noted within 20 to 60 minutes and can last for 1 to 3 hours. In some patients, a rebound effect, observed as a rise in ICP, may occur after administration.

Mannitol can cause fluid (dehydration) and electrolyte imbalance (especially hypokalemia). Serum osmolality, glucose, electrolytes, and the intake and output record must be monitored. An indwelling catheter is necessary to monitor urinary diuresis. Hypokalemia is common after days of mannitol therapy; potassium replacement is necessary. Mannitol is not administered to patients with hypovolemic shock, congestive heart failure, dehydration, or kidney disease.

Furosemide, a loop diuretic, may be used to manage the rebound effect from mannitol, but it is not a mainstay drug for the primary management of increased ICP.

Corticosteroids. Corticosteroids have no demonstrated benefit for treatment of increased ICP in cerebral infarction with edema or traumatic brain injury.[21] It is generally accepted that the use of corticosteroids in the management of vasogenic edema associated with brain tumors is effective.

NEUROMUSCULAR BLOCKADE AND SEDATION

Neuromuscular blockade (paralysis) and sedation are used to control activities associated with elevations of ICP. The goal is to prevent increases in intrathoracic and venous pressure that may occur with coughing, straining, or "bucking" of the ventilator, which initiate the Valsalva's maneuver. It also controls other activities, such as agitation, that increase cerebral metabolism and blood pressure, thus contributing to an increase in ICP. Many different drugs are used for paralysis. The most common include benzodiazepines (lorazepam, midazolam); opioids (morphine, meperidine); neuroleptics (haloperidol); and others (pancuronium, propofol, ketamine). Each drug has special management implications. For example, in patients receiving propofol, triglycerides must be monitored. With this deep sedation or paralysis, the patient's neurological signs, the most sensitive indicator of neurological status, are lost.

Although neuromuscular blocking drugs are administered for extended periods in ICUs, there are no real standards of care. There are wide variations in individual responses to neuromuscular blockade and a number of side effects, such as prolonged weakness. Side effects may be minimized by precise monitoring of the degree of blockage for correlation with drug titration. Using a peripheral nerve stimulator and monitoring clinical signs of muscle movement are safe ways of periodically monitoring degree of blockade by the nurse and other care providers.[22]

In a recent review of the literature, the conclusion about sedation in critically ill neurological patients was that preservation of the neurological examination is paramount in documenting clinical improvement or deterioration. Pharmacological sedation of this population requires careful consideration of the underlying neurophysiological disturbances and potential adverse effects introduced by sedative drugs.[23]

TEMPERATURE CONTROL

The cerebral metabolic rate increases when body temperature is elevated. In the patient with existing cerebral hypertension, the increase in systemic blood pressure and CBF exacerbates the existing increase in ICP. Therefore, it is important to treat hyperthermia aggressively.

This is accomplished with antipyretic drugs, such as acetaminophen, used alone or in combination with a hypothermia blanket. If a cooling blanket is used, cool the patient slowly to prevent shivering because this will increase ICP.

SEIZURE CONTROL

Cerebral metabolic rates are increased with seizures; this results in increased CBF, CBV, and ICP. The underlying cause of seizures should be treated. Seizure prophylaxis should be instituted for patients who are high risk for seizures. The drug of choice is phenytoin (Dilantin). A loading dose of phenytoin can be given intravenously over 1 hour for the seizing patient. If drug reaction or allergy to phenytoin is noted, phenobarbital can be used. The average maintenance dosage of phenytoin is 100 mg orally or intravenously, three to four times daily. See Chapters 11 and 31 for further discussion of anticonvulsants.

FLUIDS AND FLUID RESTRICTION

Rigid fluid restriction is no longer followed because of concern for dehydration and hypotension. Hypotension is a dangerous consequence of decreased cerebral perfusion pressure and cerebral ischemia. The concurrent cerebral hypoxia can result in further increases in ICP. The goal is adequate fluid management with *saline*. Monitoring of serum osmolality, electrolytes, and glucose is necessary to guide clinical decisions regarding electrolyte replacement, selection of saline concentration of fluids, rate of fluid administration, and glucose management. Hypoglycemia and hyperglycemia can produce neurological changes, so they are to be avoided. Hypotonic glucose intravenous solutions are avoided. Hyperglycemia is controlled with a sliding scale of regular insulin according to periodic finger sticks and if needed, a regular insulin intravenous drip.

CEREBROSPINAL FLUID DRAINAGE

The insertion of a catheter into a lateral ventricle for CSF drainage is called a **ventriculostomy**. The catheter is inserted through a burr hole made into the skull as a temporary method to reduce ICP rapidly. Ventriculostomy can sustain the patient through spikes in ICP or during acute hydrocephalus associated with subarachnoid hemorrhage. For patients who are undergoing continuous ICP monitoring, the nurse can periodically drain the CSF when the ICP exceeds a predetermined level established by the physician. Insertion of a ventricular catheter is invasive and places the patient at high risk for infection. Controversy exists about antibiotic prophylaxis for patients with ventriculostomies. The drainage system is maintained as a closed system with an inclusive dressing to decrease the risk of infection. The level of the drainage bag is calibrated according to agency policy.

In some instances, CSF drainage occurs through the insertion of a lumbar catheter to a drainage bag. This is used for chronic drainage needs. Again, concern for infection is present. Positioning of the drainage bag is according to agency policy.

SURGERY

If there is a localized mass, such as a hematoma, tumor, or abscess, removal or debulking of the lesion will help to reduce intracranial hypertension. In addition, in patients with intracranial hypertension that is resistant to control by the usual methods, decompression by debulking of infarcted and necrotic cerebral tissue may improve control of intracranial hypertension.

BARBITURATE COMA

Barbiturate coma therapy is a controversial treatment modality developed to manage uncontrolled intracranial hypertension that is resistant to conventional therapy. It has been useful in reducing increased ICP in patients with head injuries, Reye's syndrome, encephalitis, and cerebral hemorrhage. The underlying therapeutic principle is a rapid decrease in cerebral metabolism and CBF, which leads to a decrease in CBV and ICP. Barbiturates also have a vasoconstriction effect.

Barbiturate therapy consists of administering a loading dose and maintenance doses of a short-acting barbiturate. The drug most often used is pentobarbital (Nembutal), although some physicians prefer thiopental. The following are expected outcomes from barbiturate therapy:

- Cerebral vasoconstriction, which decreases CBF and CBV
- Decreased cerebral metabolism, which promotes stabilization of the cell membrane
- Preservation of ischemic cerebral cells from irreversible damage by improving and stabilizing the blood supply throughout the entire cerebral arterial system
- Lowered ICP to an acceptable level

Once barbiturate coma is induced, the usual parameters of neurological assessment, such as the pupillary, gag, and swallowing reflexes, are lost. Cortical activity, as measured by electroencephalogram, is depressed, although brain stem-evoked responses may remain intact. Continuous invasive monitoring of ICP, cardiac, and pulmonary function is necessary. Peripheral and central lines for fluid and drug administration are also needed. The patient is maintained on a ventilator with an endotracheal or tracheostomy tube and a urinary catheter in place.

There is controversy regarding the best approach to barbiturate coma, that is, low-dose or high-dose barbiturates. Induction of coma is accomplished by administering a loading dose of intravenous pentobarbital, 3 to 10 mg/kg, over 15 to 30 minutes, depending on dose. After that, smaller maintenance doses—about 1 to 2 mg/kg per hour—are given. Maintenance doses are adjusted to maintain the serum level in the range of 3 to 4 mg/dL or the target therapeutic concentration set by the physician. A typical protocol is to administer a loading dose of 200 to 300 mg of pentobarbital and observe the patient for improvement. Pentobarbital, 100 mg, is then administered every hour for 24 to 48 hours for maintenance.[24]

Barbiturate coma should have an almost immediate effect of lowering the ICP. After the patient has maintained an ICP of less than 20 mm Hg pressure (or whatever the level prescribed by protocol) for 24 to 72 hours, the drug is gradually tapered. If there is no response to therapy, the physician must decide how long the trial period should continue before the therapy is declared unsuccessful.

The major problems associated with barbiturate coma are hypotension, dehydration, cardiac depression, and erratic dose response. Vasopressors may be administered to maintain blood pressure within targeted ranges. Phenylephrine hydrochloride or dopamine, administered intravenously, are frequent choices. Albumin and other fluids are given to provide adequate volume and prevent dehydration. The other drugs used in the conventional management of increased ICP are also continued (*e.g.*, mannitol, steroids). Therapeutic ranges for physiological parameters, such as blood pressure and CPP, must be set to guide practice.

The barbiturate, which is usually pentobarbital, is stored in body fat. The decision to discontinue barbiturate coma is not followed by declaring the patient brain dead. The brain death criteria followed by physicians in the United States are based on the absence of spontaneous respirations and brain stem reflexes. Barbiturates could be responsible for the loss of these activities. Therefore, these criteria cannot be established until the drug is cleared from the body. It can be difficult to wait, especially if organ donation is a consideration. However, there are serious medicolegal implications if this is rushed.

HYPOTHERMIA

Use of hypothermia to decrease central metabolism and oxygen consumption is being used experimentally to preserve neuronal tissue and improve outcomes. The body temperature is dropped to 35°C and the patient monitored. Clinical trials are currently in progress.

MEASURING AND MONITORING INCREASED INTRACRANIAL PRESSURE

Continuous ICP monitoring has become common in neurological ICUs for patients with intracranial hypertension associated with conditions such as head injuries, Reye's syndrome, subarachnoid hemorrhage, stroke, and herpes encephalitis. Monitoring of ICP provides data for making treatment decisions and assists the nurse in observing the patient's responses to nursing interventions and medical treatment.

The major components of an ICP monitor are the sensor, transducer, and recording device. The intracranial sensor, once implanted, transmits changes in ICP to the transducer, which converts the impulses to electrical or light signals. The recording device converts the electrical impulses into visible tracings on an oscilloscope or graph paper or to digital values that appear on a screen.

Types of Monitoring Techniques

Four basic devices are used for continuous ICP monitoring: the intraventricular catheter, subarachnoid bolt, epidural or subdural catheter or sensor, and fiberoptic transducer-tipped catheter (FTC; Fig. 17-7). Table 17-4 presents a summary of the advantages and disadvantages associated with each device. A few additional comments are made about the FTC because it is the most popular and widely used catheter.

FIBEROPTIC TRANSDUCER-TIPPED CATHETER

The FTC, developed by Camino Laboratories, is a frequently used catheter. The FTC is a 4-French catheter with a miniature fiberoptic transducer located at the catheter tip. Light fibers within the catheter convey light impulses created by movement of a mirrored diaphragm, which reflects pressure changes. The light signal is converted into electrical signals in the amplifier connector. Mean pressures are displayed on a digital monitor that can interface with an additional analog monitor for display of continuous waveforms (Fig. 17-8).

The FTC is calibrated by the manufacturer before shipping. Just before insertion, the catheter is zero (atmospheric) balanced. There is no further need to recalibrate during use. The FTC can be inserted easily into the ventricle (ventriculostomy), subarachnoid space, subdural space, brain parenchyma, or under a bone flap. A scalp stab wound is made, and a small twist drill is used to drill a small hole through bone. A housing device (a small bolt) is then screwed in place. The dura is perforated, and the transducer probe is threaded through the housing device to the desired depth and fixed in position by tightening the ring unit over the housing device. Finally, a protective sheath is snapped into position.

Pressure Waves

With continuous ICP monitoring, the fluctuations in waveforms correlate with specific physiological events. Waveforms, which can be examined individually or in trend recordings, are helpful in identifying changes in the patient's condition. The morphology of each waveform has been discussed previously in relation to compliance.

Trend recordings compress continuous ICP recording data into time periods (*e.g.*, 5- to 60-minute blocks) to reflect general trends in ICP over longer periods. Three distinct pressure waves have been identified: A (plateau) waves, B waves, and C waves (Fig. 17-9).

A Waves (Plateau Waves)

- Derive their name from the "plateau" shape of the trended waves forms
- Sudden, transient waves that begin from an *already* elevated ICP (>20 mm Hg) and last 5 to 20 minutes
- Seen in patients with *already* elevated ICP who have decreased cerebral compliance
- Elevations in pressure noted to levels of 50 to 100 mm Hg
- Often cause transient or paroxysmal symptoms, sometimes called *pressure signs* (see discussion that follows)
- Reflect cerebral ischemia and "pressure signs," which do not reverse

B Waves

- Sharp spikes occurring every 30 seconds to 2 minutes
- Peak ICP of 20 to 50 mm Hg but pressure level not sustained
- Seen in relation to fluctuations in the respiratory cycle, as in Cheyne-Stokes respirations
- Not considered clinically significant

C Waves

- Relate to normal changes of the systemic arterial pressure
- Occur four to eight times per minute
- Pressure of up to 20 mm Hg
- Not considered clinically significant

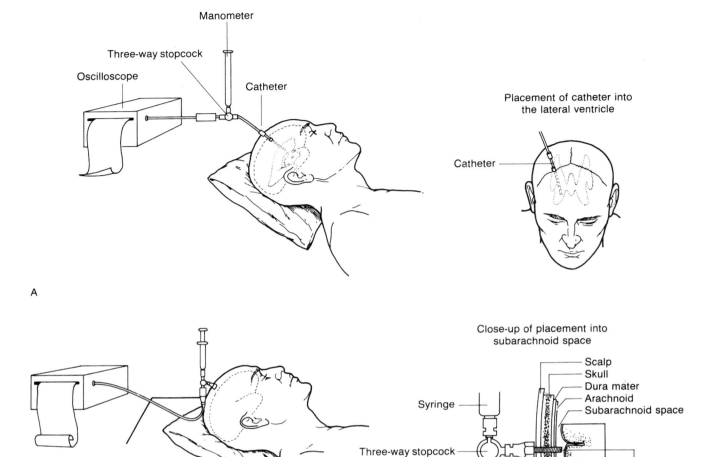

FIGURE 17-7
Major intracranial pressure monitoring devices. (*A*) Vetricular catheter monitor. (*B*) Subarachnoid screw or bolt monitor. (From Smeltzer, S., & Bare, B. [1996]. *Brunner and Suddarth's textbook of medical-surgical nursing* [8th ed.]. Philadelphia: Lippincott-Raven Publishers.)

CLINICAL IMPLICATIONS OF PLATEAU WAVES

Plateau waves are clinically significant because they peak to levels of 50 to 100 mm Hg from an **already elevated base ICP**. Plateau waves correlate physiologically with cerebral hypoxia, ischemia, and possible infarction to selected areas. Because cerebral tissue is sensitive to decreased O_2, symptoms of cerebral dysfunction may be evident.

The degree of dysfunction may be subtle (*e.g.*, confusion, restlessness) or pronounced (*e.g.*, hemiplegia). "**Pressure signs**" may include deterioration in LOC; abnormal pupillary reaction; paresis, paralysis, or decortication or decerebration; aphasia; headache; changes in respiratory pattern (*e.g.*, Cheyne-Stokes); and other changes in vital signs. Although pressure symptoms are paroxysmal, transient manifestations, they may last for a prolonged period

after the plateau waves have subsided. Early recognition of a tendency toward plateau waves or the presence of factors that trigger plateau waves should be followed by early intervention to prevent or control these dangerous waves.

Infection Control and the Intracranial Pressure Monitor

Any invasive monitoring, such as ICP monitoring, increases the risk of infection. This risk is further increased if a patient is immunosuppressed as a result of steroid therapy. Some physicians order prophylactic antibiotics for these patients, and others do not. Vancomycin is a common choice for prophylaxis and treatment of an infection.

Incidence rates for infection related to ICP invasive mon-

TABLE 17-4
Advantages and Disadvantages of the Various Intracranial Pressure Monitoring Devices

TYPE/COMMENT	ADVANTAGES	DISADVANTAGES
Intraventricular catheter (IVC) (Pioneered by Lundberg, 1960) See Fig. 17-7A	• Gold standard for accuracy • Drains excess CSF fractionally to reduce ICP • Collects CSF specimens for analysis • Injects contrast media for roentgenographic studies • Evaluates cerebral compliance by injection of fluid (rarely done)	• Insertion may be difficult if ventricles are small (owing to lateral mass effect from edema). • A large burr hole is needed for catheter insertion. • The nurse must zero and recalibrate frequently. • CSF leakage may occur around insertion site. • Catheter can become plugged with blood or cerebral tissue. • It is associated with a high risk of infection.
Subarachnoid screw/bolt (Developed by Vires, 1973) See Fig. 17-7B	• Collects CSF specimens for analysis • Decreased CSF drainage around catheter site • Insertion easier and quicker than IVC.	• Possible occlusion of bolt from herniation of cerebral tissue, especially when pressure is high or hematoma present • Less accurate at high ICPs because of occlusion • Must zero and recalibrate frequently (*e.g.*, when repositioning patient and at least every 4 h) • Tendency for dampened waveforms and baseline drift • Requires frequent flushing to maintain patency • High risk for infection
Epidural/subdural catheter or sensor (Fiberoptic sensor uses light to ascertain position of diaphragm, which moves in response to internal pressure)	• Depending on specific type, recalibration not necessary • The brain or subarachnoid space not penetrated, so chance of infection lessened • Ease of insertion • Decreased risk of infection	• Does not allow for collection of CSF samples • Does not allow for drainage of CSF • "Wedge effect" as a result of pressure from adjacent dura; can lead to inaccurate readings over time, so accuracy questioned • Baseline drift
Fiberoptic transducer-tipped catheter (Developed by Camino Laboratories)	• Easy to insert; requires a very small hole • Versatile; can insert into ventricle, subarachnoid space, subdural space, or brain parenchyma • Zero-balancing required once, at time of insertion • Baseline drift minimal over time • Has own monitor; patient can be transported while being monitored • Waveform without artifacts • Decreased risk of infection	• Does not allow for CSF sampling • Fragile fiberoptic cable that can break as a result of patient movement or during care; replacement of the probe necessary periodically.

itoring vary widely, with reported ranges of 1.7% to 64%.[25,26] The variables identified as influencing these rates follow:

• Type of catheter (highest rate with intraventricular catheters; lowest with FTCs)
• Length of time of monitoring (rates increase greatly after 4 days)
• Flushing of the system (increases the infection rate)
• Open versus closed systems (open, air-vented systems have increased infection rate)

Nursing Management of the Patient During Intracranial Pressure Monitoring

Continuous ICP monitoring provides a means for the nurse to assess the effect that patient and nursing activities have on the patient's ICP. Most patients undergoing ICP monitoring also have central lines for hemodynamic monitoring that supply continuous data on MAP. These data are used to calculate

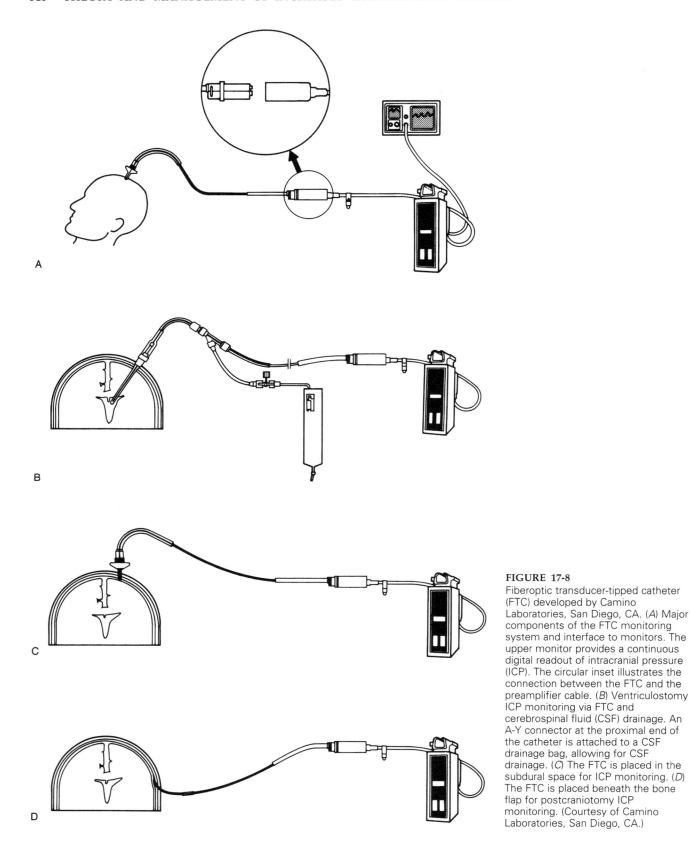

FIGURE 17-8
Fiberoptic transducer-tipped catheter (FTC) developed by Camino Laboratories, San Diego, CA. (*A*) Major components of the FTC monitoring system and interface to monitors. The upper monitor provides a continuous digital readout of intracranial pressure (ICP). The circular inset illustrates the connection between the FTC and the preamplifier cable. (*B*) Ventriculostomy ICP monitoring via FTC and cerebrospinal fluid (CSF) drainage. An A-Y connector at the proximal end of the catheter is attached to a CSF drainage bag, allowing for CSF drainage. (*C*) The FTC is placed in the subdural space for ICP monitoring. (*D*) The FTC is placed beneath the bone flap for postcraniotomy ICP monitoring. (Courtesy of Camino Laboratories, San Diego, CA.)

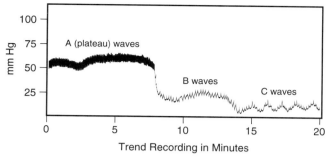

FIGURE 17-9
Intracranial pressure waves. Composite diagram of A (plateau) waves, B waves, and C waves.

CPP. Normal range is 60 to 90 mm Hg, although the target goal may be set higher than the minimum for certain patients. CPP is a direct indicator of the adequacy of cerebral perfusion pressure, so monitoring the CPP is just as important as monitoring ICP. The ability to interpret accurately continuous waveforms and trends in waveforms (previously discussed in this chapter) assists the nurse in monitoring the dynamics of ICP and hemodynamics.

Special considerations in the nursing management of a patient with an ICP monitor include the following:

- Maintain an occlusive dry sterile dressing around the insertion site, and change it on a prescribed schedule according to agency policy (usually every 24 to 72 hours).
- Monitor the insertion site for signs of infection, drainage, or CSF leakage.
- Position the equipment and patient properly; this means periodic zeroing for some types of catheters.
- Handle the FTC carefully to prevent breakage.
- Interpret the data for increased ICP, and alert the physician as necessary.
- Monitor pressure waveforms for dampening effect.
- Follow the manufacturer's specific instructions for use of monitoring system.
- Develop skill in basic troubleshooting of the equipment.

NURSING MANAGEMENT OF THE PATIENT WITH ACUTE INCREASED INTRACRANIAL PRESSURE

The nursing management of the patient with increased ICP is complex because the mechanisms that control ICP are not well understood, and the theoretical basis for treatment is still not well established. *Increased ICP is a collaborative problem* and requires a collaborative effort by physician and nurse to manage the patient successfully.

The research of Mitchell, Parsons, Rudy, and others has contributed to the body and knowledge for research-based practice in the management of patients with increased ICP (see bibliography for citations). These data have identified some correlations between independent nursing activities (*e.g.*, turning, positioning) and changes in ICP. Although many ques-

tions are unanswered, neuroscience nurses must incorporate knowledge for research-based practice.

General Nursing Management Principles

The nursing management of patients with acute increased ICP is directed toward identifying the patient at risk, managing factors known to increase ICP, supporting all body systems, controlling intracranial hypertension, and preventing complications. A summary of general nursing management is found in Chart 17-3.

NEUROLOGICAL ASSESSMENT

Frequent assessment of neurological and vital signs must be undertaken to ascertain any changes in neurological status. This means that at frequent intervals (every 15 minutes to every 4 hours, depending on the patient's situation), a neurological assessment is performed that includes the following:

- LOC
- Pupillary size and direct light reaction
- Eye movement
- Motor function
- Selected reflexes (*e.g.*, corneal, gag) as necessary
- Vital signs

Changes in findings are often subtle and may be detected only by performing serial evaluations and comparing those findings to previous assessments. For example, if the nurse notices that a previously alert and oriented patient is now confused, this is a significant finding. The nurse may need to consider other explanations of confusion, such as response to drugs, but alterations in consciousness are often apparent *before* changes in pupillary size or reaction to light, eye movement, motor or sensory function, or vital signs occur.

Vigilant nursing observation is still the most sensitive indicator of early change. Early recognition allows for definitive action to be taken to reverse the deterioration process. Once the pupillary and other signs become apparent, the downhill course of events can occur rapidly, allowing little time for intervention.

Noting trends of subtle changes applies not only to the LOC, pupillary size and reaction, eye movement, and motor function, but also to vital signs. It is most important to note trends in vital signs because deterioration in neurological status can herald a change from a compensatory neurological state to one of decompensation. Slowing of the pulse, widening of the pulse pressure, and an elevated systolic reading are signs of deterioration, although these are late signs. (The nurse should not wait until these signs are present before acting on evidence of change identified from subtle, earlier signs and symptoms.) In summary, periodic neurological assessment is the basis for identifying neurological change.

IDENTIFYING THE PATIENT AT RISK

The patient at risk is one who has an elevated ICP. Such patients are at risk for decreased intracranial compliance and
(text continues on page 322)

CHART 17-3
Summary of Nursing Management of the Patient With Increased Intracranial Pressure (ICP)

Principles of nursing management for the patient with increased ICP incorporate concepts of physiology and pathophysiology and objectives of medical management. In a patient with cerebral hypertension and increased ICP, a major objective is to protect the patient at risk from sudden increases in ICP and decreased CPP. The specific points of nursing care outline the nurse's role in providing care.

Nursing Responsibilities	Rationale
Neurological Assessment	
1. Assess baseline neurological signs, then reassess periodically and compare to previous findings. (Assess level of consciousness, pupillary size and reaction to light, eye movement, and motor and sensory function.)	1. Subtle changes in neurological signs can indicate deterioration or improvement in neurological status. These changes can only be detected by frequent monitoring and comparison with previous findings.
2. Assess vital signs. (Compare findings with previous recordings to note trends.)	2. Note trends. Vital signs correlate poorly with early neurological deterioration.
3. Assess temperature; initiate treatment for elevations. Guard against shivering; if on a cooling blanket, remove patient when a temperature 1°C or 2°F above normal body temperature is reached because temperature drifts downward even after the blanket has been discontinued.	3. Elevated temperature, increased oxygen consumption, and increased production of byproducts of metabolism exacerbate increased ICP.
Establishing and Maintaining a Patent Airway and Adequate Ventilation	
1. Assess rate, depth, and pattern of respirations. (Respirations should be regular and in a normal range.)	1. Indicates the patency of the airway and neurological basis of respirations
2. Assess skin for cyanosis (check around mouth, nail beds, and ear lobes).	2. Indicates adequacy of respirations and the oxygen–carbon dioxide exchange
3. Auscultate chest for breath sounds. (Normal breath sounds should be heard in all lobes without rales.)	3. Indicates proper lung expansion and presence of adventitious sounds
4. Suction, as necessary, for no more than 15 seconds per catheter insertion.	4. The time limit prevents increased CO_2, which is a potent cerebral vasolidator that can exacerbate increased ICP.
5. Preoxygenate with 100% O_2 for 30 sec to 1 min before suctioning, if high O_2 concentration is not contraindicated.	5. Provides adequate oxygenation so elevation of CO_2 will be minimized
6. If ventilator does not have a "sigh" setting for periodic hyperinflation, use an Ambu bag for a few minutes periodically to expand all areas of the lungs.	6. Preventive measures to control atelectasis.
7. If a tracheostomy is present, provide tracheostomy care every 4–8 h.	7. Maintains patency of airway
8. Monitor blood gases.	8. Reliable indicator of hemodynamics of respiratory function
9. Administer O_2 as ordered.	9. Supplements O_2 as needed
10. Apply pulse oximeter to a finger or earlobe.	10. Monitors SaO_2 on a continuous basis and alerts nurse to low level
Positioning and Moving Patients	
1. The head of the bed should be elevated to 30° or flat if ordered by physician; avoid a prone position, or extreme hip flexion.	1. Elevating the head of the bed facilitates venous return from the brain. Recognize the underlying principle if the flat position is ordered; monitor the

(continued)

CHART 17-3 Summary of Nursing Management of the Patient With Increased Intracranial Pressure (ICP)
(Continued)

Nursing Responsibilities	Rationale
	ICP and CPP if ICP monitoring is being used. Avoiding the prohibited positions averts increased intraabdominal or intrathoracic pressure interference with drainage from the venous vessels from the head and brain.
2. Maintain the head in neutral position. Avoid lateral neck flexin or constricting bands (tracheostomy tube tapes) around the neck.	2. Facilitates venous drainage from the brain.
3. Turn the patient every 2 h, and give skin care.	3. Prevents skin breakdown from pressure and moisture; also aids in respiration by preventing hypostatic pneumonia and atelectasis
4. Patients who are able to follow simple directions should be instructed to exhale on turning or moving.	4. Prevents initiation of the Valsalva's maneuver and attendant increases in ICP
5. Assist in moving up in bed. *Do not* ask the patient to push with his or her heels or arms or to push against the footboard.	5. Prevents initiation of the Valsalva's maneuver and attendant increases in ICP
6. Do not suggest isometric exercises for alert patients. However, passive range-of-motion exercises *should* be incorporated into the nuring care plan.	6. Isometric contractions initiate the Valsalva's maneuver, whereas passive range-of-motion exercises do not. Muscle tone, atrophy, and contractures are prevented by administering passive range-of-motion exercises.

Management of Urinary Elimination and Bowel Function

1. Monitor fractional urinary output and periodic specific gravity of urine.	1. Indicates the amount of diuresis and urinary dilution. Trauma may precipitate diabetes insipidus, which would be evidenced by specific gravity of 1.001 to 1.005 and an output of 200 mL or more for 2 consecutive h.
2. Administer stool softeners. Avoid enemas or straining at stool.	2. Prevents initiation of the Valsalva's maneuver, which occurs when straining at stool or as a result of an enema

Ventricular Drainage

1. With ventriculostomy drainage, head-of-the-bed elevation will depend on the physician. The nurse should know how high the drainage bottle should be kept above the level of insertion.	1. Placing the collection bag too low provides for too-rapid removal of drainage and can lead to brain herniation; placing the collection bag too high will restrict drainage.
2. Maintain strict aseptic techniques at all times.	2. Prevents infection
3. Maintain a closed system.	3. Prevents infection

Continuous Intracranial Monitoring

1. If used, the nurse must be familiar with the specific type of ICP monitoring device in use.	1. Ability to use equipment safely and to troubleshoot the system
2. The nurse must assume responsibility for interpreting the readings and should know what to do about atypical readings.	2. Guides initiation of appropriate interventions
3. Maintain strict aseptic technique.	3. Prevents infection

General Nursing Management

1. Plan nursing care so that activities that are apt to produce spikes in ICP are not clustered together.	1. Contrary to what has previously been considered good organizational skills in patient management, *do not* cluster activities, such as turning and

(continued)

CHART 17-3 Summary of Nursing Management of the Patient With Increased Intracranial Pressure (ICP)
(Continued)

Nursing Responsibilities	Rationale
	pulling the patient, getting the patient on and off a bedpan, or suctioning within the same time period. Individually, these activities may not cause ICP spikes in the patient at risk, but collectively, such spikes can be precipitated.
2. Review laboratory data (BUN, electrolytes, blood gases, osmolality, creatinine).	2. Identifies abnormal findings for collaboration with physician
3. Check stools for occult blood daily.	3. These patients are high risk for GI bleeding.
4. Monitor serum glucose every 4–6 h.	4. A side effect of Decadron therapy is hyperglycemia.
5. Monitor blood level of anticonvulsive drug.	5. A therapeutic drug level must be maintained for control of potential seizure activity.
6. Maintain seizure precautions.	6. Prevents injury, should a seizure occur
7. Apply elastic stockings and consecutive sequential air boots; monitor the patient for development of deep vein thrombosis.	7. Thrombophlebitis is a common complication for patients maintained on bed rest. Pulmonary emboli can result from dislodged thrombi.
8. Administer basic hygienic care and basic preventive interventions to control consequences of immobility.	8. Measures designed to meet basic needs, prevent complications from developing, and reverse the signs and symptoms of increased ICP

Drug Therapy

1. The nurse must be well versed as to the action, dosage, preparation, route, side effects, contraindications, and interactions of each drug prescribed.	1. Provides for safety of the patient and ensures optimal therapeutic value from drugs
2. Common drugs used include:	
• Osmotic diuretics: mannitol, 20%–25%, IV, small doses	• Decreases cerebral edema and ICP
• Anticonvulsants: phenytoin (Dilantin), 100 mg t.i.d., PO	• Prevents seizure activity
• Stool softeners: Colace, 100 mg t.i.d., PO	• Prevents straining at stool (Valsalva's maneuver)
• Antacid: Maalox or another antacid, 30 mL PO, with Decadron	• Prevents GI irritation
• Histamine blockers: cimetidine (e.g., Tagamet), 300 mg q.i.d., PO or IV	• Prevents stimulation of gastric secretions and increased acidity
• Antipyretics: Tylenol, 650 mg, PO or PR	• Controls elevated temperatures

subsequent compromised CPP, ischemia, hypoxia, neurological deficits, and further exacerbation of the already increased ICP to higher levels of intracranial hypertension. By identifying the patient at risk early, the nurse can modify the planned care to prevent spikes in ICP and control the already present intracranial hypertension.

MANAGING FACTORS KNOWN TO INCREASE INTRACRANIAL PRESSURE

Table 17-2 summarizes the factors known to cause an increase in ICP. Much of the information included is supported by nursing research. Within the realm of independent nursing practice, the nurse can apply this knowledge to assist in man-

aging activities that have the potential for increasing ICP, some of which are described in the following sections.

Positioning and Turning. **Valsalva's maneuver** is the forceful expiration of air against a closed glottis, which increases intra abdominal and intrathoracic pressure, impedes venous return from the brain, and impedes venous return to the heart. Changing position when lying down is an example of an activity that may precipitate Valsalva's maneuver. Because the nurse is responsible for positioning and turning the patient on a regular basis, steps must be taken to avoid triggering Valsalva's maneuver.

To avoid stimulating the Valsalva's maneuver, the patient is turned and positioned in proper body alignment, avoiding angulation of body parts. The proper technique can be compared to rolling a log, which actually facilitates alignment when turning. Special attention must be given to the neck and hips. The neck is maintained in a neutral position at all times. A soft collar, towel roll, or small pillow may be helpful. The following positions should be avoided:

- Lateral flexion of the neck
- Trendelenburg or prone position
- Extreme hip flexion or flexion of the upper legs on a pendulous abdomen

The head of the bed is usually elevated 30 degrees to facilitate cerebral venous drainage (see Fig. 16-1). In recent years, there has been discussion about elevation of the head and its effect on CPP. Some physicians prefer to keep the head of the bed flat because arguing that this position better facilitates adequate CPP.[27] The flat position is maintained within preset ICP and CPP parameters; once these parameters are exceeded, the decision may be made to elevate the head of the bed. Elevation of the head of the bed to 30 degrees is the general practice by a majority of physicians. However, the nurse should be aware that in some circumstances, the head of the bed may be maintained in the flat position.

The patient should be positioned in good body alignment in the lateral position. This also facilitates oropharyngeal drainage. Pillows are useful to position the patient properly. If able to follow instructions, the patient should be instructed to exhale when being turned.

Bowel Management. A bowel program should be initiated to prevent constipation, which increases intra-abdominal pressure and causes straining at stool, both of which increase ICP. Stool softeners are usually administered once the patient is stabilized and able to tolerate intake through a feeding tube or gastrostomy tube. Chapter 14 covers the components of a bowel program. Because they increase intra-abdominal pressure, enemas are not administered.

Isometric Muscle Contractions. An **isometric muscle contraction** is an increase in muscle tension without changes in the length of the muscle. With this in mind, foot boards are not used. Canvas or running shoes can be applied to maintain foot position in the postacute phase if air boots, used to prevent deep vein thrombosis (commonly in comatose patients), are not in the way. Other activities that cause isometric contractions follow:

- Pushing oneself up using the feet or elbows to push against the mattress
- Shivering
- Decerebration, decortication, or pulling on arm restraints

For agitated patients who tend to pull on their tubes, judicious use of sedation may be appropriate. Additionally, soft restraints may be needed to protect the patient. Medications may also be used to control shivering (chlorpromazine hydrochloride) and abnormal posturing if these are contributing to an increase in ICP. Medication to blunt the effects of suc-

tioning (lidocaine) or to buck the ventilator (*e.g.,* morphine sulfate) is used in some institutions.

Emotional Upset and Noxious Stimuli. Conversation that may be emotionally stimulating to the patient, such as a discussion of prognosis, condition, deficits, legal proceedings, restraints, or pain, should not be conducted within the patient's hearing range. Studies have shown that such conversations, when overheard by the patient, cause an elevation in ICP. Families should also be cautioned about refraining from unpleasant or stimulating conversations.

Soft stimuli are useful, such as a soft, soothing voice; pleasant conversation; soft music; the voices of loved ones being played on a tape recorder; or gentle therapeutic touching of the skin. The nurse should guard the patient from emotional upset. Even though certain patients may be classified as comatose, there is no way of knowing whether their hearing is intact or whether they can understand what is being said. The most reasonable approach for the nurse and others to take is to assume that patients can hear and understand.

Noxious stimuli, which are unpleasant or painful stimuli, increase ICP. Common noxious stimuli that the patient might experience follow:

- Plugging of a drainage tube (*e.g.,* urinary catheter), which causes pressure and pain from bladder distention
- Painful nursing or medical procedures (*e.g.,* removing tape from the skin)
- Loud noises or sudden jarring of the bed
- Parts of the neurological examination, especially motor response to painful stimuli

Noxious stimuli should be prevented, if possible, or minimized by technique or avoiding the need to perform multiple uncomfortable procedures. Soft stimuli, such as those mentioned previously, are useful to decrease the input of noxious stimuli when an uncomfortable procedure must be performed. The value of therapeutic touch cannot be overemphasized.

Clustering of Nursing Activities. In patients at risk, clustering of activities and procedures known to increase ICP often has a cumulative effect, causing spikes in ICP that can result in ischemia. For example, bathing, turning, and other common activities involved in routine care when clustered together may cause a rise in ICP. Even arousing the patient to assess neurological signs increases ICP. Suctioning and other respiratory procedures that are provided frequently for the acutely ill patient are notorious for their effect of increasing ICP.

The nurse should plan care to avoid clustering of activities. In patients who are undergoing continuous ICP monitoring, the nurse should watch the monitor to determine the effect each activity has on ICP. Rest periods between procedures need to be planned so that the ICP is allowed to return to the baseline level.

SUPPORTING ALL BODY SYSTEMS

When planning patient management, one must recognize the interrelationship of the functions of all body systems and their effects on the brain and increased ICP. Therefore, supporting of all body systems is important in controlling increased ICP.

Specific Nursing Management for Increased Intracranial Pressure Control

Various forms of medical therapy, both conventional and controversial, are discussed in a previous section. This section focuses on the independent and collaborative roles of the nurse in controlling intracranial hypertension and managing increased ICP.

NURSING DIAGNOSES AND COLLABORATIVE PROBLEMS

The following lists the major nursing diagnoses and collaborative problems associated with management of patients with intracranial hypertension and increased ICP.

The following are possible nursing diagnoses:

- Ineffective Airway Clearance
- Risk for Aspiration
- Impaired Environmental Interpretation Syndrome
- Total Incontinence
- Constipation
- Risk for Infection
- Risk for Injury
- Ineffective Respiratory Function
- Sleep Pattern Disturbance
- Ineffective Thermoregulation
- Hyperthermia
- Altered Cerebral Tissue Perfusion
- Impaired Physical Mobility (see Chap. 16)

The following are possible collaborative problems:

- Increased ICP
- Pulmonary embolism
- Decreased cardiac output
- Dysrhythmias
- Neurogenic pulmonary edema
- Deep vein thrombosis
- Hypoxemia
- Atelectasis, pneumonia
- Electrolyte imbalance
- Sepsis
- Acidosis (respiratory or metabolic)
- Alkalosis (respiratory or metabolic)
- Seizures
- Anticonvulsant therapy, adverse effects
- GI bleeding

RESPIRATORY MANAGEMENT

A focus of nursing management is maintaining a patent airway and adequate ventilation. If the patient cannot protect his or her airway, an endotracheal tube will be inserted. Oxygen therapy and ventilatory support with a ventilator may be ordered. If hyperventilation is ordered, the nurse will manage the patient within prescribed parameters.

Assessment. The patency of the airway and ventilation adequacy can be determined by the following:

- Observing the airway for mucus or other drainage
- Auscultating the chest for breath sounds
- Observing the respiratory pattern
- Observing chest and abdominal movement for evidence of respiratory distress
- Noting the presence of restlessness or a change in color (slight cyanosis)
- Reviewing blood gases and complete blood count (hemoglobin, hematocrit, red blood cells)

Interventions. The patent airway is often maintained with an endotracheal tube. Suctioning of the airway is also necessary to maintain patency. Oxygen therapy can be administered in various concentrations. The goal is to prevent hypercapnia and hypoxemia, which contribute to increased ICP. Ventilation support is provided with a respirator. Chest physical therapy should be provided for all patients. The following summarizes respiratory management in the patient with increased ICP.

Preventing Hypercapnia and Hypoxemia. To prevent situations that contribute to the development of hypercapnia and hypoxemia, certain principles of patient management can be implemented.

- Sedatives should be avoided or given guardedly in reduced doses, because they can have adverse effects, such as altered consciousness, hypotension, and respiratory distress in the at-risk patient.
- Maintain supplemental oxygen therapy as ordered; adjust according to blood gases.
- Suction to maintain patency (follow 15-second limitation discussed in next section).
- Before and after suctioning, preoxygenate for 30 seconds. (Some ventilators have a manual control to provide oxygenation with 100% oxygen.) If preoxygenation is administered with an Ambu bag, then squeezing of the Ambu bag must be synchronized with the inspiratory phase of the respiratory cycle. If this is not done, intrathoracic pressure is significantly increased, obstructing the valveless venous drainage from the brain and increasing CBV and ICP.

For ventilated patients, the following points should be considered:

- Patients who are out of sync with their ventilator are not being ventilated properly; also, their intrathoracic pressure is raised, impeding venous drainage from the brain and raising ICP.
- Patients who are "bucking" the ventilator (asynchrony) may have to be medicated to decrease the respiratory drive or paralyze the respiratory muscles. Morphine sulfate, pentobarbital, propofol, and others are used for this purpose.
- Monitor mode, pressure support, and PEEP.
- PEEP is associated with increased ICP in some patients, particularly at moderate to high levels (see previous discussion about respiratory management). The benefit of PEEP for "stiff lungs" has to be evaluated against the risk of a further increase in ICP.

Suctioning. The need to suction is determined by observing the patient's color, chest and abdominal movement, presence of secretions within the upper respiratory pathways, and chest auscultation. Slight cyanosis or duskiness around the mouth, nail beds, or ear lobes suggests hypoxia. Natural or artificial light should be sufficient to determine subtle changes. Observing chest and abdominal movements during the respiratory cycle may reveal use of auxiliary muscles related to dyspnea. The increased abdominal muscle tone increases intraabdominal pressure. This pressure is referred to the thorax and then to the head as an increase in ICP. Adventitious lung sounds or decreased lung sounds in particular areas, such as the bases of the lungs. The rasping sound of mucus in the upper respiratory tract is obvious to the ear without auscultation. It is critical for the nurse to be alert for the subtle signs of respiratory distress, which can be caused by partial obstruction of the respiratory tract. These subtle symptoms include an increase in pulse rate, perspiration, and restlessness.

Evaluate the patient frequently for any obvious or subtle indications of the need for suctioning. The usual protocol for suctioning includes the following measures:

- Preoxygenate lungs before and after suctioning. (Some ventilators can do this with a manual control.) This helps to maintain levels of oxygen. However, in certain respiratory conditions, such as chronic obstructive pulmonary disease, this therapy may be contraindicated. This should be discussed with the physician.
- Suction as necessary to remove secretions and maintain a patent airway; suction gently. Limit catheter insertion to **no more than 15 seconds** for each insertion, and oxygenate between each catheter insertion.
- In the at-risk patient, suctioning can cause plateau waves in patients who already have an elevated ICP. Suction gently according to the previous procedure. If ordered, instill 1 to 2 mL of lidocaine elixir into the endotracheal tube.

Positioning to Enhance Respiratory Function. In addition to suctioning, respiratory function can be enhanced by changing the patient's position periodically (turning every 2 hours) and asking the conscious, cooperative patient to take a few deep breaths hourly. Both procedures are well-accepted methods for improving aeration of lung tissue and expulsion of drainage.

Positioning patients on their side allows for drainage of secretions from the mouth to promote an adequate airway. The patient should be turned from side to side at least every 2 hours so that secretions do not pool in the upper or lower respiratory tract and so atelectasis can be prevented. The neck should be maintained in a neutral position to facilitate cerebral venous drainage.

Hyperventilation. The purpose of ventilator-controlled hyperventilation is to "blow off" CO_2, promoting vasoconstriction, as previously discussed. Hyperventilation is a very effective means for rapidly reducing increased ICP.

The physician sets the desired level of CO_2 to be achieved. This is usually an arterial PCO_2 blood level of 25 to 35 mm Hg. The respirator settings are adjusted as necessary by the respiratory therapist to maintain the appropriate level. The nurse should follow these care measures:

- Review blood gas to determine achievement of target levels.
- If the patient is agitated or is bucking the ventilator, try to determine the cause and treat; if the agitation continues, report it to the physician, who may wish to order neuromuscular blockade drugs to synchronize the patient with the ventilator.
- Monitor degree of neuromuscular blockade with a peripheral nerve stimulator.
- Do not let the arterial CO_2 drop below the prescribed lower level because decreased cardiac output and hypoxia can result.

For a patient who is not on a ventilator, the physician may order hyperventilation if there are any spikes in ICP. This can be accomplished by attaching the Ambu bag to the endotracheal tube or tracheostomy tube and continuing use of the Ambu bag until the spikes in ICP disappear on the monitor.

DRUG THERAPY FOR INCREASED INTRACRANIAL PRESSURE

Osmotic diuretics are often used for the management of patients with increased ICP. **Corticosteroids** are not effective with increased ICP unless it is associated with vasogenic cerebral edema. The following nursing responsibilities relate to the use of mannitol, the osmotic diuretic most commonly used:

- Monitor serum osmolarity; the desired target range is set by the physician. It is usually desirable to maintain the osmolarity below 310 to 320 mOsm.
- When mannitol is ordered, it is usually ordered as 50 to 100 g (20%–25%) every 3 to 5 hours, depending on serum osmolarity and ICP readings.
- Intravenous mannitol must be administered with a filter to prevent crystallization.
- An indwelling catheter is needed to measure hourly urinary output.
- Dehydration hypotension, and electrolyte imbalance are possible problems associated with the use of mannitol. Therefore, central venous pressure, urinary output, and electrolytes should be monitored periodically.

GI Prophylaxis. Patients with intracranial lesions and injury, such as increased ICP, are at high risk for peptic ulcers and GI hemorrhage. GI prophylaxis is provided with H_2 blockers, such as ranitidine (Zantac), famotidine (Pepcid), or cimetidine (Tagamet). Cimetidine is used less frequently because it may cause confusion in patients older than 50 years. It is used with caution in kidney or liver failure. Sucralfate (Carafate) is another drug that forms a protective coating in the stomach. It is not useful if continuous feedings are administered by a gastric feeding tube. If a gastric tube is in place, periodic monitoring of gastric aspirations for pH is useful. A 30-mL dose of magnesium hydroxide (Maalox) may be given every 3 to 4 hours to protect the gastric mucosa for a low pH.

BLOOD PRESSURE CONTROL

The nurse must monitor MAP and ICP to maintain an adequate CPP. (CPP is calculated as MAP minus the ICP, as previously discussed.) Maintaining an adequate CPP (approximately 70 mm Hg) is critical in preventing cerebral ischemia. To maintain an adequate CPP, the systolic blood pressure is usually maintained at a higher level (a systolic pressure of 140–150 mm Hg) to compensate for an elevated ICP. Antihypertensive agents, such as beta blockers or labetalol, if the blood pressure is high or vasopressors if systolic is low, may be ordered.

The following nursing responsibilities are involved in controlling blood pressure:

- Monitor the MAP and ICP to ensure that an adequate CPP is maintained.
- Maintain the arterial blood pressure and CPP within the target ranges set for systolic, diastolic, and CPP.
- Titrate drugs as necessary to maintain target ranges.
- Prevent the development of hypotension; if it occurs, treat with a bolus of fluid, and use drugs as necessary.

NEUROMUSCULAR BLOCKADE AND SEDATION

Muscle relaxation or paralysis or sedation may be necessary in the agitated patient or in the patient who is bucking the respirator. The drugs that are commonly used have already been discussed in the section on respiratory management. Monitor sedation using an objective means, such as the Ramsey Scale.[28] Use a peripheral nerve stimulator to monitor degree of sedation.

TEMPERATURE CONTROL

CBF increases approximately 6% for each degree centigrade increase in temperature. The increased CBF also increases CBV and contributes to a rise in ICP. In addition, the general metabolism rate of the body and the cellular metabolic rate increase when the body temperature is elevated. As a result, there is an increase in the end-products of cellular metabolism (CO_2 and organic acids, such as lactic acid), causing vasodilation and a rise in systemic blood pressure. These factors contribute to a rise in ICP. Therefore, it is important to control elevations in temperature.

This is accomplished with antipyretic drugs, such as acetaminophen, which may be used alone or in combination with a cooling blanket. If shivering occurs, ICP will increase; thus, the patient must be monitored closely to prevent this adverse effect. Chlorpromazine (Thorazine) may be given to control shivering. The nursing responsibilities related to temperature control include the following:

- Monitor the core body temperature every 2 to 4 hours.
- Administer antipyretics as ordered.
- If a cooling blanket is used, turn off the blanket when the temperature is approximately 1° above the desired level. (Temperature will continue to drift downward because the blanket will remain cool.)
- Lower the temperature gradually to prevent shivering.

SEIZURE CONTROL

Seizure activity increases cerebral metabolism and can cause an increase in ICP. For this reason, patients at risk for seizures will receive prophylactic anticonvulsants. The drug ordered

most often is phenytoin, 100 mg three or four times daily. The nursing responsibilities involved in seizure control include the following:

- Monitor serum levels to ensure therapeutic drug level.
- Because phenytoin binds to albumin, monitor albumin level if serum values drop.
- Once tube feedings are started, the protein may decrease a previously therapeutic phenytoin level, requiring a bolus dose.

FLUID RESTRICTION

Strict fluid restriction is now considered dangerous because dehydration and hypotension may result. The goal is now fluid maintenance for euvolemia.

CEREBROSPINAL FLUID DRAINAGE

Because CSF provides a favorable environment for an infection to develop rapidly, absolutely flawless aseptic technique must be maintained. A scalp incision and burr hole are made to provide an access route for insertion of the catheter into the ventricle. Regardless of how carefully sutured, drainage from the incision, especially around the catheter, frequently occurs. This saturates the dry sterile dressing and creates an ideal site for infection; therefore, the dressing must be monitored.

The level of the collection bag is adjusted as indicated by the physician. Lowering the collection container increases the amount of CSF drainage; raising it diminishes the amount of drainage. Too-rapid removal of drainage could lead to brain stem herniation and is contraindicated if the clamp is open.

The drainage tubing necessary for ventricular drainage is fine and pliable and prone to kinking. Check the tubing frequently to ensure patency. The amount of drainage is observed and recorded at frequent intervals. As mentioned previously, too-rapid removal of drainage could lead to brain stem herniation and deterioration of the patient's neurological status. The physician may want to send specimens of CSF drainage for culture and sensitivity or other analysis. Specimens must be obtained under sterile conditions.

The nursing responsibilities that relate to CSF drainage include the following:

- Maintain an occlusive, dry sterile dressing around the ventriculostomy site.
- Maintain a closed sterile system.
- "Level" the drainage bag to the prescribed height.
- Maintain the collection bag at the prescribed level.
- Take precautions neither to raise nor lower the collection bag when draining the CSF.
- Observe the drainage tubing to ensure an intact drainage system without kinks.
- Monitor the amount and color of drainage; bright red blood may indicate *rebleeding*, which should be reported immediately to the physician.

SURGERY

Patients who have had a decompression craniotomy and those who have undergone craniectomy to reduce intracranial bulk are managed in a similar manner (see Chap. 18). An ICP monitor may be placed under the bone flap. If a craniectomy has been performed, the patient is kept off the operative site to prevent pressure on the brain.

BARBITURATE COMA

The usual parameters of neurological assessment are severely diminished or lost when the patient is receiving barbiturate coma therapy. Therefore, such patients are managed by invasive monitoring of hemodynamics, vital signs, and ICP; central lines for administration of fluids and drugs; and a ventilator. Blood is drawn to monitor electrolyte, glucose, and barbiturate levels and osmolarity. The nurse must coordinate and interpret data to make clinical decisions for patient management.

Summary

The management of increased ICP is a fundamental problem in clinical practice. A review of the physiological basis for ICP, independent and collaborative nursing roles, and major management concerns has been provided.

References

1. Marmarou, A., & Tabaddor, K. (1993). Intracranial pressure: Physiology and pathophysiology. In P. R. Cooper (Ed.), *Head injury* (3rd ed.) (pp. 203–224). Baltimore: Williams & Wilkins.
2. Germon K. (1988). Interpretation of ICP pulse waves to determine intracerebral compliance. *Journal of Neuroscience Nursing, 20*(6), 346.
3. Cardosa, E. R., Rowan, J. O., & Galbraith, S. (1983). Analysis of cerebrospinal fluid pulse wave in intracranial pressure. *Journal of Neurosurgery, 59*, 817–821.
4. Ibid, p. 818.
5. Westmoreland, B. F., Benarroch, E. E., Daube, J. R., Reagan, T. J., & Sandok, B. A. (1994). *Medical neurosciences: An approach to anatomy, pathophysiology, and physiology by systems and levels* (p. 283). Boston: Little, Brown.
6. Ibid, p. 284.
7. Ibid, pp. 284–186.
8. Ropper, A. H., & Kennedy, S. K. (1993). Physiology and clinical aspects of raised intracranial pressure. In A. H. Ropper, (Ed.), *Neurological and neurosurgical intensive care* (3rd ed.) (pp. 11–28). New York: Raven Press.
9. Ibid, Westmoreland et al., p. 285.
10. Eisenberg, H. M., Frankowski, R. F., Conant, L. P., Marshall, L. F., & Walker, M. D. (1988). High dose barbiiturate control of elevated intracranial prssure in patients with severe head injury. *Journal of Neurosurgery, 69*, 15–23.
11. Ropper, A. H., & Rockoff, M. A. (1993). Physiology and clinical aspects of raised intracranial pressure. In A. H. Ropper (Ed.), *Neurolgical and neurosurgical intensive care* (3rd ed.) (pp. 15–16). New York: Raven Press.
12. Rosner, M. J., & Daughton, S. (1990). Cerebral perfusion pressure management in head injury. *Journal of Trauma, 30*(8), 933–941.
13. Ropper & Rockoff, ibid, p. 287–288.
14. Klatzo, I. (1967). Neuropathological aspects of brain edema. *Journal of Neuropathology and Experimental Neurology, 20*, 1.
15. Adams, R. D., & Victor, M. (1989). *Principles of neurology* (4th ed.) (p. 501). New York: McGraw-Hill.
16. Plum, F., & Posner, J. (1980). *The diagnosis of stupor and coma* (3rd ed.). Philadelphia: F.A. Davis.
17. Ibid, pp. 60–120.
18. Koch, S. M., & Allen, S. J. (1995). Invasive neurologic monitoring. In R. L. Levine & R. E. Fromm Jr. (Eds.), *Critical care monitoring: From pre-hospital to the ICU* (pp. 265–285). St. Louis: C.V. Mosby.
19. Frank, J. (1993). Management of intracranial hypertension. *Medical Clinics of North America, 77*(1), 63.
20. Ropper, A. H., & Rockoff, M. A. (1993). Treatment of intracranial hypertension. In A. H. Ropper, (Ed.), *Neurological and neurosurgical intensive care* (3rd ed.) (pp. 29–52). New York: Raven Press.
21. Kelley, D. F. (1995). Steroid in head injury. *New Horizons, 3*(3), 453–455.
22. Ford, E. V. (1995). Monitoring neuromuscular blockade in the adult ICU. *American Journal of Critical Care, 4*(2), 122–130.
23. Mirski, M. A., Muffelman, B., Ulatowski, J. A., & Hanley, D. F. (1995). Sedation for the critically ill neurologic patient. *Critical Care Medicine, 23*(12), 2038–2053.
24. Eisenberg, H. M., Frankowski, R. F., Contant, C. F. et al. (1988). High-dose barbiturate control of elevated intracranial pressure in patients with severe head injury. *Journal of Neurosurgery, 69*, 15–23.
25. Yablon, J. S., Lantner, H. J., McCormack, T. M., et al. (1993). Experience with a fiiberoptic intracranial pressure monitor. *Journal of Clinical Monitoring, 9*, 171–175.
26. Aucoin, P. J., Kotilainen, H., R., Gantz, N. M., et al. (1986). Intracranial pressure monitoring: Epidemiological study of risk factors and infections. *American Journal of Medicine, 80*, 369–376.
27. Rosner, M. J., & Coley, I. B. (1986). Cerebral perfusion pressure, intracranial pressure, and head elevation. *Journal of Neurosurgery, 65*, 636–641.
28. Ramsey, M. A. E., Savage, T. M., Simpson, B. R. J., et al. (1974). Controlled sedation with alphaxalone/alphadolone. *British Journal of Medicine, 2*, 656–659.

Bibliography

Books

Cooper, P. R. (Ed.) (1993). *Head injury* (3rd ed.). Baltimore: Williams & Wilkins.

Ropper, A. H. (Ed.) (1993). *Neurological and neurosurgical intensive care* (3rd ed.). New York: Raven Press.

Periodicals

Bader, M. K., Littlejohns, L., & Palmer, S. (1995). Ventriculostomy and intracranial pressure monitoring: In search of a 0% infection rate. *Heart & Lung, 24*, 166–172.

Bell, S. D., Guyer, D., Synder, M. A., & Miner, M. (1994). Cerebral hemodynamics: Monitoring arteriojugular oxygen content differences. *Journal of Neuroscience Nursing, 26*, 270–277.

Bingaman, W. E., & Frank, J. (1995). Malignant cerebral edema and intracranial hypertension. *Neurologic Clinics, 13*(3), 479–510.

Borel, C. O., & Guy, J. (1995). Ventilatory management in critical neurologic illness. *Neurologic Clinics, 13*(3), 627–645.

Clifton, G. L. (1995). Hypothermia and hyperbaric oxygen as treatment modalities for severe head injury. *New Horizons, 3*(3), 474–478.

Cody, C. M. (1992). Benign intracranial hypertension. *American Family Physician, 45*(4), 1671–1678.

Cummings, R. (1992). Understanding external ventricular drainage. *Journal of Neuroscience Nursing, 24*, 84–87.

Davis, M., & Lucatorto, M. (1994). Manitol revisited. *Journal of Neuroscience Nursing, 26*, 1700–174.

Diringer, M. N. (1992). Management of sodium abnormalities in patients with CNS disease. *Clinical Neuropharmacology, 15*, 427–447.

Doyle, D. J., & Mark, P. W. S. (1992). Analysis of intracranial pressure. *Journal of Clinical Monitoring, 8*, 81–90.

Feldman, Z., Kanter, M. J., Robertson, C. S., Contant, C. F., Hayes, C., & Sheinberg, M. A. (1992). Effect of head elevation on intracranial pressure, cerebral perfusion pressure, and cerebral blood flow in head-injured patients. *Journal of Neurosurgery, 76,* 207–211.

Ford, E. V. (1995). Monitoring neuromuscular blockage in the adult ICU. *American Journal of Critical Care, 4,* 122–132.

Frank, J. I. (1993). Management of intracranial pressure. *Contemporary Clinical Neurology, 77,* 61–77.

Gambardella, G., d'Avella, D., & Tomasello, F. (1992). Monitoring of brain tissue pressure with a fiberoptic device. *Neurosurgery, 31,* 918–922.

Germon, K. (1994). Intracranial monitoring in the 1990s. *Critical Care Nursing Quarterly, 17*(1), 21–32.

Hubner, C., & Jain, U. (1996). Caring for the ICU patient receiving propofol. *Dimensions of Critical Care Nursing, 15*(3), 133–141.

Johnston, I., Besser, M., & Morgan, M. K. (1988). Cerebrospinal fluid diversion in the treatment of benign intracranial hypertension. *Journal of Neurosurgery, 69,* 195–202.

Jordon, K. G. (1995). Neuropysiologic monitoring in the neuroscience intensive care unit. *Neurologic Clinics, 13*(3), 579–626.

Kalisch, B. J., Kalisch, P. A., Burns, S. M., Kocan, M. J., & Prendergast, V. (1995). Intrahospital transport of neruo ICU patients. *Journal of Neuroscience Nursing, 27*(2), 69–77.

Kanter, M. J. (1991). Intracranial pressure monitoring. *Neurosurgery Clinics of North America, 2,* 257–265.

Kerr, M. E., & Brucia, J. (1993). Hyperventilation in the head-injured patient: An effective treatment modality. *Heart & Lung, 22,* 516–521.

Kerr, M. E., Lovasik, D., & Darby, J. (1995). Evaluating cerebral oxygenation using jugular venous oximetry in head injuries. *AACN Clinical Issues, 6,* 1, 11–20.

Miriski, M. A., Muffelman, B., Ulatowski, J. A., & Hanley, D. F. (1995). Sedation for the critically ill neurologic patient. *Critical Care Medicine, 23,* 2038–2053.

Mitchell, P. H. (1986). Intracranial hypertension: Influence of nursing care activities. *Nursing Clinics of North America, 21*(4), 563–574.

Mollman, H. D., Rockswold, G. L., & Ford, S. E. (1988). A clinical comparison of subarachnoid catheters to ventriculostomy and subarachnoid bolts: A prospective study. *Journal of Neurosurgery, 68,* 737.

Muizelaar, J. P., Marmarou, A., Ward, J. D., Kontos, H. A., Chol, S. C., & Becker, D. P. (1991). Adverse effects of prolonged hyperventilation in patients with severe head injury: A randomized clinical trial. *Journal of Neurosurgery, 75,* 731–739.

Myles, G. L., Perry, A. G., Malkoff, M. D., Shatto, B. J., & Scott-Killmade, M. C. (1995). Quantifying nursing care in barbiturate-induced coma with the therapeutic intervention scoring system. *Journal of Neuroscience Nursing, 27,* 35–42.

Parsons, L. C., & Wilson, M. M. (1984). Cerebrovascular status of severe closed head injured patients following passive position changes. *Nursing Research, 33*(2), 68–75.

Parsons, L. C., Peard, A. L., & Page, M. C. (1985). The effects of hygiene interventions on the cerebrovascular status of severe closed head injured persons. *Research in Nursing Health, 8,* 173–181.

Riekem K., Schwab, S., Krieger, D., Kummer, R., Aschoff, A., Schuchardt, V., & Hacke, W. (1995). Decompressive surgery in space-occupying hemispheric infarction: Results of an open, prospective trial. *Critical Care Medicine, 23*(9), 1576–1587.

Rising, C. J. (1993). The relationship of selected nursing activities to ICP. *Journal of Neuroscience Nursing, 25,* 302–308.

Rosner, M. J., & Coley, I. B. (1986). Cerebral perfusion pressure, intracranial pressure, and head elevation. *Journal of Neurosurgery, 65,* 636–641.

Rudy, E., Baan, M., Stone, K., & Turner, B. (1986). The relationship between endotracheal suctioning and changes in intracranial pressure: A review of the literature. *Heart & Lung, 15,* 488–494.

Shanker, S. (1995). Neurologic intensive care unit management and economic issues. *Neurologic Clinics, 13*(3), 679–694.

Schicker, D. J., & Young, R. F. (1992). Intracranial pressure monitoring: Fiberoptic monitor compared with the ventricular catheter. *Surgical Neurology, 37,* 251–254.

Sharpiro, B. A., Warren, J., Egol, A. B., Greenbaum, D. M., Jacobi, J., Nasraway, S. A., Schein, R. M., Spevetz, A., & Stone, J. R. (1995). Practice parameters for sustained neuromuscular blokage in the adult critically ill patient: An executieve summary. *Critical Care Medicine, 23*(9), 1596–1600.

Sharpiro, B. A., Warren, J., Egol, A. B., Greenbaum, D. M., Jacobi, J., Nasraway, S. A., Schein, R. M., Spevetz, A., & Stone, J. R. (1995). Practice parameters for intravenous analgesia and sedation for adult patients in the intensive care unit: An executive summary. *Critical Care Medicine, 23*(9), 1601–1605.

Sieber, F., & Traystman, R. J. (1992). Special issues: Glucose and the brain. *Critical Care Medicine, 20*(1), 104–114.

Sikes, P. J., & Segal, J. (1994). Jugular bulb oxygen saturation monitoring for evaluating cerebral ischemia. *Critical Care Nursing Quarterly, 117,* 9–20.

Wilberger, J. E., & Cantella, D. (1995). High-dose barbiturates for intracranial pressure control. *New Horizons, 3*(3), 469–473.

Williams, A., & Coyne, S. M. (1993). Effects of neck position on intracranial pressure. *American Journal of Critical Care, 3,* 68–71.

Wisinger, D., & Mest-Beck, L. (1990). Ventriculostomy: A guide to nursing management. *Journal of Neuroscience Nursing, 22,* 365–369.

Young, G. B. (1995). Neurologic complications of systemic critical illness. *Neurologic Clinics, 13*(3), 645–646.

CHAPTER 18

Management of Patients Undergoing Neurosurgical Procedures

Joanne V. Hickey

THE PREOPERATIVE PHASE

For the patient undergoing intracranial surgery, the circumstances of admission influence preoperative preparation. Admission is either unplanned or planned. Unplanned emergent admissions are usually related to trauma or a sudden, life-threatening event, such as an aneurysmal rupture. Immediate intracranial surgery may be necessary as a life-saving measure. The immediacy of the situation compresses all preoperative preparation, but the family still needs information concerning what is happening and what can be expected postoperatively. With planned admissions, or postponed surgery, there is time for planned preoperative teaching. In a managed care environment, preparation may occur by telephone, videocassette, or printed material. The nurse does hold the primary responsibility to be sure patients and families are adequately prepared. Before preoperative teaching is discussed, the issue of informed consent is considered.

Informed Consent

It is the physician's responsibility to provide the patient and family with enough information so that the decision for surgery is based on informed consent. Altered consciousness, impaired cognition, or both can severely influence the patient's level of understanding. A responsible family member should be present during the discussion, and in some instances, the responsible family member will give consent for surgery.

For informed consent, the role of the physician is to discuss the purpose of surgery, the possibility of alternative treatment (if any), the potential risks, and the expected outcomes.

Discussing these points honestly and answering questions posed by the patient or family will reduce the possibility of misunderstandings and litigation. Ideally, the nurse should be present for the discussion. At a minimum, the nurse must be aware of what information was given to the patient and family and what concerns were raised. This knowledge is helpful in clarifying and reinforcing the information provided. The nurse incorporates this information into patient and family teaching.

Assessment of the Patient and Family

The nursing admission history and ongoing assessments provide a database for planning care. Psychosocial information about the patient and family is part of this database and is helpful for modifying the preoperative teaching plan to meet their needs.

For the patient who is conscious and oriented, the prospect of cranial surgery is often associated with overwhelming anxiety and fear. Paramount is the fear of loss of life, permanent disability, and loss of independence. Of equal concern is the prospect of loss of mental ability, self-control, and personality characteristics that make an individual unique. Additional stress is stirred by thoughts of what effect this illness will have on relationships with family and friends and of concern about being a burden to loved ones. On the other hand, patients with an altered level of consciousness or impaired cognitive function may be unable to grasp the seriousness of the situation and may express little response. In all cases, the family usually experiences many of the same feelings as the patient. The following nursing diagnoses are frequently made:

- Knowledge Deficit
- Anxiety
- Fear

The teaching plan is directed toward providing information about what is happening and what can be expected and is intended to control fear and anxiety. The process is also intended to provide a supportive environment that will assist the patient and family in coping with the crisis.

Preoperative Teaching Plan

The teaching plan is tailored to the needs of the patient and family. However, several points are addressed in all cases, and these are detailed in Table 18-1.

The patient's comprehension and memory are first assessed. In addition, the family is assessed to determine the best teaching approach. In all instances, the family should be involved. For the cognitively intact patient, information is reinforced, and misconceptions are clarified. Subsequently, questions are encouraged, and learning is evaluated by assessing comprehension of concepts discussed. Written material is useful and is a focus for discussion. If slight to moderate cognitive deficits are present, the teaching approach is modified to include use of simple sentences, visual aids, and written and pictorial material. With severe deficits, the family becomes the major focus of preoperative teaching. The patient is included with a very simple explanation. Family members are encouraged to take care of themselves with adequate rest, nutrition, and support.

Prior to Surgery

In planned admissions, routine tests for any surgical patient are often completed on an outpatient basis. Specific neurological diagnostics have probably been performed to establish a diagnosis that warrants intracranial surgery. Home preparation instructions are provided. Many patients are now admitted the day of surgery after some home preparation. However, regardless of the time line, certain preoperative activities are conducted to collect baseline data and prepare the patient for surgery. A neurological assessment, which is a history of medical problems, risk factors, and current medications, is recorded. (An enema is usually *not* ordered.)

When the hair is prepared, a special cleaning soap (such as pHisoHex) may be used for washing to decrease the count of microorganisms on the hair and scalp. Long hair is neatly braided. The minimum amount of hair and scalp shaving is usually done in the operating room. The need to cut some of the hair can be upsetting to some patients.

In addition to the nothing by mouth status after midnight, other specific preparation is directed to special needs of the neurosurgical patient. Thigh-high elastic (TED) stockings are applied. The patient is sent to the operating room with sequential compression air boots that will be functional during the surgery. The purpose of the boots is to decrease the risk of deep vein thrombosis and pulmonary emboli. The results of the final preoperative neurological assessment and vital sign check are recorded on the flow sheet and sent to the operating room with the patient.

Depending on the circumstances, the family may be allowed to visit the patient briefly before surgery. The patient and family often need considerable emotional support. If desired, a visit from the clergy may be comforting. Any other special preoperative orders are completed, and the patient is transported to the operating room.

THE INTRAOPERATIVE PHASE

Arrival at the Operating Room Suite

Once the patient arrives in the operating room, monitoring equipment is attached, and the anesthesiologist begins intravenous (IV) induction of anesthetics. When the patient loses consciousness, several other pieces of monitoring equipment are attached, including the following:

TABLE 18-1
General Preoperative Teaching Plan for Intracranial Surgery

*Patient and Family**
- Clarify and reinforce the information provided by the physician related to surgery.
- Provide written material about the specific type of surgery or a general preoperative teaching guide.
- Describe preparatory events before surgery: blood work, electrocardiogram, chest x-ray study, shampoo, elastic stockings and air boots, visit from anesthesiologist, NPO before surgery, and so forth.
- Inform them where the patient will go after surgery (recovery room; neurological intensive care unit).
- Prepare them for a change in the appearance of the patient after the surgery (*e.g.,* periorbital ecchymosis, dry sterile dressing).
- Collaborate with the physician to provide more information or to clarify the information already given, if needed.

Patient
- Teach leg exercises and deep-breathing exercises, if possible.

Family
- Inform the family of visiting hours before surgery and on the intensive care unit.
- Inform the family that cranial surgery often takes several hours and that this is to be expected.
- Inform the family where they can wait or where the physician can reach them by telephone when the surgery is completed.
- With long surgeries, provisions may be made to update the family periodically.
- Prepare the family for how the patient will look in the intensive care unit (*e.g.,* tubes, monitors, intravenous lines).

* Be prepared to repeat and reinforce some of the information provided (people under severe stress have difficulty retaining all of the information given).

- Sequential compression air boots are plugged in to prevent pooling of blood in the lower extremities.
- A urinary catheter is inserted if one is not already in place; this is necessary if hyperosmotic diuretics will be administered or if surgery will be long in duration.
- The eyes are protected from corneal abrasions with the application of a bland eye ointment; they are then taped closed, and sterile eye pads are applied.
- Other monitoring devices may be added at this time, such as a Swan-Ganz catheter, esophageal temperature probe, arterial line for continual monitoring of arterial blood pressure, Doppler ultrasonographic chest piece (to detect venous air emboli if the sitting position is used), and other equipment as necessary.
- The patient is intubated after the larynx is sprayed with lidocaine to prevent coughing or retching, which increases intracranial pressure (ICP).
- The head is shaved carefully so that no scalp abrasions occur; these would increase the possibility of postoperative infection. The hair is saved and placed in a labeled envelope.
- The patient is placed in the position (lateral, prone, or sitting) that the surgeon has selected as most advantageous for the surgical procedure planned; the sitting position is used for posterior fossa surgery because it affords optimal visualization of the operative field.
- Various body supports, such as the headrest and armrests, are carefully put into place and padded so that no undue pressure is exerted that will cause ischemia or injury.

Positioning is often complex, and it may take from 1 to 1.5 hours to position the patient and to pad pressure areas. Intracranial surgery may last a few hours to 24 hours, depending on the surgical procedure. Maintaining the patient in one position for a long time can easily lead to pressure ulcers unless special attention is paid to positioning and padding.

Neuroanesthesia

There is no ideal anesthetic agent for neurosurgical procedures. Of the several drugs available, all have actions and side effects that may cause problems or be unpredictable. An important consideration when choosing anesthetic drugs is their effect on cerebral metabolism (cerebral metabolic oxygen requirement), cerebral blood flow, ICP, and vasomotor tone (cerebral vasoconstrictors or vasodilators). Other considerations when selecting anesthetic agents are nonflammability (which is especially important if cautery instruments will be used), ease of administration, effect on hemostasis and blood pressure, adequate brain relaxation, nonirritability so that coughing and retching are not precipitated, and minimal side effects and adverse reactions on the various body systems.

For neurosurgical procedures, a combination of drugs is given so that one drug offsets the negative side effects of another. A common combination of drugs is nitrous oxide, oxygen, narcotics (fentanyl citrate), barbiturates (thiopental sodium [Pentothal] or pentobarbital), and possibly muscle relaxants (*e.g.,* pancuronium).

A mannitol solution (20%–25%) is usually begun to reduce brain volume. Cerebrospinal fluid (CSF) may also be removed to reduce ICP and provide the neurosurgeon with a larger work area. Dexamethasone to control cerebral edema,

phenytoin (Dilantin) to control seizures, and antibiotics to control risk of infection may be administered periodically throughout the surgery. Cardiac drugs may also be given to control hypotension or hypertension.

Other Intraoperative Concerns

During surgery, controlled hypotension, hypothermia, and hyperventilation may be indicated. Also, one special consideration when the sitting position is used is venous air embolus.

HYPOTENSION

In some surgical procedures in which vascularity is increased, induction of controlled hypotension is advantageous. Hypotension is particularly helpful during the dissection of an aneurysm because the lowered intraluminal pressure reduces the pressure on the aneurysmal sac. This lessens bleeding if rupture occurs and increases the plasticity of the aneurysm to facilitate application of a secure clip or other materials. Drug therapy, the sitting position, and the effects of anesthetic agents, such as halothane, can induce hypotension. The desired level of hypotension depends on the procedure. The arterial pressure is monitored by use of the arterial monitoring cannula.

HYPOTHERMIA

The purpose of hypothermia is to decrease cellular metabolism and the need for oxygen. The less oxygen needed, the less metabolic end-products produced. For every degree lowered from 37° to 25°C (98.6°–77.0°F), there is a 6% reduction in oxygen consumption by the brain. The reduction in oxygen consumption and cerebral metabolism results in vasoconstriction. If the temperature drops below 28°C (82.4°F), cardiac irritability increases and extracorporeal support of the systemic circulation becomes necessary.

HYPERVENTILATION

Controlled hyperventilation can be maintained during surgery with a ventilator. It is an effective means of reducing brain bulk ICP. The reduced production of carbon dioxide results in a reduction in cerebral blood flow and subsequent vasoconstriction. This causes a reduction in brain bulk and ICP.

VENOUS AIR EMBOLUS

A potential problem associated with the sitting operative position is an air embolus. When the head is higher than the heart, a negative pressure is produced in the dural venous sinuses and veins draining the brain and head. If air is introduced into the venous system, it is quickly carried to the right side of the heart. The patient must be monitored with a Doppler sensor. A change in the Doppler signal indicates the presence of air in the heart. When an air embolus is suspected, the surgeon is notified so that an attempt can be made to identify and occlude the possible site of air entry. When the problem site has been occluded, the anesthesiologist aspirates air through the central venous catheter using a 20-mL syringe and an airtight stopcock. Once the air has been aspirated, the entry site closed, and the patient stabilized, surgery can continue. If the entry site cannot be located, the patient is placed in the supine position, and the surgery is terminated. The patient is observed for transient neurological deficits. A **mill-wheel murmur** heard through an esophageal stethoscope is a late sign of intracardiac air. Air embolus is a serious problem that can lead to death.

NEUROSURGICAL PROCEDURES AND OTHER RELATED THERAPEUTIC TECHNIQUES

Development of instrumentation, lasers, and radiation therapies has increased the options that the neurosurgeon can offer patients. A craniotomy may be combined with laser treatment of some conditions previously managed by craniotomy alone. Other nonsurgical treatment modalities have been introduced into practice and may decrease the need for surgery in the future.

Definition of Terms and Basic Concepts

The following is an explanation of several common terms and neurosurgical procedures:

- **Surgery** can be classified by anatomical location. Two terms differentiate the areas of the brain on which surgery is performed (Fig. 18-1):
  Supratentorial is the area above the tentorium that includes the cerebrum. The tentorium cerebelli is a double fold of the dura mater that forms a partition between the cerebrum and the brain stem and cerebellum. The supratentorial approach is used to gain access to space-occupying lesions in the frontal, parietal, temporal, and occipital lobes of the cerebral hemispheres. Occasionally, temporal or occipital lobe lesions located close to the tentorial margin may be excised through the infratentorial approach.
  Infratentorial is the area below the tentorium that includes the brain stem (midbrain, pons, medulla) and cerebellum; this area includes the posterior fossa. The infratentorial approach is used to gain access to the brain stem area and cerebellum space-occupying lesions.
- A **burr hole** is a hole made in the cranium with a special drill for evacuation of an extracerebral clot or in preparation for craniotomy. In the case of a craniotomy, a series of burr holes is made. The bone between the holes is cut with a special saw, allowing removal of the piece of bone.
- A **craniotomy** is a surgical opening of the skull to provide access to the intracranial contents for reasons such as removal of a tumor, clipping of an aneurysm, or repair of a cerebral injury. It is usually performed for supratentorial procedures and involves making a scalp flap around the area below the lesion. The flap created is either a free flap or an osteoplastic flap. With a **free flap**, the bone is completely removed and preserved for later replacement. With an **osteoplastic flap**, the muscle is left attached to the skull to maintain the vascular supply (Fig. 18-2).
- A **craniectomy** is excision of a portion of the skull without replacement. This procedure may be done to achieve decompression after cerebral debulking or removal of bone fragments from skull fracture. In addition, the posterior fossa is a much smaller region than the supratentorial space. The posterior fossa (infratentorial space) is defined by the large transverse venous sinuses superiorly and the foramen magnum inferiorly. Because of the small areas and increased risk of dural tearing, a craniectomy or bone removal without replacement is usually performed for surgical access.[1]
- A **cranioplasty** is repair of the skull to reestablish the contour and integrity of the skull. This procedure involves the replacement of part of the cranium with a synthetic material.

Use of Stereotaxis for Precise Positioning

The first practical instruments for stereotactic surgery were developed in 1947. **Stereotaxis** pertains to precise localization of a specific target point based on three-dimensional coordinates derived with the use of stereotaxis frame and instrumentation. Figure 18-3 illustrates representative stereotactic equipment. Various types of stereotactic frames and instruments have been developed and are constantly being updated. Stereotactic surgery is used in neurosurgery for the precise localization of deep brain lesions for surgical biopsy and removal. The advantage of the technique is that small lesions can be localized and removed from areas that were previously surgically inaccessible, with minimal trauma to the adjacent tissue.

Once the stereotactic frame is applied to the patient's head, the target site within the brain is located by determining the X (anteroposterior), Y (superior-inferior), and Z (left to right) coordinates in relation to the stereotactic frame.

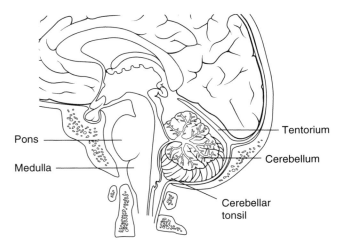

FIGURE 18-1
Surgery on the area of the brain above the tentorium is called *supratentorial;* surgery below the tentorium is *infratentorial.*

Pons

Medulla

Tentorium

Cerebellum

Cerebellar tonsil

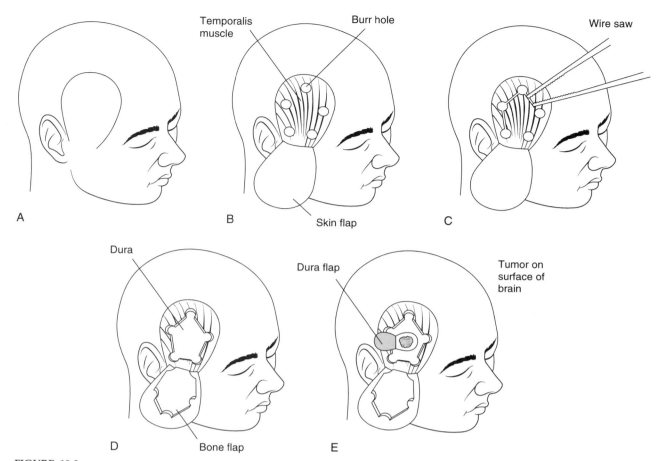

FIGURE 18-2

Craniotomy. A number of steps are involved in a craniotomy to gain access to the brain. An incision is made into the scalp over the area of the brain to be explored. This creates a skin flap, which is retracted (*A*). Burr holes are made through the cranium (*B*); a saw is used to connect the burr holes and cut through the bone (*C*). The bone flap remains attached to the muscle, creating a "hinge" that is turned back for access to the brain. The dura mater is exposed, incised, and retracted (*D*). Access to the cerebral tissue is gained, and surgery proceeds (*E*). When the surgery is completed, the dura is sutured, the bone flap replaced, and the muscle and scalp realigned and sutured.

The point of intersection of all three coordinates identifies the target tissue. Traditional x-ray films of anatomical landmarks have been used to identify the target zone, but newer approaches use the computed tomography (CT) scanner and a computer for target point identification.

Microsurgery

Microsurgery can be defined as any surgery performed with the assistance of an operating microscope that provides magnification of various intensities. The surgical technique (micro-operative technique), instruments (microinstrumentation), illumination for visualization, and magnification (operating microscopes), along with a host of other equipment, are specifically designed for this use. Microsurgery has improved several standard neurosurgical procedures, such as the removal of brain tumors (acoustic neuromas, aneurysm obliteration, and cervical and lumbar diskectomy). It also provides the means for various neurosurgical procedures, such as transsphenoidal removal of pituitary tumors without violating the integrity of the pituitary gland; cerebral anastomosis

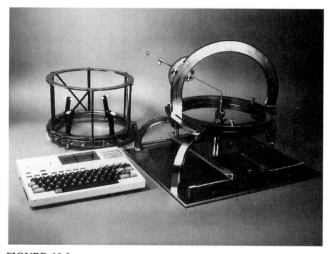

FIGURE 18-3

Some of the components of the BRW CT stereotactic system. (Courtesy of Radionics, Burlington, MA)

of intracranial and extracranial arteries previously considered too small to identify or suture with standard surgical procedures; obliteration of previously inaccessible aneurysms; and various brain and spinal cord procedures that require precise structural identification of microscopic neural and vascular areas, delicate dissection of structures, and management of hemostasis.

One of the necessary conditions for microsurgery is a means for accurate and effective coagulation of small cerebral vessels. The bipolar electrocoagulator has been used for this purpose. There are several technical requirements for any piece of electrocoagulation equipment, but the precision required for microsurgery places added demands on the instrumentation design (e.g., dissection instruments, retractors, drills, curettes, forceps, needles, and needle holders). In addition, head fixation devices, operative tables, and suction equipment must be designed specifically for microsurgery.

Once the target area has been identified, the stereotactic electrode or probe is passed through the slide carrier, which is attached to the stereotactic frame to the target area. It is necessary to verify by x-ray studies or CT scans that the target area has been reached. Once placement of instruments is verified, the procedure can continue. Because most procedures are conducted using local anesthesia, the cooperation of the patient must be gained. This is accomplished through a thorough patient teaching program on admission to the hospital.

Stereotactic neurosurgery is indicated for the removal or biopsy of deep, small, subcortical brain tumors. However, this technique has also been suggested for or applied to implantation of radioactive seeds into brain tumors; aspiration of intracerebral hematomas, colloid cysts, and abscesses; ablative procedures for extrapyramidal diseases (tremors, rigidity, and others); chronic pain control; and removal of craniopharyngiomas. Additional uses will probably be developed as experience with the technique increases.

Lasers

Surgical lasers were first introduced in the early 1960s, but it was not until 1979 that laser neurosurgery began to come into vogue in the United States. The word **laser** is an acronym for *light amplification by stimulated emission of radiation*. The basic properties of light and electromagnetic radiation govern laser technology. A laser is a device that concentrates a single wavelength of light into an intense, narrow beam of coherent monochromatic light energy that can be accurately focused on specific tissue. The selected body tissue absorbs the laser beam. The laser beam is transformed into immense heat energy, and the thermal energy of the laser beam allows simultaneous surgical dissection and coagulation.

Three types of surgical lasers are available to the neurosurgeon: the carbon dioxide, argon, and neodymium: yttrium-aluminum-garnet (Nd: YAG) laser. Each type uses a different light energy and allows different options for controlling and applying the laser beam. The beam can be applied directly to tissue, or it can be used to heat microprobes, which are then applied to tissue.

The value of lasers in neurosurgery is that the surgeon, using microscopic visualization, can dissect a precise structure without causing trauma to surrounding tissue, a consequence of traditional surgical techniques. This technique provides an approach for removing tumors from delicate and formerly inaccessible areas of the brain and spinal cord.

The use of lasers for neurosurgical procedures is still relatively new. Because of limited clinical application, patient selection is important. Patients with tumors that are extrinsic to brain tissue but proximal to delicate cerebral tissue are considered good candidates for laser surgery. Acoustic neuromas, craniopharyngiomas, certain brain stem gliomas, pinealomas, ventricular tumors, and meningiomas have been removed successfully with laser surgery. The removal of selected intradural and extradural spinal cord tumors has also been successful. These tumors include astrocytomas, ependymomas, meningiomas, and neuromas.

To summarize, the value of laser surgery is to provide accessibility to neurosurgical sites that were previously inaccessible. Lasers can dissect tissue by vaporization (while leaving adjacent tissue uninjured), coagulate blood vessels, and in some instances, shrink tumors. The clinical application of lasers is limited, but this so-called bloodless surgery is certain to become more refined in the foreseeable future. (See Chap. 25 for additional information.)

Radiosurgery: The Gamma Knife

The gamma knife, which is not a knife at all, was developed at the Karolinska Institute in Stockholm in 1968. It consists of a heavily shielded helmet containing 201 radially distributed, sealed, radioactive sources containing curies of cobalt-60. These are focused with precision on a central common target in the brain. Unlike conventional radiation therapy, this stereotactic radiosurgery is capable of destroying deep and inaccessible lesions in a single treatment session. This closed cell destruction of a focal point is possible because the target point has been determined by minute measurements and precise positioning of the patient.

Because of the extremely high levels of radiation involved, the Nuclear Regulatory Commission imposes strict guidelines that must be met by each facility using this technique. Purchase of the gamma knife requires a capital investment of a few million dollars, not including the site preparation costs. It is found in selected major medical centers.

The gamma knife is used for arteriovenous malformations (AVMs), brain tumors (e.g., acoustic neuromas, malignant tumors), and a variety of other intracranial conditions for which conventional surgery is inappropriate. In Sweden, the gamma knife has also been used for psychiatric and movement disorders. The criteria for selection of patients usually include excessive risk for conventional surgery, prior surgical failure, surgical inaccessibility of the lesion, and refusal of the patient to submit to a craniotomy. The cost-benefit ratio associated with the gamma knife is attractive.

A few major concerns relating to use of the gamma knife include the following:

• The lag time between treatment and result (AVMs take 1–3 years for maximal shrinkage; acoustic neuromas can take up to 4 years for maximal shrinkage).

- The lag time before side effects may appear (For example, hearing loss after treatment for an acoustic neuroma may not be noted for a year).

The gamma knife offers a new technology for treatment of patients who previously had no treatment options. Additional uses for the gamma knife will undoubtedly be found as experience is gained.

POSTOPERATIVE NURSING MANAGEMENT

After surgery, the patient is taken to the recovery room or at some hospitals, immediately to the neurological intensive care unit (NICU). Regardless of the hospital or physician preference, patients are admitted to the surgical or NICU after recovery from anesthesia, where they remain until well stabilized. The stay in the NICU allows close observation and extensive physiological monitoring.

Admission to the Neurological Intensive Care Unit

During transfer to the NICU, the nurse should expect a complete report, which will include the following:

- Overview of surgery (reason for surgery, anatomical approach, length of surgery, and specific area of the brain involved)
- History of preoperative neurological deficits
- Pre-existing medical problems
- Current baseline neurological signs
- Information provided to the family
- Review of the postoperative orders

This database is a basis for planning care. Chart 18-1 provides a summary of nursing diagnoses and interventions for postoperative patient management. The approach to care will depend on whether the patient has undergone supratentorial or infratentorial surgery. A comparison of the nursing focus for each approach is found in Chart 18-2.

Objectives of Nursing Management

The overall objectives of nursing management in the early postoperative period following a craniotomy are directed toward the following:

- Extensive physiological monitoring
- Frequent assessment and monitoring of neurological signs for early recognition of increased ICP
- Control of factors known to contribute to increased ICP
- Prevention and early recognition of other complications
- Administration of supportive care
- Emotional support of patient and family
- Early rehabilitation
- Beginning focused discharge planning

These objectives are appropriate throughout the patient's hospitalization, although emphasis may change as the patient is transferred from the NICU to the intermediate care unit. Specific protocols are outlined in Charts 18-1 and 18-2. The basic maintenance and supportive nursing care provided, regardless of procedure or anatomical location, are summarized in Chart 18-3. Chart 18-4 summarizes important information pertinent to postoperative drug therapy.

Assessment and Monitoring

Hemodynamic, respiratory, metabolic, and neurological assessment and monitoring are frequent and ongoing. The knowledge that the patient has recently undergone surgical insult is reason enough to draw the conclusion that increased ICP may be present. However, the nurse, when assessing the neurological signs, should identify changes in condition that may be subtle or rapid. Current findings are compared with baseline findings to determine trends.

The frequency with which the assessment is conducted will depend on how stable the patient's condition is and how soon after surgery it is performed. Neurological signs should be assessed every 15 to 30 minutes for the first 8 to 12 hours postoperatively, then every hour for the next 12 hours. As the patient stabilizes, the frequency of assessment will eventually be reduced to every 4 hours. Blood chemistries, complete blood count, and other laboratory monitoring are frequent. Chest x-ray, CT scans, electroencephalogram monitoring, and other diagnostics may be necessary to monitor progress.

Transfer from the Intensive Care Unit to the Acute Care Unit

As mentioned previously, the objectives of nursing management remain the same throughout the patient's hospitalization. To maintain continuity of care, the NICU nurse communicates with the nurse accepting the patient on the intermediate care unit to plan for a smooth transition. The patient and family need reassurance that the patient is stable and ready for this transfer. If possible, it is helpful for the receiving nurse to meet the patient and family before the transfer to relieve anxiety and fear.

POSTOPERATIVE COMPLICATIONS

Numerous complications and problems can develop after a craniotomy, including hemorrhage, hypovolemic shock, cardiac arrhythmias, increased ICP, cerebral edema, respiratory problems, gastric ulceration and hemorrhage, tension pneumocephalus, hydrocephalus, seizures, CSF leakage, meningitis, wound infection, thrombophlebitis, electrolyte imbalance, and diabetes insipidus (DI). Certain complications usually occur earlier in the postoperative period (*e.g.*, hypovolemic shock), whereas others (*e.g.*, wound infection) are apt to appear later in the postoperative course. The nurse is responsible for monitoring the patient for the development of complications and implementing preventive measures when possible. For example, strict aseptic technique is followed in the care of the incision to prevent wound infection.

(text continues on page 340)

CHART 18-1
Nursing Care Plan for the Patient Undergoing Intracranial Surgery

Nursing Diagnoses	Nursing Interventions	Expected Outcome(s)
Preoperative Phase		

• Knowledge Deficit related to (R/T) upcoming surgery	• Institute preoperative teaching.	• The patient/family will:
		  • State the reason for the surgery.
		  • Be aware of the preoperative and postoperative care that will be administered.
		  • State the anticipated outcome of surgery.

• Fear R/T upcoming surgery	• Allow the patient to express feelings. • Correct any misconceptions. • Provide emotional and psychological support. • Help patient to identify fears and discuss them. • Institute preoperative teaching.	• There will be a decrease in observable signs and symptoms of fear.
• Anxiety R/T upcoming surgery	• Institute preoperative teaching. • Reassure the patient and be supportive. • Allow the patient to express feelings. • Help patient and family mobilize their support systems.	• There will be a decrease in observable signs and symptoms of anxiety. • The patient will verbalize that he or she is feeling less anxious.
• Spiritual Distress R/T illness and surgery	• Allow the patient to express feelings. • Refer the patient to clergy or other appropriate person. • Be supportive.	• The patient will verbalize acceptance of the situation and will acknowledge feeling some sense of control.
• Ineffective Individual Coping R/T illness and surgery	• Help mobilize the patient's coping skills. • Assess how the patient has dealt with problems in the past. • Recognize ineffective use of defense mechanisms; do not reinforce use of these mechanisms. • Help the patient substitute adaptive coping mechanisms for maladaptive ones. • Set limits.	• The patient will be able to use adaptive coping skills.

(continued)

CHART 18-1 Nursing Care Plan for the Patient Undergoing Intracranial Surgery (Continued)

Immediate and Early Postoperative Phase

- Ineffective Airway Clearance R/T altered consciousness, altered respiratory function, or neuromuscular deficits

  - Assess the patient for abnormal breath sounds (rales, rhonchi, wheezing, snoring).
  - Observe O_2 saturation; monitor the patient for adequate saturation.
  - Note any increase in respiratory rate and pulse.
  - Note the presence of dyspnea or cyanosis.
  - Suction the patient's airway to maintain patency.
  - Encourage expectoration of sputum if the patient is conscious.
  - Elevate the head of the bed 30 degrees.
  - Keep the patient's neck in a neutral position.
  - Do not position an unconscious patient in the supine position.
  - Position the patient on one side to facilitate drainage of secretions.
  - Provide chest physical therapy.

  - Patency of the patient's airway will be maintained.

- Impaired Gas Exchange R/T ineffective breathing pattern and altered respiratory function
  Note: The patient may be intubated, on a ventilator, or in the process of being weaned from a ventilator.

  - Monitor the patient's blood gas levels to maintain levels set by the physician (levels may reflect a need for a decrease in CO_2).
  - Hyperventilate the patient before suctioning.
  - Position the patient to facilitate respirations.
  - Monitor ventilation settings.

  - Adequate O_2–CO_2 gas exchange will be maintained as evidenced by blood gas values that are within normal limits or that fall within the levels set by the physician.
  Note: The Po_2 is often set at a lower than normal limit (*e.g.,* 28) based on the new lower intracranial pressure (ICP).

- Pain: headache R/T intracranial surgery, discomfort R/T positioning, or oral discomfort
  Note: After operation, mouth care and lip gel *greatly* alleviate discomfort.

  - Assess the patient for signs and symptoms of pain (*e.g.,* restlessness, pulling on head dressing, change in vital signs).
  - Apply ice packs to the patient's eyes.
  - Provide mouth care frequently.
  - Apply lip gel as needed.

  - Pain or discomfort will be alleviated or eliminated; patient will appear to be comfortable.

- Risk for Electrolyte Imbalance R/T:
  - Fluid Volume Deficit secondary to use of osmotic diuretics (mannitol)

  - Monitor electrolyte levels and serum osmolality.
  - Administer mannitol, as ordered, if osmolality is less than the limits set by the physician.

  - Electrolyte balance will be maintained within normal limits.

(continued)

CHART 18-1 Nursing Care Plan for the Patient Undergoing Intracranial Surgery (Continued)

• Fluid Volume Excess secondary to cerebral edema	• Observe the patient for signs and symptoms of electrolyte imbalance. • Administer replacement therapy as ordered.	
• Risk for Fluid Volume Deficit or Excess R/T diabetes insipidus (DI), syndrome of inappropriate secretion of antidiuretic hormone (SIADH), use of diuretics, or cerebral edema	• Maintain an intake and output record. • Monitor serum osmolarity and electrolyte levels. • Monitor urine-specific gravity. • Weigh the patient twice a week. • Observe the patient for signs and symptoms of DI and SIADH. • Observe the patient for signs and symptoms of overhydration or underhydration. • Albumin (IV) is often ordered for patients who have undergone cerebrovascular surgery to maintain adequate volume and cerebral perfusion pressure.	• Fluid balance will be maintained. The patient will be euvolemic.
• Altered Urinary Elimination R/T decreased level of consciousness, development of DI or SIADH, or indwelling catheter	• Maintain intake and output record. • Monitor hourly urinary output and specific gravity of urine. • Report a urinary output of 200 mL/h or more for 2 consecutive hours (DI). • Report diminished urinary output (<30 mL/h). • Maintain patency of the catheter.	• Urinary elimination will be maintained at a level of 60 mL/h as a baseline.
• Altered Nutrition: Less than body requirements R/T altered consciousnes, inability to swallow, or inability to tolerate feedings	• Monitor the patient's dietary intake. • Calculate the daily calorie count. • Monitor the patient's body weight and compare it with the patient's weight on admission. • Assess the patient's swallowing ability before initiating oral intake. • If the patient is receiving tube feedings, maintain the food pump at the desired rate; limit the time the pump is off (*e.g.,* for suctioning). • Request a nutritional consultation as necessary.	• Adequate nutrition will be maintained. • Protein will be available for tissue repair. • Body weight will be maintained within a normal range.

(continued)

CHART 18-1 Nursing Care Plan for the Patient Undergoing Intracranial Surgery (Continued)

- Constipation R/T altered diet, drug side effects, and dehydration

  - Monitor the characteristics of the patient's stools and the pattern of elimination.
  - Initiate a bowel program.
  - Administer stool softeners as ordered.
  - Assess the patient for peristalsis.
  - Administer a mild laxative as necessary.
  - Include roughage in the patient's diet, if possible.

  - Bowel function will be maintained without constipation or straining at stool; stool will be soft and formed.

- Altered Cerebral Tissue Perfusion R/T cerebral edema, hypoxia, or ischemia and resulting in altered thought processes, impaired physical mobility, impaired verbal communication, and self-care deficits

  - Maintain the head of the bed at 30 degrees.
  - Maintain the patient's head in a neutral position.
  - Arrange for consultation (physical, occupational, or speech therapy), as necessary.
  Note: The physician often writes these orders as part of the postoperative orders.

  - Assessment of neurological deficits will be arranged with other health professionals as ordered.
  - Through collaboration, continuity of care will be supported.

- Risk for Injury R/T altered consciousness, altered thought processes, and neuromuscular deficits

  - Assess the patient's safety needs.
  - Observe the patient frequently.
  - Pull up side rails on the top and bottom of the bed.
  - Maintain the bed in a low position when not at the bedside.
  - Restrain patients when necessary to protect them from injury. (A physician's order will be necessary.)
  - Ensure that the call light is within the patient's reach.

  - Injury and falls will be prevented.

Collaborative Problem:
↑ **ICP**

  - Monitor neurological signs for changes and trends.
  - Observe ICP monitoring data for spikes and waveform changes.
  - Maintain specified fluid restrictions.
  - Elevate the head of the bed 30 degrees.
  - Monitor the patient's body temperature and maintain within the normal range; administer antipyretics as ordered.

  - Factors known to increase ICP will be controlled.
  - Spikes in ICP will be noted, and interventions ordered by the physician will be implemented.

(continued)

CHART 18-1 Nursing Care Plan for the Patient Undergoing Intracranial Surgery (Continued)

- Monitor the patient for pain, agitation, or restlessness; administer medications to treat these conditions as ordered.
- Monitor the patient's blood pressure; maintain blood pressure within the limits set by the physician.
- Prevent the Valsalva's maneuver.
- Calculate cerebral perfusion pressure, and maintain it within the limits set by the physician.

Hemorrhage

Intracranial hemorrhage is a serious postoperative complication in the neurological patient, resulting in bleeding into the subdural, epidural, intracerebral, or intraventricular space. Unlike bleeding that is visible externally, bleeding within the cranial vault is characterized by signs or symptoms of rapidly increasing ICP. A rapid deterioration in neurological status is often associated with intracranial bleeding; this condition requires immediate intervention to prevent irreversible cerebral damage and death. Intracranial hemorrhage is diagnosed on a clinical basis and confirmed by CT scan.

Hemorrhagic shock is caused by blood loss during surgery. Postoperative hemorrhage from the surgical site is uncommon. Hemorrhagic shock may also be attributable to gastrointestinal (GI) bleeding. Prophylaxis of the GI tract with histamine H_2 blockers is given. The nurse should monitor the patient for signs and symptoms of hemorrhagic shock, including tachycardia (perhaps the first sign of shock); a thready pulse; decreased blood pressure; pallor; cold, clammy skin; and restlessness. Blood replacement therapy may be required if blood loss is significant.

Hypovolemic Shock

Hypovolemic shock results from general fluid loss (blood, plasma, or water), particularly if osmotic diuretics have been used. The result is a decreased amount of circulating volume. The characteristics of hypovolemic shock include a decline in venous pressure. Common signs and symptoms include tachycardia; decreasing blood pressure; shallow and rapid respirations; cool, pale skin; low urinary output (10–25 mL/h); and restlessness to coma.

Treatment is directed toward fluid replacement using a bolus of saline; fluid expanders, such as plasmanate, lactated Ringer's solution; or blood products. Vasopressor drugs (*e.g.,* NeoSynephrine or dopamine) may be given. Hemodynamics (e.g., central venous pressure, cardiac output), oxygenation (ABGs, SaO_2), and vital signs should be monitored frequently.

Cardiac Arrhythmias

Cardiac arrhythmias are not unusual, especially after posterior fossa surgery or if blood has entered the CSF. Continuous cardiac monitoring is important for at least the first 24 to 48 hours after surgery. Periodically observe the rate, rhythm, and pattern on the monitor to determine the presence of an arrhythmia.

If a monitor is not available, the apical pulse should be checked during the postoperative period to identify abnormalities in the heart rate or rhythm. Any abnormalities should be reported to the physician immediately. In addition, serum potassium levels should be monitored for depletion secondary to diuresis.

Increased Intracranial Pressure

Although some increase in ICP is expected (with the peak occurring about 72 hours after surgery), great spikes in ICP are life threatening. Great increases in ICP can result from conditions such as cerebral edema, hemorrhage, meningitis, and surgical trauma. Treatment includes management of the underlying cause, judicious use of osmotic diuretics, and possible ventricular drainage. See Chapter 17 for a more detailed discussion of increased ICP.

Cerebral Edema

In the neurosurgical patient, the major cause of increased ICP is cerebral edema. Cerebral edema may have been present before surgery, or it can develop or increase as a result of surgical trauma. Postoperative cerebral edema can be controlled by head elevation to 30 degrees, euvolemia, possible use of steroids if vasogenic edema is present (*e.g.,* brain tumor resection), osmotic diuretics, and possible CSF drainage. (Elevation of the head of the bed to 30 degrees facilitates drainage of blood from the brain. Gravity can be used to enhance drainage because the venous vessels from the brain are valveless.) An

(text continues on page 344)

CHART 18-2
Nursing Management Following Supratentorial and Infratentorial Surgery

Supratentorial	Infratentorial

Incision

Supratentorial

- The scalp incision is made within the boundaries of the hairline, directly over the area to be explored on the cerebral hemisphere. The incision creates a skin flap. The actual location and shape of the skin flap can vary from one that appears horseshoe-shaped to one that follows the hairline in the frontal region.
- Sutures are usually removed within 7–10 d.

Infratentorial

- The incision (skin flap) is made above the nape of the neck around the occipital area or posterolaterally in the occipitotemporal region.
- Sutures are usually removed 7–10 d after surgery.

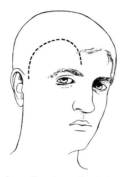
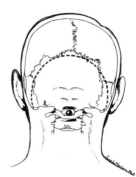

(Figures above are from Smeltzer, S., & Bare, B. [1996]. *Brunner and Suddarth's Textbook of medical-surgical nursing* [8th ed.]. Philadelphia: Lippincott-Raven Publishers.)

Head Dressing

- A turban-style dressing is applied initially.
- Many physicians remove the dressing completely after 24 h.
- The dressing is monitored for evidence of blood or cerebrospinal fluid (CSF) drainage.
- The incision is monitored for redness, drainage, or signs of wound infection.

- A turban-style dressing is applied initially.
- Many physicians remove the dressing completely after 24 h.
- The dressing is monitored for evidence of blood or CSF drainage.
- The incision is monitored for redness, drainage, or signs of wound infection.

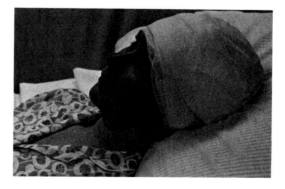

(continued)

CHART 18-2 Nursing Management Following Supratentorial and Infratentorial Surgery (Continued)

Positioning of the Head of the Bed

The position of the head of the bed (HOB) depends on the specific surgical procedure and the preference of the physician. Review the doctor's order sheet for any specific instructions. If there are any position restrictions for the HOB, a sign should be posted conspicuously at the HOB and in the nursing care plan.

Some physicians follow a protocol of gradual elevation of the HOB for postoperative management of ventricular shunts and chronic subdural hematomas to prevent cerebral hemorrhage. An example of a protocol followed for postoperative management of both shunts and evacuation of a chronic subdural hematoma is as follows: keep the HOB flat for 24 h; then elevate the HOB 15 degrees for the next 24 h; then elevate the HOB 30 degrees for the next 24 h; then elevate the HOB 45 degrees for the next 24 h; finally elevate the HOB to 90 degrees.

Supratentorial	Infratentorial
• The HOB is elevated 30 degrees. (This position facilitates venous blood return from the brain and promotes a decrease in intracranial pressure [ICP].) • A pillow may be placed under the patient's head and shoulders. The neck should be maintained in a neutral position.	• The HOB may be elevated at a 30-degree angle or lowered flat, depending on the preference of the physician. • *Do not angulate the neck anteriorly or laterally.* A small pillow is placed under the head for comfort. • For the patient who experiences dizziness or orthostatic hypotension, the HOB is elevated gradually while concurrently monitoring vital signs.

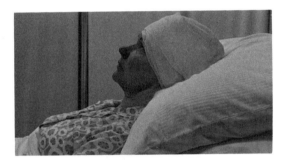

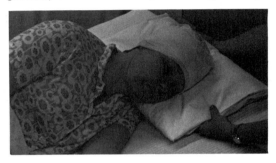

Turning and Positioning

• There is usually no restriction on turning. • If a large tumor has been removed from a cerebral hemisphere, the physician may write an order to avoid positioning on the operative site to prevent shifting of cranial contents secondary to gravity. • Positioning an unconscious patient or one who is recovering from anesthesia on the side facilitates drainage of oral secretions and promotes a patent airway. • When positioning a patient, avoid extreme flexion of the upper legs or lateral or anterior flexion of the neck. A soft collar may be applied to keep the neck in a neutral position.	• There is usually no restriction on turning. • If a large tumor has been removed from a cerebral hemisphere, the physician may write an order to avoid positioning on the operative site to prevent shifting of cranial contents secondary to gravity. • Positioning an unconscious patient or one who is recovering from anesthesia on the side facilitates drainage of oral secretions and promotes a patent airway. • When positioning a patient, avoid extreme flexion of the upper legs or lateral or anterior flexion of the neck. A soft collar may be applied to keep the neck in a neutral position.

Ambulation

The patient is allowed out of bed as soon as tolerated, which will depend on general condition and the judgment of the physician and nurse.	The patient is allowed out of bed as soon as the vertical position is tolerated. Patients undergoing infratentorial procedures are often maintained on bed rest longer than those undergoing supratentorial procedures because of the frequency of dizziness experienced by these patients. This dizziness is caused by transient edema in the area of cranial nerve VIII.

(continued)

CHART 18-2 Nursing Management Following Supratentorial and Infratentorial Surgery (Continued)

Supratentorial	**Infratentorial**

Nutrition

- The patient is given nothing by mouth (NPO) for 24 h; IV fluids are administered slowly.
- If the patient is not experiencing nausea or vomiting and can protect his airway, clear fluids are started.

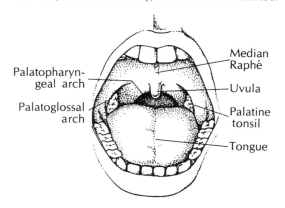

- The diet is progressed as tolerated.
- If fluid restriction is ordered, the daily allowance is adhered to strictly.

- The patient is NPO for at least the first 24 h; IV fluids are administered slowly. Nausea tends to be more of a problem with surgery in this region than in the supratentorial area. Presence of the gag reflex and ability to protect the airway must be evident before food and fluids are given.
- Edema of cranial nerves IX and X may affect the swallowing and gag reflexes.
- If no nausea or vomiting is noted, and the gag and swallowing reflexes are present, the patient may sip water using a straw. Ask the patient to take a small sip and swallow it.
- The gag reflex is checked by touching the posterior wall of the pharynx. The normal response is contraction of the pharynx.
- If nausea or vomiting occurs, continue the patient's NPO status and IV therapy; after nausea or vomiting has subsided, ingestion of oral fluids may be attempted again.
- Once the patient is able to tolerate fluids, progress from clear liquids to a diet as tolerated.
- If fluid restriction is ordered, the daily allowance is adhered to strictly.

Elimination

- An indwelling urinary catheter is inserted for most neurosurgical procedures. The catheter is removed as soon as possible. If there is difficulty with voiding, a bladder retraining program is begun.
- Constipation can occur as a result of diuretics and pain medication (*e.g.*, morphine or codeine). Straining at stool initiates the Valsalva's maneuver, which can increase ICP. A bowel program is begun to avoid constipation.

- An indwelling urinary catheter is inserted for most neurosurgical procedures. The catheter is removed as soon as possible. If there is difficulty with voiding, begin a bladder retraining program.
- Constipation can occur as a result of medication (*e.g.*, morphine or codeine). Straining at stool initiates the Valsalva's maneuver, which can increase ICP. A bowel program is begun to avoid constipation.

Fluid and Electrolyte Balance

- Most patients are maintained euvolemic. Intake is balanced with output.
- An intake and output record is maintained, and the fluid restriction is adhered to strictly.
- Serum electrolyte and osmolarity levels are monitored.
- If surgery is performed in the area of the pituitary gland or hypothalamus, transient diabetes insipidus may develop. Urinary output and specific gravity are monitored every 1–4 h.

- Most patients are maintained euvolemic. Intake is balanced with output.
- An intake and output record is maintained, and the fluid restriction is adhered to strictly.
- Serum electrolyte and osmolarity levels are monitored.

(continued)

CHART 18-2 Nursing Management Following Supratentorial and Infratentorial Surgery (Continued)

Special Focus of Neurological Assessment

The nurse monitors the patient's neurological status, performing an assessment at frequent intervals. Based on an understanding of specific neurological functions controlled by the supratentorial region and infratentorial region, the nurse places special emphasis on the following areas of assessment:

Supratentorial	**Infratentorial**

• Potential cranial nerve dysfunction
  —Optic nerve (II): visual deficits, homonymous hemianopia
  —Oculomotor nerve (III): ptosis
  —Oculomotor, trochlear, abducens (III, IV, VI): deficits in extraocular movement
	• Potential cranial nerve dysfunction
	  —Oculomotor, trochlear, abducens (III, IV, VI): deficits in extraocular movement
	  —Facial (VII): lower lid deficit, absent corneal reflex, weakness or paralysis of the facial muscles
	  —Acoustic (VIII): decreased hearing, dizziness, nystagmus
	  —Glossopharyngeal and vagus (IX, X): diminished or absent gag or swallowing reflex, orthostatic hypotension
	• Potential cerebellar dysfunction
	  —Ataxia, difficulty with fine motor movement, difficulty with coordination

indwelling catheter should be in place if osmotic diuretics are ordered. The urinary output should be measured to quantify the amount of diuresis and calculate fluid intake to maintain euvolemia or slight negative balance.

Respiratory Complications

Partial or complete obstruction of the airway can occur from improper positioning or accumulation of mucus or other drainage.

• Unconscious patients should never be positioned on their back because the tongue can easily slip backward and obstruct the airway.
• The neck should be maintained in a neutral position.

If an unconscious patient begins to snore, it is most likely attributable to obstruction of the airway. This situation must be corrected immediately to prevent not only respiratory failure, but secondary brain injury from cerebral hypoxia as well. This could easily lead to an increase in ICP. If obstruction is suspected, the jaw is pulled forward and downward to relieve the obstruction. The patient should be positioned laterally, with the head elevated to facilitate drainage. Elevating the head of the bed 30 degrees is helpful for maintaining a patent airway.

Respiratory difficulty may also result from edema in and around the brain stem, particularly following infratentorial surgery. Aspiration caused by diminished or absent gag and swallowing reflexes can be minimized by properly positioning the patient on the side with the head elevated. Also, oral intake should be withheld until the presence of the gag and swallow-ing reflexes has been verified and the patient is able to protect his or her own airway.

The nurse should be aware that adult respiratory distress syndrome and neurogenic pulmonary edema (NPE) can develop. (See Chap. 12 for a discussion of both conditions.) A sudden, massive increase in ICP can trigger a pressor response, which results in the development of NPE. The signs and symptoms are the same as those associated with acute pulmonary edema caused by cardiac decompensation, although in the neurological patient, there is no evidence of cardiac disease to which acute pulmonary edema can be attributed.

Other pulmonary complications include pneumonia, atelectasis, and pulmonary emboli. Pneumonia and atelectasis have already been discussed. However, pulmonary emboli are possible complications in any surgical patient, especially if surgery is prolonged and hypothermia has been used. Frequent turning, suctioning, deep breathing techniques, and chest physical therapy help to prevent respiratory complications.

GASTRIC ULCERATION AND HEMORRHAGE

Gastric ulceration (Cushing's ulcer) accompanied by GI hemorrhage has frequently been observed in neurological patients. Neurological procedures and acute and chronic central nervous system diseases (e.g., craniocerebral trauma, tumors) have been associated with symptoms of active gastric bleeding. An increased incidence of gastric ulcers is associated with lesions around the anterior hypothalamus. Although the underlying pathophysiology is controversial, it is thought that the stress response is the probable cause.

CHART 18-3
Basic Nursing Management Following Cranial Surgery

Nursing Management

- Give basic hygienic care until the patient is able to participate in self-care (*e.g.*, bath, oral hygiene, hair combing, nail cutting).
- Apply thigh-high elastic stockings and sequential compression air boots, and inspect legs daily. Note any signs of thrombophlebitis (redness, tenderness, warmth, swelling).
- Provide skin care every 4 h.

- Turn patient every 2 h, being careful to maintain the patient's body alignment. (It may be necessary to use pillows and other similar devices to maintain good body alignment.)
- Carry out range-of-motion exercises four times daily.

- Provide urinary catheter care daily using soap and water. Pin the catheter to prevent undue traction on the meatus. Remove the catheter as soon as possible.
- Apply warm or cold moist compresses to the eye area.
- Inspect eyes every 4 h for signs of irritation or dryness. Lubricate the eye with normal saline, commercially prepared eye lubricant, or ointment, as prescribed by the physician. To protect the eye from injury (corneal ulcerations or abrasions) if the lids do not tightly, cover the eye, use an eye shield, or tape the eye closed.
- Pull up the side rails of the bed, and apply a jacket restraint as necessary.
- Evaluate periods of restlessness for an underlying cause (check for patency of the airway, evidence of pain, or distention of the bladder).

- Administer analgesics as ordered (the drug selected should not mask neurological signs).

- Do not cluster together nursing activities that are known to increase intracranial pressure (ICP) in the patient at risk.

- Monitor routine vital signs.

Rationale

- Maintains cleanliness and encourages independence in activities of daily living

- Improves blood return to the heart and decreases the risk of thrombophlebitis

- Cleanses, lubricates, and provides the opportunity for an inspection of the skin to note irritation or skin breakdown
- Prevents prolonged pressure on specific areas of the skin, pooling of secretions, and development of musculoskeletal abnormalities; decreases the risk of pneumonia and atelectasis
- Maintains muscle tone to prevent atrophy and contractures
- Reduces the incidence of urinary tract infection

- Relieves periocular edema

- Decreases the risk of corneal ulceration, eye infections, or injury

- Provides for patient's safety

- In the neurological patient, restlessness may be caused by an obstructed airway, pain, or a distended bladder; the nurse should identify the underlying cause and provide the appropriate intervention.
- Provides for the comfort of the patient and helps to control restlessness

- Prevents dangerous spikes in ICP

- Provides baseline data and data for comparison

(continued)

CHART 18-3 Basic Nursing Management Following Cranial Surgery (Continued)

Nursing Management	Rationale
• Assess neurological signs at prescribed intervals: —Level of consciousness —Pupillary reaction —Eye movement —Motor function —Sensory function	• Provides data about the patient's neurological condition and for comparison with previous signs to detect any change in the patient's condition
• Review laboratory reports. Conventional normal values for some studies are as follows: —Hemoglobin: 12.0–16.0 g in females 13.5–18.0 g in males —Hematocrit: 37%–48% in females 42%–50% in males —BUN: 8–25 mg —Potassium: 3.5–5.0 mEq —Calcium: 8.5–10.5 mg —Sodium: 135–145 mEq —Fasting blood sugar: 70–110 mg —Creatinine: 0.6–0.9 mg/dL in females 0.8–1.2 mg/dL in males —Serum osmolarity: 275–295 mOsm/L	• Identifies abnormal levels that signal the need for intervention. Also, some medical orders may set parameters for treatment (*e.g.*, maintain the serum osmolarity at 305–310 mOsm/kg). A review of the laboratory data also provides guidelines for interventions.

Some of the drugs used in neurological treatment protocols also contribute to gastric irritation. Examples of such drugs are dexamethasone (Decadron), phenytoin, and certain antibiotics. For this reason, acetaminophen (Tylenol) is preferred to aspirin for the treatment of mild discomfort or as an antipyretic drug. When dexamethasone is administered, magnesium hydroxide (Maalox) is often given to reduce gastric irritation. A histamine H_2-blocker is administered prophylactically to reduce gastric secretions and protect against gastric hemorrhage. Sucralfate (Carafate) is another gastric protector.

The nurse should monitor the patient's hematocrit and hemoglobin. Complaints of gastric distress should be evaluated. Additionally, the stools should be monitored daily for occult blood, which would indicate bleeding somewhere in the GI tract. Symptoms of gastric ulceration are those of gastric distress. Bleeding may be acute and massive or slow and painless. A gradual decline in the hematocrit or hemoglobin suggests bleeding somewhere in the body. Treatment of active gastric bleeding includes nasogastric suction, fluid and blood replacement, and possibly surgical intervention if bleeding is diagnosed.

Tension Pneumocephalus

Pneumocephalus is the entry of air into the subdural, extradural, subarachnoid, intracerebral, or intraventricular compartments. Pneumocephalus is a postoperative complication associated with posterior fossa craniotomy, burr hole for evacuation of a chronic subdural hematoma, and transsphenoidal hypophysectomy. The sitting position assumed during postoperative surgery is a risk factor. During hypophysectomy, air enters the subarachnoid space through the pituitary fossa and is gradually absorbed. However, in the presence of CSF rhinorrhea, additional air can enter the intracranial space, creating a pneumocephalus.

The trapped air, when warmed within the body, expands. A small amount of air can usually be reabsorbed and is not problematic. However, if the air pocket is of sufficient volume, it acts as a space-occupying lesion, causing neurological deterioration. The time frame for pneumocephalus to develop is either early (within 24 hours after surgery) or late (1 week following surgery). Signs and symptoms include drowsiness, decreased level of consciousness, and focal or lateral deficits. The diagnosis is established by CT scan. Treatment includes evacuation of the air.

Hydrocephalus

The postoperative complication of hydrocephalus can develop early or late in the postoperative course as a result of edema or bleeding into the subarachnoid space. Bleeding can interfere with the normal absorption of CSF by plugging the arachnoid villi. Such plugging of the arachnoid villi is also associated with primary disease processes, such as a ruptured cerebral aneurysm or head trauma. Scarring or obstruction in the ventricular system can also lead to hydrocephalus.

The signs and symptoms of hydrocephalus are outlined in Chapter 17. The usual treatment involves a ventriculostomy to drain CSF temporarily. If the hydrocephalus does not resolve, then a surgical shunting procedure is warranted. This is necessary to relieve the brain of excessive CSF and to prevent cerebral atrophy.

CHART 18-4
Possible Drug Therapy in the Postoperative Period

Classification and Drugs	Purpose	Comments
Anticonvulsants		
• Phenytoin (Dilantin) is the drug of choice—100 mg t.i.d. or q.i.d. PO or IV or in liquid form for administration through a feeding tube • Phenobarbital or carbamazepine (Tegretol)	• Used in patients at high risk for seizures secondary to cerebral edema and surgical trauma • Given prophylactically to prevent seizures • Ordered if Dilantin is not tolerated	• Observe the patient for Dilantin rash. • The drug may be continued after surgery for some patients. • Monitor the blood levels of the drug to maintain a therapeutic range.
Cortocosteroids (controversial)		
• Dexamethasone (Decadron), PO or IV • Solu-Medrol sometimes preferred	• Used to decrease cerebral edema after brain tumor resection • Drug tapered gradually (usually over 7–10 d)	• Monitor the patient for GI bleeding; check stools for occult blood. • Patients are usually maintained on a histamine blocker (*e.g.,* Tagamet) to prevent GI irritation. • Monitor blood glucose levels for elevation.
Osmotic Diuretics		
• Mannitol (20%–25%), IV in small doses	• Used to decrease cerebral edema • Furosemide (Lasix) may be administered to treat the rebound effect of Mannitol.	• Administer the drug with a filter (to guard against crystallization) • Monitor serum osmolarity (the physician usually sets parameters of <310); urinary output; and serum K^+ for depletion.
Antibiotics		
• Broad-spectrum antibiotics are used, such as Keflin, IV q6–8h for 3–5 d.	• Used in patients at high risk for infection; prophylactic antibiotics may be given.	• Monitor the results of cultures. • Monitor the patient for signs and symptoms of infection.
Antipyretics		
• Acetaminophen (Tylenol), PO or PR or through feeding tube q4–6h	• Used to maintain normothermia	• Aspirin is not used because it is known to irritate the GI system.
Antiemetics		
• Metoclopramide hydrochloride (Reglan), PO or IV • Trimethobenzamide hydrochloride (Tigan), PO, PR, or IM	• Used to control nausea	• Nausea may be related to vertigo; it is seen most often with posterior fossa surgery.

(continued)

CHART 18-4 Possible Drug Therapy in the Postoperative Period (Continued)

Histamine (H₂) Receptor Antagonist and Other Gastric Protectors

• Ranitidine (Zantac)	• Used to decrease risk of gastrointestinal (GI) bleeding • Blocks the action of histamine at receptors in the acid-secreting parietal cells of the gastric mucosal glands	• Monitor patients for thrombocytopenia, neutropenia, and increased prothrombin times.
• Sucralfate (Carafate)	• Coats stomach	

Analgesics

• Tylenol (plain), 650 mg PO or PR q4–6h • Tylenol with codeine, 1 to 2 tablets q4–6h (Tylenol #3 contains 30 mg of codeine) • Morphine sulfate, 10 mg parenterally q4h	• Used to control headache; the drug used will depend on the severity of the headache, which the nurse should assess. • Morphine is used in small doses in the intensive care unit because it can easily be reversed.	• If receiving codeine or morphine, monitor the patient for constipation. • Note that morphine causes constriction of the pupils as a side effect.

Antacids

• Maalox, 30 mL q3–4h PO or through feeding tube	• Used to coat the gastric mucosa to protect it from gastric irritation	• If a feeding tube is in place, monitor the pH of GI aspirations for acidity. • Monitor the patient for GI bleeding.

Seizures

Seizures following intracranial surgery may take the form of generalized convulsions or focal seizure activity. Seizures can be an early or late postoperative complication. Focal seizures in the form of twitching of selected muscles, particularly of the face or hand, are also common. Focal seizures in these two areas are common because both occupy large areas on the motor strip of the cerebral cortex; therefore, irritation from surgery or cerebral edema can easily initiate such seizure activity.

Because seizures are common after intracranial surgery, patients undergoing craniotomy may receive prophylactic anticonvulsants, most commonly phenytoin, to prevent seizure activity. Other physicians give prophylactic anticonvulsants only to patients who are high risk for seizure. For patients receiving anticonvulsants, blood levels must be monitored to maintain a therapeutic range.

Cerebrospinal Fluid Leakage

Postoperative leakage of CSF can occur early or late in the postoperative course and is caused by an opening in the subarachnoid space. It is seen most often with CSF leakage from the operative site. A CSF leak can also be associated with head trauma, especially a basal skull fracture. A CSF leak will often seal over spontaneously. Serial lumbar punctures or a CSF lumbar drain may be necessary to keep CSF pressure low. If these measures are not successful, surgical repair may be in-

dicated. A patient usually receives prophylactic antibiotics to prevent infection when a CSF leak is discovered. (See the following section on meningitis for further discussion.)

Meningitis

Microorganisms responsible for meningitis can be introduced into the meninges or CSF by spreading from a wound infection, from a head injury in which the dura mater has been punctured, or by contamination during surgery. Contamination of the head dressing is another possible cause of meningitis. Presence of a dural tear, a prime site for entrance of microorganisms, is indicated by clear drainage on the head dressing or from the ear or nose. Drainage on the dressing that is clear or yellowish suggests CSF drainage.

CSF may also be noticed draining from the ear or nose. To determine whether the drainage is CSF, a Dextrostix can be used to test the fluid. If the drainage is CSF, the fluid will test positive for glucose. Mucus does not contain glucose, although blood does contain glucose. If more conclusive evidence is required and CSF can be collected, it can also be checked for chloride. CSF will show a glucose level of approximately 60% to 80% of the blood level, and a chloride level greater than the serum level.

• If CSF is present in drainage from the nose, patients must *not* be suctioned nasally or blow their nose.

- The physician should be notified at once if meningitis is suspected.

Meningitis is treated with antibiotics and a quiet environment.

Other signs and symptoms associated with meningitis include the following:

- Positive Kernig's and Brudzinski's signs
- Stiff neck
- Photophobia
- Restlessness and hyperirritability
- Elevated temperature

Prophylactic measures should be taken to prevent the development of meningitis, and strict aseptic technique should be followed in the management of the surgical site. Most neurosurgeons routinely order prophylactic antibiotics during and after all intracranial surgery and continue antibiotic therapy for a few days to prevent meningitis. Part of the nursing responsibility is checking for drainage on the dressing and observing its character. A wet head dressing should be reinforced immediately and the physician notified. Because moisture provides organisms with a transport system, a wet head dressing is an ideal medium on which organisms can grow. The gauze used in most dressings absorbs drainage by capillary attraction. The wicking action helps to remove drainage from the skin. If a wet dressing is allowed to remain on the incision, the incision will become contaminated from organisms in the air or on bedclothes by the wicking action of the moist dressing.

When head dressings are changed, strict aseptic technique should be followed. Usually, the initial dressing is not touched until the sutures are removed or unless it has become wet. Many physicians remove the dressing completely after 24 hours. The policy of the hospital and physician should be followed concerning who may change an initial dressing.

Wound Infection

Wound infections can result from poor aseptic technique during surgery or dressing changes. Patients may also contaminate the incision by touching it with their hands. To avoid this, patients must be cautioned against such action and restrained if necessary. The most frequent causative organisms for wound infections are the various staphylococcal organisms. Redness and drainage from the wound are the usual early symptoms. Thus, the nurse should observe the incision and dressing for evidence of drainage. A foul odor from the wound or an elevated white blood count (may be slight if receiving steroids) raise suspicion of a wound infection. Strict aseptic technique should be followed in the management of the wound or dressing.

Thrombophlebitis

Any patient who is maintained on bed rest for even short periods is prone to the development of thrombophlebitis. In addition, techniques used in surgery, such as hypothermia and keeping the patient in certain positions for extended periods, are also risk factors. Thrombophlebitis is a serious concern because it can lead to a life-threatening pulmonary embolism.

Treatment of thrombophlebitis follows the usual medical protocol of bed rest, application of elastic stockings, and elevation of the involved limb. Discretion is used when instituting anticoagulation therapy, a common treatment modality, because such drugs may cause bleeding at the surgical site.

The following principles for the prevention of thrombophlebitis should be incorporated into the nursing care plan:

- Application of thigh-high elastic stockings, which are valuable in preventing stasis of blood in the lower legs and improving the venous blood return to the heart
- Continued use of sequential compression air boots at all times
- Observation of the legs for signs and symptoms of thrombophlebitis (redness, swelling, pain)

Electrolyte Imbalance

The most common electrolyte imbalance seen in neurosurgical patients is hyponatremia. Hypokalemia is also common. Hyponatremia must be corrected slowly with saline solutions. Potassium supplements are used for hypokalemia.

Diabetes Insipidus

Supratentorial surgery, particularly in and around the pituitary fossa, can lead to temporary DI. DI is caused by a disturbance of the posterior lobe of the pituitary gland, which produces antidiuretic hormone (ADH). If this hormone is not secreted in sufficient quantity, the patient will produce large amounts of urine with a low specific gravity. The danger is fluid and electrolyte imbalance with dehydration, a serious concern that can affect all body systems.

The development of DI is often a transient problem requiring no specific treatment other than adjusting IV therapy to correlate with urinary output. If the condition does not correct itself, desmopressin acetate (DDAVP), is the drug of choice for DI. The dosage is 0.1 to 0.4 mL intranasally one or two times daily. The duration of the drug is 12 to 24 hours; it has minimal effects of irritation or vasoconstriction of the nasal mucosa. Aqueous vasopressin (Pitressin), 5 to 10 U, may be given subcutaneously every 3 to 6 hours.

An accurate intake and output record and fractional urinary output must be maintained. This is a simple task if an indwelling catheter is in place, as is often the case in the early postoperative period when DI is most apt to appear. The specific gravity of the urine should also be checked every 1 to 4 hours. A reading of 1.005 or less is considered low. Large amounts of urine, coupled with low specific gravity, suggest DI.

The hydration level, electrolytes, and serum osmolarity should be monitored regularly to determine the need for replacement therapy. As mentioned previously, the DI is often temporary and corrects itself without treatment. See Chapter 10 for a discussion of DI.

POSTOPERATIVE DEFICITS RELATED TO SURGERY

As a result of surgery, various neurological deficits may be noted. The particular deficits or changes noted depend on the deficits that were present before surgery, the type of surgical procedure, and the amount of edema present. Many of these deficits will resolve completely in the postoperative period. Others may require physical therapy or rehabilitation. The nurse assesses and monitors the patient for changes. Independent and collaborative interventions also may be implemented to manage the various problems.

Diminished Level of Consciousness

As cerebral edema subsides postoperatively, ICP decreases and the level of consciousness improves. It is often surprising to find a patient who is fully alert and well oriented after surgery even though there is some cerebral edema present. Debulking of a mass, such as a brain tumor, can make a significant difference. For other patients, improvement in the level of consciousness will occur as cerebral edema gradually subsides.

Deficits in Communications

Patients' ability to express themselves verbally and to understand the spoken word will depend on what deficits were present before surgery and what part of the brain was the site of the surgery. If deficits are associated with cerebral edema, they will most likely improve as cerebral edema subsides. If the deficit was prominent before surgery or if surgical dissection was close to the language area, recovery will be much slower, perhaps requiring referral to a speech therapist.

The nurse should evaluate the type of communication deficit and develop an alternative method of communication. If the patient requires only that the nurse speak more slowly and use simple rather than complex sentences, such an adjustment can easily be made if the nursing diagnosis of the problem has been accurate. The nursing care plan should include a notation describing what alterations in communication patterns are necessary. If these adjustments are made by all personnel, it will greatly reduce the frustration of the patient and staff when communicating.

Motor and Sensory Deficits

As with consciousness and communication deficits, a decrease in cerebral edema results in an improvement in motor and sensory function. The level of improvement is contingent on the neurological deficit present before surgery and the surgical site.

For patients with motor deficits, a physical therapy program is usually implemented to facilitate return of motor function. The nurse must be aware of specific deficits experienced by the patient and should participate in and support the principles of the physiotherapeutic program, thereby promoting continuity of care. Adaptations of nursing care may be necessary to meet the needs of the patient.

The nurse can participate by encouraging the patient to use a weak limb in the activities of daily living (ADLs), administering range-of-motion exercises, ensuring proper positioning, applying special braces and splints if these devices are part of the program, and helping the patient ambulate. Most of all, the nurse often provides emotional support as the patient deals with loss of body function and alterations in body image and self-concept.

Headache

Postoperatively, headache is expected in the first 24 to 48 hours, and it may be moderate to severe. Much of the pain originates from surgical stretching or irritation of the nerves of the scalp. Pain can also result from traction on the dura, falx, or large blood vessels within the intracranial space. A headache can be intensified by a head dressing that has been applied too tightly. The snugness of the dressing should be assessed for comfort. If a dressing becomes too tight (as evidenced by swelling), the dressing will need to be loosened, cut, or changed.

Codeine sulfate or acetaminophen are the drugs most commonly ordered to alleviate headache. In some facilities, morphine is used more often than codeine because it can easily be reversed. The drug selected will depend on the severity of the headache. A quiet environment with limited direct light or a dimly lit room is soothing.

Hyperthermia

Some elevation in temperature is expected in the early postoperative period. A rectal temperature is taken at prescribed intervals to monitor the patient's body temperature. Elevation of body temperature may indicate the presence of infection or irritation of the hypothalamus, the area of the brain responsible for regulation of the body temperature; the specific cause of the hyperthermia must be determined (neurogenic hyperthermia versus infection). Traction or petechial hemorrhage of the hypothalamus or pons can cause major elevations in body temperature (105°F; 40.6°C). Surgery in or around the third or fourth ventricle can also cause dramatic spikes in body temperature because of the proximity to the hypothalamus.

As body temperature becomes elevated, there is an increase in blood pressure, cerebral blood flow, and cerebral metabolic rate. The metabolism of glucose, the major nutrient of the brain, is directly proportional to the rate of oxygen consumption. As cerebral metabolism increases, production of the metabolic by-products (carbon dioxide and lactic acid) increases. Both carbon dioxide and lactic acid are potent vasodilating agents that contribute to an increase in ICP. It is important to control elevations of body temperature in the neurosurgical patient because hyperthermia may result in increased ICP.

Hyperthermia is controlled by using antipyretic drugs, such as acetaminophen, which is administered by mouth, feeding tube, or rectally. Drug therapy may be used in conjunction with a hypothermia blanket, control of the environment, removal of excess bedclothes, or sponging of the body with cool water. The lowering of body temperature is achieved gradually to prevent shivering. If shivering occurs, chlorpromazine (Thorazine) may be ordered to control it, because shivering causes an increase in ICP.

Periocular Edema

Swelling around the eyes (periocular edema) is common after cranial surgery because of the manipulation of scalp, skull, and intracranial contents. Periocular edema is usually accompanied by discoloration and ecchymosis. Edema peaks at about 48 to 72 hours postoperatively.

Alternating warm and cold saline or water compresses or applying cold compresses initially followed by warm saline compresses after 24 hours can be helpful. The eyes should be cleansed to prevent crusting and lubricated with saline eye drops. Periocular edema will disappear in 5 to 6 days. Discoloration and ecchymosis will take 10 to 14 days to resolve.

Diminished Gag and Swallowing Reflexes

The gag and swallowing reflexes are controlled by cranial nerves (CN) IX and X. Both nerves emit from the brain stem at the medulla. Surgery in the posterior fossa (infratentorial area) may cause edema to the CNs proximal to the operative site, resulting in temporary loss or diminished response of both reflexes. As edema subsides, the reflexes will return.

The danger of a temporary loss of either reflex is difficulty in swallowing and increased risk of aspiration. Aspiration with consequent aspiration pneumonia and respiratory difficulty are serious concerns. Therefore, oral intake should not be started unless the patient is able to protect his or her airway. Suction equipment should be readily available for use should the need arise.

Visual Disturbances

Vision should be assessed if the patient is sufficiently conscious to provide information. Temporary visual field deficits in one-half or one-quarter of the visual field are common after surgery because of increased ICP or surgical trauma. Diplopia (double vision) and dimness of vision can also be evaluated by asking the patient to describe changes in vision. If diplopia is evident, an eye patch can be worn.

Even in noncommunicative patients the nurse can often draw a presumptive conclusion about visual loss by observation. For example, the nurse may observe that the patient does not notice environmental objects on one side of the bed or reacts only when someone approaches from a specific side. Both situations suggest visual deficits.

Loss of Corneal Reflex

The presence of the corneal reflex is determined by lightly touching the cornea of the eye with a wisp of cotton. Immediate blinking should be noted. If the corneal reflex is absent, the affected eye must be protected from injury. Corneal abrasion and ulceration can develop from direct injury or from depriving the eye of proper lubrication with moisture. Blindness can be the unfortunate and permanent consequence of corneal ulceration. Applying an eye shield or taping the lids closed can prevent corneal abrasion. Periodic inspection and administration of artificial tears or saline solution (four times per day) can moisten the eye and prevent drying of the cornea.

The corneal reflex is controlled by CN V and VII. Other functional deficits in these CNs may be present. In CN V, loss of facial sensation to touch or weakness of the masseter and temporal muscles may be noted. The facial nerve (VII) controls the ability to wrinkle the brow, show the teeth, open the mouth, close the eyes, smile, and whistle. In addition, taste in the anterior two-thirds of the tongue is innervated by CN VII. Although these nerves need not be evaluated with every assessment, the nurse should periodically ascertain their functional levels.

Personality Changes

Changes in the baseline personality may be temporary or permanent. Permanent changes can occur from cerebral anoxia or surgery in the frontal area, whereas temporary personality changes can result from cerebral edema, surgery, drugs, or emotional stress.

The reason for any assessed personality change may be difficult to determine, because the cause may be singular or multiple. If personality changes continue after cerebral edema has subsided, a psychological evaluation may be indicated.

Personality changes, although common after cranial surgery, are most disturbing for the patient and the family. The nurse should be supportive, answer questions as honestly as possible, and provide encouragement.

THE NURSE'S ROLE IN REHABILITATION AND DISCHARGE PLANNING

Although a craniotomy is a conventional neurosurgical treatment for many underlying problems, the degree and time of recovery and the need for further treatment and rehabilitation will depend on the particular needs of the patient. For example, the discharge planning for a young patient who has had a craniotomy for a benign pituitary tumor will be quite different than the plan for an elderly person undergoing craniotomy for a malignant tumor. The neurological deficits in these two patients are probably quite different, as is the impact of surgery on the patients and their families. The need for individual planning thus becomes quite apparent. Ongoing neurological assessment and monitoring of neurological deficits provide a database for discharge planning and identification of rehabilitation needs. As cerebral edema subsides, a more accurate profile of neurological deficits emerges. Some deficits recover spontaneously with time, whereas other deficits need treatment and rehabilitation to achieve the optimal level of recovery. The human impact is assessed by talking to the patient and family and assessing their responses.

Independent Role

As part of the independent nursing role, the nurse assesses the patient's functional level and collects the following data, which will be used for planning nursing care and for discharge planning:

- Level of consciousness, orientation, and cognitive function
- Presence of neurological deficits
- Independence in performing ADLs and instrumental ADLs
- Verbal communication skills (ability to participate in a conversation, any word-finding difficulty)

- Emotional response to surgery and the underlying problem (*e.g.*, depression)
- Safety concerns (Is the patient at risk for injury or falls?)
- Support systems and living situation (Could the patient manage at home safely? If the patient needs assistance, will a family member be available to assist the patient?)

Integration of the principles of rehabilitation into the plan of nursing care is designed to help the patient achieve the highest level of independence possible. Depending on the level of consciousness, the nurse should involve the patient with the environment and ADLs as much as possible. Many patients have an intolerance for activity and are easily fatigued after surgery. Rest periods are planned to prevent exhaustion and to build tolerance for activity. Chart 18-5 summarizes the major nursing responsibilities in the postacute phase of recovery.

Supporting the patient and family throughout the hospitalization and preparing them for discharge are major nursing responsibilities. Patient and family teaching begun earlier in the course of hospitalization is now expanded. The family is encouraged to participate in basic care and ADL routines to develop skill and confidence in posthospital care.

Feelings of anxiety, ambivalence, hostility, and depression are common in the postoperative period and continue even after the transition to home. One interesting cause of depression relates to the degree of progress made postoperatively. During the hospital stay and initially after discharge, recovery and improvement are very rapid. If one were to chart this on a graph, it would be represented initially by a steeply ascending line; a plateau would then be reached, marking a period of minuscule improvement or no apparent improvement. If patients are unable to perform activities that they believe are realistic and feasible, they may become upset. Discouragement is further augmented by fatigue, which causes these patients to abandon certain activities. This sequence of events reinforces discouragement and depression and elicits complaints of constant fatigue or a low energy level. In these circumstances, the patient needs to be helped to set more realistic goals in view of the major insult experienced from surgery. A sympathetic approach and explanation of the postoperative course can be very supportive.

Collaborative Role

Early in the postoperative period, the nurse and physician collaborate in identifying neurological deficits that need further evaluation by other health professionals. These data, discussed previously, are the basis for collaboration. Although the needs of each patient vary, the most frequent referrals are

---

CHART 18-5
Rehabilitative Aspects of Nursing Management in the Postacute Period

Nursing Management	Rationale
• Encourage the patient to begin taking responsibility for activities of daily living (ADLs) based on individual ability.	• Promotes independence in ADLs
• Prepare meal trays (*e.g.*, pour milk, cut up food) so that patients with motor deficits can feed themselves.	• Promotes independence in ADLs
• Encourage progressive ambulation if loss of motor function is not prohibitive.	• Improves general well-being of all body systems and motor function; supports independence
• Help the patient to set realistic short- and long-range goals.	• Patient less apt to be discouraged and depressed if goals realistic
• Help female patients improve their body image by encouraging use of makeup and wigs.	• Improves body image and self-image; helps maintain sense of self-worth and dignity
• Talk to patients, play the radio, open the shades so that they can see activity around them, show them pictures or cards that might be in the room, and so forth.	• Provides reality orientation and can distract the patient from anxiety-provoking thoughts
• For the confused and disoriented patient, present reality through the use of as many senses as possible; correct misconceptions.	• Provides reality orientation
• Carry out range-of-motion exercises four times daily; position the patient carefully, and position to prevent dependent edema.	• Maintains motor function; prevents deformities; prevents dependent edema
• Involve the family in giving basic care, if appropriate.	• Provides the family with an opportunity to learn how to give care and to feel a part of the team
• Collaborate with other health team members (*e.g.*, physical, occupational, or speech therapists).	• Supports continuity of care

made to physical therapy, occupational therapy, speech therapy, social service, and sometimes psychiatry. The physician may also make a referral to another physician, such as the neuro-oncologist or neuroradiologist. Once the patient is evaluated and patient needs are identified in concrete terms, a discharge plan is formalized and implemented.

It is impossible to generalize about typical responses to a craniotomy. The experience is unique. For some patients, a craniotomy provides a cure for a treatable condition, such as a subdural hematoma. For others, intracranial surgery ameliorates symptoms of cerebral compression so that an extension of time can be offered the patient with a terminal prognosis. The implications of the craniotomy in terms of the patient's life can only be assessed individually. Depending on the reason for surgery and the prognosis, the patient or family may need to make major decisions about postacute care facilities and choice of treatment.

SELECTED NEUROSURGICAL PROCEDURES

A few surgical procedures are discussed in this section: transsphenoidal hypophysectomy, carotid endarterectomy, and placement of a ventricular shunt.

Transsphenoidal Hypophysectomy

DESCRIPTION

The transsphenoidal approach for access to the pituitary gland is possible because of the development of microsurgical techniques and equipment. Visual and surgical access is provided to areas that were formerly accessible only by the intracranial approach (Fig. 18-4).

Pituitary adenomas, craniopharyngiomas, and a complete hypophysectomy for control of bone pain in metastatic

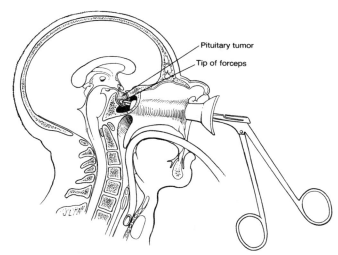
Pituitary tumor

Tip of forceps

FIGURE 18-4
Transsphenoidal approach in pituitary surgery. (From Smeltzer, S. C. & Bare, B. G. [1996]. *Brunner and Suddarth's textbook of medical-surgical nursing* [8th ed.] [p. 1738]. Philadelphia: Lippincott-Raven Publishers.)

cancer are the usual conditions for which a transsphenoidal surgical approach is used. The transsphenoidal surgical approach affords access to the pituitary gland by means of an incision in the upper pancuronium gum area or nasal submucosa, which bilaterally extends to the nasal septum. After the sphenoid sinus floor is resected, the sella turcica is visible. A portion of the sella floor is removed, and the dura is incised. With the aid of a surgical microscope, the pituitary is partially or completely removed, or the impinging tumor is excised. A graft of muscle taken from the anterior surface of the thigh or a fat pad (taken from the abdomen or thigh) is then applied to the surgical site as a patch to prevent CSF leakage. Nasal Vaseline packings are inserted to control bleeding and to replace the septal mucosa. A dry, sterile dressing is firmly applied to the donor site (abdomen or thigh). The specific tissue that is surgically excised depends on the reason for surgery. If surgery was scheduled for removal of a pituitary adenoma, the pituitary gland would be left intact, if possible, and the tumor excised. In a patient who undergoes craniopharyngioma, only the tumor would be excised. Removal of this tumor prevents or alleviates damage to the pituitary, hypothalamus, and optic chiasma.

PALLIATIVE SURGERY FOR PAIN SECONDARY TO CANCER

Palliative hypophysectomy in patients with cancer necessitates total removal of the pituitary. The surgeon attempts to excise the pituitary in one piece, because cells left at the surgical site continue to secrete hormones and decrease the anticipated relief of pain. It is unclear why a hypophysectomy can alleviate pain or further metastasis. It is thought that the removal of the anterior lobe, with the resultant cessation of prolactin and the growth-stimulating hormone, helps to control breast and prostatic cancer.

PREOPERATIVE PREPARATION

Preoperative preparation begins with patient teaching. The patient should have a realistic expectation of the procedure if it is planned for alleviation of pain from cancer. If the surgery is planned for removal of a pituitary tumor, the patient should know that some of the signs and symptoms associated with the tumor will gradually be alleviated.

Another aspect of the preoperative teaching plan is education of the patient and family about the need for drug replacement therapy. This should be discussed with the physician so that the specifics of the drugs that the patient will need to take on a regular basis can be presented to the patient. Beginning 2 days before surgery, cortisone acetate, 100 mg intramuscularly, is administered daily.

POSTOPERATIVE COMPLICATIONS

Few and infrequent postoperative complications are associated with transsphenoidal hypophysectomy. They include CSF leakage (rhinorrhea), DI, sinusitis, and delayed epistaxis. In addition, postoperative hematomas, meningitis, hydrocephalus, and deep venous thrombosis are seen in less than 1% of the patients. Therefore, the patient should be monitored for the development of these complications. Of these complications, only DI is discussed.

Postsurgical Diabetes Insipidus. **Central DI** is defined as the cessation of ADH secretion by the pituitary gland as a result of damage from disease or injury of the hypothalamus, the supraopticohypophysial tract, or the posterior pituitary. The most common cause of central DI is neurosurgery. Postsurgical DI can occur at any time up to 2 weeks postoperatively.

Monitoring the patient for development of DI is a major postoperative nursing responsibility. (See Chap. 10 for further discussion.) The symptoms of DI are copious amounts of pale urine (>200 mL/h for 2 consecutive hours) and a low urinary specific gravity (<1.005). Fractional urinary output, specific gravity, and serum osmolality must be monitored every 1 to 2 hours.

Others may experience a transient period of copious urinary output and low specific gravity. If the patient is able to drink enough fluid to quench thirst and maintain fluid and electrolyte balance, no medical treatment is indicated. This routine is followed to determine whether the DI is transient or permanent. Some patients may also experience a period of low urinary output 2 or 3 days postoperatively before permanent DI develops.

If a total hypophysectomy has been performed, permanent DI is expected, whereas with partial resection or removal of an adenoma from the pituitary, permanent DI is not anticipated. Instead, transient DI may develop, which may or may not require treatment. In the immediate postoperative period, aqueous vasopressin (Pitressin) may be administered because of its short duration of action (3–6 hours) until the DI can be evaluated to determine if it is transient or permanent. For long-term management, a special nasal spray or snuff called lypressin (Diapid) may be used. This drug is inhaled and absorbed from the nasal mucous membranes. Lypressin increases the reabsorption rate of water from the distal renal tubules.

The patient must be instructed in the safe use of lypressin, especially if self-administration of the drug is planned. The patient should know the following:

- Nasal mucosal irritation may occur; this will interfere with absorption of the drug.
- Overuse of the drug will cause water intoxication (mental confusion, drowsiness). For some patients, it may be more convenient and safer to use vasopressin in oil, 2.5 to 5.0 mg intramuscularly every 2 to 3 days, to control the DI.
- Daily weight must be recorded and monitored.
- Oral intake must be balanced with daily output.

The newest addition to the drugs used for treatment of severe permanent or transient complete central DI is DDAVP. It is administered intranasally, 0.1 to 0.4 mL, in nasal drops one or two times daily. The drug has a duration of 12 to 24 hours and has minimal side effects, which include nasal irritation or vasoconstriction of the nasal mucosa. DDAVP is currently the drug of choice.

Hormonal Replacement. In the case of total hypophysectomy, hormonal replacement is necessary. The usual drugs ordered include (1) adrenocorticotropic hormone (ACTH), 25 mg in-

tramuscularly in the morning and 12.5 mg intramuscularly at night, beginning immediately after surgery, and (2) thyroxin, 0.2 to 0.3 mg daily. Thyroid replacement therapy is delayed for 3 to 4 weeks following surgery. The patient is also fortified against adrenal insufficiency through the administration of cortisone acetate, 100 mg/d intramuscularly, beginning 2 days before surgery. The drug is continued postoperatively but at a lower dose than that indicated previously.

Patient Teaching for Drug Replacement. If replacement drug therapy is needed as a result of complete surgical excision of the pituitary gland, it is most important that the patient and family understand the purposes of drug therapy. The nurse should begin with a basic overview of the function of the pituitary gland to foster an understanding of the rationale for drug replacement therapy. The sophistication with which this information is presented will depend on the learner's level of understanding. To reinforce the verbal explanation, visual aids are helpful. Written material regarding home care is helpful because verbal instructions are easily forgotten or misunderstood. Written material also reinforces areas covered during patient teaching. The teaching plan should include the following:

- Specific information to record and submit to the physician, such as daily weight
- Signs and symptoms of undermedication or overmedication
- Side effects of drugs
- Lifestyle alterations necessitated as a result of drug therapy

Adrenocorticotropic Hormone. Certain cells of the anterior pituitary gland produce ACTH, which is stored until the hypothalamus secretes corticotropin-releasing hormone (CRH), a hormone that signals the pituitary gland to release ACTH. The target organ of ACTH is the cortex of the adrenal glands that affects the sensitive adrenal cortex by way of the blood stream. The following hormones are secreted by the adrenal cortex:

- The glucocorticoids, such as cortisol (hydrocortisone) and cortisone, are its major secretion. They are absolutely necessary for (1) carbohydrate metabolism, which promotes glucose production from amino acids; (2) protein metabolism into amino acids for use in tissue repair and cell anabolism; and (3) fat metabolism. At the same time, the glucocorticoids help the body cope with physical and emotional environmental stresses. Cortisone is a hormone that requires daily replacement for the patient to survive.
- The mineralocorticoids (particularly aldosterone) control salt and water metabolism by reabsorbing sodium ions in exchange for potassium in the kidney. This hormone does not require replacement on a daily basis.
- Certain male and female hormones play a minor role in comparison to the secretions of the ovaries and the testes. Replacement therapy is contraindicated if a hypophysectomy was done to control breast or prostatic cancer. In other patients, replacement therapy on a monthly basis may or may not be necessary, depending on the patient's age and other considerations. This determination will be made by the physician.

High levels of corticotropic hormone in the blood inhibit the secretion of CRH so that no more ACTH is secreted by the pituitary gland. The body normally produces the largest amount of ACTH in the early morning hours so that the glucocorticoids necessary for carbohydrate, protein, and fat metabolism are available during the day.

During times of physical and emotional stress, individuals require large amounts of cortisol. ACTH is continually produced to meet this need. Under severe stress, ten times the normal amount of cortisol may be required; approximately 25 mg is the daily requirement under normal circumstances.

Following hypophysectomy, the adrenal gland is deprived of stimulation because the ACTH that is normally produced by the pituitary gland is absent. The patient therefore requires ACTH replacement or administration of hydrocortisone, the natural glucocorticoid secreted by the adrenal cortex. This drug also has some of the mineralocorticoid properties provided by adrenal secretion.

The patient receiving cortisone therapy should know the following:

- The drug must be taken daily as ordered; failure to take the drug can be life threatening.
- The dosage of the cortisone must be increased for periods of emotional stress, illness, excessive exercise, major changes in daily routine, exposure to high altitudes, tooth extraction, fever, or infection.
- Gastric irritation, a side effect of steroid therapy, can be minimized by taking an antacid (30 mL of magnesium hydroxide) with each dose of the drug.
- The presence of tarry stools should be reported to the physician immediately.
- Blood pressure must be checked periodically for hypertension (an elevation in blood pressure is common with cortisone therapy); adjustments in the dosage of antihypertensive drugs may be necessary if the patient has been taking such a drug.
- Urine and blood should be checked periodically for glucose; ACTH is associated with diabetes mellitus.
- Behavioral changes are common with cortisone therapy and should be reported to the physician. Common behavioral manifestations may include euphoria, restlessness, sleeplessness, agitation, and depression.
- The following are signs and symptoms of undermedication (addisonian crisis):
  Weakness, dizziness, orthostatic hypotension
  Nausea and vomiting
  Sodium and water retention
  Decreased blood pressure
- Management of cortisone insufficiency requires the parenteral administration of hydrocortisone sodium succinate (Solu-Cortef). Failure to treat this condition will lead to circulatory collapse.
- The following are signs and symptoms of overmedication:
  Cushingoid signs (moon face, fat pads, buffalo hump, acne, hirsutism, and weight gain)
  Psychic disturbances
  Peptic ulcers
  Headache, vertigo, cataracts, and increased ICP and intraocular pressure
- A medical alert bracelet must be worn at all times.
- An emergency kit of hydrocortisone sodium succinate must be carried at all times.

NURSING MANAGEMENT AFTER TRANSSPHENOIDAL SURGERY

Specific points regarding the nursing management of the patient undergoing surgery by the transsphenoidal approach are outlined Charts 18-6, 18-7, and 18-8. The areas to be addressed include (1) early postoperative management, (2) prevention of complications, (3) supportive care, and (4) patient teaching.

Pain. After surgery, the patient is relatively free from pain at the oronasal suture line because the pain receptor fibers have been cut, resulting in loss of pain perception. Regeneration of the fibers will occur, but by that time, the suture line will have healed. If the oral route was used, sutures will be absorbed in about 7 to 10 days. The nasal mucosa requires at least 1 month to heal satisfactorily. Nasal packings are removed in 3 to 4 days. The sense of smell and taste will return in 2 or 3 weeks. Patients may have a headache as a result of sinus congestion or ear discomfort related to the nasal packings.

In a patient who has undergone hypophysectomy for the control of metastasis and bone pain, relief of pain may be evident within hours after surgery; in other patients, it may take days to a few weeks to reverse the patient's psychological response to the physical perception of pain. In this instance, a gradual improvement in the response to pain will be noted over several days. Survival rates for these patients may be extended to 2.5 years after surgery.

Psychosocial Aspects of Patient Management. A patient with an endocrine disorder precipitated by a pituitary adenoma will be concerned about alterations in body function and appearance. Patients with chromophobe adenomas complain of loss of libido, amenorrhea, and low basal metabolism rates. Males develop female characteristics. The threat to sexuality, body image, and self-esteem is apparent. Behavioral and personality changes caused by hormonal imbalance are common; as a result, disturbances in normal interpersonal relationships may develop, and patients may feel that they are losing control of their lives and their minds.

For the patient with metastatic cancer, the surgery is usually a "last chance" effort to control severe, unbearable pain that has made the activities of daily life impossible. The patient may have elected to undergo this surgery in the hope of being able to maintain some quality of life for the time remaining. Many patients will express a desire for their families to see them comfortable without the use of drugs and to fulfill certain life goals before death.

The nurse's role in such cases is supportive. Clarifying misinformation and providing necessary information are vital roles. Any activities that improve the patient's body image and self-esteem are worthwhile endeavors.

Carotid Artery Surgery

Cerebrovascular insufficiency can result from occlusion of the carotid artery secondary to atherosclerosis. If untreated, this can lead to transient ischemia attacks (TIAs) or stroke. In some instances, even though the internal carotid artery is occluded, the external carotid artery will remain patent as a result of collateral blood flow from the contralateral external carotid

(text continues on page 358)

CHART 18-6
Nursing Management After Transsphenoidal Surgery

Nursing Management	Rationale
Early Postoperative Management	
• Frequently monitor vital and neurological signs.	• Provides information for baseline comparisons to indicate trends, deterioration, or complications
• Maintain the head of bed at 30 degrees.	• Promotes venous drainage from the brain, controls intracranial pressure, and prevents hemorrhage at the operative site
• Check the dressing at the donor site on the thigh for evidence of bleeding.	• Detects bleeding for early intervention
• Frequently check nasal drains and packing; observe for hemorrhage or cerebrospinal fluid (CSF) drainage from the operative site; the mustache dressing should be observed and changed as necessary.	• Promotes early detection of hemorrhage or CSF and subsequent early intervention
Prevention of Complications	
• Monitor urinary output and specific gravity frequently.	• Monitor for evidence of diabetes insipidus
• Monitor electrolyte and osmolarity laboratory values for abnormally high or low readings (serum and urine osmolarity, serum sodium). Normal values are as follows: —Serum osmolarity: 280–295 mOsm/L —Urine osmolarity: 500–800 mOsm/L —Serum sodium: 135–145 mEq/L	• In diabetes insipidus, the serum sodium level is increased, serum osmolarity is increased, and urine osmolarity is decreased; also, serum electrolyte testing can indicate an electrolyte imbalance.
• Give frequent mouth care, but do not allow the patient to brush teeth if the oral approach was used.	• Prevents injury at the suture line, yet allows the mouth to be refreshed and cleansed
• Progress diet from liquid to soft as necessary.	• Prevents injury to the suture line
• After packings are removed, caution the patient against blowing the nose or sneezing for at least 1 mo.	• Prevents hemorrhage from fragile nasal tissue at operative site
Supportive Care	
• Provide for routine hygienic care, such as bathing, hair combing, and nail cutting.	• Maintains general well-being
• Offer fluids frequently, as ordered.	• Maintains hydration and moistens the oral mucous membrane, which becomes dry from mouth breathing (required when nasal packings are in place)
• Provide eye care (clean and lubricate).	• Prevents infection, inflammation, and drying of the cornea
• Apply compresses to the periocular region if periocular edema occurs.	• Controls and alleviates periocular edema
Patient Teaching	
• Prepare and implement a patient teaching plan to outline any adjustments in lifestyle, precautions necessary with the drug protocol, and general information about the patient's health problem.	• Provides for the safety and well-being of the patient and includes the patient as an involved, informed participant in health management
• Provide written material to summarize the major points of home management for the patient.	• Reinforces the major points of the teaching plan and reduces the possibility of confusion or questions about home protocol
• Include the family in the teaching plan.	• Includes the family in the plan of care so that they can become a knowledgeable support system for the patient

CHART 18-7
Nursing Care Plan for the Patient After Transsphenoidal Surgery

Nursing Diagnoses	Nursing Interventions	Expected Outcome(s)
Risk for Fluid Volume Deficit related to (R/T) large amounts of urine secondary to diabetes insipidus	• Assess the patient for signs and symptoms of diabetes insipidus. • Maintain an intake and output record. • Monitor fractional urinary output frequently. • Report a urinary output of 200 mL/h or more for 2 consecutive h. • Monitor urine-specific gravity as necessary (every 1–4 h). • Review serum and urine osmolarity studies and electrolyte levels. • Observe the patient for signs and symptoms of dehydration. • If the patient is able to consume fluids orally, encourage fluid intake.	• Fluid balance will be maintained.
Altered Oral Mucous Membrane R/T mouth breathing	• Offer mouth care frequently. • Assess the suture line at least every 4 h. • Do not allow the patient to brush teeth or place hard objects in the mouth if the oral approach was used for surgery. • Provide a soft diet.	• The oral cavity will be moist. • The suture line will remain intact.
Knowledge Deficit R/T surgery and drug therapy	• Develop a teaching plan that includes information about drugs, their possible side effects, and the need to take drugs daily on a permanent basis. • Assess the patient's understanding and knowledge as he or she is being taught. • Assess the patient's retention of the information provided. • Provide written material on drugs, their side effects, and other pertinent information. • For patients who will need permanent daily drug replacement, stress the importance of adhering to the plan.	• The patient will learn about his or her condition and the drug treatment program that will be necessary for management at home. • The patient will be able to verbalize the consequences of noncompliance to the drug program.
Body Image Disturbance R/T periocular edema and ecchymosis	• Apply cold or warm compresses under the patient's eyes. • Tell the patient that the periocular edema is expected and that it will disappear eventually. • Encourage female patients to use cosmetics and wear their own clothes.	• Edema will be alleviated. • A positive body image will be supported.
Pain (sinus/ears) R/T nasal packings and postoperative discomfort	• Monitor the patient for pain. • Provide comfort measures as necessary. • Administer pain medication as ordered.	• The patient will report feeling comfortable.

CHART 18-8
Potential Complications of Transsphenoidal Surgery and Appropriate Nursing Interventions

Complication	Nursing Interventions	Outcome(s)
• Hemorrhage • Leakage of cerebrospinal fluid • Infection (sinusitis and meningitis) • Deterioration of vision (secondary to slippage of nasal packings)	• Caution patients against blowing their nose. • Monitor vital signs. • Note the amount and color of drainage on the mustache dressing; note the number of times the dressing has to be changed. • Observe the patient for excess swallowing (which may indicate bloody drainage). • Monitor the status of the patient's vision; report any deterioration to the physician.	Abnormal findings will be reported to the physician.

---

artery. In this event, the external carotid artery becomes extremely important in maintaining an adequate blood supply to the brain. Thus, a patient with occlusion of a carotid artery may be asymptomatic because of continued collateral circulation.

PATHOPHYSIOLOGY OF ATHEROSCLEROSIS

For reasons unknown, common atherosclerotic sites are the large cerebral arteries, including the common carotid artery (especially at the bifurcation), the internal carotid artery, and the external carotid artery. Arterial walls are composed of three layers:

- Adventitia—the outermost layer, composed of connective tissue
- Media—the middle layer, composed of smooth muscular tissue
- Intima—the innermost layer, a smooth endothelial layer that comes in contact with blood

The pathophysiological process underlying atherosclerosis begins with lipids entering the vessel through the intimal layer. This occurs as a result of elevated blood pressure or unknown chemical substances. Blood-borne cells that stimulate smooth muscle growth in the medial layer act on the lipids. The process continues toward the adventitia. As the confines of the vessel are exhausted, a narrowing of the vessel lumen occurs. In addition, platelets accumulate in areas on the injured intimal layer, forming an atheroma (atherosclerotic plaque) or thrombus. These plaques can then break off, acting as an embolus. These processes further compromise the cerebral blood flow and can lead to stenosis, cerebral ischemia, and cerebral infarction.

DIAGNOSIS

Diagnosis of cerebral vascular insufficiency is made on the basis of a history of TIAs, CT scan, transcranial Doppler studies, cerebral arteriogram (sometimes), and noninvasive cerebral blood flow studies.

TREATMENT

The most common cerebral revascularization surgical procedure is the carotid endarterectomy (CEA). Other surgical procedures include the superior temporal artery-middle cerebral artery (STA-MCA) anastomosis and the subclavian artery-external carotid artery (SA-ECA) bypass graft.

CAROTID ENDARTERECTOMY

A **CEA** is a surgical procedure that is performed to remove the atheroma from the lining of the innermost layer of the carotid arteries. Depending on the severity of the occlusion and the degree of collateral circulation, a bypass graft may be necessary. The graft may come from the saphenous vein in the leg. An occlusion of 70% or more is an indication for grafting to be considered.

Preoperative Concerns. Many patients who have cerebrovascular atherosclerosis also have other concurrent conditions, such as coronary artery disease, kidney disease, or diabetes mellitus. Treatment and stabilization of other medical conditions are necessary before surgery. Hypertension must be controlled before surgery.

Postoperative Management. Patients are usually admitted to the NICU for a short stay following CEA because a number of cardiovascular and cerebrovascular complications can occur. Thus, close monitoring and careful medical management of these patients are necessary. The major postoperative complications are hemodynamic instability seen as hypotension and hypertension, intracerebral hemorrhage, stroke, myocardial infarction, and hypoperfusion syndromes.

Hypotension. The most common postoperative complication of CEA is hypotension. It is suggested that hypotension is related to stimulation of the carotid body baroreceptors that are exposed at surgery, thus causing hypotension and bradycardia. Maintaining an adequate CVP during the preoperative and intraoperative period may minimize these complications. In the postoperative period, it may be necessary to treat hypotension with vasopressors, such as Neo-Synephrine, and bradycardia with atropine. The physician needs to set parameters for blood pressure and pulse. A possible consequence of hypotension is cerebral hypoxia and ischemic stroke.

Hypertension. Hypertension is a poorly understood occurrence in approximately 20% to 50% of patients.[2] The underlying cause of the hypertension is thought to be surgical denervation of the carotid sinus. Postoperative hypertension has been associated with intracranial hemorrhage and hemorrhagic stroke. Hypertension is treated with titrated infusions of nitroglycerin or another antihypertensive. Again, parameters for blood pressure need to be set. Blood pressure and pulse usually return to normal within several hours to 36 hours after surgery.

Postoperative Nursing Management. Frequent assessments should be conducted and should include monitoring of vital signs and neurological signs, observation of the dressing, and monitoring of the amount of drainage. Some physicians insert a Jackson-Pratt drain at the operative site, whereas others order continuous suction of a drainage catheter placed at the operative site. The purpose of the drain is to prevent development of a hematoma, which could compress the airway. Although the heparinization used during surgery is reversed, the operative site is observed for bleeding. Some physicians order minidoses of heparin in the immediate postoperative period to prevent clot formation at the operative site.

The physician sets the parameters for maintenance of systolic and diastolic blood pressure. The usual range is 120 to 180 mm Hg for systolic and 80 to 100 mm Hg for diastolic pressure, based on a reasonable baseline before surgery. Vasopressors or antihypertensives may be ordered to maintain the desired blood pressure levels.

Frequent monitoring of neurological signs is necessary to determine any neurological changes associated with cerebral ischemia or stroke. In addition, the CNs, especially V, VII, IX, X, XI, and XII, are assessed for deficits (facial drooping, hoarseness, diminished or lost gag and swallowing reflexes, and weakness of the tongue).

In the immediate postoperative period, the head of the bed may be flat or elevated, depending on the preference of the physician. The patient is positioned off of the operative site. A central venous line, peripheral IV line, urinary catheter, cardiac monitor, drain with or without suction at the operative site, and oxygen therapy are usually used. The drain and suction are removed after 24 hours. Other tubes and equipment are removed when the patient is stable, at which time clear liquids are begun, and the diet is advanced as tolerated.

Most patients are discharged on or about the third postoperative day on a daily dose of aspirin (5 g), an antiplatelet drug, or sodium warfarin (Coumadin), an anticoagulant. The medication is usually continued for approximately 3 to 6 months after surgery. Periodic blood studies to monitor coagulation times are necessary. If aspirin is well tolerated, it is often continued indefinitely.

Other Cerebrovascular Procedures

The following are other surgical procedures used for cerebral revascularization. In both cases, the postoperative management is similar to that described for carotid endarterectomy.

SUPERIOR TEMPORAL ARTERY-MIDDLE CEREBRAL ARTERY ANASTOMOSIS

STA-MCA is a microneurosurgical bypass procedure that is used to provide collateral circulation to the areas of the brain supplied by the middle cerebral artery. It involves the anastomosis of the superior temporal artery, a branch of the external carotid artery, to the middle cerebral artery. The desired result of an STA-MCA anastomosis is improved collateral circulation to the brain, thereby correcting preoperative TIAs.

SUBCLAVIAN ARTERY-EXTERNAL CAROTID ARTERY BYPASS GRAFT

The SA-ECA bypass graft consists of a bypass graft from the subclavian artery to the external carotid artery. Once the arteries have been isolated, clamps are placed proximal and distal to the area where the anastomosis will be made. Once the subclavian graft is anastomosed, blood flow is gradually restored, first through the carotid artery and then through the subclavian artery.

Ventricular Shunts

A ventricular shunt is used to treat hydrocephalus. It consists of a primary catheter, a reservoir, a one-way valve, and a terminal catheter. It is implanted surgically to provide for drainage of excessive CSF from the brain to decrease or prevent increased ICP. The primary catheter is implanted into the lateral ventricle through a burr hole. An incision is made under the scalp, and the catheter is pulled through so that the reservoir rests on the mastoid bone. CSF flows from the catheter to the reservoir, which collects the CSF. The one-way valve at the reservoir prevents CSF reflux. A special instrument is used to pull the terminal catheter under the skin to the terminal point, which is the subarachnoid space or another body cavity (peritoneum, vena cava). The terminal catheter is then secured into position. In the adult, the peritoneal cavity is often used. The shunt is left in place permanently unless it becomes dislodged, plugged, or infected. In these situations, the shunt would be removed surgically and replaced.

The postoperative nursing management for patients with a ventricular shunt is similar to that provided for other intracranial procedures. See Chart 18-2 for possible restrictions concerning raising the head of the bed.

Depending on the type of shunt placed, the physician may write an order to pump the shunt a certain number of times at prescribed intervals (*e.g.*, 10 times every 6 hours). The purpose of pumping a shunt is to flush the system of exudate that could plug the small tubing. To pump the shunt, lightly palpate the mastoid process with the index and middle fingers until the reservoir is felt. It will feel bouncy to the touch. Next, with the index or middle finger, compress and gently release the reservoir the prescribed number of times. Documentation and any changes in neurological function are recorded in the patient's chart.

References

1. Turner, D. A. (1994). Neurosurgery. In D. C. Sabiston, Jr. & H. K. Lyerly (Eds.), *Sabiston essential of surgery* (2nd ed.) (p. 497). Philadelphia: W.B. Saunders.
2. Ropper, A. H., & Kennedy, S. K. (1993). Postoperative neurosurgical care. In A. H. Ropper (Ed.), *Neurological and neurosurgical intensive care* (3rd ed.) (pp. 185–201). New York: Raven Press.

Bibliography

Books

Ojemann R. G., Ogilvy, C. G., Crowell, R. M., & Heros, R. C. (1995). *Surgical management of cerebrovascular disease* (3rd ed.). Baltimore: Williams & Wilkins.

Cottrell, J. E., & Smith, D. S. (Eds.) (1994). *Anesthesia and neurosurgery* (3rd ed.). St. Louis: C.V. Mosby.

Rengachary, S. S., & Wilkins, R. H. (Eds.) (1994). *Principles of neurosurgery.* (3rd ed.) Baltimore: Wolfe.

Ropper A. H. (Ed.) (1993). *Neurological and neurosurgical intensive care.* New York: Raven Press.

Schmidek, H. H., & Sweet, W. H. (Eds.) (1988). *Operative neurosurgical techniques: Indications, Methods and Results.* Orlando: Grune & Stratton.

Turner, D. A. (1994). Neurosurgery. In D. C. Sabiston, Jr. & H. K. Lyerly (Eds.), *Sabiston essential of surgery* (2nd ed.). (pp. 478–496). Philadelphia: W.B. Saunders.

Periodicals

Cunha, B. A., & Tu, R. P. (1988). Fever in the neurosurgical patent. *Heart & Lung, 17*(6, Pt. 1), 608–611.

Donald, P. J. (1992). Combined middle fossa/intratemporal fossa surgery. *AORN, 55*(2), 480–489.

Fode, N. C. (1990). Carotid endarterectomy: Nursing care and controversies. *Journal of Neuroscience Nursing, 22*(1), 25–31.

Saper, C. B., & Breder, C. D. (1994). The neurologic basis of fever. *New England Journal of Medicine, 330*(30), 1880–1886.

CHAPTER 19

Management of Chronic Pain: A Neuroscience Perspective

Joanne V. Hickey
Rosemary P. Brown

Pain is the most universal of all afflictions. Chronic pain is a complex multidimensional phenomenon that is a significant problem faced by millions of Americans. For many, living with severe pain affects the quality of life of the person and his or her family. The economic impact from traditional and nontraditional treatment, over-the-counter drugs, and loss of productivity in the work environment is estimated at millions of dollars annually. The human misery and suffering caused by chronic pain are immeasurable. The causes of chronic pain are varied, just as the character of chronic pain in an individual is varied. Nurses and other health care professionals involved in neuroscience practice see people with chronic pain. Managing people with chronic pain is one of the greatest challenges in health care today. This chapter provides a brief overview of chronic pain management with an emphasis on the role of the nurse as a member of an interdisciplinary team providing medical and surgical management to people with chronic pain.

Pain is an "unpleasant sensory and emotional experience associated with actual or potential tissue damage or described in terms of such damage."[1] Pain is a universal sensation that has plagued mankind since the beginning of time. From medicine men to priests to physicians, relief of pain has been the goal for which generations have searched. Pain refers to the mechanisms by which noxious stimuli are detected. Pain, however, is more than just detection of noxious stimuli. Noxious stimuli may initiate the pain processes, but the experience of pain depends on many factors, such as experience with the stimuli, the stress or anxiety at the time, and the affective state.

In addition to the general definition of pain, there are separate definitions for acute and chronic pain. **Acute pain** is defined as "a complex constellation of unpleasant sensory, perceptual, and emotional experiences and certain associated autonomic, psychological, emotional and behavioral responses."[2] Acute pain has the biological function of protecting and alerting the person of potential or real tissue damage. **Chronic pain**, on the other hand, is described as pain that persists beyond the time when the acute disease course or reasonable time for healing has passed.[3] This time frame is generally considered to be 1 month to 6 weeks. Chronic pain includes pain that is continuous or that recurs at intervals for months or years. "Chronic pain has no biologic function and causes great social, financial, emotional and physical stress on the patient and family."[4,5] Developing universally accepted terms to describe pain has been difficult, but the International Association for the Study of Pain has attempted to define many of these terms (see Definition of Terms below).

Typically, patients with chronic pain have suffered for years and often present with chronic disability, fear, depression, and pain behavior. **Pain behavior** is a "collection of misdirected activities that are superficially linked to pain but are, often unconsciously, directed at ends other than pain relief."[6] One example of this behavior is exaggerated complaints of pain to obtain more narcotic medication.

The type of pain treated through neurosurgical procedures is neurogenic pain. **Neurogenic pain** occurs as a result of damage to nerves; it can be peripheral or central in origin. Generally, neurosurgical pain procedures are performed for chronic pain only after all other avenues of pain relief or control have been exhausted.

Neurogenic chronic pain can be caused by a number of conditions and diseases (Chart 19-1). Headache is discussed in Chapter 30, peripheral nerve injuries in Chapter 24, and cranial nerve diseases in Chapter 35.

CHART 19-1
Common Causes of Chronic Neurogenic Pain

- Spinal cord tumors
- Traumatic spinal injuries
- Intervertebral disc disease
- Spinal stenosis with root compression
- Compression of plexuses
- Thalamic pain syndrome
- Metastatic bone pain (*e.g.*, vertebra)
- Cauda equina disease
- Referred pain
- Peripheral nerve diseases
- Entrapment syndromes
- Mononeuropathy
- Polyneuropathy
- Reflex sympathetic dystrophy
- Causalgia
- Crushing nerve injuries
- Phantom pain

Definition of Terms

The following are definitions of frequently used terms related to pain:

- **Anesthesia dolorosa:** pain in an area or region that is anesthetic
- **Causalgia:** a syndrome of sustained burning pain and hyperpathia after a traumatic nerve lesion, often combined with vasomotor and psychomotor dysfunction and later trophic changes
- **Central pain:** pain associated with a lesion of the central nervous system
- **Deafferentation pain:** pain due to loss of sensory input into the central nervous system, as occurs with avulsion of the brachial plexus or other types of lesions of peripheral nerves or due to pathology of the central nervous system
- **Dysasthesia:** an unpleasant abnormal sensation, whether spontaneous or evoked
- **Hyperpathia:** excruciating sensitivity to touch
- **Hyperesthesia:** an increased sensitivity to stimulation, excluding special senses
- **Hypoesthesia:** a diminished sensitivity to stimulation, excluding special senses
- **Neuralgia:** pain in distribution of nerve or nerves
- **Neuritis:** inflammation of a nerve or nerves
- **Nociceptor:** a receptor that is preferentially sensitive to a noxious stimulus or to a stimulus that would become noxious if prolonged
- **Pain threshold:** the least experience of pain that a subject can recognize
- **Paresthesia:** an abnormal sensation, whether spontaneous or evoked

- **Reflex sympathetic dystrophy:** a variety of syndromes that involve sympathetic hyperactivity associated with persistent pain
- **Trigger point:** a hypersensitive area or site in muscle or connective tissue, usually associated with myofascial pain syndromes

PAIN THEORIES

Humans have struggled to understand and explain pain since the beginning of time. Some of the earliest pain theories, such as those from ancient Egypt and India, believed that the heart was the center of all sensation and that pain was associated with demons and gods. This belief lasted almost 2,000 years. It was not until the 17th century that Descartes described some of the beginning concepts of pain pathways from the periphery to the brain (Fig. 19-1). According to Descartes, when the foot comes near a fire, this sensation enters the body and travels up threads to the brain (Fig. 19-1).

The 19th century heralded the study of pain physiology as an experimental science. This research led to the discovery that the dorsal root of the spinal cord was involved with sensory function and the ventral root with motor function. In 1840, Muller wrote that the brain could only receive information about the external environment by way of the sensory nerves. This information plus discoveries in pain management with morphine, codeine, regional anesthesia, and radiation therapy paved the way for several physiological pain theories. The *specificity theory* noted that there were different afferent

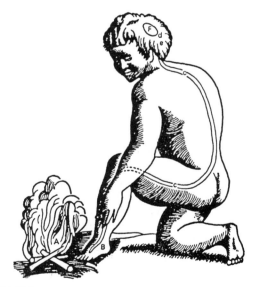

FIGURE 19-1
Descartes' (1664) concept of the pain pathway. He writes: "If for example fire (*A*) comes near the foot (*B*), the minute particles of this fire, which as you know move with great velocity, have the power to set in motion this spot of the skin of the foot which they touch, and by this means pulling upon the delicate thread (c.c.) which is attached to the spot of the skin, they open up at the same instant the pore (d.e.) against which the delicate thread ends, just as by pulling at one end of a rope makes to strike at the same instant a bell which hangs at the other end." (From Melzack, R. & Wall, P. D. [1965] *Pain mechanisms: A new theory.* Science)

sensory neurons for pain and touch. The *intensive theory* supported the idea that any sensory stimulus could become painful if it becomes intense enough.

Debate about these theories and development of several new theories continued into the 20th century. One theory that has become the most widely accepted theory is *the gate control theory* developed by Melzack and Wall in 1965. According to this theory, the central nervous system is surrounded by a barrier that can only be entered by a gate (Fig. 19-2). Pain enters through the gate, and the more pain that is present, the wider the gate opens. The gate can be closed, however, by pulling it shut from the outside (peripheral) or by pushing it shut from the inside (centrally by the brain and spinal cord). This theory takes into account the effect of the person's motivational, cognitive, and affective state during the pain experience. According to the gate control theory, the gate can be opened wider by increasing noxious stimulation, anxiety, and depression. The gate can be pushed closed by higher centers of the brain through distraction, relaxation, high levels of endorphins, and enkephalins. The gate can be pulled shut from the periphery through activities such as rubbing and transcutaneous nerve stimulation or vibration.

MECHANISMS OF PAIN

The body has specialized nerve endings involved in the transmission of light, sound, touch, and tissue damage. The nerve endings that recognize tissue damage are called **nociceptors**. Pain can result from stimulation of nociceptors in the skin, viscera, and musculoskeletal structures.

Visceral pain and musculoskeletal pain are not as clearly understood as the physiology behind cutaneous nociception. The cutaneous receptors are affected by thermal, chemical, or mechanical stimulation, which is transmitted through their axons to the spinal cord. These cutaneous receptors have different types of axons: A-beta, A-delta, and C fibers (Fig. 19-3). A-beta axons are large, heavily myelinated, and respond to light touch. A-delta are smaller, thinly myelinated fibers that conduct ''pinprick'' or ''sharp'' pain rapidly. C fibers are thin and unmyelinated and transmit burning, aching type pain slowly. For example, a person who burns his or her finger feels immediate pain from stimulation of the A-delta fibers (first pain), followed by a longer lasting burning sensation from the stimulation of C fibers (second pain).

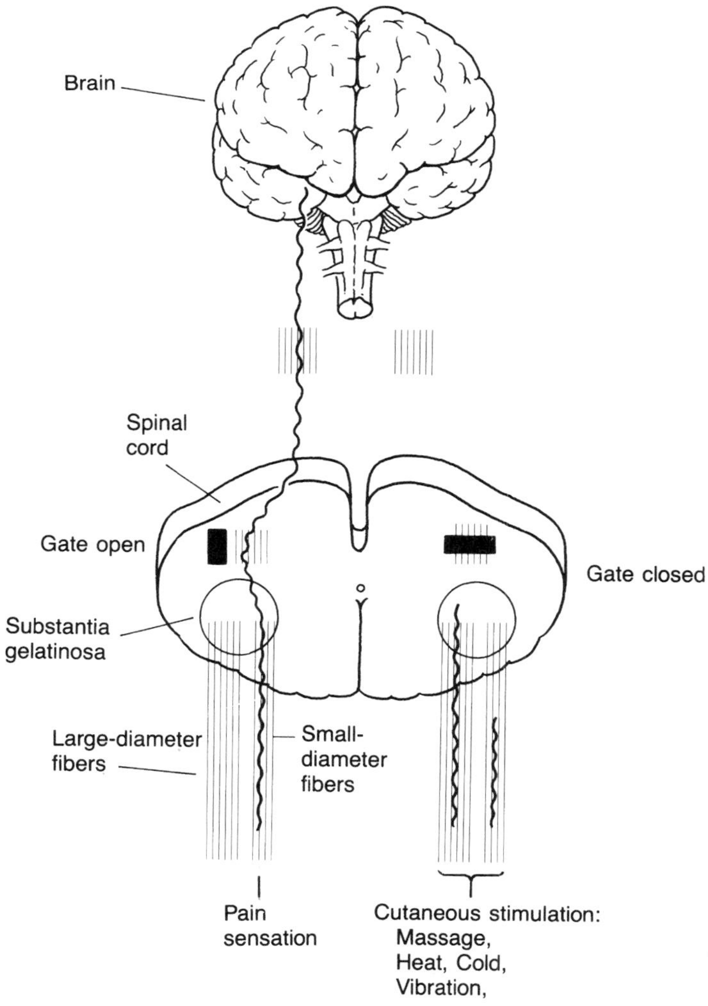

FIGURE 19-2
Gate control theory. This shows how thin (tissue damage responding) fibers force open the ''gate'' into the central nervous system, bringing pain to consciousness. The gate can be pulled shut from the outside, reducing pain, by the activation of large A-beta fibers, rubbing/massage, transcutaneous electrical nerve stimulation, or vibration. The gate can also be pushed shut from inside the central nervous system by various inhibitory systems descending from the brain; some of these inhibitory systems are activated by acupuncture, others by drugs. (From Hudak, C. M. & Gallo, B. M. [1994]. *Critical care nursing: A holistic approach.* [6th ed.] [p. 647]. Philadelphia: J. B. Lippincott.)

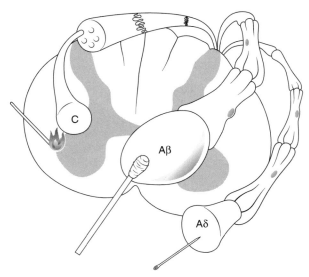

FIGURE 19-3
Primary afferent fibers from skin to spinal cord. The largest (Aβ) and most rapidly conducting myelinated fibers are activated by light touch (illustrated by a cotton bud); these are the fibers that are activated by transcutaneous electrical nerve stimulation and vibration. Smaller, more slowly conducting (Aδ) myelinated fibers are activated by pinprick and are involved in acupuncture stimulation. The smallest and slowest fibers (C) are unmyelinated and are excited by tissue damage, here illustrated by a lighted match; they are often called *nociceptors*. (From Carroll, D., & Bowsher, D. [1993]. *Pain management and nursing care* [p. 9]. Boston: Butterworth & Heineman.)

Tissue damage also causes cell disruption, which leads to release of chemical substances known as arachidonic acid metabolites. Prostaglandins and leukotrienes are two of these metabolites. These chemicals result in sensitization of the area and cause previously innocuous stimuli to be perceived as painful. Damaged tissue also releases serotonin, bradykinin, and substance P, which activate nociceptors and further contribute to the pain and inflammation.

Pain impulses enter the spinal cord through the dorsal root synapse in lamina I, II, or V and then cross through the gray matter to the spinothalamic tract. Next, the spinothalamic tract transmits pain to the thalamus. Pain impulses finally proceed to the sensory cortex, frontal lobes, and reticular formation.

MANAGEMENT OF CHRONIC PAIN

The following section examines approaches to chronic pain management and then reviews options in the medical and surgical management of pain.

An Approach to Chronic Pain Management

MULTIDISCIPLINARY APPROACH

A collaborative, interdisciplinary approach to pain control is emphasized in the clinical practice guidelines for pain management.[7] Active participation of the patient and family is re-

quired. The goal is to develop an individualized pain control plan that is agreed on by the patient, family, and health providers. Nonpharmacological and pharmacological therapies to prevent or control pain must be included. Once a plan is developed, the patient's pain must be assessed frequently so that modifications in the plan of care can be made as necessary. Many patients are initially seen and followed in a pain clinic that offers a comprehensive, interdisciplinary approach to patient management. Other patients are referred to a pain clinic for an evaluation and recommendations that provide the primary care provider with suggestions for management.

ASSESSMENT, EVALUATION, AND DEVELOPING A PLAN OF CARE

Because pain is a subjective phenomenon, it can be challenging to evaluate patients with chronic pain. Instruments such as the McGill Pain Questionnaire (MPQ) may be useful for assessing pain. The MPQ includes 20 categories of descriptive terms addressing the sensory, affective, and evaluative characteristics of pain.[8] In addition to a general and complete neurological assessment, a pain history must be collected. The following components are included in a pain history:

- **Onset**: Collect a historical sequence of the onset of pain: Were there any precipitating injuries? If so, describe the circumstances and mechanism of injury. Was pain onset gradual or acute?
- **Location**: Draw with your finger where the pain is located. (This can be done as a paper and pencil report on which the patient colors the body areas involved on an anterior and posterior anatomical figure.)
- **Characteristics**: What is the pattern of the pain with time? Is it constant or periodic? What makes it come and go? Does it spread? If so, where? Has it changed with time?
- **Quality**: What does the pain feel like (*e.g.*, stabbing, sharp, dull, "pins and needles," throbbing)?
- **Aggravating circumstances**: What makes the pain worse? What makes it better?
- **Quantity**: How intense is the pain? (Many instruments are available for quantifying the intensity and distress of pain; Fig. 19-4).
- **Impact**: How does the pain affect your ability to function (activities of daily living [ADLs], job requirements, role and responsibilities in the home, family, and community)? Are related physiological events associated with the pain (*e.g.*, nausea, vomiting, dizziness, sensory loss)? How do you feel emotionally in response to the pain (*e.g.*, irritable, teary)?
- **Treatment**: How do you treat the pain? Does it work? How much relief do you achieve? What else have you tried in the past? Did it work? If not, why not? If yes, why did you stop using it?

Once a complete medical history, pain history, and physical examination are completed, other discipline specific data may be added. For example, an evaluation by the pharmacist or physical therapist may be helpful in understanding the pain experience for the individual. Once data collection is complete, the interdisciplinary team can develop a pain control plan with the patient and family.

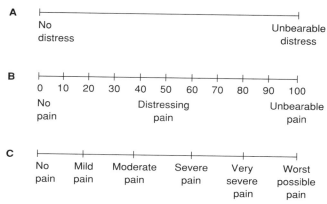

FIGURE 19-4

Pain rating scales. Rating scales for measuring pain: (*A*) Visual analog scale; (*B*) numeric pain distress scale; and (*C*) simple descriptive pain intensity scale. (From Acute Pain Management Guideline Panel [1992]. *Acute pain management: Operative or medical procedures and trauma. Clinical practice guideline.* AHCPR Pub. No. 92-0032. Rockville, MD: Agency for Health Care Policy and Research, Public Health Service, U.S. Department of Health and Human Services.)

The nurse as a member of the interdisciplinary collaborative team conducts, collects, and analyzes data to identify nursing diagnoses and develop a nursing treatment plan. The major nursing diagnoses include the following:

- Acute Pain
- Chronic Pain
- Sensory/Perceptual Alterations

Treatment decisions must be considered in the context of the individual's life and the effect of pain on the quality of life. Many possible combinations of medical and surgical therapies may be helpful for the patient. They are discussed below.

MEDICAL MANAGEMENT OF CHRONIC PAIN

Medical management of chronic pain can include nonpharmacological management and pharmacological modalities. In the nonpharmacological approach, there are a number of traditional and nontraditional methods of managing chronic pain. These are briefly discussed in this section. Often, use of multiple nonpharmacological modalities and pharmacological agents is necessary to optimize patient comfort.

Nonpharmacological Management: Physical and Psychosocial Modalities

The Agency for Health Care Policy and Research has published clinical guidelines for the management of acute pain (1992) and management of cancer pain (1994). The 1994 publication has information related to chronic pain that is helpful.[9,10] Physical modalities include physical therapy, local electrical stimulation, and acupuncture. The major psychosocial modalities include relaxation therapy and imagery, distraction

and reframing, biofeedback, patient education, psychotherapy, counseling, and emotional support.

PHYSICAL MODALITIES

Physical Therapy. Physical therapy uses a number of therapies, such as cutaneous stimulation and exercises designed to decrease discomfort, promote successful engagement in ADLs, and maintain or restore function. Thermotherapy, cryotherapy, massage, and therapeutic exercise are modalities that may be incorporated into the pain management protocol.

Application of dry or moist heat, called **thermotherapy,** can provide analgesic, antispasmodic, and sedative effects.[11] Increasing the temperature of tissue causes increased blood flow, relaxation of motor tone, and increased local cellular metabolism; therefore, this aids in restoring blood flow to tissues and removing waste products. Stretching and active and passive exercise usually follow heat application; this can lengthen and strengthen muscles and tendons, thereby decreasing pain. Heat application should be used cautiously in patients with loss of sensation, circulatory compromise, acute inflammation or injury, and malignancy because heat may accelerate cell growth and metastasis.[12]

Cryotherapy, the application of cold, has analgesic, anti-inflammatory effects, decreased neuromuscular transmission, and antipyretic effects. Initially, cold causes vasoconstriction and decreased nerve conduction, which means fewer noxious stimuli transmissions. This means that the "gate" will not be opened, and pain will not be transmitted to the brain. After the initial response to cold comes the burning sensation that competes with the other pain transmissions to enter the gate. The vasoconstriction caused by the cold also reduces blood flow, which leads to decreased edema, bleeding, and leukocytosis. Cryotherapy should be used cautiously with patients who have circulatory compromise, Raynaud's syndrome, loss of sensation, and cryoglobulinemia.

The primary physiological effect of **massage** is by stimulation of peripheral receptors through repetitive and irritative movements of the therapist's hands or massage device. This type of stimulation produces impulses that transmit to the higher brain centers, producing sensations of pleasure or well-being.

Therapeutic exercise is a critical component of all treatment for acute and chronic pain. During the acute phase, exercise is usually limited to range of motion (ROM). However, during the subacute and chronic phase of illness, exercise programs are designed to restore function; increase ROM; decrease muscle spasticity, tension, and contracture; and increase strength and endurance.

Local Electrical Stimulation. The major local electrical stimulation therapy used is called transcutaneous electrical nerve stimulation (TENS). **TENS** is a method of applying controlled, low-voltage electrical stimulation to large, myelinated peripheral nerve fibers through cutaneous electrodes for the purpose of modulating stimulus transmission and relieving pain.[13]

Acupuncture. Acupuncture is an ancient method for the treatment of disease, including pain, that dates back more than 5,000 years in Chinese history. **Acupuncture** is a neurostimulatory technique that involves the insertion of small, solid needles into the skin at varying depths and at specified areas. This drugless, nontoxic, and economical technique has gained acceptance by some as a nontraditional method of managing a variety of pain, including chronic pain of various types. Why it works is unclear.

PSYCHOSOCIAL MODALITIES

Relaxation Therapy. **Relaxation therapy** is a strategy that can be used to decrease stress and pain and regain self-control. It is believed to decrease pain by causing production of endorphins. Physiologically, relaxation lowers blood pressure, respiratory rate, heart rate, and muscle tension and contraction. There are two categories of mental and physical relaxation. The first category involves muscle relaxation, which then facilitates the response of mental relaxation. Examples of this approach are deep breathing, yoga, and progressive muscle relaxation. Twenty minutes, free of distraction, are necessary for relaxation to occur. A sample of relaxation therapy is as follows:

We begin by closing our eyes and concentrating on feeling what our body is like when it is at rest. Secondly, we impose tension upon it and feel the difference. Then we relax the body and feel a third quality, that of deep relaxation. Finally, it is possible to discover another state, what we call a ''letting go,'' when the body feels different again.[14]

Relaxation tapes can be purchased in book stores and health centers for use at home or in health care facilities.

Meditation and Imagery. The second category of relaxation focuses mental relaxation to achieve physical relaxation. **Meditation** requires the ability to concentrate and takes practice. **Imagery** is a cognitive-behavioral strategy of focusing on a personalized pleasant mental image to aid in relaxation. Relaxation techniques are most helpful when combined with personalized imagery.[15]

Distraction and Reframing. **Distraction** is a cognitive strategy of focusing attention on stimuli other than pain or the accompanying negative emotions.[16] Distraction may be internal (*e.g.,* praying) or external (*e.g.,* listening to music, watching television). **Reframing** is a cognitive strategy that teaches the person to monitor and evaluate negative thoughts and images and replace them with more positive ones. For example, if the person is preoccupied with thoughts of being unable to conduct his or her normal business because of pain, substituting self-messages that remind the person that often activities are not negated by pain increases personal control.

Biofeedback. **Biofeedback** is a process in which a person learns to influence two types of physiological responses: those that are not ordinarily under voluntary control and those that are ordinarily regulated, but as a result of disease or trauma, regulation has been interrupted.[17]

Patient Education. Patient education is a cognitive strategy of providing the patient and family with comprehensive and accurate information about pain, pain assessment, and the use of drugs and other methods of pain control with an emphasis on effective management. The goal of patient education is to involve the patient actively in his or her pain management and reaffirm the control of the person to successfully manage self and pain.[18] In addition, providing patients with the names and addresses of community resources can enhance sources of information and support for the patient and family.

Psychotherapy, Counseling, and Emotional Support. Depression, anxiety, and maladaptive coping or behavior are often related to chronic pain. A short or long course of physiotherapy, counseling, structured support, and peer support groups may be helpful to support the person and develop effective coping strategies.

Pharmacological Management: Nonnarcotics, Opioid-Narcotics, and Adjuvant Analgesics

The pain experience is highly individualized; therefore, drug therapy to decrease the pain experience must also be individualized. Analgesics are the pharmacological mainstay of pain management for acute and chronic pain. Analgesics can be broadly divided into nonnarcotics and opioid-narcotics. Generally opioid-narcotic analgesics relieve acute pain or cancer pain, while non-narcotics are recommended for chronic pain. Also, adjuvant analgesic drugs have analgesic properties or can enhance the effect of the analgesics. The drug classifications included in the adjuvant analgesic drug category are antidepressants, anticonvulsants, and anxiolytics.

NON-NARCOTIC ANALGESICS

Aspirin and aspirin-like drugs, such as acetaminophen and nonsteroidal anti-inflammatory drugs, are the major non-narcotic analgesics. In addition to their analgesic properties, these drugs have antipyretic and anti-inflammatory effects. The one current exception is acetaminophen, which has no anti-inflammatory properties. These drugs relieve pain by inhibiting the release of prostaglandins and thromboxane 2, which are associated with pain. Non-narcotic analgesics are most effective for mild to moderate levels of pain.

OPIOID-NARCOTIC ANALGESICS

Opioid by definition is any drug, either natural or synthetic, that has similar actions to morphine. Narcotic can mean an analgesic that has central nervous system depressant effects and can cause physical dependence. Narcotic has also been associated with a group of illegal drugs, such as marijuana and cocaine. For this reason, opioid is a better term to describe this group of drugs. Opioids act on receptors within and outside the central nervous system. Their effects are analgesia, respiratory depression, sedation, and euphoria. These drugs are effective against moderate to severe pain, but there are many side effects, some of which are life threatening. Side effects include respiratory depression, orthostatic hypotension, cough suppression, nausea, vomiting, constipation, and urinary retention. Physical tolerance, dependency, and abuse occur with prolonged use of opioids.

It is generally believed that opioids are best suited for acute pain, but under certain conditions, opioids can be beneficial for chronic pain. Some guidelines have been proposed for selection of patients for long-term use of opioid-narcotics:[19]

- Persistent pain is the major impediment to function (pain is disabling).
- Psychological problems are not present or considered pertinent.
- All other analgesic (non-narcotic) medications have failed.
- There is no history of substance abuse.
- A primary physician will assume responsibility for monitoring the patient and the response to the drug.

A frequent drug of choice is methadone (Dolophine) for the following reasons: It has properties similar to those of morphine, a long duration of action, and good oral absorption. Methadone is, therefore, a good opioid choice for long-term chronic pain management.

ADJUVANT ANALGESICS

The adjuvant analgesic drugs that enhance the effect of analgesics are antidepressants, anticonvulsants, and anxiolytics.

Antidepressants. Depression and chronic pain go hand in hand with one reinforcing the other. Lack of sufficient norepinephrine and serotonin may be the cause of depression, and these substances play a role in pain transmission. Therefore, depression enhances the pain experience. Amitriptyline (Elavil), doxepin (Sinequan), imipramine (Tofranil), and nortriptyline (Pamelor) are a few of the widely used antidepressants.

Anticonvulsants. Anticonvulsants stabilize the neuronal membrane, reducing neuronal excitability. These drugs are used most frequently for pain that has a sharp, electrical, shooting quality, such as that of tic douloureux. Carbamazepine (Tegretol) and phenytoin (Dilantin) are two common anticonvulsants used in conjunction with analgesics.

Anxiolytics. Anxiety can increase the perception of pain and can prevent the individual from tolerating pain. The benzodiazepines, such as alprazolam (Xanax), clorazepate (Tranxene), and diazepam (Valium), are common anxiolytic drugs. Baclofen (Lioresal) is a muscle relaxant used to relieve some types of pain associated with spasm and muscle tension.

Surgical Management of Chronic Pain

Surgical procedures for neurogenic pain are directed toward interrupting input of nociceptors. This interruption can occur at different neuron levels. Pain sensations are transmitted by delta type A and type C fibers from peripheral receptors to the spinal cord. This peripheral tract contains the **first-order neurons**. The pain transmission continues through the dorsal root of the spinal nerve into the dorsal root entry zone gray matter of the spinal cord. The pain transmission pathways in the spinal cord are composed of the **second-order neurons**. The **third-order neurons** transmit the pain sensation from the thalamus to the cortex.

FIRST-ORDER NEURONS

Neurosurgical procedures directed at first-order neurons include neurectomy and rhizotomy. A **neurectomy** is the resection of one or more peripheral branches of cranial or spinal nerves. Neurectomy is a safe, quick procedure requiring only local or regional anesthesia. However, there are several problems with neurectomies. First, peripheral nerves contain motor and sensory input, so motor loss accompanies the loss of pain sensation. Pain relief is often only temporary following neurectomies, and the return of pain can include a new pain syndrome, such as anesthesia dolorosa. Also, the specific peripheral nerves are often difficult to isolate.

For these reasons, neurectomies are infrequent today. One exception is the peripheral neurectomy for treatment of trigeminal neuralgia (tic douloureux) when gangliolysis has failed or when microvascular decompression is not possible. See Table 19-1 for postneurectomy assessment and monitoring.

A **rhizotomy** is the selective destruction of the spinal nerve dorsal root to relieve pain. Indications for a rhizotomy are a limited area of pain and a normal life expectancy. Gen-

---

TABLE 19-1
Postoperative Observations and Assessment After Specific Neurosurgical Procedures

PROCEDURE	OBSERVATIONS/ASSESSMENT
Neurectomy	Hematoma, ecchymosis, signs and symptoms of infections, wound drainage, motor and sensory function to the involved area
Rhizotomy	Cerebrospinal fluid (CSF) leakage, wound drainage, signs and symptoms of infection or meningitis, motor and sensory function, respiratory depression (especially in bilateral cervical rhizotomy), and bowel, bladder, and sexual dysfunction (especially in sacral rhizotomy)
Cordotomy	CSF leakage, wound drainage, signs and symptoms of infection or meningitis, hypotension, respiratory depression, urinary dysfunction, ipsilateral motor loss, and Horner's syndrome (complications most frequent with bilateral, open cordotomies)
Dorsal root entry zone	CSF leakage, wound drainage, signs and symptoms of infection or meningitis, and motor and sensory dysfunction

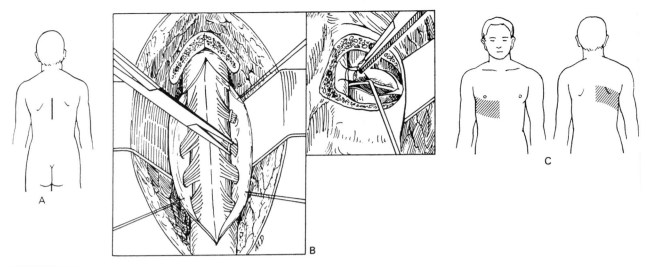

FIGURE 19-5
Dorsal rhizotomy. (*A*) Location of midline dorsal incision for T4–T7 dorsal rhizotomy. (*B*) Intradural dorsal rhizotomy with application of metal clip on the rootlets of a root already transected above and being applied to the rootlets of a root below just prior to resectioning them. Inset on the right depicts extradural dorsal rhizotomy showing division of the dorsal root central to the ganglion prior to extirpation of the ganglion by a lesion which will be made just distal to the ganglion. (*C*) Expected area of sensory loss following right T4 to T7 dorsal rhizotomy. (From Bonica, J. J. [1990]. *The management of pain.* [2nd ed.] [p. 2049]. Philadelphia: Lea & Febiger.)

erally, selective nerve blocks are performed to determine if a rhizotomy *will* be effective. If a patient obtains relief from a selective nerve block, then a rhizotomy should be effective to relieve pain. Because only the dorsal root is affected, the ventral motor fibers are spared. The open rhizotomy procedure requires laminectomies and is performed on the same side as the pain. The dura is opened, and the nerve rootlets are identified. The rootlets are then transected (Fig. 19-5). As a result of a rhizotomy, there is complete sensory loss; therefore, no pain, temperature, or pressure sensations remain intact.

Although these procedures interrupt only sensory input, movements of joints and muscles, a motor function, frequently depend on sensory information. Loss of sensory input can directly result in loss of motor function. For this reason, rhizotomies are generally indicated for thoracic and high cervical pain relief and not recommended for extremities or low lumbar areas. Rhizotomies have been successful in relieving sacral pain due to malignancy or postradiation pain. See Table 19-1 for postoperative rhizotomy assessment and monitoring.

SECOND-ORDER NEURONS

Neurosurgical procedures on the second-order neurons involve interruption of the lateral spinothalamic tract within the spinal cord. Cordotomy and dorsal root entry zone lesion surgeries are examples of second-order neuron procedures.

A **cordotomy** is the operative procedure by which the spinothalamic tract is interrupted for the relief of pain. Cordotomies are considered for patients with intractable malignant and nonmalignant pain below the level of the mandible. Cor-

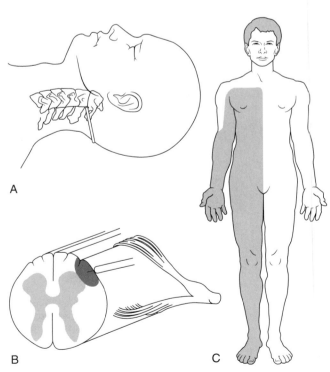

FIGURE 19-6
(*A*) Site of percutaneous C1–C2 cordotomy. (*B*) Lesion produced by percutaneous C1–C2 cordotomy. (*C*) Extent of analgesia produced by left C1–C2 percutaneous cordotomy.

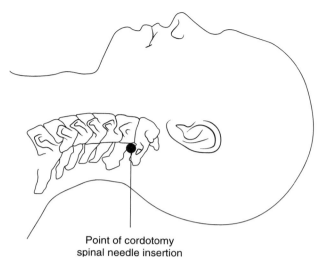

FIGURE 19-7
Site of insertion of needle for percutaneous C1–C2 cordotomy.

dotomies can be performed as a percutaneous or open procedure. The percutaneous cordotomy can be successfully performed on cancer patients who cannot undergo major surgery (Fig. 19-6). This procedure involves introducing a spinal needle at the level of C1–C2 with guidance from a myelogram. The anterior border of the spinal cord is visualized and an electrode inserted through the spinal needle; lesions are produced (Fig. 19-7). Access for an open cordotomy can be through an anterior or a posterior approach (Fig. 19-8). General anesthesia and a laminectomy are necessary. The complication rate is higher for the open cordotomy. The most common complications are hypotension, respiratory depression, urinary tract dysfunction, and ipsilateral motor loss. The result

of the percutaneous and open cordotomy is anesthesia below the level of the lesions.

A **dorsal root entry zone (DREZ)** is an operative procedure that involves making a series of lesions in the DREZ of the spinal cord (Fig. 19-9). These lesions are usually made in the substantia gelatinosa and surrounding fibers. This procedure is indicated for central pain disorders, such as brachial plexus avulsion, postherpetic neuralgia, phantom limb pain, postparaplegia pain, and severe facial pain. This surgery requires laminectomies and general anesthesia. The postoperative period requires 2 to 4 days of bed rest followed by intensive physical therapy and discharge on day 5 or 6. The main complications are wound infection, cerebrospinal fluid leak, and ataxia. Patients who have pain in an extremity with intact motor function may suffer a transient incoordination postoperatively because the spinal cerebellar tract is crossed by the electrode. This usually resolves in weeks to months, but with repeat DREZ procedures, this may become a permanent problem. See Table 19-1 for assessment and monitoring after a DREZ procedure.

THIRD-ORDER NEURONS

Neurosurgical procedures to relieve pain at the level of third-order neurons are directed at the frontal lobe of the cerebral cortex or thalamus. Cingulotomy and thalamotomy are examples of these procedures. These procedures are done stereotactically or with electrical stimulation.

Cingulotomy. The cingulum is an area in the frontal lobe that is connected with the limbic system. Pathophysiology in this area has been associated with the suffering part of pain. Surgical procedures with the creation of lesions in this area are associated with pain relief without measurable deterioration in personality or intellect. The procedure is performed stereotactically through burr holes, in which lesions are created

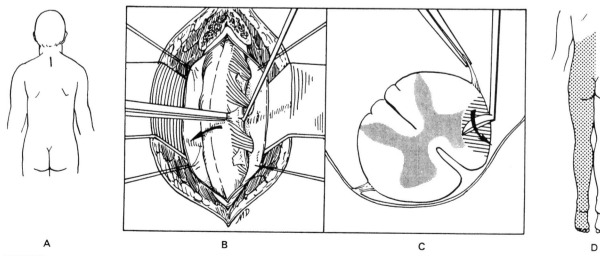

A   **B**   **C**   **D**

FIGURE 19-8
(*A*) Site of open thoracic cordotomy. (*B*) and (*C*). Method of performing open thoracic cordotomy. (*B*) After T1–T2 laminectomy, the dura is opened and the dentate ligaments sectioned. The linea alba is grasped in a hemostat and the spinal cord is rotated 45°. (*C*) A special cordotomy knife is used to section the anterolateral quadrant. (*D*) Extent of analgesia on dorsal surface produced by right T1–T2 open cordotomy. (From Bonica, J. J. [1990]. *The management of pain*. [2nd ed.] [p. 2049]. Philadelphia: Lea & Febiger.)

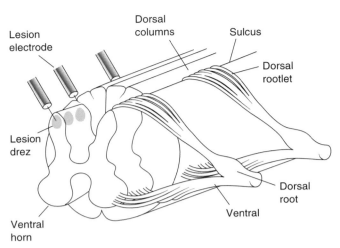

FIGURE 19-9
Schematic drawing showing the dorsal root entry zone (DREZ) and the region for DREZ lesions.

using a radiofrequency technique (Fig. 19-10). The most common indication for a cingulotomy is neoplastic pain associated with depression and suffering. The surgery is contraindicated in patients with bleeding disorders or uncontrolled hypertension. Headache and fever often occur postoperatively, but the greatest danger of the procedure is postoperative intracranial hemorrhage. Other complications include seizures and urinary incontinence.

A **thalamotomy** involves making lesions stereotactically in the thalamus, resulting in interruption of the spinothalamic tract and the absence of pain and temperature opposite to and below the level of the lesions (Fig. 19-11). The most common indication for a thalamotomy is cancer pain. Pain relief is excellent in the early postoperative period, but the relief diminishes with time. Intracranial hemorrhage and infection are rare but dangerous complications of this procedure. Ataxia and mild apathy may occur postoperatively.

GENERAL PREOPERATIVE MANAGEMENT

Patients hospitalized for a neurosurgical pain procedure must be managed by a multidisciplinary team because chronic pain is a complex phenomenon of physical, psychological, and emotional components. Typically, neurosurgical pain procedures are not considered the first-line treatment for pain. Therefore, years of a pain syndrome and pain behavior reinforcement may occur before the patient is finally recommended for the surgery. People with chronic pain, therefore, often have a history of addiction to pain medications; alteration in functional level; loss of self-esteem, social, and financial support; and a history of repeated failed procedures to relieve pain. Patients must often travel to distant centers where these neurosurgical procedures are performed, so their support systems may be limited.

A preadmission contact is helpful to provide information about local lodging, the hospital admitting procedure, and a brief description of the hospitalization. This contact can be made by phone, letter, or a patient education brochure. In ad-

dition, a clinical pathway can be created for these neurosurgical procedures. This pathway can be shared with the patient and assists greatly in developing realistic expectations and outlining day by day activities.

The usual preoperative routines and preparation common for any surgical procedure are followed. In addition, the following baseline data are collected:

- Baseline functional assessment by physical and occupational therapy
- In-depth pain assessment, including pattern, location, associated symptoms, and relieving and aggravating factors (conducted by a professional familiar with detailed pain assessment and patient management)
- Psychological testing (required by some physicians), which can assist with screening for psychiatric diagnosis and as a baseline measure for assessing the treatment protocol

Other specific teaching and points of care include the following:

- Preoperative teaching is essential; patients need to understand what to expect, including an explanation about the procedure and immediate postoperative management. Realistic expectations about outcomes from the procedure within a time frame must be clear to the patient and family.
- Skin preparation depends on the area of the surgery. Typically, skin preparation for stereotactic procedures is done in the operating room. Because the dura is often opened during the procedure, it is common to administer steroids before and often during surgery to decrease swelling and inflammation. High-dose methylprednisolone is commonly used for the DREZ procedure.
- Application of elastic stockings and sequential compression boots is necessary to prevent deep vein thrombosis and pulmonary emboli.

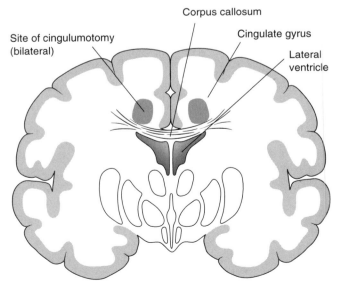

FIGURE 19-10
Coronal section of brain indicating sites of lesions for cingulotomy.

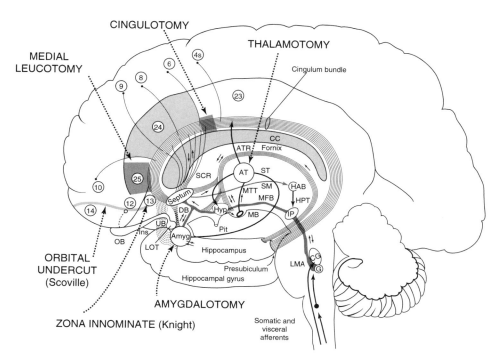

FIGURE 19-11
Sites of limbic system surgery. (OB = olfactory bulb; LOT = lateral olfactory striae; INS = insula; UB = uncinate bundle; DB = diagonal band of Broca; AMYG = amygdala; SCR = subcallosal radiations; HYP = hypothalamus; AT = anterior thalamus; MB = mammillary body; MTT = mammillothalamic tract [Vicq d'Azyr's tract]; ATR = anterior thalamic radiations; ST = stria terminalis; HAB = habenula; MFB = medial forebrain bundle; SM = stria medullaris; HPT = habenulointerpeduncular tract [fasciculus retroflexus of Meynert]; IP = interpeduncular nucleus; LMA = limbic midbrain area of Nauta; G = nucleus of Gudden; CG = central gray; CC = corpus callosum.)

- Patients undergoing lumbar or sacral laminectomies should expect some spasms in the lower back, thigh, or abdominal region.
- The following should be explained to patients:
  Log-rolling technique
  Postoperative pain medication administration
  Incentive spirometry or deep breathing exercises
  Postoperative monitoring (vital signs, dressing checks, turning)
  Importance of maintaining proper body alignment after surgery
  Pain scale used to quantify the severity of pain
  Neurological assessment, especially of motor and sensory function

An understanding of what to expect after surgery and the patient's role is important to pain control in the postoperative period because anxiety and fear contribute to pain perception.

GENERAL POSTOPERATIVE MANAGEMENT

After the postanesthesia recovery period, some patients may be transferred to the surgical or neuroscience intensive care unit for 24 hours for respiratory monitoring and pain control. Pain medication is administered during the postoperative period, and pain assessments are made regarding the level of postoperative pain compared with the original pain. Pain control is often best managed by a multidisciplinary pain team, which includes the clinical pharmacist. Some patients experience complete relief immediately after surgery, but for others, pain subsides gradually.

Bed rest may be maintained for 2 to 4 days depending on the type of surgery. For example, after a DREZ procedure, patients typically remain on bed rest for 3 to 4 days. The elevation of the head of the bed also depends on the area of the surgery. After a lumbar procedure, elevation of the head of the bed is restricted for 24 to 48 hours to encourage dural healing. All postlaminectomy patients need to be log rolled and wear antiembolic stockings with sequential compression boots. Physical therapy will initially begin on the first postoperative day with gentle ROM and isometric exercises. As the patient is mobilized, physical therapy will increase the level of exercise. Occupational therapy should re-evaluate the patient prior to discharge. The physical and occupational therapists should make recommendations for equipment, home therapy, and a continued exercise program.

Pain control during the postoperative period can be complex because the patient has acute pain from the operative site and remnants of chronic pain. The goal must be to control the postoperative pain. As hospitalization progresses, the question of weaning from previous analgesics for chronic pain must be addressed. Hospitalization time is short, and patients are often discharged with considerable postoperative discomfort. Prior to discharge, patients should ideally be on oral pain medication and should have a physician who will assist them through the pain medication withdrawal process. Some patients will require admission to a pain withdrawal center; others will wean quickly as their original pain is relieved.

PAIN AND PAIN MANAGEMENT: THE FUTURE

Research into the understanding of the pain phenomenon, the human impact, and treatment options is exciting and blazing new frontiers of inquiry. The age of molecular biology and neuroimmunology has opened the doors to new understandings about the interplay of the mind on the body and the ability to control pain. These breakthroughs come at a time of a changing health care system and a managed care environment in which treatment options to patients are increasingly controlled by third party payers. The real challenge is for health care providers to demonstrate the cost-effectiveness and health outcomes that can be achieved for people who suffer from chronic pain.

References

1. International Association for the Study of Pain Task Force on Chronic Pain, Ready, L. B. (chair) (1992). Seattle: IASP Publications.
2. Bonica, J. J. (1990). *The management of pain* (Vols. I & II) (2nd ed.). Philadelphia: Lea & Febiger.
3. Ibid,
4. Carroll, D., & Bowsher, D. (1993). *Pain management and nursing care.* Boston: Butterworth-Heinemann.
5. Mersky, H. (1986). Classification of chronic pain: Description of chronic pain syndromes and definitions. *Pain, 3*(Suppl.), SI 225.
6. Hyman, S. E., & Cassem, N. H. (1995). Pain. In D. C. Dale & D. D. Federman, (Eds.), *Scientific American medicine* (Vol. III) (p. 1).
7. Jacox, A., Carr, D. B., Payne, R., et al. (1994). *Management of cancer pain. Clinical practice guideline.* AHCPR Pub. No. 94-0592. Rockville, MD: Agency for Health Care Policy and Research, Public Health Service, U. S. Department of Health and Human Services.
8. Melzak, R. (1975). The McGill pain questionnaire: Major properties and scoring methods. *Pain, 1,* 277.
9. Acute Pain Management Guideline Panel (1992). *Acute pain management: Operative or medical procedures and trauma. Clinical practice guideline.* AHCPR Pub. No. 92-0032. Rockville, MD: Agency for Health Care Policy and Research, Public Health Service, U. S. Department of Health and Human Services.
10. Ibid, Jacox et al., p. 2.
11. Ibid, Bonica, p. 1770.
12. Ibid, Bonica, p. 1770.
13. Ibid, Jacox et al., p. 79.
14. Ibid, Carroll & Bowsher, p. 133.
15. Ibid, Jacox et al., p. 82.
16. McCaffery, M., & Beebe, A. (1989). *Pain: Clinical manual for nursing practice.* St. Louis: C.V. Mosby.
17. Ibid, Jacox et al., p. 185.
18. Ibid, Jacox et al., p. 83.
19. Portenoy, R. K. (1989). Opioid therapy in the management of chronic low back pain. In C. D. Tollidon (Ed.), *Interdisciplinary rehabilitation of low back pain* (pp. 137–157). Baltimore: Williams & Wilkins.

Bibliography

Books

(1985). *Application of TENS in the management of patients with pain.* Alexandria, VA: American Physical Therapy Association.

Blumenkopf, B. (1994). Chronic pain. In S. S. Rengachary & R. H. Wilkins (Eds.), *Principles of neurosurgery* (pp. 48-1–48-9). St. Louis: Wolfe.

Bonica, J. J. (1990). *The management of pain* (Vols. I & II). (2nd ed.). Philadelphia: Lea & Febiger.

Borysenko, J. (1987). *Minding the body, mending the mind.* Reading, MA: Addison-Wesley.

Caillet, R. (1993). *Pain: Mechanisms and management.* Philadelphia: F.A. Davis.

Carroll, D., & Bowsher, D. (1993). *Pain management and nursing care.* Boston: Butterworth-Heinemann.

Nashold, B. S., Jr., & Ovelmen-Levitt, J. (Eds.) (1991). *Deafferentation pain syndromes: Pathophysiology and treatment.* New York: Raven Press.

Philips, H. C., & Rachman, S. (1996). *The psychological management of chronic pain: Treatment manual.* (2nd ed.), New York: Springer.

Portency, R. K. & Kanner, R. M. (1996). *Pain management: Theory and practice.* Philadelphia: F. A. Davis.

Periodicals

Gilbert, M., Counsell, C. M., Martin, P., & Snively, C. (1994). Spinal ctable pain: Nursing implications. *Journal of Neuroscience Nursing, 26*(6), 347–351.

Iacono, R. P., Guthkelch, A. N., & Boswell, M. V. (1991). Dorsal root entry zone stimulation for deafferentation pain. *Stereotactic Functional Neurosurgery, 59,* 56–61.

Kost, R. G. & Straus, S. E. (1996). Posthepatic neurologic-pathogenesis treatment and prevention. *New England Journal of Medicine, 335*(1), 32–42.

Nashold, B. S., Jr., El-Naggar, A. O., Ovelmen-Levitt, J., & Abdul-Hak, M. (1994). A new design of radiofrequency lesion electrodes for use in the cudalis nucleus DREZ operation. *Journal of Neurosurgery, 80,* 1116–1120.

Rawlings, C., III, Rossitch, E., & Nashold, B. S., Jr. (1992). The history of neurosurgical procedures for the relief of pain. *Surgical Neurology, 38,* 454–463.

Richardson, D. R. (1995). Deep brain stimulation for the relief of chronic pain. *Neurosurgery Clinics of North America, 6*(1), 135–144.

Segatore, M. (1994). Understanding chronic pain after spinal cord injury. *Journal of Neuroscience Nursing, 26*(4), 230–236.

Tasker, R. R., DeCarvalho, G. T. C., & Dolan, E. J. (1992). Intractable pain of spinal cord origin: Clinical features and implications for surgery. *Journal of Neurosurgery, 77,* 373–378.

Thomas, D. G. T. (1993). Brachial plexus injury: Deafferentation pain and dorsal root entry zone (DREZ) coagulation. *Clinical Neurology and Neurosurgery, 95*(Suppl.), S48–S49

Section 5

Nursing Management of Patients With Injury to the Neurological System

CHAPTER 20

Multiple Trauma

Donna Nayduch
Joanne V. Hickey

Trauma remains the leading cause of death among young adults in the United States. As the population of elderly increases, the incidence of trauma in those older than 65 years is also increasing. However, this expensive disease, trauma, remains the most preventable health care problem.[1] The most important impact of trauma on society is the loss of years of productive life, a loss that exceeds the total of life-years lost due to cancer and heart disease combined.[1] The purpose of this chapter is to provide the neuroscience nurse with a comprehensive, priorities-of-care approach to the assessment and early management of patients who have sustained multiple trauma. This information is included because the nurse caring for the neuroscience patient must also manage injuries to other body systems that result from trauma. Expansive knowledge and skill are required to manage the patient safely and cost effectively. Details of the management of specific conditions or problems are not included in this chapter.

Multiple trauma refers to injuries involving more than one body system as a result of vehicular, occupational, or household injuries; sporting events; or acts of violence. Mortality, morbidity, and the optimal rehabilitative level achieved by the patient depend on the severity of injury, time elapsed from injury to the initiation of health care, and the quality of care provided. The development of critical care medicine, emergency medicine, and traumatology as specialties has been paralleled by the development of critical care nursing, trauma nursing, and emergency nursing. Critical care nursing has piqued the interest of many nurses, as evidenced by the popularity of seminars and workshops that focus on various issues in critical care, the growth of critical care nursing organizations, and the ever-increasing number of periodicals and textbooks addressing critical care practice. Although this textbook focuses on neuroscience nursing, the concept of critical care management of the patient sustaining multiple trauma is important because the neuroscience nurse cares for many patients with injuries to the nervous system and to several other body systems.

No body system is an isolated functional unit. Because the human body is a composite of interrelated physiological and psychosocial systems, every patient must be managed holistically. However, the nervous system has direct responsibility for controlling functions in all body systems, and many feedback loops control the interaction of the nervous system with each body system. Not only will injury to the nervous system affect other body systems, but dysfunction of a body system will often affect the normal physiology of the nervous system. For example, a patent airway and adequate respirations will support cerebral oxygenation and adequate perfusion and decrease the possibility of the development of secondary injury to the brain, such as cerebral ischemia, cerebral hypertension, and increased intracranial pressure (ICP). Therefore, the nurse caring for the critically ill trauma patient with neurological injury must accept the awesome responsibility of caring for the patient holistically, while recognizing and appreciating the interrelatedness of body systems. With this approach, the nurse is better able to consider the probability of the development of particular problems and associated nursing diagnoses.

TRAUMA CARE SYSTEMS

How the trauma victim is managed depends on the organizational structure of the *trauma system* in the area. Access, resources, and protocols are addressed within the organizational structure. Significant differences exist throughout the country because the United States is an urban and a rural nation, with variations in population distribution, topography, and health care resources. It is impossible to generalize, except to note that the management of trauma must be organized to meet the needs of the particular area and people served. The continuum of trauma care necessitates a trauma system to be efficient and effective in achieving optimal outcomes from resuscitation through rehabilitation and reintegration into society.

Trauma care systems involve community awareness of prevention and first responder care of the injured, emergency medical services (prehospital care), community hospitals and designated trauma centers, and rehabilitation and home care services. Certainly, the primary goal is to reduce preventable deaths. Studies have demonstrated significant decreases in preventable deaths when a system was implemented.[3,4] Preventable deaths that did occur as a result of postoperative problems instead of delays to definitive care or inadequate resuscitation.[3] Trauma systems have also resulted in more effective triage and use of resources within a state or community. A system is only complete if all components participate. The goal of optimal functional outcome for each patient is paramount. Measurement of this goal occurs in region-wide quality management activities.

Prehospital Management

The most critical time for the outcome of a patient who has sustained injury is the time from injury until admission to an acute care facility. The faster a patient is immobilized, resuscitated, and safely transported to the definitive care facility, the less chance there is of death, complications, and extension of injuries. Appropriate triage of trauma patients at the scene is the most effective means of providing the best possible outcome for the patient. It is most important that the emergency medical personnel who attend the patient at the injury site be well trained and knowledgeable in rapid assessment and triage, airway and cardiovascular stabilization, immobilization, and safe transportation of the patient. A mechanism for communication between the emergency medical personnel at the injury site and a physician at an acute care hospital should be available for assessment and instruction concerning patient management. A short-wave radio is often used for this purpose. Protocols that can be initiated at the trauma site provide guidance for rapid intervention without delays. The hour after injury has been called the "golden hour"; it is the period that makes the critical difference in patient outcomes. Secondary injuries and complications will rapidly develop without swift and skilled intervention.

Admission to the Definitive Care Setting

The decision concerning the facility to which the patient should be transported is critical because valuable time can be lost if the patient is taken to a facility that is not staffed or equipped to provide the necessary management. The personnel treating the patient at the injury site must triage the patient independently or seek advice from a physician by way of radio contact about the destination of transport. A critically ill patient may be transported immediately by land vehicle or air evacuation to a trauma center, regional head injury center, or spinal cord injury center.

Once patients arrive at an acute care setting, they are rapidly triaged and assessed again. Patients may be admitted immediately to the trauma service (if in a trauma center), stabilized, and managed by a team of specialists coordinated by the trauma surgeon. Such patients remain on the trauma service until they are discharged or have only a single system injury remaining that requires hospitalization. At that point, they are then transferred to the service that can best manage their remaining injuries. Management includes any necessary surgery, invasive procedures, ongoing monitoring, and early

rehabilitation. Patients are usually admitted to an intensive care unit (ICU) when they require intensive nursing and medical management. In hospitals that do not have a trauma service, patients are stabilized in the emergency department and then transferred to a trauma center that can adequately provide for the patient's needs. Some patients may not require transfer and can be managed safely in a local facility. These patients may also be admitted to the ICU for stabilization, management, and ongoing monitoring. A serious review of a facility's capabilities and limitations should guide triage considerations for these patients to ensure admission to the correct facility, not just the nearest facility.

The nursing management required is challenging because the patient's needs for ongoing monitoring and management to support life are enormously complex, missed injuries may become evident, and serious complications from the injury can begin to develop. The catastrophic event that has critically injured the patient's body has also had a tremendous impact on his or her family system, independence in making critical decisions, and financial resources. In addressing the problems precipitated by injury, the focus of care includes rehabilitation and discharge planning for the multidisciplinary needs and extended care necessary for achieving the highest level of rehabilitation possible for the patient. All of these processes tend to be complex and demanding.

SCORING SYSTEMS

The complexity of the multisystem trauma patient requires a care management methodology. The first of these is to assess acuity and the potential for survival. The second is case management of patients to guide care and effectively use resources. There are many scoring systems with different applications. The initial and most important for planning the trauma resuscitation response team is the Revised Trauma Score[5] (RTS). The RTS is a physiological score with respiratory rate, systolic blood pressure, and converted Glasgow Coma Scale (GCS) components. The score's range is from 0 to 12 with an optimal score of 12 (Chart 20-1). Patients with scores of 8 or less are the potentially more seriously injured admissions. It has been demonstrated that patients with low RTS scores (0–3) have a lower survival rate, shorter length of stay, and therefore less nursing acuity hours of care. Extensive nursing care hours are required for patients with a score of 4 to 9, who have a lower incidence of death and are more seriously ill.[6]

The GCS score is meant to be repeated and compared for trends to identify patient progress. The GCS ranges from 3 to 15, with a score of 15 considered a normal response[7] (see Chap. 8). Nursing acuity hours are highest for patients with a score of 5 to 6 and significantly lower for patients with GCS scores of 3 to 4 due to the higher incidence of early death in this group.[6]

An Injury Severity Score (ISS) is an anatomical score calculated retrospectively but helpful in identifying an injured patient's probability of survival, especially when compared with the RTS.[8] The ISS is based on six body areas with weighted scores for degree of severity of the injury. A detailed knowledge of the actual injuries is necessary to calculate this score. It is usually used as a quality improvement tool and monitor for preventable deaths. The range for ISS is 1 to 75

CHART 20-1
Revised Trauma Score

Respirations 10–29	4		
>29	3		
6–9	2		
1–5	1		
0	0		
Systolic blood pressure			
>89	4		
76–89	3		
50–75	2		
1–49	1		
0	0		
Glasgow Coma Scale (GCS)			
Eye opening			
Spontaneous	4		
To verbal	3		
To pain	2		
None	1		
Verbal response			
Oriented	5		
Confused	4	GCS Conversion	
Inappropriate words	3	13–15	4
Inappropriate sounds	2	9–12	3
None	1	6–8	2
Motor response		4–5	1
Follows commands	6	3	0
Purposeful	5		
Withdrawals to pain	4		
Abnormal flexion	3		
Extension	2		
None	1		
Total		*Total points*	__

with a score of 1 being the least injured and a score of 75 essentially unsurvivable. Nursing acuity hours increase as the ISS increases, except for the high extreme (66–75), in which the death rate is high.[6]

A well-known system of measuring acuity and potential for survival (at-risk patient identification) is the Acute Physiology, Age, Chronic Health Evaluation (APACHE) score. Presently, the APACHE III prognostic system is being used in many facilities.[9] The APACHE III includes vital signs, laboratory values, acid–base abnormalities, neurological status, comorbidity, and age components. Its ability to predict at-risk for hospital death patients has been demonstrated at 95%, which was within 3% of that actually observed.

CASE MANAGEMENT

With the need to control expenses yet continue to provide quality management of patients, health care has had to become more efficient in its approach to patients. Case manage-

ment enables provision of quality care, organization, better outcome and quality of life, and containing costs.[10] This method of patient care, through an episode of illness, provides specific clinical and fiscal outcomes achieved in an allotted time frame. The structure includes a work design (case management plans and critical paths), clinical roles as case managers, and monitoring with immediate feedback.[11] Case management plans are detailed protocols for the patient's entire episode. Length of stay, outcomes, and activities to accomplish these outcomes are detailed throughout the protocol. The critical path is an abbreviated version of the key elements of care.

There are five key factors in case management. Expected outcomes, or an alternative set of negotiated expectations, is the first. The second is that collaborative practice is necessary to complete successfully the outcome objectives. The practice must be well coordinated and organized. Third, effective use of resources is imperative to decrease waste of time, energy, and money. Discharge should be timely and within the expected length of stay as the fourth key factor. The professional development of the staff and improved staff morale will only improve the effectiveness of the plans as the fifth and final factor in case management.

The protocol for the particular illness or event must be adapted to the patient's needs and responses.[12] Goals are determined and evaluated daily for patient progress. The primary nurse is the optimal case manager, because he or she has the closest relationship to the patient and family. There should be frequent group meetings with the multidisciplinary team involved to monitor trends and variances (deviations from the plan) and to develop care strategies or identify new, acceptable outcomes. Families and patients must be involved with the decision making and outcome determination.

Professional outcomes include the opportunity for research activities, concurrent quality management, and identification of educational needs. With successful patient outcomes, shorter lengths of stay, and more effective management of resources, the multidisciplinary staff will be more effective in patient management and more satisfied in their positions. Case management for the multisystem trauma patient is extremely complex and requires the cooperation of all members of the team to be effective. Management protocols must focus on immediate needs and prevention of complications. As variances occur, changes must be made rapidly. Occasionally, outcome goals must change if the patient is unable to achieve the initial discharge goals.

ASSESSMENT AND MANAGEMENT OF THE TRAUMA PATIENT

The assessment and management of the multitrauma patient are concurrent processes because the potentially life-threatening problems involved often require immediate intervention. Appropriate interventions to stabilize and treat the patient are conducted as needed while the assessment process proceeds. Assessment is an ongoing process that is imperative for unstable patients because their condition changes so rapidly.

The nurse functions as a team member in the early assessment and management of the patient. In most emergency departments and trauma centers, each member of the team assumes a prescribed role that has been practiced in simulated drills. Although each team member assumes a different role and responsibilities, the activities as a whole are designed to complement each other in a coordinated effort to meet the complex needs of the patient.

Priorities in the Management of Trauma Patients

The multitrauma patient has multiple, complex problems and needs that can be overwhelming unless the patient is viewed in perspective. The complex catastrophic situation presented by a multitrauma patient can be viewed as a series of interrelated, less complex components. Once the various components are recognized, they can be organized systematically based on priorities of management that address the most critical and life-threatening problems first to prevent needless loss of life and rehabilitative potential.

Although the nurse is a collaborative team member, and a team approach is most effective in managing the patient, the nurse should be able to approach the patient independently with a conceptualization of the assessment and management process. Nurses are familiar with the priority for assessing and maintaining the ABCs of life support in emergency care—*air*way, *b*reathing, and *c*irculation. A patent airway while maintaining cervical spine immobilization, adequate respiratory function, and support of circulation are imperative for supporting cardiopulmonary function to maintain life. Without maintenance of these conditions, irreversible brain damage and death will occur in minutes. However, when managing multitrauma patients, a more extensive approach is necessary for assessing the overall needs of the patient. A well-known systematic approach to the assessment of the multitrauma patient is the ABC approach, which addresses the priorities in which body systems and functions should be assessed. The priorities of care are listed in alphabetical order from A through E so that the higher priorities are managed first and then other priorities are handled in descending order of urgency.[13] Chart 20-2 provides a description of the approach.

Diagnostic Tests and Procedures

Laboratory, radiographic, technologically generated, and other diagnostic data are valuable in assessing, diagnosing, and monitoring the patient with multiple injuries. The nurse must include these parameters when assessing, planning, implementing, and evaluating nursing care. Although the diagnostic protocol will depend on the type of injuries sustained, common tests and procedures include the following:

- SMA-7 (glucose, blood urea nitrogen, sodium, potassium, chloride, creatinine, and carbon dioxide) plus alkaline phosphatase, amylase, and lipase
- Arterial blood gases
- Complete blood count (CBC)
- Type and screen (unless blood transfusion is expected, then cross-match)

- Coagulation studies: prothrombin time, partial thromboplastin time
- Toxicology screen: alcohol, barbiturates, amphetamines, and street drugs, such as tetrahydrocannabinol, cocaine, opiates, and phencyclidine hydrochloride
- Chest x-ray, cross-table lateral cervical spine film, pelvis radiographs
- Diagnostic peritoneal lavage
- Computerized tomography: abdomen, single-cut thoracic, head
- Aortogram or arteriogram studies
- Any necessary long bone films
- Swan-Ganz monitoring for any patient older than 65 years or with a significant past medical history
- Ventriculostomy for increased ICP management

Tests may be repeated periodically as necessary to monitor and treat the patient. The assessment and evaluation of the patient are ongoing.

THE STABILIZED PATIENT AND NURSING MANAGEMENT

Once stabilized, the patient will be transferred to the appropriate nursing unit or the operating suite. The same nursing process is used to provide care whether the patient is admitted to the ICU or a general care unit.

Assessment

The nurse should review all of the information that has been documented in the patient's record, beginning with the prehospital report for mechanism of injury through the emergency department and operative events. The nurse begins to compile the nursing history, which is based on available information. Because the patient is often unable to provide information, family members may be interviewed to obtain necessary information. A complete assessment of the patient is the basis for the multidisciplinary plan for the patient.

All parameters should be monitored, including vital signs, neurological signs, respiratory function, urinary output, hemodynamics, fluid intake (which is usually administered through a peripheral intravenous or central line), SVO2 and pulse oximetry readings, nutritional variables, and output from thoracostomies, nasogastric tube, and other drainage tubes. Careful documentation of the data is essential to note trends in the findings. Laboratory data (*e.g.*, blood gas values, CBC and coagulation studies, electrolyte levels, cultures, and urinalyses) are also monitored. Various equipment (*e.g.*, a ventilator, traction devices, cooling blanket, cardiac monitor, or ICP monitor) should be checked periodically to ensure that settings are correct and the equipment is functioning properly.

Information about the medications that the patient is receiving needs to be correlated to understand their effects on the patient. For example, patients receiving steroids may have a systemic infection without exhibiting the classical signs and symptoms of infection because steroids are anti-inflammatory drugs that can mask infections. Drug interactions are more

CHART 20-2
Priorities in the Assessment of the Multitrauma Patient According to Body Systems

In the ABC approach, the letters A through E each stand for a significant body system that can present with life-threatening injury:

A: Airway and cervical spine immobilization
B: Breathing
C: Circulation
D: Deficit (neurological assessment)
E: Expose

The application of this system as the primary survey involves the following: When considering each category of the ABCs, assume the presence of every possible life-threatening injury or problem until it has been ruled out.

Each system is assessed and stabilized before going on to the next system.

Do not deviate from the prescribed order of assessment. The prescribed order addresses the most life-threatening injuries first. It is imperative that each is managed in order or simultaneously.

A report from the person(s) who brought the patient to the hospital is helpful in determining the circumstances of injury, potential injuries, treatment already in progress, and time from injury to definitive care. A written report will be available later. This information is helpful in identifying injuries that may have been incurred. A report prior to arrival is most helpful in anticipating injuries.

Collect as much information as possible about the patient's medical history; note whether any medication or indication of health problems, such as a medical alert bracelet, was found on the patient. This should be done during the secondary survey, unless there is someone available to spend time with the family to gather this information (or if the patients can provide this information themselves).

Recognize that the information about the patient and injury may be incomplete and fragmented because of the circumstances of injury; try to fill in the gaps in information as soon as possible.

Initial Assessment Using the ABC Approach

A. Airway

1. Patent airway (highest priority of care): Immediately provide an airway by whatever means is necessary—simple airway adjuncts, intubation, or cricothyrotomy
   Note: If there is any question of cervical fracture, the neck must be kept in a neutral position and immobilized; do not hyperflex, hyperextend, laterally flex, or rotate the head or neck.

B. Breathing

1. Assess the breathing pattern, and ventilate the patient if necessary (with 100% oxygen). Note the rate, rhythm, and characteristics of respirations.
2. Observe the chest for symmetry of movement; note any uneven movements or retractions.
3. Auscultate the chest for bilateral breath sounds; note the absence of breath sound or the presence of rales or rhonchi. Immediately manage hemothorax or pneumothorax to avoid a tension pneumothorax from occurring or to treat one. Placement of a tube thoracostomy will be necessary. Provide a large tube, 32–36 Fr.
4. Note the presence of cyanosis, air hunger, or dyspnea.
5. Check the chest for open wounds, lacerations, contusions, or fractures of the ribs or sternum. Possible injuries or problems commonly seen in multitrauma patients include the following:
   Obstruction (partial or complete) of the airway
   Pneumothorax, hemopneumothorax, open pneumothorax, lacerated lung
   Flail chest, fractured ribs

C. Circulation

1. Assess the pulses and capillary refill. Initiate at least two large bore IVs (14–16g) with warm lactated Ringer's solution. Have blood products available for transfusion if unresponsive to crystalloid solutions. It has been demonstrated that infusion of fluids, blood, and inotropic agents does not affect intracranial pressure. Many patients appear normotensive but have evidence of impaired perfusion.

(continued)

CHART 20-2 Priorities in the Assessment of the Multitrauma Patient According to Body Systems (Continued)

2. Assess the patient for the signs and symptoms of hypovolemic shock.
3. Assess the patient for obvious signs of hemorrhage, and apply pressure.
4. Impalement injuries—Do not remove the impaling object until surgical hemostasis can be provided; support the object with a dressing to prevent further tissue trauma.
5. Limb-threatening dislocations (decreased or lack of pulses) require immediate reduction by orthopedics while the primary survey is continued by the lead physician. Possible injuries or problems commonly seen with multitrauma patients include the following:
   Hypovolemic shock caused by frank or occult hemorrhage
   Laceration of viscera or blood vessels; gunshot wounds or impalement objects with subsequent hemorrhage

D. Deficit

1. Brief neurological assessment (alert; responds to verbal; responds to pain; unresponsive). Assess pupils and brain stem reflexes. Possible injuries and problems commonly seen in multitrauma patients include the following:
   Epidural, subdural, intracerebral, or subarachnoid hemorrhage
   Cerebral concussion, contusion, or laceration, diffuse axonal injury (shear)
   Fracture of the facial bones, skull, or vertebral column (including fracture dislocation of the vertebral column and basal skull fracture)
   Spinal cord injury
   Dural tears

E. Expose

1. Observe the patient for contusions, lacerations, or ecchymosis from head to toe, including the back.
2. Keep the patient warm.
3. Remove the backboard if at the definitive care facility (use a padded board if nursing prefers the presence of a board. This *must* be removed on arrival to the final destination—intensive care unit, operating room, unit)

Secondary Survey

A complete head to toe survey and reassessment of all previously assessed systems is needed. If intervention is necessary, proceed.

Head:

1. Reassess airway.
2. Reassess neurological response.
3. Palpate the face (if not already done prior to intubation) for fractures, especially beneath lacerations.
4. Note any drainage from the nose or mouth and check for CSF.

Neck:

1. Assess for jugular venous distention, subcutaneous emphysema, discomfort.
2. Replace the cervical collar.
3. Maintain manual immobilization while assessing the neck.

Chest:

1. Reassess breath sounds.
2. Palpate and observe for flail chest.
3. Listen to heart sounds, note muffling.

Abdomen:

1. Insert nasogastric or orogastric tube to decompress the stomach and prevent vomiting.
2. If vomiting occurs, tilt the backboard to the left.
3. Assess genitourinary system. Note blood at the urinary meatus or a high riding prostate; do not insert a Foley catheter in this case. Consult urology for SPT placement. If negative, insert a Foley catheter, monitor output, and send a UA.

(continued)

CHART 20-2 Priorities in the Assessment of the Multitrauma Patient According to Body Systems (Continued)

3. Palpate the abdomen for tenderness or distention.
4. If unable to assess tenderness due to the patient's level of consciousness or spinal cord injury, consider abdominal computed tomography or diagnostic peritoneal lavage.
5. Note contusions or abrasions.
6. While assessing the abdomen, press on the pelvic wings and symphysis pubis to assess instability.
7. A rectal examination should include tone, gross blood, and prostate position.
8. Examination of the female should include a brief vaginal examination to assess for open fracture and bleeding.

Extremities:

1. Palpate all extremities; note position, attitude, symmetry.
2. Palpate all pulses again; note symmetry.
3. Provide traction for reduction of femur and hip fractures. Use splints for upper extremity and tibial fractures. Splint upper extremities in functional position.
4. Note open wounds over joints or deformities as possible open fractures.

Gunshot wounds:

1. Note sites, appearance.
2. Photograph or diagram if possible before cleansing the area.

Definitive care:

1. Priorities are based on the most life-threatening injuries. The abdomen has priority because hemorrhage will lead to rapid decompensation. Head injuries with operative lesions (SDH, EDH) also have priority to prevent herniation and brain death from increased intracranial pressure (volume-occupying lesions).
2. Radiographic studies occur after the primary and secondary surveys are complete.
3. Rapid transfer to the trauma center is imperative before extensive radiographic studies occur.
4. Within the trauma center, rapid transfer to the operating room or intensive care unit is necessary to optimize outcome.
5. Laboratory tests and arterial blood gases (ABGs) should be drawn at the time of IV sticks or during the secondary survey.

likely to occur when patients receive several drugs. In some instances, as with phenytoin, several drug interactions have been well documented. Anticonvulsants have also been noted to decrease the functional outcome of the head-injured patient and are recommended only when necessary. To ensure the therapeutic level of some drugs, blood levels should be assessed periodically and the dosage of the drug adjusted accordingly.

All of the information about the patient must be considered together to ascertain a complete and accurate picture of his or her status. The nurse also assesses each body system for normal function. Oxygenation, hemodynamics, skin integrity, nutrition, fluid and electrolyte balance, elimination, and emotional response are a few of the areas of assessment. Assessment and monitoring are ongoing processes, as are all the steps of the nursing process.

Planning

Planning nursing management can be difficult because of the multitrauma patient's complex needs and physiological instability. For example, turning the patient for back care may be difficult in the event of a fractured pelvis or spine injury. Pa-

tient care goals need to be met by protocols adapted for individual patients. The nurse should also remember that such patients are prone to infections because they are compromised hosts. Attention should be directed to preventing sepsis when planning care. Nutritional concerns are foremost, because the trauma patient is hypermetabolic, especially when a head injury is involved. Timing and route of feeding need early consideration. Primary concerns are pulmonary, nutrition, immobility, pain, and coping. To manage these areas successfully, multiple disciplines must work collaboratively, including nursing, medicine, social services, chaplain, physical therapy, occupational therapy, speech therapy, and nutritional services. Frequently, the traumatic event involved substance abuse, and these services should also be included in the multidisciplinary team.

Implementation

The care that the patient requires is often very complex and time consuming. The nurse should document the implementation of the care plan and the patient's response to that care. The goal of all management is resuscitation and then optimal functional outcome. Mortality and morbidity can be significantly reduced by collaborative, efficient, and cost-effective care.

Evaluation

As with every other step in the nursing process, the nursing management of the patient must be evaluated to determine whether it is meeting the patient's needs or whether a change is indicated. Variances that occur in the patient's episode of illness must be identified and dealt with immediately. Prevention of these deviations from the plan is the focus of evaluation. Participation of the patient and family is necessary to accomplish goals acceptable to all parties. Evaluation of care should hinge on these parameters as outcome criteria.

PROBABILITY AND EARLY RECOGNITION OF COMPLICATIONS

Probability is defined as the chance of an event occurring or its projected occurrence based on the history of occurrences and the laws of probability. This concept can be applied to the multitrauma patient to anticipate the possibility of the development of particular complications. A baseline assessment, also called primary survey, and subsequent assessment, called secondary survey, are critical sources of data about the possibility of ensuing problems. The data collected through patient assessment; information about contributing factors, such as the mechanism of injury, the circumstances surrounding the event, and pre-existing health problems; and the nurse's knowledge, skills, and experience help the nurse to predict the development of potential problems. Appreciation of the interrelatedness of various physiological systems helps focus the nurse's assessment on particular information. At times, it is difficult to identify potential complications and systems failure because so many physiological events occur simultaneously. The usual signs and symptoms that the nurse expects to find may be absent, or they may be masked by other conditions. For example, a patient may develop acute pancreatitis from an injury. The predominant symptom is upper abdominal pain that radiates to the left shoulder and becomes worse when the patient lies flat on the back, but if the patient is unconscious, it will not be possible to localize pain to these specific areas. The nurse may notice that the patient is restless, but the cause of the restlessness may remain a mystery. Laboratory data and possibly jaundice may provide the first objective evidence of this problem.

Timing is also important when considering the potential development of problems and complications. For example, if an acute subdural hematoma is not present on the initial computed tomography scan or one taken within 24 to 48 hours of an acute head injury, a subdural hematoma will probably not develop. On the other hand, one would not expect to find evidence of normal-pressure hydrocephalus within the first few days after injury, because the probability of its development increases with time after a cerebral hemorrhage.

The goal of management of the multitrauma patient is early recognition of the development of problems and complications before acute, life-threatening events occur.

MULTIPLE ORGAN FAILURE SYNDROME

When considering the nursing management of the patient who has sustained multiple trauma, the nurse should be familiar with the concept of multiple organ failure. Multiple organ failure syndrome is defined as life-threatening failure of two or more physiological systems, requiring definitive intervention for the survival of the patient. Physiological complications superimposed on the original problems, especially adult respiratory distress syndrome, sepsis, and disseminated intravascular coagulation (DIC), can produce secondary insult and injury that result in the failure of multiple organ systems. For example, a patient with a severe head injury can rapidly develop respiratory complications, such as neurogenic pulmonary edema, DIC, aspiration pneumonia, and atelectasis; cardiovascular complications, such as life-threatening arrhythmias and systemic hypertension; endocrine disorders, such as diabetes insipidus or syndrome of inappropriate secretion of antidiuretic hormone; and an unlimited number of other problems. Combine this potential for complications with problems of immobility, a hypermetabolic state, and actual injury to the other systems and the potential for significant life-threatening complications becomes apparent.

The development of multiple systems failure depends on several overriding factors, such as the following:

- Circumstances of injury (e.g., direction of impact of injury, such as a head-on collision; wearing of seat belts; speed of impact; drug abuse)
- Extent and type of multiple trauma sustained
- Time elapsed before arrival of emergency medical care
- Time elapsed before transport to a hospital and level of care available en route
- Patency of the airway and adequacy of respiratory function
- Immobilization during transport
- Hemorrhage
- Pre-existing health problems (e.g., heart disease, chronic lung disease, diabetes mellitus)
- Patient's age

Prevention of multiple organ failure requires the prevention or successful management of other complications that further deplete the body's ability to heal. Careful attention to all systems will result in a functional outcome with minimal to no complications despite the severity of injury.

DISCHARGE PLANNING

The patient sustaining multiple trauma will need extensive discharge planning. As soon as possible after the patient is stabilized, discharge planning should commence, with input from all team members involved in the care of the patient (see Chap. 15). Discharge planning options for the multisystem trauma patient most often include rehabilitation or a short-stay skilled nursing facility placement for therapy. Home health options are increasingly important, because patients are discharged earlier in their management. Outpatient services serve the same purpose, except some degree of mobility of the patient is necessary. Vocational rehabilitation and the opportunity for drug and alcohol rehabilitation cannot be overlooked.

Summary

Few patients are as complicated and difficult to manage as the multisystem trauma patient. The implementation of a statewide trauma system provides an organized initial approach to the injured patient and methods for rapid transport of the patient to the appropriate facility. After the initial assessment and resuscitation, use of case management and acuity scoring systems combines technology with efficient care of the patient and family. The goal of management is to obtain the optimal functional outcome for the injuries. Services must be coordinated for a timely discharge, efficient use of resources, and optimal choice of discharge facility. Certainly, a discharge to home with return to previous roles is the goal. Rehabilitation services provide the opportunity for the patient to achieve that return to preinjury lifestyle. The ultimate goal is the prevention of injury. Each nurse has the responsibility to promote safety and health, including injury prevention. The key to eradicating the disease, trauma, is the prevention efforts of each individual.

References

1. Institute on Medicine (1985). *Injury in America: A continuing health problem*. Washington, DC: National Academy Press.
2. American College of Emergency Physicians (1987). Guidelines for trauma care systems. *Annals of Emergency Medicine, 16*, 459–463.
3. Thoburn, E. et al. (1993). System care improves trauma outcome: Patient care errors dominate reduced preventable death rate. *Journal of Emergency Medicine, 11*, 135–139.
4. Mullins, R. J. et al. (1994). Outcome of hospitalized injured patients after institution of a trauma system in an urban area. *Journal of the American Medical Association, 271*, 1919–1924.
5. Champion, H. R., Sacco, W. J., Copes, W. S., Gann, D. S., Gennarelli, T. A., & Flanigan, M. E. (1989). A revision of the trauma score. *Journal of Trauma, 29*, 623–629.
6. Bond, E., Thomas, F. O., Menlove, R. L., MacFarlane, P., & Petersen, P. (1993). Scoring acuity hours and costs of nursing for trauma care. *American Journal of Critical Care, 2*, 436–443.
7. Teasdale, G., & Jennett, B. (1974). Assessment of coma and impaired consciousness, a practical scale. *Lancet, 2*, 81–83.
8. Association for the Advancement of Automotive Medicine (1990). *The abbreviated injury scale*. Des Plaines, IL: .
9. Knaus, W. A. et al. (1991). The APACHE III prognostic system, risk prediction of hospital mortality for critically ill hospitalized adults. *Chest, 100*, 1619–1636.
10. Harrahill, M. A. (1995). Trauma case management: An extension of the trauma coordinator role. *International Journal of Trauma Nursing, 1*, 70–73.
11. Zander, K. (1988). Nursing case management: Strategic management of cost and quality outcomes. *JONA, 18*, 23–30.
12. Giuliano, K. K., & Poirier, C. E. (1991). Nursing case management: Critical pathways to desirable outcomes. *Nursing Management, 22*, 52–55.
13. American College of Surgeons (1993). *Advanced trauma life support*. Chicago: IL, American College of Surgeons.
14. Scalea, T. M., Maltz, S., Yelon, J., Trooskin, S. Z., Duncan, A. O., & Sclafani, S. J. (1994). Resuscitation of multiple trauma and head injury: Role of crystalloid fluids and inotropes. *Critical Care Medicine, 22*, 1610–1615.

Bibliography

Goldstein, L. B. (1995). Common drugs may influence motor recovery after stroke. The Sygen In Acute Stroke Study Investigations. *Neurology, 45(5)*, 865–871.

Goldstein, L. B. (1995). Prescribing of potentially harmful drugs to patients admitted to hospitals after head injury. *Journal of Neurology, Neurosurgery, and Psychiatry 58(6)*: 753–755.

Rauen, C. (1993). The complicated elderly trauma patient: A case study analysis. *Critical Care Nurse, June*, 63–69.

Scalea, T. M. et al. (1990). Geriatric blunt multiple trauma: Improved survival with early invasive monitoring. *Journal of Trauma, 30*, 129–136.

Schwab, C. W. (1992). Trauma in the geriatric patient. *Archives of Surgery, 127*, 701–706.

Stamatos, C. A. (1994). Geriatric trauma patients: Assessment and management of shock. *Journal of Trauma Nursing, 1*, 45–54.

Zeitlow, S. P., Capizzi, P. J., Bannon, M. P., & Farnell, M. B. (1994). Multisystem geriatric trauma. *Journal of Trauma, 37*, 985–988.

CHAPTER 21

Craniocerebral Injuries

Joanne V. Hickey

A PERSPECTIVE

More than 2 million head injuries occur each year in the United States; about 1.5 million are mild injuries, and 500,000 are severe enough to require hospitalization. About 120,000 are classified as severe brain injuries, and about half of these people die before reaching the hospital. Motor vehicle accidents account for 50% of all traumatic brain injuries; falls, 21%, assaults and violence, 12%; and sports and recreation, 10%. The highest incidence of head injuries is in people 15 to 24 years old, with occurrences in males two to three times higher than in females. A second peak incidence occurs in the elderly. Of the survivors of head injury, 70,000 to 90,000 will have lifelong serious functional loss, 5,000 will develop epilepsy, and 2,000 will remain in a persistent vegetative state. The cost of treatment and rehabilitation of one severe brain-injured person is estimated to be $310,000 based on 1990 costs; this does not reflect lifetime care.[1] The loss of human potential and impact on physical, emotional, psychosocial, vocational, and family function is immeasurable and devastating, thus creating the need for many health-related and community services.

GENERAL OVERVIEW OF HEAD INJURIES

Definitions and Classification

Head injury refers to any injury to the scalp, skull (cranium or facial bones), or brain. The terms **head injury** and **craniocerebral trauma** are used to denote injury to the skull or brain or both that is of sufficient magnitude to interfere with normal function and to require treatment. The more accurate term that describes the major traumatic event is **brain injury**.

Several different classification criteria are cited, including descriptors of location and types of injuries (Chart 21-1), Glasgow Coma Scale (GCS) severity of injury (Chart 21-2), and the mechanism of injury. Mechanisms of injury are discussed further in the chapter.

Anatomical Considerations

The cranial vault is a closed box with only one major opening at the base of the foramen magnum. The three compartments (anterior, middle, and posterior fossae) within the cranial vault are divided by irregularly shaped, bony buttresses (see Chap. 5, Fig. 5-6). The contour of the intracranial vault is smooth in some areas (*e.g.*, occipital area) and highly irregular in other areas (*e.g.*, frontal-orbital and temporal areas). Within the bones are etched tracts for some major blood vessels, such as the middle meningeal artery located on the inside plate of the temporal bone in an area where the skull is the thinnest. With temporal bone fractures, this artery may be torn, causing an epidural hematoma (EDH).

Mechanisms of Craniocerebral Injury

Classification of the mechanisms of craniocerebral injury includes the following (Fig. 21-1):

- **Deformation**: distortion of the skull either by indentation (bending inward) or outward rebound of the skull contour
- **Acceleration-deceleration**: the rapid changes in velocity of the brain within the cranial vault along a straight line from forward movement to an abrupt stop
- **Rotation** (sometimes called **angular acceleration**): angular acceleration-deceleration of the brain

Direct blows to the head are most often associated with deformation injuries. The velocity (low or high) of the impact determines whether injury is restricted to the skull (low velocity) or includes the brain (high velocity). Deformation can result in *focal* injuries (skull fractures, dural tears, contusions, lacerations, and intracranial hemorrhage). Direct blows may also result in acceleration-deceleration injuries with *diffuse* cerebral injury (*e.g.*, concussions and diffuse axonal injury [DAI]) without concurrent skull injury. Acceleration-deceleration can produce *strains* on cerebral tissue that result in injury. These strains include **compression** (pushing together of tissue), **tension** (traction on tissue), and **shearing**

CHART 21-1
Classification of Head Injuries by Location and Type

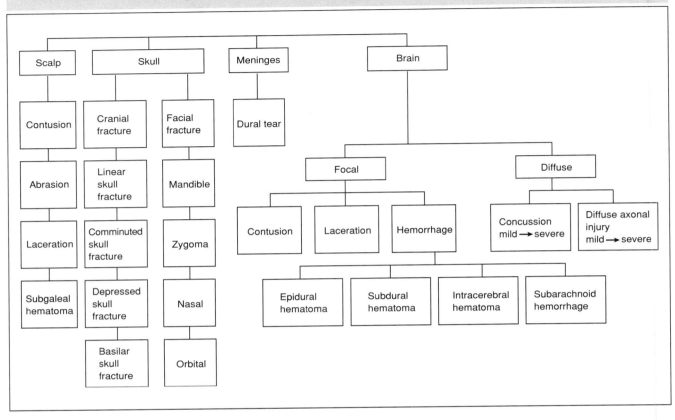

(sliding of portions of tissue over another portion). These strains often operate simultaneously or in rapid succession to produce injury. Penetrating injuries due to bullets from gunshots and blunt objects of impalement can cause injury by the previous mechanisms.

A focal cerebral injury directly under the area of impact (deformation) is called a **coup injury**. In contrast, a **contrecoup injury** is a cerebral injury sustained to the opposite pole of direct impact. The contrecoup injury, which is most often a contusion and occasionally a laceration, is caused by the rapid acceleration-deceleration of the semisolid brain within the rigid cranial vault (see discussion of contusions later in this chapter).

SCALP INJURIES

The velocity and characteristics of the impacting object determine the extent of scalp injury. The object may cause compression, tension, or tearing of the scalp.

SKULL INJURIES

The mechanism of skull injury is deformation. Factors that determine the degree of injury include the skull thickness at the point of impact and the weight, velocity, and angle of impact of the intruding object. At impact, several actions are set in motion in split-second sequence: At the point of impact, there is a relative indentation that may be temporary or permanent (depending on the velocity), and stress waves are set into motion, radiating throughout the entire skull. With *high-velocity impact*, a depressed skull fracture with or without a dural tear and cerebral laceration can occur. With *low-velocity impact*, the area of indentation rebounds outward and may result in no fracture, a linear fracture, or comminuted fractures

CHART 21-2
Classification of Brain Injury According to Glasgow Coma Scale

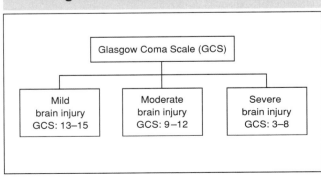

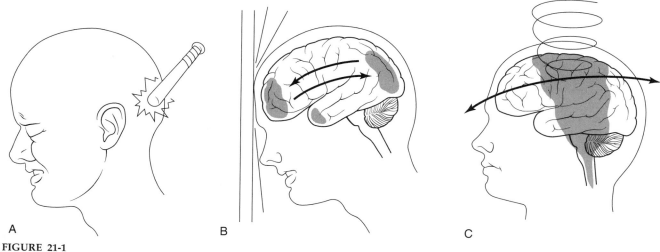

FIGURE 21-1
Mechanisms of injury: (*A*) deformation, (*B*) acceleration-deceleration, and (*C*) rotation.

(Fig. 21-2). The fracture line extends toward the point of impact and toward the base of the skull (bony buttresses direct the fracture toward the base of the skull).

BRAIN INJURIES

The two mechanisms responsible for brain injury are acceleration-deceleration and concurrent rotational movement. At the time of impact to the skull, there is *always* a certain amount of acceleration-deceleration to the head, whether the head is fixed or free. The difference in density between the skull (a solid substance) and the brain (a semisolid substance) causes the skull to move faster than the intracranial contents. The brain located within the rigid skull (compartmentalized by the dura and bony buttresses) responds to force exerted on the skull by gliding forward and then rotating within the compartment. The rotational force produces distortion of the brain

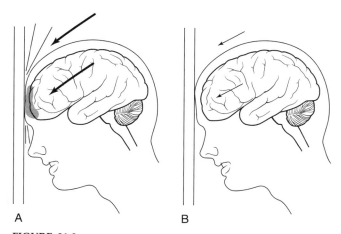

FIGURE 21-2
(*A*) A high-velocity impact damages the brain and skull. (*B*) A low-velocity impact damages only the skull.

and tension, stretching, and shearing of involved tissue. The maximal amount of injury is usually found at the tips of the frontal and temporal lobes. Shearing or sliding of cerebral tissue over another portion implies stresses on two different planes. With rotational acceleration, the stress of shearing is directed toward areas where tough, fibrous tissue and cerebral tissue meet. These high-risk areas include the crista galli, the sphenoid wing, the margins of the tentorium or falx, and the foramen magnum. The degree of injury will depend on the extent and direction of the angular acceleration. Rotational movement in the brain can cause damage to axons, leading to a fatal outcome, even without gross lesions visible.[2]

Pathophysiology of Head Injuries

PRIMARY AND SECONDARY INJURIES

Many factors are responsible for the pathophysiological events and ultimate functional outcomes associated with head injury. Head injury can be divided into primary and secondary injury. **Primary injury** is the purely *mechanical* injury to the brain. The cerebral injury may be focal (contusion or laceration) or diffuse (concussion or DAI), but the injury is a direct result of the initial insult. **Secondary injury** is caused by a flow-metabolism mismatch, resulting in cerebral *ischemia* that unleashes the ischemic cascade and biochemical changes on the cellular level that can result in neuronal infarction and degeneration.[3] The secondary injury may occur in seconds, hours, or days after injury and may result from a single event, series of events, or multisystem complications (respiratory, cardiac, renal, endocrine) that precipitate additional pathophysiological effects on the brain. Causes of secondary injury include hypoxemia, systemic hypotension, focal hypoperfusion, sustained increased intracranial pressure (ICP), respiratory complications, electrolyte imbalance, and infections. These problems compromise the supply of oxygen and nutrients (flow-metabolism mismatch) necessary for adequate cerebral cell metabolism and contribute to poor patient outcomes or even death.

MAJOR PATHOPHYSIOLOGICAL CHANGES ASSOCIATED WITH BRAIN INJURY

The understanding of pathophysiological processes associated with primary and secondary brain injury, neuronal recovery, and degeneration following traumatic injury are incompletely understood. However complex the processes, because of multiple concurrent reactions and interactions, there are molecular and cellular changes, altered cerebral hemodynamics, cerebral edema, increased ICP, and potential for herniation in response to brain injury. Discussions of these general areas follow.

Molecular and Cellular Level. The first responses are failure of anaerobic glycolysis, phosphocreatine production, high-energy cellular functions, and adenosine triphosphate (ATP) production. Failure of anaerobic glycolysis causes a fall in intracellular pH due to the production of lactate with resulting cellular acidosis. Failure of ATP production means the sodium-potassium pump can no longer maintain the homeostatic balance of intracellular ions with higher intracellular concentrations of K+ and higher extracellular concentrations of Na+. As a result, extracellular K+ increases as K+ leaks out of the cell, and Na+, Ca2+, and water move into the cell from the extracellular space.[4] As a result of ATP energy failure and disturbance of acid–base and ionic homeostasis, several mechanisms are activated that can cause cellular damage[5] (Fig. 21-3).

A major final common pathway for cell death is loss of *calcium homeostasis.*[6] Loss of calcium homeostasis causes inhibition of cellular metabolism, which results in an increased breakdown of protein and lipids, increased breakdown of cell membrane from phospholipids hydrolysis, and the production of toxins (eiconsanoid, platelet-activating factor, and free radicals). Concurrently, following trauma, there is immediate severe cellular energy failure. Consequently, there is a striking increased level of extracellular excitatory neurotransmitters, called excitatory amino acids (EAA). EAAs include glutamate,

asparate, and acetylcholine. The source of EAA is believed to be injured, energy depleted, and depolarized neural cells (neurons and glia) that release their glutamate. Escalating levels of glutamate (perhaps the most well known EAA) and asparate stimulate specific EAA receptors that normally mediate excitatory synaptic transmission between neurons. The three subclasses of glutamate receptors are *N*-methyl-D-aspartate (NMDA), kainate (K), and quisqualate (Q) subtypes. Excessive stimulation of glutamate receptors opens ionic channels, thus causing sodium-mediated cellular swelling and calcium-mediated neuronal disintegration from membrane lipid hydrolysis and protease activation.[7] Thus, overstimulated EAA receptors have been implicated as a final common pathway of neurotoxicity in numerous central nervous system problems, including traumatic injury.[8]

Free radicals disrupt the cellular membrane. Various pathophysiological processes lead to the formation of free radicals. Three free oxygen radicals, superoxide, hydroperoxyl, and hydroxyl, occur with injury. Their activity varies with tissue pH and the availability of superoxide dismutase (SOD) that converts superoxide to hydrogen peroxide, which in turn is converted to water by catalase. As a result of free radicals, cellular membranes are disrupted, leading to a vicious cycle of further generation of free radicals and ongoing cellular damage.[9]

If tissue injury results in blood and breakdown products within the brain, this becomes another source of oxygen free radicals. Hemoglobin breakdown results in free iron, which can transfer an electron to oxygen-forming superoxide molecules or to hydrogen peroxide to form hydroxyl. These free radicals can overwhelm cytoplasmic defenses and begin to oxidize cellular membrane by *lipid peroxidation.* Through lipid peroxidation, electrons are transferred to unsaturated fatty acids, which form free radicals called lipid peroxyl or alkoxyl moieties.[10] Ongoing lipid peroxidation causes eventual loss of integrity of the

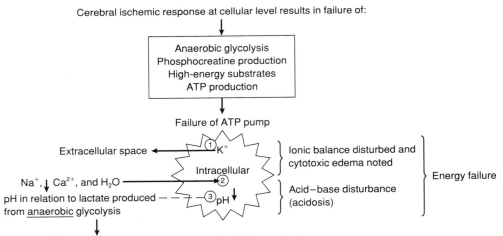

FIGURE 21-3
Ischemia: final common pathway in all central nervous system injuries.

cellular membrane and oxidation of membrane lipoproteins. The process also spreads to adjacent cells and perpetuates cell death and edema.[11]

Altered Cerebral Hemodynamics. After cerebral injury, microscopic examination of a contused or lacerated area reveals small hemorrhagic areas, ischemia, infarction, and necrosis of adjacent brain tissue. The brain is particularly vulnerable to deprivation of adequate cerebral blood flow (CBF) and cerebral oxygen delivery. Normally, vascular autoregulatory mechanisms maintain a constant CBF that is closely matched to metabolic needs. CBF is maintained over a wide range of cerebral perfusion pressures (CPPs) and within a wide range of mean arterial pressure (MAP; 50 and 150 mm Hg). Beyond these parameters, CBF is linearly and passively related to blood pressure. CBF is also particularly sensitive to carbon dioxide partial pressure, so hypoxia and hypercarbia produce cerebral vasodilation and increase CBF. CPP, the difference between MAP and cerebral venous pressure, exerts a strong influence on CBF. When CPP decreases, cerebral vasodilation occurs to maintain CBF until the lower limits of autoregulation are reached, at which point CBF declines. With brain trauma, injured areas may lose vasomotor tone, resulting in regional CBF that directly depends on MAP and ICP. Increased focal blood flow and focal dilation increase the pressure in the capillaries and venules. With cerebral injury, there is also focal injury to the blood–brain barrier. The altered blood–brain barrier and vasomotor tone result in movement of fluid into the extracellular space, causing vasogenic edema.

Cerebral Edema. Cerebral edema can be localized or global, appearing in unpredictable and unquantifiable patterns. Hypercapnia from inadequately perfused areas contributes to local acidosis and vasodilation, which increases edema. A vicious cycle develops as the biochemical and vascular alterations perpetuate and increase cerebral edema, which can lead to a mass effect, significant increase in ICP, and cerebral herniation syndromes (see Chap. 17). The clinical importance of increased ICP is its negative effect on CBF, CPP, and the viability of neurons. When CPP is sustained at a low level, irreversible neuronal changes occur, and cell death results.

Cerebral Ischemia. Cerebral ischemia has a profound effect on cerebral function. Normal CBF is about 50 to 55 mL/100 g per minute. **Ischemic penumbra** (Fig. 21-4) is a clinical concept introduced by Astrup[12] to describe brain tissue characterized by compromised CBF between the upper limits of the threshold for electrical failure and the lower limits of the threshold for membrane failure.[13] The **threshold of electrical failure** is a point in CBF (about 15–20 mL/100 g per minute) when the electroencephalogram (EEG) becomes isoelectric, and synaptic transmission ceases.[14] The **threshold of membrane failure** is a lower level of CBF (about 6–10 mL/100 g per minute) in which there is failure of the ionic pump, K+ leaves the cell, Ca2+ enters the cell, and ATP is depleted; cell death is the outcome (Fig. 21-5). What is critically important about the penumbra is that even though the tissue is electrically silent and nonfunctional, it is *viable*. Tissue functional recovery is possible if an adequate blood supply is restored, or irreversible damage (cell death) will occur with sus-

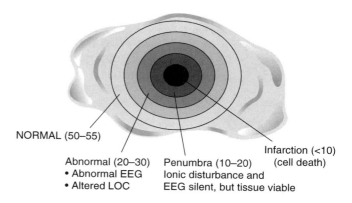

NORMAL (50–55)

Abnormal (20–30)
• Abnormal EEG
• Altered LOC

Penumbra (10–20)
Ionic disturbance and
EEG silent, but tissue viable

Infarction (<10)
(cell death)

Ischemic Penumbra: Normal CBF = 50–55 ml/100g/min. Variations in CBF noted. Penumbra is the critical area for salvage or death of cells: Potential for treatment.

FIGURE 21-4
Ischemic penumbra. (EEG = electroencephalogram; LOC = level of consciousness; CBF = cerebral blood flow)

tained compromised CBF. As Hayek and Veremakis point out, the potential salvagability of the ischemic penumbra provides a conceptual basis for brain resuscitation to prevent or minimize secondary brain injury.[15]

In summary, multiple concurrent molecular and cellular effects are mediated by primary and secondary brain injury. Cerebral hemodynamics, cerebral edema, and increased ICP all have a role in the ischemic cascade that causes neuronal demise. In addition to providing the reader with a cursory overview of key components of neuronal injury, the discussion also provides a basis for understanding the role of neuroprotective drugs currently in clinical trials. These are discussed later in this chapter.

SPECIFIC TYPES OF HEAD INJURIES

Injuries to the Scalp

The scalp is composed of five layers that cover the bone of the top of the skull (calvarium): (1) the dermal (skin) layer, (2) the subcutaneous fascia, (3) the galea aponeurotica, (4) layer of loose areolar tissue, and (5) the periosteum. The **dermal layer** has hair and protects the scalp from injury. The **subcutaneous fascia** is a tough fibrotic tissue with a vascular fatty layer that can bleed profusely when the scalp is lacerated. The **galea aponeurotica**, a sheetlike tendon layer, connects the frontalis and occipitalis muscles. Below the galea is the **subgaleal areolar space**, which contains emissary veins that empty into the venous sinus. It is a potential area for the development of hematomas. If an infection develops in this space, it can spread to the brain. The **periosteum**, located below the subgaleal space, is a very thin layer of tissue that can be stripped away from the skull.

Injuries to the scalp can be classified as follows:

- **Abrasion**: The top layer of the scalp is scraped away; this is a minor injury that may cause slight bleeding. The area is

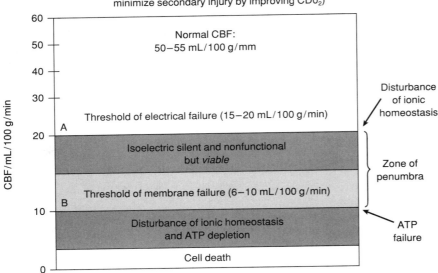

Ischemic penumbra: Conceptual Basis for Brain Resuscitation (Prevent or minimize secondary injury by improving CḊO₂)

FIGURE 21-5
Ischemic penumbra: conceptual basis for brain resuscitation (prevent or minimize secondary injury by improving CḊO₂).

cleaned and possibly dressed, and no other treatment is required.
- **Contusion**: The scalp is bruised with possible effusion of blood into the subcutaneous layer without a break in the integrity of the skin; there is no specific treatment.
- **Laceration**: The scalp is torn and may bleed profusely; suturing may be necessary.
- **Subgaleal hematoma**: This hematoma in the subgaleal layer of the scalp will usually absorb on its own.

DIAGNOSIS AND TREATMENT

The diagnosis of scalp injury is made by physical inspection. Abrasions require no specific treatment. A scalp contusion may benefit from the application of ice initially to prevent a hematoma from forming. Skull films may be ordered to rule out a skull fracture, but otherwise, no treatment is required.

All scalp lacerations are irrigated with saline and explored with a sterile gloved finger to determine whether a fracture or a foreign body is present. Severely contused tissue may need to be débrided. The subgaleal area is examined for hematomas. Small fractures are not always seen on x-ray studies but may be found by visualization and palpation. Evidence of bone fragments or a depressed skull fracture warrants surgical exploration in the operating room. Scalp lacerations often require suturing and aseptic management.

Injuries to the Skull

The skull is the bony framework of the head. The **cranium (calvarium)** is the part of the skull that encloses the brain; it is composed of the frontal, parietal, temporal, occipital, sphenoid, and ethmoid bones. The facial bones provide a framework for the face and include the maxillary, zygomatic, nasal, lacrimal, and palatine bones and the inferior nasal concha, vomer, mandible, and part of the ethmoid and sphenoid bones

(see Chap. 5, Fig. 5-6). The mandible is the only movable bone in the facial portion of the skull.

TYPES OF CRANIAL FRACTURES

Classification of skull fractures include **linear, comminuted, depressed,** and **basal** skull fractures. If there is an overlying scalp laceration, the fracture is considered open. The type of fracture produced depends on the velocity, direction, and momentum of the object causing the impact. With a *depressed skull fracture*, hair, dirt, and other debris may be found within the wound. The dura may or may not be torn. A *basal skull fracture* involves the base of the skull and may be a linear or a depressed fracture. Most often, a basal skull fracture arises from the extension of a linear fracture into the base of the skull. The frontal and temporal bones are usually affected so that the fracture involves the anterior or middle fossae.

Basal Skull Fracture. When considering fractures of the skull, it is important to distinguish between fractures of the cranial vault and those of the base of the skull. Although the mechanism by which the fractures arise is similar, the consequences of basilar fractures are more serious than those of cranial vault fractures.

A consequence of basal skull fractures is the frequency with which fractures traverse the paranasal air sinuses (frontal, maxillary, or ethmoid) of the frontal bone or the air sinuses located in the petrous portion of the temporal bone. The fragility of the bones in these areas and the intimate adherence of delicate dura account for the frequency of the lesion and the consequent leakage of cerebrospinal fluid (CSF) through the dural tear. Drainage of CSF from the nose is called **rhinorrhea,** whereas drainage of similar components from the ear is called **otorrhea.** When CSF drains from the paranasal sinuses, it drains into the postnasal area and is felt as a postnasal drip. The appearance of blood encircled by a yellowish stain on the dressing or bed linen is called the **halo sign** and is highly suggestive of blood encircled by CSF. Continued leakage of CSF is a serious problem because of the associated high risk for meningitis or abscess formation, which can result from organisms gaining entry by way of the ear, nose, or paranasal sinuses through the dural tear. In addition, osteomyelitis is another infection-related complication.

Two additional complications associated with basal skull fractures are worth mentioning. The first possible complication is associated with cerebrovascular injuries, including injury to the internal carotid artery at the point of entrance through the foramen in the base of the skull. Fracture in or around the foramen can result in cerebral hemorrhage from laceration, thrombosis, development of a traumatic aneurysm, a carotid-cavernous sinus fistula, or carotid-cavernous sinus compression. A carotid-cavernous sinus fistula is characterized by chemosis, bruit, and pulsating exophthalmos. The oculomotor, trochlear, trigeminal, and abducens cranial nerves pass through the cavernous sinus. Compression of the sinus may be evidenced by ophthalmoplegia or trigeminal dysfunction.

The second possible complication is the trapping of portions of the frontal arachnoid and dura between the fracture edges, creating a permanent route for leakage of CSF. Radiographical and surgical identification of the exact area of the dural tear is extremely difficult, yet such identification is necessary to facilitate surgical repair.

Diagnosis. A computed tomography (CT) scan and sometimes plain radiographs are used to diagnose skull fractures. The ease with which a diagnosis of skull fracture is made depends on the site of the fracture. If a fracture is found on x-ray, then there is always the question of associated brain injury and the need for a CT scan. For example, a linear fracture of the parietal bone may be readily evident on an x-ray, whereas thin-slice CT may be necessary to find a basal skull fracture. If the paranasal sinuses are fractured, air may be evident in the sinuses on x-ray studies. With fracture of the temporal bone, the mastoid sinuses may be opaque. Common physical findings include the following:

Anterior Fossa Fracture (Fracture of the Paranasal Sinuses)

- Rhinorrhea: CSF and blood
- Subconjunctival hemorrhage
- Periorbital ecchymosis (raccoon's eyes)

Middle Fossa (Associated With Fracture of the Temporal Petrous Bone)

- Otorrhea: CSF and blood
- Hemotympanum
- Battle's sign (ecchymosis over mastoid bone); does not usually develop for 12 to 24 hours
- Conductive hearing loss (may be associated with signs of vestibular dysfunction, such as vertigo, nausea, and nystagmus)
- Facial nerve palsy (Bell's palsy); appears 5 to 7 days after injury

Treatment. Treatment depends on the type of fracture. Generally, a linear skull fracture will not require special medical management other than observation for underlying cerebral injury. In the past, surgical débridement and elevation of depressed skull fractures were the norm. The aims of surgery were reduction of post-traumatic epilepsy, amelioration of associated neurological deficits, prevention of infection, and correction of cosmetic deformity. The indications for surgery continue to be refined, with the suggestion that conservative management is possible in all but the most contaminated wounds and comminuted and cosmetically deforming depressed fractures.[16] If a craniectomy is necessary, a cranioplasty with insertion of a bone or artificial graft may be done immediately or postponed for a few months (approximately 3–6 months) if cerebral edema is present.

Use of prophylactic antibiotics with basal skull fractures is controversial; many argue that prophylactic use allows for proliferation of other virulent organisms. Most CSF leaks resolve spontaneously within 7 to 10 days. To aid resolution of leakage lasting more than 4 to 5 days, a lumbar catheter for continual drainage of CSF may be inserted.[17] If leakage of CSF continues, a craniotomy may be necessary to repair the tear surgically or to repair the leakage with graphs.

TYPES OF FACIAL FRACTURES

Facial fracture is not uncommon with vehicular trauma, especially if the patient was an unrestrained driver or passenger. Injuries may involve the soft tissue (contusions, lacerations), the facial bones (fractures), or both. The facial bones include most of the paranasal sinuses and the primary receptor organs for the senses of vision, hearing, taste, and smell. Facial injuries can result in disfigurement, motor and sensory dysfunction, and deficits in communication. Table 21-1 summarizes the common facial fractures.

CRANIAL NERVE INJURIES ASSOCIATED WITH SKULL FRACTURES

Specific cranial nerves tend to be compressed or injured because of anatomical location, transection, and attachments. *Frontal bone fractures* are associated with olfactory nerve (most vulnerable) and sometimes optic nerve injury. Cribriform plate fractures often produce anosmia because of injury of the olfactory nerve. Orbital plate fractures may affect the optic and oculomotor nerves, resulting in loss of vision and impaired eye movement. The orbits are created by many bones that may be fractured in a head injury. Isolated lesions of the trochlear or abducens nerves are rare. *Temporal bone fractures* often result in facial nerve paralysis, the most commonly injured motor cranial nerve. Auditory nerve dysfunction of the cochlear or vestibular branches is seen with less frequency.

TREATMENT

Many facial fractures require surgical repair and reconstruction for cosmetic effects. A series of surgical procedures may be necessary to achieve the desired outcome. Timing of surgery depends on stabilization and management of other higher priority needs. Some studies have shown that early craniofacial repair can be performed safely with appropriate gen-

TABLE 21-1
Common Facial Fractures

BONE	FRACTURE	SIGNS AND SYMPTOMS
MANDIBLE • Only movable bone of the face • Composed of lower jaw and ramus portions • Lower jaw or chin, portion that contains the teeth • Ramus portion vertical with condyloid processes that fit into the temporomandibular joint	• Most frequently fractured facial bone • Because of its arched shape, fractures common in two places	• Malalignment of the teeth • Pain • Bruising and laceration over the fracture site • Ecchymosis in the floor of the mouth • Palpation of a "shelf" defect in the inferior border • Inability to palpate condylar movement when the little finger is placed in the external ear canal and the jaw is opened
MAXILLA • Holds upper teeth • Includes the palate • Forms a portion of the floor of the orbits • Forms part of the floor and outer wall of the nasal fossa • Meets the temporal and zygoma bones laterally • Contains maxillary sinus	• Involved in midface fractures (involves the maxillae, naso-orbital bones, and the zygomatic bones) • Midface fractures classified using the system devised by René Le Fort: —**Le Fort I** fracture—horizontal detachment of the maxilla at the nasal floor; leaves maxillary alveolar ridge of the hard palate mobile —**Le Fort II** fracture—pyramid-shaped fracture of the central part of the face; includes transverse fractures across the medial maxillae and nasal bones, medial half of the infraorbital rim, and the medial part of the orbit and orbital floor —**Le Fort III** fracture—separates the cranial and facial bones; includes a Le Fort II fracture along with fractures of both zygomatic bones so that the fracture line cuts through both orbits transversely	*Midface fractures* • Distortion of facial symmetry (elongated face, flattened naso-orbital area) • Possible pushing of the upper and lower molar teeth together • Inability to close jaw • Pain • Edema • Ecchymosis of the buccal mucosa in the lateral portions • Abnormal movement (free-floating maxillary segment) • Possible respiratory obstruction • Hemorrhage
ZYGOMA • Forms the prominence of the cheekbone • Forms part of the outer wall and floor of the orbit • Part of temporal and zygomatic fossa	• Often involved in midface fractures • Fractures of the zygoma often called tripod fractures because of their shape • Fracture of the zygoma always involves the orbits	• Flatness of the cheek • Loss of sensation on the side of the face of the fracture • Diplopia • Ophthalmoplegia
NASAL • Forms bridge of nose • Forms part of upper inner orbit	• May occur alone or in conjunction with orbital or Le Fort fractures	• Ecchymosis and edema of the dorsum of the nose • Nosebleed • Laceration
ORBITAL • Seven facial and cranial bones that form the orbits (frontal, maxillary, zygomatic, lacrimal, sphenoid, ethmoid, and palatine)	• Fracture with Le Fort fractures or, less frequently, as an orbital blow-out fracture • Blow-out fractures, result of a spike in intraorbital pressure caused by a blunt object (fist, baseball) directed at the globe; spike in pressure, fracture at the weakest point—the orbital floor or medial wall; the orbital contents may protrude into the maxillary sinus	*Blow-out fractures* • Sinking of the globe • Diplopia (secondary to injury of the extraocular muscles) • Ophthalmoplegia • Possible blindness (secondary to detached retina) • Edema • Ecchymosis of the eyelid • Conjunctival hemorrhage • Paresthesia

(Data from Bertz, J. [1981]. Maxillofacial injuries. Clinical Symposia 33(4), 1–32; Black, J., & Arnold, P. G. [1982]. Facial fractures. American Journal of Nursing, 82(7), 1086; and Lower, J. [1986]. Maxillofacial trauma. Nursing Clinics of North America, 21(4), 611–28.)

eral surgical and neurosurgical support in selected patients, avoiding costly delay and complications.[18]

Injuries to the Meninges

A tear of the dura mater can result from a basal skull fracture, depressed fractures involving the temporal or frontal bones, or some facial fractures. Leakage of CSF may occur from the ear or nose or postnasally. There may also be blood behind the tympanic membrane (hemotympanum). The diagnosis and treatment of dural injuries are discussed in a previous section.

Injuries to the Brain

Injuries to the brain can be divided into diffuse injuries and focal injuries.

DIFFUSE INJURIES

Diffuse injuries include concussion and DAI.

Concussions. The word **concussion** means to shake violently. A **cerebral concussion** is defined as a transient, temporary, neurogenic dysfunction caused by mechanical force to the brain. Signs and symptoms may include immediate unconsciousness lasting a few seconds, minutes, or hours; momentary loss of reflexes; and momentary (few seconds) and possible retrograde or antegrade amnesia (loss of memory for events immediately before and after the injury, respectively). Other common signs and symptoms include headache, drowsiness, confusion, dizziness, irritability, giddiness, visual disturbances (seeing stars), and gait disturbances.

Acceleration-deceleration (with shearing stress on the reticular formation) is the mechanism of injury. Patients who have sustained other head injuries, such as contusions, lacerations, and hematomas, have also sustained a concussion in most instances. Concussions are classified as mild or classic, based on the degree of symptoms, particularly those of unconsciousness and memory loss. **Mild concussion** is defined as temporary neurological dysfunction without loss of consciousness or memory. By contrast, a **classic concussion** includes temporary neurological dysfunction, unconsciousness, and memory loss. Recovery of consciousness usually takes minutes to hours. Some patients will develop a postconcussion syndrome (described later in this section).

DIAGNOSIS AND TREATMENT. The diagnosis of concussion is based on the patient's history, neurological examination, and absence of any focal lesion on a CT scan, if a CT scan is done. The patient is supported and observed to ensure that no other focal lesion, such as a subdural hematoma (SDH), has been overlooked.

Diffuse Axonal Injury. The important concept of DAI has undergone marked refinement in the last several years. **DAI** is a primary injury of diffuse microscopic damage to axons in the cerebral hemispheres, corpus callosum, and brain stem (Fig. 21-6). Axonal damage is further defined as balloonings (formerly termed retraction balls), microglial stars, long tract degeneration, and diffuse gliosis. Because of the gradient acceleration difference on certain areas during primary impact, shearing forces at the white-gray junction, corpus callosum, brain stem, and sometimes cerebellum result in diffuse tearing of axons and small blood vessels.[19,20] In addition, unilateral contusion is often associated with DAI. Two mechanisms help to explain the contusions. First, during angular acceleration, there is more movement and displacement of the gray cortical matter so that most of the tissue injury occurs at the white-gray junction with the resultant contusion. Second,

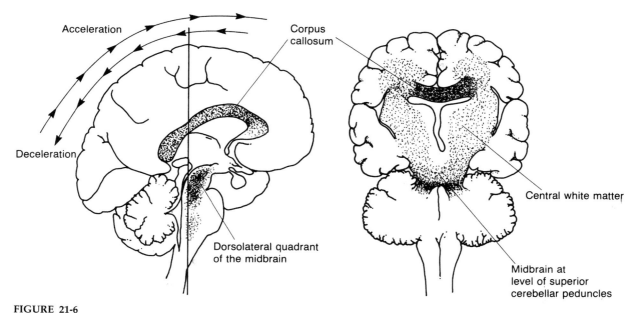

FIGURE 21-6
Diffuse axonal injury. Diffuse axonal injury results from acceleration-deceleration and shearing force on the brain. Depending on the severity of the injury, the areas of the brain most often affected are the corpus callosum, the dorsolateral area of the midbrain, and the parasagittal white matter.

the bridging veins are displaced during acceleration, which causes rupture and SDH.[21]

Of interest is the timeline for the development of particular microscopic axonal changes identified previously. *Axonal ballooning* takes 12 to 24 hours to develop and may persist for some time. The numbers and distribution vary with the severity of the head injury and survival time. *Microglial stars* are small clusters of hypertrophied microglia seen in intermediate survival (several days to weeks) and are associated with axonal ballooning. In long survival (several weeks to months) *long tract degeneration* of the wallerian type is seen. These three degenerative effects are finally replaced by *diffuse white matter gliosis*. Gliosis is the chief finding in long-term survivors (*e.g.,* 6 years).[22] Although these changes are microscopic events, the knowledge is helpful to appreciate the basis of severe, permanent disability in survivors of severe head injury. DAI can be classified as mild, moderate, or severe, depending on the amount of damage sustained; a three-stage severity grading system has been proposed. Patients who sustain mild DAI may have only mild long-term disability, while severe DAI is a cause of significant mortality and morbidity.

In the past, references had been made to brain stem injuries based on the clinical findings of immediate unconsciousness. It is now recognized that exclusive injury to the brain stem is rare and is probably more likely part of DAI.

DIAGNOSIS AND TREATMENT. Clinically, the patient presents with immediate coma, decortication or decerebration, and an initially low ICP. A magnetic resonance imaging (MRI) scan is more efficacious than a CT scan in detecting small DAI lesions.[23]

FOCAL INJURIES

Focal injuries include cerebral contusion, cerebral laceration, and intracerebral hemorrhage. The following anatomical considerations help to explain focal injuries to the brain.

The anterior and middle fossae at the base of the skull have irregular, bony buttresses that are capable of contusing or lacerating the brain on impact. The distribution of *contusions* in these particular areas is explained by the movement of the brain within the skull (Fig. 21-7). The frontal-temporal regions are most sensitive to shearing stress injury because of the relatively greater restraint created by the sphenoidal ridges and other irregularities of the base of the skull. The rotational forces created by movement of the brain cause shearing, tearing, and compression of cerebral tissue. Less common sites of injury are the inferolateral angles of the occipital lobes, the medial surfaces of the hemispheres, and the corpus callosum. The presence of the firm, membranous falx cerebri and tentorium cerebelli restrict movement of the brain. With a lateral blow in the frontal-temporal area, the brain may be contused or lacerated by the falx and tentorium so that surface contusion of the contralateral temporal lobe and corpus callosum can also be sustained. Injury to the inferolateral angles of the occipital lobe and less commonly, the inferior surface of the cerebellar and cerebral peduncles can occur as a result of impact by the tentorium. A blow to the vertex of the head may cause cerebellar, cerebellar tonsillar, and brain stem contusions initiated by the downward thrust of the brain toward the foramen magnum.

Cerebral Contusions. A **cerebral contusion** is a bruising of the surface of the brain (cerebral parenchyma). Contusions may occur from blunt trauma, causing depressed skull fractures beneath which contusion or intracerebral hematoma (ICH) occur; penetrating wounds; or acceleration-deceleration closed injuries. With acceleration-deceleration, the sites of injury are generally predictable and are located where the brain impacts on the bony protuberances of the skull (see Fig. 21-7). These areas include the frontal poles, frontal-orbital areas, the frontal-temporal junction around the Sylvian fissure (where the brain is close to the lesser sphenoidal wings), and the temporal poles (the inferior and lateral surfaces of the temporal lobes

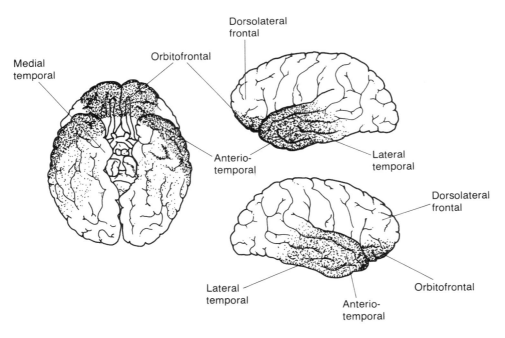

FIGURE 21-7
Cerebral contusions. The most frequently involved areas of the brain for cerebral contusions are the orbitofrontal and anteriotemporal regions. These are the areas that come in direct contact with the irregular bony surfaces in the inside frontal skull area.

where there is a shelflike separation between the anterior and middle fossae). Contusions may be coup or contrecoup depending on the degree of acceleration-deceleration and area involved. ICHs and contusions are sometimes difficult to differentiate. The mechanisms by which traumatic ICHs and large contusions are predicted are similar.

The clinical effect of a contusion depends on its size and related cerebral edema. Small, unilateral, frontal lesions may be asymptomatic, whereas larger lesions may result in a frontal lobe syndrome of inappropriate behavior and cognitive deficits. Contusions can cause secondary mass effect from edema, a subsequent increased ICP, and possible herniation syndromes when cerebral edema is reached.

DIAGNOSIS AND TREATMENT. The CT scan will identify most contusions. Increased ICP and specific conditions related to the lesion are treated. Depending on the degree of injury, some patients will develop post-traumatic seizures or functional deficits, requiring rehabilitation.

Cerebral Laceration. **Cerebral laceration** refers to a traumatic tearing of the cortical surface of the brain. The circumstances surrounding a contusion and laceration are similar, and they may be found together.

DIAGNOSIS AND TREATMENT. The diagnosis and treatment of cerebral laceration are similar to those described for contusions.

Intracranial Hemorrhage. Traumatic intracranial hemorrhage is a common complication of head injury. Hemorrhage can occur beneath a fracture (either a depressed fracture or nondepressed fracture) or from an acceleration-deceleration injury in which there is shearing of the bridging veins or of a cortical artery. As a result, hemorrhage into the epidural, subdural, or subarachnoid spaces or ventricles can occur.

Although bleeding may begin immediately after injury, its presence may not be clinically apparent until the bleeding is of a sufficient amount to cause signs and symptoms of a space-occupying lesion and mass effect. The interval between bleeding and the appearance of clinical symptoms may be minutes or weeks, depending on the site and rate of bleeding. Intracranial hemorrhage may be an occult development in a patient who has sustained a seemingly minor head injury in which consciousness has been maintained or quickly restored. Other patients with hemorrhage may be unconscious from the moment of impact.

The following describes the major types of bleeding associated with head trauma: EDH, SDH, ICH, and subarachnoid and intraventricular hemorrhage. It is useful to think of these lesions as distinct clinical entities, but two or more types of hemorrhagic lesions can coexist.[24]

Epidural Hematoma. An **EDH**, also known as an extradural hematoma, refers to bleeding into the potential space between the inner table of the skull (inner periosteum) and the dura mater (Fig. 21-8A). As the hematoma enlarges, it gradually strips away the dura from the inner table of the skull, and a large, ovoid mass develops, creating pressure on the underlying brain and causing a mass effect. Most patients who develop an EDH have sustained a skull fracture to the thin, squamous portion of the temporal bone, under which is located the middle meningeal artery. A lacerated middle meningeal artery or one of its branches is the source of hemorrhage, although venous injury can also cause this hematoma. EDHs are seen most often in children and young people because the dura is less firmly attached to the bone table than it is in older people. EDHs account for about 2% to 6% of post-traumatic intracranial lesions.

SIGNS AND SYMPTOMS. Clinically, the classic description of an EDH is that of momentary unconsciousness followed by a lucid period lasting for minutes to a few hours. Rarely, the

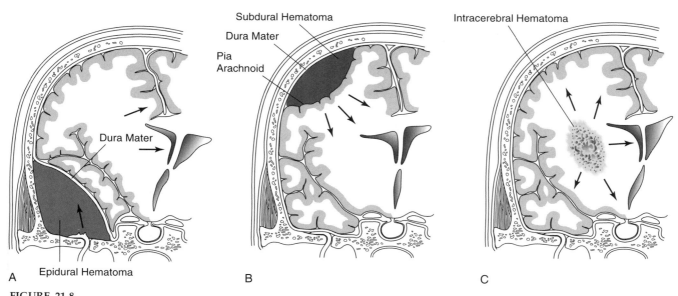

FIGURE 21-8
Cerebral hematomas: (*A*) an epidural hematoma, (*B*) a subdural hemotoma, and (*C*) an intracerebral hematoma.

interval can last for a few days when venous bleeding is involved. The lucid period is followed by rapid deterioration in the level of consciousness (drowsiness, confusion, coma) as mass effect and herniation develop. Other symptoms include pupillary signs (ipsilateral dilated, sluggish, fixed), headache, possible seizures, hemiparesis or hemiplegia, and decortication or decerebration. Although the lucid interval is generally considered to be characteristic of an EDH, in at least 15% of patients, there is no lucid period.

DIAGNOSIS AND TREATMENT. Diagnosis is by CT scan; MRI is also accurate. These clots often produce a large mass effect and a neurosurgical emergency.[25] Small EDHs may reabsorb spontaneously and not require surgery.

Subdural Hematoma. SDH refers to bleeding between the dura mater and arachnoid or pial layer (see Fig. 21-8*B*). Approximately 29% of patients with post-traumatic intracranial lesions have SDHs. A majority of SDHs are caused by tearing of the bridging veins located over the convexity of the brain. Other causes include tearing of small cortical arteries, cerebral contusions, and acute bleeding into chronic SDHs.[26] Bilateral SDHs are not uncommon. SDHs are subdivided into three categories based on the interval between injury and the appearance of signs and symptoms. The classifications and approximate intervals for the appearance of symptoms are as follows:

- *Acute*—up to 48 hours. This consists of clotted blood that is hypodense on CT.
- *Subacute*—2 days to about 3 weeks. The clot now lyses, and blood products and fluid are present.
- *Chronic*—about 3 weeks to several months. The clot is a fluid and is hypodense on CT.

SIGNS AND SYMPTOMS. The most common signs and symptoms associated with *acute SDH* are gradual deterioration of the level of consciousness from drowsiness, slow cerebration, and confusion to coma; pupillary signs; and hemiparesis or hemiplegia. *Subacute SDHs* are associated with less severe underlying contusions. Failure of a patient to regain consciousness raises the suspicion of an SDH. The level of consciousness is not improved when an SDH is present because of unrelenting cerebral pressure. Signs and symptoms correspond closely to those of the acute SDH.

Chronic SDHs can develop from seemingly minor head injuries. The lapse of time between injury and the development of symptoms may be months, so the initial injury may not be recalled. The lesion becomes encased within a membrane that is easily separated from the arachnoid and dura. The SDH slowly increases in size, probably due to repeated small bleeding, until a mass effect occurs. The most common symptoms of a chronic SDH include headache (progressing in severity), slow cerebration, confusion, drowsiness, and possibly a seizure. Papilledema, sluggish ipsilateral pupillary response, and finally hemiparesis may develop.

Elderly patients, because of the cerebral atrophy associated with the normal aging process, are prone to develop SDHs because of traction on the fragile bridging veins that are increasingly prone to tear and rupture with cerebral trauma. Atrophy also provides more free space into which bleeding can occur before symptoms are evident from a mass effect.

With chronic SDHs, the development of symptoms can be subtle because of gradual spatial compensation. The same can be said for chronic alcoholic patients, because they undergo a process of cerebral atrophy and are especially prone to SDHs.

DIAGNOSIS AND TREATMENT. The diagnosis of SDH is established by CT scan. A small SDH may be treated medically because they frequently reabsorb without surgical intervention. With large SDHs, surgical evacuation is necessary because of mass effect, increased ICP, and impending herniation. Elderly patients and people with long-term alcohol abuse who have had an evacuation of an SDH tend to rebleed.

Burr holes for the hematoma evacuation are usually created for an acute SDH. However, with some subacute and all chronic SDHs, a craniotomy will be necessary because the SDH has become gelatinous and encased in a membrane that must be dissected away from the dura and arachnoid layers.

Intracerebral Hematoma. An **ICH** refers to bleeding into the cerebral parenchyma, a complication seen in 4% to 15% of brain-injured patients[27] (see Fig. 21-8*C*). Most ICHs are related to contusions and therefore tend to occur in the frontal and temporal lobes and by the same mechanisms as contusions. Clinically, ICHs behave as expanding, space-occupying lesions. Serial CT scanning has demonstrated recognition of delayed traumatic ICHs in about 1% to 7% of patients. **Delayed traumatic ICHs** occur hours to days after head injury following an interval during which no hematoma was present.[28] The pathogenesis of these lesions is controversial, but it is generally believed that the bleeding is into existent traumatized areas, such as a contusion. ICHs are associated with poor outcomes and mortality.

SIGNS AND SYMPTOMS. Unconsciousness, which occurs at the onset of bleeding, may also be attributable to the accompanying serious contusions and lacerations. Signs and symptoms include headache, deteriorating consciousness progressing to deep coma, hemiplegia on the contralateral side, and a dilated pupil on the side of the clot. As ICP increases, there is evidence of developing tentorial herniation with accompanying changes in pupils, respirations, and other vital signs.

DIAGNOSIS AND TREATMENT. Diagnosis is established by CT scan. Treatment is individualized. A craniotomy with ICH evacuation has been beneficial in a few cases, primarily because widespread cerebral contusion is usually present.

Subarachnoid and Intraventricular Hemorrhage. A traumatic subarachnoid hematoma is rare; however, subarachnoid hemorrhage is a common finding in severe head injury. Intraventricular hemorrhage occurs secondary to subarachnoid hemorrhage or as an extension from an ICH.

Signs and symptoms are related to increased ICP and irritation of the meninges. Nuchal rigidity, headache, a deteriorating level of consciousness, hemiparesis or hemiplegia, and an ipsilateral dilated pupil are the signs and symptoms commonly seen. Hemorrhage is evident on CT scan. Treatment includes drainage of CSF with a ventriculostomy.

Injury to Blood Vessels. In addition to intracranial hemorrhage (hematomas, subarachnoid hemorrhage), injury to and tears of cerebral blood vessels can cause vasospasm, resulting in focal ischemia. Subsequent to an intracranial hematoma, vessels can also be compressed from the traumatic mass or from localized cerebral edema. In addition, cerebral blood vessels may become thrombosed or occluded or may give rise to traumatic aneurysms from being stretched or torn at the time of injury.

PENETRATING INJURIES

Missile Injuries. Missile injuries are most often inflicted by guns and bullets. The wound created by the bullet depends on the ballistics, that is, the size, shape, velocity, direction, and effect of the bullet. As the bullet is propelled and penetrates the skull, it compresses the air in front of it, thereby increasing the destruction of brain tissue locally and remotely. Missile injuries have been described as *tangential injuries*, in which the missile does not enter the cranial cavity but produces a depressed skull fracture, scalp laceration, and meningeal and cerebral contusion-laceration; *penetrating injuries*, in which the missile enters the cranial cavity but does not pass through it, resulting in the presence of metal, bone fragments, hair, and skin within the brain; and *through-and-through injuries*, in which the missile perforates the cranial contents and leaves through an exit wound. Usually, one tract is created from a missile entering the brain, while several tracts are possible intracranially if the bullet ricochets.

The major effects of missile injuries are cerebral contusions and lacerations, focal tissue necrosis, hemorrhage from tearing of blood vessels, and focal or generalized cerebral edema. Hemorrhage and edema may produce increased ICP and possible herniation associated with rapid expansion during impact and in response to a space-occupying lesion. The severity of injury sustained depends on the structures involved and herniation. Infections, such as meningitis and brain abscess, are postinjury concerns.

DIAGNOSIS AND TREATMENT. The history and evidence of an entrance and possible exit gunshot wounds are important indicators of injury. Skull films and CT scan are necessary to determine the amount of injury, identify bone fragments and site of the bullet if it did not exit, and plan the surgical approach if contemplated. Emergency surgical intervention is common for the following reasons: to evacuate hematomas, such as EDH or SDH; to débride the wound and remove the bullet and necrotic tissue; and to treat other system injuries caused by bullets or trauma. Secondary brain injury can occur as a result of hypoxia and hypotension related to hemorrhage in other body systems. Antibiotics are ordered because of the risk of infection.

Impalement Injuries. To *impale* means to pierce with something pointed. **Impalement injuries** of the head refer to piercing of the scalp, skull, or brain by a foreign object, such as an ice pick.

·DIAGNOSIS AND TREATMENT. Skull films are necessary to determine the object's angle and depth or penetration, and a CT assesses intracranial trauma. Any foreign object protruding from the skull should be left in place until it can be removed by a neurosurgeon in a setting where bleeding can be controlled. In the meantime, the object should be supported

to prevent further damage to the tissue. Because the patient is at high risk for infection, antibiotics are ordered.

MANAGEMENT OF THE HEAD-INJURED PATIENT: THE CONTINUUM OF CARE

The continuum of care begins at the trauma scene and continues until the final outcome. Care is along a continuum regardless of setting, and continuity between settings and transitions is key to optimal, cost-effective outcomes. The guiding conceptual basis for care is prevention of secondary brain injury through nervous system and other body system support and interventions.

Prehospital Management

Prehospital management refers to the initial resuscitation and stabilization interventions at the injury scene and en route to the hospital; it has profound impact on the subsequent course of events and outcomes. The conceptual basis for timely and effective brain resuscitation is the minimal reserve of the brain to meet ongoing metabolic needs. When faced with insufficient substrates as a result of insufficient CBF and cerebral oxygen delivery, ischemia and hypoxia precipitate the pathophysiological processes described previously in this chapter. As a result, secondary injury causes further injury to the brain. Therefore, timely, skillful, and thorough resuscitation measures are critical for salvaging brain tissue, preventing secondary injury, and promoting optimal outcomes.

The American College of Surgeons has set national standards and developed Advanced Trauma Life Support (ATLS) training programs to manage trauma victims effectively. Emergency medical services systems are designed to provide timely resuscitation and stabilization by well trained personnel who can rapidly triage and transport victims to the *appropriate* health care facility. The emergency medical system includes telecommunication linkages with personnel at the health care facility where collaborative data analysis and clinical decision making occur through consultation that guides patient management at the trauma site and during transport. Because many head-injured patients sustain multisystem trauma, patients must be assessed systematically for evidence of these injuries.

Emergency management is directed toward maintaining cerebral metabolic needs, preventing and treating intracranial hypertension (induced hypocarbia, fluid control, and diuretics), and supporting other body systems. Establishing and maintaining a patent airway (possible intubation) and circulation to meet cerebral metabolic needs by preventing cerebral hypoxia and cerebral ischemia are critical. Maneuvers to maintain airway patency must be modified to prevent cervical injuries. Treating all head-injured patients for possible cervical fractures or spinal injury by immediate head and neck immobilization cannot be overemphasized. All emergency medical personnel must be mindful of the disastrous consequences (cord transection, quadriplegia, death) associated with neck manipulation.

Emergency Department or Trauma Center Management

On arrival at the health care facility, many concurrent and simultaneous activities are initiated by a well trained team of health professionals. Activity includes inserting peripheral and central lines and an indwelling urinary catheter, attaching monitoring equipment, and conducting primary and secondary trauma surveys. The history and circumstances of injury and previous treatment are verified, clarified, and amplified. The following are examples of important information to consider:

- Circumstances of injury (direct blow to head, thrown from car, fell off bar stool)
- Seat belt or helmet worn (type of seat belt: lap or shoulder)
- How patient was found (*e.g.*, lying face down)
- Unconsciousness (immediate; lucid period)
- Documented apnea or cyanosis and length of time
- Significant blood loss at the scene

PRIMARY AND SECONDARY SURVEY

The ATLS manual[29] provides a framework for primary and secondary trauma surveys and for assessment of head injuries. Primary and secondary surveys are conducted according to ATLS standards. The following cautions need to be considered with head-injured patients when conducting primary surveys:

Patent Airway Maintenance

- All *unconscious* head-injured patients are intubated to prevent aspiration. Note: Tracheal intubation may be contraindicated in cases of midface trauma and sometimes with basal skull fractures.
- Intubation technique reflects consideration of potential cervical fracture or spinal cord injury and should be done only by trained personnel.
- The nose and mouth are suctioned of blood, mucus, and drainage to ensure airway patency; nasal suctioning is not done if a basal skull fracture is suspected.
- The airway is suctioned as necessary; suctioning is limited to 15 seconds or less per pass.
- Aspiration related to trauma is very common. Aspiration may be present even with negative early chest x-rays.

Breathing. Once an airway is established, breathing is assessed, and measures are instituted to support respirations and adequate oxygenation. Oxygen therapy is implemented, and often a ventilator is needed.

Circulation. Pulses, capillary refill, continuous electrocardiographic (EKG) monitoring, and arterial pressure are assessed. Hypotension is disastrous to the brain and must be aggressively treated. The underlying cause must be determined, such as occult bleeding. If hypertension is present, it is usually related to the head injury and is managed with an increased ICP protocol (Chart 21-3).

Once the patient is stabilized, the **secondary survey** is conducted.

ASSESSMENT FOR HEAD INJURES

The following are key elements for assessment of head injuries:

- History and circumstances of injury
- Initial assessment (**a**irway with cervical spine control, **b**reathing, and **c**irculation)
- Assessment of vital signs (hypotension, often related to other system injuries, is disastrous); patterns such as Cushing's response associated with increased ICP (see Chart 21-3)
- AVPU (the level of consciousness: **A**, alert; **V**, response to **v**ocal stimuli; **P**, response to **p**ainful stimuli; and **U**, **u**nresponsive)
- Minineurological examination
GCS (see Chart 21-3 for severity of injury)
Pupillary size and response
Motor function (lateralization suggests focal lesion)

LABORATORY STUDIES AND OTHER DIAGNOSTICS

The following lists laboratory studies for the initial resuscitation and treatment of *severe head-injured people* (GCS 8 or less):

- Complete blood count (CBC), arterial blood gases, electrolytes, glucose, creatinine, and blood urea nitrogen
- Drug screen, optional
- Chest x-ray
- Cervical spine films (to rule out cervical fractures or unstable vertebral column)
- CT scan (done as soon as possible)
- Peritoneal lavage
- Other emergent diagnostic studies

The CT scan is the gold standard for head injury diagnosis, and most patients will require at CT at some time. It will be done immediately on admission or postponed until the patient is stabilized. A CT scan can identify a depressed skull fracture, EDH, SDH, ICH, contusion, and most DAIs. If a lesion is found, the patient will go to the operating room emergently for burr holes, a craniotomy, elevation of a depressed fracture, or craniectomy. If there is no lesion requiring surgery, transfer is to the intensive care unit (ICU).

RESUSCITATION

The initial brain resuscitation[30] treatment for severe head injury is directed at controlling the intracranial hypertension caused by cerebral edema, cerebral ischemia, cerebral hyperemia, and an expanding lesion, if present. The management includes endotracheal intubation to protect the airway and facilitate hyperventilation. In addition, drainage of CSF if a ventriculostomy is in place, mannitol, and hyperventilation are the key interventions available for emergency management of intracranial hypertension. Use of oxygen, sedation or neuromuscular blockade, seizure management, and hyperthermia control are all designed to optimize oxygen supply by controlling activities known to increase cerebral metabolic rate of oxygen consumption ($CMRO_2$) and therefore increase demand for oxygen by the brain.

CHART 21-3
Vital Signs and Their Significance in a Head-Injured Patient

Respirations

- Head injuries can result in abnormal respiratory patterns that roughly correlate with the level of neurological dysfunction (see Chap. 8 for a discussion of abnormal patterns and level of injury).
- In general, an initial increase in intracranial pressure (ICP) results in slowing of respirations. If the rise in ICP continues, the pattern becomes rapid and noisy until the end, when respirations cease.
- A few conditions can affect respirations:
  —Complications of metabolic disorders, such as diabetic acidosis, can change respiratory patterns (Kussmaul's respirations).
  —Injuries to the cervical spine below C-4 can cause respiratory difficulty, whereas injuries above C-4, the site of phrenic nerve innervation, can cause total arrest.

Blood Pressure

- Hypotension is rarely attributable to cerebral injury.
  —*Hypotension and tachycardia* are seen as terminal events in head injury.
  —*Hypotension and tachycardia* in a patient who is not terminal is usually related to occult bleeding, most likely in the abdominal, pelvic, or thoracic cavity.
  —*Note:* The inherent risk of hypotension involves its relationship to CBF, CPP, and subsequent hypoperfusion and ischemia CCP. Hypoperfusion is associated with CPP.
  —*Hypotension and bradycardia* may be a secondary response to cervical cord injury if the descending sympathetic pathways have been interrupted.
- Hypertension is commonly associated with ↑ ICP; it may also be associated with pain, fear, or anxiety.
  —*Hypertension and bradycardia* are associated with ↑ ICP; they are late signs that correlate with pressure on the brain stem.
  - *Cushing's response* is an ischemic response of the body that maintains cerebral blood flow in the presence of rising ICP. Cushing's response includes hypertension, bradycardia, and a widening pulse pressure.
  - *Cushing's triad* includes hypertension, bradycardia, and an irregular respiratory pattern; it reflects a rising ICP in which there is direct pressure on the medullary center of the brain stem. It is often seen in the terminal stage and is associated with irreversible brain stem damage.

Pulse

- Pulse has been discussed in conjunction with blood pressure.
- *Bradycardia* is associated with increasing ICP or cervical injury.
- *Tachycardia* is associated with the following:
  —Occult (non-neurological) hemorrhage or hypovolemic shock
  —An autonomic response to injury of the hypothalamus or its connections
  —A terminal event in severe head injury

Temperature

- *Hypothermia* can occur as a result of hypothalamic injury, because the hypothalamus is the heat regulatory center of the brain. The patient will assume the temperature of the ambient room air; if it is cold, body temperature will drop. Hypothermia (96°–97°F) is also seen early in cervical cord injuries.
- *Hyperthermia* in the head-injured patient can be associated with direct injury to the hypothalamus or petechial bleeding into the hypothalamus or pons. Hyperthermia must be controlled because it *increases* the metabolic rate of all body cells, including the brain.
  —Oxygen consumption rises 10% for every 1°C rise in temperature.
  - A rise from 37°C (98.6°F) to 40.5°C (105°F) results in a 35% increase in oxygen consumption.
  - This can result in ischemia for the injured brain that was barely meeting metabolic needs when the temperature was within normal range.

(CBF = cerebral blood flow; CPP = cerebral prefusion pressure.)

In summary, the management of the head-injured patient in the emergency department is directed at resuscitation, stabilization, and establishment of a diagnosis. Once these steps have been completed, a decision is made regarding immediate surgical intervention for life-threatening problems or transfer to the ICU for medical management.

Intensive Care Unit Management of Severe Head-Injured Patients

The patient with a severe head injury (GCS of 8 or less) who does not require immediate surgery will be admitted to the ICU. Patients who go to surgery are admitted to the ICU postoperatively. Those who are physiologically unstable or need frequent monitoring and observation need to be managed in an ICU environment. The goals of care are to manage intracranial hypertension, maintain adequate cerebral oxygen delivery to meet cerebral metabolic needs, improve CBF, and manage other systemic problems.

Patients are usually admitted to an interdisciplinary severe head trauma care map to guide care. The case manager or discharge planner, nurse, and physician must work closely together to move the patient along in the continuum of care. By using the interdisciplinary collaboration model, comprehensive assessment and treatment are provided. In addition to the nursing staff, other disciplines may be involved, including physical therapy, occupational therapy, speech therapy, pharmacy, nutritional support, and social services. As the various disciplines work with the patient, identification of care needs following discharge from the acute care setting are formulated (see Chap. 15 for transitions and discharge). In the ICU environment, management is directed toward prevention of secondary brain injury and prevention of other system complications that can contribute to morbidity, mortality, and increased costs.

INTRAHOSPITAL TRANSPORT OF INTENSIVE CARE UNIT PATIENTS

Nurses in clinical practice all have stories of patients "going bad" either during transport for diagnostic procedures or during the actual procedure at a distance from equipment and resources to stabilize the patients. "Going bad" means that some significant physiological deterioration occurs that may be life threatening. A number of articles have recently appeared addressing the risks associated with intrahospital transport.[31] Patients who are not physiologically stable should not be transported without sufficient personnel, monitoring, and resuscitative equipment to manage changes.

MONITORING AND TECHNOLOGY

On admission to the ICU, the patient may be placed on a special therapeutic bed and will be connected to a physiological monitoring system. A number of possible invasive monitoring lines may be used, including an arterial line, central venous pressure catheter, pulmonary catheter, ventriculostomy, ICP catheter, and possibly a retrograde jugular catheter; they will probably be inserted at this time.

The nurse is responsible for knowing how to use and troubleshoot the equipment, interpret the data collected, and use this information in clinical reasoning and decision making. The patient will also be connected to a mechanical ventilator using the endotracheal tube, cardiac monitoring leads, sequential compression boots, peripheral oximeter, and rectal temperature probe. If the cervical spine has not already been cleared, then that will be done as soon as possible. (Precautions should be taken to treat as a cervical spinal injury until cleared.) A nasogastric (NG) tube is inserted unless there is an anterior fossa basilar skull or midface fracture. With an anterior fossa basilar skull fracture, an NG tube can be inserted through the mouth and guided by a laryngoscope to avoid passing the tube through the fracture area into the brain. The NG tube should be inserted after the endotracheal tube is in position because the insertion of an NG tube may cause vomiting and aspiration.

Maintaining physiological parameters to achieve therapeutic target goals is a *collaborative* effort. Each physiological target goal is set either as a range, such as maintaining the MAP between 90 and 100 mm Hg, or as a critical threshold, such as maintaining CPP at 70 mm Hg or above. To maintain the targeted goals, the nurse many need to titrate drugs (*e.g.*, dopamine to a set cardiac output), suction in response to a declining systemic arterial oxygen saturation (SaO_2), or reposition the patient's neck in response to noisy respirations (partial obstructed airway). The goal of setting and maintaining physiological targets is to optimize physiological function and prevent complications that can lead to secondary brain injury.

TITRATION TO DESIRED TARGETED PHYSIOLOGICAL GOALS

The central goal of therapy is to maintain an adequate CBF and CPP to meet the $CMRO_2$ and cerebral oxygen delivery (CDO_2) needs (Table 21-2). The CPP is calculated as MAP − ICP = CPP. Typically, the critical threshold for CPP is >70 mm Hg. To achieve it, the MAP will need to be manipulated to be high enough to account for an elevated ICP. Titration of drug to desired effect is the usual therapeutic approach. When selecting drugs for use with any type of brain injury, its effects on autoregulation, CBF, $CMRO_2$, CPP, and effects on other organs need to be carefully considered. Some drugs should not be used for this patient population. Consultation with the pharmacist is very helpful in drug selection.

NEWER MONITORING TECHNIQUES

Arterial and central lines and pulmonary and ICP catheters are a mainstay of the ICU monitoring options. Newer monitoring techniques include jugular venous oxygen saturation ($SjvO_2$) monitoring, transcranial Doppler studies, and evoked potentials.

Jugular Venous Oxygen Saturation. The goal of treatment for severe head injury is to provide a continuous and adequate oxygen supply to meet cerebral metabolic needs. Insertion of a retrograde catheter into the bulb of the internal jugular vein for continuous $SjvO_2$ saturation monitoring provides data about the saturation of the venous blood leaving the brain and

TABLE 21-2
Cerebral Oxygen Determinants and Values

Determinants	Approximate Values
• Cerebral flood flow (CBF)	50–55 mL/100 g/min
• Systemic arterial oxygen saturation (SaO$_2$)	20 mL/100 mL
• Cerebral oxygen delivery (CDO$_2$) = CBF × SaO$_2$	10 mL/100 g/min
• Cerebral arterial-venous oxygen content difference (AVDO$_2$) = CBF/CMRO$_2$	5.0–7.5 mL/100 mL
• Cerebral metabolic rate of oxygen conmsumption (CMRO$_2$) = CBF × AVDO$_2$	3.2 mL/100 g/min
• Jugular venous oxygen content (CjvO$_2$)	13 mL/100 mL
• Jugular venous oxygen saturation (SjvO$_2$)	60%–80%
• Cerebral perfusion pressure (CPP) desired level CPP = MAP – ICP	>70 mm Hg
• Mean arterial pressure (MAP) desired level set to maintain adequate CPP $$Map = \frac{systolic - diastolic}{3} + diastolic$$	

the arterial-jugular oxygen content difference to identify cerebral ischemia or increased CBF (hyperemia). The catheter is oximetric and may be inserted into the jugular bulb on the dominant side, side of injury, or bilaterally. The jugular bulb receives venous blood from the brain with minimal contamination for extracerebral origins.[32] The retrograde jugular catheter provides a means for monitoring consumption and delivery of oxygen by monitoring oxygen extraction in three ways: *calculating* cerebral oxygen extraction; *calculating* arteriovenous difference in oxygen; or *monitoring* SjvO$_2$. Continuous monitoring of jugular venous oxygen saturation provides the earliest identification of cerebral hypoxia or ischemia.[33-35] Normal values for SjvO$_2$ are about 60% to 80%.

Transcranial Doppler Studies. One of the newer technologies gaining acceptance for bedside assessment is transcranial Doppler studies. This is a noninvasive technique that will examine the flow of cerebral blood through the major cerebral arteries, most frequently the middle cerebral artery. It measures flow velocities, determines the pulse index, and can determine the presence of vasospasm. By collecting baseline data followed by a series of daily or every other day data collection, a determination of adequacy of blood flow, response to therapy, and prognosis can be made.

Electroencephalogram. The role of electrophysiological monitoring has grown—the continuous EEG monitoring is gaining acceptance at the bedside. Several EEG patterns have been described that have been correlated with distinct levels of coma and prognostic information. Using compressed spectral array technology, EEG data are compressed into an array of tracings that illustrate a spectrum of frequencies and power. This makes it easier to manage and analyze data. In head-injured patients, particularly those who are sedated or neuromuscularly blocked, seizure activity may be present without accompanying motor activity. The EEG is useful to identify these patients. In the future, the application of EEG monitoring is expected to expand and be used to identify early trends of ischemia and vasospasm.

Other Studies. Evoked potential, like EEG, is an indirect way of assessing the neurophysiological function of the nervous system after head injury. The use of evoked potentials hinges on continued refinement of recording and analytic methods to use the data effectively. Evoked potentials continue to be used in clinical practice. Although the Kety-Schmidt method is still the standard by which all other methods are compared, recently two continuous measurements of local CBF have become available. One uses thermal diffusion technology, and the other uses laser Doppler technology. Bedside use will provide a way for repeated measures of CBF that will help in calculating CMRO$_2$. This will be helpful for monitoring progress; response to interventions, such as hyperventilation and drugs; and prognostic outcomes.[36]

MANAGEMENT OF INTRACRANIAL HYPERTENSION

The basic strategies for ICU management of intracranial hypertension are summarized in Table 21-3. Medical therapeutics are the domain of medical practice, maintaining physiological target goals is a collaborative effort, and specific nursing interventions are within the independent domain of the nursing practice.

Medical management strategies are organized into two categories: conventional treatments and treatments for intracranial hypertension refractory to conventional therapies. The conventional therapies are organized in a sequence based on a risk-benefit ratio as suggested by Chestnut.[37] The following briefly discusses the management of increased ICP and maintenance of adequate cerebral oxygen delivery. A thorough discussion of increased ICP management is found in Chapter 17; therapies for refractory ICP are also found in Chapter 17 and are not discussed here.

Cerebrospinal Fluid Drainage. Many patients with severe head injuries will have a ventriculostomy inserted for drainage of CSF. Concurrently, the patient has an ICP monitor in place. The order to drain CSF is set to a particular ICP, most

TABLE 21-3
Early Management of Severe Brain Injury (GCS 8 or less) Focus on Increased ICP Management

Medical Therapeutics: Medical Management	Maintain Physiological Parameters: Collaborative Effort	Nursing Interventions: Independent Nursing Practice
• Mechanical ventalatory support • Oxygen 20%–40% • Hyperventilation: $PaCO_2$ 30–35 • Mannitol (0.25–1.0 g/kg) bolus • Indwelling urinary catheter • Sedation • Analgesics • Neuromuscular blockage • Treat seizures or prophylaxis for high risk • Fluid replacement with saline • Intracranial pressure (ICP) monitoring • Possible ventriculostomy for drainage if ICP >20 mm Hg	• PaO_2: 90–100 mm Hg • $PaCO_2$: 27–30 mm Hg • SaO_2: 92–100 • MAP: 90–100 mm Hg; to support CPP > 70 mm Hg • Maintain systolic 140–160 mm Hg • CPP: >70 mm Hg • ICP <20 mm Hg • CO: 4–6 L/min • CI: >3.0 L/min • SVR: • CVP: 8–10 mm Hg • PWCP: 14–16 • Serum Osm: <320 • Hct: <320 • Normal glucose • Normal electrolytes • Hgb: >10 g • Normothermia • Urine-specific gravity • Adequate urinary output/h • Tightly controlled intake and output balance for euvolemia • Arterial blood gases	• Elevate head of bed to 30 degrees. • Maintain neutral head position. • Maintain patent airway: suction prn (<15 sec/insertion). • Turn q2h from side to side. • Control noxious stimuli. • Oxygenate before and after suctioning. • Perform chest PT q2h. • Prevent Valsalva's maneuver. • Do not hyperventilate when suction; maintain normal $PaCO_2$. • Possible blockade when suction. • Frequently monitor vital neurological signs; look for deviation trends. • Treat ↑ temperature aggressively. • Control coughing. • Control asynchrony with vent. • Prevent shivering.

SECOND LINE: REFRACTORY TO CONVENTIONAL RX
• Hyperventilation: $PaCO_2$ 27–30
• Barbiturate coma
• Hypothermia
• Decompression craniectomy
• Hypertensive therapy

often, 20 mm Hg. Some physicians may set a lower level for drainage, such as 15 mm Hg. Unit protocol for draining should be followed. The protocol should identify the duration of time to drain (*e.g.*, 5 minutes) and points of documentation. During drainage, the ICP waveform is lost with some types of ventriculostomy systems. The color of the drainage should be monitored (*e.g.*, very bloody, pinkish).

Sedation, Analgesics, Neuromuscular Blockade. When evaluating potential drugs, effect on $CMRO_2$, CBF, ICP, cardiovascular function, respiratory function, toxicity, side effects, time to awakening after discontinuation, incidence of prolonged weakness after discontinuation, efficacy, effect on outcome, and cost must be considered.[38]

SEDATION. Many protocols include sedatives and analgesics as part of the therapy for severely head-injured patients (GCS <8) as a means of limiting increased ICP related to agitation, restlessness, posturing, asynchrony with the mechan-

ical ventilator, and painful interventions that increase $CMRO_2$ and oxygen needs.

For sedation, benzodiazepines are the most commonly used sedatives and do not affect $CMRO_2$, CBF, or ICP. Lorazepam (Ativan) or midazolam (Versed) are frequently used. Propofol (Diprivan) is a sedative-hypnotic agent that is supplied in an intralipid emulsion for intravenous (IV) use. Propofol decreases $CMRO_2$, CBF, ICP, and CPP. A major advantage of propofol is that it is ultrashort acting, so the IV infusion can be stopped and a neurological assessment conducted in about 5 to 10 minutes without the masking of the drug. The disadvantages are cost, dose-dependent hypotension, potential of bacterial or fungal infection associated with use of a preservative-free emulsion, and muscle weakness with prolonged use. Because it is a lipid emulsion, triglycerides need to be monitored.

ANALGESICS. Sedative medications do not possess analgesic properties. Sedation without analgesia administration to patients with pain may lead to increased agitation and combativeness. Therefore, need for analgesics must be considered.[39] For analgesia, parenteral narcotics, such as fentanyl or morphine, are frequent choices for pain control. They do not increase $CMRO_2$, CBF, or ICP in conventional doses. A low-dose continuous infusion of morphine is a frequently used method of administration. Respiratory depression is the major side effect to consider.

NEUROMUSCULAR BLOCKADE. From 1% to 10% of ICU patients now receive continuous administration of neuromuscular blockade drugs for more than 24 hours.[40] The neuromuscular blockade protocol uses selected drugs to induce paralysis to counteract the increase in ICP to interventions such as suctioning and ventilation. Drugs commonly used include pancuronium, vecuronium, and pipecuronium. It is difficult to judge the depth of paralysis and overdose. Recent literature advocates the routine use of peripheral twitch monitoring to evaluate response.[41] **Peripheral nerve stimulation** is the application of low-voltage electrical stimulation to a peripheral nerve, such as the ulnar nerve, to elicit a twitch response. A series of four stimulations are administered (train of four) and response noted. A complete blockade (0 of 4) response suggests deep paralysis. However, some question the validity and reliability of this technique. The major complication is prolonged weakness or myopathy after prolonged use (more than 24 hours).

Steroids. The use of steroids to manage severe head injury is considered ineffective and is no longer used.[42] (It is useful for vasogenic cerebral edema associated with brain tumors.) The risk of complications with steroid therapy is significant and includes elevated serum glucose, gastrointestinal (GI) bleeding, immunosupression, and infection. Therefore, steroids are not used indiscriminately.

Seizure Management. Post-traumatic seizures are classified into three groups according to the time of occurrence: **immediate seizures** occur within the first 24 hours after the trauma (most occur in the first few hours), **delayed early seizures** occur more than 24 hours to 7 days after trauma, and **late seizures** occur more than 1 week after trauma.[43] Immediate and delayed early seizures are considered reactions to the trauma, and only the late seizures are considered post-traumatic epilepsy. Most seizures classified as early seizures are focal with or without generalization.[44]

The role of *prophylactic anticonvulsants* to prevent seizures is unclear. One study found that phenytoin exerts a beneficial effect by reducing seizures only during the first week after severe head injury.[45] However, seizures greatly increase $CMRO_2$ and ICP. In patients who are receiving neuromuscular blockade, seizure activity or even status epilepticus may occur without the usual motor activity typical of a seizure. Tachycardia, blood pressure instability, and intracranial hypertension may be the only occult evidence of seizure activity.[46] The high risk of secondary injury from clinical undetected seizures is the rationale given for seizure prophylaxis by many. Patients who do not "wake up" when other clinical data suggest improved neurological status may be having undetected seizures. Use of compressed spectral array EEG bedside monitoring for seizure activity is becoming common in ICUs. In the

future, nurses will assess and monitor these data as part of their ongoing assessment.

If seizures do occur, aggressive treatment is necessary to control the seizure to prevent cerebral hypoxia. The most common drug used is phenytoin. A loading dose (1 g) of IV phenytoin, with subsequent maintenance doses, is given to maintain a therapeutic level.

IV phenytoin should not be given any faster than 50 mg/min because of the possibility of hypotension and cardiac arrhythmias. It must also be administered in normal saline to prevent precipitation in solution. Many drugs interact with phenytoin (see Chap. 31).

Phenytoin can be administered through a nasogastric tube at a later time. The usual dose is 300 to 400 mg daily. It is necessary to monitor blood levels of phenytoin to maintain a therapeutic range (10–20 mg/mL). Adjustment in the dosage of phenytoin may be necessary when a tube feeding is started, because phenytoin binds to the protein within the feeding. A patient who has been in a therapeutic range may now be subtherapeutic and will need adjustment of the dose. When administering the drug IV, the manufacturer's instructions should be followed.

Nursing responsibilities related to seizures include maintaining seizure precautions, observing for seizure activity, and monitoring anticonvulsant drug blood level. As mentioned previously, motor signs of seizure activity may not be evident in a sedated or neuromuscular blocked patient. The only clinical evidence may be tachycardia, blood pressure instability, and intracranial hypertension. If there is suspicion of seizure activity, continuous EEG monitoring is diagnostic.

In the ICU environment, seizure precautions are integrated into care. The patient's airway is maintained with an endotracheal tube or other airway, and suctioning equipment is readily available. Side rails are usually up when the nurse is not at the bedside. Padding can be easily added to the side rails. When the patient is transferred to an intermediate unit, any equipment not routinely available at the bedside needs to be added. Protection from injury needs to be considered in an awake and ambulatory patient.

Hyperthermia Management. Hyperthermia can result from local or systemic infections, a central injury to the hypothalamus, cerebral irritation from hemorrhage, or drug response, particularly to anticonvulsants. For each degree rise in temperature (centigrade), there is an approximate 10% increase in $CMRO_2$. This puts the patient at high risk for inadequate oxygen (every 2 hours) supply at the cellular level and secondary injury. Therefore, frequent monitoring of temperature and aggressive management of hyperthermia are critical. It is important to identify the cause of the elevated temperature and treat the primary cause. The patient should be pan-cultured (screening for the sites of infection) to determine the cause of the elevation. Treatment includes acetaminophen (650 mg every 4–6 hours, as needed) and other cooling measures (*e.g.,* cooling blanket, removal of excess bed covers, environmental control). The goal is to maintain normothermia.

Diuretics. To control acute increased ICP caused by cerebral edema, osmotic diuretics, a loop diuretic, or both are administered. The osmotic diuretic of choice is mannitol, 0.25 to 1.0 g/kg through IV bolus (usual adult dose is 25–50 g) every 3 hours to decrease extracellular fluid and cerebral edema. The trigger for administering mannitol is an elevated mean ICP (>20 mm Hg). If furosemide (Lasix), a loop diuretic, is used, the dosage is 0.5 to 1.0 mg/kg. The indication for furosemide is a persistent ICP elevation, even with the use of mannitol. An indwelling urinary catheter is necessary to monitor urinary output and diuresis. Serum should be maintained at less than 320 osm. The blood pressure and electrolytes should be monitored carefully. A danger with diuresis is hypotension, which would result in cerebral hypoperfusion and ischemia. Electrolyte imbalance is also common and needs to be monitored and treated as necessary.

Hyperventilation. Serious risks are involved with the use of hyperventilation, and it should be used with caution. The therapeutic effect of hyperventilation is that hypocapnia (lowered PCO_2) causes vasoconstriction and improves cellular and CSF acidosis. In the injured brain, not all areas are perfused equally nor is vasoconstriction homogeneous. A $PaCO_2$ of 20 to 25 mm Hg will cause cerebral ischemia; with variations within the brain, some areas may be injured when other areas will have a therapeutic effect. Currently, there is no direct way to monitor for the focal ischemia in the brain. Use of jugular venous oxygen saturation monitoring is helpful but provides a global value of cerebral oxygenation.

The patient with a severe head injury will be intubated for airway protection and respiratory management. Hyperventilation is achieved with mechanical ventilation. There is much discussion about the therapeutic target range for PCO_2. An initial target range is 30 to 35 mm Hg for most severe head-injured patients. If this is not effective in lowering the ICP, a target range of PCO_2 to 27 to 30 mm Hg may be considered with caution.

It is unclear for how long hyperventilation is effective and how long it should be used as a therapy for increased ICP. Most sources consulted say hyperventilation is effective for about 3 to 4 days,[47] while a few say 24 hours is the limit. Abrupt cessation can cause a rebound effect of ICP. The effect on cerebral and CSF acidosis is short lived. Use of a buffer, tromethamine (THAM), has been reported to sustain the buffer effect on the acidosis.[48] Although research is promising, use of THAM is currently not a standard of management.

Fluid Management. Fluid restriction has fallen out of favor. It was previously used to control cerebral edema, but current thinking is that fluid restriction has little effect on cerebral edema, can be harmful by causing hypotension, and *should be abandoned in favor of euvolemia.* Movement of water between the brain and the intravascular space depends on osmotic gradients. Hypertonic saline solutions decrease brain water and ICP while temporarily increasing systolic blood pressure and cardiac output.[49] Saline solutions from 0.9% to 3.0% are commonly used. The higher saline concentration is used when concurrent hyponatremia is present.

Hypotonic glucose and other hypotonic solutions (0.45 saline) should not be given rapidly or in large volumes to patients with intracranial hypertension because excess free water from these solutions will lower plasma osmolality and drive water across the blood–brain barrier, thus increasing cerebral water content and ICP. With ischemia and brain injury, plasma glucose is metabolized to lactic acid, thereby lowering tissue pH (acidosis).[50] An elevated serum glucose may aggravate ischemic insult in head-injured patients and worsens neurological outcome; therefore, glucose solutions should be avoided.[51,52] A normal glucose serum level should be maintained.

Colloids Used as Volume Expanders. Human albumin solutions are available either as 5% or 25% concentrations. Albumin (Plasmanate) is an effective volume expander and has no intrinsic effects on clotting. There are also synthetic colloid volume expanders, including hetastarch, pentastarch, and pentafraction. Of these, hetastarch is used most frequently, although its use is limited due to its effect on prolonging clotting time.[53] Packed red blood cells may also be given to expand volume if the hematocrit or hemoglobin is low.

Gastric Prophylaxis. The risk of gastric irritation, gastric ulcers, and GI hemorrhage is increased with severe head trauma (called Cushing's ulcer). Common drugs to prevent bleeding are H2 receptor antagonists, such as ranitidine (Zantac) 150 mg twice a day through an NG tube or 50 mg every 6 to 8 hours IV or famotidine (Pepcid) 20 mg twice a day through an NG tube or 20 mg every 12 hours IV. Sucralfate (Carafate) 1 g every 4 to 6 hours through an NG tube is an aluminum salt that is only minimally absorbed from the GI tract. It coats the stomach, protecting it from attack, but it needs to be taken on an empty stomach. If the NG tube is being used for continuous feedings, sucralfate will be washed away and therefore ineffective.

An antacid, such as Maalox (30 mL every 3–4 hours), may be given through an NG tube as a standing order or in response to assessment of gastric contents for pH. The goal is to maintain the pH above 5.0. Stools should be monitored for occult blood and the hemoglobin for a drop.

Bowel Management. To prevent constipation and stimulation of the Valsalva's maneuver, a bowel program is instituted. A stool softener, such as docusate (Colace) 150 mg twice a day through an NG tube is useful. Cisapride (Propulsid) 20 mg twice a day through an NG tube or 10 mg IV is useful as a stimulant. A laxative of choice, often Milk of Magnesia, 30 mL through an NG tube at hour of sleep, is helpful. The frequency and consistency of bowel movements are monitored. The abdomen should be assessed for peristalsis.

ASSESSMENT AND CLINICAL REASONING: KEY ROLE OF THE NEUROSCIENCE NURSE

The following reviews a few key points of assessment and clinical reasoning as they apply to head-injured patients.

Vital Signs

The significance of vital signs as they relate to neurological function and other body systems is found in Chart 21-3. The frequency with which vital signs are monitored will depend on the stability of the patient's condition. In the ICU setting, they are monitored at least every 2 hours.

Neurological Signs

An initial baseline assessment and frequent subsequent assessments are conducted to determine trends in neurological status (stability, deterioration, or improvement). Impending cerebral herniation and onset of new intracranial hemorrhage are the major problems of acute deterioration that are life threatening. The importance of frequent, serial assessments cannot be overstated. The frequency with which a serial neurological assessment is conducted depends on the patient's condition and degree of stability. In the unstable patient, neurological signs may be monitored as frequently as every 5 to 15 minutes. Once the patient is well stabilized, monitoring every 2 to 4 hours may be sufficient. The following are specific areas of the neurological assessment:

- Level of consciousness and cognition (if responding verbally); if comatose, GCS used
- Size, shape, and reaction of pupils to light (asymmetry seen with a focal lesion)
- Brain stem function, as evidenced by corneal and gag reflexes and extraocular movement
- Motor function (focal mass indicated by asymmetry or lateralization)

LEVEL OF CONSCIOUSNESS

Level of consciousness is the most sensitive indicator of neurological change. If the patient is able to respond verbally, orientation to time, place, and person is assessed. Cognition is assessed by asking simple questions, such as: "Show me two fingers." "Show me your left thumb." "Raise your left arm." "Why are you here?" If comatose, the GCS is used.

Assessing and monitoring brain stem function begins with the pupils. *Pupils* are normally equal in size and midposition, round, and briskly reactive to direct light. Any *new* change in the size or reaction of one or both of the pupils needs to be evaluated. With lateral transtentorial herniation caused by localized cerebral edema (peaks 72 hours after injury) or a focal lesion, one pupil will become dilated and progressively unresponsive to light. This is attributable to unilateral compression of the oculomotor nerve by the edematous herniating brain. An oval or ovoid pupil is also considered to be an early sign of beginning transtentorial herniation. Immediate intervention may be necessary to prevent herniation and irreversible neurological deterioration. Also, when looking into the eyes, observe the position of the eyes for spontaneous asynchronous movement or deviation.

OTHER BRAIN STEM REFLEXES

The corneal and gag reflexes can be assessed easily at the bedside. If the reflexes are absent, it is a poor prognostic sign. Special protective eye care and lubrication should be applied if the corneal reflex is absent. Symmetry of the facial nerve can be checked by inserting a cotton-tipped applicator in one nostril and then the other. By observing each side for grimacing, one can tell if there is a facial nerve deficit.

With an absent gag reflex, the patient is at high risk for aspiration pneumonia. Before consideration is given to removal of an endotracheal tube, one criterion is the ability to protect the airway and an intact gag reflex. Provided there is no cervical fracture or dislocation, confirmed by cervical spine films, the eyes can be checked for doll's eye reflex (oculocephalic reflex).

MOTOR FUNCTION

The patient is observed for spontaneous movement. Asymmetry of movement or lateralization suggests a focal mass lesion on one side of the brain. Hemiparesis and hemiplegia are signs of lateralization because they involve only one side of the body. The lesion will be located in the hemisphere opposite the side of motor weakness. Decortication or decerebration posturing is observed in comatose patients who have suffered severe head injury. Also, bilateral or unilateral flaccidity may be associated with spinal injuries.

OTHER OBSERVATIONS

The patient's face and scalp are examined for signs of other injury because abrasions or contusions may have been missed. Note the presence of ecchymosis on the mastoid bone (Battle's sign), periorbital ecchymosis (raccoon's eye), conjunctival hemorrhage, or clear or bloody drainage from the ear, nose, or postnasal area. These signs are related to a basal skull fracture. The neck is assessed for evidence of nuchal rigidity, a sign of meningeal irritation. The rigidity can be caused by meningitis or blood in the CSF from subarachnoid hemorrhage.

If an ICP monitor is in place, the nurse observes for elevations in pressure and the shape of the P1, P2, and P3 components. There are often standing orders for interventions to be implemented when a certain degree of pressure elevation is reached. The monitor is also helpful in allowing the nurse to observe the effect of various nursing interventions on ICP. If the ICP is elevated, planned activities may be postponed until the pressure decreases.

Nursing Management of Multisystem Complications of Head Injury

A management focus for head-injured patients is prevention, early recognition, and nursing management of multisystem problems (Table 21-4). Again, management is directed at optimizing cerebral perfusion and prevention of secondary brain injury from systems problems. Some complications are more apt to occur in the first few days after injury, and others are delayed. The following is organized to address each system as it relates to head injury (see also Chap. 12).

RESPIRATORY COMPLICATIONS

Respiratory management of the patient with a severe head injury has developed rapidly in the last few years. Newer mechanical ventilators with positive end-expiratory pressure (PEEP) and pressure support are standard methods of managing patients. PEEP increases PaO_2 in patients with *decreased* functional residual capacity (FRC) resulting from interstitial edema or alveolar col-

(text continues on page 408)

TABLE 21-4
Summary of the Nursing Management of Multisystem Problems in Acute Head Injury

System-Specific Considerations	Nursing Diagnoses	Assessment Data	Management/Interventions
NEUROLOGICAL SYSTEM • Severe head injury will result in unconsciousness and will alter many neurological functions. • All body functions must be supported. • Increased intracranial pressure (ICP) and herniation syndromes are life threatening. • Institute measures to control elevated ICP.	• Altered Cerebral Tissue Perfusion • Ineffective Thermoregulation • Risk for Secondary Brain Injury • Sensory/Perceptual alterations • Self-Care Deficits • Risk for Injury	**Clinical data** • Assessment of neurological signs • Assessment for signs and symptoms of ICP elevations • Calculation of cerebral perfusion pressure (CPP) if ICP monitor is in place **Laboratory data** • Monitoring of anticonvulsant blood levels	See Table 21-2 for nursing interventions.
RESPIRATORY SYSTEM • Complete or partial airway obstruction will compromise the oxygen supply to the brain. • An altered respiratory pattern can result in cerebral hypoxia. • A short period of apnea at the time of impact can result in spotty atelectasis. • Systemic disturbances from head injury can cause hypoxemia. • Brain injury can alter brain stem respiratory function. • Shunting of blood to the lungs as a result of a sympathetic discharge at the time of injury can cause neurogenic pulmonary edema.	• Risk for Aspiration • Ineffective Airway Clearance • Impaired Gas Exchange • Ineffective Breathing Pattern • Risk for Infection	**Clinical data** • Assessment of respiratory function —Auscultate chest for breath sounds. —Note the respiratory pattern if possible (not possible if a ventilator is being used). —Note the respiratory rate. —Note whether the cough reflex is intact. **Laboratory data** • Blood gas levels • Complete blood count • Chest x-ray studies • Sputum cultures • O_2 saturation using pulse oximetry	• Monitor respiratory function for changes. • Suction the patient as necessary to maintain a patent airway. • Instill lidocaine into the endotracheal tube to blunt increases in ICP secondary to suctioning. • Oxygenate the patient before suctioning. • Use an Ambu bag periodically to hyperinflate all lung tissue; the sigh function on the ventilator may also be used for this purpose. • Provide tracheostomy care every 4–8 h to maintain patency. • See Chapter 12 for information on ventilator management. • Turn the patient every 2 h to prevent stasis of secretions. • Administer supplemental oxygen, as ordered, if a ventilator is not being used. • Observe the patient for signs of respiratory distress (*e.g.*, neurogenic pulmonary edema).
CARDIOVASCULAR SYSTEM • The patient may develop cardiac arrhythmias, tachycardia, or bradycardia. • The patient may develop hypotension or hypertension (see Chart 17-2). • Because of immobility and unconsciousness, the patient is at high risk for deep vein thromboses (DVTs) and pulmonary emboli.	• Altered Peripheral Tissue Perfusion • Altered Cerebral Tissue Perfusion • Impaired Tissue Integrity (venous stasis)	**Clinical data** • Assessment of vital signs • Monitoring for cardiac arrhythmias • Assessment for DVTs of legs **Laboratory data** • Electrocardiogram • Electrolyte studies • Blood coagulation studies • I^{125} fibrinogen scan of legs	• Apply thigh-high elastic antiembolic hose • Maintain sequential compression air boots, as ordered. • Monitor vital signs. • Observe cardiac monitor for arrhythmias. • Monitor legs for signs of DVTs. • Monitor the patient for signs of pulmonary emboli.

(continued)

TABLE 21-4
Summary of the Nursing Management of Multisystem Problems in Acute Head Injury Continued

System-Specific Considerations	Nursing Diagnoses	Assessment Data	Management/Interventions
INTEGUMENTARY SYSTEM (SKIN)			
• Immobility secondary to injury and unconsciousness contributes to the development of pressure areas and skin breakdown. • Intubation causes irritation of the mucous membrane.	• Risk for Impaired Skin Integrity • Altered Peripheral Tissue Perfusion • Altered Oral Mucous Membrane	**Clinical data** • Assessment of skin integrity and character of the skin	• Provide skin care every 4 h. • Turn the patient every 2–4 h. • Provide mouth care every 2–4 h. • Monitor the patient for signs and symptoms of skin irritation or breakdown. • Institute special skin precautions and treatment as needed.
MUSCULOSKELETAL SYSTEM			
• Immobility contributes to musculoskeletal changes. • Decerebrate or decorticate posturing makes proper positioning difficult.	• Impaired Physical Mobility • Risk for Disuse Syndrome	**Clinical data** • Assessment of range of motion (ROM) of joints and development of deformities or spasticity	• Monitor joint ROM, and note alterations in muscle tone. • Provide ROM exercises once daily. • Position the patient in proper body alignment; use rolls, pillows, and other aids to maintain the position. • Collaborate with physical and occupational therapists (PT/OT) regarding splints or positioning and ROM in the rigid or spastic patient. • Control noxious stimuli (which accentuate abnormal posturing).
GASTROINTESTINAL (GI) SYSTEM			
• Administration of steroids places the patient at high risk for GI hemorrhage. • Injury to the GI tract can result in paralytic ileus. • Constipation can result from bed rest, NPO status, fluid restriction, and opiate derivatives given for pain control. • Incontinence is related to the patient's unconscious state or altered mental state.	• Risk for Injury (gastric ulceration and bleeding) • Constipation • Bowel Incontinence	**Clinical data** • Assessment of abdomen for bowel sounds and distention **Laboratory data** • Monitoring for decreased hemoglobin	• Monitor stools for occult blood daily. • Monitor the pH of gastric contents by nasogastric tube aspiration every 4–6 h. • Auscultate the abdomen for bowel sounds in all four quadrants every shift. • Observe the patient for changes in vital signs that may indicate hemorrhage. • Establish a bowel program.
GENITOURINARY SYSTEM			
• Fluid restriction or use of diuretics can alter the amount of urinary output. • Urinary incontinence is related to the patient's unconscious state.	• Altered Urinary Elimination • Urinary Incontinence	**Clinical data** • Intake and output (I&O) record	• Maintain an indwelling catheter or condom catheter as ordered. • Monitor the 24-h I&O record for signs of imbalance (fluid retention or dehydration).
METABOLIC (NUTRITIONAL) SYSTEM			
• The patient receives all fluids intravenously (IV) for the first few days until the GI tract is usable. • A nutritional consultation is ordered within the first 24–48 h; total parenteral nutrition may be started.	• Fluid Volume Deficit • Altered Nutrition: less than body requirements	**Clinical data** • Assessment of fluid and electrolyte balance • Recording of weight, if possible **Laboratory data** • Hematocrit • Electrolyte studies	• Monitor I&O record for excessive output. • Monitor fractional urinary output every 1–2 h for excessive output. • Monitor central venous pressure readings. • Check urine-specific gravity every 1–4 h.

(continued)

TABLE 21-4
Summary of the Nursing Management of Multisystem Problems
in Acute Head Injury Continued

System-Specific Considerations	Nursing Diagnoses	Assessment Data	Management/Interventions
• Fluid and electrolyte imbalance can be related to several problems, including alterations in antidiuretic hormone (ADH) secretion, the stress response, or fluid restriction. • Specific conditions may occur: —Diabetes insipidus —Syndrome of inappropriate secretion of ADH (SIADH) —Electrolyte imbalance —Hyperosmolar nonketotic hyperglycemia		• Glucose level • Acetone level • Osmolality	• Monitor body weight twice a week.
PSYCHOLOGICAL/EMOTIONAL RESPONSE			
• The severely head-injured patient is unconscious. • The family needs much support to deal with the crisis.	• Altered Family Processes • Fear • Ineffective Family Coping • Decisional Conflict • Knowledge Deficit • Spiritual Distress • Ineffective Family Coping: Disabling	**Clinical data** • Collection of information about the family unit and the role of the head-injured person within that unit. • Assessment of the family unit to determine how functional it was before the injury occurred	• Establish rapport with the family. • Provide orientation material pertaining to the unit (*e.g.*, visiting hours, where to eat, location of bathrooms). • Provide a synopsis of what has happened since the family last visited. • Help the family to identify and mobilize their supports (*e.g.*, clergy, friends). • Help the family to appoint a family spokesperson to whom information can be directed. • Provide information and support. • Request a consultation for family support and crisis intervention from a psychiatric clinical nurse specialist or social worker.

lapse, such as adult respiratory distress syndrome (ARDS). It is ineffective in conditions with a high FRC, such as emphysema. PEEP elevates ICP only when mean airway pressures are increased, causing transmission to the mediastinum. When pulmonary compliance is reduced, as occurs in ARDS, the effect of PEEP or ICP is attenuated.[54] Complications associated with PEEP are barotrauma and cardiovascular decompensation. Withdrawal of PEEP must occur gradually. Oxygen therapy is delivered at an FIO_2 from 20% to 40%.

Monitoring SaO_2 saturation, blood gases, CBC, sputum cultures, and chest x-rays assists in evaluating respiratory function. Chest auscultation and quality of respirations are the major clinical guides for assessment.

Airway Patency. A patent airway is the common pathway to the respiratory system and is the top priority in management. In the acute phase of head injury, head-injured patients are neither able to manage their own secretions nor able to position themselves in the most expeditious way for adequate drainage of secretions. Meeting these needs becomes an objec-

tive of nursing care of the highest priority. Follow precautions to suction as needed to prevent an increase in carbon dioxide and subsequent hypercapnia, which contributes to cerebral vasodilation, cerebral edema, and increased ICP.

- Position the patient on the side to facilitate drainage of secretions and prevent aspiration.
- Preoxygenate with 100% oxygen before suctioning (with physician's approval).
- Limit the catheter insertion to 15 seconds or less to prevent an increase of CO_2.
- If a tracheostomy is present, provide tracheostomy care frequently to prevent crusting and buildup of secretions that can obstruct the airway.
- Do not hyperextend or hyperflex the neck, because such maneuvers create a partial obstruction of the airway.

Hypoxemia, defined as less than the normal amount of arterial blood oxygen, is a common early systemic finding in head-injured patients and is probably the direct result of the head injury. At the time of injury, there is a short period of apnea, followed by spontaneous respirations. However, spotty atelectasis may result from incomplete alveoli expansion. Supplemental oxygen should be provided as soon as possible. **Hypoxia** is defined as a diminished tissue oxygen. As a result of pathophysiological changes in cerebral autoregulation and neuronal metabolism, hypoxia of the cerebral tissue occurs. Hypoxia results in cerebral ischemia and neuronal death of involved cells.

A respiratory problem that can develop rapidly is atelectasis. **Atelectasis** is defined as a collapsed or airless state that may involve any part of the lung. It is, therefore, important to be sure that all areas of the lungs are expanded. To assess the lungs for atelectasis, the nurse auscultates the chest for breath sounds, making sure to listen to the entire chest, especially the bases. Nursing management is directed at preventing atelectasis and includes the following:

- If the patient is being ventilated on a system that can be adjusted for sighs, this should be included.
- If the patient is on a special bed for pulmonary percussion, this should be used.
- In the conscious patient, encourage deep breathing exercises to expand the lungs and loosen secretions.

Pneumonias. The patient can develop a number of different types of pneumonias. *Aspiration pneumonia* can result from aspiration at the time of injury or at any other time. Bacterial invasion and stasis of fluid in the lungs also commonly cause *bacterial pneumonia* and hypostatic pneumonia, respectively. *Nosocomial pneumonias* are also common and are usually caused by gram-positive organisms (*Staphylococcus aureus, Streptococcus pneumonia*, and *Haemophilus influenzae*) and sometimes gram-negative organisms (enteric bacteria or *Pseudomonas*). The patient is assessed for signs and symptoms of pneumonia, and nursing measures are incorporated to prevent its development. To assess the lungs for the development of pneumonia, the nurse should auscultate the chest for breath sounds and adventitious sounds, monitor the character of the sputum for color and foul odor, and monitor the temperature and white blood count for elevation.

Nursing management to prevent pneumonia incorporates the following:

- Maintain a patent airway.
- Turn from side to side every 2 hours to prevent stasis of fluid in the lungs.
- Do not position on the back, because this increases the possibility of aspiration.
- Administer chest physiotherapy to loosen and drain pulmonary secretions.
- The intubated or tracheotomized patient is immunocompromised and prone to infection; use meticulous aseptic technique when delivering care.
- Maintain inflated cuffs on the endotracheal tube or the tracheostomy tube to prevent aspiration.
- Confirm that the gag reflex is intact before feeding a patient.

Neurogenic pulmonary edema is a poorly understood, common complication seen with severe head injury and increased ICP and sometimes after a major generalized seizure. As the name implies, it is acute pulmonary edema that is non-

cardiogenic and not related to damaged alveolar epithelium or capillary endothelium that occurs minutes to days after injury. The pathophysiology is poorly understood and is probably due to a combination of hydrostatic forces and permeability changes. At the time of impact, there is shunting of blood into the lungs as a result of an abrupt rise in ICP and sympathetic discharge. The clinical findings are nonspecific (dyspnea, tachypnea, tachycardia, hypoxemia, and mild elevation in leukocytes). On a chest x-ray, "fluffy" infiltrates are seen. Neurogenic pulmonary edema can progress to respiratory failure and a condition similar to ARDS, or it can be self-limiting, resolving in hours to days. Treatment consists of treating the underlying increased ICP with medical and nursing strategies and providing ventilatory support with PEEP.

Pulmonary emboli can result from deep vein thromboses (DVT) in the immobilized head-injured patient. Signs and symptoms include a cough, often with hemoptysis; dyspnea; tachypnea; and chest pain. Nursing management is directed at the prevention of DVT and includes the application of elastic stockings or sequential compression boots to improve blood return to the heart.

CARDIOVASCULAR COMPLICATIONS

Cardiac arrhythmias are often reported in head injury. Some life-threatening arrhythmias are associated with myocardial ischemia. Other arrhythmias are more common if there was bleeding into the subarachnoid space. The cause of the cardiac problems is thought to be the autonomic discharge at injury and the ensuing hyperdynamic state.

Cardiovascular function is assessed by monitoring the patient's vital signs and observing the continuous pattern on a cardiac monitor for arrhythmias. In addition, electrolytes, coagulation studies, CBC, creatine kinase isoenzymes for myocardial infarction, perhaps a echocardiogram if cardiac mechanics are questioned, and a 12-lead EKG may be ordered. These abnormalities should be treated promptly and aggressively with a search for identifying and treating the underlying cause.

Nursing management is directed toward monitoring for arrhythmias and other abnormalities through chest auscultation, pulse and blood pressure monitoring, and observing the EKG pattern on the cardiac monitor. Treatment is usually pharmacological, guided by targeted physiological values for hemodynamic variables, such as cardiac output and MAP, for which to titrate the drug administration.

Many drug options are available to maintain higher blood pressure for patients with intracranial pathology. Alpha- and beta-adrenergic blockers do not directly affect CBF and have no effect on ICP in patients with intracranial hypertension; therefore, they may be the preferred agents for control of blood pressure in brain-injured people.[55] Adequate MAP is facilitated with vasopressor drugs progressing from dopamine (Intropin) to phenylephrine (Neo-Synephrine) to labetolol (Normodyne). *Dopamine*, the precursor of norepinephrine, increases kidney perfusion at lower doses (2–5 μg/kg per minute) and causes alpha effects at 10 to 20 μg/kg per minute with peripheral vasoconstriction and increased cerebral perfusion. It is often titrated to cardiac output. *Phenylephrine* is a vasopressor by stimulating alpha-adrenergic receptors. *Labe-*

tolol has mixed alpha- and beta-adrenergic antagonists, and it increases CPP and lowers ICP.

Hypertensive crisis requires immediate attention to prevent a stroke. These drugs decrease CPP by lowering MAP and increasing ICP. Passive dilation of cerebral capacitance vessels increases ICP. This, combined with lowered cerebral arterial flow, diminishes CPP.[56] There is no ideal drug for treatment. *Sodium nitroprusside* (Nipride) has a rapid onset (within seconds) and lasts 1 to 3 minutes. It decreases cerebral vascular resistance and increases ICP by dilating arterial and venous smooth muscles so that CPP falls by as much as 50%. *Nitroglycerin* has an even worse effect on CPP and a rise in ICP. The major calcium channel blockers are nimodipine, nifedipine, and verapamil. *Nimodipine* has a varied effect on ICP, CBF, and CPP. It is useful for cerebral vasospasm. *Verapamil* lowers systemic blood pressure and CPP significantly (about 33%) and increases ICP by up to 67%.[57] *Nifedipine* lowers CPP and increases ICP. Of these drugs, there are no ideal drugs, but a nitroprusside drip is the drug of choice for hypertensive crisis.

HEMATOLOGICAL COMPLICATIONS

Many head-injured patients develop some problem with clotting without bleeding. Some will develop disseminated intravascular coagulation (DIC), a catastrophic insult in brain injury that is due to the release of large amounts of thromboplastin and the presence of tissue emboli from the circulating factor XII from the vascular endothelial lining.[58]

Accurate diagnosis is important, and abnormal findings on the activated partial thromboplastin time (aPTT), prothrombin time (PT), platelet count, and plasma fibrinogen level are not the complete picture. Highly suggestive of DIC are fibrin split products and thrombin time. The double-D-dimer degradation product is used to confirm the diagnosis. Other available tests include the plasma prothrombin, ethanol gelatin tests, and the fibrinopeptide-A level. If the patient survives, DIC corrects in hours. The mainstay of treatment is replacement of clotting factors and maintenance of adequate blood volume. Replacement of clotting factors includes fresh frozen plasma (replaces fibrinogen and factor VIII) and cryoprecipitate (replaces factor V).

Clotting Abnormalities Without Bleeding. Abnormalities may be found in the aPTT, PT, platelet count, or plasma fibrinogen levels. These do not necessarily need to be tested. However, they should be monitored and a search conducted for underlying correctable causes, such as changing an anticonvulsant drug that is causing thrombocytopenia.

Deep Vein Thrombosis. About 40% of patients with head injury develop DVT.[59] For neurosurgical patients in general, the incidence of calf DVT is 29% to 43%. The incidence of DVT is related to surgery, immobility, motor deficits, lower extremity trauma, and gram-negative sepsis, which are common to head-injured patients.[60] Diagnosis is by contrast venogram, but this is invasive. Clinical evidence is found in only a small number of patients. DVT can lead to pulmonary embolus and therefore needs to be treated if suspected. Treatment includes heparin therapy and possible insertion of a vena cava filter.

However, prevention is a better alternative. Prophylaxis includes antiembolic elastic stockings and sequential compression boots. If not contraindicated, minidoses of heparin, 5,000 U subcutaneously every 12 hours, are helpful.

GASTROINTESTINAL COMPLICATIONS

In the early acute phase of serious head injury, two major concerns for the nurse are gastric hemorrhage and gastric atony. Cushing's ulcer is common in head-injured patients, occurring in the upper GI tract, whereas stress-related ulcerations are usually located in the duodenum. The use of sucralfate and H₂ blockers has decreased the incidence of Cushing's ulcers. Gastric atony, another common problem, delays beginning feeding and may increase the risk of aspiration.[61] See previous section on GI prophylaxis.

METABOLIC COMPLICATIONS

Electrolyte and neuroendocrine disturbances are common in head-injured patients. The most common electrolyte problem is hyponatremia. It is often associated with diabetes insipidus and syndrome of inappropriate secretion of antidiuretic hormone (SIADH). When potassium is affected, hypokalemia is most common and is associated with aldosterone, hyperventilation, and diuretics. Common neuroendocrine problems include diabetes insipidus, SIADH, and sometimes nonketotic hyperosmolar hyperglycemia (see Chap. 10 for a detailed discussion). Some of these problems will correct themselves as long as supportive therapy is provided, such as maintaining fluid and electrolyte balance and replacement.

Hyponatremia. With hyponatremia, early recognition and correction of a downward trend is important.[62] A higher concentration of IV saline solution, extra salt added to the tube feeding, and drug therapy, such as fludrocortisone acetate (Florinef) are used. Fludrocortisone is a mineralocorticoid that increases sodium reabsorption in renal tubules and increases potassium and hydrogen excretion. Dosage is 0.1 to 0.2 mg/d. With hypokalemia, replacement with potassium chloride, 20 to 40 mEq/1,000 mL IV unit is the practice.

Hyperglycemia. What should be done about elevated serum glucose? The serum glucose may be related to a stress response to head trauma, or the patient may be a borderline or known diabetic. As discussed with fluid management previously in this chapter, an elevated serum glucose may aggravate ischemic insult in head-injured patients and worsen neurological outcome; therefore, glucose solutions should be avoided.[63] In addition, serum glucose should be maintained in a normal range. If the serum glucose is elevated, a regular insulin drip can be started. If the glucose remains high, then a divided schedule of regular insulin and NPH insulin given subcutaneously should be started. Glucose management must be aggressively controlled.

Fluid Replacement. The goal of fluid balance is euvolemia. See the section on fluid replacement in this chapter.

Nursing management is directed toward monitoring serum electrolytes, glucose, osmolality, urine-specific gravity, fractional urinary output, and overall fluid and electrolyte balance. A negative fluid balance can cause hypotension and secondary brain injury. (See Chap. 10 for further discussion of the nurse's role.)

NUTRITION ISSUES

Undernutrition is a common problem with head-injured patients. The metabolic response to severe head injury is similar to the needs of patients with severe burns (5,000–6,000 kcal/d). Caloric and nutritional needs of the patient should be discussed with the nutritionist. Feeding should begin as soon as possible (within 24 hours of admission). Insertion of a Dobhoff feeding tube into the jejunum of the small intestines is common because it avoids the problem of gastric regurgitation and aspiration common with an NG tube. Early feeding is important to maintain the integrity of the mucosal lining of the intestines; a beginning rate of 10 to 20 mL is a reasonable start. A nutrition consultation for recommendations of type of feeding and goal is important. Feeding rate is gradually increased to goal based on tolerance and response. The gut may be a trigger for the development of multiple organ failure syndrome, and postponement of feeding may increase the risk of this syndrome.

Nursing management includes making sure that nutrition is addressed early and feeding is begun without interruptions. Serum calcium, potassium, phosphorus, blood urea nitrogen, creatinine, and other laboratory values related to nutrition should be monitored. Interruptions in feeding schedules can decrease the daily intake.[64] (See Chap. 9 for a discussion of nutritional needs.)

SEPSIS AND SEPSIS SYNDROMES

Sepsis can result from injuries sustained at the time of injury (open head wounds, bullets) or invasive procedures (ICP monitor, indwelling urinary catheter, pulmonary catheter, surgery), or it may be nosocomial. Universal precautions, strict aseptic technique, and adherence to culture and dressing protocols are critical to prevention. See previous section on hyperthermia management and respiratory complications. The ICU nurse needs to be familiar with signs and symptoms of septic syndromes (*e.g.*, decreased systemic vascular resistance and increased cardiac index) for early identification and management.

Nursing Management for Special Problems

BASAL SKULL FRACTURES

Clinical evidence of a basal skull fracture depends on the particular basal skull fossa involved. Signs and symptoms may include ecchymosis of the mastoid process (Battle's sign), periorbital hemorrhage (raccoon's eyes) and ecchymosis, blood behind the eardrum (hemotympanum), decreased hearing, drainage from the nose (rhinorrhea) or ear (otorrhea), and postnasal drainage (postnasal drip). Nursing management is directed at reducing the risk of meningitis, as follows:

- Never suction through the nose if there is question of a basal skull fracture; the catheter could slip into the dural tear and become a source of contamination.
- Caution against blowing the nose; this could introduce organisms into a dural tear.
- Do not introduce anything into the orifice (nose or ear) or irrigate the area; sterile cotton or other absorbent material should be placed loosely around the orifice and changed frequently.

If there is any question as to whether the drainage is CSF, laboratory analysis of a test tube specimen for detection of chloride is helpful. CSF chloride will be greater than the serum chloride level. Testing for glucose is unreliable, because nasal secretions can yield a positive reaction. The presence of drainage from the nose or ear is highly suggestive of CSF leakage. In clinical practice, drainage is often a combination of CSF and blood. A characteristic stain with a dark center and a lighter outer area (halo sign) is often seen. Depending on the patient's condition, he or she may be out of bed. Most CSF leaks will heal spontaneously within days. In rare instances, surgery is necessary to find and patch the tear. Use of prophylactic antibiotics for basal skull fractures is controversial.

A basal skull fracture is considered to be a serious injury because of the proximity of the fracture line to vital brain stem structures. Local edema can rapidly develop, leading to respiratory problems. Nursing management includes monitoring for deterioration in vital or neurological signs and signs of meningeal irritation.

CAROTID-CAVERNOUS FISTULA

A carotid-cavernous fistula is an uncommon complication of head trauma due to a laceration of the carotid artery resulting in direct communication between the high-pressure arterial blood of the internal carotid artery (ICA) and the low venous pressure of the cavernous sinus. The cavernous sinuses are located at the basal skull on either side of the sphenoid body. The ICA and several of its branches of the oculomotor, the trochlear, two divisions of the trigeminal, and the abducens nerves pass through the cavernous sinus. A bruit over the affected orbit, pulsating proptosis, conjunctival edema, orbital pain and chemosis, facial pain, limitation of extraocular movement, headache, and visual deficits (diplopia, photophobia, and decreased visual acuity that can lead to blindness) are common findings. The definitive diagnostic procedure is carotid angiography. Although spontaneous resolution may occur in a few patients, surgery is necessary for most. Surgical procedures include ligation of the ICA above and below the fistula or embolization. Nursing management includes neurological assessment, including all cranial nerves, auscultation of the bruit, assessment of pain, and presence of conjunctival edema. Special eye care, control of pain, and eye injury prevention, such as corneal ulcerations, are needed.

HYDROCEPHALUS

As a result of intracranial bleeding, communicating or normal pressure hydrocephalus may develop, as evidenced by enlarged ventricles on CT scan. In such cases, serial removal of

CSF, temporary external ventricular drainage, or a surgical shunting procedure may be performed.

HYGROMA

A **hygroma** is an encapsulated collection of CSF, caused by a tear in the arachnoid, which allows fluid to escape into the subdural space. Concurrent cerebral edema locks the fluid into the space and creates pressure on the brain. A **subdural hygroma** is a collection of clear or yellowish fluid (CSF and blood). The total accumulation of fluid may range from a few milliliters to, in rare cases, as much as 50 mL. The subdural hygroma is unilateral and may extend over the entire hemisphere, or it may become encapsulated. The fluid has a high protein content, which may be why it coagulates occasionally. Symptoms corresponding to a slowly developing SDH occur, beginning with headache, which becomes severe and persistent. The only effective treatment is surgical removal.

NURSING MANAGEMENT DURING THE INTERMEDIATE PHASE OF SEVERE HEAD INJURY

Once the patient is physiologically stabilized and no longer needs continuous monitoring, the collaborative team, working closely with the case manager, will make the decision to transfer the patient to an intermediate unit. The interdisciplinary care map that guided care in the ICU environment now continues in this next phase. The goals of nursing management are basically the same, except that rehabilitation and discharge planning are the major focus.

Assessment and Ongoing Monitoring

The frequency with which vital signs and neurological signs are assessed depends on the patient's condition and varies from 4 to 8 hours. If the patient is awake and able to follow commands, a much more complete assessment, especially a cognitive assessment, will be possible. Ability to respond to questions and participate in higher level skills (*e.g.*, doing calculations, identifying similarities between concepts, memory retrieval and problem solving) should be evaluated.

General nursing management principles include the following:

- Assess level of consciousness frequently to note any changes.
- Consider causes other than neurological for altered consciousness.
- Reorient the patient to time, place, and person; use the patient's name.
- For patients who are classified as level I to III on the Rancho Los Amigo Scale (RLAS), provide environmental stimuli or a sensory stimulation program;[65] talk to the patient, turn on the radio, open the shades, place family pictures in their visual field, and so forth.
- For patients who are at level IV to VI on the RLAS, provide structure and control stimulation.

- For patients who are at level VII to VIII on the RLAS, provide for practice in higher cognitive skills needed to integrate back to the community.

See Chapter 14 for a discussion of cognitive rehabilitation and the RLAS.

Cranial nerve, motor, sensory, and cerebellar function are assessed to determine functional deficits and their effect on activities of daily living. Collaboration with the case manager, social worker, physical therapist, occupational therapist, speech therapist, and others will refine the discharge plan. In the managed care environment, patients move through the system rapidly. Any education and teaching of the patient or family occur in a compressed time frame.

The patient is monitored for evidence of medical complications and risks associated with secondary injury.

MINOR AND MODERATE BRAIN INJURIES

The incidence of mild and moderate head injury is difficult to determine because of lack of contact with the health care system, varying definitions and classifications of mild and moderate head injury, absence of data sets, and coexistence of the head injury with other problems.

The definitions of mild and moderate head injury are imprecise. Practitioners may be able to discriminate intuitively, but there are no good instruments to discriminate reliably among injury types. Also, victims are often seen at a doctor's office, emergency room, or not seen at all, and they are often excluded from epidemiological databases. The head injury may be concurrent with other injuries that are more prominent, serious, and receive primary attention. The GCS is one widely used method for classification. However, it may not be sensitive enough to capture the deficits common to these injuries.

What is unclear is the influence of a managed care environment on how the person with a mild head injury will be treated and what options for diagnostics and hospitalization will be authorized.

Mild brain injury (GCS = 13–15) is a transient event in which there may be a dazed appearance, unsteady gait, and short-term confusion after a blow to the head. The patient feels well after a few minutes; most patients have full recovery without problems. Some will have a post-traumatic amnesia and a postconcussion syndrome. There is also a subgroup who seem perfectly fine when seen and then have serious problems from secondary brain injury and die. It is unclear how to identify and manage these patients.

There are no clear criteria for diagnosis or management of these patients. It is unclear if a CT scan should be ordered for all patients or if only certain patients should receive scans. This continues to be a clinical judgment of the caregiver. What is clear is that all patients with a mild head injury need to be observed and monitored for evidence of deterioration. For patients with loss of consciousness, neurological deficits, CSF leak or drainage from the nose or ear, alcohol consumption or other medical condition that makes assessment difficult, or absence of a support person, admission is warranted. People who seem perfectly fine may be sent home with a responsible person. Written instructions should outline signs and symptoms and what should be done if they appear.

Moderate brain injury (GS = 9–12) is a more serious brain injury often concurrent with other organ system problems. These patients are initially managed as multisystem trauma patients with all the precautions, such as cervical neck injury immobilization, outlined for severe head injury. Once stabilized, a CT scan should be done as soon as possible. These patients often require an ICU admission. If they are admitted to other than a neurological ICU, the concern is that the brain injury may be underestimated and not treated appropriately. Patients with moderate brain injury need frequent observation and the same management as outlined for severe head injury. There may be serious deficits postinjury that affect the person's ability to work and function effectively in roles previously assumed before injury, such as parent, spouse, or community member. Personality disorders are not uncommon. These patients need to be monitored after discharge and provided with appropriate rehabilitation services and counseling.

Postconcussion syndrome consists of complaints of irritability, fatigue, headache, difficulty concentrating, dizziness, and memory problems. Anxiety and depression are also frequently noted, especially later in the course. The cause of these symptoms was believed to be psychological, but current evidence supports the idea of a physiological basis of injury. Treatment consists of educating the patient and family and supportive counseling related to emerging problems at work or at home. Symptoms usually subside with time, but it may take months before resolution is complete.

REHABILITATION

A number of physical, behavioral, cognitive, and psychosocial problems can result from head injury. Based on individual patient needs, a plan of care is developed. Where the rehabilitation will occur depends on a number of factors, including functional deficits, managed care options, and available resources. Many of these activities related to discharge planning are now handled by the case manager and discharge planner. It is the nurse's responsibility to contribute to the database and work with the case manager and discharge planner as an advocate for patient and family needs. See Chapter 15 for a discussion of discharge planning and transitions in care.

Community Resources

A number of community resources provide information and support groups for head-injured patients and their families. Information about these resources should be made available within the hospital setting. They include the following:

National Head Injury Foundation
1776 Massachusetts Avenue, NW
Suite 100
Washington, DC 20036
800-444-6443

Coma Recovery Association
377 Jerusalem Avenue
Hempstead, NY 11550
516-486-2847

Predicting Outcome From Head Injury

Predicting outcomes following head injury continues to be one of the mysteries of neuroscience practice. Prognostic indicators of outcome are many, but no individual variable or cluster of variables is sufficiently reliable to predict outcome accurately. Outcome from head injury has been expanded to include cognitive and neurobehavioral measures and functional assessment. Interest in enhancing the accuracy of outcome prediction has led to the development of a number of models for determining probability of a particular outcome in a clinical situation. Work continues, but thus far, predicting outcome is not well developed.

One outcome scale, the **Glasgow Outcome Scale**, is a well known scale that assesses the outcome of patients sustaining central nervous system trauma (Chart 21-4). Survivors are assigned to one of four levels, depending on the degree of function and independence that they maintain. The scale does not evaluate cognitive impairment; it conveys only a general opinion of the examiner as to how the patient is doing.

Quality of life has become an important framework in describing outcome. However, the means for defining and measuring this concept have not been established. Indicators for quality of life are independence in performing activities of daily living, social relationships, roles, gainful employment, and control of one's life. Other scales have been developed to assess particular deficits related to head injury.

Personality and Behavioral Deficits

Factors that contribute to the presence and persistence of behavioral problems include site of injury, the severity, premorbid personality, and the environment. Personality changes

---

CHART 21-4
Glasgow Outcome Scale

- *Good outcome*—may have minimal disabling sequelae but returns to independent functioning and a full-time job comparable to preinjury level
- *Moderate disability*—capable of independent functioning but not returned to full-time employment
- *Severe disability*—dependent on others for some aspect of daily living
- *Persistent vegetative state*—no obvious cortical function
- Dead

(Jennett, B., & Bond, M. [1975]. Assessment of outcome after severe brain damage: A practical scale. *Journal of Neurosurgery, 4*, 673.)

may include silly, childlike behavior, as characterized by self-centeredness, an inability to show empathy, impatience, and impulsiveness. Injuries predominantly involving the frontal lobe are characterized by decreased drive and initiative, flat affect, disinhibition, disregard for social protocols, apathy, lethargy, lack of goal-directed behavior, difficulty with impulse control, and an impaired sense of self-identity. Lesions of the temporal lobe are characterized by episodes of violent behavior and possibly seizure disorders. Early intervention is helpful in modifying behavioral patterns and assisting the patient and family in managing such behaviors before the behavior becomes established.

Family Relationship Deficits

The psychosocial and personality deficits affecting the patient, alterations in the patient's roles and responsibilities, and the tremendous burden placed on the family resulting from injury contribute to disrupted family function. If the family was dysfunctional before the injury, the added stress of a severely head-injured family member compounds that stress. The stress on a marriage is significant when a spouse is a victim. The uninjured spouse must assume the caregiver role to a person who is now quite different than when they were married. The stresses of the caregiver role and the role of fatigue are well documented in the literature.

Summary

The consequences of head injury are multifaceted and can be devastating, especially with severe head injury. Many of these problems are addressed initially in the rehabilitation setting, and their resolution is continued in the community. The rehabilitation literature should be consulted for a further in-depth discussion of this phase of recovery.

THE FUTURE: TRENDS AND BREAKTHROUGHS

At the forefront of cerebral injury research breakthroughs is the exciting initiative of neuroprotective agents. With a better understanding of the neurochemical basis of cellular injury, new models of pharmacological cellular neuroprotection are rapidly developing. Many drugs are currently in clinical trials, and they are expected to become available for clinical use in the future. Free radical scavengers, EAA antagonists, and antioxidants are the focus of investigations. Trilazad is the first of a series of synthetic nonglucocorticoid steroids to protect the cell membrane from the damaging effects of lipid peroxidation.[66] Polyethylene glycol-bound superoxide dismutase (PEG-SOD) is another free-radical scavenger that is given to increase the SOD level noted with ischemic brain injury.[67] Of the EAAs, glutamate is an excitatory neurotransmitter, and NMDA-antagonist drugs have been developed to block the effects of glutamate.

Another line of investigation has focused on cytokines; elevated in tissue after head injury, they play a role in a cascade of events resulting in cell death. In the laboratory, cytokines alter the blood–brain barrier, which produces cerebral edema. Although not completely understood, interleukin (IL)-1, IL-6, tumor necrosis factor, and IL-8 play a role in cellular injury.[68] Further investigation many suggest pharmacological interventions to ameliorate the cascade.

In practice, the goal of research-based practice is emerging. Many of the practices in patient management are being questioned, and validation is being sought from well designed prospective studies. As practices are examined, it is evident that the scientific basis is not always congruent with the practices that have been the routine. It is also apparent that all head injuries are not the same, and a distinction must be made among multifactorial pathophysiological processes, such as cerebral ischemia, cerebral hyperemia, and cytotoxic edema, and vasogenic edema to choose the most appropriate and effective treatment. More care is being targeted to maintaining certain critical physiological thresholds, such as CPP, and keeping physiological parameters within certain therapeutic ranges to optimize cerebral oxygen delivery and meet the metabolic needs of cerebral tissue. In addition, a better understanding of the development of cerebral pathophysiology over a time line assists the clinician to know when to target certain therapies to be most effective.[69] Understanding that the peak of cerebral edema occurs about 72 hours postinjury will assist in administering specific therapies to optimize effect.

Finally, there have been a number of therapeutic interventions for managing increased ICP in head-injured patients. These interventions have been treated as a pool of possibilities without any assignment of order for use or risk-benefit ratio. As a result of clinical research, an order of when and under what circumstances particular interventions should be given is emerging, and the random use or use based on personal preference is being replace by new paradigms and algorithms to guide practice. The most important contribution to care brought to the bedside by the clinician is the clinical reasoning and decision-making skills. A refined understanding of when and how to use particular interventions, such as hyperventilation, will improve the clinical reasoning and decision-making skills and thus improve outcomes for patients. It is possible that the refinement of treatment strategies will continue in the next few years, resulting in major strides as the decade of the brain comes to a close.

References

1. U.S. Department of Health and Human Services, Public Health Service (1990). *Healthy people 2000: National health promotion and disease prevention objectives*. Washington, DC: DHHS Publication No. (PHS) 91-50212. Washington, DC: US Government Printing Office.
2. Valsamis, M. P. (1994). Pathology of trauma. *Neurosurgery Clinics of North American, 5*(1), 175–183.
3. Olshaker, J. S., & Whye, D. W. (1994). Head injury. *Emergency Medicine Clinics of North America, 11*(1), 165–186.
4. Siesjo, B. K. (1988). Mechanisms of ischemic brain damage. *Critical Care Medicine, 16*, 954–963.
5. Hayek, D. A., & Veremakis, C. (1992). Physiologic concerns during brain resuscitation. In Civetta, J. M., Taylor, R. W., Kirby, R. R. (Eds.), *Critical care* (pp. 1449–1466). Philadelphia: J.B. Lippincott.
6. Siesjo. B. K. (1993). Basic mechanisms of traumatic brain damage. *Annals of Emergency Medicine, 22*, 959–969.
7. Caron, M. J., Hovda, D. A., & Becker, D. P. (1991). Changes in the treatment of head injury. *Neurosurgery Clinics of North America, 2*(2), 483–491.

8. Lipton, S. A. (1993). Molecular mechanisms of trauma-induced neuronal degeneration. *Current Opinion in Neurology and Neurosurgery, 6,* 588–596.

9. Ibid, Caron et al., p. 487.

10. Ibid, p. 488.

11. Ibid, p. 488.

12. Astrup, J. (1982). Energy-requiring cell functions in the ischemic brain. *Journal of Neurosurgery, 56,* 482.

13. Ibid, Hayek & Vermakis, p. 1450.

14. Symon, L. (1985). Flow thresholds in brain ischaemia and the effects of drugs. *British Journal of Anesthesia, 57,* 34.

15. Ibid, Hayek & Vermakis, p. 1450.

16. Wilberger, J, & Chen, D. A. (1991). The skull and meninges. *Neurosurgery Clinics of North America, 2*(2), 341–350.

17. Chestnut, R. M., & Marshall, L. F. (1993). Management of severe head injury. In A. H. Ropper (Ed.), *Neurological and neurosurgical intensive care* (3rd ed.) (pp. 203–246). New York: Raven.

18. Brandt, K. E., Burruss, G. L., Hickerson, W. I., White, C. E., & DeLozier, J. B. (1991). The management of mid-face fractures with intracranial injury. *The Journal of Trauma, 31*(1), 15–19.

19. Adams, J. H., Doyle, D., Ford, I., Gennarelli, T. A., Graham, D. I., & McLellan D. R. (1989). Diffuse axonal injury in head injury: Definition, diagnosis, and grading. *Histopathololgy, 15,* 49–59.

20. Chedid, M. K., & Flannery, A. M. (1995). Head trauma. In J. E. Parrillo & R. C. Bone (Eds.), *Critical care medicine: Principles of diagnosis and management* (pp. 1235–1259). St. Louis: C.V. Mosby.

21. Ibid, p. 1240.

22. Crooks, D. A. (1991). The pathological concept of diffuse axonal injury; Its pathogenesis and the assessment of severity. *Journal of Pathology, 165,* 5–10.

23. Slazinski, T., & Johnson, M. C. (1994). Severe diffuse axonal injury in adults and children. *Journal of Neuroscience Nursing, 26*(3), 151–154.

24. Aldrich, E. F. (1991). Surgical management of traumatic intracerebral hematomas. *Neurosurgical Clinics of North America, 2*(2), 373–385.

25. Ibid, Chedid & Flannery, p. 1240.

26. Drake, C. G. (1961). Subdural hematoma from arterial rupture. *Journal of Neurosurgery, 8,* 597.

27. Ibid, Aldrich, p. 373.

28. Cooper, P. R. (1992). Delayed traumatic intracererbral hemorrhage. *Neurosurgery Clinics of North America, 3*(3), 659–665.

29. Committee on Trauma, American College of Surgeons (1993). *Advanced trauma life support: Course for physicians* (5th ed.) (pp. 161–183). Chicago: American College of Surgeons.

30. Rosomoff, H. L., Kochanek, P. M., Clark, R., DeKosky, S. T., Ebmeyer, U., Grenvik, A. N., Marion, D. W., Palmer, A., Safar, P., & White, R. J. (1996). Resuscitation from severe brain trauma. *Critical Care Medicine, 24*(Suppl.), S48–S56.

31. Kalisch, B. J., Kalisch, P. A., Burns, S. M., Kocan, M. J., & Presdergast, V. (1995). Intrahospital transport of neuro ICU patients. *Journal of Neuroscience Nursing, 27*(2), 69–77.

32. Eisenhart, K. (1994). New perspectives in the management of adults with severe head injury. *Critical Care Nursing Quarterly, 17*(2), 1–12.

33. Bell, S. D., Guyer, D., Snyder, M. A., & Miner, M. (1994). Cerebral hemodynamics: Monitoring arteriojugular oxygen content differences. *Journal of Neuroscience Nursing, 26*(5), 270–277.

34. Kerr, M. E., Lovasik, D., & Darby, J. (1995). Evaluating cerebral oxygenation using jugular venous oximetry in head injuries. *AACN Clinical Issues, 6*(1), 11–20.

35. March, K. (1994). Retrograde jugular catheter: Monitoring SjO2. *Journal of Neuroscience Nursing, 26*(1), 48–51.

36. Robertson, C. S., & Simpson, R. K. (1991). Neurophysiologic monitoring of patients with head injuries. *Neurosurgery Clinics of North American, 2*(2), 285–299.

37. Chestnut, R. M. (1995). Medical management of severe head injury: Present and future. *New Horizons, 3*(3), 581–593.

38. Prielipp, R. C., & Coursin, D. B. (1995). Sedative and neuromuscular blocking drug use in critically ill patients with head injuries. *New Horizons, 3*(3), 456–468.

39. Ibid, p. 456.

40. Murray, M. J., Strickland, R. A., & Weiler, C. (1993). The use of neuromuscular blocking drugs in the intensive care unit: A US perspective. *Intensive Care Medicine, 19,* S40–S44.

41. Ford, E. V. (1995). Monitoring neuromuscular blockade in the adult ICU. *American Journal of Critical Care, 4*(2), 122–130.

42. Kelly, D. F. (1995). Steroids in head injury. *New Horizons, 3*(3), 453–455.

43. Elvidge, A. R. (1939). Remarks on post-traumatic convulsive state. *Transactions of the American Neurology Association, 65,* 125–129.

44. Temkin, N. R., Dikmen, S. S., & Winn, H. R. (1991). Posttraumatic seizures. *Neurosurgery Clinics of North American, 2*(2), 425–435.

45. Temkin, N. R., Dikmen, S. S., Wilensky, A. J., Keihm, J., Chabal, S., & Winn, H. R. (1990). A randomized, double-blind study of phenytoin for the prevention of post-traumatic seizures. *New England Journal of Medicine, 323*(8), 497–502.

46. Ibid, Chestnut, p. 219.

47. Ibid, Chedid & Flannery, p. 1249.

48. Muizelaar, J. P., Marmarou, A., Ward, J. D., Kontos, H. A., Choi, A. C., Becker, D. P., Gruemer, H., & Young, H. F. (1991). Adverse effects of prolonged hyperventilation in patients with severe head injury: A randomized clinical trial. *Journal of Neurosurgery, 75,* 731–739.

49. Zornow, M. H., & Prough, D. S. (1995). Fluid management in patients with traumatic brain injury. *New Horizons, 3*(3), 488–498.

50. Pulsinelli, W. A., Waldman, S., Rawlinson, D. et al. (1982). Moderate hyperglycemia agents ischemia brain damage: a neuropathologic study in the rat. *Neurology, 32,* 1239–1246.

51. Ibid, p. 491.

52. Lanier, W. L., Stangland, K. J., Scheithauer, B. W. et al. (1987). The effects of dextrose infusion and head position on neurologic outcome after complete cerebral ischemia in primates: Examination of a model. *Anesthesiology, 66,* 39–48.

53. Zornow, M. H., & Prough, D. S. (1995). Fluid management in patients with traumatic brain. *New Horizons, 3*(3), 492.

54. Bingaman, W. E., & Frank, J. I. (1995). Malignant cerebral edema and intracranial hypertension. *Neurologic Clinics, 13*(3), 479–509.

55. Tietjen, C. S., Hurn, P. D., Ulatowski, J. A., & Kirsch, J. R. (1996). Treatment modalities for hypertensive patients with intracranial pathology: Options and risks. *Critical Care Medicine, 24*(2), 311–322.

56. Rose, B. A. Neurological therapies in critical care. *Critical Care Nursing Clinics of North America, 5*(2), 237–246.

57. Bedford, R., Darcey, R., Winn, R. et al. (1983). Adverse impact of a calcium entry-blocker (verapamil) on intracranial pressure in patients with brain tumors. *Journal of Neurosurgery, 59,* 800–802.

58. Chestnut, R. M. (1993). Medical complications of the head-injured patient. In P. R. Cooper (Ed.), *Head injury* (pp. 476–478). Baltimore: Williams & Wilkins.

59. Nih, C. R. (1986). Prevention of venous thrombosis and pulmonary embolism. *Journal of the American Medical Association, 256,* 744–749.

60. Ibid, Chestnut (1993), p. 472.

61. Kaufman, H. H., Timberlake, G., Voelker J., & Pait, T. G. (1993). Medical complications of head injury. *Medical Clinics of North America, 77*(1), 43–60.

62. Ibid, Chestnut (1993), pp. 481–482.

63. Lam, A. M., Winn, H. R., Cullen, B. F., & Sundling, N. (1991). Hyperglycemia and neurological outcome in patients with head injury. *Journal of Neurosurgery, 75,* 5445–5551.

64. Stechmiller, J., Treloar, D. M., Derrico, D., Yarandi, H., & Guin, P. (1994). Interruption of enteral feedings in head injured patients. *Journal of Neuroscience Nursing, 26*(4), 224–229.

65. Davis, A. E., & White, J. J. (1995). Innovative sensory input for the comatose brain-injured patient. *Critical Care Nursing Clinics of North America, 7*(2), 351–361.

66. Hall, E. D., Yonkers, P. A., McCall, J. M. et al. (1988). Effects of the 21-aminosteroid U-74, 006F on experimental head injury in mice. *Journal of Neurosurgery, 68,* 456–461.

67. Meldrum, B., Millan, M. H., & Obrenovitch, T. P. (1992). Excitatory amino acid release induced by injury. In M. Y. Globus & W. D. Dietrich (Eds.), *The role of neurotransmitters in brain injury.* New York: Plenum Press.

68. Ott, L., McCain, C. J., Gilespe, M. et al. (1994). Cytokines in metabolic dysfunction after severe head injury. *Journal of Neurotrauma, 11,* 447–472.

69. Chestnut, R. M. (1995). Medical management of severe head injury: Present and future. *New Horizons, 3*(3), 589–593.

Bibliography

Books

Alexander, M. P. (1993). Survivors of traumatic brain injury. In R. T. Johnson & J. W. Griffin (Eds.), *Current therapy in neurologic disease* (4th ed.) (pp. 202–206). St. Louis: B.C. Decker.

Chestnut, R. M. (1993). Medical complications of the head-injured patient. In P. R. Cooper (Ed.), *Head injury* (3rd ed.) (pp. 459–501). Baltimore: Williams & Wilkins.

Chestnut, R. M., & Marshall, L. F. (1993). Management of Severe Head Injury. In H. A. Ropper (Ed.), *Neurological and neurosurgical intensive care* (3rd ed.) (pp. 203–246). New York: Raven Press.

Kraus, J. F. (1993). Epidemiology of head injury. In P. R. Cooper (Ed.), *Head injury* (3rd ed.) (pp. 1–25). Baltimore: Williams & Wilkins.

McQuillan, K. A. (1995). Traumatic brain injury. In N. Urban, K. Greenlee, J. Krumberger, & C. Winkelman (Eds.), *Guidelines for critical care nursing* (pp. 24–51). St. Louis: C.V. Mosby.

Periodicals

Bergquist, T. F., & Jacket, M. P. (1993). Awareness and goal setting with the traumatically brain injured. *Brain Injury, 7*(3), 275–282.

Bontke, C. F., & Boake, C. (1991). Traumatic brain injury rehabilitation. *Neurosurgery Clinics of North America, 2*(2), 473–482.

Borel, C. O., & Guy, J. (1995). Ventilatory management in critical neurologic illness. *Neurologic Clinics, 13*(3), 627–644.

Brust, J. C. M. (1995). Neurological effects of illicit drug abuse. *The Neurologist, 1,* 105–114.

Cervos-Navarro, J., & Lafuente, J. V. (1991). Traumatic brain injuries: Structural changes. *Journal of the Neurological Sciences, 103,* S3–S14.

Chestnut, R. M., Marshall, L. F., Klauber, M. R., Blunt, B. A., Baldwin, N., Eisenberg, H. M., Jane, J. A., Marmarou, A., & Fooulkes, M. A. (1993). The role of secondary brain injury in determining outcome from severe head injury. *The Journal of Trauma, 34*(3), 216–222.

Coburn, K. (1992). Traumatic brain injury: The silent epidemic. *AACN Clinical Issues, 3*(1), 9–18.

Condeluci, A. (1992). Brain injury rehabilitation: The need to bridge paradigms. *Brain Injury, 6*(6), 543–551.

Cooper, P. R. (1992). Delayed traumatic intracerebral hemorrhage. *Neurosurgery Clinics of North America, 3*(3), 659–665.

Crosby, L. J., & Parsons, L. C. (1992). Cerebrovascular response of closed head-injured patients to a standardized endotracheal tube suctioning and manual hyperventilation procedure. *Journal of Neuroscience Nursing, 24*(1), 40–49.

Davis, M., & Lucatorto, M. (1994). Mannitol revisited. *Journal of Neuroscience Nursing, 26*(3), 170–174.

Diringer, M. N. (1992). Management of sodium abnormalities in patients with CNS disease. *Clinical Neuropharmacology, 15*(6), 427–447.

Godbole, K. B., Berbiglia, V. A., & Goddard, L. (1991). A head-injured patient: Caloric needs, clinical progress and nursing care priorities. *Journal of Neuroscience Nursing, 23*(5), 290–294.

Grinspun, D. (1993). Bladder management for adults following head injury. *Rehabilitation Nursing, 18*(5), 300–305.

Gualtieri, T., & Cox, D. R. (1991). The delayed neurobehavioural sequelae of traumatic brain injury. *Brain Injury, 5*(32), 219–232.

Guin, P. R., & Freudenberger, K. (1992). The elderly neuroscience patient: Implications for the critical care nurse. *AACN Clinical Issues, 3*(1), 98–105.

Gurnery, J. G., Rivara, F. P., Mueller, B. A., Newell, D. W., Copass, M. K., & Jorovich, G. J. (1994). The effects of alcohol intoxication on the initial treatment and hospital course of patients with acute brain injury. *Journal of Trauma, 33,* 709–713.

Hall, E. D. (1992). The neuroprotective pharmacology of methylprednisolone. *Journal of Neurosurgery, 76,* 13–22.

Hall, E. D., McCall, J. M., & Means, E. D. (1994). Therapeutic potential of the lazaroids (21-aminosteroids) in acute central nervous system trauma, ischemia and subarachnoid hemorrhage. *Advances in Pharmacology, 28,* 221–268.

Hilton, G. (1994). Secondary brain injury and the role of neuroprotective agents. *Journal of Neuroscience Nursing, 26*(4), 251–255.

Jastremski, C. A. (1994). Traumatic brain injury: Assessment and treatment. *Critical Care Nursing Clinics of North America, 6*(3), 473–481.

Johnston, M. V., & Hall, K. M. (1994). Outcomes evaluation in TBI rehabilitation. Part I: Overview and system principles. *Archives of Physical Medicine & Rehabilitation, 75*(SC), 2–9.

Kreutzer, J. S., Marwitz, J. H., & Kepler, K. (1992). Traumatic brain injury: Family response and outcome. *Archives of Physical Medicine & Rehabilitation, 73,* 771–778.

Leaf, L. E. (1993). Traumatic brain injury: Affecting family recovery. *Brain Injury, 7*(6), 543–546.

Kerr, M. E., & Brucia, J. (1993). Hyperventilation in the head-injured patient: An effective treatment modality? *Heart & Lung, 22,* 516–521.

Lehmkuhl, L. D., Hall, K. M., Mann, N., & Gordon, W. A. (1993). Factors that influence costs and length of stay of persons with traumatic brain injury in acute care and inpatient rehabilitation. *Journal of Health Trauma Rehabilitation, 8*(2), 88–100.

Levin, H. S., & Eisenberg, H. M. (1991). Neurobehavioral outcome. *Neurosurgery Clinics of North America, 2*(2), 457–472.

Marion, D. W. (1991). Complications of head injury and their therapy. *Neurosurgery Clinics of North America, 2*(2), 411–424.

Marmarou, A. (1994). Traumatic brain edema: An overview. *Acta Neurochir, 60*(Suppl), 421–424.

Massagli, T. L. (1991). Neurobehavioral effects of phenytoin, carbamazepine, and valproic acid: Implications for use in traumatic brain injury. *Archives of Physical Medicine & Rehabilitation, 72,* 219–226.

McIntosh, T. K. (1994). Neurochemical sequelae of traumatic brain injury: Therapeutic implications. *Cerebrovascular and Brain Metabolism Reviews, 6,* 109–162.

Obana, W. G., & Pitts, L. H. (1991). Extracerebral lesions. *Neurosurgery Clinics of North America, 2*(2), 351–372.

Rimel, R. W., Giordani, B., Barth, J. T., Boll, T. J., & Jane, J.A. (1981). Diasbility caused by minor head injury. *Neurosurgery, 9,* 221–228.

Rosenthal, M. (1993). Mild traumatic brain injury syndrome. *Annals of Emergency Medicine, 22*(6), 1048–1051.

Siesjo, B. K. (1993). Basic mechanisms of traumatic brain damage. *Annals of Emergency Medicine, 22*(6), 959–969.

Stratton, M., & Gregory, R. J. (1994). After traumatic brain injury: A discussion of consequences. *Brain Injury, 8*(7), 631–345.

Sundrani, S. (1995). Neurologic intensive care unit management and economic issues. *Neurologic Critical Care, 13*(3), 679–693.

Szymanski, H. V., & Linn, R. (1992). A review of the postconcussion syndrome. *International Journal of Psychiatry in Medicine, 22*(4), 357–375.

Torner, J. C. (1992). Outcome evaluation in acute neurological injury. *Current Opinion in Neurology and Neurosurgery, 5,* 831–839.

Vollmer, D. G., & Dacey, R. G. (1991). The management of mild and moderate head injuries. *Neurosurgery Clinics of North America, 2*(2), 437–455.

Ward, J. D. (1991). Prehospital care. *Neurosurgery Clinics of North America, 2*(2), 251–255.

White, B. C., & Krause, G. S. (1993). Brain injury and repair mechanisms: The potential for pharmacologic therapy in closed-head trauma. *Annals of Emergency Medicine, 22*(6), 970–979.

Young, B., Ott, L., Phillips, R., & McClain, C. (1991). Metabolic management of the patient with head injury. *Neurosurgery Clinics of North America, 2*(2), 301–320.

Young, G. B. (1995). Neurologic complications of systemic critical illness. *Neurologic Clinics, 13*(3), 645–658.

CHAPTER 22

Vertebral and Spinal Cord Injuries

Joanne V. Hickey

This chapter has been divided into two parts to organize better the large volume of information. Part I presents background material on vertebral and spinal cord injury and interdisciplinary management to help the nurse understand the basis for care. Part II focuses on the nursing management of patients in the acute and postacute phases of care. The nurse's role in a rehabilitation facility is beyond the scope of this text. However, a discussion of the continuum of care will provide the acute care nurse with an understanding of acute care management and outcomes in the rehabilitation phase.

Part One
Background and
Interdisciplinary Management

A PERSPECTIVE

Statistics and Facts

Recent information from the National Institute of Neurological Disorders and Stroke provides the following information on spinal cord injury:[1]

- Incidence: About 10,000 Americans are paralyzed by spinal cord injury each year.
- Prevalence: Estimates of the number of people living with spinal cord injuries vary from 200,000 to 500,000.
- Age: Sixty percent of spinal cord injuries occur in people 16 to 30 years old.
- Gender: Eighty-two percent of those affected are males.
- Etiology: Motor vehicle accidents (47.7%) remain the number one cause of spinal cord injuries, followed by falls, gunshot wounds, and recreational sports, particularly diving accidents. In some areas, gunshot wounds can exceed motor vehicle accidents for cause of injury.

- Greatest risk for injury: In the summer, Americans spend the most time on the road, hiking, swimming, and participating in other recreational activities.
- Cost: Care and services for severely disabled survivors are constantly increasing; estimates for 200,000 severely disabled survivors now exceed $10 billion a year.

A Philosophy of Care

The lessons learned from the Model Regional Spinal Cord Injury (SCI) Care System program established in 1970 by the Rehabilitation Services Administration have been effective in providing a comprehensive model for managing patients with spinal cord injuries across the continuum of care. The best patient and cost effective outcomes have been achieved when a well developed system from management of patients from injury site through rehabilitation is in place. The most important change in the care of acute spinal cord injured patients is the use of the high-dose steroid protocol established in 1991. This is discussed in the treatment section.

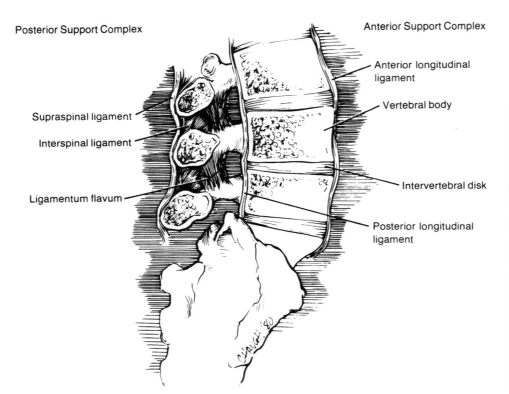

Cervical Nerves
- C1
- C2 — Head and Neck
- C3 — Diaphragm
- C4 — Deltoids, Biceps
- C5 — Wrist Extensors
- C6
- C7 — Triceps
- C8 — Hand

Thoracic Nerves
- T1
- T2
- T3
- T4 — Chest muscles
- T5
- T6
- T7
- T8
- T9
- T10 — Abdominal muscles
- T11
- T12

Tetraplegia

Paraplegia

Lumbar Nerves
- L1
- L2
- L3 — Leg muscles
- L4
- L5

Sacral Nerves
- S1
- S2
- S3
- S4 — Bowel, Bladder, Sexual Function
- S5

FIGURE 22-1
The higher the injury on the spinal cord, the more extensive the paralysis.

GENERAL INFORMATION

Anatomical Considerations

To appreciate the potential injuries to the spinal axis and its surrounding structures, a few points should be made about the relationship of anatomical structures. The vertebral column, the spinal cord, the supporting soft tissue, and the intervertebral discs are all interrelated. The vertebrae are the irregularly shaped bones that support the muscles and protect the spinal cord. There are 33 vertebrae in the vertebral column: 7 cervical, 12 thoracic or dorsal, 5 lumbar, 5 sacral (fused into one), and 4 coccygeal (fused into one). The vertebrae of each area have a distinctive shape. Stacked one on another to form the vertebral column, the vertebrae are laced into position by a series of supporting structures called ligaments. The ligaments, muscles, and other supporting structures are considered to be soft-tissue components (Figs. 22-1 and 22-2; see also Chap. 5).

There are two main parts to a vertebra: the body and the arch. The vertebral bodies are separated by intervertebral discs that serve as shock absorbers for the vertebral column during movement. The arch of the vertebra is created by a series of irregularly shaped projections—that is, the fusion of two pedicles and two laminae along with seven articular processes that create a bony ring. The various projections of the vertebral arch allow for alignment, flexion, and movement of the vertebral column. The soft, vulnerable spinal cord passes through the bony arch of the vertebrae, which offers it protection.

The close anatomical relationship of the vertebrae, ligaments and other soft tissue structures, intervertebral discs, and spinal cord increases the probability that injury to any one of these structures can cause concurrent injury to any one or all

Posterior Support Complex

- Supraspinal ligament
- Interspinal ligament
- Ligamentum flavum

Anterior Support Complex

- Anterior longitudinal ligament
- Vertebral body
- Intervertebral disk
- Posterior longitudinal ligament

FIGURE 22-2
Soft-tissue supporting structures of the spine. Two basic soft-tissue units constitute each spinal segment: the *anterior support complex*, formed by the anterior and posterior longitudinal ligaments, the disc, and the annulus, and the *posterior support complex*, formed by the supraspinal ligament and interspinal ligament, the ligamentum flavum, and the facet capsules. When the posterior complex is disrupted, the spine is unstable, and surgical fusion is necessary. When the anterior complex is disrupted, the spine is usually more stable and can heal with use of a rigid brace. (From Weiner, W. J., & Goetz, C. G. [eds] [1989]. *Neurology for the non-neurologist* [2nd ed.] [p. 261]. (Fig. 21-1). Philadelphia: J. B. Lippincott.)

of the other structures. In other instances, injury to one structure, such as a vertebral fracture, can create the potential of injury to another structure, such as the spinal cord, if the primary injury is not treated promptly and effectively. Therefore, when discussing injury to the vertebral column and spinal cord, one must consider the interrelatedness of not only these two structures, but also the supporting soft-tissue structures and the intervertebral discs.

Vertebral, spinal cord, and soft-tissue injuries are discussed in this chapter. Intervertebral disc disease is the focus of Chapter 23.

Kinetics of Movement

Beginning at the top, the seven cervical vertebrae support the head, which weighs 8 to 10 lb. These vertebrae provide substantial movement of the neck and head in various directions, including flexion, extension, and rotation. The total amount of flexion and extension possible at the cervical spine is an 80-degree arc, 75% of which is extension. Rotation is made possible by the uniquely shaped atlas (C-1) and axis (C-2). Beneath the cervical vertebrae are the 12 thoracic vertebrae, which move very little because of the anchoring of the ribs. Because the cervical spine is not fixed like the thoracic spine, it is extremely vulnerable to injury as a result of acceleration-deceleration.

Mechanics of Injury

Spinal injuries result when excessive forces are exerted on the spinal column. These forces are most often the result of acceleration-deceleration events that result in hyperflexion, hyperextension, deformation, axial loading, and excessive rotation.

ACCELERATION-DECELERATION

Acceleration and deceleration are discussed together because they often occur in rapid sequence. At the moment of impact in a rear-end collision (in which external force is applied from the rear), there is sudden **acceleration** of the portion of the body that is in contact with the seat. The head and upper back that are not in contact with the seat or headrest are violently thrust backward (hyperextension). Once the head strikes the back of the seat or has hyperextended to its limit, it is then thrust forward. The head may strike the steering wheel or dashboard as it slows down or decelerates.

Deceleration is often the major mechanism implicated in head-on collisions. The outside force is exerted from the front, causing the head and body to continue moving forward until contact is made, usually with the dashboard. The person is forcibly hyperflexed while moving forward, hits the dashboard, and then snaps back into a forced hyperextension position.

CATEGORIES OF RESPONSE TO EXTREME ACCELERATION-DECELERATION EVENTS

Acceleration-deceleration can produce simultaneous or successive actions, or both, as detailed in the following descriptions:

- Hyperflexion. **Hyperflexion** tends to produce compression of the vertebral bodies with disruption of the posterior longitudinal ligaments and the intervertebral discs.
- Hyperextension. **Hyperextension** usually causes fractures of the posterior elements of the spinal column and disruption of the anterior longitudinal ligaments.
- Deformation. **Deformation** refers to the various alterations in the spinal cord and supporting soft-tissue structures that are necessary to accommodate abnormal movements, such as hyperflexion, hyperextension, and excessive rotation. For example, in hyperextension of the cervical neck, the spinal canal shortens, the anterior longitudinal ligaments elongate, and the ligamenta flava are compressed and may bulge into the spinal canal, resulting in injury to the involved tissue.
- Axial loading. **Axial loading**, also known as **vertical compression**, occurs when a vertical force is exerted on the spinal column. Examples of incidents in which axial loading is seen are diving accidents, landing on the feet when jumping from a height, or landing on the buttocks when falling from a height.
- Excessive rotation. **Excessive rotation** refers to turning of the head beyond the normal range on the horizontal axis, resulting in compression fractures, tearing or rupture of the posterior ligament, dislocation at the facet joint, and fracture at the articular processes.

Classification of Injuries

The velocity, angle of impact, and type of exaggerated mechanical movement produced affect the type of injury sustained. These factors are considered in the classification of injuries.

Patients who have anatomical abnormalities or disease processes of the spinal column are much more vulnerable to injury than those who do not. Chronic conditions, such as cervical spondylosis, spinal stenosis, arthritis, and scoliosis, are examples of conditions that increase the probability of injury.

A basic classification of the causes of injury to the vertebral column, spinal cord, and soft tissue includes the following categories and their characteristics.

HYPERFLEXION INJURIES

Hyperflexion injuries (Figs. 22-3 and 22-4) are caused by hyperflexion of the head and neck, as in sudden deceleration; they are seen in head-on collisions and in diving accidents.

If the posterior ligaments are intact, a **wedge** or **compression fracture** of the vertebral body is common; this is considered to be a relatively stable fracture that does not usually require surgery. A flexion-extension fluoroscopic study may be ordered to rule out a fracture not seen on plain x-rays.

If the posterior ligaments are torn, the facets are usually disengaged and dislocated; this is considered an unstable fracture, probably requiring surgical stabilization.

There is a high probability of cord damage with fracture dislocations or bilateral jumped locked facet fractures. These injuries occur most often in the cervical region and involve the greatest areas of stress, levels C-5 and C-6. A lateral hyperflexion injury can occur as a result of extreme lateral flexion or rotation of the head and neck.

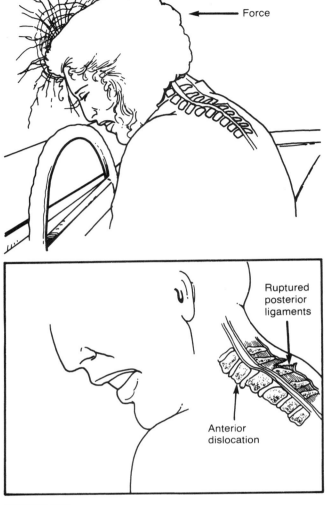

FIGURE 22-3
Hyperflexion injury. With hyperflexion to the cervical spine, there may be tearing of the posterior ligamentous complex, resulting in anterior dislocation.

HYPEREXTENSION INJURIES

Hyperextension injuries (Fig. 22-5) are caused by hyperextension of the head and neck, such as that which occurs in a rear-end vehicular collision. Hyperextension injuries tend to cause the greatest amount of injury because backward and downward movement involves a larger arc than flexion. If the head flexes forward, the chin strikes the chest and limits the arc. If the head flexes laterally, the head strikes the shoulder.

The spinal cord is stretched and lies against the ligamenta flava. This type of injury can cause contusion and ischemia to part of the spinal cord, resulting in neurological deficits even if the x-ray examination proves negative. As a rule, ligaments remain intact; no fractures or dislocations occur. The greatest area of stress for a hyperextension injury is at the level of C-4 and C-5; respiratory compromise, either from direct injury or ascending edema, is a concern.

These injuries are commonly seen in elderly people if they fall and strike their chin. A less severe form of a hyperextension injury is called a "whiplash" or acceleration injury. It is a stress and strain injury to the soft tissue (muscles and ligaments), but there is no vertebral or spinal cord injury.

COMPRESSION INJURIES

Compression injuries (Figs. 22-6 and 22-7) are caused by axial loading or vertical pressure, such as occurs when a person falls from a height and lands on the feet or buttocks; they can also result from lateral flexion. Compression fractures cause wedging, crushing, or bursting of the vertebral body. Compression fractures are sometimes subdivided into **simple wedge fracture, burst fracture,** and **teardrop fracture,** depending on the degree of compression or fracture line as noted on x-ray films.

ROTATIONAL INJURIES

Rotational injuries (Fig. 22-8) are caused by extreme lateral flexion or twisting of the head and neck. The posterior ligaments are torn or ruptured so that the rotational force causes

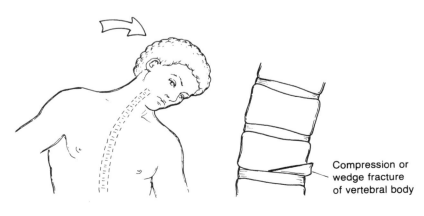

Compression or wedge fracture of vertebral body

FIGURE 22-4
Lateral hyperflexion injury. Compression or wedge fracture of the vertebral body.

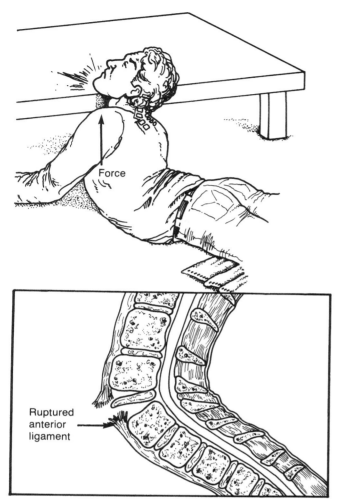

FIGURE 22-5
Hyperextension injury in the cervical area. Injuries related to falls in which the chin is struck, forcing the neck to hyperextend, may cause rupture of the anterior ligament.

SPECIFIC INFORMATION ABOUT INJURIES

Soft-Tissue Injuries

WHIPLASH

Whiplash is a lay term used to describe an acceleration injury that causes the head to hyperextend as a result of a rear-end vehicular collision. The ligaments and muscles of the neck sustain stress and strain injury. The usual signs and symptoms—stiff neck, pain in the neck and shoulder, limitation of movement, and muscle spasms—may not begin until 12 to 48 hours after injury. Other signs and symptoms may include headache, parenthesia, dizziness, vertigo, and tinnitus. The findings on physical examination are normal except for the previous signs and symptoms. The radiological examination is negative. The diagnosis is based on the history of injury and the presence of the characteristic signs and symptoms. This is a common injury causing much pain and suffering to the patient, even though no abnormalities are noted on radiographical examination.

The pain caused by whiplash is thought to be attributable to the tearing, stretching, microhemorrhage, and edema incurred by the anterior neck muscles (sternocleidomastoid, sca-

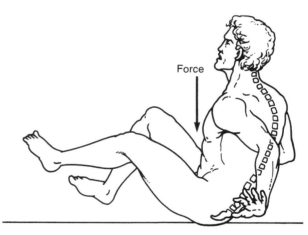

dislocation at the facet joint and fracture at the articular processes.

One or two facets may be involved. If one facet is dislocated or locked, there are usually no neurological deficits. More than half of the patients with two facets locked will have neurological deficits. Reduction of the fracture is achieved by traction (cervical traction or halo with or without a jacket) or surgery to disengage the facets and stabilize the vertebral column (Cotrel-Dubousset [CD] rods; see surgical management section later in this chapter).

PENETRATING INJURIES

Penetrating injuries occur when missiles, such as bullets or shrapnel, or impalement instruments (knives, ice picks) penetrate the spinal column or supporting soft tissue. The object may shatter bone, create bone fragments, or transect a portion or complete plane of the spinal cord or soft tissue.

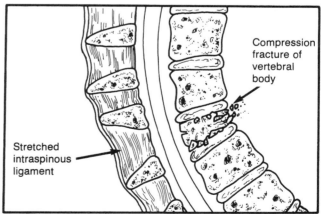

FIGURE 22-6
Hyperflexion injury in the lumbar area. Injury can be caused by falling onto the buttocks. Note the compression fracture and the stretching of the intraspinious ligament.

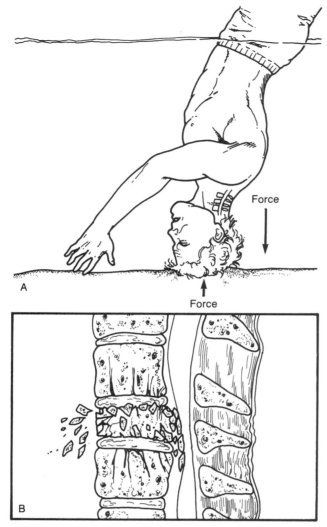

FIGURE 22-7
Compression fracture secondary to axial loading.

lenus, and longus colli muscles). The muscles, and possibly the ligaments, are strained. Patients with pre-existing cervical spondylosis and some other conditions are at greater risk of developing problems if a whiplash injury occurs because of narrowing of the foramina and osteophytes and increased rigidity of the spinal column.

Treatment. Treatment includes measures directed at comfort. Mild injuries are treated with mild analgesics (*e.g.*, aspirin, acetaminophen), local heat, and rest. More severe injuries are treated with short-term use of a soft collar, heat and cold application, analgesics, muscle relaxants, and anti-inflammatory agents.

Non-narcotic analgesics should be used as much as possible. Ibuprofen (Motrin) is a common choice because it also has an anti-inflammatory effect. It inhibits prostaglandin synthesis, a substance known to be related to pain. Narcotic analgesics are reserved for severe pain and should be used sparingly to prevent dependency. One of the most popular muscle relaxants is cyclobenzaprine hydrochloride (Flexeril). In ad-

dition to Motrin, other anti-inflammatory agents used are phenylbutazone (Butazolidin) and indomethacin (Indocin).

Extended use of a cervical collar is controversial. Some physicians believe that collars hinder recovery of involved muscles if worn for more than a few days (Fig. 22-9).

OTHER SOFT-TISSUE INJURIES

Other soft-tissue trauma (see Fig. 22-2) may occur simultaneously with vertebral injury. Soft-tissue trauma is important when considering the stability versus the instability of the vertebral column and thus is discussed with vertebral and spinal cord injuries.

Vertebral Injuries
CLASSIFICATION

Although fractures can occur singularly in any part of the vertebral arch, most injuries occur in combination with vertebral body injuries. The "ends" of the vertebral column—the cervical and lumbar portions—have the greatest built-in mobility, thereby predisposing them to injury. The thoracic region

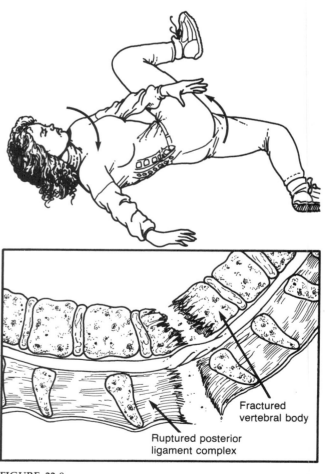

FIGURE 22-8
Rotational injury. When rotational force occurs, there is concurrent fracture and tearing of the posterior ligamentous complex.

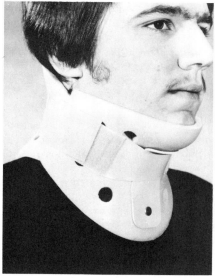

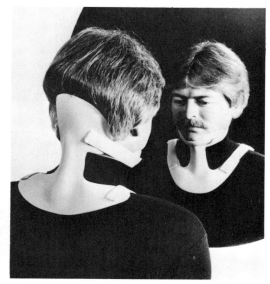

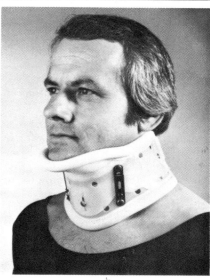

FIGURE 22-9
Types of rigid cervical collars.

is less prone to trauma because of the rigidity imparted to it by the rib cage.

Vertebral injuries can be classified according to criteria based on a perspective of injury:

- **Types of fractures**: simple or compression fractures
- **Fracture or dislocation**: pure fracture, dislocation, and fracture-dislocation
- **Stability or instability of injury**: according to a three-column framework
- **Segmental involvement**: upper cervical, subaxial cervical, thoracic or lumbar, and sacral

Each criterion offers a special practical perspective and is discussed in the following section.

Type of Fractures. For the purposes of this discussion, vertebral fractures are subdivided into simple and compression fractures.

Simple fractures appear as a singular break, and the alignment of the vertebral parts remains intact. These types of fractures usually occur to the spinous or transverse process, facets, pedicles, and vertebral body. There is usually no neural compression.

Compression fractures are sometimes further subclassified as *simple wedge fractures, burst fractures,* and *teardrop fractures.* They are caused by axial loading and hyperflexion.

Simple (wedge) compression fractures are caused by vertical compression when the cervical vertebral column is flexed, whereas the burst fracture is caused by the same mechanical force but when the vertebral column is straight. The posterior ligaments are intact; therefore the fracture is stable. No surgery is required; they heal well with hard collar immobilization for about 2 months.[2]

Burst fractures are explosive fractures caused by severe axial loading on a straight cervical column. They shatter the vertebral body into several pieces; these fragments then have the potential for being driven into the spinal cord, resulting in serious injury. If there is no neurological damage and the posterior ligaments are stable, then wearing a hard collar for 2 months may be warranted. However, burst fractures often require a combined neurosurgical-orthopedic procedure for the removal of bone fragments, cord decompression, and vertebral column stabilization by insertion of CD rods, a type of segmental rodding that can be accommodated to the individual's level of injury. This approach has rapidly replaced Harrington rods.

Teardrop fractures are caused by extreme flexion with axial loading so that one vertebral body is crushed by the vertebral body superior to it, causing the anterior portion of the compressed body to break away. These fractures are usually unstable (involving disruption of the posterior ligaments, resulting in forward dislocation) and are managed with anterior decompression and fusion with halo immobilization.

Fracture or Dislocation. As described previously, one type of injury sustained can be a vertebral fracture only. Another type of injury, dislocation, can occur without a fracture.

Dislocation occurs when one vertebra overrides another, and there is unilateral or bilateral facet dislocation. X-ray studies reveal a disruption in the established alignment of the vertebral column. Usually, the supporting ligaments are also injured, and the spinal cord may or may not be involved.

Subluxation is a partial or incomplete dislocation of one vertebra over another. Damage to the cord and supporting ligaments may or may not be present. With dislocation, reestablishment of alignment is necessary. This may be accomplished by traction followed by immobilization or by surgical stabilization (fusion or sometimes insertion of CD rods if the posterior ligaments are injured).

Fracture-dislocation, as the name implies, denotes a combined injury of a fracture and a dislocation that is usually accompanied by ligament and cord injury. As with simple dislocation, realignment is necessary. The fracture must be allowed to heal, and any bone fragments impinging on the cord must be removed. Therefore, surgery is indicated.

Stability or Instability of Injury. When considering vertebral fractures, it is critical to distinguish between fractures and dislocations that are stable from those that are unstable. To make this distinction, many base their opinion on the posterior ligaments. If the posterior ligaments are intact, the injury is considered stable; if they have been torn, usually by a rotational force, they are considered unstable. Stability of the vertebral-spinal elements is also considered using a three-column theoretical framework. This approach is discussed in Chart 22-1. A stable fracture or dislocation is not apt to displace beyond what was caused at the time of the injury, whereas unstable fracture or dislocation is highly probable for further displacement with extension of injury to the spinal cord. External immobilization or internal fixation may be unnecessary for stable injuries, whereas it is essential for unstable injuries. In addition, when ligaments heal, scar tissue forms. The scarred tissue is weaker than the preinjury tissue and may result in chronic instability, which can lead to spinal cord injury.

Segmental Vertebral Level. According to Lenke, O'Brien, and Bridwell, vertebral injuries are divided into four groups based on the involved segmental level: upper cervical, subaxial cervical, thoracic and lumbar, and sacral.[3]

UPPER CERVICAL SEGMENT. There are three types of upper cervical segment injuries. The four most commonly encountered are the atlas fractures, atlantoaxial subluxation, odontoid fractures, and hangman's fractures. The four less common injuries include occipital condyle fractures, atlanto-occipital dislocation, atlantoaxial rotary subluxation, and the C-2 lateral mass fractures. A summary of upper cervical fractures and lower cervical fractures is presented respectively in Tables 22-1 and 22-2.

SUBAXIAL CERVICAL SEGMENTS. An important differentiation between upper cervical spine and subaxial (below C-2) cervical spinal injuries is the increased risk of cervical cord injury in the lower (subaxial) cervical vertebrae. Two factors account for this finding: the size of the spinal canal decreased in the lower spine and the increased prevalence of injuries that narrow rather than expand the canal. Five types of subaxial cervical vertebrae injuries are discussed:

- **Isolated posterior element fractures** of the lamina, articular process, or spinous process occur as a result of compression-extension with impact of the posterior elements on one another.
- **Minor avulsion and compression fractures** of the subaxial cervical vertebrae include anterior compression or avulsion injuries of the vertebral body. Additionally, anterior and posterior concurrent bone injuries with minimal displacement and angulation are noted.
- **Vertebral body-burst fractures**, common in diving accidents, result from axial loading and flexion. The anterior and middle columns are involved, creating instability; bone may protrude into the spinal canal.
- **Teardrop fractures** occur from flexion and axial loading, resulting in a teardrop fragment on the anteroinferior aspect of the affected body. Spinal cord injury and three-column instability are usual.
- **Facet injuries causing spinal malalignment** occur with a variety of biomechanical forces. Reduction may have to be done in stages to prevent additional injury. If it cannot be done with traction, surgery will be necessary. Traumatic disc herniation may also be present and usually requires an anterior discectomy and fusion.

The treatment for subaxial cervical vertebral injuries includes immobilization with sternal-occipital-mandibular orthonic device, halo vest, posterior fusion and stabilization with wires or instrumentation, anterior approaches for decompression and fusion with or without instrumentation, and a combination of the above. Treatment choices will depend on the specifics of the fracture or malalignment and the stability of the ligaments.

(text continues on page 430)

CHART 22-1
*The Three-Column Framework: Spinal Stability and Instability**

Spinal stability refers to the ability of the vertebral support column to protect adequately the neural elements from injury during inactivity and activity. This determination is critical in managing patients because an unstable injury can result in extension of or new neurological deficits. Currently, criteria for determining spinal stability or instability are controversial.

Some physicians consider only the condition of the posterior ligaments when determining stability. Another approach is the three-column framework. The three-column approach provides an anatomical framework for considering stability. The cross-section of the spine is organized into three anatomical columns:

- The **anterior column** consists of the anterior longitudinal ligament, anterior half of the vertebral body, annulus fibrosis, and disc.
- The **middle column** consists of the posterior half of the vertebral body, annulus, disc, and posterior longitudinal ligament.
- The **posterior column** consists of the facet joints, ligamentum flavum, posterior elements, and interconnecting ligaments.

Applying this classification system to spinal injuries results in four classification categories, which are determined by the specific column(s) injured.

Type of Injury	Columns Injured		
	Anterior	*Middle*	*Posterior*
Compression fractures	Yes	No	No
Burst fractures	Yes	Yes	No
Flexion-distraction fractures	Yes/no	Yes	Yes
Fracture-dislocations	Yes	Yes	Yes

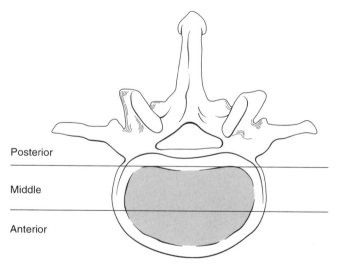

The rule of thumb is when one column is injured, the spine is usually stable; when two or three columns are injured, the sustained injury is considered unstable.

(Reference: Lenke, L. G., O'Brien, M. F., & Bridwell, K. H. [1995]. Fractures and dislocations of the spine. In C. R. Perry, J. A. Elstrom, & A. M. Pankovich (Eds.). The handbook of fractures [pp. 157–189]. New York: McGraw-Hill.)

TABLE 22-1
Upper Cervical Vertebral Injuries (Occiput to C-2)*

TYPE	DESCRIPTION	TREATMENT

Atlas (C-1) fractures 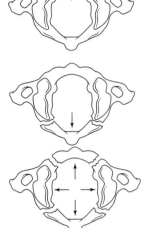	• Result from vertical compression of the occipital condyles on the arch of C-1; cause single or multiple fractures of the C-1 ring; bony pieces thrust away from the center, increasing the space for the spinal cord; thus neurological injury is rare.
	• There are four types of atlas fractures:
	  (1) **Isolated anterior arch fractures:** avulsion from anterior part of ring (usually stable)
	  (2) **Isolated posterior arch fracture:** hyperextension with compression of posterior arch of C-1 between occiput and C-2 (usually stable)
	  (3) **Lateral mass fracture:** fracture (fx) anterior-posterior to articular surface of C-1 with unilateral displacement; stable fx
	  (4) **Jefferson's fracture:** burst fx into three or four pieces; can result in concurrent rupture of transverse ligament, resulting in instability
		• Isolated *anterior or posterior arch fx:* usually no neural injury; about 3 mo in cervical hard collar or halo vest
		• *Lateral mass fx:* hard collar or halo vest
		• *Jefferson's fx:* If transverse ligament strong, halo and vest; if weak, cervical traction followed by halo vest for 3–4 mo

Atlantoaxial subluxation	• Caused by a weak or ruptured transverse ligament that stabilizes dens to anterior ring of atlas. • Produces atlantoaxial instability; high risk for spinal injury due to compression of upper cervical cord against the posterior arch of C-1	• Halo vest for 3 mo, only ligament injuries need a C-1 to C-1 posterior fusion

Odontoid fractures 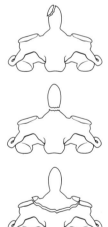	• Need to rule out in all patients with neck pain following a motor vehicle accident (MVA) or elderly with even minor injury to head or neck
	• Displacement, anterior or more often, posterior with rare (10%) neurological injury
	• Odontoid fractures classified into three types:
	  (1) **Type I:** chip avulsion fx through the tip of the odontoid; stable fracture; heals well
	  (2) **Type II:** fx through the base of the dens with separation, usually anteriorly, from the body of C-2; most common; poor blood supply to area; nonunion in 40%–50%; treatment depends on severity and response to treatment options
	  (3) **Type III:** fx line extends into the body of C-2
		• *Type 1:* halo vest or hard collar.
		• *Type II:* difficult to treat; there are 4 options: traction to align then 3 mo in halo vest; halo vest; surgical fixation and fusion; or traction and surgery.
		• *Type III:* if reduced adequately, halo vest for 3 mo; if not, cervical traction first, then halo vest

Hangman's fractures 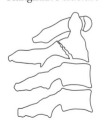	• Bipedicular fx with disruption of the disc and ligaments between C-2 and C-3 resulting from hyperextension and distraction
	• Named for injury seen in judicial hangings
	• Further classified according to amount of displacement and angulation of the C-2 body in relation to the posterior elements:
	  (1) **Type I:** fx of neural arch without angulation and with up to 3 mm of anterior C-2 displacement on C-3; stable fx
	  (2) **Type II:** <5 mm anterior displacement or angulation of C-2 on C-3
		• *Type I:* managed with a hard collar
		• *Type II:* <5 mm, halo vest if reduction maintained; if >5 mm, skeletal traction for 3–6 wk followed by halo vest
		• *Type IIA:* traction contraindicated; halo vest
		• *Type III:* open reduction when closed reduction not possible and posterior fusion of C2-3; then halo vest for 3 mo

(continued)

TABLE 22-1
Upper Cervical Vertebral Injuries (Occiput to C-2)* Continued

TYPE	DESCRIPTION	TREATMENT
	(3) **Type IIA:** severe angulation of C-2 on C-3 with minimal displacement because anterior longitudinal ligament is hinge (4) **Type III:** bipedicle fx associated with unilateral or bilateral facet dislocations; unstable; often neurological deficits present • Most types unstable; may or may not include neurological deficits depending on amount of displacement or angulation. • Important to know type of fx to determine treatment	
Occipital condyle fractures	• Rare injury caused by concurrent axial loading and lateral flexion • Associated with severe head injury • Two types: avulsion or comminuted compression fx	• Cervical collar, such as a Philadelphia collar
Atlanto-occipital dislocations	• Rare injury caused by extension or flexion injury • Results in an avulsion of the atlas (C-1) body from the occipital bone and all ligaments • Almost always immediately fatal	• Traction contraindicated; halo vest
Atlantoaxial rotary subluxation	• Rare injury associated with MVAs • Diagnosis often missed	• Cervical traction for alignment, then a halo vest
Lateral mass fractures	• Rare injury associated with a combined axial loading and lateral flexion forces	• Usually hard collar

(Based on: Lenke, L. G., O'Brien, M. F., & Bridwell, K. H. [1995]. Fractures and dislocations of the spine. In C. R. Perry, J. A. Elstrom, & A. M. Pankovich (Eds.). The handbook of fractures [pp. 166–189]. New York: McGraw-Hill; Adams, J. C., & Hamblen, D. L. [1992]. Outline of fractures [pp. 79–108]. [10th ed]. Edinburgh: Churchill Livingstone.)

TABLE 22-2
Lower Cervical Vertebral Injuries (C-3 to T-1)

TYPE	DESCRIPTION	TREATMENT
Hyperflexion dislocation of C-3 to T-1	Most common cause of paralysis; only neck pain and no neurological deficits may be present	Reduction of the dislocation, then halo immobilization (for 3–6 mos) or a posterior fusion
Flexion-rotational injuries of C-3 to T-1	Usually, anterior subluxation with a unilateral subluxated facet	Reduction of the dislocation with traction; if unstable, posterior fusion
Hyperextension fractures	Usually involves only ligamental and muscle injury; often associated with central cord syndrome	Usually stable fractures; treated with a hard collar for 6–10 wk until the patient is pain-free
Compression fraction of C-3 to T-1	Results from flexion and significant axial loading; may be a simple wedge, burst, or teardrop fracture (see vertebral classification)	Treatment depends on the stability of the fracture; hard collar may be effective for stable fractures, whereas unstable ones may require surgical fusion.

THORACIC AND LUMBAR SEGMENTS. Injuries in the thoracic and lumbar regions account for paralysis of the trunk and lower extremities. Normally, little movement is possible in the vertebrae of the thoracic region compared with the lumbar region because of the inherent structural stability provided by the rib cage. The spinal cord ends at the upper border of the first lumbar vertebra. The cord gradually tapers, beginning at the lower two thoracic vertebrae. As the cord tapers, it forms a cone called the conus medullaris, which continues at the filum terminale. The nerve roots coming off the lower segments of the spinal cord, termed the cauda equina, hang loosely and are susceptible to injury. However, injury to these nerves is more likely to result in recovery than is injury to the spinal cord. Also, it is less likely to require the emergency procedures of decompression because the roots tolerate trauma far better than the spinal cord itself.

Vertebral fractures of the thoracic, thoracolumbar, and lumbar spine are classified into four general categories:

- **Compression fractures**, caused by axial loading and hyperflexion, are common in the thoracic and upper lumbar regions of the vertebral column. Significant direct force must be applied to produce a fracture in the thoracic area. Injury is usually the result of a direct force being applied to one vertebra, with subsequent force and compromise of the underlying cord. When this happens, there is hyperflexion of the vertebra. A compression fracture in the thoracic or lumbar region may be compressed anteriorly with or without subluxation of the vertebra. The other possibility is total compression of the vertebral body with anteroposterior protrusion.
- **Burst fractures** include injury to the anterior and middle columns and possibly the posterior column, creating an unstable fracture. Axial loading with flexion is the biomechanical force responsible for the injury. The vertebral body explodes or ''bursts'' as a result of the energy associated with injury, and often the vertebral body protrudes into the spinal canal.
- **Flexion-distraction injuries** involve three columns and are thus unstable. The fracture extends through the posterior elements, pedicle, and vertebral body. The mechanism of injury is acute flexion of the torso usually on the lap belt.
- **Fracture-dislocations** of the thoracic and lumbar areas are of three general categories: anterior or posterior dislocation of the whole vertebral body with fracture of the bony parts; comminuted fractures of the vertebral body with anterior or posterior displacement and rotation so that the rotational force usually tears the supporting ligaments; and lateral dislocation of the vertebra with fracture. All three columns are involved so that the fracture is unstable, making the patient high risk for neurological injury.

SACRAL SEGMENTS. Fractures of the sacrum and coccyx usually result from direct trauma. These injuries are most frequently caused by falls. Any fall in the sitting position, such as falling on ice or being thrown from a horse and landing on the buttocks, can result in a fracture. Nerve injury in this region can cause bladder, bowel, or sexual dysfunction and saddle anesthesia.

Lesions of the conus medullaris can occur with fractures in the lumbar region. These lesions can have confusing clinical presentations. Injury to the conus usually results in lower motor neuron symptoms (muscle flaccidity, muscle atrophy, hyporeflexia) because of the disruption of the anterior gray horn cells. A decompression laminectomy may be necessary if there is pressure on the neural elements. Lesions involving the cauda equina produce selected root syndromes. A decompression laminectomy may also be necessary.

Spinal Cord Injuries

Injury to the spinal cord can cause a devastating loss of many body functions that allow independence in functioning. The loss of function may be permanent or temporary, depending on the type of injury. Several syndromes relate to spinal cord injury (Chart 22-2); injuries to the spinal cord can be classified by type of injury and by syndrome.

CLASSIFICATION BY CAUSE

The spinal cord can be injured by concussion, contusion, laceration, transection, hemorrhage, or damage to the blood vessels that supply the cord.

- **Concussion—Spinal shock** or jarring can cause temporary loss of function lasting 24 to 48 hours; this is attributable to a severe shaking of the spinal cord. No identifiable neuropathological changes are noted on examination of the cord.
- **Contusion**—A bruising of the cord includes bleeding into the cord, subsequent edema, and possible necrosis from the compression of the edema or damage to the tissue. The extent of neurological deficits depends on the severity of the contusion and the presence of necrosis. Fractures, dislocations, and direct trauma to the cord can cause a contusion.
- **Laceration**—An actual tear in the cord results in permanent injury to the cord. Contusion, edema, and cord compression accompany a laceration.
- **Transection**—A severing of the cord can be complete or incomplete. Complete transection is rare, although as a clinical presentation, it is frequently seen.
- **Hemorrhage**—Bleeding into or around the spinal cord acts as an irritant to the delicate tissue, resulting in changes in the neurochemical components, edema, and neurological deficits.
- Damage to the blood vessels that supply the cord—Interference or damage to the vessels that supply the spinal cord, the anterior spinal artery, or the two posterior spinal arteries results in ischemia and possible necrosis. Episodes of ischemia can cause temporary neurological deficits. Prolonged ischemia and necrosis will cause permanent deficits.

PATHOPHYSIOLOGY

In most instances, the spinal cord is not severed at the time of injury; rather, it is bruised or compressed. However, in the first few hours after injury, several chemical and vascular changes occur, causing the spinal cord to initiate an intrinsic process of self-destruction and the injury to worsen.

The pathophysiology of spinal cord injury can be divided into primary and secondary injuries. The **primary injury** occurs at the time of mechanical injury and is irrevers-

(text continues on page 434)

CHART 22-2
Selected Syndromes Related to Spinal Cord Injury

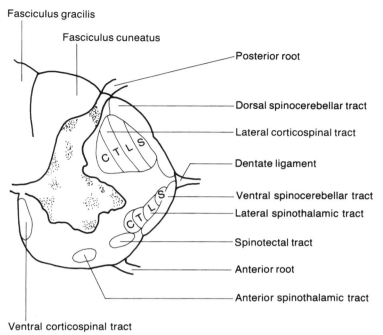

Cross-section of spinal cord with sensory and motor tracts identified.

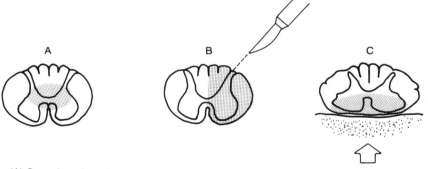

(A) Central cord syndrome. (B) Brown-Séquard syndrome. (C) Anterior cord syndrome.

Several terms related to spinal cord injury are defined.

- Tetraplegia (quadriplegia) refers to a lesion involving one of the cervical segments of the spinal cord that results in dysfunction of both arms, both legs, bowel, and bladder.
- Paraplegia refers to a lesion involving the thoracic lumbar or sacral regions of the spinal cord that results in dysfunction of the lower extremities, bowel, or bladder.
- A complete lesion (*e.g.,* complete quadriplegia or complete paraplegia) implies total loss of sensation and voluntary muscle control below the injury.
- An incomplete lesion implies preservation of the sensory or motor fibers, or both, below the lesion. Incomplete lesions are classified according to the area of damage: central, lateral, anterior, or peripheral.

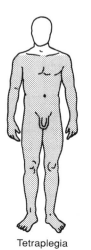

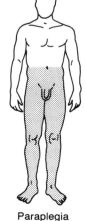

Tetraplegia   Paraplegia

The shaded area shows the extent of motor and sensory loss.

(continued)

CHART 22-2 Selected Syndromes Related to Spinal Cord Injury (Continued)

Central Cord Syndrome

- Presentation: There are more motor deficits in the upper extremities than the lower extremities; sensory loss varies but is more pronounced in the upper extremities; bowel/bladder dysfunction is variable, or function may be completely preserved.
- Cause: Injury or edema of the central cord, usually of the cervical area, is the underlying cause; hyperextension injuries, particularly if bony spurs are noted, can be causative.
- Result: Edema in the central cord exerts pressure on the anterior horn cells. The cervical fibers of the corticospinal tract are located in a more central position in the cord than the sacral fibers, which are located in the periphery. As a result, motor deficits are less severe in the lower extremities than in the upper extremities.
- Treatment: High-dose steroid (methylprednisolone) protocol for acute cord injury (see pp 438–440); immobilization or bed rest is the treatment of choice; steroids may be used to reduce the edema. Flexion-extension x-rays are usually obtained. The prognosis varies.

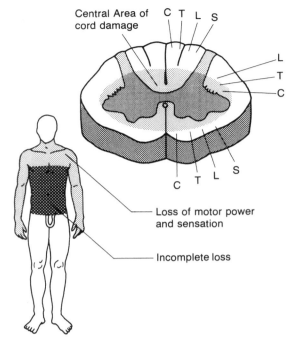

Central Cord Syndrome
A cross section of the cord shows central damage and the associated motor and sensory loss (C, cervical; T, thoracic; L, lumbar; S, sacral).

Anterior Cord Syndrome

- Presentation: Loss of pain, temperature, and motor function is noted below the level of the lesion; light touch, position, and vibration sensation remain intact.
- Cause: The syndrome may be caused by acute disc herniation or hyperflexion injuries associated with fracture-dislocation of a vertebra. It also may occur as a result of injury to the anterior spinal artery, which supplies the anterior two thirds of the spinal cord.
- Result: Injury to the anterior part of the spinal cord, which includes the spinothalamic tracts (pain), corticospinal tracts (temperature), and anterior gray horn motor neurons, is noted.
- Treatment: High-dose steroid (methylprednisolone) protocol for acute cord injury (see pp 438–440); surgical decompression is usually necessary to manage fracture-dislocation. The prognosis varies.

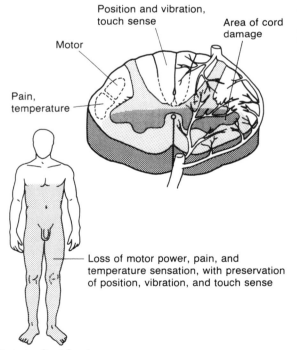

Anterior Cord Syndrome
Cord damage and associated motor and sensory loss are illustrated.

(continued)

CHART 22-2 Selected Syndromes Related to Spinal Cord Injury (Continued)

Brown-Séquard Syndrome (Lateral Cord Syndrome)

- Presentation: Ipsilateral paralysis or paresis is noted, together with ipsilateral loss of touch, pressure, and vibration and contralateral loss of pain and temperature.
- Cause: The lesion is caused by a transverse hemisection of the cord (half of the cord is transected from north to south), usually as a result of a knife or missile injury, fracture-dislocation of a unilateral articular process, or possibly an acute ruptured disc.
- Result: With right-sided cord transection, for example, the following would occur: paralysis of all voluntary muscles below the level of injury on the right side of the body (lateral corticospinal tract); loss of perception of touch, vibration, and position on the right side of the body below the level of injury (posterior columns, which include the fasciculus gracilis and fasciculus cuneatus); and loss of pain and temperature perception on the left side of the body below the injury (lateral spinothalamic tracts). Fibers that carry pain and temperature cross to the opposite side of the cord immediately after entering the cord and then ascend. The other tracts mentioned do not cross until they reach the brain stem.
- Treatment: High-dose steroid (methylprednisolone) protocol for acute cord injury (see pp 439–440); no specific treatment is undertaken except fracture-dislocation management.

Posterior Cord Syndrome

- This is a rare syndrome in which the position and vibration senses of the posterior columns are involved.

Root Syndromes (Peripheral Syndromes)

- Presentation: Root syndromes cause tingling, pain, motor weakness of an isolated muscle or muscle group, and absent or diminished reflexes in the involved area. The spinal cord terminates at T-12 or L-1. The nerve roots that extend from the conus medullaris are collectively called the cauda equina. Lesions of L-1 through L-5 denote paraplegia. Patients with this level of involvement can move readily and walk with the assistance of various types of bracing. Lesions of the lumbrosacral region may involve multiple roots of the cauda equina with a varying pattern of motor and sensory loss. Deep tendon reflexes are usually diminished or absent. Isolated nerve root involvement is common in the lumbrosacral region so that saddle hypalgesia—diminished or absence of sensation in the saddle

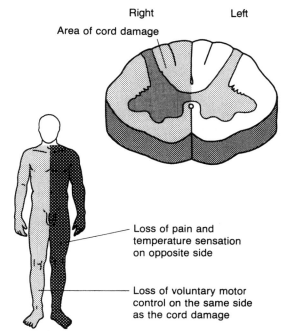

Right Left

Area of cord damage

Loss of pain and temperature sensation on opposite side

Loss of voluntary motor control on the same side as the cord damage

Brown-Séquard Syndrome
Cord damage and associated motor and sensory loss are illustrated.

region—is possible. Therefore, careful examination of the patient is necessary to identify the erratic sensory or motor loss. When the sacral roots are involved, the patient may experience bladder or bowel dysfunction. If the cervical region is involved, there is usually tingling in the arm, muscle weakness in the arm or shoulder, and pain radiating down the arm and into the shoulder.
- Cause: Compression secondary to intervertebral disc herniation or vertebral subluxation is the cause of these syndromes. Any area of the cord can be involved.
- Result: Compression of one or more nerve roots coming off the spinal cord, rather than compression or injury to the cord itself, occurs. The compression can also cause edema.
- Treatment: Nonsurgical treatment with traction is initiated to release the compressed nerve roots, and drugs may be prescribed to control the associated edema, pain, and muscle spasms. In some cases, surgery for decompression of the nerve roots may be necessary.

(continued)

CHART 22-2 Selected Syndromes Related to Spinal Cord Injury (Continued)

Horner's Syndrome

- Presentation: Horner's syndrome, which may be seen with partial spinal cord transection at the level of T-1 or above, may be associated with miosis, ptosis, and loss of sweating on the ipsilateral side.

- Cause: The syndrome is caused by a lesion involving either the preganglionic sympathetic trunk or the cervical postganglionic sympathetic neurons.

(Cross-sections of spinal cord in this chart are from Kitt, S. & J. Kaiser. [1990]. Emergency nursing: A physiological and clinical perspective. Philadelphia: W.B Saunders.)

---

ible. Small hemorrhages in the gray matter occur in minutes as the spinal cord blood flow falls and hypoxia ensues. Edema of the white matter occurs and leads to necrosis of tissue. The **secondary injury** occurs as a result of the vascular and neuronal pathological changes and the release of vasoactive agents and cellular enzymes. The injury to the blood vessels results in ischemia, increased vascular permeability, and edema. Hypoxia of the gray matter stimulates the release of catecholamines, which contribute to the hemorrhage and necrosis and cause further spinal cord dysfunction. The release of catecholamines and vasoactive substances (norepinephrine, serotonin, dopamine, and histamine) from the injured tissue can cause vasospasm and impede microcirculation. These events further extend necrosis of blood vessels and neurons. The release of proteolytic and lipolytic enzymes from the injured cells causes delayed swelling and necrosis in the spinal cord.[4]

Function of the highly specialized central nervous system cells is affected as a result of the ischemia and hypoxia (noted within 30 minutes). Irreversible nerve damage develops as a result of the replacement of normal neural elements with glial and fibrotic scar tissue; neurological deficits become permanent.

ACUTE SPINAL CORD TRAUMA

Immediate Signs and Symptoms of Spinal Cord Trauma

When the spinal cord is suddenly transected, spinal shock occurs in the portion of the cord severed, resulting in complete loss of motor, sensory, reflex, and autonomic function below the level of injury. The term **flaccid paralysis** is used to describe the clinical signs seen at this time because the muscles are flaccid. Specific functional losses resulting from spinal cord injury are listed in Table 22-3.

Sudden, complete transection of the spinal cord results in immediate spinal shock, manifested by the following:

- Flaccid paralysis of all skeletal muscles below the level of injury
- Loss of all spinal reflexes below the level of injury

- Loss of pain, proprioception, and the sensations of touch, temperature, and pressure below the level of injury. (Pain may be felt at the site of the injury because of a zone of heightened sensitivity [hyperesthesia] immediately above the level of the lesion.)
- Absence of somatic and visceral sensations below the level of injury
- Loss of the ability to perspire below the level of injury
- Bowel and bladder dysfunction

Spinal cord transection can also be partial. The extent of loss of function with partial transections is less than that found with complete transections. The symptoms of spinal shock can also occur in portions of the cord that have been injured by causes other than transection, such as concussion, contusion, compression, laceration, hemorrhage, and damage to the blood supply.

Special Considerations
SPINAL SHOCK

Definition and Description. An immediate response to acute spinal cord injury is called spinal shock. **Spinal shock** is the temporary suppression of reflexes controlled by segments below the level of injury. The normal activity of the spinal cord is dependent on the continual tonic discharge of impulses from the higher centers of the brain. With acute injury, the input of impulses from these higher centers abruptly ceases, resulting in spinal shock. After a period that may vary from hours to months, the spinal neurons gradually regain their excitability, ending the period of spinal shock.

The earliest indication heralding the end of spinal shock is the return of the perianal reflexes (bulbocavernous and anal reflexes). The bulbocavernous reflex is tested by squeezing the glans penis or pulling the indwelling catheter and observing for slight muscle contraction and retraction of the scrotum. The anal reflex is present if there is a puckering of the anal sphincter ("anal wink") during digital examination of the rectum or scratching of the skin around the anal region. Muscle contraction may also be noted when inserting a rectal thermometer. Perianal reflexes return before deep tendon reflexes. Weeks may elapse between the appearance of the two reflexes. Acute spinal injury does not always produce complete loss of function, so varying degrees of spinal shock are possible.

TABLE 22-3
Functional Loss From Spinal Cord Injury (Based on Complete Lesions)

LEVEL OF SPINAL INJURY	MOTOR FUNCTION	DEEP TENDON REFLEXES	SENSORY FUNCTION	RESPIRATORY FUNCTION	VOLUNTARY BOWEL AND BLADDER FUNCTION	REHABILITATIVE POTENTIAL
C1-4	• Tetraplegia: loss of all motor function from the neck down		• Loss of all sensory function in the neck and below (C-4 supplies the clavicles.)	• Loss of involuntary (phrenic) and voluntary (intercostals) respiratory function; ventilatory support and a tracheostomy needed	• No bowel or bladder control	• Can be discharged home on a ventilator with home care
C-5	• Tetraplegia: loss of all function below the upper shoulders • **Intact:** sternomastoids, cervical paraspinal muscles, and the trapezius; can control head	C-5, C-6 biceps	• Loss of sensation below the clavicle and most portions of arms, hands, chest, abdomen, and lower extremities • **Intact:** head, shoulders, deltoid, clavicle, portion of forearms (C-5 supplies the lateral aspect of the arm.)	• Phrenic nerve intact, but not intercostal muscles	• No bowel or bladder control	• Use of extremity-powered devices to achieve some upper limb control • Head control facilitates wheelchair balance • Adaptive tools, held in mouth, for typing and writing
C-6	• Tetraplegia: loss of all function below the shoulders and upper arms; lacks elbow, forearm, and hand control • **Intact:** deltoid, biceps, and external rotator muscles of shoulders	C-5, C-6 brachio-radials	• Loss of everything listed for a C-5 lesion, but greater arm and thumb sensation • **Intact:** head, shoulders, arms, palms of hands, and thumbs (C-6 supplies the forearm and thumb.)	• Phrenic nerve intact, but not intercostal muscles	• No bowel or bladder control	• Needs assistive devices to use arms (may be able to help feed, groom, and dress self) • Needs a motorized wheelchair • Dependent for all transfers
C-7	• Tetraplegia: loss of motor control to portions of the arm and hands • **Intact:** voluntary strength in shoulder depressors, shoulder abductors, internal rotators, and radial wrist extensors	C-7, C-8 triceps	• Loss of sensation below the clavicle and portions of arms and hands • **Intact:** head, shoulders, most of arms and hands (C-7 supplies the middle finger.)	• Phrenic nerve intact, but not intercostal muscles	• No bowel or bladder function	• Can perform some activities of daily living (ADLs) • Can use wrist extensor with a special splint to induce finger flexion • Can push a wheelchair with special handgrasps • May be able to drive a specially equipped car
C-8	• Tetraplegia: loss of motor control to portions of arms and hands		• Loss of sensation below the chest and in portions of hands	• Phrenic nerve intact, but not intercostal muscles	• No bowel or bladder function	• Able to do push-ups in the wheelchair • Improved sitting tolerance

(continued)

TABLE 22-3
Functional Loss From Spinal Cord Injury (Based on Complete Lesions)
Continued

LEVEL OF SPINAL INJURY	MOTOR FUNCTION	DEEP TENDON REFLEXES	SENSORY FUNCTION	RESPIRATORY FUNCTION	VOLUNTARY BOWEL AND BLADDER FUNCTION	REHABILITATIVE POTENTIAL
	• **Intact:** some voluntary control of elbow extensors, wrist, finger extension and finger flexors		• **Intact:** sensation to face, shoulders, arms, hands, and part of chest (C-8 supplies the little finger.)			• Can grasp and release hands voluntarily. • Independent in most ADLs • Independent in use of wheelchair • Can use hands for catheterization and rectal stimulation for bowel movements
T1-6	• Paraplegia: loss of everything below the midchest region, including the trunk muscles • **Intact:** control of function to the shoulders, upper chest, arms, and hands		• Loss of sensation below the midchest area • **Intact:** everything to the midchest region, including the arms and hands (T-1 and T-2 supply the inner aspect of the arm; T-4 supplies the nipple area.)	• Phrenic nerve functions independently • Some impairment of intercostal muscles	• No bowel or bladder function	• Full control of upper extremities and completely independent in wheelchair • Full-time employment possible. • Independent in managing urinary drainage and inserting suppositories • Able to live in a dwelling without major architectural changes
T6-12	• Paraplegia: loss of motor control below the waist • **Intact:** shoulders, arms, hands, and long trunk muscles		• Loss of everything below the waist • **Intact:** shoulders, chest, arms, and hands (T-10 supplies the umbilicus; T-12 supplies the groin area.)	• No interference with respiratory function	• No bowel or bladder control	• In addition to the previously described capabilities, there is complete abdominal and upper back control. • Good sitting balance (allows for greater ease of wheelchair operation and athletics)
L1-3	• Paraplegia: loss of most control of legs and pelvis • **Intact:** shoulders, arms, hands, torso, hip rotation and flexion, and some leg flexion	L2-4 (knee jerk)	• Loss of sensation to the lower abdomen and legs • **Intact:** all of the above plus some sensation to the inner and anterior thigh (L-3 supplies the knee.)	• No interference with respiratory function	• No bowel or bladder control	• Independent for most activities from wheelchair
L3-4	• Paraplegia: loss of control of portions of lower legs, ankles, and feet		Loss of sensation to portions of the lower legs, feet, and ankles	• No interference with respiratory function	• No bowel or bladder control	• Voluntary control of hip extensors; weak abductors • Walking with braces possible

(continued)

TABLE 22-3
Functional Loss From Spinal Cord Injury (Based on Complete Lesions)
Continued

LEVEL OF SPINAL INJURY	MOTOR FUNCTION	DEEP TENDON REFLEXES	SENSORY FUNCTION	RESPIRATORY FUNCTION	VOLUNTARY BOWEL AND BLADDER FUNCTION	REHABILITATIVE POTENTIAL
L-4 to S-5	• **Intact:** all of the above, plus increased knee extension • Paraplegia: degree varies • Segmental motor control L-4 to S-1: abduction and internal rotation of hip, ankle dorsiflexion, and foot inversion L-5 to S-1: foot eversion L-4 to S-2: knee flexion S1-2: plantar flexion S1-2: (ankle jerk) S2-5: bowel/bladder control	S1-2 (ankle jerk)	**Intact:** all of the above, plus sensation to the upper legs • Lumbar sensory nerves innervate the upper legs and portions of the lower legs L-5: medial aspect of foot S-1: lateral aspect of foot S-2: posterior aspect of calf/thigh • Sacral sensory nerves innervate the lower legs, feet, and perineum	• No interference with respiratory function	• Bowel and bladder control possibly impaired • S2-4 segments control urinary continence • S3-5 segments control bowel continence (perianal muscles)	• Can walk with braces or may use wheelchair • Can be relatively independent

Recovery From Spinal Shock. Spinal shock may last a few days to several weeks (1–6 weeks after injury), depending on the severity of the injury. Recovery from spinal shock is a gradual process in which the spinal neurons slowly regain their excitability. Throughout the nervous system, neurons that have lost the source of their facilitory impulses seem to compensate by increasing the degree of their excitability.

Depending on the completeness of the cord transection, one of two possibilities will eventually occur. The first possibility is that the transmission of impulses will resume, resulting in the return of motor, sensory, reflex, and autonomic function below the level of injury. The second possibility is that the isolated cord segment, devoid of any suprasegmental control, will develop its own reflex activity. This autonomous neural activity is divided into a sequence of phases of variable lengths, including minimal reflex activity, flexor spasm activity (superficial reflexes), alternating flexor and extensor spasm activities, and predominant extensor spasm activity (deep reflexes).

NEUROGENIC SHOCK

Under normal conditions, the sympathetic nervous system, which has its origins in the thoracolumbar region of the spinal cord, receives impulses from the brain stem. The input from the brain stem contributes to basic reflex control of vital signs through the cardiac accelerator and vasoconstriction reflexes. With cervical cord injury, the modulation of control from the higher centers is lost, and a condition called **neurogenic shock** results.

Neurogenic (vasomotor) shock is the temporary loss or disruption of autonomic nervous system innervation below the level of injury, resulting in cardiovascular changes. It is characterized by **orthostatic hypotension** secondary to the vasodilation of the vascular beds below the level of injury, **bradycardia** resulting from the suppression of the cardiac accelerator reflex, and **loss of the ability to sweat** below the level of injury because of lack of innervation of the sweat glands. The patient's temperature tends to be lower than normal (96°–98°F, 35.5°–36.5°C) because of the break in the connection between the hypothalamus and the sympathetic nervous system. Body heat is lost by way of the passively dilated vascular bed of the skin.

ORTHOSTATIC HYPOTENSION

Immediately after cord injury, the blood pressure tends to be unstable and lowered. After 1 to 2 weeks, it gradually rises until it is stabilized at a reading that corresponds to the preinjury norm for the patient. However, problems of orthostatic hypotension can impede the rehabilitative process because the patient cannot be raised in bed or assume the vertical position.

Orthostatic hypotension is defined as a rapid drop in blood pressure when the vertical position is assumed. Because the blood supply to the brain is inadequate, syncope results. Brain damage and even death can result if the condition is not rectified. This condition is seen in patients who have been bedridden for a prolonged period, are postoperative from a lumbar sympathectomy, or are new paraplegics or tetraplegics.

Physiologically, the drop in arterial blood pressure is attributable to the loss of arteriole vasomotor tone below the level of the lesion so that there is pooling of blood in the abdomen and lower extremities when the patient assumes an upright position. Orthostatic hypotension is seen particularly in cord-injured patients with lesions above the T-7 level. Even slightly raising the head of the bed for a new tetraplegic patient can result in a drastic lowering of blood pressure.

RESPIRATORY INSUFFICIENCY

The diaphragm is innervated by C-1 to C-4. If a high cervical injury is sustained, the innervation to the diaphragm is affected, and the patient will suffer respiratory arrest. Mechanical ventilation will be necessary. If the cord injury is below the innervation to the phrenic nerve and above the innervation to the intercostal muscles, diaphragmatic breathing will be noted. This patient will also need varying degrees of respiratory support.

COMPLICATIONS

After recovery from spinal shock, various complications can develop, depending on the type and level of injury. Examples of such problems include autonomic hyperreflexia, sexual dysfunction, bladder dysfunction, and autonomic dysfunctions. These topics and others are discussed in the section on the postacute phases.

OVERVIEW OF EARLY MANAGEMENT OF PATIENTS WITH SPINAL CORD INJURY

Prehospital Management

The prehospital management of spinal cord injuries is critical to the patient's ultimate neurological outcome. Until proven otherwise, every trauma patient should be treated as if he or she had a spinal cord injury. This rule applies to any patient with a head injury and to the inebriated trauma victim whose sensory and cognitive functions are impaired (see Chap. 21).

The basic objectives of management at the injury site include (1) rapid assessment to determine the extent of vertebral or spinal cord injury; (2) immobilization and stabilization of the head and neck to prevent extension of injury; (3) extrication of the patient from the vehicle or injury site; (4) stabilization and control of any other life-threatening injuries; (5) triage to the appropriate facility; and (6) rapid and safe transport. The rescue personnel must be well trained because improper handling at the injury site can turn a minor vertebral injury into a major, irreversible spinal cord injury. Of critical importance is immediate institution of the **high-dose steroid protocol** (Chart 22-3).

Emergency Department Management

On admission to the emergency department, a report of the prehospital management and a history of the injury are collected rapidly. Critical information includes the details of beginning the high-dose steroid (intravenous [IV] methylprednisolone) protocol. The patient is maintained in neural

position. On arrival, the patient may be safely log-rolled off the spine board by well trained emergency room personnel. Pressure areas from being on the board are of great concern even in the very early phase of acute spinal injury.

HISTORY OF ACCIDENT

The history of the accident can be obtained from a variety of sources—the patient, a family member, another accident victim, or rescue personnel. Information about the circumstances of the injury, the neurological status of the patient immediately after injury, the treatment at the accident site, and the mode of transport are all vital data. At the same time, a baseline assessment (primary survey) is conducted.

ASSESSMENT

For victims of trauma, a complete primary and secondary survey must be conducted (see Chap. 21). The medical history, including drugs and drug allergy, should be collected. Routine laboratory data will be ordered.

The few special considerations related to the spinal-vertebral injury are mentioned in the following sections.

Adequacy of Respiratory Function. The airway is checked for patency, and respirations are evaluated to determine whether the diaphragm and intercostal muscles are functional. Skin color, nail beds, and earlobes are also checked for evidence of proper oxygenation. If there is a cervical injury and respiratory assistance is necessary, special techniques carried out by a specially trained anesthesiologist are necessary to prevent extension of the injury. A tracheostomy or endotracheal tube may be necessary if an endotracheal tube is not already in place. Any injury compromising ventilation must be treated promptly and effectively. The patient must be observed carefully for ascending edema, which may rapidly compromise respirations.

Vital Sign Evaluation. Patients with spinal cord injuries (particularly those in the cervical region) may show signs of hypotension, bradycardia, and lowered body temperature. These are symptoms of spinal shock. The lowered blood pressure is attributable to vasodilation, which results from the loss of vasomotor tone below the level of injury. In most instances, treatment will not be necessary unless the hypotension is compounded by hemorrhagic shock. Adding blankets will usually control the lowered body temperature. Once the primary survey is completed and the patient is stabilized, the secondary survey is concluded.

Minineurological Examination. Two goals are accomplished by the minineurological examination: an estimation of cord involvement is ascertained, and a baseline assessment is made so that future neurological examinations can be compared with previous findings. The patient is also evaluated for possible head injury.

The physician in the emergency department conducts the neurological examination with a focus on determining the presence, absence, or diminished sensory and motor function of reflexes.

CHART 22-3
High-Dose Methylprednisolone Treatment of Acute Spinal Cord Injury (Sample)*

Suggested Physician Orders for High-Dose Methylprednisolone Administration

1. Record patient weight: _____ kg

2. In the emergency department begin: methylprednisolone _____ mg (30 mg/kg) IV over 15 minutes
   Record start time _____
   ❑ Check when given

3. Pause 45 minutes. Administer NSS, KVO.

4. Dosage calculation only:
   Methylprednisolone _____ mg
   IV over 23 hours (5.4 mg/kg/h × 23 hours)

5. Start methylprednisolone 3,000 mg IV to run at _____ mg/h (5.4 mg/kg/h)
   Record start time _____
   Record end time _____
   ❑ Check when started

Administer the IV bolus using the chart below. (Sample of Selected Weights)					Initiate maintenance therapy by **first hanging a 3-g methylprednisolone IV bag** as a 62.5 mg/mL solution. Administration rate is found below by weight. Rate calculated for a 5.4 mg/kg/h infusion.		
Patient Weight		30 mg/kg IV Bolus over 15 min	For 62.5 mg/mL Solutions		Remaining dose **after 3 g given**		For 62.5 mg/mL Solutions
lb	kg	Dose (mg)	Dose (mL)	Pause for 45 min	Dose (mg)	Rate (mg/h)	Rate (mL/h)
165.0	75	2,250	36.0		6,315	405.0	6.48
167.2	76	2,280	36.5		6,439	410.4	6.57
169.4	77	2,310	37.0		6,563	415.8	6.65
171.6	78	2,340	37.4		6,688	421.2	6.74
173.8	79	2,370	37.9		6,812	426.6	6.83
176.0	80	2,400	38.4		6,936	432.0	6.91
178.2	81	2,430	38.9		7,060	437.4	7.00
180.4	82	2,460	39.4		7,184	442.8	7.08
182.6	83	2,490	39.8		7,309	448.2	7.17
184.8	84	2,520	40.3		7,433	453.6	7.26
187.0	85	2,550	40.8		7,557	459.0	7.34
189.2	86	2,580	41.3		7,681	464.4	7.43
191.4	87	2,610	41.8		7,805	469.8	7.52
193.6	88	2,640	42.2		7,930	475.2	7.60
195.8	89	2,670	42.7		8,054	480.6	7.69
198.0	90	2,700	43.2		8,178	486.0	7.78
200.2	91	2,730	43.7		8,302	491.4	7.86
202.4	92	2,760	44.2		8,426	496.8	7.95
204.6	93	2,790	44.6		8,551	502.2	8.04
206.8	94	2,820	45.1		8,675	507.6	8.12
209.0	95	2,850	45.6		8,799	513.0	8.21
211.2	96	2,880	46.1		8,923	518.4	8.29
213.4	97	2,910	46.6		9,047	523.8	8.38
215.6	98	2,940	47.0		9,172	529.2	8.47
217.8	99	2,970	47.5		9,296	534.6	8.55
220.0	100	3,000	48.0		9,420	540.0	8.64
222.2	101	3,030	48.5		9,544	545.4	8.73
224.4	102	3,060	49.0		9,668	550.8	8.81
226.6	103	3,090	49.4		9,793	556.2	8.90

(Dosage chart based on NASCIS2 guidelines. Bracken, D, et al. [1990]. *New England Journal of Medicine, 322,* 1405–1411.)
*Solu-Medrol® (methylprednisolone)—Upjohn 1 g/16 mL = 62.5 mg/mL

Other Organ Systems. Trauma patients frequently have multiple injuries, including cardiac, intrathoracic, or abdominal injuries. The patient should be assessed for possible cardiac complications. Cardiac contusion is another serious possibility. An electrocardiogram (EKG) can be helpful in diagnosing cardiac injury. The presence of tachycardia with hypotension and cool and clammy skin should raise suspicion of visceral hemorrhage and a search for signs of intra-abdominal or intrathoracic injury. Because of diminished or absent pain perception, pain will not draw attention to a salient, life-threatening, ruptured viscera. Neurogenic and hemorrhagic shock can be simultaneously present. Careful assessment and clinical reasoning must be used to recognize the problem and quickly institute appropriate treatment. Failure to find and treat the injury can be life threatening.

Radiographic Examination. Anteroposterior and especially lateral films of the spine and any other possible areas of involvement should be obtained. Careful movement to prevent extension of injury is critical. A physician should accompany the patient to supervise the handling of the patient. The C-7 to T-1 vertebral level is normally difficult to visualize, but it is particularly difficult in obese or heavily muscled patients. To visualize C-7 and T-1, it may be necessary to pull the patient's shoulders downward toward the foot of the bed while the radiographic examination is conducted. If these x-ray studies are not satisfactory, the patient may be placed in the swimmer's position. The C1-2 level, especially the odontoid process, is also difficult to visualize. X-ray films are taken with the patient's mouth open to visualize the odontoid process. The physician must decide the specific type of x-ray studies necessary while considering the risk to the patient.

MEASURES INITIATED IN THE EMERGENCY DEPARTMENT

Respiratory Support. Respiratory support in the form of a ventilator for patients with cervical injuries or oxygen for those with thoracic injuries may be ordered. Observation of the patient for signs of ascending cord edema, which can rapidly compromise respirations, is a priority.

Management of Paralytic Ileus. An acute paralytic ileus, which is characterized by the absence of normal peristalsis, abdominal distention, nausea, and vomiting, occurs with spinal cord injuries. A nasogastric tube is inserted and connected to suction to decompress the stomach and prevent vomiting and aspiration and to facilitate free diaphragmatic movement. Paralytic ileus is not only a sign of spinal shock, but also can indicate intra-abdominal injury. Normally, the patient with an intra-abdominal injury will experience pain, but with a cord injury, the sensation of pain may be lost.

Management of an Atonic Bladder. The patient with a spinal cord injury and spinal shock will have an atonic bladder that will become overdistended. Urine may be retained and may overflow, and the bladder may be distended on palpation. An indwelling urinary catheter is inserted to manage the urinary output and to prevent injury to the bladder from overdistention.

Drug Therapy. High-dose steroid protocol (IV methyprednisolone) is now the standard of practice in managing acute spinal cord injury (see Chart 22-3). The following outlines the patient selection and considerations:

- **Purpose** of the protocol is to improve neurological recovery.
- **Indications** are a complete or incomplete spinal cord injury less than 8 hours old.
- **Absolute contraindications** follow:
  Injury more than 8 hours old
  Spinal lesion below lumbar 2
  A cauda equina lesion
- **Special considerations** follow:
  Pregnancy
  Age less than 13 years
  Penetrating wounds to the spinal cord
  Fulminating infections, such as tuberculosis
  Human immunodeficiency virus infection
  Severe diabetes mellitus
- **Monitoring parameters** follow:
  Routine assessment parameters for spinal cord injury
  EKG monitoring
  Evidence of acute hyperglycemic, psychiatric, gastrointestinal (GI), or infectious complications
  Dysrhythmias or cardiovascular collapse (rare)

Within the first 8 hours after injury (the sooner the better) patients are given a loading dose of 3 g of methylprednisolone (30 mg/kg body weight) over 15 minutes, followed by a pause in which normal saline is run as a "keep open" for 45 minutes. This is followed by 5.4 mg/kg every hour for the next 23 hours. Statistically significant improvement is noted in sensory and motor function in most patients compared with outcomes for those who do not receive the protocol. The usual precautions for steroid use should be followed: administering an H2 blocker (*e.g.*, cimetidine) to decrease gastric secretions and checking the gastric pH for excessive acidity, stools for occult blood, and urine for glucose.

Invasive and Noninvasive Monitoring. A peripheral IV line is routinely inserted if one is not already in place. A central line is also common. Depending on the patient's condition, invasive monitoring devices, such as a Swan-Ganz catheter, may be inserted. A cardiac monitor is used to monitor for bradycardia related to spinal shock or possible arrhythmias associated with cardiac contusion.

Early Medical Management of Spinal Cord Injury

After initial stabilization and assessment, the patient may be admitted to the intensive care unit (ICU) or other unit depending on his or her condition.

SELECTION OF TREATMENT APPROACH: SURGICAL OR NONSURGICAL

The basic goals of spinal cord injury management are decompression, realignment, and stabilization. Decompression-stabilization may be done emergently, especially if neurological deterioration is noted on serial neurological assessment.

Decompression of the spinal cord or spinal nerves prevents pain, loss of neurological function, ischemia, and necrosis to the involved tissue. Decompression can be achieved through the use of skeletal traction or surgery. If surgery is chosen, a decompression laminectomy is the usual procedure.

Realignment of the vertebral column is necessary to optimize intact function. Realignment is often associated with decompression management. Skeletal traction, a halo and vest application, braces, or surgery are methods of achieving alignment, depending on the type of problem. If the vertebral facets are locked, then surgical intervention will be necessary to unlock the facets and align the vertebrae.

Stabilization of the spinal column is accomplished with surgery instrumentation or by spontaneous fusion during the natural healing process. Skeletal traction and immobilization promote the natural healing process. These treatment methods can be used singularly or in combination with surgery to achieve the desired outcome. If surgery is indicated, stabilization is achieved with fusion using an analogous bone graft or insertion of stabilization rods instrumentation (see below).

The management of the patient will depend on the type of spinal cord injury and any associated injuries or health problems.

SURGICAL MANAGEMENT OF SPINAL CORD INJURIES

If surgery is indicated, selecting the best time for surgery is critical. Early surgery (within the first 12–24 hours) can preserve, improve, or restore spinal cord function. The following are reasons for early surgery:

- Evidence of cord compression
- Progressive neurological deficit
- Compound fracture of the vertebra (potential for bony fragments to dislodge and penetrate the cord)
- Penetrating wounds of the spinal cord or surrounding structures
- A bone fragment evident in the spinal canal

Early surgery is usually postponed in the following circumstances:

- When rapid and significant improvement in neurological function is demonstrated
- When staging is necessary, as in the need first for traction or immobilization to realign the vertebral column or reduce dislocations or fracture-dislocations before surgery
- When a life-threatening injury or disease exists elsewhere in the body. With severe trauma, the patient may have other injuries such as a head injury, contused kidney, cardiac contusion, intestinal rupture, or other problems in addition to spinal cord injury. Emergent surgery for life-threatening injuries, such as a ruptured spleen, may be necessary. The patient may not be stable enough to tolerate prolonged anesthesia and surgery that would be necessary for the spinal surgery.

Types of Procedures. Surgery is the selected mode of stabilization when the physician determines that the nature of the injury requires this form of intervention. The following are among the most common procedures performed:

- Posterior approach, open reduction internal fixation with interspinous wiring in cervical spine with fusion using autologous iliac bone graft
- Decompression laminectomy by anterior cervical or thoracic approach with fusion
- In the thoracic area a posterior approach with an autologous fusion graft, rod placement, or other instrumentation

Laminectomies and spinal fusion, along with nursing care, are discussed in Chapter 23. There have been a few additions to the surgical procedures performed for spinal stabilization. **Harrington rods** developed in the early 1960s were the cornerstone of spinal surgery instrumentation until recently. The Harrington rod system consisted of a rod or rods and wires affixed to the base of spinous processes and then attached to the rod. This provided multiple fixation points for stabilization.[5]

In the early 1990s, **CD rods** were introduced; they are used in conjunction with lamina hooks or pedicle screws and are the current approach for thoracic lumbar instrumentation.[6] This system provides for multiple points of fixation and greater stabilization. CD rod placement is technically more difficult, but it does not usually require postoperative immobility. Ideally, the use of CD instrumentation facilitates mobility of the patient. However, in some instances, such as with multiple, complex burst fractures, the physician may order an external orthosis (molded brace or corset) and bed rest for a few days after surgery. Patient care after surgery is based on the patient, extent of injury, and physician preference.

NONSURGICAL MANAGEMENT OF SPINAL CORD INJURIES

Immobilization with a halo vest or brace and traction for reduction and realignment are common approaches, singularly or more often in combination, in the nonsurgical management of the patient with a spinal cord injury. Vertebral subluxation with or without cord involvement is often managed with immobilization with a halo vest and traction.

Specialized Approaches to Management Based on the Level of Injury
CERVICAL INJURIES

Cervical Traction. Cervical traction is used much less frequently today than in the past because of the advent of early and better surgical stabilization. When cervical traction is used, its purpose is realignment or reduction of cervical vertebral dislocations. Crutchfield, Vinke, Gardner-Wells, and other types of cervical tongs have been almost eliminated in favor of the versatile halo traction. The most common type of cervical traction is provided by the halo system (described below). Skeletal traction greatly facilitates care and enhances patient comfort. Once the traction is in place, pain is greatly decreased or completely obliterated. Traction relieves pain by separating and aligning the injured vertebrae and reduces or eliminates spasms in the distracted muscles.

A regular, firm, hospital bed is used with cervical traction. Some physicians prefer using a special bed, such as a Roto Rest. Depending on the type of injury and method of immobilization, other special beds may be used to decrease the possibility of pressure areas. When in traction, the patient can be turned safely with a special turning technique to allow for skin care and changes in position to reduce pressure.

The Halo System. The halo is the most frequently ordered method for cervical and high thoracic vertebral injuries. Following are two uses for the halo:

- Direct skeletal traction involving the application of hanging weights; the patient is maintained on complete bed rest and managed with special nursing care techniques (Fig. 22-10).
- Use with a special body vest to stabilize the spine, thereby allowing healing and stabilization; ambulation is possible if the patient is neurologically intact (Fig. 22-11).

The halo is applied with the use of local anesthesia. The halo (metal ring) is inserted into the external bony table of the cranium by four pins—two posterior and two anterior. If direct traction is desired, then a rope with hanging weights is applied. If immobilization and stabilization are desired, then

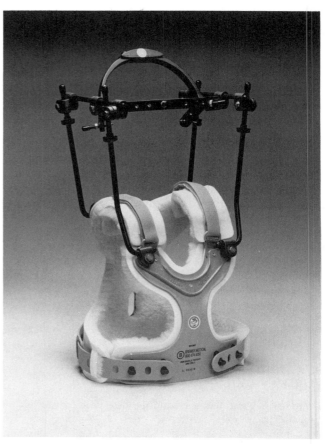

FIGURE 22-11
Halo and vest. A lightweight, fleece-lined vest with a halo may be used to stabilize cervical vertebrae. Note that the vest comes in various sizes and does not need to be removed for magnetic resonance imaging studies. (Courtesy of Bremer Medical, Inc., Dawin Road, Jacksonville, FL 32207.)

a vest with external metal rods attaching to the halo ring is applied. Small, dry, sterile dressings are placed around the pin sites (see Fig. 22-10). The halo is fairly comfortable despite its appearance, although some patients may develop a headache initially. In addition, any sound caused by bumping the halo can result in annoying vibrations. Rubber tips added to the pins reduce this problem.

One outstanding cost advantage of using the halo for immobilization and fixation or stabilization is that it allows for a shorter period of hospitalization. If no paralysis exists, the patient is able to ambulate, thereby counteracting the multitude of potential problems associated with bed rest and immobility. The halo with vest is beneficial in cervical and very high thoracic fractures.

Another feature of the halo is that surgery can be performed while the patient is in halo traction. This avoids the risk of malalignment of the injured area or extension of cord injury that could occur with removal of the traction device. One should remember that the physician often applies skeletal traction prior to surgery to reduce the injury. When the best alignment possible is achieved, surgery (usually spinal fusion) is scheduled.

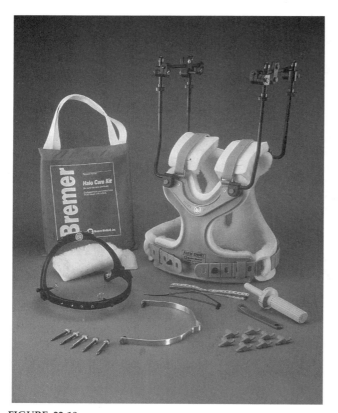

FIGURE 22-10
Halo cervical skeletal traction. (Courtesy of Acromed Corp., Cleveland, OH)

THORACIC AND LUMBAR INJURIES

When a patient sustains a thoracic or lumbar fracture or fracture-dislocation, various treatment options are possible, depending on the specific type of injury. If surgery is indicated, procedures frequently performed include laminectomy, with or without a fusion, and insertion of CD rods. To maintain thoracic or lumbar alignment as an adjunct to surgery or as the only management protocol for the injury, the following may be used:

- A fiberglass or plastic vest (The vest, which is fitted to the patient, provides immobilization and support to the injured area; see Fig. 22-11.)
- A canvas corset
- A Jewett brace, which extends the spinal column (providing support to the lower thoracic and lumbar region)
- Other specially designed braces or orthotics

SACRAL AND COCCYGEAL INJURIES

The usual treatment for sacral and coccygeal fractures is bed rest. The affected area is supported by a low support corset or special brace. A rubber ring can provide relief from pain and discomfort in the supine position. Pain is increased by sitting on a hard surface, so this is avoided. The patient should be evaluated for bowel, bladder, and sexual dysfunction.

FOCUS ON THE COLLABORATIVE MANAGEMENT IN THE ACUTE AND POSTACUTE PHASES

Acute Phase

There are several areas to consider in the acute phase of spinal cord injury, when the priority is stabilizing the patient. The major areas of focus are included in Tables 22-4 and 22-5.

Postacute Phase

The postacute phase begins after the patient is well, physiologically stabilized, and spinal shock has begun to reverse. An increasingly precise picture of the extent of the patient's overall deficits and how they will affect his or her former lifestyle begins to emerge. The focus at this time is no longer on surviving the injuries, but on coping with the alterations that the injury has imposed on the patient's daily life. Early rehabilitation efforts are integrated into the plan of care. A systematic assessment for discharge planning is a priority.

The problems that typically arise are presented in Table 22-6. During the postacute phase, several phenomena can develop that require special patient management. They include autonomic hyperreflexia, spasticity, bladder dysfunction, bowel dysfunction, sexual dysfunction, and psychological response to injury.

AUTONOMIC HYPERREFLEXIA

Autonomic hyperreflexia, also termed autonomic dysreflexia, is a serious emergency hypertensive event that arises in the postacute or rehabilitation phase of spinal cord injury. If left untreated, it can lead to a stroke, seizures (including status epilepticus), or myocardial infarction. Autonomic hyperreflexia is seen only **after** recovery from spinal shock when reflex activity has returned.

Autonomic hyperreflexia is caused by noxious stimuli that create an exaggerated sympathetic response (involving the thoracolumbar outflow of the autonomic nervous system) because of a lack of control from higher centers. It is seen only in patients with spinal cord lesions at or above T-6. In lesions below this level, more of the sympathetic nervous system is intact, so this abnormal response is avoided.

Noxious stimuli, which may occur from a distended bladder, ascend the spinal cord. Because of the spinal lesion, upward ascension to higher centers is interrupted. As a result, a mass reflex stimulation of the sympathetic nerves *below* the lesion occurs. This causes arteriolar spasms of the pelvic and abdominal viscera and of the skin, resulting in vasoconstriction *below* the lesion. The vasoconstriction produces cold skin and goose flesh in the involved area and causes a rise in blood pressure. Baroreceptors in the aortic arch and carotid sinus are stimulated, and a message is sent through the vagus nerve to the vasomotor center (in the medulla), causing reflex slowing of the heart (bradycardia) and vasodilation *above* the lesion. The bradycardia represents an attempt by the body to cause vasodilation and lower the blood pressure. Because the descending impulses are blocked by the spinal lesion, the skin *above* the lesion is warm and moist (owing to vasodilation and sweating) but cold with goose flesh *below* the lesion.

Noxious stimuli are most often caused by a distended bladder secondary to a plugged catheter. Other noxious stimuli originate from constipation or fecal impaction, urinary calculi, cystitis, acute abdominal lesions, operative incisions, uterine labor contractions, pressure on the glans penis, and stimulation from skin lesions, such as inguinal rash, pressure ulcers, or ingrown toenails.

Clinically, the patient suddenly becomes hypertensive and develops a severe, pounding headache secondary to the hypertension. The rise in blood pressure may reach levels as high as 240/120 or higher, or there may be a significant rise in blood pressure for that patient compared with his or her usual baseline (*e.g.*, a rise from a normal blood pressure of 100/70 to 140/90). The patient may appear anxious, with a flushed face, neck, and upper chest moistened with perspiration and with lower extremities exhibiting goose flesh and feeling cold. Complaints of nasal congestion and nausea are also common.

Management. Treatment is directed toward removal of the noxious stimuli and lowering of the blood pressure. Management includes elevation of the head, rapid assessment to find the cause of the condition, replacement of the catheter if irrigation does not dislodge a plug, application of a topical anesthetic to the rectum before attempting to disimpact, and removal of pressure from areas of irritated or broken skin. Antihypertensive drugs may also be ordered. This situation represents a medical emergency and should be treated as such.

(text continues on page 447)

TABLE 22-4
Summary of the Collaborative Management of Multisystem Problems in the Acute Phase After Spinal Cord Injury

SYSTEM-SPECIFIC CONSIDERATIONS	NURSING DIAGNOSES AND COLLABORATIVE PROBLEMS	ASSESSMENT AND MONITORING DATA	MANAGEMENT AND INTERVENTIONS
NEUROLOGICAL SYSTEM • The level and pattern of neurological loss depend on the level of injury and need to be assessed and monitored for change; change can occur as a result of extension of injury or ascending edema. • As a result of spinal shock, many motor, sensory, and reflex functions are lost. Many of the specific deficits are listed under the body system that they primarily affect. • Hypothermia and orthostatic hypotension are commonly seen in the acute phase. • The patient who is tetraplegic is completely dependent on the care provider for self-care and mobility. • Often a cerebral concussion was also sustained at the time of injury; often memory is impaired for the circumstance of injury.	**Nursing diagnoses** • Risk for Altered Body Temperature • Hypothermia • Knowledge Deficit • Impaired Memory • Pain, acute • Impaired Physical Mobility • Self Care Deficit, complete • Self Care Deficit, instrumental • Sensory/Perceptual Alterations • Sexual Dysfunction • Sleep Pattern Disturbance • Impaired Swallowing • Risk for Injury **Collaborative problems** • Increased intracranial pressure if also sustained a head injury	**Clinical data** • Assess baseline and monitor highest sensory level, motor function, and reflexes. • Monitor vital signs. • Assess baseline and monitor routine neurological signs for evidence of a concomitant head injury. **Laboratory data** • Magnetic resonance imaging (MRI) or computed tomography (CT) scan • X-rays of spine	• Provide for total care needs of patient. • Make sure that the patient is on the right type of bed based on the stability of the fracture and personal characteristics of the patient, such as weight. • Provide information to patient and family as requested; recognize that information will need to be repeated because of inability to comprehend fully the impact of the injury. • Be alert for decreased neurological function as a result of edema.
RESPIRATORY SYSTEM • Can develop varying degrees of respiratory difficulty depending on the level of injury: Injury at C-4 or above: Paralysis of diaphragm requires ventilator support. C-5 to T-6: Diaphragm is spared, but intercostals (T1-6) are involved; patient is at high risk for respiratory problems and may need oxygen and other special respiratory support. Even with lower injuries (T6-12 innervating the abdominal muscles), there may be minor respiratory deficits. Also, immobilization and bed rest will decrease respiratory function (*e.g.*, vital capacity), regardless of the level of injury. • The probability of certain respiratory complications decreases the lower the injury because the diaphragm and intercostals are spared. • Patients who cannot cough or manage their own secretions need a special respiratory management program. • Cervical surgery (both the procedure itself and the associated anesthesia) increases the risk of postoperative respiratory complications; thus, an optimal time for surgery (when the respiratory system is in the best condition possible) must be chosen.	**Nursing diagnoses** • Ineffective Airway Clearance • Risk for Aspiration • Ineffective Breathing Pattern • Impaired Gas Exchange • Inability to Sustain Spontaneous Ventilation • Risk for Respiratory Infection • Risk for Altered Respiratory Function **Collaborative problems** • Hypoxemia • Atelectasis, pneumonia • Pneumothorax • Respiratory arrest	**Clinical data** • Determine baseline respiratory status. (Auscultate the chest; note the breathing pattern; assess the patient's ability to cough and deep breathe effectively.) **Laboratory data** • Chest x-ray studies • Blood gas levels • Complete blood count (CBC) • Sputum cultures • Pulmonary function studies (*e.g.*, vital capacity)	• Intubate and provide ventilator support if the diaphragm is paralyzed or if respiratory function is ineffective. (The mode setting will depend on the needs of the patient.) • Provide supplementary oxygen as necessary. • Perform respiratory regimen (chest percussion; respiratory toilet; suctioning for patency; deep breathing if on a ventilator or sighing on ventilator setting). • Consult with a pulmonary physician as necessary. • Provide tracheostomy care every 4 h to maintain patency. • See Chap. 12 for ventilator management. • Provide chest physical therapy (PT) and deep breathing exercises every 2–4 h; if the patient is unable to cough effectively, assist with coughing by firmly depressing the abdomen when the patient coughs (place hands below the rib cage and above the umbilicus.)[1]

(continued)

TABLE 22-4
Summary of the Collaborative Management of Multisystem Problems in the Acute Phase After Spinal Cord Injury Continued

SYSTEM-SPECIFIC CONSIDERATIONS	NURSING DIAGNOSES AND COLLABORATIVE PROBLEMS	ASSESSMENT AND MONITORING DATA	MANAGEMENT AND INTERVENTIONS
• Other risk factors contributing to altered respiratory function include immobilization; bed rest; smoking; pre-existing pulmonary disease (*e.g.*, chronic obstructive pulmonary disease); concurrent chest trauma (*e.g.*, fractured ribs, contused lungs); anemia; and gastric distention or paralytic ileus. Gastric distention may be associated with vomiting, aspiration, and compromised lung expansion. • Alert: Ascending edema can rapidly cause respiratory difficulty that requires immediate intervention; monitor rate and pattern frequently.			• Provide for intermittent positive pressure breathing (IPPB) every 4 h. • Provide for use of incentive spirometer every 4 h.
CARDIOVASCULAR SYSTEM • Loss of sympathetic input from the higher brain centers results in bradycardia and vasomotor paralysis (vasodilation of blood vessels below the level of injury), so blood pressure is lowered. • Orthostatic hypotension results in pooling of blood below the level of injury because of vasodilation; this causes hypotension and decreased blood return to the heart. • Pooling of blood, coupled with immobility, greatly increases the risk of vascular stasis and orthostatic hypotension.	**Nursing diagnoses** • Impaired Gas Exchange • Decreased Cardiac Output • Altered Tissue Perfusion • Risk for Peripheral Neurovascular Dysfunction **Collaborative problems** • Decreased cardiac output • Dysrhythmias • Deep vein thrombosis • Hypovolemia	**Clinical data** • Monitor vital signs. • Provide cardiac monitoring. • Monitor response to elevation of head (orthostatic hypotension). • Observe for signs and symptoms of thrombophlebitis, DVT, and pulmonary embolus. **Laboratory data** • Electrocardiogram • Electrolyte, coagulation studies	• Treat any life-threatening arrhythmias. • Apply sequential compression boots. • Prophylactic use of heparin (5,000 μ every 12 hs) helps prevent DVTs; this is *contraindicated* if any internal bleeding is present or if surgery has been performed. • Use vasopressors as necessary. • Cardiology consult may be necessary, especially if a cardiac contusion is suspected. • Assess for arrhythmias by observing the cardiac monitor. • Monitor patient's response to elevation of the head (orthostatic hypotension). • Observe for signs and symptoms of DVT and pulmonary embolus.
INTEGUMENTARY SYSTEM (SKIN) • Loss of vasomotor tone, paralysis, and bed rest contribute to the development of pressure areas and skin breakdown. • Once developed, broken areas of skin are very difficult to heal; therefore, use of a bed to relieve continuous pressure while maintaining alignment should be considered.	**Nursing diagnoses** • Risk for Peripheral Neurovascular Dysfunction • Impaired Skin Integrity • Impaired Tissue Integrity • Altered Peripheral Tissue Perfusion **Collaborative problems** • Pressure ulcers	**Clinical data** • Monitor for signs and symptoms of redness or breakdown.	• Provide skin care and turn the patient every 2–4 h. • When a special bed (*e.g.*, a Roto Rest bed) is in use, adapt care measures appropriately.

(continued)

TABLE 22-4
Summary of the Collaborative Management of Multisystem Problems in the Acute Phase After Spinal Cord Injury Continued

SYSTEM-SPECIFIC CONSIDERATIONS	NURSING DIAGNOSES AND COLLABORATIVE PROBLEMS	ASSESSMENT AND MONITORING DATA	MANAGEMENT AND INTERVENTIONS
MUSCULOSKELETAL SYSTEM • Prolonged immobility and paralysis have significant effects on bone, joints, and muscles (see Table 22-5).	**Nursing diagnoses** • Disuse Syndrome • Impaired Physical Mobility • Altered Protection **Collaborative problems** • Contractures • Ankylosis • Muscle atrophy • Osteoporosis	**Clinical data** • Monitor range of motion of joints for development of deformities, spasticity, or ankylosis.	• Consult with physical therapist to develop individualized physical therapy (PT) program. • Provide range-of-motion exercises once daily. • Position the patient's extremities in proper body alignment.
GASTROINTESTINAL (GI) SYSTEM • Peristalsis is lost with spinal shock, resulting in paralytic ileus. • A distended abdomen interferes with adequate respirations. • Stress ulcers and gastric hemorrhage can also occur; because sensation is lost, the patient cannot feel the pain of ulceration. • Monitor for constipation.	**Nursing diagnoses** • Ineffective Breathing Pattern • Risk for Altered Respiratory Function • Risk for Injury • Bowel Incontinence • Constipation **Collaborative problems** • Paralytic ileus • GI bleeding • Constipation	**Clinical data** • Perform abdominal auscultation for bowel sounds. • Monitor stools for occult blood. • Monitor gastric pH. **Laboratory data** • CBC • Decreased hemoglobin	• Immediately insert a nasogastric tube to intermittent suction (low) for GI decompression. • Maintain NPO status until bowel sounds return and the nasogastric tube is removed. • Initiate a bowel program as soon as possible. • Maintain a pH >5.0 by using Maalox, 30 mL every 3 h. • Administer drugs (*e.g.,* cimetidine) to decrease gastric secretions. • Stool softeners/laxatives to facilitate a bowel program.
GENITOURINARY SYSTEM • Bladder reflexes and control of micturition from higher brain centers are lost with cord injury; atonic bladder results. • An atonic bladder (loss of bladder tone) is distended and predisposes the patient to urinary tract infections (UTIs).	**Nursing diagnoses** • Reflex Incontinence • Altered Pattern of Urinary Elimination • Urinary Retention • Risk for Infection **Collaborative problems** • Acute urinary retention • Urinary tract infection	**Clinical Data** • Palpate suprapubic area for bladder distention. • Review intake and output record. **Laboratory Data** • Urine C&S, UIA, BUN, and creatinine	• Insert an indwelling urinary catheter immediately. • Remove catheter and initiate intermittent catheterization program every 8–10 h once the patient is stable. • Aggressively treat UTI. • Maintain an intake and output record. • Use aseptic technique when managing the indwelling catheter.
METABOLIC (NUTRITIONAL) SYSTEM • The method of providing nutrition will depend on the associated injuries, level of consciousness, and the presence or absence of peristalsis. • The body needs sufficient fluid, carbohydrates, and protein for energy and tissue repair.	**Nursing diagnoses** • Altered Nutrition: Less than body requirements • Fluid Volume Deficit • Fluid Volume Excess **Collaborative problems** • Negative nitrogen balance • Electrolyte imbalances • Acidosis • Alkalosis • Hypoglycemia, hyperglycemia	**Clinical data** • Assess skin turgor and mucous membranes for adequacy of hydration. • Monitor weight two times a week. • Monitor muscle mass of extremities. **Laboratory data** • Albumin, electrolytes, and other indications of nutritional levels	• Maintain NPO status until peristalsis returns. • Nutrition consult is necessary as soon as possible. • May need to consider total parenteral nutrition. • Use GI tract, if not contraindicated, as soon as peristalsis returns.

(continued)

TABLE 22-4
Summary of the Collaborative Management of Multisystem Problems in the Acute Phase After Spinal Cord Injury Continued

SYSTEM-SPECIFIC CONSIDERATIONS	NURSING DIAGNOSES AND COLLABORATIVE PROBLEMS	ASSESSMENT AND MONITORING DATA	MANAGEMENT AND INTERVENTIONS
PSYCHOLOGICAL OR EMOTIONAL RESPONSE			
• If the patient is conscious, he or she is usually in a state of shock and denial of what has happened and the impact on lifestyle. • Allow the patient to ask questions when ready. • The family may require the most support as they begin to comprehend what has happened and what it means to the patient and to them.	**Nursing diagnoses** • Impaired Adjustment • Anxiety • Body Image Disturbance • Confusion • Decisional Conflict • Defensive Coping • Ineffective Denial • Diversional Activity Deficit • Grieving • Ineffective Individual Coping • Personal Identity Disturbance • Powerlessness • Impaired Social Interaction **Collaborative Problems** • Depression • Anxiety	**Clinical data** • Assess the patient to determine what he or she is ready to hear. • Assess the family unit and their response to the injury and its ramifications.	• Be supportive of the patient and family. • Provide information • Make appropriate referrals for support.

SPASTICITY

After a few weeks of spinal shock, a state of flaccidity and areflexia, spasticity develops. **Spasticity** is a state of excessive muscular tonus of selected muscles and of exaggerated deep tendon reflexes. The antigravity muscles, the flexors of the arms and the extensors of the legs, are predominantly affected.

The most common position assumed by the patient is one in which the arms are flexed and pronated and the legs are extended and adducted. When the limb is moved very slowly, there may be little or no change in the tonus. However, if the muscle is stretched rapidly, the "clasp-knife" phenomenon is seen. **Clonus**, a series of involuntary muscle contractions, describes a hyperreflexic response to abrupt stimuli that is also seen in spasticity. The clasp-knife analogy has been used to explain spasticity; the action of the muscles is compared with the "catch" and "give" of a spring-loaded knife blade. Through the initial phase of passive movement on a spastic limb, there is palpable resistance to stretching, as with the opening of a knife blade. Toward the end phase, abrupt loss of muscle resistance occurs, with the muscle completely submitting to the movement, similar to the final phase of blade action.

The pathophysiological basis for spasticity is an interruption of the descending inhibitory pathways through spindle afferent impulses (increased tonic activity of gamma motor neurons) and centrally through reticulospinal and vestibulospinal pathways that act mainly on alpha motor neurons.

Spasticity can occur any time from a few weeks (4–6) to several months (7–8) after cord injury. The magnitude of spasticity can gradually increase, reaching its height in $1\frac{1}{2}$ to 2 years, at which time it gradually diminishes in magnitude. Spasticity occurs in a predominant pattern of flexion or extension. In **extensor spasticity**, which affects approximately two thirds of patients, extensor spasms predominate over flexor spasms. In **flexor spasticity**, the reverse is true—flexor spasms

(text continues on page 450)

TABLE 22-5
Musculoskeletal Changes Caused by Prolonged Immobilization

	INITIAL	ADVANCED
BONE	Skeletal malalignment; loss of calcium	Skeletal deformities and generalized osteoporosis, which can result in an increased amount of cavities and pathological fractures
JOINTS	Joint stiffness; shortening or stretching of ligaments	Ankylosis
MUSCLES	Muscle weakness; shortening or stretching of muscles	Muscle atrophy; fibrotic changes; muscle contractures

TABLE 22-6
Summary of the Collaborative Management of Multisystem Problems in the Subacute Phase After Spinal Cord Injury

SYSTEM-SPECIFIC CONSIDERATIONS	NURSING DIAGNOSES AND COLLABORATIVE PROBLEMS	ASSESSMENT/ MONITORING DATA	MANAGEMENT/ INTERVENTIONS
NEUROLOGICAL SYSTEM • With recovery from spinal shock, autonomic hyperreflexia can occur with cord injuries at the level of T6 or above. • Initially, pain may be experienced at the level of injury. • As spinal shock resolves, some sensations may return if the lesion is incomplete; these sensations range from mild tingling to severe, intractable pain. • Pain may be caused by scar tissue or posttraumatic sympathetic dystrophy • Paresthesias and hyperesthesias may also be noted.	**Nursing diagnoses** • Hypothermia • Knowledge Deficit • Impaired Physical Mobility • Self-Care Deficit, complete • Self-Care Deficit, instrumental • Sensory/Perceptual Alterations • Sexual Dysfunction • Sleep Pattern Disturbance • Impaired Swallowing • Risk of Injury **Collaborative problems** • Autonomic hyperreflexia • Pain	**Clinical data** • Assess baseline and monitor highest sensory level, motor function, and reflexes. • Monitor vital signs. • Monitor for signs and symptoms of autonomic hyperreflexia. • Monitor for complaints of pain or abnormal sensations. **Laboratory data** • MRI or CT scan • X-rays of spine	• Provide for total care needs of patient. • Provide information to patient and family. • Treat for autonomic hyperreflexia (see text). • Evaluate pain and pain control via drugs, surgery, or other methods. • Assess pain and use pain control strategies. • Begin patient/family teaching related to: —Prevention of autonomic hyperreflexia —Comfort measures —Prevention of injury to tissue
RESPIRATORY SYSTEM • If possible, wean the patient from the ventilator (start by changing mode, and so forth) • For patients who cannot be weaned, consider long-term management options (*e.g.,* discharge home on a ventilator; diaphragmatic pacer; or other options) • Patients with cervical injuries usually have decreased: —Volumes of air exchange in tidal volumes —Movement of the chest with each respiration —Forced expiration volume	**Nursing diagnoses** • Ineffective Airway Clearance • Risk of Aspiration • Impaired Gas Exchange • Risk of Respiratory Infection • Risk of Altered Respiratory Function **Collaborative problems** • Hypoxemia • Atelectasis, pneumonia	**Clinical data** • Observe respiratory effort • Perform chest auscultation **Laboratory data** • Blood gas levels • Chest x-ray studies • Pulmonary function studies to plan for long-term management	• Provide respiratory care (chest physical therapy [PT]; intermittent positive pressure breathing treatments [IPPB]; oxygen therapy; ventilator support) • Provide vigorous treatment of infections • Provide permanent airway (tracheostomy) if necessary • Begin a patient/family teaching program: —Respiratory care —Breathing exercises —Assisted coughing —Suction technique —Oxygen, intermittent positive pressure breathing (IPPB) and other therapy treatments
CARDIOVASCULAR SYSTEM • As in the acute phase, bradycardia and orthostatic hypotension may occur. • Problems with orthostatic hypotension may arise when the head of the bed is raised.	**Nursing diagnoses** • Impaired Gas Exchange • Risk of Peripheral Neurovascular Dysfunction **Collaborative problems** • Dysrhythmias • Deep vein thrombosis • Pulmonary embolism • Hypovolemia • Orthostatic hypotension	**Clinical data** • Monitor for signs and symptoms of deep vein thromboses (DVTs), pulmonary embolus, and orthostatic hypotension • Monitor vital signs **Laboratory data** • Chest x-ray studies	• Continue use of air boots • Continue administration of heparin if not contraindicated • Provide PT with use of tilt table if orthostatic hypotension is a problem • Apply abdominal binder and thigh-high elastic (TED) stockings.

(continued)

TABLE 22-6
Summary of the Collaborative Management of Multisystem Problems in the Subacute Phase After Spinal Cord Injury Continued

SYSTEM-SPECIFIC CONSIDERATIONS	NURSING DIAGNOSES AND COLLABORATIVE PROBLEMS	ASSESSMENT/ MONITORING DATA	MANAGEMENT/ INTERVENTIONS
INTEGUMENTARY SYSTEM (SKIN)			
• Skin pressure problems continue to be a concern, although anesthesia is present below the level of injury.	**Nursing diagnoses** • Risk of Peripheral Neurovascular Dysfunction • Impaired Skin Integrity • Impaired Tissue Integrity • Altered Peripheral Tissue Perfusion **Collaborative problems** • Pressure ulcers • Osteomyelitis	**Clinical data** • Assess for signs and symptoms of skin breakdown	• Apply strategies for prevention of skin breakdown. • Provide skin care and turn the patient every 2 to 4 hours. • Provide for range-of-motion exercises once daily. • If a special bed is used, adapt care accordingly.
MUSCULOSKELETAL SYSTEM			
• Prolonged immobility and paralysis have significant effects on bone, joints, and muscles (see Table 22-5). • Spasticity becomes a problem as recovery from spinal shock occurs.	**Nursing diagnoses** • Disuse Syndrome • Impaired Physical Mobility • Altered Protection **Collaborative problems** • Contractures • Ankylosis • Muscle atrophy • Osteoporosis • Spasticity	**Clinical data** • Provide assessment with PT **Laboratory data** • Long bone x-ray studies	• Consult with physical medicine department • Implement aggressive PT program • Implement prevention strategies. • Provide for range-of-motion exercises once daily. • Position the patient's extremities in proper body alignment.
GASTROINTESTINAL (GI) SYSTEM			
• Peristalsis recurs, but is sluggish. • GI reflexes are sluggish. • The development of gastric ulcers or hemorrhage remains a concern.	**Nursing diagnosis** • Risk of Injury • Bowel Incontinence • Constipation **Collaborative problems** • Paralytic ileus • GI bleeding • Constipation	**Clinical data** • Monitor bowel sounds and rigidity of abdomen, as well as blood in stools or hematemesis • Monitor vital signs • Monitor bowel movements • Assess for rigid abdomen • Assess for hematemesis **Laboratory data** • Decreased hemoglobin level • Occult blood in stool • Upper GI series • Barium enema	• Administer drugs to decrease gastric irritation • Administer drug therapy to facilitate a bowel program
GENITOURINARY SYSTEM			
• As spinal shock resolves, an atonic bladder may change to a spastic bladder. • There are several possible variations of bladder dysfunction (see Chapter 14). • Altered sexual function is also noted.	**Nursing diagnoses** • Reflex Incontinence • Altered Pattern of Urinary Elimination • Urinary Retention • Risk of Infection • Sexual Dysfunction **Collaborative problems** • Renal calculi • Urinary tract infection (UTI) • Atonic or spastic bladder • Kidney disease • Priapism	**Clinical data** • Assess voiding pattern (large or small amounts) • Monitor for hematuria • Monitor for foul-smelling urine • Monitor intake and output (I&O) record **Laboratory data** • Blood urea nitrogen (BUN) and creatinine tests, urinalysis, and urine culture • Kidney-ureter-bladder (KUB) films; intravenous pyelogram	• Continue with the intermittent catheterization protocol. • Begin a bladder retraining program as soon as possible. • Use meticulous aseptic technique. • Force fluids, if possible. • Listen to the patient's concerns about sexual dysfunction. • Provide information and initiate teaching when the patient is ready. • Provide urology consult as needed.

(continued)

TABLE 22-6
Summary of the Collaborative Management of Multisystem Problems in the Subacute Phase After Spinal Cord Injury Continued

SYSTEM-SPECIFIC CONSIDERATIONS	NURSING DIAGNOSES AND COLLABORATIVE PROBLEMS	ASSESSMENT/ MONITORING DATA	MANAGEMENT/ INTERVENTIONS
	• Sexual dysfunction	• Cystometric studies	• Begin frank discussion of the impact of the injury on sexual function • Provide vitamin C, 500 mg t.i.d., or another drug to acidify the urine
METABOLIC SYSTEM • A high-fluid, high-carbohydrate and high-protein diet is still needed to fuel energy and tissue repair.	**Nursing diagnoses** • Altered Nutrition: Less than body requirements • Fluid volume deficit **Collaborative problems** • Negative nitrogen balance • Electrolyte imbalances	**Clinical data** • Assess hydration, nutrition, skin, and muscle mass • Monitor I&O record • Weigh patient and record weight two times a week, if possible **Laboratory data** • Serum albumin level • Complete nutritional assay	• Provide for nutrition consult • Provide therapeutic diet • Provide for adequate fluid and nutritional intake.
PSYCHOLOGICAL/EMOTIONAL RESPONSE • The impact of the injury on the patient's previous functional level and lifestyle begin to be realized. • The patient begins the loss, grief, and bereavement process. • The impact of the injury on family and significant other(s) begins to be realized.	**Nursing diagnoses** • Impaired Adjustment • Anxiety • Body Image Disturbance • Decisional Conflict • Defensive Coping • Ineffective Denial • Diversional Activity Deficit • Grieving • Ineffective Individual Coping • Personal Identity Disturbance • Powerlessness • Impaired Social Interaction • Caregiver Role Strain • Fear • Altered Family Processes • Hopelessness • Social isolation • Spiritual distress **Collaborative problems** • Depression • Anxiety	**Clinical data** • Assess for behavior consistent with denial, anger, or depression • Monitor for suicidal themes	• Communicate with patient; be supportive • Communicate with family; be supportive • Set realistic goals • Provide for psychiatric consult, as necessary

predominate over extensor spasms. The spasticity patterns occur in incomplete and complete cord transection.

Management. Management of spasticity includes control of aggravating factors and medical management. Factors known to trigger spasticity in patients prone to this condition include cold, anxiety, fatigue, emotional distress, infections, impaction, and decubital ulcers.

Medical management involves various physical therapy techniques, such as application of cold and heat, passive range-of-motion exercises, stretching exercises, and electrical

stimulation. Temporary relief has been attained with alcohol or phenol nerve injection. Pharmacological interventions include the administration of antispasmodics, such as baclofen (Lioresal) and dantrolene sodium (Dantrium).

BLADDER DYSFUNCTION

Early removal of the urinary catheter decreases a major risk factor for urinary tract infections. An intermittent catheterization protocol is begun as soon as possible. As spinal shock resolves, a bladder retraining program is instituted. Cystometric studies to evaluate bladder function are scheduled. Drug therapy to acidify the urine and treat any urinary tract infection may be ordered.

BOWEL DYSFUNCTION

Institution of a bowel program is necessary in the postacute phase of spinal cord injury. This is managed by the nursing staff. (See the appropriate sections in Chap. 14 and Part II of this chapter for further information.)

SEXUAL DYSFUNCTION

Although sexuality and sexual adjustment should be an integral part of the patient's overall rehabilitation, this basic need has been grossly neglected. Health personnel often avoid this issue by assuming that the patient is too concerned with other health problems to care about sex. The truth is that sex, as a basic need, is a concern to all human beings. Gratification of sexual needs covers a wide range of behaviors and attitudes and is important to the individual.

Sexual function is controlled by spinal levels S-2, S-3, and S-4. Several articles have been published about sexual function among patients with cord injury or cauda equina lesions. In general, the findings suggest the following:

- **Men with upper motor neuron lesions**: Seventy percent of male patients with complete lesions and 80% of those with incomplete lesions can consummate coitus; most patients cannot ejaculate or have orgasm.
- **Men with lower motor neuron lesions**: Seventy-five percent of male patients with complete lesions are unable to have erections of any kind, whereas 25% have psychogenic erections. (Neither can achieve coitus, ejaculation, or orgasm.) Eighty-three percent of patients with incomplete lesions have psychogenic erections; 90% are able to have coitus (70% of this group are able to ejaculate, and of these, 10% may be able to father a child).
- **Women, regardless of type of lesion**: A woman with a spinal cord injury lacks sensation during intercourse. Women of the childbearing age can become pregnant. Most patients regain menses; 50% do not miss a single menstrual period. Vaginal delivery is possible if the pelvic measurements are adequate. Early cesarean section may be selected for patients prone to autonomic hyperreflexia.

Sexually active patients need birth control counseling. Because of the correlation of thrombophlebitis and the "pill," oral contraception may be contraindicated for a woman with a spinal cord injury. If she does not want to become pregnant, another form of contraception or contraception by her partner should be used.

PSYCHOLOGICAL RESPONSE TO INJURY

The impact of catastrophic illness coupled with devastating loss is overwhelming to the patient and family. Much patient and family education and support are required, as are sensitivity and compassion. The nurse should acknowledge the losses while being optimistic for the future. The patient and family will need much information to make appropri-

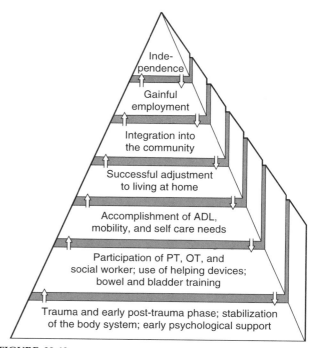

FIGURE 22-12
The rehabilitation process following spinal cord injury. (PT = physical therapy; OT = occupational therapy; ADL = activities of daily living.)

ate decisions. However, such information will be heard only when they are ready to hear it. In addition to the support provided by the individual practitioner, patient-centered conferences or family meetings incorporating an interdisciplinary team approach may be helpful in supporting the patient and family. A psychiatric consultation may be helpful for some patients.

Interdisciplinary Management During the Postacute Phase

Collaboration among all professionals involved with the care of the patient and family is essential to create a smooth transition from the acute phase of spinal cord injury to the rehabilitation phase (see Chart 22-6). A multidisciplinary team composed of physicians, nurses, social workers, physical therapists, occupational therapists, and others is needed to achieve this goal.

DISCHARGE PLANNING

The recognition that patients with spinal cord injuries have better outcomes when treated in spinal cord injury centers has prompted a trend toward rapid transfer to these centers. For this reason, more patients with spinal cord injuries are being referred at an earlier postinjury stage. Therefore, major decisions related to discharge planning are being made almost immediately on initial evaluation of the patient. The assessments of the interdisciplinary team provide a comprehensive data base for matching patient needs with available resources (see Chap. 15).

THE REHABILITATION PHASE

Rehabilitation is a complex relearning process that addresses the holistic needs of the person. The continuum of care from critical care to rehabilitation is designed to help the patient achieve the highest level of independence and quality of life possible. The goal of the rehabilitation phase is reintegration of the patient into the community. The recovery of a patient with a spinal cord injury can be viewed as analogous to Maslow's hierarchy of needs (Fig. 22-12).

Transfer of a patient to a rehabilitation facility, if not already at a spinal cord injury center, offers an opportunity for a comprehensive and individualized program for the patient.

The program may take several weeks to months. The core of the multidisciplinary staff includes physicians, nurses, physical therapists, occupational therapists, social workers, psychologists, vocational counselors, and other specialists. Depending on the needs of the patient, sexual counseling or marriage counseling may also be provided. Individual, group, and family counseling help the patient and family to accept and adjust to disabilities and changes in lifestyle resulting from the injury. Advice on necessary environmental modifications that would allow the patient to return home to live is also offered. The social worker can help identify special funds that may be available to help meet the needs of the person with a spinal cord injury. (For example, some states and private agencies provide funds to build ramps and purchase special equipment for the home.)

The care within a rehabilitation facility is beyond the scope of this text. The reader is directed to other sources in the rehabilitation literature for this information.

Part Two
Nursing Management
in the Acute
and Postacute Phase

NURSING MANAGEMENT DURING THE ACUTE CARE PHASE OF SPINAL CORD TRAUMA

Setting

After being stabilized in the emergency department, the patient will be admitted to a clinical unit (ICU, neuromedical-neurosurgical unit, or medical-surgical unit). Because the benefits of care in a spinal cord injury center have been well documented, many patients are triaged immediately to these centers. Others may be transferred in the postacute phase. Regardless of the setting, the nurse has the responsibility of caring for a patient with extremely complex needs who will probably need long-term rehabilitation.

Selection of a Bed

The physician may order a special trauma bed for the patient that is designed to facilitate vertebral stability, combat the multisystem problems associated with immobility, and facilitate patient care. One bed that may be selected for the patient with spinal cord injuries is the Roto Rest bed (Kinetic Treatment Table), a motor-powered bed that provides for continual turning of the patient through a maximal arc of 124 degrees at a minimal rate of 3.5 minutes. It also has three hatches at the underneath surface, cervical, thoracic, and lumbosacral (rectal), that allows easy access to all parts of the patient's body, including the entire back and rectal area for providing

back care and rectal care (Fig. 22-13). However, with the trend toward earlier surgery for spinal stabilization, other bed options are available for the stabilized patient. Physician and nursing staff preference and cost dictate the choice of bed for patients.

Signs and Symptoms of Spinal Cord Trauma

The signs and symptoms of spinal cord trauma are discussed in the previous section. The higher the level of injury, the greater the loss of motor, sensory, and reflex function. See Table 22-3 for a description of the functional loss that relates to specific levels of injury.

Special Considerations in Acute Spinal Cord Trauma

A number of conditions unique to spinal cord trauma warrant special consideration in the acute phase. These include spinal shock, neurogenic shock, ascending spinal cord edema, and respiratory insufficiency.

SPINAL SHOCK

Spinal shock is the temporary loss of reflex control below the level of injury secondary to the loss of descending pathway impulses. It begins 30 to 60 minutes after injury and can last for approximately 4 months or less. As a result, the patient can present with paralytic ileus or an atonic bladder.

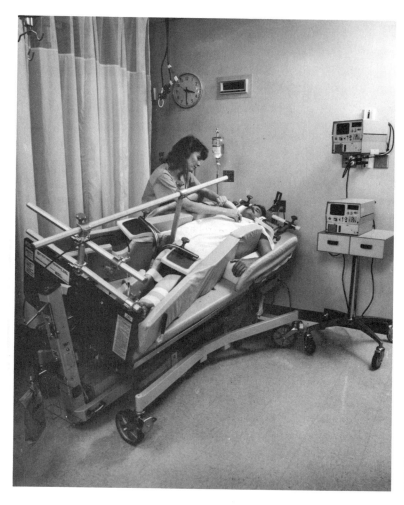

FIGURE 22-13
Roto Rest bed. (Courtesy of Kinetic Concepts, San Antonio, TX.)

Paralytic ileus is treated with insertion of a nasogastric tube to allow intermittent suctioning and withholding of all intake by mouth. The physician will order IV fluid administration or total parenteral nutrition. Once peristalsis returns, the GI tract can be used for nutrition. Related nursing diagnoses include *Altered nutrition: Less than body requirements; Risk for Fluid Volume Deficit;* and *Constipation.*

An atonic bladder is managed with an indwelling catheter initially. The nurse should follow meticulous aseptic technique in managing the catheter to prevent infections. As soon as possible, the catheter is removed, and an intermittent catheterization program is initiated. The reason for the urgency for catheter removal is that extended use of an indwelling catheter predisposes the patient to urinary tract infection. Therefore, It is important to remove this risk factor for infection as soon as possible. Related nursing diagnoses include *Altered Urinary Elimination* and *Risk for Infection.*

NEUROGENIC SHOCK

The temporary loss of autonomic function, termed **neurogenic shock,** affects vital signs. The blood pressure is low (especially with cervical injuries), and bradycardia is present. A cardiac monitor may be ordered to monitor the patient for cardiac arrhythmias. The low blood pressure is related, in part, to or-

thostatic hypotension. Because there is pooling of blood in the lower parts of the body below the level of injury, the blood return to the heart is decreased. Orthostatic hypotension is a major consideration in cervical injuries. The nursing diagnosis of *Decreased Cardiac Output* is appropriate in such patients.

The ability to perspire is lost below the level of injury, so body temperature is equivalent to the ambient room temperature. Most often, the temperature will be low (possibly dropping to 95°F), although in hot weather, the body temperature may be high. The related nursing diagnosis is *Ineffective Thermoregulation.*

ASCENDING SPINAL CORD EDEMA

With spinal cord trauma, one can expect cord edema to develop soon after injury as a physiological response to injury. The swelling results in cord compression and compounds the functional loss. It is also potentially life threatening, especially in the case of cervical or high thoracic injury. Edema can ascend the cord quickly, so a patient with previously adequate respirations may develop respiratory difficulty rapidly because C-4 and above (the phrenic nerve innervates the diaphragm) are now affected.

The spinal cord tolerates cord compression poorly. Permanent loss of function may be the result of frank damage to the cord itself or temporary loss related to exaggerated edema. With resolution of the edema, some functional return is possible, provided that irreversible damage has not been sustained. It is of critical importance for the nurse to observe the patient's status frequently for signs of deterioration from baseline function, especially in the early, acute phase of injury (during the first 72 hours or so). The related nursing diagnoses are *Altered Spinal Tissue Perfusion* and *Risk for Injury*.

RESPIRATORY INSUFFICIENCY

With C1-4 injuries, the intercostal muscles and often the diaphragm are paralyzed. The patient is dependent on a ventilator for respiratory support. Although the diaphragm is spared in injuries at C-5 or below, a ventilator may be necessary in the acute phase owing to ascending cord edema. Related nursing diagnoses include *Ineffective Breathing Pattern, Ineffective Airway Clearance,* and *Impaired Gas Exchange.*

Nursing Assessment

The nursing data base begins with the nursing history and assessment at the time of admission. The data collected in the history are part of the data base for discharge planning, which is initiated on admission of the patient. Information about the family unit, work and leisure activities, and previous coping patterns is helpful in individualizing the plan of care.

The physical assessment of the patient includes vital signs, neurological signs, spinal cord assessment, monitoring of laboratory data, and a body systems review. Much of the physiological assessment data are from invasive monitoring and a computer interface.

VITAL SIGNS

The nurse will monitor vital signs frequently. A lower than expected blood pressure, bradycardia, and a low temperature may be noted, especially with cervical cord injuries. The basis for these changes in relationship to spinal cord trauma is discussed in the previous section. However, changes in the vital signs may also reflect injuries to other body systems. Patients with spinal cord injuries are trauma patients who have often sustained trauma to other body systems. Some injuries may not be noted immediately. A change in vital signs may be the first sign of occult internal hemorrhage or other potentially life-threatening problems. Therefore, the nurse must frequently monitor vital signs for change.

NEUROLOGICAL SIGNS

An abbreviated neurological assessment is conducted periodically, including evaluation of the level of consciousness and pupillary response. Patients with spinal cord injuries often have concurrent head injuries of varying degrees of severity. A standard neurological assessment sheet may be used.

SPINAL CORD ASSESSMENT SHEET

To conduct a detailed assessment to determine exactly what functional level is intact, an extensive motor, sensory, and reflex assessment is necessary (Chart 22-4). This data base will

not only help the nurse monitor the patient for neurological change, but also will facilitate development of an individualized plan of care.

BODY SYSTEMS REVIEW

There are two reasons for conducting a systematic assessment of body systems in the patient with spinal cord injury. The first is to determine the location and extent of injuries to body systems other than the neurological system. The second is to determine the impact of the neurological injuries on other body systems (see Table 22-4).

Injuries to Other Body Systems

As discussed previously, patients with spinal cord injuries often sustain injury to other body systems. It is therefore important to consider the possibility of other injuries when assessing the patient.

Assessment of the patient is complicated by the fact that all sensations are lost, including pain (often an indicator of a problem), below the level of injury. Because pain cannot be used as a subjective indicator of dysfunction in these patients, the nurse must rely on other indicators, such as laboratory data, to assess the patient. For example, gastric hemorrhage is often heralded by pain, a decreased hematocrit and hemoglobin, and a decline in central venous pressure. The nurse will need to concentrate on parameters other than pain to monitor the patient for hemorrhage. See Chapter 20 for management of the patient sustaining multiple trauma.

Impact of Neurological Injury on Other Body Systems

Assessment data for problems arising in the acute phase of spinal cord injury are included in Table 22-4.

LABORATORY DATA

The laboratory data obtained during the acute phase of spinal cord injury include blood chemistry values (*e.g.,* electrolyte studies, glucose and blood gas levels), microbiological tests (*e.g.,* cultures), and hematological studies (*e.g.,* complete blood count, hematocrit, hemoglobin). Also included among the diagnostic data are results from radiology (*e.g.,* chest x-ray films, spinal films), special procedures (*e.g.,* myelography, computed tomography scanning, magnetic resonance imaging), and other sources. Review of this data base is helpful to the nurse in correlating observed clinical signs and symptoms with laboratory findings, identifying the need for special assessment and monitoring, and determining specific, appropriate nursing interventions.

Summary

Sources of data are numerous, and the needs of the patient can change dramatically, especially in the acute phase of spinal cord injury. Therefore, ongoing comprehensive assessment is the basis for analysis and establishment of appropriate nursing diagnoses to meet patient needs.

CHART 22-4
Nursing Assessment of Spinal Cord Function

Part I. Motor Function			Part II. Reflexes		
Left	Muscle Action	Right	Left	Deep Tendon Reflexes	Right
	Abduct upper arm			Ankle Jerk—S-1, S-2	
	Adduct upper arm			Knee Jerk—L-3, L-4	
	Extend upper arm			Biceps—C-5, C-6	
	Flex elbow			Triceps—C-7, C-8	
	Extend elbow			Superficial Reflexes	
	Flex wrist			Perineal—S3-5	
	Extend wrist			Abdominals, upper—T8-10	
	Flex fingers			Abdominals, lower—T10-12	
	Extend fingers			Gag—cranial nerve IX and X	
	Thumb opposition				
	Upper abdominals				
	Lower abdominals				
	Flex upper leg				
	Extend upper leg				
	Flex knee				
	Extend knee				
	Dorsiflex foot				
	Plantarflex foot				
	Extend big toe				

A few selected reflexes are assessed.

The grading of deep tendon reflexes is assessed using the following scale:

- 4+ = very brisk; hyperactive
- 3+ = more brisk than average
- 2+ = average or normal
- 1+ = diminished response
- 0 = no response

The grading of superficial reflexes is assessed using the following scale:

- + = present
- 0 = absent

Motor function is assessed using the following scale:

- 5 = normal strength
- 4 = slight weakness; can tolerate only a moderate amount of resistance
- 3 = moderate weakness; full range of movement against gravity only (no resistance)
- 2 = severe weakness; can move only when gravity is eliminated
- 1 = very severe weakness; a weak muscle contraction palpated but no visible movement noted
- 0 = complete paralysis

(continued)

CHART 22-4 Nursing Assessment of Spinal Cord Function (Continued)

Part III. Sensory Function

Left		Level	Right		Left		Level	Right	
Pain	POS/VIB	Cervical	Pain	POS/VIB	Pain	POS/VIB	Sacral	Pain	POS/VIB
		1					1		
		2					2		
		3					3		
		4					4		
		5					5		
		6							
		7							
		8							
		Thoracic							
		1							
		2							
		3							
		4							
		5							
		6							
		7							
		8							
		9							
		10							
		11							
		12							
		Lumbar							
		1							
		2							
		3							
		4							
		5							

Two sensory modalities are assessed: pain (pinprick), which is conducted by the lateral spinothalamic tract, and position (or vibration), which is controlled by the posterior columns. Pain sense is tested with a pin. Position is tested by asking patients to close their eyes and move the big toe, fingers, or extremities in various positions. If vibration is tested, a 256-Hz tuning fork is used. Using a dermatome, dermatomic areas are tested on each side of the body separately.

Sensory function is assessed using the following scale:

- 2 = normal
- 1 = present but abnormal
- 0 = absent

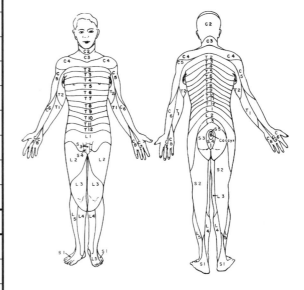

Dermatomes

Cutaneous distribution of the spinal nerves (See Figure 2-33, page 40). (From Barr, M.L., and J.A. Kiernan 1988. The human nervous system, 5th ed. Philadelphia: J. B. Lippincott.)

Nursing Interventions

GENERAL CONSIDERATIONS

Patients who are admitted to the hospital with spinal cord injuries will have self-care deficits. The nurse will assess the patient for independence in bathing and hygiene, dressing and grooming, feeding, and toileting to determine whether the patient can perform these functions independently, needs assistance, or is completely dependent. Care will be provided to meet basic needs. Other appropriate nursing interventions are included in Table 22-4.

LEVEL OF INJURY

Based on the level of injury, the nurse can make some assumptions about patient needs (see Table 22-3).

SPECIAL NEEDS

Special protocols are used to manage patients who are being treated with halo cervical skeletal traction and the halo with a vest (Charts 22-5 and 22-6). Patients maintained in cervical traction are on complete bed rest and are at high risk for the multiple problems associated with immobility.

NURSING MANAGEMENT DURING THE POSTACUTE CARE PHASE OF SPINAL CORD TRAUMA

Clarifying Patient Needs: An Interdisciplinary Approach

The postacute phase of spinal cord trauma begins when the patient is well stabilized. By this time, reversal of spinal shock has begun, and a clearer clinical picture emerges of the patient's intact functions and deficits. This information is useful in identifying rehabilitative needs.

It is also the time when referrals are made to interdisciplinary team members to provide a comprehensive needs assessment for immediate treatment and rehabilitation. Referrals are often made to social service personnel, physical therapists, and occupational therapists. These specialists form a basic core of health professionals who work with the physician and nurse to manage care. Other disciplines are included as necessary. It is often the nurse's responsibility to coordinate the assessment and care provided by the various disciplines.

Nursing Management in the Postacute Phase

ASSESSMENT AND INTERVENTIONS

Nursing assessment is ongoing as the patient is stabilized and specific deficits and needs become apparent. Table 22-6 includes a summary of assessment techniques and interventions for specific body systems during the postacute phase of care.

Special Considerations in the Postacute Phase

Some special considerations are unique to the postacute phase of spinal cord trauma. These include autonomic hyperreflexia, spasticity, bladder retraining, bowel retraining, and psychological response to injury.

AUTONOMIC HYPERREFLEXIA

The pathophysiology of autonomic hyperreflexia is discussed in Part I of this chapter. As spinal shock reverses, the potential for dysreflexia should be considered for patients with injuries at the T-6 level or above. Nursing interventions should be aimed at preventing the conditions that are known to trigger autonomic hyperreflexia. The causative noxious stimulus that is most often implicated is a distended bladder secondary to a plugged catheter or kinked drainage tubing. Other forms of noxious stimuli include constipation or fecal impaction, urinary calculi, cystitis, acute abdominal lesions, operative incisions, uterine labor contractions, pressure on the glans penis, and stimulation from skin lesions, such as inguinal rash, pressure ulcers, or ingrown toenails.

The nurse should be aware of the signs and symptoms of autonomic dysreflexia. These include paroxysmal hypertension, pounding headache, bradycardia, profuse sweating above the level of injury, flushing of the face and neck, and goose flesh. Treatment is directed toward removing the noxious stimuli and lowering the blood pressure. Should autonomic hyperreflexia occur, appropriate interventions include the following:

- Immediately elevate the head of the bed to a sitting position (to induce postural hypotension).
- Assess the bladder for distention. If a catheter is in place, check it for evidence of obstructed flow, such as a kink in the tubing. If the catheter is plugged, immediately irrigate it with a small amount (about 30 mL) of solution. If it still does not drain, replace the catheter immediately.
- In patients who are being catheterized intermittently, it is important to catheterize the patient immediately, regardless of the time that has elapsed since the last catheterization.
- Symptoms of autonomic hyperreflexia often occur during bowel care or attempts at defecation. If this is the case, all such activities should cease until symptoms subside. Assess the lower bowel for the presence of stool. Apply a topical anesthetic ointment (*e.g.*, Nupercaine) to the anus, and insert the ointment 1 in into the rectum. Wait 5 to 10 minutes, then try to disimpact the bowel.
- If a pressure ulcer is the noxious stimulus, spray the ulcer with a topical anesthetic agent.
- Monitor vital signs every 5 minutes.
- Drugs may be ordered to lower the blood pressure. The nursing diagnosis related to this condition is *Dysreflexia.*

SPASTICITY

Spasticity is a difficult problem that is best managed with the collaboration of a physical therapist. A combined regimen of

(text continues on page 460)

CHART 22-5
Summary of the Nursing Management of a Patient in Cervical Skeletal Halo Traction

Nursing Diagnoses	Nursing Interventions	Expected Outcome(s)
Orthopedic Traction Equipment		
• Risk for Injury	• Check the orthopedic frame and traction daily to ensure that nuts and bolts are secure. • Check tongs daily to be sure that they are secure. • Be sure that traction weights are hanging freely and not resting on the floor or frame. (Releasing the traction is dangerous because cord injury could be extended.)	• The orthopedic frame will remain intact. • Tongs will not slip. • Traction weights will hang freely. • There will not be any extension of cord injury secondary to slippage of the traction apparatus.
Skin Integrity		
• Risk for Infection • Impaired Skin Integrity	• Inspect tong sites, and clean and dress daily as ordered (may be referred to as "pin care"). • Turn the patient every 2 h from side to back to other side using a triple log roll technique as described below if a patient is on a regular hospital bed.	• The pin site will remain free of infection. • Skin integrity will be maintained. • The vertebral column will be maintained in a neutral position and in proper alignment.
	• Nurse # 1 stands behind the head of the bed and places hands firmly on the patient's head and neck, maintaining it in a neutral position; the head and neck are turned as a unit. Nurse #2 stands at the patient's side and moves the patient's shoulders. Nurse #3 stands at the patient's side and moves the patient's hips and legs. • Plan ahead, identifying desired position and pillow placement *before* moving the patient. When all three nurses are ready, turn the patient as a log on the count of three. Leave the patient positioned in the middle of the bed (if not, he or she will be uncomfortable); use pillows to support the patient's body in alignment. • Nurse #1 should hold the head and neck until the patient is supported adequately (if traction slips, manual traction can be supplied by Nurse # 1).	
Basic Care		
• Self-Care Deficits	• Provide for basic care needs that the patient cannot do for self.	• Basic care needs will be met.

(continued)

CHART 22-5 Summary of the Nursing Management of a Patient in Cervical Skeletal Halo Traction (Continued)

Nursing Diagnoses	Nursing Interventions	Expected Outcome(s)
Respiratory System		
• Risk for Aspiration • Ineffective Airway Clearance • Risk for Infection • Impaired Gas Exchange • *Note:* The patient on a ventilator will need special care.	• Have suction available to maintain a patent airway. • Provide respiratory care. • Provide for deep-breathing, assistive coughing, and incentive spirometer exercises every 1 to 2 h.	• Airway patency will be maintained. • The patient will not aspirate. • The patient will not develop a respiratory infection.
Cardiovascular System		
• Impaired Tissue Integrity (venous stasis) • Altered Peripheral Tissue Perfusion • Decreased Cardiac Output	• Maintain thigh-high elastic (TED) stockings and sequential compression boots. • If the patient is receiving heparin, observe for signs and symptoms of bleeding. • Monitor for deep vein thrombosis (DVTs) and pulmonary emboli. (May be on minidoses of subcutaneous heparin q 12 h, if not contraindicated.)	• Air boots and TEDs will be worn at all times. • Vital signs will be maintained within normal limits. • The patient will be observed for DVTs and pulmonary emboli.
Musculoskeletal System		
• Risk for Disuse Syndrome • Pain (related to muscle spasm) • Sensory Perceptual Alterations: Visual and tactile	• Provide comfort measures. • Provide range-of-motion exercises once daily. • Position the patient in proper body alignment. • Reposition the patient frequently. • Stretch the patient's heel cord with exercises.	• The patient will be free of pain. • Contractures will not develop. • Strategies will be used to manage spasticity if it occurs.
Gastrointestinal System		
• Colonic Constipation	• Institute a bowel retraining program. • Auscultate the abdomen for bowel sounds. • Record the frequency and consistency of stool.	• Pattern of bowel evacuation every 1 to 2 d will be established.
Genitourinary System		
• Altered Urinary Elimination • Risk for Infection • Sexual Dysfunction	• Monitor intake and output • Force fluids. • If an intermittent catheterization protocol is initiated, use aseptic technique. • If the patient is voiding on his or her own, monitor postvoid residuals. • Provide information about sexual function.	• Intake will be 3,000 mL unless contraindicated. • Postvoid residuals will be less than 100 mL. • Strict aseptic technique will be used for catheter protocols. • Sexual function and spinal cord injury will be discussed with the patient when he or she is ready.
Nutrition		
• Altered Nutrition: Less than body requirements • Fluid Volume Deficit	• Encourage an adequate diet. • Ask the dietician to see the patient. • Provide for adequate fluid intake up to 3,000 mL daily.	• A diet that is high in protein and carbohydrate, and that includes a fluid intake of up to 3,000 mL will be provided.

(continued)

CHART 22-5 Summary of the Nursing Management of a Patient in Cervical Skeletal Halo Traction (Continued)

Nursing Diagnoses	Nursing Interventions	Expected Outcome(s)
	• Encourage the patient to take small portions of food into the mouth and chew well to prevent aspiration. • Keep suction equipment handy.	• Aspiration will be prevented.
Emotional and Psychological Support		
• Powerlessness • Social Isolation • Ineffective Individual Coping • Diversional Activity Deficit • Body Image Disturbance • Knowledge Deficit	• Provide for social interaction and diversion based on the patient's functional level. • Reinforce a positive self-image. • Allow the patient to participate in decision making as much as possible. • Provide for patient teaching.	• The patient's mental health will be supported. • Social interaction and diversion will be provided based on the patient's ability to participate. • A positive body image will be supported. • Necessary information will be provided.

proper positioning, physical therapy, and drug therapy is usually effective, depending on the severity of the spasticity. Related nursing diagnoses are *Risk for Disuse Syndrome* and *Risk for Injury*.

The initial appearance of spasticity can be a false ray of hope for the patient. The "movement" noted is often misinterpreted by the patient or family as a return of normal voluntary function, rather than a heightened reflex response. Spasticity must be explained clearly and concisely to prevent any misunderstanding of its significance.

Management of spasticity by the nurse includes various nursing actions and procedures directed at preventing, controlling, or reducing spasticity while limiting debilitating effects and complications, such as contractures, pressure ulcers, and bowel and bladder dysfunction. The major nursing problems encountered on a day-to-day basis are the difficulty of positioning the patient and his or her lack of mobility. Because flexor spasticity develops first, the patient's extremities assume a flexed position. The development of contractures further compounds the problems of positioning.

Several nursing interventions and responsibilities are important in the management of the spastic patient:

• Provide passive range-of-motion exercises at least four times a day, because stiffness increases spasticity.
• Prevent the development of contractures; flexor spasticity and contractures gravely limit the patient's ability to participate in activities of daily living (ADLs). Use positioning and consult with the physical therapist for splints and so forth.
• When touching the patient, limit the amount of tactile stimuli; be gentle, yet firm and steady.
• Avoid circumstances that precipitate noxious stimuli known to increase spasticity (*e.g.*, extremes in temperature, remaining in one position for an extended period, anxiety, pain, bladder or bowel distention, tight clothing or equipment, decubital ulcers).

• Assume an unhurried manner when working with the patient; allow plenty of time for transfer activities, ambulation, dressing, and so forth.
• Turn and reposition the patient at least every 2 hours; prevent rubbing or irritating the skin.
• A sudden increase in spasticity should be viewed as a sign of an underlying factor that is precipitating noxious stimuli. Examples of such underlying causes include a kink in the urinary drainage, fecal impaction, a skin abrasion or pressure ulcer, and stiffness. The underlying cause should be treated or eliminated promptly.

BLADDER RETRAINING

Based on an assessment of bladder function, the nurse may establish the nursing diagnoses of *Altered Urinary Elimination* or *Urinary Retention*. The indwelling urinary catheter is removed as soon as possible, and an intermittent catheterization protocol is begun. Bladder retraining is considered when spinal shock begins to diminish and the specific type of bladder dysfunction can be identified.

Bladder retraining is initiated during the postacute phase. To increase the possibility of success, the urinary tract must be maintained in the best possible condition during the acute phase. This is accomplished by careful attention to aseptic technique when managing the catheter, which represents a potential source of infection and trauma.

A urinary antiseptic, such as methenamine mandelate (Mandelamine), is often administered. A urine pH of 5.5 must be maintained for the drug to be effective; therefore, a urinary acidifier, such as vitamin C, is often prescribed. The average adult dose is 1 to 2 g four times daily. The patient is instructed about the necessity for consuming large amounts of liquid (3,000–5,000 mL every 24 hours). Because cranberry juice and apple juice are urinary acidifiers, they should be included as part of the fluid intake. (Vitamin C must be incorporated into the pharmacological plan for most patients, because one would have to drink $2\frac{1}{2}$ quarts of cranberry or apple juice

CHART 22-6
Summary of Nursing Management of the Patient in a Halo With Vest

Nursing Responsibilities	Rationale
Management of the Halo Device and the Body Vest	
• Check the pins on the halo ring to be sure they are secure and tight.	• Ensures safety and integrity of the treatment
• Check the edges of the fiberglass vest for comfort and fit by inserting the small finger or index finger between the vest and the patient's skin. If the vest is too tight, skin breakdown, edema, and possible nerve injury can occur.	• Provides for comfort and prevents skin irritation
• The vest should be supported while the patient is in bed.	• Maintains proper body alignment
• Place a rubber cork over the tips of the halo device to diminish magnification of sound if the pin is bumped.	• Provides for comfort
Meticulous Skin Care	
• Inspect and cleanse the pin site once or twice daily, as prescribed, to prevent infection.	• Maintains skin integrity and monitors the patient for infections
• Turn the patient in bed every 2 h by means of the triple log roll technique to prevent the development of hypostatic pneumonia, atelectasis, and skin breakdown.	• Maintains proper body alignment and prevents injury
• Provide sponge pads to prevent pressure on prominent body areas, such as the forehead and shoulder, while the patient is in bed.	• Prevents injury and irritation to the skin
• Inspect under the vest, and keep dry all areas of skin	• Provides early identification of skin irritation or breakdown
Altered Body Image	
• Help the patient adjust to the distorted body image that the halo device can create.	• Supports the patient's emotional well-being.
Control of Pain: Comfort	
• Administer mild analgesics to control headache and discomfort around the pin site, which are common.	• Provides for comfort
• Provide a soft diet, because many patients have jaw pain if they attempt to chew.	• Provides for comfort
Basic Hygienic Care	
• Allow the patient to care for himself or herself as much as possible.	• Maintains the patient's independence and supports self-esteem
Support of Body Systems	
• Maintain an intake and output record.	• Provides information on urinary tract function and adequacy of fluid intake
• Provide for a bowel program.	• Prevents constipation and maintains a normal pattern of bowel evacuation
• Provide for range-of-motion exercises for all extremities.	• Maintains muscle tone
• Provide for deep-breathing exercises at least four times a day.	• Encourages hyperinflation of the lungs and prevents infections and atelectasis

(continued)

CHART 22-6 Summary of Nursing Management of the Patient in a Halo With Vest (Continued)

- Apply thigh-high elastic (TED) stockings to the legs to improve blood return to the heart.
- Observe the legs for development of thrombophlebitis or deep vein thrombosis.

- Decreases the possibility of thrombus or embolus formation
- Allows early identification of potential problems so that treatment can be initiated

Assessment Data

- Monitor neurological signs, vital signs, and vital capacity.

- Establishes a baseline and indicates change

Ambulation

If the patient's neurological function is intact, he or she will be able to ambulate in the halo ring and vest.

- Start to assess the patient's tolerance of the upright position by having him or her sit on the edge of the bed ("dangle"). Check vital signs. (Orthostatic hypotension may be a problem to overcome in the early stages.)
- Teach the patient to compensate for lost head and neck movement by making increased use of eye movement to scan the area.
- Accompany patients when ambulating because they are more accident-prone owing to a displaced center of gravity, a tendency for loss of balance, and decreased peripheral vision.
- Consider the patient's use of a walker for ambulation as a means of support and greater safety.

- Prevents development of untoward side effects

- Provides for safety needs

- Same as above

- Same as above

Patient Teaching

- If the patient is to go home with the halo and vest, begin a patient and family teaching plan using a booklet or other printed material. Review any written material prepared by the manufacturer for accuracy before giving it to the patient or family.

- Provides for safety and independence
- Meets the patient's and family's knowledge needs

---

daily to acidify the urine. See Chapter 14 for a further discussion of bladder retraining.

BOWEL RETRAINING

A bowel program is instituted and managed by the nurse. The related nursing diagnosis is *Constipation.* Most patients with spinal cord injuries are able to regain bowel control with an appropriate bowel training program. The large bowel musculature has its own neural center within the intestinal wall that responds to distention caused by the fecal contents. Dietary intake and digestive activities from the upper intestinal tract also influence bowel evacuation. There can be reflex expulsion, as in the infant, or defecation can be postponed by the conscious voluntary inhibition of the reflex. At the appropriate time and place, the bowel can be evacuated by voluntary relaxation of the rectal sphincter and contraction of the abdominal and pelvic muscles.

The neural innervation of the bowel, located in the lower intestinal wall, is usually not greatly affected by spinal cord injury. The neurological injuries affecting bowel evacuation may cause the following:

- Loss of the sensation of fullness in the lower bowel
- Loss of awareness of bowel evacuation
- Loss of the ability to control the rectal sphincter
- Loss of the ability to contract the abdominal muscles and to expel the stool

These points are important to note because nursing is directed toward helping the patient find alternate means of creating conditions conducive to bowel evacuation.

Most people have a bowel movement about every 1 to 3 days, frequently after a meal. If the bowel is evacuated routinely, then the possibility of spontaneous defecation is greatly reduced. Defecation should be accomplished as normally as possible. To use the abdominal muscles and diaphragm, the patient should be in a comfortable position with feet flat on the floor. If the abdominal muscles are impaired, the patient may be taught to exert pressure on the abdomen with the hands, or an abdominal belt may be recommended for a patient who cannot strain at stool.

Prevention of constipation and fecal impaction is important for many reasons; for instance, such a problem could trigger autonomic hyperreflexia and aggravate spasticity. A well balanced diet that is high in roughage, combined with sufficient fluid intake, helps to forestall such problems by producing a soft stool and stimulating peristalsis. Medications, such as stool softeners, bulk producers, and lubricants, are also helpful. Mild cathartics and suppositories may be ordered. Digital dilation may be recommended. If these methods are not successful, then a mild enema of limited fluid content can be administered.

A final important consideration is that selected body rhythms can be effectively used to help achieve bowel evacuation at predictable times. For example, the stimulus for defecation commonly occurs after meals because food is a stimulus for peristalsis, and peristalsis aids in moving the contents of the GI tract. The gastrocolic reflex responsible for strong contractions and peristalsis in the GI tract can be initiated by feeding the patient warm fluids and food at any time of the day. Therefore, planning for bowel evacuation and retraining should capitalize on normal body rhythms.

Bowel training must be a planned activity and must be individualized. Collaboration among the patient, nurse, and physician is necessary for successful outcomes. Patience and an optimistic attitude on the part of the nurse are necessary to provide a climate for success. (See Chap. 14 for a more in-depth discussion of bowel retraining.)

PSYCHOLOGICAL RESPONSE TO INJURY

The rapidity with which patients move from acute care settings to rehabilitation is accelerated by managed care. Patients often do not have sufficient time to begin to process what has happened to them and what it means to their personhood. A wide range of emotional responses are experienced by the patient with a spinal cord injury as he or she progresses from the acute postinjury phase to the rehabilitation phase. The sensory losses associated with spinal cord injury and the subsequent immobilization create sensory and perceptual alterations. Immobilization and confinement to bed by traction or paralysis limit and distort visual and auditory stimuli. For instance, vision may be distorted for the patient on bed rest who may be fully aware of the ceiling, the upper half of the walls, and people from the waist up but who cannot visualize most objects in their totality.

Immobility is an extreme hardship for a paralyzed patient who may not even be able to scratch his or her nose. Confinement represents limited territoriality, with lack of control over access to one's surroundings. For those accustomed to exercise and physical activity to relieve stress, immobility negates the use of this stress reduction strategy. As a result, physical immobility can lead to psychological distress.

As the nurse assesses the patient and family, any number of the following nursing diagnoses may be applicable:

- Anxiety
- Impaired Adjustment
- Body Image Disturbance
- Decisional Conflict
- Diversional Activity Deficit
- Ineffective Individual Coping
- Fear
- Loneliness
- Dysfunctional Grieving
- Personal Identity Disturbance
- Powerlessness
- Self Esteem Disturbance
- Hopelessness
- Social Isolation
- Impaired Social Interaction
- Spiritual Distress

In addition, the emotional and psychological responses of the family may require intervention. Some family-focused nursing diagnoses include the following:

- Ineffective Family Coping
- Anticipatory Grieving
- Parental Role Conflict
- Altered Family Processes
- Caregiver Role Strain

Psychological Response: A Model for Intervention. Sudden, catastrophic injury precipitates a crisis. Crisis theory and adjustment to long-term disability provide the nurse with a framework for viewing spinal cord injury and an approach to intervention.

Spinal trauma, a catastrophic event, is met with shock, disbelief, and denial. Initially, much of the activity is directed toward life-saving measures and stabilization of the patient. The focus is on survival. If the patient is conscious, he or she is in a state of emotional shock. Shock and disbelief then evolve into denial. Patients who are experiencing denial do not believe that what they are being told has any bearing on their life. They may acknowledge some of their injuries but may deny or downplay the seriousness of others. For example, a patient may recognize and acknowledge that his or her legs are dysfunctional but may believe that this is just a temporary state. Such patients may be convinced that next week or the week after, they will be back to normal. The nurse should listen but give no false hope. Focusing on the present helps to keep the patient firmly grounded in reality.

The next stage is one of reaction, and it often lasts for a long time. There may be an acknowledgment that significant losses of body function have occurred that affect degree of independence and lifestyle. Reactions are varied, and may include anger, rage, depression, bargaining, verbal abuse of caregivers and family, ideation of suicide, and inappropriate sexual behavior. Listening, gentle reminders of intact functions, and support are helpful during this stage. Any suggestions of suicide should be taken seriously and the patient protected from self-harm.

Next, the person begins to seek information about the injury and what can be expected in terms of outcome and approach to management. He or she thus becomes an active participant in care and in rehabilitation. The nurse should allow the patient as much independence as possible, allowing him or her to maintain control by making decisions.

Finally, the person begins to cope effectively if adaptation has progressed. During this phase, the patient develops a plan for a productive life, considering the limitations imposed by the injury. At this time, the patient can be integrated into the community.

The entire adjustment process just described can take many years to achieve. The nurse should be aware that because many patients are transferred almost immediately to specialized care centers from other hospitals, they may be only at the stage of denial or early reaction at the time of transfer.

A Nursing Approach. Caring for a patient who has sustained a spinal cord injury requires an awareness of the impact that the illness has had on the patient's emotional and psychological equilibrium. The following general suggestions are offered as an approach to providing patient care:

- Establish a therapeutic nurse–patient relationship.
- Cultivate a climate of trust.
- Allow the patient to verbalize feelings.
- Accept the patient's behavior without being judgmental.
- Let the patient know that it will take time to adjust to the disability.
- Answer questions, referring those that you are unable to answer to the appropriate resource.
- Include written documentation of the patient's emotional and psychological reactions in the chart.
- Incorporate steps for meeting the emotional and psychological needs of the patient into the care plan.
- Promote a good self-concept and body image by encouraging the patient to use good grooming habits.
- Use team conferences to discuss the patient's emotional and psychological status.
- Involve the patient in the decision-making process related to his or her care to foster a feeling of self-control on the part of the patient.

DISCHARGE PLANNING

Given the current trend toward transferring injured patients to a spinal cord injury center, discharge planning must begin immediately on admission. The nurse often is the coordinator for this multidisciplinary process. The responsibilities of the nurse related to discharge planning include the following:

- Initiate the formal discharge plan and referral for rehabilitation in collaboration with the physician.
- Involve the patient and family in planning for discharge from the acute care facility to a rehabilitation hospital or other extended care facility.
- Answer questions and clarify information for the patient and family.
- Assess and document the patient's functional level in terms of ADLs.

- Document nursing diagnoses and issues that remain unresolved in the acute care setting.
- Work collaboratively with other health team members in planning for discharge.

See Chapter 15 for a more in-depth discussion of discharge planning.

REHABILITATION: THE ROAD AHEAD

Most patients who are paraplegic or tetraplegic will need a long-term rehabilitation program. How this need is met will vary from patient to patient, based on individual needs and the availability of resources. In addition to an initial rehabilitation program, resources for comprehensive follow-up care will be necessary. In the era of managed care, patients are transferred from acute care hospitals early. Some of the considerations in the postacute phase, such as bladder and bowel retraining, will occur in a rehabilitation facility.

Tetraplegic and paraplegic patients represent special categories in rehabilitation. Although patients in other rehabilitation programs are helped to achieve an optimal level of function and then usually remain at that level, patients with tetraplegic and paraplegic disabilities are at increased risk for medical, social, psychological, and vocational deterioration. Therefore, lifelong follow-up care is an absolute necessity for maintaining their rehabilitative status and preventing problems and complications.

References

1. Hingley, A. T. (1993). Spinal cord injuries: Science meets challenge. *FDA Consumer, July-August,* 17–23.
2. Lenke, L. G., O'Brien, M. F., & Bridwell, K. H. (1995). Fractures and dislocatons of the spine. In C. R. Perry, J. A. Elstrom, & A. M. Pankovich (Eds.), *The handbook of fractures* (pp. 166–189). New York: McGraw-Hill.
3. Porth, C. M. (1994). *Pathophysiology: Concepts of altered health states* (4th ed.) (pp. 1052–1053). Philadelphia: J.B. Lippincott.
4. Adams, J. C., & Hamblen, D. L. (1992). *Outline of fractures* (10th ed.) (pp. 81–85). Edinburgh: Churchill Livingstone.
5. Maher, A. B., Salmond, S. W., & Pellino, T. A. (1994). *Orthopedic nursing* (pp. 581–616). Philadelphia: W.B. Saunders.
6. Cotrel, Y., Dubousset, J., & Guillaumat, M. (1988). New universal instrumentation in spinal surgery. *Clinical Orthopaedics and Related Research, 277,* 10–23.

Bibliography

Books

Bridwell, K., & DeWald, R. (Eds.) (1991). *The textbook of spinal surgery.* Philadelphia: J.B. Lippincott.
Buchanan, L. (1987). *Comprehensive management of spinal cord injury.* Baltimore: Williams & Wilkins.
Danielson, C. B., Hamel-Bissell, B., & Winstead-Fry, P. (1993). *Families, health, and illness* (pp. 275–311). St. Louis: C.V. Mosby.
Errico, T. J., Bauer, R. D., & Waugh, T. (1991). *Spinal trauma.* Philadelphia: J.B. Lippincott.

Fogel, C. I., & Lauver, D. (1990). *Sexual health promotion.* Philadelphia: W.B. Saunders.

Kitt, S., & Kaiser, J. (1990). *Emergency nursing: A physiologic and clinical perspective.* Philadelphia: W.B. Saunders.

Maher, A. B., Salmond, S. W., & Pellino, T. A. (1994). *Orthopedic nursing* (pp. 581–616). Philadelphia: W.B. Saunders.

Pitts. L. H., & Wagner, F. C. (Ed.) (1990). *Craniospinal trauma.* New York: Thieme Medical Publishers.

Whiteneck, G. G. (Eds.) (1993). *Aging with spinal cord injury.* New York: Demos.

Wilkins, R. H., & Rengachary, S. S. (Eds) (1994). *Principles of neurosurgery.* St. Louis: Mosby Wolfe.

Zejdlik, C. P. (1992). *Management of spinal cord injury* (2nd ed.). Boston: Jones and Bartlett.

Periodicals

Anson, C., & Gray, M. (1993). Secondary complications after spinal cord injury. *Urologic Nursing, 13*(4), 107–112.

Battle, F. J., & Northrup, B. E. (1993). Pathophysiology of acute spinal cord injury. *Trauma Quarterly, 9*(2), 29–37.

Bejciy-Spring, S. M., Neutzling, E., & Newton, C. (1994). Nursing case management: Enhancing interdisciplinary care of the spinal cord injured patient. *SCI Nursing, 11*(3), 70–73.

Bracken, D., Shepard, M., Collins, W. et al. (1990). Randomized controlled trial of methylprednisolone or naloxone in the treatment of acute spinal cord injury. *New England Journal of Medicine, 322,* 1405–1411.

Bracken, M. B. (1992). Pharmacological treatment of acute spinal cord injury: Current status and future prospects. *Paraplegia, 30,* 102–107.

Campbell, S. K., Almeida, G. L., Penn, R. D., & Corcos, D. M. (1995). The effects of intrathecally administered baclofen on function in patients with spasticity. *Physical Therapy, 75*(5), 352–362.

Chancellor, M. B. (1993). Urodynamic evaluation after spinal cord injury. *Physical Medicine and Rehabilitation Clinics of North America, 4*(2), 272–298.

Chin, D. E., & Kearns, P. (1991). Nutrition in the spinal-injured patient. *Nutrition in Clinical Practice, 6*(6), 213–222, 231–233.

Cohen, M. (1993). Initial resuscitation of the patient with spinal cord injury. *Trauma Quarterly, 9*(2), 38–43.

Cohn, J. R. (1993). Pulmonary management of the patient with spinal cord injury. *Trauma Quarterly, 9*(2), 65–71.

Cotrel, Y., Dubousset, J., & Guillaumat, M. (1988). New universal instrumentation in spinal surgery. *Clinical Orthopaedics and Related Research, 277,* 10–23.

Dalton, J. R. (1993). Urologic management of the patina with spinal cord injury. *Trauma Quarterly, 9*(2), 72–81.

Ditunno, J. F. Jr., Marino, R. J., & Crozier, K. S. (1993). Neurologic and functional assessments in acute spinal cord injury: Uses in prognosis and management. *Trauma Quarterly, 9*(2), 44–52.

Ducker, T. B. (1990). Treatment of spinal cord injury. *New England Journal of Medicine, 322*(20), 1459–1461.

Ducker, T. B., & Zeidman, S. M. (1994). Spinal cord injury. *Spine, 19*(20), 2281–2287.

Formal, C. (1992). Metabolic and neurologic changes after spinal cord injury. *Physical Medicine and Rehabilitation Clinics of North America, 3*(4), 783–795.

Gibson, C. J. (1992). Overview of spinal cord injury. *Physical Medicine and Rehabilitation Clinics of North American, 3*(4), 699–709.

Green, B. G., Foote, J. E., & Gray, M. (1993). Urologic management during acute care and rehabilitation of the spinal cord-injured patient. *Physical Medicine and Rehabilitation Clinics of North America, 4*(2), 249–272.

Green, D., Twardowski, P., Wei, R., & Rademaker, A. W. (1994). Fatal pulmonary embolism in spinal cord injury. *Chest: The cardiopulmonary Journal, 105*(3), 853–855.

Houda, B. (1993). Evaluation of nutritional status in persons with spinal cord injury: A prerequisite for successful rehabilitation. *SCI Nursing, 10*(1), 4–7.

Hughes, M. C. (1990). Critical care nursing for the patient with a spinal cord injury. *Critical Care Nursing Clinics of North America, 2*(1), 33–40.

Jackson, A. B., & Groomes, T. E. (1994). Incidence of respiratory complications following spinal cord injury. *Archives of Physical Medicine and Rehabilitation, 75*(3), 270–275.

King, R. B., Carlson, C. E., Mervine, J., Wu, Y., & Yarkony, G. M. (1992). Clean and sterile intermittent catheterization methods in hospitalized patients with spinal cord injury. *Archives of Physical Medicine and Rehabilitation, 73*(9), 798–802.

Laskowski-Jones, J. (1993). Acute SCI. . . . spinal cord injuries. *American Journal of Nursing, 93*(12), 22–32.

Lemons, V. R., & Wagner, F. C., Jr. (1994). Respiratory complications after cervical spinal cord injury. *Spine, 19*(20), 2315–2320/

Marino, R. J., & Crozier, K. S. (1992). Neurologic examination and functional assessment after spinal cord injury. *Physical Medicine and Rehabilitation Clinics of North America, 3*(4), 829–852.

Merli, G. J., Crabble, S., Paluzzi, R. G., & Fritz, D. (1993). Etiology, incidence, and prevention of deep vein thrombosis in acute spinal cord injury. *Archives of Physical Medicine & Rehabilitation, 74*(11), 1199–1205.

Nayduch, D., Lee, A., & Butler, D. (1994). High-dose methylprednisolone after spinal cord injury. *Critical Care Nurse, 14*(4), 69–72, 77–78.

Nolan, S. (1994). Current trends in the management of acute spinal cord injury. *Critical Care Nursing Quarterly, 17*(1), 64–78.

Rapp, J. (1993). Discharge of a ventilator-dependent quadriplegic patient from a critical care unit to home. *Rehabilitation Nursing, 18*(3), 185.

Reich, S. M., & Cotler, J. M. (1993). Mechanisms and patterns of spine and spinal cord injuries. *Trauma Quarterly, 9*(2), 7–28.

Saboe, L. A., Reid, D. C., Davis, L. A., Warren, S. A., & Grace, M. G. (1991). Spine trauma and associated injuries. *The Journal of Trauma, 31*(1), 43–48.

Segatore, M. (1994). Understanding chronic pain after spinal cord injury. *Journal of Neuroscience Nursing, 26*(4), 230–236.

Segatore, M., & Miller, M. (1995). The pharmacotherapy of spinal spasticity, A decade of progress. I. Theoretical aspects. *SCI Nursing, 11*(3), 66–69.

Segatore, M., & Miller, M. (1995). The pharmacotherapy of spinal spasticity, A decade of progress. II. Therapeutics. *SCI Nursing, 12*(1), 2–7.

St. George, C. L. (1993). Spasticity: Mechanisms and nursing care. *Nursing Clinics of North America, 28*(4), 819–827.

Staas, W. E., & Ditunno, J. F., Jr. (1992). A system of spinal cord injury care. *Physical Medicine and Rehabilitation Clinics of North America, 3*(4), 893–902.

Weingarden, S. I. (1992). The gastrointestinal system and spinal cord injury. *Physical Medicine and Rehabilitation Clinics of North America, 3*(4), 765–781.

Worthington, P., Crowe, M. A., & Armenti, V. T. (1993). Nutritional support for patients with spinal cord injury. *Trauma Quarterly, 9*(2), 82–92.

CHAPTER 23

Back Pain and Intervertebral Disc Injury

Joanne V. Hickey

Managing patients with back pain is challenging. Low back pain, for example, affects virtually everyone at some time during their life and is a common cause of disability and pain. It ranks high among reasons for seeking health care and consumes a large portion of health care dollars. The lost productivity and disability of sufferers add to the toll from back problems. Acute back problems are not always "cured" following treatment. Rather, they may become chronic conditions characterized by periods of exacerbation and temporary relief. Even after surgical intervention, some patients continue to experience symptoms of varying severity. How to manage acute back pain is a controversial issue.

CONDITIONS RELATED TO BACK PAIN

Several conditions are related to back pain, including the following:

- Degenerative changes of aging
- Neoplasms of the vertebral column and spinal cord
- Infections of the vertebral column and spinal cord
- Degenerative diseases of the vertebral column (spondylosis and osteoarthritis)
- Inflammatory diseases (Marie-Strümpell spondylitis, rheumatoid arthritis)
- Trauma (sprains and strains, spondylosis, spondylolisthesis, ruptured intervertebral disc disease)

Degenerative changes of aging are discussed below. Other conditions mentioned previously are summarized in Table 23-1 (see also Figs. 23-1 and 23-2).

Degenerative Changes Associated With Aging

As a result of the normal aging process, several changes affect the vertebrae and supporting soft tissue (ligaments, intervertebral discs). For example, the fluid content of the nucleus pulposus gradually decreases from 88% in people in their early 30s to 66% in later years. As a result, the discs become less efficient shock absorbers for stress from movement and become somewhat smaller so that they can more easily slip from their normal anatomical position. In addition, the aging process causes degeneration of the annulus fibrosus and the posterior longitudinal ligaments that secure the vertebral bodies together. As these ligaments degenerate, they are less able to respond to the various alterations required in movement so that stresses, strains, and injuries are much more easily precipitated. The normal anatomical degeneration of aging, plus the cumulative effects of everyday activity, make the back vulnerable to injury.

Osteoporosis is demineralization of the bone matrix related to hormonal changes that occur during the postmenopausal period in women. It is also seen in patients with Cushing's syndrome and in those receiving long-term steroidal therapy. The vertebrae are particularly vulnerable. The patient may be completely asymptomatic or may complain of back pain. Slight trauma can cause collapse, dislocation, or fracture of the fragile, demineralized vertebrae. Compression of the spinal cord or nerve roots by the collapsed vertebrae can result, and surgical decompression may be necessary.

Low Back Pain

The *Quick Reference Guide for Clinicians: Acute Low Back Problems in Adults: Assessment and Treatment* (1994) published by

TABLE 23-1
Conditions Related to Back Pain

CONDITIONS	DESCRIPTION, SIGNS AND SYMPTOMS	MANAGEMENT OR TREATMENT
DEVELOPMENTAL PROBLEMS • Scoliosis; kyphosis —Predispose the patient to disc and vertebral disease	Cause anatomical alterations; may result in • Malalignment of one vertebra with the next • Disproportionate stress to selected areas of the vertebral column • A narrowed space within the spinal canal	Possible management approaches depend on the degree of dysfunction: • Physical therapy • Braces • Harrington rods • Fusion
NEOPLASMS • Metastatic lesions involving the vertebrae or spinal cord • Primary tumors of the dura or spinal cord	• Metastases are most often from prostate, lungs, breast, or gastrointestinal tract; deficits depend on the level of the lesion. —They cause pain, neurological deficits (*e.g.,* bowel or bladder dysfunction, paresis, paresthesia). • With primary tumors, the deficits depend on the spinal level involved; signs and symptoms are the same as for metastatic lesions.	Surgical decompression may be necessary; alternatively, irradiation with or without surgery (see Chapter 23) may be advised.
INFECTIONS • Abscess secondary to infections elsewhere in the body, especially the lungs • Infections possibly related to surgical procedures • Possible organisms include *Staphylococcus,* tubercle bacillus, *Aspergillus,* and *Streptococcus*	• Pain is the chief complaint; other deficits relate to the dermatome level.	Management may include: • Bed rest • Immobilization • IV antibiotics for 4–6 wk • Surgical drainage • Spinal fusion, if necessary
DEGENERATIVE DISEASES OF THE VERTEBRAL COLUMN		

• *Spondylosis:* degeneration of the vertebral bodies or of the intervertebral discs with abnormal fusion of two or more vertebrae and narrowing of the intervertebral space
  —An *osteophyte* (bone spur) can develop as a result of the irritation.
  —The cervical region is commonly involved.
	• Pain results from fatigue and additional stress on the vertebral column.
	• This is most common in cervical region.
	• Disc protrusion can cause collapse of the disc space, resulting in narrowing of the intervertebral foramen and compression of the nerve roots.
		Conservative management (effective in more than 50% of patients):
		• Bed rest and immobility
		• Cervical traction
		• Drug therapy (non-narcotic analgesics; nonsteroidal agents [ibuprofen]; other anti-inflammatory drugs)
		Surgical approach:
		• If conservative treatment is ineffective, a laminectomy is performed to remove osteophytes and decompress any neural elements.

• *Osteoarthritis:* a degenerative process of the articular cartilages
  —Most frequently the cervical region is involved; the next most common site is the lumbar region
  —It is related to long-term stress on the back and is seen in older people.
	• Clinical symptoms relate poorly to x-ray findings.
	• Signs and symptoms include stiffness, limitation of movement, and pain aggravated by movement.
	• Marked osteophytic overgrowth with osteophyte development occurs.
	• Nerve root spinal cord compression, or both, occur, resulting in myelopathy.
		• Treatment is the same as for spondylosis.

INFLAMMATORY DISEASES
• *Marie-Strümpell spondylitis:* also known as ankylosing spondylitis
  —Predominantly affects young men
  —Sacroiliac joints primary sites
  —Involves destruction of the joints and ankylosis
  —Slowly progressive disease; can result in complete calcification of the anterior longitudinal ligament with resulting immobilization of the spine
	• The chief symptom is pain in the center lower back. Morning stiffness is common, and decreased hip mobility may also occur.
	• Slow, progressive course lasts several years.
	• In early disease, symptoms precede roentgenographical changes; as the disease advances, the spine looks like a "bamboo spine" on x-ray studies.
	• Back pain, stiffness, and limitation of movement are the most common symptoms.
		Management is symptomatic:
		• Pain control
		• Physical therapy
		• Other approaches, depending on the age of the patient and the degree of disability
		
		Treatment is the same as for Marie-Strümpell spondylitis.

(continued)

TABLE 23-1

Conditions Related to Back Pain Continued

CONDITIONS	DESCRIPTION, SIGNS AND SYMPTOMS	MANAGEMENT OR TREATMENT
• *Rheumatoid arthritis:* a generalized disease process affecting the connective tissue of the spine, hips, and hands —Cervical atlantoaxial area commonly affected —Women aged 25 to 45 years affected three times more often than men	• As the disease progresses, pain occurs in the lower back owing to disc displacement or possible cord compression.	
TRAUMA		
• *Sprains and strains,* including whiplash (see Chap. 22) • *Spondylolysis:* breakdown of the structure of the vertebra; usually involves a fracture of the isthmus • *Spondylolisthesis:* a defect on both sides of the vertebra through the isthmus, with the anterior section displacing forward and the posterior elements (spinous process and laminae) remaining in place • *Intervertebral disc disease:* discussed in the next section of this chapter	• Spondylolysis precedes spondylolisthesis. • The most frequent affected area is L-5, followed by L-4. • Symptoms are mild early in the course of the disease, then progress (lower back pain radiating to the thighs and legs; tenderness over L-4 and L-5; sensory and motor weakness). • Narrowing of the spinal canal and cord compression are possible as a result of disc displacement.	• Management includes conservative pain control and physical therapy. • In slippage of a vertebra or disc, surgery for cord decompression or laminectomy for disc displacement may be necessary.
REFERRED PAIN FROM VISCERA		
• A patient may have back pain secondary to referral from viscera, such as the gallbladder, kidneys, and other organs.	• A thorough physical examination will reveal the underlying cause.	Treatment depends on the underlying cause.

the Agency for Health Care Policy and Research is an excellent resource that sets national standards for patient management. The recommendations from the panel are based on a review of the literature and consensus of expert practitioners. According to the Guidelines, acute low back problems are defined as activity intolerance due to lower back or back-related leg symptoms of less than 3 months' duration. About 90% of pa-

tients spontaneously recover activity tolerance within 1 month. Subsequent episodes of low back problems for a patient are managed similarly to that of a new acute episode.[1] The Guidelines have shifted the focus of management from managing pain to helping patients improve activity tolerance.

Diagnosis of Back Problems

Back pain can be the result of many conditions and disease processes. The initial assessment is directed at the following:

- Collecting a detail-focused history about the current problem and how it limits normal lifestyle
- A regional back examination (deformity, vertebral point tenderness, muscle spasm)
- A neurological examination with particular attention to muscle strength, sensory dermatomes (pinprick and light touch), reflexes, and observations of the patient walking (posture, walking tandem, on toes, on heels, squat)
- Straight leg raising test
- Identification of any potentially dangerous underlying conditions, such as a tumor, infection, spinal fracture, or cauda equina syndrome

The Guidelines state that in the absence of signs of serious problems, there is no need for special diagnostic studies because 90% of patients will recovery spontaneously within 4 weeks. However, if a *serious underlying condition* is found or if there is *rapid progression of neurological deficits*, immediate consultation for emergency studies and definitive care should be sought.

FIGURE 23-1
Axial view of the lumbar spine, showing an intervertebral disc, the contents of the spinal canal, and the elements of the poserior bony arch.

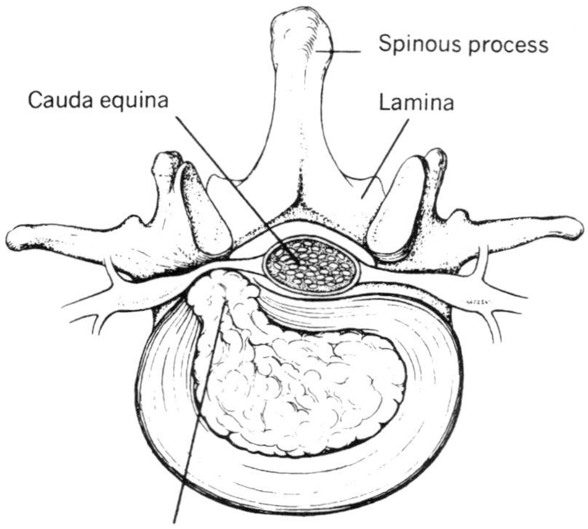

FIGURE 23-2
Ruptured vertebral disc. (From Chaffee, E. E., & Lytle, I. M. [1980]. *Basic physiology and anatomy.* Philadelphia: J. B. Lippincott.)

Initial Management

Patients with back problems are almost always treated on an outpatient basis. The cornerstones of early management are education and reassurance, patient comfort, and activity alterations.

EDUCATION AND REASSURANCE

Patients need to be reassured that most people recover from back problems within 4 weeks. Education is a key element to recovery and prevention of future problems. The nurse often assumes the role of educator.

PATIENT COMFORT

Pain and discomfort are the usual reasons for seeking health care. The safest effective medication for acute low back problems is acetaminophen. Nonsteroidal anti-inflammatory drugs (NSAIDs), such as ibuprofen or aspirin, are also recommended but cause gastric irritation and renal and allergic side effects. Narcotics are avoided if at all possible because of possible dependency. Muscle relaxants may also be ordered. About 30% of patients experience drowsiness, which interferes with daytime activities. Application of heat or cold to the concentrated area of pain may provide some relief. No evidence supports the use of skin traction or massage as treatment modalities.

ACTIVITY ALTERATION

The purpose of alteration in activity is to avoid undue back irritation and debilitation from inactivity. Most patients will not require bed rest. Prolonged bed rest (more than 4 days) has potential debilitating effects, and its efficacy in the treatment of acute back problems is unproven. For people with severe limitations due to leg pain, 2 to 4 days of bed rest may be helpful.

To avoid undue stress to the back, patients need education on body mechanics (how to lift, sit, walk, bend). Lifting more than 5 lb is discouraged. Avoiding debilitation is accomplished by low stress aerobic conditioning, such as walking, stationary biking, and swimming, with the time of exercise gradually increasing. Temporary activity restrictions for the workplace may be necessary, depending on the type of work an individual performs.

After One Month

If after 1 month, the patient has not recovered and there is a question of an underlying problem or physiological evidence of tissue insult or neurological dysfunction, imaging and possibly conduction studies are ordered.

- Magnetic resonance imaging (MRI) is now the gold standard for diagnosis; myelograms are rarely ordered any more.
- Computed tomography (CT) scans are also common.
- Nerve conduction studies are ordered in special circumstances.

If surgery is a consideration, the patient needs to be advised of options and the probable outcome of surgery. More specific information is found in the Guidelines as cited previously in this section.

HERNIATED INTERVERTEBRAL DISCS

The herniation of intervertebral discs is the major cause of severe acute and chronic back pain. The cervical and lumbar regions are the most flexible areas of the spine and thus are most susceptible to injury and stress, with the lumbar area being most frequently affected by herniated disc disease. Thoracic herniations are uncommon. Patients may present with complaints of arm or leg pain and have a diagnosis of **radiculopathy,** defined as disease of the spinal nerve roots.

Men suffer from intervertebral herniation much more frequently than women. Most patients with disc disease are 30 to 50 years old. About 90% to 95% of lumbar herniations occur at the L4-5 to S-1 levels. When the cervical region is involved, the most common levels are C6-7 and then C5-6. Multiple herniations occur in 10% of patients.

Etiology

Trauma accounts for approximately 50% of disc herniations. Examples of traumatic incidents include lifting heavy objects while in a flexed position (most common), slipping, falling on the buttocks or back, and suppressing a sneeze. In a number of patients, no history of trauma can be identified. Injuries are minor but have a cumulative effect, resulting in a chronic condition that makes the patient high risk for herniation. The herniation syndrome can also occur with other degenerative processes, such as osteoarthritis or ankylosing spondylitis

(Marie-Strümpell spondylitis). Patients with congenital anomalies, such as scoliosis, appear to be predisposed to disc injury because of the malalignment of the vertebral column.

Pathophysiology

As mentioned previously, degenerative changes of the posterior longitudinal ligaments and the annulus fibrosis occur in middle and later life. Simultaneously, degenerative changes begin to occur in the intervertebral discs after a peak level of development is reached in the early 30s. Fraying and tearing of the annulus fibrosis make the disc vulnerable to posterior displacement in response to a prolapse of the nucleus pulposus. This can occur with slight provocation, such as making an awkward movement, sneezing, or lurching forward. The nucleus pulposus can also protrude through the annulus fibrosus. A fragment may be laterally or centrally thrust into the spinal canal, where it encroaches on nerve roots (see Fig. 23-2). The herniation may be spontaneously reduced or reabsorbed, but most often it persists as a source of chronic root irritation. The presence of symptoms, particularly pain, depends on the quantity of disc material that has herniated into the spinal canal, the degree of narrowing of the spinal canal from herniation and edema, the number of discs involved, and the degree of encroachment on nerve roots.

Signs and Symptoms by Location

LUMBAR AREA

Herniation of a lumbar disc is usually lateral and only occasionally central. More than 90% of all clinically significant lower extremity radiculopathy is due to disc herniation at the L4-5 or L5 to S1 level. The signs and symptoms of herniated lumbar discs are categorized into the following general areas: pain, postural deformity, motor changes, sensory changes, alterations of reflexes, and specific diagnostic signs.

Pain. Pain is the first and most characteristic symptom of a herniated disc. Initially after the injury, pain is present, varying in terms of the severity of aching and sharpness. The alleged etiology of the pain is stimulation of the pain fibers of the posterior annulus and the posterior longitudinal ligament. The low back pain persists for varying periods, with radiation across the buttock, thigh, and one entire leg. In some patients, buttock and leg pain develops without back pain. The term **sciatica** is sometimes used to describe a syndrome of lumbar back pain that spreads down one leg to the ankle and is intensified by coughing and sneezing. The nerve roots L-4, L-5, S-1, S-2, and S-3 give rise to the sciatic nerve. The pain in the buttocks is described as deep, aching, or gnawing. The intensity of pain is influenced by leg position.

Pain from a herniated disc is aggravated and intensified by coughing, sneezing, straining, stooping, standing, sitting, blowing the nose, spasms of the paravertebral muscles, and any jarring movement while walking or riding. The character of pain can range from mild discomfort to excruciating agony. Sitting is particularly painful. In the acute phase, the patient is most comfortable lying in bed on the back with knees flexed and a small pillow at the head. Other patients prefer the lateral recumbent position, lying on the unaffected side with the knee flexed on the affected side.

Postural Deformity. On physical examination, the normal lumbar lordosis is absent in about 60% of patients with herniated discs. This sign is also accompanied by lumbar scoliosis and spasms of the paravertebral muscles. Movement of the lumbar spine is limited, and lateral flexion is restricted.

In the standing position, the patient exhibits a typically flattened lumbar spine (Fig. 23-3), slight tilting forward of the trunk, and slight flexion on the affected side of the hip and knee. The alterations of normal posture are defense mechanisms to compensate for the pathophysiological changes. The paravertebral muscles contract to prevent traction on the affected nerve roots, which would intensify the pain if the spine were extended. The patient walks cautiously, bearing as little weight as possible on the affected side. The gait may be described as stiff, and movement is deliberate to prevent jarring. Climbing stairs is particularly painful.

Motor Deficits. Hypotonia is common with motor root compression. Slight motor weakness may be experienced, although major weakness is rare. Motor weakness is difficult to evaluate because of the defensive reaction precipitated by pain. Weakness may be evident on plantar flexion or dorsiflexion of the foot and occasionally of the hamstring and quadriceps muscles. Atrophy of the affected muscles may develop, although it is not a usual finding and can be minimal. Footdrop has been evident in some patients. Motor weakness is sometimes accompanied by difficulty with micturition and sexual activity.

Sensory Deficits. The most common sensory impairments from root compression are paresthesias and numbness, particularly of the leg and foot. Note the specific areas of decreased sensation in the foot and leg using the pinprick method of sensory testing. Tenderness is noted over the L-5 and S-1 vertebral spines and along the tracking of the sciatic nerve (Fig. 23-4).

Alterations of Reflexes. With herniated discs, depending on the level of the disc herniation, the knee or ankle reflexes are absent or diminished.

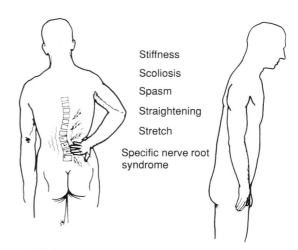

Stiffness
Scoliosis
Spasm
Straightening
Stretch
Specific nerve root syndrome

FIGURE 23-3
The spinal signs of lumbar disc herniation.

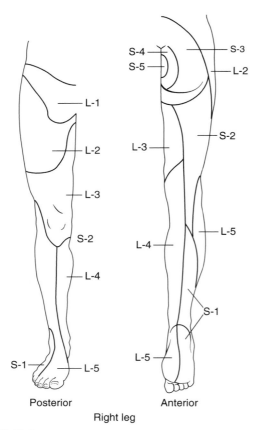

FIGURE 23-4
Dermatomes of the leg.

Other Diagnostic Signs. Other signs associated with lumbar herniated disc disease include straight leg raising test, Neri's sign, Naffziger's test, and Kernig's sign.

Straight leg raising test (Lasègue's sign) is helpful in determining limitations of lower limb range of motion and pain location. Normally, it is possible when lying on the back to move the straightened leg about 90 degrees with only some slight discomfort in the hamstring muscles. The sciatic nerve becomes stretched with movement and creates traction on the proximal nerve roots. Traction and stretching of the nerve roots begin when the leg is at a 30 to 40 degree angle. In the patient with a herniated low back disc, the stretching of the sciatic nerve during passive, straight leg raising creates traction on the irritated nerve roots, thereby producing severe pain. Patients with severe sciatica will not be able to raise their legs beyond 20 to 30 degrees. Less severe involvement allows straight leg raising to 50 or 60 degrees. Repeating the Lasègue's maneuver on the unaffected leg produces pain of decreased severity on the contralateral side.

Neri's sign is elicited when the patient bends forward, resulting in knee flexion on the affected side. This is a protective mechanism to prevent stretching of the sciatic nerve.

Naffziger's test is done by compressing both jugular veins while the patient is in a standing position (Fig. 23-5). This maneuver will produce pain in the patient with a herniated disc. Physiologically, compression of the jugular veins obliterates venous drainage from the brain, thereby increasing intraventricular pressure of the cerebrospinal fluid (CSF). The

result is an increase in intraspinal pressure, which will produce pain if a herniated disc is present.

Kernig's sign is carried out by attempting to flex the hip and knee while the patient is in the dorsal recumbent position (Fig. 23-6). When the hip is flexed 90 degrees, the knee is slowly extended. In the normal patient, the knee should be able to be extended about 90 degrees. In a patient with a low-back herniated disc, severe pain will be precipitated by stretching the nerve roots with knee extension. Therefore, it will not be possible to extend the knee the normal range in the patient with a herniated disc. Any manipulation of the leg is painful.

SPECIFIC LUMBAR LEVELS

The most common sites for lumbar disc herniation are the L4-5 and the L-5 to S-1 levels in that order. Lesions at the L3-4 level are rare.

Each level presents a characteristic syndrome of symptoms that is distinct from that of other levels.

L4-5 Level. Pain is felt in the hip, groin, posterolateral thigh, lateral calf, dorsal surface of the foot, and the first or second and third toes. Paresthesias may be experienced over the lateral leg and web of the great toe. There is tenderness at the femoral head and lateral gluteal region. There is some weakness with dorsiflexion of the great toe and foot. Footdrop can occur. The patient has difficulty walking on the heels. Atrophy, if present, is minor. Reflexes are usually not diminished.

L-5 to S-1 Level. Pain is felt in the midgluteal region, posterior thigh, and calf region down to the heel and the outer surface

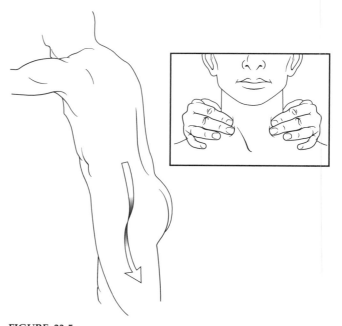

FIGURE 23-5
In Naffziger's test, the jugular veins are compressed simultaneously while the patient is standing erect. Radiating components of the pain are usually accentuated by this maneuver. The examiner must avoid bilateral compression of the carotid arteries when performing Naffziger's test.

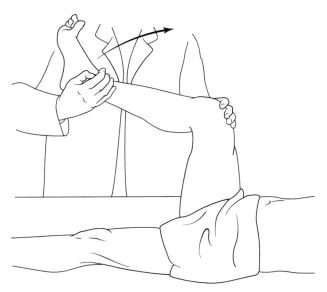

FIGURE 23-6
Testing for Kernig's sign. Flex one of the patient's legs at hip and knee, then straighten the knee. Note resistance or pain.

of the foot on the side of the fourth and fifth toes. Paresthesias are found in the posterior calf and lateral heel, foot, and toe. Tenderness is especially apparent in the area of the sacroiliac joint. Weakness in plantar flexion of the foot and the great toe is noted. The patient has difficulty walking on the toes. The hamstring muscles may also show signs of weakness. If atro-

phy is present, the gastrocnemius and the soleus muscles are affected. The ankle jerk reflex is diminished or absent.

L3-4 Level. Pain is located in the lower back, hip, posterolateral thigh, and anterior leg. Paresthesias are experienced in the middle section of the anterior thigh. Weakness is noted in the quadriceps muscles, which may also demonstrate atrophic changes. The knee-jerk reflex is diminished.

Remission of Pain. The pain associated with herniated disc disease is recurrent. Patients typically present a history of one or several episodes of low back pain radiating across the buttocks and into one leg to the ankle. Between acute episodes, pain may be completely absent or at least substantially diminished so that the patient is able to cope with the discomfort. Remissions of acute episodes are probably attributable to recovery of the protruding disc, decreased local edema, relief of root compression, and reabsorption of disc exudate.

CERVICAL AREA

The cervical region of the spine is also prone to trauma, degeneration, and spondylitic changes, which predispose the affected person to a wider range of pathological conditions. A serious consequence of nerve root or spinal cord compression is possible interference with vital respiratory functions.

One of the most common causes of neck, shoulder, and arm pain in the middle-aged and older population is disc herniation of the lower cervical region. Symptoms can develop without any apparent injury, or they may follow trauma, such

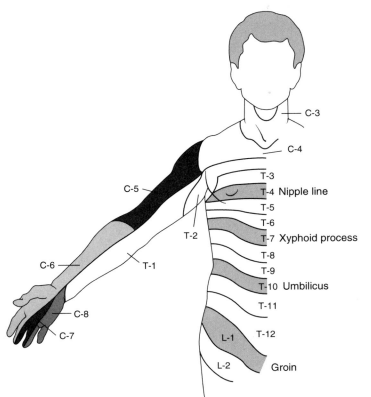

FIGURE 23-7
Sensory dermatomes of the cervical nerves, including all overlap, can be used to document the lowest functioning nerve root in a traumatic complete tetraplegia.

as whiplash or hyperextension injuries. On radiological investigation, salient disc degeneration, arthritis, or spondylitis are frequently identified. The most common sites of cervical herniation are at the C5-6 and C6-7 levels, with pain along the affected sensory dermatomes (Fig. 23-7). Herniation may be lateral or central.

Anatomically, there is little free room within the spinal canal to accommodate any extraneous material. The cervical spinal cord is firmly positioned by the ligamenta denticulata. Disc protrusion in the cervical area can result not only in root compression, but also in cord compression because of the lack of free space. The particular presenting symptoms depend on the anatomical point of disc protrusion. The possible locations of disc protrusion include lateral, paracentral, or central herniation.

Lateral Herniation. Symptoms of lateral cervical disc herniation include root pain in the shoulders, neck, and arm (Fig. 23-8) and paresthesias along the dermatome of the compressed nerve root. Paravertebral muscle spasms, which cause a stiff neck, accompany the pain. Reflex loss and possible motor weakness follow. Neck movement is often restricted to some degree in all directions. Tenderness may be experienced when pressure is exerted over the involved cervical spine. Weakness of the hand muscles and forearm may be noted. Atrophy may also be detected on physical examination. Arm reflexes are absent or diminished.

Paracentral or Central Herniations. Symptoms of herniation of paracentral or central regions can be contrasted with those of lateral herniations. Pain, if present, is usually mild, insidious, and intermittent (Fig. 23-9). An acute or gradual onset of spinal cord compression occurs. Weakness of the lower extremities and an unsteady gait become apparent. As the compression increases, spasticity is noted. There may be difficulty with voiding and sexual function. Reflexes of the lower extremities become hyperactive, whereas those in the upper extremities vary.

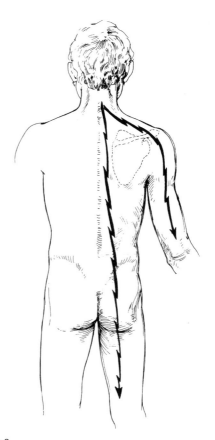

FIGURE 23-9
Pattern of pain radiation with a midline herniated cervical disc. (From Hoppenfeld, S. [1977]. *Orthopaedic neurology.* Philadelphia: J. B. Lippincott.)

SPECIFIC CERVICAL LEVELS

The most common cervical herniations are at C5-6 and C6-7. Each level presents a characteristic syndrome of symptoms that is distinct from that of other levels.

C5-6 Level (Lateral Herniation). Pain is experienced in the neck, shoulder, anterior portion of the upper part of the arm, radial forearm, and possibly the thumb and forefinger. Less frequently, pain extends to the scapular and clavicular regions. The paresthesias and sensory loss are found in the thumb, forefinger, radial and lateral forearm, and lateral aspects of the upper arm. Weakness is noted with flexion of the forearm (biceps). Tenderness is found in the supraspinal area of the scapula and the biceps region. Reflexes that are diminished or absent include the biceps and supinator reflexes. The triceps reflex is either exaggerated or left intact.

C6-7 Level (Lateral Herniation). Pain is experienced in the neck, shoulder blade, and lateral surfaces of the upper arm and forearm. The index finger, the little finger, and sometimes the ring finger are plagued by pain, although all of the fingers may be involved. Paresthesias and sensory loss are most prominent in the second and third fingers and lateral forearm. Weakness is found in the triceps and extensor carpi radialis (extensors for forearm and handgrips). Occasionally, wrist-

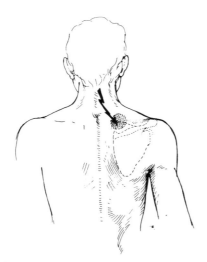

FIGURE 23-8
Pattern of pain radiation accompanying lateral protrusion of a cervical disc. (From Hoppenfeld, S. [1977]. *Orthopaedic neurology.* Philadelphia: J. B. Lippincott.)

drop may result. Tenderness is most apparent in the area over the medial shoulder blade. Reflexes that are preserved include the biceps and supinator, whereas the triceps reflex is diminished or absent.

Diagnosis

Intervertebral disc herniation must be differentiated from other diseases, such as primary metastatic neoplasms, and from all of the other causes of back pain previously mentioned. Making a diagnosis on clinical examination is difficult, if not impossible. Usual diagnostic procedures are ordered to provide additional information. The diagnosis of a herniated disc is based on physical findings, pain, a history of trauma, and an abnormal MRI or CT scan. The MRI is preferred because it provides better visualization of the soft tissue in contrast to bone. X-ray films are not specific but can indicate a narrowing of the intervertebral disc space, osteophytes (spurs), or hypertrophic osteoarthritis. In special cases, an electromyography may be performed to differentiate between neural and muscle injury. Myelograms, previously the mainstay of diagnosis, have been replaced by the MRI scan.

Treatment

Treatment of herniated disc disease follows two possible paths: *conservative treatment* or *surgery*. The belief that disc disease is caused by repeated trauma with degenerative changes is generally accepted. Most physicians, therefore, propose a course of treatment that will protect the involved area from added trauma and provide an environment that will allow for healing of the injured degenerative discs by fibrosis. This two-pronged approach, together with pain control, constitutes conservative treatment.

CONSERVATIVE TREATMENT

As discussed previously, conservative treatment may be tried for 4 weeks. The three cornerstones of management are education and reassurance, patient comfort, and activity intolerance. The need for bed rest and restriction of activity depends on the severity of symptoms. A patient with mild or moderate symptoms is generally advised to do the following:

- Decrease general activity for a short time.
- Avoid any flexion of the spine, such as lifting, bending, or twisting.
- Use a firm mattress.
- Participate in physiotherapy—hot (hydroculator packs) or cold packs.
- Take drugs (non-narcotic analgesics, anti-inflammatory drugs, muscle relaxants).

The patient with severe symptoms is treated with bed rest for a short time. Resumption of light activity is advised compared with prolonged bed rest. Use of skin traction, an ineffective treatment, is no longer ordered. Drug therapy and physiotherapy are also included.

NURSING MANAGEMENT DURING CONSERVATIVE TREATMENT

With the advent of diagnosis-related groupings and managed care, conservative management of the patient with disc disease often takes place in the home with the assistance of the family and possibly the home care nurse. Hospitalization is reserved for the patient with extreme symptoms who will likely be taken to surgery in the near future. The focus of care for this population, as with all patients, is education and reassurance, patient comfort, and activity alterations. Goals of care are maintaining altered activity restrictions, administering medications, and preventing complications. See Chart 23-1 for a summary of nursing management during conservative treatment.

Bed Rest. **Bed rest** for patients with pain in the lumbar region is limited to a short course (less than 4 days), followed by resumption of light activity. When on bed rest, proper positioning on the back with knees flexed is recommended. A pillow may be placed under the knees to prevent excess tension on the nerve roots. In addition, pressure must not be allowed to build up on the popliteal nerve. A small pillow may be placed under the head for comfort. For a patient with cervical pain, a small pillow may be placed in the nape of the neck. Because the purpose of bed rest is to reduce strain and pulling on the nerves, any items the patient may need should be within easy reach to avoid any undue stretching or moving. The nurse should discuss the overall purpose and goals of the bed rest regimen and the expected amount of bed rest prescribed by the physician. Most physicians want the patient to resume walking; proper body mechanics should be reviewed and stressed during ambulation.

Activity Restrictions. Following a period of bed rest, the length of the which is determined by the patient's progress, gentle mobilization is indicated. The patient may begin by walking short distances within the home, being careful to use good body mechanics. Bending, stooping, pushing, and pulling should be avoided. The patient should be advised not to lift objects heavier than 5 lb. If symptoms and pain subside, activity restriction can be decreased as the patient progresses.

Drug Therapy. Analgesics, anti-inflammatory drugs, muscle relaxants, and sedative-tranquilizers are the major categories of drugs ordered to control the symptoms associated with back pain and intervertebral disc disease. All of the drugs have side effects for which the patient should be monitored.

Analgesics. Analgesics are often necessary to manage mild to severe pain. Analgesics are classified as non-narcotics or narcotics. For mild to moderate pain, non-narcotic drugs are usually ordered. The following drugs are commonly used:

- NSAIDs
- Propoxyphene hydrochloride (Darvon)
- Narcotics for severe pain:
  Acetaminophen with codeine (30 mg)
  Oxycodone hydrochloride (Tylox)
  Hydrocodone bitartrate (Vicodin)

(text continues on page 478)

CHART 23-1
Summary of Nursing Management During Conservative Treatment of the Patient With a Herniated Intervertebral Disc*

Nursing Diagnosis	Nursing Interventions
Acute or Chronic Pain related to (R/T) inflammation or rupture of an intervertebral disc	• Maintain a regimen of bed rest (patient usually retains bathroom privileges). • Instruct family to apply heat or hydroculator packs as ordered. —Protect skin from burns. —There is often decreased sensation to the involved area, and burns can easily occur. • Use pain-relieving strategies, such as imagery, relaxation technique. • Administer analgesics and muscle relaxants as necessary; assess the patient's severity of pain to decide which pain medication to give if more than one is prescribed. • Monitor the patient's response to pain-reducing treatments; use the visual analogue scale (scale of 1–10) for the patient to rate pain before and after interventions.
Risk for Trauma: extension of back injury R/T environmental factors and improper body mechanics	• Provide a firm mattress. • Use a log rolling technique when turning the patient. • Teach proper body mechanics; caution the patient against twisting, stretching, pulling, or bending. • Maintain the patient in proper body alignment to decrease stress and strain. • For those with a herniated *cervical* disc, provide a small pillow in the nape of the neck. • For those with a herniated *lumbar* disc, provide a small pillow under the knees to relieve pressure; a small pillow can also be placed under the head (avoid pressure on the popliteal areas).
Risk for Constipation related to decreased activity, bed rest, and drugs that decrease peristalsis	• Provide a diet high in bulk. • Increase fluid intake. • Monitor the frequency of bowel movements and their consistency. • Institute a bowel program according to the physician's preference (*e.g.,* stool softeners, laxatives.)
Impaired Physical Mobility R/T pain, numbness/tingling, fatigue, and muscle weakness	• Monitor the degree of motor function that is intact. • Teach the patient to perform range-of-motion exercises at least four times daily. • Provide for progressive mobilization. • Assist patient with ambulation as necessary. • Monitor the patient for use of proper body mechanics. • Provide assistive devices (*e.g.,* brace, walker) as necessary.

(continued)

CHART 23-1 Summary of Nursing Management During Conservative Treatment of the Patient With a Herniated Intervertebral Disc (Continued)

Nursing Diagnosis	Nursing Interventions
Sensory/Perceptual Alterations: tactile, R/T diminished interpretation of tactile sensation secondary to inflammation or injury of the spinal nerves.	• Monitor the degree of tactile perception that is intact in the affected areas. In patients with *cervical* discs, monitor sensation to arms, upper back, shoulders, and neck; in those with *lumbar* discs, monitor sensation to the lower back, buttocks, and legs. • Protect the involved area from injury. • Teach the patient to compensate for diminished function, such as by visually checking the position of an extremity.
Knowledge Deficit R/T body mechanics, modification of lifestyle, treatment plan, or use of braces, traction, or drugs	• Develop a teaching program tailored to the patient's needs; include proper body mechanics, a discussion of lifestyle adjustments, use of equipment, the prescribed treatment plan, use of drugs, and exercises, such as semi-situps, pelvic tilt, knee-chest bends, and gluteal setting (Fig. 23-10) when the patient is ready.

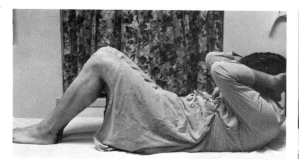 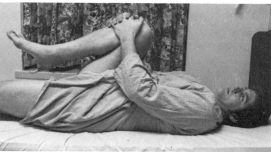

FIGURE 23-10
An exercise program for patients with a herniated disc may include semi-sit-ups (left) and knee–chest exercises (right).

Risk for Disuse Syndrome R/T bed rest and immobility	• Provide for basic maintenance interventions. • Monitor vital signs and neurological signs periodically. • Apply elastic stockings to prevent deep vein thrombosis. • Encourage deep breathing exercises at least four times a day. • Monitor urinary output for urinary retention or urinary stasis. • Monitor for musculoskeletal changes, such as atrophy, contracture, footdrop.
Anxiety R/T pain, immobility, hospitalization, uncertainty of outcome, and interference with previous lifestyle	• Explore areas of concern with the patient. • Help the patient develop strategies to reduce stress and anxiety. • Teach relaxation techniques and imagery techniques to control anxiety. • Help the patient set realistic goals. • Contact appropriate resources, such as a social worker, to assist in special problem solving.

*Differences in the management of a patient with a cervical or lumbar disc are noted when there is a variation.

Pain is best controlled with a multifaceted treatment approach. Pain-relieving protocols include positioning, anxiety reduction, relaxation therapy, imagery, heat and cold, and analgesics. Analgesics are most effective when given before the pain becomes severe. Pain should be treated appropriately; it should not be undertreated because of fear of drug addiction. When chronic pain cannot be controlled adequately and interferes with a person's quality of life, referral to a multidisciplinary pain clinic may be helpful.

Anti-inflammatory Drugs. Inflammation is triggered as part of a normal response to tissue injury. In the last decade, complex chemical substances, known as prostaglandins, have been identified as important mediators in the inflammatory process. Prostaglandins are synthesized and released in the presence of cellular injury. Drugs that treat inflammation are classified as steroidal or nonsteroidal.

Steroidal agents are chemically related to cortisone (a hormone excreted by the adrenal cortex). Nonsteroidal agents are synthetic compounds that are *not* chemically related to substances produced by the body. NSAIDs are now the most important class of drugs used to treat inflammatory processes. These drugs have varying degrees of analgesic and antipyretic effects. They act by inhibiting the synthesis of prostaglandins.

NSAIDs are classified into salicylates and nonsalicylates. Aspirin is the most common and most prescribed of the salicylate group. In the nonsalicylate group, the following drugs are commonly used:

- Ibuprofen (Motrin, Advil)
- Naproxen (Anaprox, Naprosyn)

Muscle Relaxants. A number of muscle relaxants are used. A few of the more frequently ordered drugs follow:

- Cyclobenzaprine (Flexeril)
- Methocarbamol (Robaxin)
- Carisoprodol (Soma)
- Chlorzoxazone (Paraflex)
- Metaxalone (Skelaxin)

Most drugs are given orally, although in the hospitalized patient, rapid intravenous (IV) administration of certain muscle relaxants, such as diazepam (Valium) and methocarbamol (Robaxin), is possible. For example, IV methocarbamol 500 mg in 5% dextrose in water may be given because its dilution in solution decreases the highly irritative quality of the drug. The nurse who is administering any drugs should be familiar with the many side effects and precautions for each.

Sedative-Tranquilizers. Sedative-tranquilizers are administered to decrease anxiety, which results in a decrease in muscle tension and pain. One of the drugs frequently used is diazepam.

Summary of Nursing Management. The expected outcomes for the patient who is being managed conservatively for intervertebral disc disease include the following:

- Control of pain
- Improved mobility to meet the patient's needs
- Progressive exercise program to strengthen muscles and improve posture
- Patient teaching and education to reduce the risk factors for additional disc trauma (such as going to a back school program)
- Resumption of the patient's previous lifestyle with some modifications

A majority of patients treated conservatively will have a good recovery (see Chart 23-1). Unfortunately, some will have recurrences and may require surgery.

SURGICAL INTERVENTION

Surgery is in order for patients who do not respond to conservative treatment or for those who, by the nature of the herniation or symptoms, require immediate surgical intervention. This latter group includes patients with massive central herniations that compress the cauda equina, resulting in motor and sensory paresis along with the loss of sphincter control; compression, resulting in quadriceps weakness or footdrop; severe and unrelenting pain; and prolonged and recurrent sciatica that interferes with normal life, job security, and weekly income.

The surgical procedure selected will depend on the location of the herniation (cervical, thoracic, or lumbar), the stability of the spine, and the findings on diagnostic workup.

Possible surgical procedures for a ruptured intervertebral disc include the following:

- **Discectomy**: This is removal of the nuclear disc material of an intervertebral disc; it is done with or without a laminectomy.
- Lumbar region
  A **posterior approach** is always used; the entire disc and cartilaginous plate are usually removed (to prevent recurrent disc protrusion).
- Cervical region
  If a **posterior discectomy** is performed, only the extruded disc fragments are removed (the annulus is not entered).
  If an **anterior discectomy** is done, the total disc is usually removed.
- **Hemilaminectomy**: Part of the lamina and part of the posterior arch of the vertebra are excised.
- **Laminectomy**: The lamina, part of the posterior arch of the vertebra, is removed. The approaches for hemilaminectomy and laminectomy are the posterior approach (traditional method) and the anterior approach.
- **Spinal fusion**: Specific vertebrae are immobilized by insertion of a wedge-shaped piece of bone or bone chips between the vertebrae. The bone graft is usually obtained from the iliac crest (donor site) or the bone bank. The purpose of the fusion is to immobilize and thus stabilize the vertebral column that is weakened because of degenerative disease or multilevel laminectomy; as a result of a spinal fusion, the patient must become accustomed to a permanent area of stiffness.
- Lumbar spine
  When the **lumbar** spine is fused, the patient is often unaware of stiffness after a short time because motion increases above the fusion.

- Cervical spine
  When the **cervical** spine is fused, increased limitation of movement is noted.
  Anterior cervical fusion through an incision in the anterior neck is performed when the cervical spine is unstable. When an **anterior cervical discectomy with fusion** is performed, the total disc is removed, and a fusion is done.
- **Foraminotomy**: The intervertebral foramen is surgically enlarged to increase the space for exit of a spinal nerve. By enlarging the foramen, pressure on the spinal nerve that may be entrapped will be reduced, resulting in decreased pain, compression, and edema. This procedure is performed most often in the cervical region, because anatomically, the cervical foramina are smaller than the lumbar foramina.

Microsurgical Approaches to Disc Surgery. Microsurgical techniques offer improved magnification and illumination for surgery, easier identification of anatomical structures, and improved precision in removal of small fragments or exudate. Microdiscectomy can be performed through a small incision and reduces the risk of the following:

- Dural laceration (resulting in CSF leak)
- Traction on nerve roots (which can cause muscle spasm and possible nerve root injury)
- Stripping of muscle from the spinal fasciae
- Trauma to blood vessels (hematoma) by improving homeostasis

With the small incision and increased precision of microdiscectomy, there is decreased tissue trauma and pain. The patient is able to ambulate sooner, and the length of hospitalization is shorter than with conventional disc surgery.

CHEMONUCLEOLYSIS

This is a procedure that has come in and out of vogue for managing patients in the last several years. Currently, it is not a mainstay of treatment. **Chemonucleolysis** is the injection of chymopapain into the nucleus pulposus of an intervertebral disc. Chymopapain is an enzyme extracted from the papaya plant. When injected directly into a lumbar herniated intervertebral disc, the enzyme reduces the central disc components by hydrolysis, thus decreasing the size of the protruding disc. With the pressure removed from the spinal nerve roots, pain is significantly diminished in some cases. Although this procedure was popular for a few years, it has fallen out of favor partly because its success rate is less than that of open discectomy and partly because its complications are significant. Allergy to the discolytic agent is a well established risk. More importantly, studies support the effectiveness of chemonucleolysis in comparison to placebo, with not more than 80% of patients showing short-term improvement. By comparison, some of the best open discectomy series describe success rates of 90% to 100%.[2]

PERCUTANEOUS DISCECTOMY

Percutaneous discectomy is a technique sometimes used for removing "contained" lumbar disc herniations in which the outer border of the annulus fibrosis is intact. The procedure is done through a posterolateral approach with the aid of a high-power suction shaver and cutter systems. It is monitored using an endoscope and is performed with the patient under local anesthesia and an anesthesiologist available. Percutaneous discectomy is indicated only in cases of disc-related root compression accompanied by minor neurological deficits. Results are positive and indicate that percutaneous discectomy is a viable alternative to microdiscectomy for patients who fit the stringent criteria of a contained and small lumbar disc herniation.

Nursing Management of the Patient Undergoing Laminectomy

Laminectomy is the most frequent surgical intervention, so discussion will be limited to this procedure (see interdisciplinary practice guidelines for lumbar discectomy and laminectomy and anterior cervical discectomy and fusion).

GENERAL CONSIDERATIONS

By the time a patient with a herniated disc is admitted for surgery, severe, debilitating pain has usually been present for some time. Some patients may have undergone conservative treatment at home with poor results. Others may have experienced intermittent episodes of pain for months or even years. Usually, the decision to undergo surgery is made by the patient because his or her lifestyle has been seriously disturbed by the chronicity of the back problem. Other patients have already undergone one surgical procedure but have experienced continued or renewed pain. Another surgical procedure may be perceived as a blatant reminder that surgery does not always produce remission of painful symptoms. The experience shared by all patients opting for surgery is disabling pain.

Many patients have taken various analgesics at home for extended periods with unsatisfactory relief of pain. If the pain was controlled, the medication may have been a narcotic reluctantly prescribed by the physician. In many patients, a tolerance to the most common analgesics develops, and the patient may find that it takes increasingly larger doses of the drug just to "take the edge off" the pain. Sedatives and tranquilizers are often ordered to control anxiety, which enhances the perception of pain. All medications have side effects that are usually unpleasant. Drowsiness, headache, irritability, and nausea are common distressing symptoms. Side effects from drugs, compounded by chronic severe pain, deplete the patient of normal coping mechanisms. The chronicity of pain plus alterations in lifestyle create feelings of anxiety and depression. For some patients, economic security is threatened because of the inability to work as a result of back pain.

In the clinical setting, these patients are often difficult for the nurse to manage. They may be irritable, negative, and even hostile as a result of chronic pain. It is difficult to keep them comfortable because of their severe pain, anxiety, and tolerance to many drugs. It can be frustrating to the nurse not to be able to provide for the comfort needs of the patient.

The postoperative period may be overwhelmingly disappointing to the patient who experiences muscle spasms and similar or greater pain than was present before surgery. Any patient who undergoes surgery, regardless of how explicitly the physician has explained possible outcomes, expects relief.

If the patient finds that the pain is equal to or greater than it was before surgery, he or she often becomes discouraged and angry.

The nurse can do many things to help the patient. The first is to understand what has preceded hospital admission. The duration of pain, extent of disability, and effect of the disability on the patient's life should be considered. Once the nurse has an understanding of what has happened to the patient, it may be easier to understand and accept his or her behavior. It is most important to listen to the patient so that misconceptions can be corrected, and gaps in information can be filled. The patient should be asked what the physician has told him or her about the operation. The nurse can help the patient develop realistic expectations about surgery and its outcome and provide information about strategies designed to reduce the risk of recurrent back problems.

PREOPERATIVE TEACHING

Patients must understand that they are likely to experience some pain because of nerve root irritation and edema, which will gradually subside. The possibility of muscle spasms should also be discussed so that patients are not devastated when and if they occur. Tactful handling by the nurse creates a feeling of trust. The patient can be told that many patients experience uncomfortable muscle spasms in the low back, thighs, and abdomen (following lumbar laminectomy) during the early postoperative period. The nurse might say, "You may experience muscle spasms after surgery. It is a temporary occurrence that passes in a few days. It does not indicate that your surgery was not successful. You will be receiving your pain medication after surgery to keep you comfortable." The patient should be encouraged to discuss any fears.

The basics of good body mechanics and the need to avoid stress to the back should be discussed with the patient long before discharge. Most physicians will broach the subject with the patient, but it is the nurse's responsibility to reinforce this concept. This is one way to alleviate some of the anxiety and fear about the possibility of further back problems.

The preoperative patient teaching plan should include a discussion of the following:

- Basic preoperative routines, such as nothing by mouth (NPO) status before surgery and where the patient will go after the surgery
- Basic postoperative routines (*e.g.*, vital sign monitoring, frequent checking of dressing, deep breathing exercises)
- Logrolling technique for turning the patient in bed
- Rationale for maintaining proper body alignment at all times and ways in which alignment can be maintained
- The risks of twisting, pulling, stretching, or straining after surgery
- The correct technique for getting out of bed after surgery

PREOPERATIVE NURSING MANAGEMENT

In addition to the routine preoperative preparation of the patient (*e.g.*, patient teaching, maintaining NPO status after midnight, and providing psychological support), thigh-high elastic sequential compression boots will be applied. This is done to facilitate blood return to the heart and to decrease venous stasis,

which would place the patient at high risk for deep vein thrombosis. Vasomotor changes in the lower extremities secondary to autonomic stimulation can also contribute to stasis of blood.

POSTOPERATIVE NURSING MANAGEMENT

General Care. The patient should be returned to a bed with a firm, supportive mattress. A bedboard may be added if necessary. Basic postoperative nursing management, such as frequent monitoring of vital signs, care of dressings, administration of IV fluids, and monitoring of intake and output, should be instituted.

Special Assessment. Frequent nursing assessment in the postoperative period includes the evaluation of sensory and motor function in the extremities. If the operative site was proximal to the cervical region, assessment would concentrate on arm strength. With lumbar surgery, the legs would be the focus of attention. When assessing motor and sensory function, the nurse compares present motor and sensory function with preoperative function. The patient is asked to move the extremities, wiggle the fingers or toes, and identify the part of the extremity that has been touched or squeezed. If there is apparent motor weakness, paralysis, or lack of awareness of touch or temperature in the postoperative period, nerve root compression is suspected. Such deficits should be reported to the physician immediately.

Several problems may arise following a laminectomy, including urinary retention, paralytic ileus, and muscle spasms. These are discussed in Chart 23-2, in which the common nursing diagnoses associated with the postoperative laminectomy patient are discussed. In addition, many patients will have an elevated temperature (up to 102.2°F, 39°C) for a few days after surgery. This is thought to be caused by aseptic contamination of the CSF at surgery and the response of the body to the surgical incision. In such cases, the nursing diagnosis of *hyperthermia* is established. Along with administering antipyretic drugs as ordered (aspirin or acetaminophen [Tylenol] 650 mg orally or rectally every 4 hours), nursing management for hyperthermia includes increasing fluid intake and removing excess bedclothes.

Table 23-2 presents special nursing considerations for the patient who has undergone spinal fusion or an anterior cervical fusion or discectomy.

Complications of Laminectomy: Collaborative Nursing Problems

Several complications can develop following a laminectomy or spinal fusion. Some are more apt to occur in the immediate postoperative period, whereas others usually arise later. Whenever these problems occur, they become collaborative problems because medical assessment and intervention are necessary. Complications seen after a laminectomy or spinal fusion can include hematoma at the operative site, cerebrospinal fistula, arachnoiditis, nerve root injury resulting in footdrop or hand or arm weakness, and postural deformity.

HEMATOMA AT THE OPERATIVE SITE

In rare instances, a hematoma can develop postoperatively at the incision because of bleeding. The most prominent symptom is severe, localized incisional pain that may or may not

CHART 23-2
Summary of the Nursing Management of Patients Following a Posterior Laminectomy

Nursing Diagnosis

Pain related to (R/T) tissue trauma, muscle spasms, and nerve root compression associated with surgical trauma and inflammation

- *Lumbar laminectomy:* pain and spasms in lower back, abdomen, or thighs
- *Cervical laminectomy:* pain and spasms in upper back, shoulder, neck, or arms; may have sore throat after surgery as a result of intubation (medicated throat lozenges may be ordered for comfort)
- *Anterior cervical discectomy:* pain and spasms in upper back, shoulder, neck, or arms; may have sore throat and difficulty swallowing postoperatively as a result of manipulation of the esophagus during the procedure.

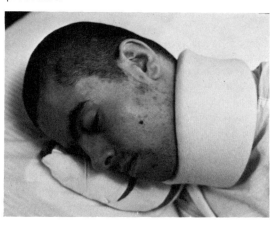

FIGURE 23-11
A Thomas collar is applied following cervical laminectomy. (From Decision Audiovisual Media [1972]. *Neurological care series.* Philadelphia: J. B. Lippincott.)

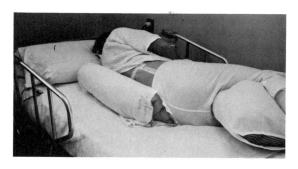

FIGURE 23-12
Position of the patient following lumbar laminectomy. (From Decision Audiovisual Media [1972]. *Neurological care series.* Philadelphia: J. B. Lippincott.)

Nursing Interventions

- Maintain the patient's bed rest regimen using a firm mattress initially.
- Position the bed to reduce stress to the operative site.
  - —*Cervical laminectomy:* The head of bed is usually elevated to a comfortable position.
  - —*Lumbar laminectomy:* Keep the bed flat or slightly elevated (5 to 10 degrees, as ordered).
  - —*Anterior cervical discectomy:* Head of bed is usually elevated to a comfortable position.
- Provide a pillow for comfort.
  - —*Cervical laminectomy:* A small pillow may be positioned under the head; a soft cervical collar is worn for comfort (Fig. 23-12).
  - —*Lumbar laminectomy:* A small pillow may be placed under the head and one may be placed under the knees periodically (Fig. 23-13) to reduce strain.
  - —*Anterior cervical discectomy:* A small pillow may be positioned under the head; a hard collar (*i.e.,* Philadelphia) is worn to prevent flexion, extension, or rotation of the neck.
- Use a log rolling technique for turning the patient during the first 12 h postoperatively.
- Maintain the patient in proper body alignment at all times so that the spine is in the neutral position.
- Reposition the patient every 2 h.
- Reinforce preoperative teaching to refrain from twisting, flexing, hyperextending, or pulling on the side rails.
- Use pain-relieving strategies, such as imagery, relaxation techniques.
- Administer analgesics as necessary; assess the severity of the patient's pain to decide which pain medication to give if more than one is prescribed.
- Monitor the patient's response to pain-reducing treatments; use the visual analogue scale (scale of 1–10) to allow the patient to rate pain before and after interventions.

(continued)

CHART 23-2 Summary of the Nursing Management of Patients Following a Posterior Laminectomy (Continued)

Nursing Diagnosis	Nursing Interventions
Urinary Retention R/T difficulty voiding in a horizontal position, the depressant effects of perioperative drugs, or sympathetic fiber stimulation during lumbar laminectomy	• Provide for privacy and comfort. Assist the patient to the bathroom, if possible • Provide male patients with an opportunity to stand for urination if the physician permits. • Palpate the bladder for distention. • Monitor the intake and output (I&O) record for adequate intake. • Intermittent catheterization may be ordered if the patient is unable to void during the early postoperative period.
Constipation R/T decreased activity, bed rest, and drugs that decrease peristalsis	• Provide a diet high in bulk. • Increase fluid intake. • Monitor the frequency of bowel movements and their consistency. • Auscultate the abdomen in all four quadrants for bowel sounds. • Institute a bowel program according to the physician's preference (stool softeners, laxatives, etc.)

Sensory/Perceptual Alterations: tactile R/T nerve root compression associated with surgical trauma and inflammation	• Monitor the patient's light touch and pain perception.
	   —*Cervical laminectomy/discectomy:* monitor sensation to the arms, upper back, shoulders, and neck
	   —*Lumbar laminectomy:* monitor sensation to the lower back, buttocks, and legs
	• Protect the involved area from injury.
	• Teach the patient to compensate for diminished function, such as by visually checking the position of the extremity.

Impaired Physical Mobility R/T pain, numbness, tingling, and muscle weakness	• Monitor the patient's ability to move legs and arms freely in bed; compare with preoperative baseline data.
	• Perform range-of-motion exercises at least 4 times daily; the patient may be taught to do this independently.
	• Provide assistive devices (brace, walker, etc.) as necessary.
	• Provide for progressive mobilization as ordered.*
	   —*Lumbar laminectomy:* the physician may write an order for the evening of surgery or the first postoperative day; follow the physician's protocol for getting the patient out of bed.†
	   —*Cervical laminectomy/discectomy:* roll the head of the bed up, align the patient at the edge of the bed, and gently assist the patient to a standing position by placing your arms across the patient's upper back and under the knees. The patient should *not* place his or her arm on the nurse's shoulder.

(continued)

CHART 23-2 Summary of the Nursing Management of Patients Following a Posterior Laminectomy (Continued)

Nursing Diagnosis	Nursing Interventions
Risk for Infection related to surgical incision	• Observe the dressing for evidence of drainage (blood or cerebrospinal fluid). • Monitor the incision for swelling, redness, drainage, irritation, or pain. • Maintain strict aseptic technique when changing the dressing. • With a lumbar laminectomy, check the dry, sterile dressing to ensure that it has not become wet; if this occurs, change the dressing immediately.
Risk for Disuse Syndrome R/T surgery, perioperative drugs, bed rest, and immobility	• Provide for basic maintenance interventions. • Monitor vital signs and neurological signs periodically. • Apply sequential compression boots to prevent deep vein thrombosis. • Encourage deep breathing exercises at least every 2 h; patients with a *cervical laminectomy* tend to have shallow respirations because of pain; these patients are at high risk for development of atelectasis and pneumonia. • Auscultate the chest for breath sounds every 4 h. • Monitor the patient for musculoskeletal changes, such as atrophy, contracture, footdrop.
Knowledge Deficit R/T body mechanics, modification of lifestyle, treatment plan, or use of braces, traction, or drugs	• Develop a discharge teaching program to decrease the risk of recurrent disc herniation by reducing stress on the back or neck; include the following information: —Proper body mechanics —Use of adequate support when on a mattress and in a chair —Maintenance of optimal weight (A weight reduction program may be necessary.) —Proper technique for any exercises prescribed by the physician, or reinforcement of exercises taught by the physical therapist, such as semi-situps, pelvic tilt, knee-chest bends, and gluteal setting (see Fig. 23-10). —Any modifications in activity, such as for climbing stairs, lifting. • Explore areas of concern with the patient. • Help the patient develop strategies to reduce stress and anxiety. • Teach relaxation techniques and imagery techniques to control anxiety. • Help the patient set realistic goals. • If possible, provide written discharge instructions.

*Differences in the management of a patient with a cervical or lumbar laminectomy are noted where there is variation.

Variations in postoperative management protocols after a laminectomy: The procedure for ambulation of patients varies from physician to physician. Some surgeons may ask that their patients dangle their feet from the edge of the bed on the evening of the day of surgery or the first postoperative day. Other surgeons do *not* allow their patients to dangle their feet at all, believing that excessive stress would be placed on the suture line. The individual protocols of the surgeon must be followed.

†*Technique for getting the laminectomy patient out of bed:* If possible, the head of the bed is raised with the patient comfortably positioned on the bed close to the edge of the side where he or she will be getting out of the bed. If the bed must remain flat, the patient is positioned on his or her side with knees and hips slightly flexed near the side of the bed from which he or she will rise. In either case, two nurses are necessary. One nurse grasps the patient under the arm and around the upper back and neck. The patient is instructed to place his or her arm around the nurse's shoulders. The other nurse grasps the patient's hips and legs. At the count of three, the nurses assist the patient to the upright position. If the patient is to walk, the support of two nurses is advisable, because weakness, dizziness, and light-headedness are common. A few steps to the door and back are sufficient for the first venture out of bed. Gradually, the patient will be able to tolerate ambulation for greater distances.

TABLE 23-2
*Special Nursing Considerations in Spinal Fusion and Anterior Cervical Fusion or Discectomy**

PROBLEM OR PROCEDURE	SPECIAL CONSIDERATIONS	POSTOPERATIVE NURSING CONSIDERATIONS
Spinal fusion (in general) • Bone graft	A bone graft will be obtained from the patient or from a bone bank. • If from the patient, the donor site is the iliac crest. • If from a bone bank, there will not be a donor site.	If a donor site is present: • Monitor the incision for bleeding or drainage. • Assess the incision daily; change the dry sterile dressing as ordered. • Position the patient so that no undue pressure is placed on the donor site.
• Immobilization of the operative site	Some form of immobilization will be ordered. • *Cervical:* a soft or rigid collar will be ordered; alternatively, a halo apparatus with jacket may be applied. • *Thoracic or lumbar:* a brace or body jacket may be ordered.	• Maintain the collar or brace as ordered. • Monitor the patient's skin for irritation. • Teach proper body mechanics. • Teach the patient the proper application of collar or brace. • If a halo apparatus has been applied, provide for patient teaching.
Anterior cervical fusion	Postoperatively, management is similar to that of posterior cervical laminectomy except that the patient may be • Out of bed on the first postoperative day wearing a cervical collar • Relatively pain-free • Bothered by a sore throat or experiencing difficulty swallowing as a result of irritation from endotracheal anesthesia	• Assess the patient for the presence of a gag and swallowing reflex before beginning oral intake. • Provide comfort measures (viscous lidocaine [Xylocaine] may be ordered by the physician).
Anterior cervical discectomy with fusion	Postoperatively, the patient is managed in a manner similar to patients undergoing anterior cervical fusion. Additional complications are related to soft-tissue injuries. The esophagus and trachea are retracted during surgery, and irritation of the laryngeal nerve and tracheal edema can result in hoarseness and difficulty coughing.	• The approach to management is the same as for anterior cervical fusion. • In addition, assess the quality of the patient's voice and the ability to cough; do not initiate oral intake if the patient cannot protect the airway adequately.

* See Chart 23-2 for general principles of postoperative care.

be described as throbbing. The nurse will note that the postoperative administration of analgesics does not keep the patient comfortable. The patient will complain bitterly about the incisional pain. On assessment, there will be a decrease in motor function of the legs or arms (depending on the location of the laminectomy) and a decrease in sensation to the involved area. The combination of severe incisional pain and decreased motor and sensory function suggests a hematoma; the physician should be notified immediately.

If an incisional hematoma is present and is causing neurological deficits (decreased motor and sensory function), the physician will probably reoperate immediately to evacuate the hematoma. A hematoma, if left untreated, could result in irreversible motor and sensory deficits, including paraplegia and bowel or bladder dysfunction.

CEREBROSPINAL FISTULA

A **cerebrospinal fistula** is an abnormal connection between the subarachnoid space and the incision, which causes CSF drainage; this will be noted on the dressing, either alone or in combination with serosanguinous drainage. The dressing is usually wet, and increased drainage occurs when the patient is lying on the back or standing. Of major concern is infection at the fistula site and meningitis, because microorganisms can ascend the fistula and flourish in the ideal environment of the cerebrospinal space.

Formation of a fistula is not an early postoperative complication. It often takes 1 week for evidence of a fistula to appear. Because CSF drainage on the dressing is the major sign of a fistula, it is important to monitor the dressing and to test the drainage with a Dextrostix strip to determine whether glucose, a component of CSF, is present. Continuous drainage on the dressing should be reported to the physician. If the fistula does not spontaneously seal itself, surgical closure will be necessary. Prophylactic antibiotics may be ordered to prevent infection. If leakage of CSF is suspected, maintaining the patient on flat bed rest, thereby decreasing pressure on the meningeal defect, may help the leak to seal spontaneously.

ARACHNOIDITIS

Arachnoiditis, an inflammation of the arachnoid layer of the spinal meninges, can result from infection caused by contamination of the surgical site at surgery or contamination of the dressing. If there is clinical evidence of infection (an increase in temperature and white blood cell count, malaise, headache, redness at the incision, or drainage on the dressing), antibiotic therapy is initiated. Arachnoiditis is a particularly worrisome complication because scar tissue and adhesions can form, causing much severe and chronic pain within weeks of surgery. The pain can be so severe that surgical intervention to remove the adhesions may be necessary.

NERVE ROOT INJURY

Footdrop or hand or arm weakness can occur as a result of sustained pressure on a nerve root (spinal nerve). If the patient has sustained nerve root injury, an aggressive program of physiotherapy will be needed, along with slings, braces, or splints, depending on the involved extremity and the extent of injury. A short course of steroids (*e.g.*, dexamethasone [Decadron]) may decrease the surrounding edema and improve function. Range-of-motion exercises will be incorporated into the nursing care plan, and careful attention must be directed toward preventing contractures, musculoskeletal deformities, and injury to the involved limb. The patient may sustain permanent disability even with an aggressive treatment program.

POSTURAL DEFORMITY

A laminectomy at more than one level of the vertebral column can cause spinal column instability and postural deformity. Such abnormalities may be noted by observing the patient while ambulating or by assessing the patient's posture in bed. When the surgeon performs a laminectomy on two or more vertebral levels, a spinal fusion may be necessary to ensure stability of the spinal column and prevent disability. If postural deformity develops after a simple laminectomy at a few levels, a spinal fusion may be necessary.

Recurrent Symptoms After Surgery

Surgery is not always synonymous with relief of symptoms. For example, a patient who has experienced long-term pain radiating down the leg before surgery will probably continue to have abated pain after surgery. It may persist for several weeks postoperatively. If there has been considerable sensory loss because of nerve root compression preoperatively, pain perception may actually increase because of improvement of the sensory deficit. Such patients may experience paresthesias for several months after surgery.

Surgery for a herniated disc does not negate the possibility of recurrence of a disc herniation at the same level on the same or opposite side or at other levels. Repeated laminectomies in the same patient are not unusual. This possibility does underscore the need for patient teaching related to body mechanics, posture, and protection from injury. However, degenerative changes may already be present that predispose the patient to future problems, even if a teaching program is judiciously followed.

References

1. Bigos, S., Bowyer, O., Braen, G. et al. (1994). *Acute low back problems in adults.* Clinical Practice Guideline, Quick Reference Guide Number 14. Rockville, MD: U.S. Department of Health and Human Services, Public Health Service, Agency for Health Care Policy and Research, AHCPR Pub. No. 95-0643.
2. Maroon, J. C., & Abla, A. A. (1986). Microlumbar discectomy. *Clinical Neurosurgery, 33*, 401–407.

Bibliography

Books

Bignami, A., & Thomas, P. K. (Eds.) (1990). *New issues in neuroscience: Cervical and lumbar compression radiculopathies.* New York: John Wiley and Sons.

Deyo, R. A. (1991). Historic perspective on conservative treatments for acute back problems. In T. G. Mayer & R. Gatchel (Eds.), *Contemporary conservative care for painful spinal disorders* (pp. 169–180). Philadelphia: Lea & Febiger.

Mourad, L. A., & Frosete, M. M. (1988). *The nursing process in the care of adults with orthopaedic problems.* New York: John Wiley and Sons.

Nussbaum, E. S., & Rengachary, S. S. (1994). Cervical disc disease and spondylosis. In S. S. Rengachary & R. W. Wilkins (Eds.), *Principles of neurosurgery* (pp. 44-1–44-16). St. Louis: Mosby Wolfe.

Ogilvy, C. S., & Heros, R. C. (1993). Spinal cord compression. In A. H Ropper (Ed.), *Neurological and neurosurgical intensive care* (3rd ed.) (pp. 437–451). Rockville, MD: Aspen Publications.

Rodts, M. F. (1994). Disorders of the spine. In A. B. Maher, S. W. Salmond, & T. A. Pellino (Eds.), *Orthopedic nursing* (pp. 581–616). Philadelphia: W.B. Saunders.

Wilkins, R. W. (1994). Lumbar intervertebral disc herniation. In S. S. Rengachary & R. W. Wilkins (Eds.), *Principles of neurosurgery* (pp. 45-1–45-9). St. Louis: Mosby Wolfe.

Periodicals

Bazzoli, A. S. (1992). Chronic back pain: A common sense approach. *American Journal of Physical Medicine & Rehabilitation, 7*(1), 53.

Chase, J. A. (1992). Outpatient management of low back pain. *Orthopaedic Nursing, 11*(1), 11–21.

Gates, S. J. (1987). Conservative management of lumbar disc herniation. *Orthopedic Nursing, 6*, 37–41.

Herzog, R. J. (1991). Selection and utilization of imaging studies for disorders of the lumbar spine. *Physical Medicine and Rehabilitation Clinics of North America, 2*(1), 7–59.

Lukert, B. P. (1994). Vertebral compression fractures: How to manage pain, avoid disability. *Geriatrics, 49*(2), 22–26.

Malmivaara, A., Hakkinen, U., Aro, T., Heinrichs, M, Kokenniemi, L., Kuosma, E., Lappi, S., Paloheimo, R., Servo, C., Vaaranen, V., & Hernerg, S. (1995). The treatment of acute low back pain—bed rest, exercises, or ordinary activity? *New England Journal of Medicine, 332*(6), 332–351.

Mayer, H., & Brock, M. (1993). Percutaneous endoscopic discectomy: Surgical technique and preliminary results compared to microsurgical discectomy. *Journal of Neurosurgery, 78*(2), 216–225.

Rodriquez, A. A., Bilkey, W. J., & Agre, J. C. (1992). Therapeutic exercise in chronic neck and back pain. *Archives of Physical Medicine & Rehabilitation, 73*(9), 870–875.

Saal, J. A., & Saal, J. S. (1991). Initial stage management of lumbar spine problems. *Physical Medicine and Rehabilitation Clinics of North America, 2*(1), 187–203.

Stankovic, R., & Johnell, O. (1990). Conservative treatment of acute low back pain: A prospective randomized trial: McKenzie method of treatment versus patient education in "mini back school." *Spine, 15*, 120–123.

Waddell, G. (1987). A new clinical model for the treatment of low-back pain. *Spine, 12*, 632–644.

CHAPTER 24

Peripheral Nerve Injuries

Joanne V. Hickey

Peripheral nerve injury is associated with trauma encountered in vehicular accidents, mechanized industry, farming, sports, and repetitive movement injuries. Injury to peripheral nerves can also develop as a result of exposure to toxic chemicals and substances used in the home and workplace. Although most cranial and all spinal nerves constitute the peripheral nervous system, this chapter concentrates on the major peripheral nerves that innervate the extremities.

MECHANISMS OF INJURY

The specific mechanisms by which peripheral nerves can be injured include complete or partial severance; contusion; stretching; compression; crushing; ischemia; electrical, thermal, and radiation injuries; and drug injection. It is possible for more than one mechanism of nerve injury to occur simultaneously.

A partially or completely **severed nerve** usually results from a sharp cutting instrument, like a chainsaw or scalpel. Regeneration of the peripheral nerve for some functional return to the involved body part is possible under certain circumstances.

With a **contusion**, the neuron remains intact structurally, but there is undetermined axonal injury. The injury can occur from a direct blow to a nerve located close to the body surface, as may occur when an elbow is bumped, causing injury to the superficial ulnar nerve, or from passage of a fast-moving object, such as a bullet or shrapnel, which may career close to the nerve.

Stretch trauma injuries result from traction exerted on the nerve. Extreme movement and excessive application of weight in orthopedic traction can cause this type of nerve injury. The shoulder joint is a common site for nerve injuries caused by extremes in movement. With traction of the hip or upper leg, the peroneal nerve may be injured by excessive pulling, which is why a major nursing responsibility involves

checking the intact motor function of the foot for inversion-eversion and plantar and dorsiflexion.

Compression injuries are caused by extreme or prolonged pressure on a peripheral nerve, such as may be exerted by tumors, herniated intervertebral discs, osteophytes, or closed fractures. A nursing concern in positioning such a patient is the prevention of pressure on the back of the knee where the peroneal nerve crosses the lateral popliteal space and the head of the fibula anteriorly, because this could cause injury to the peroneal nerve. **Entrapment syndromes** may result in compression injury in areas where peripheral nerves are encased by bone or rigid material. This is true when cranial and spinal nerves pass through narrow foramina or channels (*e.g.*, the median nerve passes between the carpal ligament and tendon sheath of the flexor arm muscles of the forearm and is involved in carpal tunnel syndrome). The narrowness of the foramina and channels, combined with edema from nearby soft-tissue trauma or pressure from a vascular lesion (hematoma or aneurysm), can easily produce a peripheral nerve entrapment syndrome.

Ischemia as a cause of peripheral nerve injury is closely associated with compression injuries because compression will eventually deprive a nerve of an adequate blood supply. In such circumstances, the etiology of nerve injury is most accurately attributed to the compression-ischemia mechanism. Occlusion of a major artery of a limb can lead to nerve injury because of ischemia.

Electrical, thermal, and radiation or traumatic injuries to the peripheral nerves are grouped together. Electrical nerve injury results from current being passed through the peripheral nerve when contact is made with electrical wires. The resulting injuries produce severe muscle and nerve coagulation, in addition to burns of the skin and destruction of bone. Prognosis for muscle reinnervation in these instances is generally poor. Thermal and radiation nerve injury cause similar types of local responses, with major damage resulting from burning and necrosis.

Drug injection into or proximal to a nerve can cause neuropathy, intraneural neuritis, and scarring. The nerves most commonly involved are the sciatic and radial nerves, which are subjected to injury as a result of improper intramuscular injection technique. Drug injection injuries are preventable if proper technique is practiced.

PATHOPHYSIOLOGY

Following transection of a nerve, three degenerative reactions occur: changes in the cell body (chromatolysis), changes in the nerve fiber segment between the cell and body and the point of transection (primary degeneration), and changes in the nerve fiber or amputated stump distal to the injury (secondary or wallerian degeneration). The effect will vary depending on whether the neuron is located entirely within the central nervous system (CNS) or partly in the peripheral nervous system. (In peripheral nerves, the cell body is located in the anterior horn of the spinal cord or in the posterior ganglion.)

A Severed Neuron Located Entirely Within the Central Nervous System

A neuron located entirely within the CNS undergoes various changes at the time of axonal transection. The effects on the cell body include swelling of the cell body; chromatolysis of the Nissl bodies in the cell body, a process by which the extranuclear ribonucleic acid (RNA) granules appear to dissolve or lose their staining characteristics; and displacement of the nucleus to the side of the cell body. As a result of these events, the cell body usually dies.

At the synaptic junction, swelling of the severed axonal fiber begins to involve the myelin sheath and axis cylinder. This is a degenerative process, called wallerian degeneration, which destroys the severed axon stump and proceeds backward toward the cell body. Neuroglial cells proliferate in the area, resulting in a phagocytic removal of the breakdown products. Breakdown of the cells and phagocytosis also extends from the point of the transection toward the cell body, a process sometimes called "dying back." Eventually, the entire cell disappears, usually over several months.

This process is replicated in each neuron of the severed nerve. (A nerve is composed of thousands of neurons.) If many nerve fibers are involved, the proliferation of neuroglial cells responsible for phagocytosis can form a dense glial scar. Neurons of the CNS do not survive axonal transection.

A Severed Peripheral Nerve (Axon Located Outside the Central Nervous System)

Peripheral nerves are composed of neurons and connective tissue. Nerve injuries are classified according to which of these components are disrupted, and these classifications are important for determining treatment and prognosis of any nerve injury. If neither the neuron nor its connective tissue covering are disrupted, then the injury is called a **neuropraxia**. This type of injury is seen in slow compressive lesions, such as carpal tunnel syndrome. Full recovery, which may take 5 to 6 weeks, is usually ensured once the compressive force is removed. If the neuronal components are disrupted but the connective tissue tracts through which the nerve travels remain intact, then the injury is called an **axonotmesis**. This type of injury is associated with wallerian degeneration of the involved neurons. Because the connective tissue tracts remain intact, the neurons are able to regenerate, albeit at a very slow rate. If the neuronal and connective tissue elements are disrupted, then the injury is called a **neurotmesis**, and recovery is unlikely, especially without surgical intervention.[1]

If a peripheral nerve has been completely severed, however, there is still a possibility for regeneration after surgical reapproximation of the severed nerve ends (Fig. 24-1). As with cell injury of the CNS, the same changes occur in the cell body of the injured peripheral nerve, that is, swelling, chromatolysis, and side displacement of the nucleus. Chromatolysis usually indicates increased RNA and protein synthesis, an example of metabolic activity necessary for the regeneration of severed axonal fibers. In the isolated axonal segment, secondary degeneration occurs (wallerian degeneration). The axis cylinder and myelin sheath degenerate and are removed by the phagocytic cells. The only remaining evidence of the severed axonal segment is the Schwann's (neurolemma) cells.

After surgical repair, the regeneration process begins with the proliferation of Schwann's cells in the proximal stump near the transection and in the distal stump. These cells divide by mitosis to form continuous cords of Schwann's cells, covering an area that encompasses the proximal stump, the gap across the transected area, the distal stump, and the area up to the sites of the sensory receptors and motor endings. The neurolemmal cords act as guidelines for the regenerating axon.

Meanwhile, the cell body is directing synthesized protein and metabolites distally to provide the nutritional machinery for axonal regeneration. The axis cylinder of the proximal axon at the transection begins to generate tiny, unmyelinated sprouts that grow longitudinally. There may be as many as 50 sprouts. The random growth of sprouts, which is accompanied by connective tissue proliferation, forms an enlargement called a *neuroma*; this can often be a source of intractable pain. Some sprouts will be misdirected and stray, but some will be successful in crossing the transected gap through the guidance of the neurolemma, finding their way to the distal stump. The rate of growth of a regenerating sprout is 1 to 4 mm/d. If the union is well aligned so that the axon will grow back into its former channel, functional return will be good.

Successfully realigned nerves will remyelinate, grow to their former size, and eventually claim a conduction velocity equivalent to 80% of their former capacity. If the nerve realignments are mismatched, functional weakness, unintentional movements of muscles, and poor sensory discrimination and localization of stimuli may result. Sprouts that are unsuccessful in making connections degenerate. Nerves proximal to the injured neurons are stimulated to produce collateral innervation to denerved areas. This process will provide innervation long before the axon has regenerated to provide innervation. Therefore, some sensory return may occur before regeneration can realistically occur. This pro-

Proximal axon

Distal axon

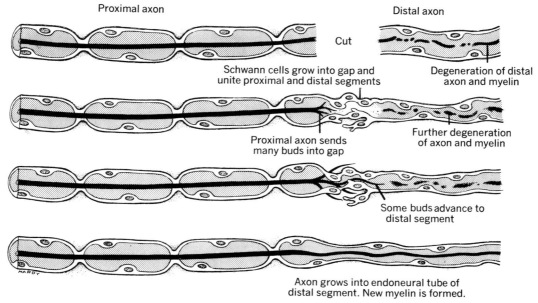

Cut

Schwann cells grow into gap and unite proximal and distal segments

Degeneration of distal axon and myelin

Proximal axon sends many buds into gap

Further degeneration of axon and myelin

Some buds advance to distal segment

Axon grows into endoneural tube of distal segment. New myelin is formed.

FIGURE 24-1

Wallerian degeneration: Diagram of changes that occur in a nerve fiber that has been cut and then regenerates.

cess is possible in the central and peripheral nervous systems.

GENERAL SIGNS AND SYMPTOMS OF PERIPHERAL NERVE TRAUMA

Motor, sensory, autonomic, and trophic signs and symptoms are the usual functional changes occurring with peripheral nerve injuries. The degree of deficit in any area depends on the type and extent of injury. Because peripheral nerves arise from spinal nerves, they are lower motor neurons and display signs and symptoms of lower motor neuron (flaccid) paralysis when injured. These signs and symptoms include the following:

- Flaccid paralysis of the muscle or muscle groups supplied by the nerve. A paresis results if some, but not all, of the lower motor neurons innervating the muscle are functional.
- Absence of deep tendon reflexes in the affected area if all neurons are affected. If some neurons are functional, deep tendon reflexes are weak.
- Atonic or hypotonic muscles
- Progressive muscle atrophy that begins early (reaches peak in several weeks)
- Fibrillations and fasciculations that peak 2 to 3 weeks after the muscle is denerved (**Fibrillations** are transitory muscle contractions caused by spontaneous stimulation of a single muscle fiber and can only be detected during electromyographic studies. **Fasciculations** are spontaneous contractions of several muscle fibers innervated by a single motor

nerve filament and can be observed during the physical examination.)
- Diminished or complete sensory loss
- Warm or dry skin (anhidrosis) caused by transection of the postganglionic sympathetic fibers
- Trophic changes

TROPHIC CHANGES

Trophic changes can be divided into a warm phase followed by a cold phase. The warm phase lasts about 3 weeks, during which time the skin in the affected areas is dry, warm, and flushed. The cold phase is characterized by cold, cyanotic skin; brittle fingernails; loss of hair; dryness and ulceration of skin; and lysis of bones and joints. The digits are affected most. In some incomplete lesions of the median, ulnar, or sciatic nerve with causalgia, the warm phase may persist and may be accompanied by sweating.

CAUSALGIA

In 1865, Weir Mitchell coined the term **causalgia** to describe a rare (except in wartime) type of peripheral neuralgia caused by partial injury to the median or ulnar nerve and occasionally the sciatic nerve. True causalgia is associated with penetrating injuries in which some sensory fibers, and usually some muscle fibers, are left intact. The pain, beginning shortly after injury, is described as a constant and intense burning. Symptoms are most pronounced in the digits, palm of the hand, or sole of the foot. Any minor stimulus, such as a draft of air, contact with clothes, or loud noise, can aggravate the pain. The patient is most comfortable when left alone with a cool moist cloth wrapped around the limb.

Abnormalities of the sweat glands and vasomotor tone in the affected area are caused by alteration of autonomic function. The involved hand (or foot) is moist, warmer or colder, and either pinker or bluer than the other hand. Trophic changes soon occur in the skin (shiny and smooth and then scaly and discolored). The underlying pathophysiology is thought to be short circuiting of the efferent sympathetic impulses to the sensory somatic fibers at the point of injury. True causalgia may respond to procaine blocks and sympathectomy but often progresses to an intractable pain syndrome.

Common Traumatic Syndromes

Specific traumatic syndromes commonly seen include brachial plexus, upper extremity injuries (median nerve [carpal tunnel syndrome], ulnar nerve, and radial nerve), and lower extremity injuries (femoral, sciatic, and common peroneal nerves).

BRACHIAL PLEXUS INJURIES

The brachial plexus is created from spinal nerves C-5, C-6, C-7, C-8, and T-1 (Fig. 24-2). (To make the difficult task of learning the anatomy of the brachial plexus easier, see the cited reference.)[2] By a series of division and recombination, three major trunks result: the upper trunk (C-5 and C-6), the middle trunk (C-7), and the lower trunk (C-8 and T-1). Again, these trunks divide and recombine to create three cords that give rise to the following nerves:

- Lateral cord (chiefly derived from C-5 and C-6)—musculocutaneous and the lateral half of the median nerve
- Median cord (chiefly derived from C-8 and T-1)—ulnar nerve and the medial half of the median nerve
- Posterior cord (C-5, C-6, and C-7)—axillary and radial nerve

Symptoms. Specific symptoms are seen with injuries involving particular trunks.

UPPER TRUNK (C-5 AND C-6) UPPER PLEXUS TYPE (DUCHENNE-ERB). Most of the shoulder muscles are involved, with the exception of the pectoralis major. There is loss or difficulty in abduction and external rotation of the arm and weak supination and flexion of the forearm. Sensory deficit is noted in the deltoid region and radial surface of the forearm.

MIDDLE TRUNK (C-7). Major but incomplete triceps loss and some involvement of the forearm flexors and extensors are seen. Symptoms include difficulty in extending the forearm. Sensory deficits are noted in the middle fingers.

LOWER TRUNK (C-8 AND T-1) LOWER PLEXUS TYPE (KLUMPKE'S OR DUCHENNE-ARAN). The forearm muscle flexors and the hand muscles are chiefly involved. There is paralysis and atrophy of the small hand muscles and wrist flexors, giving the appearance of a ''claw hand.'' Sensory deficit is noted in the medial side of the arm, forearm, and small finger.

Causes. The major cause of brachial plexus injury is traction and stretching. Traction and stretch injuries of the brachial

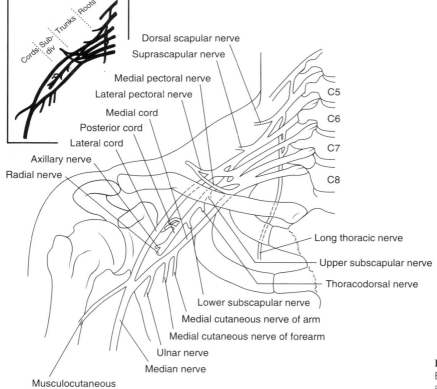

Cords; Sub-div; Trunks; Roots

Dorsal scapular nerve
Suprascapular nerve
Medial pectoral nerve
Lateral pectoral nerve
Medial cord
Posterior cord
Lateral cord
Axillary nerve
Radial nerve

C5
C6
C7
C8

Long thoracic nerve
Upper subscapular nerve
Thoracodorsal nerve
Lower subscapular nerve
Medial cutaneous nerve of arm
Medial cutaneous nerve of forearm
Ulnar nerve
Median nerve
Musculocutaneous nerve

FIGURE 24-2
Brachial plexus showing its various constituents and their relationship to structures in the region of the upper chest, axilla, and shoulder.

plexus can be caused by birth trauma and vehicular accidents. With traction injuries, there may be sensory preservation despite total motor loss. A severe traction injury usually involves avulsion of two or more spinal roots from the spinal cord. Simultaneously, other roots have probably experienced severe stretching. The result is total and permanent functional loss to both the avulsed and stretched nerves. The presence of Horner's syndrome is strongly suggestive of C-8 and T-1 avulsion. (**Horner's syndrome** refers to the sinking of the eyeball, ptosis of the upper eyelid, slight elevation of the lower eyelid, constriction of the pupil, and anhidrosis caused by paralysis of the cervical sympathetic nerve supply.)

Treatment. Each brachial plexus injury is unique. Therefore, it is impossible to generalize about the treatment protocol. Although regeneration is slow, useful recovery is generally not probable in muscles that do not begin to show function by 6 months. An intractable pain syndrome may be a part of any brachial plexus injury and may require specific medical or surgical treatment.

UPPER EXTREMITY INJURIES

Median Nerve Injuries (Derived From C-5 to T-1, but Mainly C-6)

SYMPTOMS. The following signs and symptoms are found with median nerve injury (Fig. 24-3):

- Impairment of pronation of the forearm
- Weakness of wrist flexion
- Difficulty in abducting and opposing the thumb
- Inability to flex the distal phalanges of the index finger and thumb
- Atrophy of the thenar hand muscles and the flexor-pronator group of the forearm
- Sensory loss to the radial half of the palm, the palmar surface of the thumb, index and middle fingers, and the radial half of the ring finger
- Loss of ability to sweat in affected areas

CAUSES. The median nerve may be injured in the axilla by shoulder dislocation or anywhere along its pathway by laceration, stab wounds, or gunshot wounds. However, the most frequent site of injury is at the wrist because of its vulnerable anatomical position (Fig. 24-4). The median nerves lie between the tendons of the flexor carpi radialis and palmaris longus. The flexor pollicis longus and the flexor digitorum profundus separate the median nerve from the radius. The nerve crosses the wrist level and enters the carpal tunnel, located beneath the transverse carpal ligament. The carpal tunnel is a narrow tunnel through which the median nerve passes. It is bound superiorly by the transverse carpal ligaments and laterally and inferiorly by the carpal bones, including fibrous coverings and interosseous ligaments. This syndrome commonly occurs in women between the ages of 40 and 60 years with no obvious etiological factor. If for any reason, the lumen of this channel is narrowed, the movement of the nerve and muscles is compromised. The result is the development of symptoms.

Carpal Tunnel Syndrome. The carpal tunnel syndrome, an entrapment syndrome, is caused by compression of the median

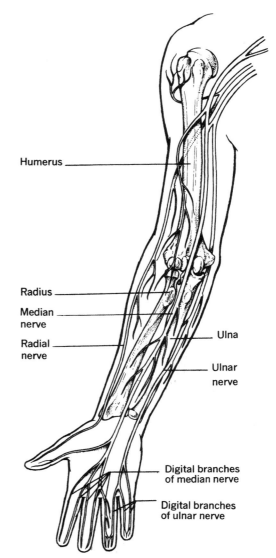

FIGURE 24-3
Distribution of peripheral nerves of the arm.

nerve because of edema of tissue in and around the carpal tunnel. Occupation-related activities that require forceful and repetitive movements of the wrists or keeping the wrists in abnormal positions for prolonged periods appear to predispose people to the carpal tunnel syndrome. Such occupational categories include press operators, construction workers who use vibrating equipment, hair dressers, typists, and pianists. A number of endocrine conditions, such as myxedema or acromegaly, pregnancy, and use of oral contraceptives, may also be a cause of the syndrome.

SYMPTOMS. Early symptoms include nocturnal dysesthesias (abnormal sensation) of the involved hand. As the disease progresses, severe dysesthesias accompany the use of the hand during daytime hours. Areas of the hand that are involved are those listed in the section on general symptoms of median nerve injury. Pain becomes constant, with motor weakness and atrophy. Vasomotor changes are intermittent.

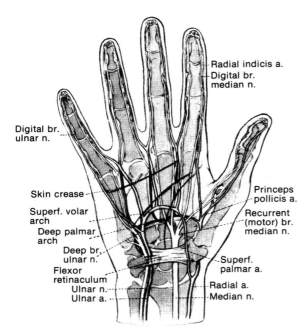

FIGURE 24-4
Distribution of peripheral nerves of the hand.

On examination, the Tinel's sign and Phalen's sign are positive. **Tinel's sign** is positive if pain and tingling are elicited by tapping over the median nerve at the wrist on the affected side. **Phalen's sign** is positive if there is tingling and pain when the wrists are flexed at right angles with the position held for at least 1 minute (Fig. 24-5).

Treatment of early carpal tunnel syndrome is directed at immobilization of the wrist with wrist splints along with use of anti-inflammatory drugs so that the inflammation and edema around the nerve can resolve. However, if nerve injury is advanced, surgery will be necessary to free the median nerve of compression. Most patients do well with surgical decompression.

Ulnar Nerve (Derived From C-8 and T-1) Injury. The ulnar nerve is most often injured at the elbow because of a fracture or dislocation of the elbow joint. Injury may also occur from a blow to the elbow that results in a contusion to the ulnar nerve. **Volkmann's contracture** refers to a muscle contraction of the arm and hand resulting from ischemic injuries at the elbow (Fig. 24-6).

SYMPTOMS. Symptoms of ulnar nerve trauma include the following:

- "Claw hand" deformity (results from wasting of the small hand muscles with hyperextension of the fingers at the metacarpophalangeal joints)
- Weakness of flexion of the wrist
- Flexion of the fourth and fifth fingers
- Inability to abduct and adduct the thumb
- Sensory loss of the fifth finger, the ulnar aspect of the fourth finger, and the ulnar border of the palm. In the instance of a contusion to the nerve, the chief symptom may be pain

with little, if any, motor deficit. As time passes, motor deficits may evolve (sometimes called tardy ulnar paralysis).

Radial Nerve (Derived From C-6, C-7, and C-8, but Mainly From C-7 Nerve Root) Injury. The radial nerve may be injured in the axilla from compression and stretching caused by crutch walking. It is most frequently compressed at the point where the nerve winds around the humerus. Fractures and compression during sleep are the usual causes.

SYMPTOMS. Symptoms of complete radial nerve injury include the following:

- Weakness in extension of the elbow, wrist, fingers, and thumb
- Possible wristdrop
- Inability to grasp an object or make a fist
- Sensory impairment over the posterior aspect of the forearm and the radial aspect of the dorsum of the hand

LOWER EXTREMITY INJURIES (FIG. 24-7)

Femoral Nerve (Derived From the L-2, L-3, and L-4 Nerve Roots) Injury. The femoral nerve may be injured from compression of a pelvic tumor or during pelvic surgery.

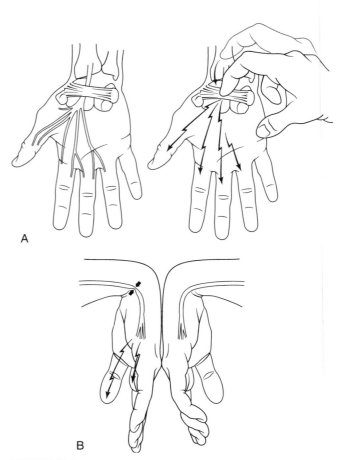

FIGURE 24-5
(A) Carpal tunnel syndrome (right) and Tinel's sign (left). (B) Phalen's sign to reproduce symptoms of carpal tunnel syndrome.

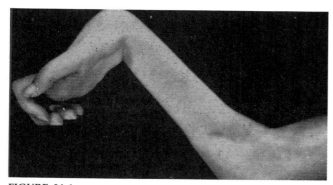

FIGURE 24-6
Volkmann's contracture. (From Boyes, J. H. [1970]. *Bunnell's surgery of the hand* [5th ed]. Philadelphia: J.B. Lippincott.)

PERIPHERAL NERVE INJURIES: DIAGNOSIS AND TREATMENT

Diagnosis of peripheral nerve injury is based on a history of injury or presence of an irritative or injurious lesion and a complete neurological examination. Electromyography and nerve conduction velocity studies are two diagnostic tests that may be ordered to give some indication that the nerve and its connection with the muscle are intact.

Treatment options must be individualized to the particular problem. If nerve injury is secondary to a primary problem, such as a tumor, attention is first directed to treatment of the primary problem. Surgery may be indicated for lacerations or transections. Ideally, any associated injuries should be clean and healed. Selecting the optimal time for surgery, however, is most important. To determine the extent of nerve injury, surgical exploration may be planned immediately after injury. Primary nerve repair is usually scheduled for 3 weeks to 2 months after injury. The judgment of the physician in selecting the proper time and surgical procedure is critical. Severed nerves may require resection and suturing to reapproximate the ends. Nerve grafts or transplantation are other options.

During surgery for anastomosis of the severed nerve, the two nerve segments will have contracted, each having formed scar tissue at the stump. Dissection of the stumps further decreases the lengths of the ends to be joined. To compensate for this, the extremity is positioned in exaggerated flexion with a cast or splint applied to maintain the position. However, healing at the suture site takes 3 or 4 weeks. After healing has been ensured, the cast or splint is revised several times, with the degree of extension gradually increased by approximately 10 degrees each time. Cable grafting with autologous nerve tissue is a newer surgical technique that allows for anastomosis of nerves over large gaps, without the need for the exaggerated flexion position.

Because denerved muscle begins to atrophy almost immediately after injury, it is important to use all available means to retard the process. As previously noted, axonal growth occurs at the rate of 1 to 4 mm/d. Some muscle atrophy will be evident before the slow process of nerve regeneration is completed.

As soon as satisfactory healing has occurred, a physiotherapy program should be implemented to deal with the problems of immobility (stiffness, atrophy, and joint ankylosis). Special spring braces should be used to prevent footdrop or wristdrop. Daily regimens of galvanic stimulation to minimize the atrophic change of muscle to fibrotic tissue may be instituted until the affected muscle demonstrates, on electromyography, that it has been reinnervated. Massage, whirlpool treatments, and an exercise program to re-educate the muscles are important components of an aggressive physiotherapy program.

The rehabilitation program is long and arduous. Depending on the type and location of the injury, the prognosis will vary. It may be necessary to offer a total rehabilitation program at a center that provides vocational rehabilitation if permanent disability will prevent the patient from assuming his or her former place in society and the job market. The patient should be kept comfortable with

SYMPTOMS. Injury to the femoral nerve results in the following:

- Weakness of extension of the knee
- Wasting of the quadriceps muscles
- Weakness of hip flexion (if injury is near the psoas muscle)
- Absence of the knee-jerk reflex
- Sensory loss of the anterolateral thigh

Sciatic Nerve (Derived From L-4 to S-3 Nerve Roots) Injury. The sciatic nerve may be injured by pelvic or femoral fractures, gunshot wounds, or injection of medication into the nerve. Pelvic tumors and herniated intervertebral discs are other possible causes of sciatic injury.

SYMPTOMS. Symptoms of complete sciatic paralysis include the following:

- Inability to flex the knee
- Weakened gluteal muscles
- Pain across the buttock and into the thigh
- Footdrop
- Sensory loss in the innervated areas

Common Peroneal Nerve (Derived From L-4 to S-3) Injury. The common peroneal nerve is injured from prolonged traction, prolonged application of a tourniquet, or compression at the lateral aspect of the knees during surgery.

SYMPTOMS. Symptoms of trauma involving the peroneal nerve include the following:

- Paralysis of dorsiflexion of foot and toes (footdrop)
- Difficulty with eversion of the foot (with involvement of the superficial peroneal nerve)
- Sensory loss of the medial part of the dorsum of the foot and outer side of the leg

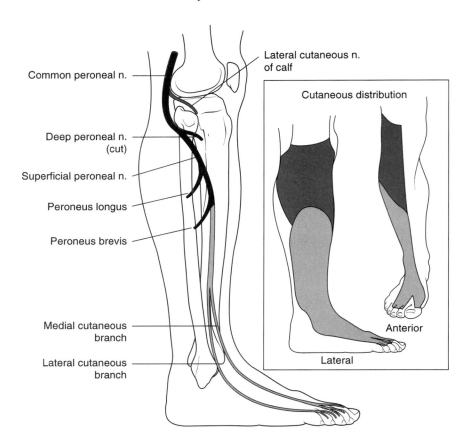

Common peroneal n.

Deep peroneal n. (cut)

Superficial peroneal n.

Peroneus longus

Peroneus brevis

Medial cutaneous branch

Lateral cutaneous branch

Lateral cutaneous n. of calf

Cutaneous distribution

Anterior

Lateral

FIGURE 24-7
Distribution of peripheral nerves of the leg.

appropriate analgesics, as necessary. The pain that sometimes accompanies peripheral nerve injury may seriously limit the functional rehabilitation of these patients and should be dealt with aggressively.[3]

NURSING MANAGEMENT OF THE PATIENT WITH PERIPHERAL NERVE TRAUMA

Specific nursing care depends on the particular problem and the type and degree of injury. The patient with a peripheral injury may be hospitalized for surgery and discharged to recuperate at home. In other instances, a peripheral injury may be only one type of injury seen in multiple trauma. The management of the peripheral injury is incorporated into the total nursing management of the patient. However, general principles can be identified and followed when caring for patients with a peripheral nerve injury. These principles can be categorized into the following areas: assessment of function, maintenance of function, and rehabilitation. See Chart 24-1 for a summary of nursing diagnoses and nursing management.

Assessment of Function

A neurological assessment of the limb is made to determine which neurological functions are intact. The assessment is initially conducted by the nurse to establish a baseline with which subsequent assessments can be compared. After the baseline has been established, subsequent assessments are conducted every 2 to 4 hours or at less frequent intervals, depending on the patient's condition.

MOTOR FUNCTION

Motor function is assessed by asking the patient to put the limb through the normal range of motion. In an acute traumatic episode, the initial injury should first be evaluated by the physician in the emergency room to determine if movement is contraindicated, as would be the case if there were danger of a broken bone severing a nerve. If movement of the involved extremity is not contraindicated, function is assessed. Any evidence of abnormal movements, such as tremors, fibrillation, or fasciculations, should be documented. Atrophy, contractions, paresis, and paralysis are abnormal findings. Deep tendon reflexes should be assessed.

SENSORY FUNCTION

The sensory innervation to the involved limb is tested by using a wisp of cotton for light touch. Pinching the skin or pricking it with a pin can test the patient's reaction to a painful stimulus. Test tubes of warm and cold water can be individually placed on the skin of the involved limb to test the patient's awareness of differences in temperature. The patient should be questioned about whether he or she has experienced any

CHART 24-1

Summary of Nursing Diagnoses and Nursing Interventions for the Patient With Peripheral Nerve Injuries

Nursing Diagnoses	Nursing Interventions	Expected Outcomes
Sensory/Perceptual Alterations: tactile related to (R/T) nerve injury and neuropathies	• Monitor thermal, positional, light touch, and painful sensation. • Teach patient to compensate with use of vision. • Use assistive devices to compensate for deficits. • Monitor and prevent injury to the affected area.	• The patient will recognize the deficit and compensate by using other perceptual modalities.
Impaired Physical Mobility R/T nerve injury	• Monitor movement of the extremities. • When ordered, provide for range-of-motion exercises. • Teach the patient the proper use of assistive devices as necessary. • Monitor the patient to prevent injury and falls.	• Injury will be avoided. • The patient will compensate for deficits by using assistive devices.
Altered Peripheral Tissue Perfusion, R/T vascular changes secondary to injury to autonomic innervation	• Monitor the skin color and temperature of the involved area. • Prevent contact with extremes in temperature to involved areas. • Teach the patient to monitor skin color and temperature.	• The patient will not sustain burns to the involved area.
Impaired Skin Integrity R/T trophic skin changes	• Monitor the skin for evidence of skin breakdown or dryness. • Provide skin care every 4 h. • Teach the patient to provide skin care.	• Skin integrity will be maintained.
Risk for Injury R/T diminished or lost sensation, proprioception, paralysis, or paresis	• Protect the involved area from injury. • Teach the patient to compensate by using vision and other senses and to inspect the involved area periodically for injury. • Provide assistive devices as necessary.	• The patient will not sustain an injury or fall.
Pain R/T nerve injury	• Monitor the patient for the presence and characteristics of pain. • Provide for pain control with distraction, imagery, positioning, and use of analgesics.	• The patient will report feeling comfortable.

Other related nursing diagnoses that may be applicable include Knowledge Deficit; Impaired Home Maintenance Management; Impaired Thermoregulation; Fear; Anxiety; Body Image Disturbance; Altered Role Performance; Anticipatory or Dysfunctional Grieving; and Social Isolation.

abnormal sensations, such as tingling, a crawling sensation, or pain. All are examples of reportable findings.

OTHER FUNCTIONAL ASSESSMENTS

The involved limb should also be assessed for color, warmth, and texture. If the skin is cool to the touch or appears cyanotic, circulatory impairment or vasomotor tone may be indicated. Warm, dry, reddish skin indicates possible early trophic changes associated with autonomic alterations. Any evidence of scaling, brittle nails, or loss of body hair should be recorded.

Maintenance of Function

Following an assessment of the involved area, the nurse plans and implements the nursing care plan with consideration of the goals of medical management.

If the physician has ordered immobilization of the involved area, the immobilization may be accomplished by a splint, cast, or traction. The purpose of immobilization is to provide rest for the involved area if an inflammatory process is present so that the process can be controlled and resolved. The second reason for immobilization is to allow for the healing of a surgical incision in which there has been a reanastomosis of a severed nerve.

SPLINT AND CAST CARE

The splint is usually held secure with an Ace wrap or Velcro. The splint and wrap can become tight because of edema. The skin around the splint or cast should be checked for tightness, warmth, and color. If the splint or cast is too tight, as evidenced by tingling, blanched color, or coolness, steps can be taken to provide a better fit. In the case of a tight cast, the physician will need to decide what adjustments need to be made to ensure a better fit. It is best to refer the need for adjustments to the department that made the splint or brace originally, because all braces and most splints are custom made to fit the contour of the wearer. A blanched appearance of the skin and coolness to the touch indicate interference with autonomic function and adequate blood supply. Any indications of drainage under the cast or splint should be addressed immediately.

POSITIONING THE EXTREMITY

If a cast or splint has been applied to the arm, a sling may be necessary to prevent edema because the arm is in a dependent position. In the case of a leg cast, the physician usually wants the leg to be supported and elevated on pillows to reduce the likelihood of edema.

SKIN CARE

Trophic changes of the skin are common signs and symptoms associated with peripheral nerve injury that make the skin susceptible to breakdown and injury. The skin should be examined for evidence of irritation or injury. Washing and careful drying are important, especially between the toes or fingers. If the skin is dry and scaly, lubrication with a lanolin preparation or cocoa butter is an effective treatment. The nails should be filed and cut straight across to prevent injury.

TEMPERATURE

The involved extremity should be carefully protected from extremes in temperature. Because of the lost or compromised sensory function, the area can be easily injured from extreme heat or cold without the patient being alerted through pain or discomfort.

AMBULATION

Depending on the extent of injury of the involved extremity, the physician may limit ambulation and other activities of daily living (ADLs). The nurse should adjust the plan of care based on the limitations imposed by the injury and the medical treatment.

Rehabilitation

The length and complexity of the rehabilitative process are based on the particular injury and the patient. The patient is encouraged to verbalize concerns about the injury. The nurse should be a good listener, correct misconceptions, and help the patient set realistic goals. Anxiety is decreased, and the patient is better able to cope with an altered body image if the nurse can be supportive of the patient. A positive, supporting nurse–patient relationship provides an ideal milieu for the active participation of the patient in the rehabilitative process.

The patient with a peripheral nerve injury requires much teaching to regain the greatest possible level of independence. Help may be needed in developing alternative methods of performing ADLs. For example, if the dominant arm and hand are encircled by a splint, the patient will need to be helped to learn to eat with the other hand. If food is adequately prepared for the patient (beverage poured, food cut, and so forth), he or she will be able to manage with practice.

When an exercise program is initiated for the involved extremity, the patient will have to learn the active and passive (prescribed) exercises. The patient should also be taught to protect the involved limb from injury. The process of regaining motor and sensory function can be so slow that the patient becomes discouraged. The nurse should encourage the patient to follow the outlined physiotherapy program to prevent skeletal deformities and slowly regain as much function as possible. The nurse's positive attitude conveys the strongest message to the patient about the progress being made.

The nurse participates in long-range planning for patient needs with other members of the health team. The rehabilitative process for peripheral nerve injury may be long. Often, the patient with the injury will be treated on an outpatient basis with physiotherapy and supervision by the physician and community health nurse.

Psychosocial Considerations

Peripheral nerve injury is usually synonymous with disability of an extremity. If the arm is involved, the patient is deprived of the normal range of motion, which will usually affect various roles: breadwinner, homemaker, handyman, child caretaker, or creative being. Thumb apposition to the index finger is a highly valued skill. Without this skill, patients are unable to pick up objects, feed themselves, or perform other ADLs. Individuals who are deprived of their ability to perform these ADLs will feel limited, especially if the injury affects their dominant side.

Peripheral nerve injury to one of the lower extremities impedes or prevents ambulation and limits the various settings in which the person can function. The inability to ambulate, drive, use public transportation, and move freely in public settings interferes with normal fulfillment of roles and responsibilities.

A decreased level of independence precipitates various emotional and psychological reactions. The patient experiences changes in body image, self-esteem, and lifestyle. Sensory deprivation, social isolation, and powerlessness result from the limitations imposed by the disability. Common behavioral manifestations from the various physical, emotional, and social disabilities include frustration, hostility, anger, and depression. Many patients go through a process of loss, grief, and bereavement over the lost function. The process of recovery is very slow (approximately 1 year with nerve transections). Physiotherapy is the major approach after surgical intervention has been completed. Anyone who has experience with patient care and physiotherapy is well aware of the painfully slow process involved in rehabilitating a limb. The process is characterized by ups and downs, so the patient can easily become discouraged with the lack of apparent improvement. If the disability is permanent, the emotional impact imposes increased demands on the person's coping skills and adjustment patterns; therefore, it is extremely important that the nurse provide the psychological and emotional support needed.

References

1. Personal communication. John Sampson, MD, March 25, 1996.
2. Peck, D. (1978). A "five-fingered" mnemonic for the brachial plexus. *Journal of Kentucky Medical Association, 76*, 70–72.
3. Personal communications. John Sampson, MD, March 20, 1996.

Bibliography

Books

Adams, R. D., & Victor, M. (1993). *Principles of neurology* (5th ed.). New York: McGraw-Hill.

Kline, D. G., & Hudson, A. R. (1995). *Nerve injuries: Operative results for major nerve injuries, entrapments, and tumors* (p. 611). Philadelphia: W.B. Saunders.

Sunderland, S. (1991). *Nerve injuries and their repair: A critical approach.* New York: Churchill Livingstone.

Terzis, J. K. (1990). *The peripheral nerves: Structure, function, and reconstruction.* New York: Raven Press.

Periodicals

Braun, R. M., & Jackson, W. J. (1994). Electrical studies as a prognostic factor in the surgical treatment of carpal tunnel syndrome. *Journal of Hand Surgery, 19A*, 893–900,

Horowitz, S. H. (1994). Peripheral nerve injury and causalgia secondary to routine venipuncture. *Neurology, 44*, 962–964.

Harter, B. T., McKiernan, J. E., Kirzinger, S. S., Archer, F. W., Paters, C. K., & Harter, K. C. (1993). Carpal tunnel syndrome: Surgical and nonsurgical treatment. *The Journal of Hand Surgery, 18A*, 734–739.

Miller, R. S., Iverson, D. C., Fried, R. A., Green, L. A., & Nutting, P. A. (1994). Carpal tunnel syndrome in primary care: A report from ASPN. *Journal of Family Practice, 38*(4), 337–344.

Section 6

Nursing Management of Patients With Tumors of the Neurological System

CHAPTER 25

Brain Tumors

Joanne V. Hickey
Terri Armstrong

OVERVIEW OF BRAIN TUMORS

The diagnosis of a brain tumor begins a journey of uncertainty, fear, and hope for the patient and his or her family. The human saga is intermingled with issues related to subtle and significant loss of neurological function, treatment options, and quality of life. A broad knowledge base provides the health professional with the information and skills to care for the patient and family in a sensitive, compassionate, and humanistic manner. Within this framework of fundamental principles, concepts related to brain tumors are explored.

Incidence and Etiology

The annual incidence of brain tumors in the United States is estimated to be 17,500 primary intracranial neoplasms and 17,400 secondary neoplasms from metastasis.[1] Intracranial tumors are found in people of all ages, with peaks of incidence occurring in early childhood and in the fifth, sixth, and seventh decades. The incidence is slightly higher in men than in women (9.6 versus 7.9 per 100,000). A higher incidence of malignant gliomas and neuromas is found in men, whereas the incidence of meningiomas and pituitary adenomas is higher in women.[2] The cause of primary brain tumors is unknown. Certain tumors appear to have a congenital basis (epidermoid, dermoid, and teratoid tumors and craniopharyngiomas). Others may be related to hereditary factors (von Recklinghausen's disease, tuberous sclerosis, and von Hippel-Lindau disease).

Classification of Brain Tumors

Brain tumors can be classified based on a number of distinguishing criteria, including primary or secondary, neuroembryonic origins, intra-axial or extra-axial, anatomical location, histological origin, malignant or benign, and childhood or adult tumors.

PRIMARY VERSUS SECONDARY BRAIN TUMORS

Primary brain tumors originate from the various cells and structures normally found within the brain. Metastatic brain tumors originate from structures outside the brain, most often from primary tumors of the lungs, breast, gastrointestinal tract, and genitourinary tract. *Carcinomatosis* is a condition in which carcinoma is widespread throughout the body. The term is sometimes used to describe multiple metastatic lesions to the brain or meninges.

NEUROEMBRYONIC ORIGINS

The nervous system originates from the ectodermal (outer) layer of the embryo. Chapter 5 briefly describes early embryonic development. At 16 days, the *neural plate* appears, changing to the *neural groove* and *neural tube* by the third week. The neuroectodermal cells not incorporated into the neural tube form *neural crests*. The neural tube and neural crests contain two types of undifferentiated cells called neuroblasts and glioblasts (spongioblasts). The *neuroblasts* become the basic unit of structure in the nervous system, and are called *neurons*. The *glioblasts* form a variety of cells that support, insulate, and metabolically assist the neurons. They are collectively called *glial cells*.[3] Glial cells are subdivided into *astrocytes* (star-shaped cells), *oligodendrocytes* (glial cells with few processes), and *ependymal cells* (line the ventricles). This is the basis for the broad category of brain tumors called *gliomas*. Gliomas are further subdivided into *astrocytomas, oligodendrogliomas,* and *ependymomas.*

INTRA-AXIAL VERSUS EXTRA-AXIAL BRAIN TUMORS

Intra-axial brain tumors are located within the central neuraxis (cerebral hemispheres, brain stem, and cerebellum). They arise from neuroglial precursor cells and are found mostly in the white matter. Extra-axial brain tumors are located outside the central neuraxis. They arise from the cranial nerves, pituitary gland, or meninges.

ANATOMICAL LOCATION

Anatomical location refers to the location of the lesion in reference to the tentorium or to cerebral tissue. One classification system that uses the tentorium as a reference point differentiates between *supratentorial,* which signifies a tumor located above the tentorium (cerebral hemispheres), and *infratentorial,* which denotes a tumor located below the tentorium (brain stem and cerebellum).

A second way of viewing anatomical location of brain tumors is by the actual site of the lesion, such as frontal lobe, temporal lobe, pons, or cerebellum (Fig. 25-1). Knowing the location of the lesion helps to predict probable deficits based on an understanding of the normal function of that anatomical area.

HISTOLOGICAL ORIGIN

The following is a histological classification of the major tumors, with their relative percentages of incidence in adults:[4]

I. Intracerebral tumors
  A. Gliomas (noncapsulated; tend to infiltrate the cerebral substance)
    1. Astrocytomas (grades I and II)—10%
    2. Glioblastoma multiforme (also called astrocytoma grades III and IV)—20%
    3. Oligodendrocytoma (grades I to IV)—5%
    4. Ependymoma (grades I to IV)—6%
    5. Medulloblastoma—4%
II. Tumors arising from the supporting structures
  A. Meningiomas—15%
  B. Neuromas (acoustic neuroma, schwannoma)—7%
  C. Pituitary adenomas—7%
III. Developmental (congenital) tumors
  A. Dermoid, epidermoid, teratoma, craniopharyngioma—4%
  B. Angiomas—4%
IV. Metastatic lesions—6%

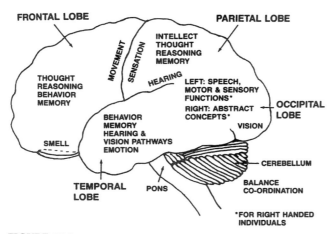

FIGURE 25-1
Cerebral function and associated anatomical areas. (Reproduced with permission from the American Brain Tumor Association.)

V. Other
  A. Unclassified (mostly gliomas)—5%
  B. Sarcomas—4%
  C. Miscellaneous (pinealoma, chordoma, granuloma)—3%

MALIGNANT VERSUS BENIGN BRAIN TUMORS

Using the word "benign" in the classification of brain tumors can be somewhat misleading. When a neoplasm is designated as benign, one concludes that a complete cure is possible; conversely, a malignant tumor would indicate a poor prognosis. This distinction is made on the basis of histological examination. Cells that are well differentiated tend to indicate a much better prognosis than do poorly differentiated cells. However, when a tumor is located within the brain, other factors take precedence. A tumor that is considered to be histologically benign may be surgically inaccessible, as with a deep tumor requiring extensive dissection of tissue or one located in a vital area, such as the pons or medulla. A benign tumor that is surgically inaccessible will continue to grow, causing an increase in intracranial pressure (ICP), neurological deficits, herniation syndromes, and finally, death. Because such a patient has lost neurological function and life, it is grossly inaccurate to suggest that the tumor was benign. There is also the possibility that such tumors can convert to more histologically malignant types as they develop.

DIFFERENCES IN BRAIN TUMORS IN CHILDREN AND ADULTS

In children (newborns to 16 years old), the incidence of brain tumors differs, with about two thirds of all childhood brain tumors located in the posterior fossa (infratentorial region). The most common childhood tumors are: astrocytomas, medulloblastomas, and ependymomas.

The percentage of total primary childhood tumors by type is as follows:

- Medulloblastoma—30%
- Astrocytoma (grades I and II)—30%
- Ependymoma—12%
- Craniopharyngioma—10%
- Optic pathway glioma (spongioblastoma)—5%
- Miscellaneous—13%

GRADING OF GLIOMAS

Grading of gliomas is based on cellular density, atypia, and tumor cell mitosis. The higher the grade, the more malignant the tumor. Currently, two grading systems are used for gliomas (Table 25-1). Astrocytomas are characterized by an increased number of cells. More malignant tumors (both the anaplastic astrocytoma and glioblastoma multiforme) not only have a marked increase in the number of cells, but display many cells undergoing mitosis (or cell division). In addition, the glioblastoma has the following characteristics: central necrosis, lining up of cells along the surrounding necrosis (pseudopallisading), and new blood vessel formation (neovascularization).

TABLE 25-1
Two Systems of Classification of Malignant Gliomas

KERNOHAN CLASSIFICATION	THREE-TIER CLASSIFICATION	MEDIAN SURVIVAL
Grades I and II	Astrocytoma	5–7 y
Grade III	Anaplastic astrocytoma	18–24 mo
Grade IV	Glioblastoma multiforme	8–10 mo

Pathophysiology of Brain Tumors

MONRO-KELLIE HYPOTHESIS

The pathophysiology of brain tumors is based on an understanding of the Monro-Kellie hypothesis, which states that the brain has limited compensatory mechanisms to maintain normal ICP by decreasing (1) the volume of brain tissue, (2) cerebrospinal fluid (CSF), and (3) cerebral blood volume (CBV). The ability to compensate also depends on how rapidly the tumor grows.

Brain Volume. In a slow-growing tumor, the brain tissue has a limited degree of compressibility. In fast-growing tumors, the brain is essentially not compressible. The volume of CSF or CBV must decrease to compensate for and prevent a rapid rise in ICP.

Displacement of Cerebrospinal Fluid Volume. First, the CSF volume within the ventricles and subarachnoid space is decreased. This is accomplished by shifting some CSF through the foramen magnum into the spinal subarachnoid space and through the optic foramen to the perioptic subarachnoid space. When limits of CSF compensation are surpassed, the pressure within the ventricles and subarachnoid space increases. This, in turn, increases pressure within the cisterns and lumbar subarachnoid space. If an ICP monitor is in place or if a lumbar puncture is performed, the pressure will be recorded as being elevated. Second, the increase in perioptic pressure impedes venous drainage from the optic head area and retina, and papilledema is noted on ophthalmological examination.[5]

Cerebral Blood Volume. The other intracranial component that has limited compensatory capability is CBV. First, the venules in the tissue surrounding the tumor are compressed. The compression elevates capillary pressure and results in *vasogenic edema.* Once the edema begins, it can perpetuate an escalating cycle of more edema. Second, for CSF absorption to occur, the pressure in the subarachnoid space must be greater than the pressure in the venous sinuses. The increased venous pressure caused by the tumor decreases CSF absorption and results in an increase in CSF volume and pressure. If increased CSF pressure occurs slowly, vasodilation of arteries and arterioles results. If ventricular pressure rises rapidly, the arterial blood pressure must also rise quickly to prevent vascular collapse. Baroreceptors in the carotid sinus trigger the carotid sinus reflex. The effect observed is a rising blood pressure, especially the systolic component, with concurrent bradycardia. (Rising systolic blood pressure, widening pulse pressure, and bradycardia are collectively known as Cushing's response.) Third, cerebral venous stasis and concurrent elevations in CO_2 levels trigger the medullary vasomotor center to cause vasodilation. The vasodilation increases the intracranial CBV. Once the limits of compensation are reached, ICP rises.

TUMOR GROWTH AND EFFECT ON BRAIN

A brain tumor will usually grow as a spherical mass until it encounters a more rigid structure, such as bone or the falx cerebri. The encounter with an aplastic substance necessitates a change in the contour of the neoplasm. Neoplastic cells can also grow diffusely, infiltrating tissue spaces as multiple cells without forming a definite mass. The size of the tumor enlarges because of cell proliferation or as a result of necrosis, fluid accumulation, hemorrhage, or accumulation of the byproducts of degeneration within the mass.

Tumors affect the brain through *compression of cerebral tissue, invasion or infiltration of cerebral tissue,* and sometimes *erosion of bone.* These mechanisms precipitate the pathophysiological changes of cerebral edema and increased ICP.

CEREBRAL EDEMA

In most patients with brain tumors, vasogenic edema develops in the surrounding tissue of the tumor because of compression. On the cellular level, the increased permeability of the capillary endothelial cells of the cerebral white matter results in seepage of plasma into the extracellular space and between the layers of the myelin sheath. This alters the electrical potential of cells and impairs cellular activity. Cerebral edema can also develop rapidly from alterations in the blood–brain barrier caused by substances released from tumor cells.[4] As cerebral edema continues to develop, it can result in signs and symptoms of increased ICP.

INCREASED INTRACRANIAL PRESSURE

Signs and symptoms of increased ICP will develop as the tumor grows and cerebral edema increases. Slowly growing tumors allow for greater compensation of intracranial contents than do rapidly growing tumors. However, as the limits of accommodation of intracranial volume and compensation are reached, ICP rises and symptoms of increased ICP become apparent. This begins the period of decompensation. The signs and symptoms of increased ICP can include any or all of the following:

- Deterioration in the level of consciousness (confusion, restlessness, stupor, coma)
- Abnormal pupillary function
- Deficits in extraocular movement
- Motor deficits (paresis, paralysis, abnormal posturing)
- Sensory deficits
- Changes in respiratory function and other vital signs

In the adult, most brain tumors are located in the supratentorial region. As ICP begins to rise, various herniation syndromes can develop (see Chap. 17). Without definitive treatment and management of increased ICP, death will result.

SIGNS AND SYMPTOMS OF BRAIN TUMORS

There are no classic signs and symptoms of brain tumors. The particular clinical presentation of a brain tumor in a patient depends on compression or infiltration of specific cerebral tissue, the related cerebral edema, and the development of increased ICP. These signs and symptoms can be classified into three general categories of clinical findings:

- General deficits of cerebral function, headaches, and seizures
- Signs and symptoms of increased ICP
- Syndromes related to specific cerebral functions

Depending on the type and location of the tumor, some patients will initially have difficulty in only one of the areas cited previously. Other patients may show signs and symptoms involving two or three areas.

General Deficits of Cerebral Function, Headache, and Seizures

The most common initial signs and symptoms of brain tumors are alterations in consciousness, cognition, or both; headache; seizures; and vomiting.

ALTERATIONS IN COGNITION OR CONSCIOUSNESS

Patients with brain tumors have varying degrees of alterations in cognition, mental function, or consciousness. Cognitive deficits include a wide range of functions, such as short- and long-term memory deficits, difficulty in concentration and vigilance, decreased mental activity, slowing of mental processes and reaction time, abulia, and difficulty with calculations, problem solving, insight, abstraction, and synthesis of ideas. Behavioral changes related to altered mental functions include irritability, emotional lability, flat affect, lack of initiative and spontaneity, and loss of social behavior. Alterations in consciousness may be subtle at first, progressing from slight confusion and somnolence to stupor and finally to coma. The blatant changes in consciousness, such as stupor and coma, are related to increased ICP. Tumors and the resultant edema, particularly in the frontal lobes, cause many of the cognitive deficits. Some patients seek medical care because of behavioral and cognitive changes noted by the patient or family. These changes make it difficult or impossible for the patient to continue with his or her usual lifestyle and interpersonal relationships.

HEADACHE

Headache is an early symptom in approximately one third of patients with brain tumors. The location and characteristics of the headache cover a wide range of possibilities. Headache, if present, is usually worse in the morning because of irritation, compression, or traction of the blood vessels. The area affected by the headache can be generalized or localized in the frontal or suboccipital regions. It is often described as intermittent

and not severe. As ICP rises, headache is generally bifrontal or bioccipital, regardless of the tumor location.

SEIZURES

Seizures are often the first sign of neurological deficit in patients with cancer. Generally, seizures were the presenting symptom in 20% of patients with metastatic brain tumors and occurred in an additional 10% during the course of their treatment. It has been reported in 40% of patients with malignant gliomas.

The workup necessary when evaluating the brain tumor patient who has seizures was recently reviewed by Gilbert and Armstrong (Fig. 25-2).[6] They divided the list into toxic or metabolic and structural factors. Metabolic factors include electrolyte abnormalities, liver or renal failure, or a direct result of chemotherapeutic agents. Structural causes include parenchymal metastases, dural metastases, or leptomeningeal disease. Additionally, hemorrhage, thrombosis, or infectious meningitis can cause seizures in the patient with known brain tumor.

The cerebral edema and alterations in the normal electrical potential of cells caused by the tumor result in hyperactive cells. This hyperactivity produces abnormal, paroxysmal discharges or seizure activity that may be generalized or focal. Focal seizures can be of diagnostic value by aiding the physician in the localization of the tumor. Seizure activity is seen primarily with supratentorial tumors. Many patients will experience seizures in the course of their illness. Please refer to

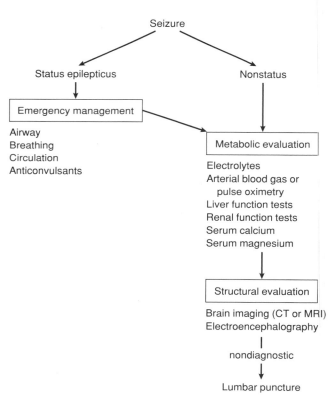

FIGURE 25-2
Algorithm for initial evaluation of patients with suspected brain tumor-based type of seizure in presenting symptoms. (MRI = magnetic resonance imaging.)

Chapter 31 for a more detailed review of seizure management and nursing implications.

VOMITING

Vomiting is most frequently seen in patients with posterior fossa tumors and is often accompanied by headache. Nausea or abdominal discomfort may accompany vomiting, although in most instances, vomiting occurs without these symptoms. Vomiting, which is unrelated to meals and occurs most commonly in the morning, can be projectile. It may be caused by direct stimulation of the vomiting center, which is located in the medulla.

TUMORS ASSOCIATED WITH GENERAL DEFICITS OF CEREBRAL FUNCTION

The tumors most likely to present with general deficits of cerebral function are astrocytoma, glioblastoma multiforme, oligodendroglioma, ependymoma, metastatic carcinoma, meningioma, and primary lymphoma.

Patients With Evidence of Increased Intracranial Pressure

Some patients with brain tumors present initially with increased ICP. The signs and symptoms associated with increased ICP are discussed in a previous section and in Chapter 17. Only localizing signs, papilledema, and obstruction to CSF flow are discussed in this section. Tumors that are likely to be associated with increased ICP are listed in Table 25-2.

LOCALIZING SIGNS

Cerebral tissue is highly specialized tissue. Encroachment on this tissue by compression or infiltration of tumor can result in localizing signs that facilitate identification of the location of the tumor within the brain. Local (focal) disturbances of normal neurological function depend on the site of the tumor. Specific limb paresis or paralysis or specific cranial nerve dysfunction (III, IV, or VI) can give the physician clues to the location of a tumor in the supratentorial area. Localizing signs of lower cranial nerve deficits (VII, VIII, IX, X, XI, or XII) relate to brain stem dysfunction. Ataxia suggests a cerebellar lesion. However, all patients will not have localizing signs, and in some instances, specific deficits can relate to increased ICP.

PAPILLEDEMA

Papilledema is seen in about 70% to 75% of patients with brain tumors. Papilledema is associated with visual changes, such as decreased visual acuity, diplopia, and deficits in the visual fields. The visual pathways extend through the lobes of the cerebral hemispheres. Therefore, it is reasonable to expect a high incidence of visual disturbances in patients with supratentorial lesions. Dysfunction of the abducens nerve (VI) is a symptom commonly seen in brain tumor lesions; it results in an inability to move the orbit outward.

It is not uncommon for a patient to state that a deterioration in vision was the main reason for referral to a neurologist. An initial appointment may have been made with the optometrist or ophthalmologist. If the examiner recognized the visual deficits as possibly reflecting a mass lesion, a referral is made to a neurologist, who would initiate a diagnostic workup.

OBSTRUCTION TO FLOW OF CEREBROSPINAL FLUID

Tumor encroachment from within or outside the ventricles or subarachnoid space interferes with the normal flow of CSF. This obstruction of CSF results in hydrocephalus. If the tumor encroachment occurs slowly, the development of an obstruction, hydrocephalus, or both will be gradual. However, rapid tumor growth produces acute precipitation of signs and symptoms, such as a massive spike in ICP with rapid deterioration in neurological status.

TUMORS ASSOCIATED WITH INCREASED INTRACRANIAL PRESSURE

Many tumors are associated with increased ICP without localizing signs. They include medulloblastoma, ependymoma of the fourth ventricle, hemangioblastoma of the cerebellum, pinealoma, colloid cyst of the third ventricle, and craniopharyngioma. These tumors are listed in Table 25-2.

Syndromes Related to Specific Cerebral Functions

Many tumors are diagnosed by the unique clinical syndrome they produce. The presenting signs and symptoms relate to dysfunction of specific anatomical areas that have unique functions, such as secretion of hormones or particular cranial nerves. Adams and Victor have identified several tumors of this type, including acoustic neuroma and other cerebellar-pontine angle tumors, pituitary adenomas, meningiomas of the sphenoid ridge and olfactory groove, glioma of the optic nerve and chiasma, pontine glioma, chordoma, and other erosive tumors of the base of the skull.[4] These tumors are listed in Table 25-2.

Signs and Symptoms Related to Tumor Areas

Regardless of the histological type, a tumor located in a specific brain area will give rise to focal signs and symptoms. The following section reviews symptoms related to specific brain areas. In addition, Table 25-3 provides nursing interventions related to brain area involved.

FRONTAL LOBE

The degree of frontal lobe deficit depends on the extent of involvement caused by the brain tumor. Unilateral involvement results in less functional loss than bilateral, and nondominant involvement produces less of a loss than if the tumor site were in the dominant hemisphere. Collectively, frontal lobe symptoms are called the *frontal lobe syndrome*. Symptoms include inappropriate behavior, inattentiveness, inability to

(text continues on page 512)

TABLE 25-2
Brain Tumors

TYPE OF TUMOR	DESCRIPTION	LOCATION OR DEMOGRAPHIC DATA	SIGNS AND SYMPTOMS	TREATMENT	PROGNOSIS
COMMON BRAIN TUMORS					
I Astrocytoma (grades I and II*) • Constitutes 25%–30% of all cerebral gliomas	• Grade I: well-defined cells • Grade II: cell differentiation less defined ↑ Cellularity	Usually found in the cerebrum, hypothalamus, and pons	Neurological deficits depend on the specific location of the tumor.	*Surgery:* complete removal is rarely possible; partial removal may prolong life; more than one excision may be done. *Irradiation:* Grade I—usually not considered because of the risk of radiation necrosis; grade II—if residual tumor is present	6–7 years on average; more years possible
II Anaplastic astrocytomas	↑ cellularity Anaplastic: cellular atypias, ↑ mitosis				* Controversial trial to compare radiation versus surgery alone closed due to poor accural
Glioblastoma multiforme (GBM) (also known as astrocytoma, grades III and IV) • Constitutes 20% of all intracranial tumors and 55% of all gliomas	• Malignant, rapidly growing • Composed of heterogenous cells (reflects frequent clinical progression from a slow- to a rapid-growing tumor) • Necrotic areas with multiple cysts and hemorrhagic areas within tumor (GBM)	Usually involves a cerebral hemisphere; more prevalent in men 40–60 years old than in women	Depend on specific location and size • Diffuse cerebral symptoms • Seizures	*Surgery:* resection and debulking to decrease ICP and relieve cerebral compression Irradiation and sometimes chemotherapy	GBM: 10-wk survival with surgery alone; 8–10 mo with XRT alone
Astrocytoma of the cerebellum (grades I–IV) • A childhood tumor	• Cystic tumor • Slow growing • Considered benign if completely excised	Cerebellar region; found in children 5–9 years old	• Paralysis of the abducens CN (outward gaze) • Paresis/paralysis of the facial CN • Hemiplegia • Sensory loss • Gaze disorders • Cerebellar dysfunction (ataxia/incoordination)	*Surgery:* removal is possible with grade I or II *Irradiation:* if the tumor is inaccessible or only partially resected *Shunting procedure:* may be necessary with ↑ ICP	Excellent with complete removal; 7–10 y for those with partial resection
Astrocytoma of the optic nerves and chiasma (spongioblastoma) • Most common in children	• As the tumor grows, it enlarges the optic foramen with little distortion of the surrounding structures • Slow-growing tumor	Found along the optic nerves; girls are affected twice as often as boys	Early symptoms include • Dimness of vision • Hemianopia • Optic atrophy • Blindness • Proptosis • Hypothalamic imbalance	*Surgery:* removal possible but the tumor often inaccessible *Irradiation:* usually a poor response	10 y or more

(continued)

TABLE 25-2
Brain Tumors Continued

TYPE OF TUMOR	DESCRIPTION	LOCATION OR DEMOGRAPHIC DATA	SIGNS AND SYMPTOMS	TREATMENT	PROGNOSIS
Ependymoma (grades I–IV) • A tumor of childhood and young adults • More benign form, astroblastoma; more malignant form, ependymoblastoma	• A glioma arising from the lining of the ventricles • Slow-growing tumor	In ventricles, particularly the fourth; can attach itself to the roof or floor of the ventricle or grow directly into the cerebral hemisphere with little or no attachment to the ventricles	Rapid elevation in ICP secondary to obstruction of CSF flow • ↓ Level of consciousness • Pupillary changes • Hemiplegia • Sensory deficits • Vital sign changes (respiration, bradycardia) • ↑ Blood pressure and widening of pulse pressure • Ataxia or incoordination (cerebellar dysfunction) • Seizures	*Surgery:* removal if surgically accessible, depending on the location *Irradiation:* for some *Chemotherapy:* for some *Shunting procedure:* may be necessary to reduce ↑ ICP from obstruction of CSF flow Interleuken 1-beta converting enzyme (ICE) regimen or high-dose cyclophosphamide	1 mo for malignant tumors; 7–8 y for benign neoplasms • About 50% of patients alive at 1 y • About 13% of patients alive at 10 y
Oligodendroglioma (grades I–IV)	• Calcification noted on radiological examination in about 50% of patients • Slow-growing tumor	Cerebral hemispheres, particularly the frontal and temporal lobes; found in patients 20–40 years old	Depend on actual location of the tumor; seizures are the first symptoms in 50% of patients	Surgery, irradiation, or both	5 y or more
Mixed gliomas • May be named for the predominant tumor cell present	• Composed histologically of two or more cell types of astrocytoma/ glioblastoma, oligodendroglioma, or ependymoma in any combination	Any place where the various glioma types can be found; if glioblastoma cells are present, tumor usually malignant	Depend on the actual location of the tumor	Depends on the type of tumor; surgery or irradiation usual treatment	1–2 y if glioblastoma cells present
Medulloblastoma • A childhood tumor	• Rapidly growing tumor that can obstruct CSF flow • Seeding into the third and lateral ventricles, cisterna magna, and along the spinal cord common	Almost exclusively in the cerebellar vermis; the tumor occupies the fourth ventricle and infiltrates its floor; males are affected most frequently; affects patients 3–5 years old	Visual disturbances first to be noted (child is squinting); rapidly elevated ICP because of obstruction of CSF; ataxia and incoordination (cerebellar dysfunction)	*Surgery:* partial dissection *Irradiation:* tumor highly radiosensitive; entire head and spinal cord irradiated because of seeding of malignant cells through CSF *Shunting procedure:* may be necessary with ↑ ICP *Chemotherapy:* with surgery or irradiation	5 y
Meningioma	• Firm, encapsulated tumor arising from arachnoid granulations/ meninges	Predilection for areas proximal to the venous sinuses.	Neurological deficits caused by compression that depend on the area involved	*Surgery:* complete removal, if possible, or partial dissection	Excellent with total removal; many years with partial excision and irradiation

(continued)

TABLE 25-2
Brain Tumors Continued

TYPE OF TUMOR	DESCRIPTION	LOCATION OR DEMOGRAPHIC DATA	SIGNS AND SYMPTOMS	TREATMENT	PROGNOSIS
	• Slow-growing; can become large before symptoms appear • Rarely malignant • Causes compression of the brain	Frequent sites include: • Superior saggital sinus • Over convexities • At sphenoid ridge • On anterior fossa floor • In posterior fossa Most common in women; average age, 50 y		*Irradiation:* with surgery if complete removal is not possible Current trials with chemotherapy for malignant meningiomas	
Metastatic brain tumors	• 10% of all brain tumors metastatic from other parts of the body (lungs, breast, stomach, lower GI tract, pancreas, and kidney) • Spread to the brain by blood • Usually well differentiated from the rest of the brain	Anywhere; individual tumor or multiple tumors throughout subarachnoid space	Depend on location	*Surgery:* resection if possible; may treat with steroids first and monitor by CT scan; if lesion is singular, surgery is considered *Irradiation:* in conjunction with surgery • Gamma knife radiosurgery (for ≤ three lesions)	Poor; however, metastatic tumors from the kidney often good prognosis
Malignant melanomas		Cerebral hemispheres from a primary lesion in the skin	Depend on location	Surgery, irradiation, chemotherapy	Unpredictable; a few months to a few years
Primary cerebral lymphoma (Note: secondary cerebral lymphomas may be seen in patients with AIDS.)	• Cellular tumor • Behaves much like a glioblastoma • Occurs in adults	May arise in any part of the brain, may be either monofocal or multifocal	• Behavioral and personality changes • Focal signs • Seen on CT scan or MRI	Radiation and steroid therapy effective • Rapid response to steroids • Current chemotherapy trials in effect (methotrexate chop)	After the initial response, a relapse occurs; average survival, 2 y
CEREBELLOPONTINE ANGLE TUMORS*					
Miscellaneous astrocytomas and meningiomas	• Can be indistinguishable from an acoustic neuroma without visualization • Meningiomas, mixed gliomas, or cerebral aneurysms also in this region • Definitive diagnosis made by surgical exposure and histological examination	Cerebellopontine angle	Variation of those seen with acoustic neuroma (below)	*Surgery:* if possible; difficult surgical access (near vital centers) *Irradiation:* may be selected over surgery	Depends on the type of tumor

(continued)

TABLE 25-2
Brain Tumors Continued

TYPE OF TUMOR	DESCRIPTION	LOCATION OR DEMOGRAPHIC DATA	SIGNS AND SYMPTOMS	TREATMENT	PROGNOSIS
Acoustic neuroma (schwannoma)	• Arises from the sheath of Schwann cells • Size of a pea to that of a walnut • Considered a benign tumor but located in an often inaccessible area • Bilateral tumors occasionally found • Slow-growing tumors • Tumor may entwine other cranial nerves that would cause *severe* deficits if the tumor were completely excised. • Bilateral tumors are possible; when they occur, they are due to a hereditary problem of chromosome 22; the tumors are part of central neurofibromatosis.	• Seen most often in the fourth or fifth decades Involves vestibular branch of CN VIII • *Small* tumors are confined to the internal auditory canal and involve CN VIII. • *Larger* tumors extend outside the internal auditory meatus. • These tumors displace CN VII and compress CN V along with CN VIII; they may also encroach on CN IX and CN X, and possibly the cerebellum.	Depend on size; deficits noted on the affected side *Small tumor (confined to internal auditory canal):* *CN VIII* • Tinnitus/vertigo • Hearing loss; most notable when using a telephone or when the source of sound is close to the affected ear • Dizziness *Large tumor (outside the auditory meatus):* Includes signs and symptoms listed above and the following: *CN VII (facial nerve)* • Loss of taste to anterior tongue • Difficulty closing lower eyelid • Facial weakness* • Decreased or absent corneal reflex *CN V (trigeminal nerve)* • Paresthesia/anesthesia to face • Difficulty chewing *CNs IX and X (glossopharyngeal and vagus nerves)* • Difficulty swallowing • Hoarseness *Cerebellar involvement* • Ataxia/incoordination • Hydrocephalus may occur with larger tumors • ↑ ICP from obstruction of CSF flow secondary to displacement of pons and medulla	*Surgery:* microsurgical technique for complete removal or debulking of larger tumors (debulking to preserve cranial nerves involved in the tumors) • Suboccipital retrosigmoid approach for smaller tumors • Translabyrinthine approach for larger tumors *Irradiation:* focused radiation (proton beam, gamma knife) alternative in older patients; scar tissue a possible problem if surgery is necessary at a later date. Also being used in other patients * *Note:* Change in facial nerve function is important to observe in the postoperative period; a *facial nerve grading system* on a scale of I (normal) to VI (total paralysis) is useful to evaluate change. (*For further information see:* House, J. W. & Brackmann, D. E. [1985]. Facial nerve grading system. *Otolaryngology, 93*(2), 146–147.)	• Excellent with small tumors that are completely removed; generally good outcome (benign tumor) • Tumor regrowth possible if removal is not complete • Some patients— permanent hearing loss, loss of facial sensation on the affected side, or facial droop
Chordoma	• Arises from remnants of the embryonic notochord • May appear as a cerebellopontine angle tumor • Affects men more frequently than women • Occurs in patients in their 30s and 40s	Found in clivus (35%) dorsum of sellae to foramen magnum and sacrococcygeal area (50%)	• Loss of vision • Paralysis of the extraocular muscle • Paralysis of the pharyngeal muscles of swallowing • Noted on MRI or CT scan	*Surgery:* excision (approach varies depending on tumor location) *Irradiation:* • Conventional • Proton beam	Tumors tend to recur; poor prognosis with aggressive and metastatic tumors

(continued)

TABLE 25-2
Brain Tumors Continued

TYPE OF TUMOR	DESCRIPTION	LOCATION OR DEMOGRAPHIC DATA	SIGNS AND SYMPTOMS	TREATMENT	PROGNOSIS
PITUITARY TUMORS					

Pituitary adenomas*	• Classified by the type of hormones(s) secreted
	—Prolactin-secreting (60%–70% of all tumor)
	—Growth hormone-secreting (10%–15% of all tumors)
	—ACTH-secreting
	• Classified by function
	—Nonfunctioning: produce symptoms as a result of pressure on adjacent structures (*e.g.,* optic nerves, bitemporal hemianopia)
	—Functioning (or hormone-secreting): cause endocrine syndromes (*e.g.,* Cushing's hyperprolactinemia, acromegaly)
	• Classified by grade of sella turcica enlargement or erosion (Hardy)
	—Enclosed adenomas
	  I—sella normal; floor may be indented
	  II—sella enlarged, floor intact
	  III—invasive adenomas; localized erosion of the floor
	  IV—entire floor diffusely eroded
	• Classified by suprasellar extension (Hardy)
	—A: no suprasellar extension
	—B: suprasellar bulge does not reach the floor of the third ventricle
	—C: Tumor reaches the third ventricle, distorting chiasmatic recess
	—D: Tumor fills the third ventricle almost to the foramen of Monro
		Pituitary gland; most pituitary tumors in the anterior lobe; both lobes can be damaged from parasellar tumors that crowd the pituitary gland	*In general:*
			• Visual disorders
			—Diminished vision (↑ scotoma)
			—Bitemporal hemianopia
			• Paresis of extraocular muscles
			• Headache
			• Various endocrine disorders (see below)
			• Abnormal sella turcica region or CT scan
			Endocrine disorders:
			• Prolactin-secreting adenoma
			—Galactorrhea
			—Amenorrhea
			—Infertility
			—Loss of pubic hair
			—Impotence
			—↑ Serum prolactin levels
			• ACTH-secreting adenoma
			—Adrenal hyperplasia
			—Cushing's syndrome
			  • Moon facies
			  • Buffalo hump
			  • Abdominal striae
			  • Pendulous abdomen
			  • Ecchymoses
			  • Hypertension
			  • Muscle weakness
			  • Osteoporosis
			  • ↑ Cortisol levels
			• Growth hormone-secreting adenoma
			—Giantism before puberty or closure of epiphyses
			—Acromegaly after puberty or closure of epiphyses
			  • Enlarged jaw, nose, tongue, hands, feet
				Depends on the size and type of the tumor, patient's age, and endocrine and visual deficits; surgery, irradiation, or drug therapy singularly or combined
				Surgery:
				• For smaller tumors, transsphenoidal microsurgery to remove total tumor and preserve or normalize pituitary; conventional radiation therapy to follow
				• For large tumors, transfrontal craniotomy for removal, follwed by irradiation
				Radiation:
				• Proton beam irradiation, if available
				• Conventional radiation therapy
				Hormonal replacement:
				• After surgery, hormonal replacement possibly necessary
				Other drug treatment:
				• Bromocriptine may be used to inhibit prolactin; in some cases, this may be all that is given for prolactin-secreting tumors.
					Very good to excellent

(continued)

TABLE 25-2
Brain Tumors Continued

TYPE OF TUMOR	DESCRIPTION	LOCATION OR DEMOGRAPHIC DATA	SIGNS AND SYMPTOMS	TREATMENT	PROGNOSIS
			• Thickening of soft tissue of facial features • Enlarged heart and pulmonary disease • Diabetes mellitus • Serum growth hormone levels >10 ng/mL *Serious complications:* • Pituitary apoplexy syndrome—acute onset of ophthalmoplegia, blindness, drowsiness, and coma; death possible		
DEVELOPMENTAL TUMORS					
Craniopharyngioma	• Thought to arise from Rathke's pouch • Solid or cystic tumors • Can compress the pituitary and may even amputate the pituitary stalk • About 75% with calcified areas • Tumor growth is directed upward, resulting in invagination of the third ventricle and possible blockage of CSF flow • Optic chiasm elevated as a result of tumor, resulting in traction on optic nerves	In or about the sella pituitary; usually affects children	• Signs and symptoms of grossly ↑ ICP because of CSF blockage • Pituitary or hypothalamic dysfunction • Visual disturbance	*Surgery:* resection by intracranial or transsphenoid approach *Irradiation:* after surgery; tumor radiosensitive	• Excellent if tumor is excised • With microsurgery, cure rate, 80% • Recurrence if only subtotal resection, even with irradiation
Epidermoid and dermoid cysts	Cysts of congenital origin arising from the ectodermal layer; cysts lined with stratified squamous epithelium; epidermoid cysts contain keratin, cellular debris, and cholesterol; dermoid cysts contain hair and sebaceous glands	On bones of skull or within brain	Depend on location	*Surgery:* complete removal is usually possible	Very good

(continued)

TABLE 25-2
Brain Tumors Continued

TYPE OF TUMOR	DESCRIPTION	LOCATION OR DEMOGRAPHIC DATA	SIGNS AND SYMPTOMS	TREATMENT	PROGNOSIS
GENETICALLY RELATED AUTOSOMAL DOMINANT DISEASES					
Von Recklinghausen's disease (neurofibromatosis)	• Genetic origin because of autosomal dominant mendelian trait • Skin, nervous system, bones, endocrine glands, and other organs are sites of congenital anomalies, in addition to the multiple tumors of skin • Firm, encapsulated lesions attach to the nerve	Benign, multiple, circumscribed dermal and neural tumors with increased skin pigmentation (cosmetically offensive); tumors late in childhood or in early adolescence	Spots of hyperpigmentation (café au lait) and cutaneous and subcutaneous tumors	*Surgery:* possible, depending on the location of the tumor *Irradiation:* tumor is radioresistant	Depends on the area involved
Hemangioblastoma (with von Hippel-Lindau disease)	• Vascular tumor • Slow-growing	• Cerebellum (as a single or multiple lesion); less common in the medulla and cerebral hemispheres; tumor in adults	• Dizziness • Unilateral ataxia • Signs and symptoms of ↑ ICP • Possible spinal cord involvement	*Surgery:* complete removal, if possible *Irradiation:* with recurrence	Usually curable

(ICP = intracranial pressure; CN = cranial nerve; ↑ = increased; ↓ = decreased; CSF = cerebrospinal fluid; GI = gastrointestinal; CT = computed tomography; AIDS = acquired immunodeficiency syndrome; MRI = magnetic resonance imaging; ACTH = adrenocorticotropic hormone.)

* Classification includes several types of tumors; the name refers to the anatomical location of the tumor.

concentrate, emotional lability, indifference, loss of self restraint, inappropriate social behavior, impairment of recent memory, difficulty with abstraction, and a quiet but flat affect.

In addition to the frontal lobe syndrome, other possible symptoms include headache (bilateral frontal region); difficulty expressing oneself in words or in writing (expressive aphasia); slowness of movement and generalized responses (abulia); incontinence caused by lack of social control; hemiparesis of hemiplegia; seizure activity, particularly focal seizures; and conjugate eye deviation. In addition, primitive reflexes, such as the grasp and sucking reflexes, may be present in patients with bifrontal tumors.

PARIETAL LOBE

The parietal lobe contains the sensory discrimination and association areas for body orientation, vision, and language. The collage of symptoms associated with parietal lobe dysfunction is called the *parietal lobe syndrome.* Common symptoms include the following:

- Hyperesthesia (impaired sensation with decreased response to tactile sensitivity)
- Paresthesia (abnormal sensation involving tingling, crawling, or burning of the skin)

- Loss of two-point discrimination (unable to determine by feeling if the skin is touched by one or two points simultaneously)
- Astereognosis (inability to recognize an object by feeling its size and shape)
- Autotopagnosia (inability to locate or recognize parts of the body)
- Anosognosia (loss of awareness or denial of the motor and sensory defect in the affected parts of the body)
- Disorientation of external environmental space (a tendency to ignore the part of the environment opposite to the cerebral lesion)
- Finger agnosia (inability to identify or select specific fingers of the hands)
- Loss of right-left discrimination
- Agraphia (loss of ability to write)
- Acalculia (difficulty in calculating numbers)
- Construction apraxia (if asked to draw an object, such as the face of a clock, ignoring the side opposite to the cerebral lesion)
- Possible homonymous hemianopia (loss of half of the visual field in each field so that the inner half is affected in one field and the outer half is involved in the other field)

If the lesion is in the dominant hemisphere and is located in the left angular gyrus of the parietal lobe, Gerstmann's syn-

TABLE 25-3
Nursing Interventions Based on Tumor Location

TUMOR LOCATION AND DEFICIT	INTERVENTIONS
Frontal lobe unilateral: Left—right hemiplegia, nonfluent dysphagia Right—left hemiplegia, mood disturbances Bifrontal—bilateral hemiplegia, impaired intellect, dementia, or emotional lability Temporal lobe: Nondominant—minor perceptual and spatial disturbances, temporal lobe seizures Dominant—dysnomia, receptive aphasia, temporal lobe seizures	—Social service consultation —Physical therapy/occupational therapy (PT/OT) consultations (for appropriate exercises, assistive devices—foot orthotics, quad cane or walker) —Education related to causes of mood disturbances; motor deficits —Psychology or psychiatry consultation for counseling or appropriate antidepressant medication —Education regarding seizure management at home, anticonvulsant medication —Speech therapy consultation
Parietal lobe: Nondominant—seizure activity, construction apraxia, astereognosis Dominant—hyperesthesia/paresthesia, agraphia, acalculi, expressive aphasia, finger agnosia, loss of right-left discrimination, seizures	—Education regarding deficits that exist —Cognitive retraining —Speech therapy consultation —Education regarding seizure management and anticonvulsants used
Occipital lobe: Contralateral homonymous hemianopsia (visual loss in half of each visual field on the side opposite the lesion) Visual hallucinations Seizures	—Education regarding existence of deficits —PT consultation to teach visual scanning techniques —Education regarding seizure management, anticonvulsants used
Cerebellum: Ataxia, incoordination Signs of increased intracranial pressure (headache, vomiting)	—Assessment for occurrence of deficits and effect on activities of daily living —PT consultation for assistive devices —Antiemetics as ordered
Brain stem: Cranial nerve deficits Dysphagia Vomiting Corticospinal/sensory tract dysfunction	—Assessment of cranial nerve (CN) function —CN II–IV and VI: Ophthalmological consultation; PT consultation for safe ambulation —CN VI: Speech therapy consultation if facial asymmetry affects speech or eating —CN IX–X: Assessment of swallowing, ability to manage secretions; speech therapy and dietary consultations —Vomiting: Assessment for timing, amount, contributing activities; changes in eating pattern; antiemetics as ordered Sensory/motor: assessment for occurrence: PT/OT consultation as needed

drome may be present (finger agnosia, loss of right-left discrimination, acalculia, and agraphia). Seizure activity is also possible with a parietal lobe lesion.

TEMPORAL LOBE

Neoplasms of the temporal lobe often result in psychomotor seizures. Focal symptoms tend to be few and uncertain, and signs and symptoms of increased ICP occur late in the illness. Loss in the upper quadrant opposite the lesion and psychomotor seizures are common findings. Psychomotor seizures may begin with an aura of peculiar sensations of the abdomen, epigastrium, or thorax. Psychomotor seizures are described as visual, auditory, or olfactory hallucinations; automatism; and amnesia for events of the attack. If the dominant lobe is involved, receptive aphasia caused by encroachment of Wernicke's area is possible. Total destruction of the temporal lobe

results in mental changes, such as irritability, depression, poor judgment, and childish behavior.

OCCIPITAL LOBE

Tumors of the occipital lobe are infrequent compared with lesions involving the other cerebral lobes. When neoplasms do occur, the symptoms tend to be associated with vision. Symptoms include contralateral homonymous hemianopia (visual loss in half of each visual field on the side opposite the lesion), visual hallucinations, and possible focal or generalized seizures.

PITUITARY AND HYPOTHALAMUS REGION

The pituitary gland and hypothalamus are closely related by location and hormonal production. Common symptoms resulting from tumors in these areas are visual deficit caused by optic atrophy and paralysis of one or more of the extraocular muscles, headache, and hormonal dysfunction of the pituitary gland with the subsequent precipitation of various syndromes, such as Cushing's syndrome, giantism, acromegaly, and hypopituitarism. In addition, tumors of the hypothalamus can affect fat and carbohydrate metabolism, water balance, sleep patterns, appetite, and sexual behavior.

LATERAL AND THIRD VENTRICLE

If the tumor remains small, the patient may be asymptomatic. If the tumor grows into the cerebral hemispheres, deficits will depend on the particular function of the area involved. Tumors that grow within the ventricle may become of sufficient size to obstruct the flow of CSF. If this occurs, headache, vomiting, and other symptoms of rapidly increased ICP will be noted. The patient may experience relief of symptoms by changing the position of the head. In this case, the position of the obstructing tumor is altered, thereby allowing the normal CSF flow pattern to be re-established.

FOURTH VENTRICLE

Tumors of the fourth ventricle obstruct the flow of CSF and infiltrate and compress the brain stem or cerebellum. Headache, vomiting, and nuchal rigidity are common symptoms. Sudden death caused by compression of the cardiorespiratory center is possible. The lower cranial nerves, which control the gag and swallowing reflexes, become impaired, making aspiration a constant concern.

MIDBRAIN

Neoplasms of the midbrain are rare. If present, they may result in occlusion of the cerebral aqueducts, cerebellar symptoms if the red nucleus is involved, Parinaud's syndrome (conjugate paralysis of upward gaze) if the quadrigeminal plate is involved, abnormal posturing, and ptosis and diminished light reflex as the tumor enlarges.

BRAIN STEM

Tumors in the brain stem tend to be invasive and to spread up and down the neural axis. Symptoms include dysfunction of the lower cranial nerves, corticospinal and sensory tract deficits, cerebellar dysfunction, dysphagia, and vomiting throughout the illness. As with fourth ventricle tumors, sudden death can occur from encroachment on vital centers (respiratory or cardiac arrest).

CEREBELLUM

Growth of a tumor in the cerebellar area is accompanied by cerebellar signs (ataxia, incoordination, cerebellar seizures), obstruction of flow of CSF, and possible brain stem compression. The usual signs of increased ICP (headache, vomiting, classical changes in vital signs) are common, particularly with CSF obstruction.

MEDICAL APPROACH TO THE PATIENT WITH A BRAIN TUMOR

Diagnosis

There are no classic signs and symptoms of a brain tumor. The clinical manifestations span a wide range of signs and symptoms, depending on the type, size, and location of the tumor. After a neurological examination, the physician usually orders a computed tomography (CT) scan (Fig. 25-3) or magnetic resonance imaging. In most instances, either one of these diag-

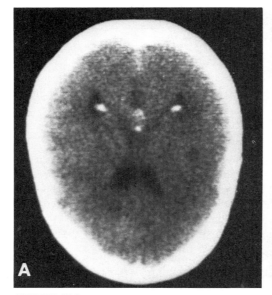 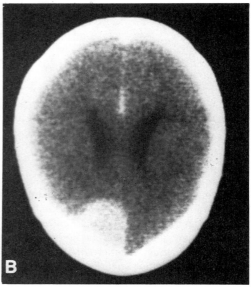

FIGURE 25-3
Computed tomography (CT) scan of brain. (*A*) Normal scan. (*B*) Scan showing a large mass in the left frontal lobe.

nostic procedures will identify a brain tumor, if present. Tissue diagnosis, either by stereotactic biopsy or open craniotomy, is most often needed to determine diagnosis.

To evaluate a brain tumor and related conditions further and to assist in selecting the best treatment, other diagnostic studies may be ordered:

- *Cerebral angiography* is helpful for outlining the vascularity within the brain. Information about encroachment of a tumor on blood vessels and the vascular pattern of a tumor can be helpful in deciding the best surgical approach.
- *Visual field and funduscopic examination* allows careful examination of the visual field and provides much information for localizing the lesion. Because the visual pathways encompass portions of the cerebral lobes, visual defects that are specific to particular areas can be detected. A funduscopic examination is included to determine evidence of papilledema, a common sign in brain tumor.
- *Audiometric studies* are helpful in determining hearing loss, especially when evaluating a tumor such as an acoustic neuroma.
- *Chest films* rule out lung cancer and detect metastatic lesions to the brain that originate in the lungs.
- *Other studies rule out a primary lesion outside the brain.* A variety of tests can be ordered before craniotomy if there is any question of a metastatic brain tumor. Some examples include chest, abdominal, or pelvic CT; bone marrow biopsy; or mammography in women.
- *Endocrine studies* are helpful when a pituitary adenoma or a craniopharyngioma is suspected; blood and urine levels of hormones controlled by the pituitary gland are evaluated. Common tests and their normal values include the following:
  Prolactin
      Premenopausal women: 2.2 to 19.2 mEq/L
      Postmenopausal women: 1.0 to 12.8 mEq/L
      Men: 1.9 to 11.7 mEq/L
  Growth hormone
      Women: 0 to 30 ng/mL
      Men: 0 to 8 ng/mL
  Cortisol
      6:00 to 8:00 AM: 10 to 25 g/L
      4:00 to 6:00 PM: less than 10 g/L
  17-ketosteroids (in urine)
      Women: 6 to 15 mg/24 h
      Men: 8 to 20 mg/24 h
  17-hydrocorticosteroids (in urine)
      4 to 12 mg/24 h

Once a brain tumor has been found, a needle biopsy may be performed to identify the specific tumor type and the grade and to make appropriate treatment decisions. Using CT-guided stereotactic technique, a needle biopsy may be attempted for tumors deep in the cerebral hemispheres or basal ganglion. Tumors that are vascular or located near vital centers may not be candidates for biopsy for fear of precipitating hemorrhage or respiratory distress. The major drawback of a needle biopsy is in the sampling of gliomas. The biopsy results may reveal a low-grade tumor when, in fact, the major portion of the tumor is of a much higher grade (glioblastomas are a mixture of low-grade and mostly high-grade cells).

Medical Treatment

Once the diagnosis of a brain tumor is established, the next major consideration is medical management. The three general methods for treatment of brain tumors are surgery, irradiation, and chemotherapy. These modalities can be used alone or in any combination. The variables that are considered when selecting appropriate treatment include the type of tumor, its location and size, related symptoms, and the general condition of the patient. Informed consent for treatment must include the patient in the decision-making process.

DRUG THERAPY

Most patients benefit from administration of a corticosteroid (dexamethasone, prednisone, or methylprednisolone), which decreases cerebral edema. The reversal of symptoms can be remarkable. In the case of a central nervous system (CNS) lymphoma, complete resolution of the enhancing tumor on scan can occur within weeks of initiating corticosteroids (although this is often a transient effect). A corticosteroid is usually begun when the tumor is diagnosed and the presence of cerebral edema and increased ICP is confirmed. If surgery is recommended, dexamethasone is administered preoperatively, continued postoperatively, and given with chemotherapy and during radiation therapy to control radiation-induced edema. Compliance with this medication is crucial, so proper education on administration and prevention of potential side effects is crucial. Known side effects include gastritis, peptic ulcer disease, alterations in healing, increased blood glucose levels, fluid retention (most commonly called "moon face" and "buffalo hump"), and steroid-induced proximal myopathy. An H2 blocker (such as Pepcid or Zantac) must be administered when a patient is on corticosteroids. Judicious dosing to ameliorate symptoms while limiting side effects is crucial.

Most patients with supratentorial lesions will be placed on anticonvulsant medications to prevent seizures. Phenytoin and carbamazepine are good first-line agents to use. If the patient is to be treated with chemotherapy, phenytoin should be used, because carbamezapene can potentiate thrombocytopenia associated with chemotherapeutic agents.[6] In some instances, polypharmacy is necessary to obtain adequate seizure control. Phenobarbital and Neurotin can both be added to the primary anticonvulsant in an attempt to obtain seizure control. Proper dosing and knowledge of signs of toxicity are important, because a toxic phenytoin level can mimic signs of increased tumor growth. Table 25-4 provides an overview of common chemotherapeutic drugs currently in use for the treatment of brain tumors.

CONVENTIONAL SURGERY

In most instances, surgery is the last step in positive diagnosis of a brain tumor. Examination of the tissue biopsy by the pathologist will identify the tumor histologically and give a clue to the prognosis. However, malignancy and surgical accessibility are equally important when judging prognosis. Some tumors, although histologically benign, cannot be completely removed; nonetheless, even a partial resection will relieve symptoms temporarily. If the tumor is a slow-growing neo-

TABLE 25-4
Chemotherapeutic Drugs Commonly Used to Treat Brain Tumors

DRUG AND CLASSIFICATION	EARLY OR DELAYED TOXICITY	LABORATORY MONITORING	NURSING RESPONSIBILITIES
Carmustine (BCNU) • Major drug used in treatment of malignant brain tumors • Cell cycle nonspecific • Nitrosourcas: causes breaks and cross-linking in DNA strands • Crosses the blood–brain barrier (BBB)	Early • Nausea and vomiting • Local phlebitis Delayed • Bone marrow depression in 3–6 wk • Pulmonary fibrosis (may be irreversible) with doses >200 mg/m² IV • Renal and liver damage • Veno-occlusive disease (hepatic or pulmonary) with high doses	Baseline data • Weekly monitoring of CBC and BUN, creatinine, uric acid, SGOT, SGPT, and alkaline phosphatase levels • Periodic chest x-ray studies	• Administer antiemetics before and during drug administration. • Apply ice to puncture site. • Protect the patient from and monitor for infections. • Monitor for respiratory, liver, and kidney dysfunction.
Lomustine (CCNU) • Cell cycle nonspecific • Nitrosourea • Similar to BCNU	Early • Nausea and vomiting Delayed • Bone marrow depression (may be prolonged) • Elevated SGOT level • Pulmonary fibrosis • Renal damage	Baseline data Same as for BCNU	• Same as for BCNU
Cisplatin (Platinol) • Heavy metal compound • Exact mechanism of action unknown; appears to bind DNA • Cell cycle nonspecific	Early • Nausea and vomiting • Anaphylactic reactions • Fever • Electrolyte imbalances Delayed • Renal damage • Ototoxicity • Peripheral neuropathy • Bone marrow depression • Electrolyte imbalance • Hypocalcemia	Baseline data Weekly monitoring of CBC and BUN, creatinine, electrolyte, and calcium levels	• Administer antiemetics as necessary. • Hydrate well. • Monitor intake and output. • Assess for hearing loss. • Assess for numbness or tingling of fingers and toes. • Monitor hearing. • Monitor the patient for electrolyte imbalance.
Procarbazine hydrochloride • Exact mechanism of action is unclear; probably inhibits protein, RNA, and DNA synthesis • Given orally • Rapidly absorbed • Crossed BBB	Early • Nausea and vomiting • CNS depression Delayed • Bone marrow depression • Stomatitis • Peripheral neuropathy • Pneumonia • Interaction with tryamine in food: hypertensive crisis	Baseline data • CBC monitored weekly • Chest x-ray studies	• This is usually given as 28-d course (usually for first 72 h). • Administer antiemetics as necessary. • Monitor for signs of neurotoxicity. • Monitor the patient for and protection from infection. • Teach avoidance of foods high in tyramine (e.g., beer, ripe and aged cheeses) • Teach avoidance of alcohol use (can cause severe GI toxicity because of Antabuse-like drug activity). • Provide for special mouth care. • Monitor peripheral nerve function. • Monitor the patient for respiratory problems.
Etoposide (VePesid) • Also called VP16 • Cell cycle nonspecific • Appears to interfere with synthesis of DNA or RNA	Early • Nausea and vomiting • Red urine (not hematuria) • Diarrhea • Fever • Hypotension	Urinalysis	• Administer antimetics as necessary. • Monitor vital signs. • Monitor the color of the urine.

(continued)

TABLE 25-4
Chemotherapeutic Drugs Commonly Used to Treat Brain Tumors Continued

DRUG AND CLASSIFICATION	EARLY OR DELAYED TOXICITY	LABORATORY MONITORING	NURSING RESPONSIBILITIES
	Delayed • Bone marrow depression • Alopecia • Peripheral neuropathy • Mucositis • Hepatic damage	CBC and SGOT and SGPT levels monitored weekly	• Monitor the patient for and protect from infection. • Prepare the patient for hair loss; support positive body image. • Monitor peripheral nerve function.

CBC = complete blood count; BUN = blood urea nitrogen; SGOT = serum glutamic-oxaloacetic transaminase; SGPT = serum glutamate pyruvate transaminase; GI = gastrointestinal; CNS = central nervous system.)

plasm, as with meningiomas, the patient may be asymptomatic for years.

The role of stereotactic biopsy versus a debulking craniotomy for malignant tumors remains controversial. No study to date shows a true survival benefit for extensive surgery. The intraoperative risks of stereotactic biopsy are extremely low (<5%). Conversely, if ICP is increased or the risk of herniation is great, biopsy will do nothing to decrease the potential for harm. Obstruction of CSF flow may require a shunting procedure to relieve CSF pressure. The nursing care is the same as for the craniotomy patient. See Chapter 18 for general principles of surgical intervention.

LASER SURGERY

Laser surgery is increasingly being used to treat brain tumors. Use of lasers may be combined with conventional surgery to treat the patient. Laser therapy alone may also be suggested.

Tumors that have been treated with lasers include acoustic neuromas, craniopharyngiomas, some brain stem gliomas, pinealomas, ventricular tumors, meningiomas of the brain and spinal cord, and neuromas of the spinal cord. The advantage of using lasers for treatment of brain tumors is that they enable the neurosurgeon to dissect or shrink tumors without inflicting injury on surrounding tissue. Areas of the brain formerly inaccessible to the neurosurgeon are now accessible by this indirect means. Although lasers have limitations, they are an important treatment modality for brain tumors.

RADIATION THERAPY

The objective of radiation therapy is to destroy tumor cells without injuring normal ones. Tumor cells are more radiosensitive than are nontumor cells. A course of radiation treatment can increase survival rates after surgery. The treatment dose for the tumor depends on several variables, including histological type, radioresponsiveness, location, and level of tolerance.

The histological identification of a tumor aids in anticipating the treatment needs and prognosis of the patient. The following types of tumors are generally amenable to radiation therapy: medulloblastoma, any metastatic lesions, deep and centrally located tumors that would create permanent major neurological deficits from dissection if surgery were attempted, and some tumors involving vital areas (*e.g.*, pons, medulla) that would cause high mortality rates if surgical resection were attempted.

Tumor resection is never complete with malignant gliomas. This tumor type is infiltrative, and even if the surgeon removes all visible tumor, there is often microscopic spread into normal parenchyma. A course of postoperative radiation therapy may be recommended for the following tumors: astrocytoma, grades II, III, and IV (grades III and IV are also known as glioblastoma multiforme); ependymoma; oligodendroglioma; sarcoma; craniopharyngioma; and chordoma.

With a conventional radiation protocol, the amount of radiation is based on individual differences previously cited. The total tumor dose range is usually from 4,000 to 7,000 rad, administered over 4 to 8 weeks. The area to be irradiated depends on the anatomical extent of the tumor. Current radiation field recommendations for malignant gliomas are to be delivered to the tumor plus edema plus a 2 cm margin. Many patients improve remarkably from their symptoms after surgical decompression and irradiation. If irradiation is not preceded by surgery, large doses of corticosteroid may be used as an adjunct to reverse temporarily and control symptoms of increased ICP.

Unfortunately, not all patients respond well to radiotherapy. In some, radiation-induced edema exacerbates an already elevated ICP. The result is an increase in symptoms, which could be falsely interpreted as the progression of tumor growth. In other patients, a recurrence of symptoms is evident within approximately 6 months. Radiation-induced necrosis can be the cause, but it may be difficult to differentiate from tumor progression.

Radiation therapy, alone or as adjunctive therapy with surgery, presents special nursing management problems. If the course of radiation therapy is to follow surgery, the incision is allowed to heal well before radiation is begun. For the patient, diagnosis and treatment of a brain tumor are a period of great physiological, emotional, and psychological stress. Irradiation is often the treatment of choice for tumors that are surgically inaccessible or for remnants of tumors that cannot be excised completely by surgery. The patient is usually advised by the physician of his or her prognosis and the benefits anticipated from radiation therapy. Also discussed are the possible side effects that might be experienced as a result of the treatment.

Proton beam irradiation has been used successfully to treat some tumors (*e.g.*, chordomas). However, only two centers have this technology available, so it is not considered a routine treatment modality. The *gamma knife* is a newer radiation therapy that can be used alone or in combination with intracranial surgery. It is available only at major centers.

Problems Related to Radiation Therapy. A problem with radiation therapy is the failure of complete annihilation of malignant cells. Persistence of malignant cells after radiation therapy has been attributed, in part, to the presence of hypoxic cells. Hypoxic cells are still viable and are approximately three times more resistant to radiation than are well-oxygenated cells.[7] Increasing the dosage of radiation to destroy these cells could cause serious damage and radiation necrosis to other tissue. To counteract the problem of hypoxia, various protocols have been developed that include use of hyperbaric oxygen during irradiation, hypoxic cell radiation sensitizers (drugs), and high linear energy transfer radiation, such as neutrons.[7] These protocols have had limited success and are not considered to be mainstream radiation management.

The limiting factor in the use of radiation therapy is cerebral cell intolerance with resulting necrosis. The total dose of radiation is administered in divided doses over 4 to 6 weeks. The incidence of radiation necrosis is inversely related to the number of fractional doses. Based on this premise, some physicians increase the number of times the patient receives treatment, thus decreasing the dosage of radiation per treatment. This means that the patient is scheduled to receive one dose of radiation therapy 5 days a week or even twice a day. For some debilitated patients, this is an intolerable schedule.

Other approaches to radiation therapy include interstitial brachytherapy and heating of the tumor. *Interstitial brachytherapy* is high-dose focal irradiation using implanted radioactive isotopes for limited periods. CT stereotactic technique is used for precise location of the implantation site. Finally, heat, at a nonlethal temperature, sensitizes cells to irradiation. Implantation of a microwave probe or electrodes provides localized heating. All of the treatment variations for radiation therapy mentioned are controversial. They are attempts to improve the outcome for patients who have few treatment options.

CHEMOTHERAPY

Although chemotherapy (see Table 25-4) has been the mainstay of treatment for a variety of other malignancies, its use in brain tumor treatment has been sporadic at best. The purpose of chemotherapy is to destroy tumor cells, either by destroying actual cells or affecting their ability to replicate. Chemotherapeutic agents are classified into cell cycle-specific agents (only active during certain phases of the cell's life cycle) and cell cycle-nonspecific (effective during all phases of the cell cycle). The dosage of drug that can safely be given to a patient is limited by how much damage is expected to be incurred by normal cells, such as bone marrow. This is called *dose-limiting toxicity.*

Special concerns when treating a malignant lesion of the brain and using chemotherapeutic agents include the following:[5,8]

- Wide excision of a brain tumor is not possible because there is no excess tissue within the brain, and regeneration is not possible within the brain.
- Wide excision of glial tumors is not possible because the tumor has infiltrated normal brain tissue, although this cannot be seen by scan.
- The location of the tumor in the brain affects choice of treatment.
- Cerebral edema affects drug entry into the tumor.
- Brain tissue has a low capacity to remove dead tissue, cell debris, fluid, and drugs because there is no lymphatic drainage in the brain.
- Tumor cell resistance (when tumor cells are no longer susceptible to damage by a particular drug) can occur.
- Brain tumors rarely metastasize outside the CNS.
- Malignant tumors (GBM) are composed of diverse (heterogeneous) cells; this results in differences in the chemosensitivity of cells within the tumor.
- Many drugs cannot cross the blood–brain barrier.

Development of New Drugs. The development of new drugs and new methods of delivery for treatment of malignant brain tumors includes preclinical testing and clinical investigation. Preclinical testing involves laboratory study on rodents. If preclinical testing indicates that a drug is probably effective and can be administered safely to humans, clinical investigation begins and is divided into four phases:

- Phase I establishes an optimal safe dose and defines toxicity.
- Phases II determines the action of the drug against specific tumors.
- Phase III compares the new drug with standard therapy for a specific tumor.
- Phase IV adopts the new treatment as part of standard treatment.

The limited use of chemotherapy in brain tumors is likely to be related to the inability of certain drugs to get through the blood–brain barrier. One group of agents, the nitrosureas, can penetrate this barrier and have formed the basis of most chemotherapeutic regimens for glial tumors. High-grade glial tumors (anaplastic astrocytomas and glioblastoma multiforme) have had the emphasis of chemotherapeutic trials due to the high incidence rate and aggressive nature.

Standard treatment has most commonly included carmustine (BCNU) or lomustine (CCNU) given either immediately following or concurrently with radiation therapy. Response rates have been reported as high as 30% to 40%. Unfortunately, a recent review by Upchurch et al. using more stringent criteria has shown this response to be 5% to 7%.[9] In an effort to increase effectiveness, other agents have been tried either with a nitrosurea or as a single agent (procarbazine, vincristine, cisplatin, and diaziquone as examples). Combination agents as listed, given in the adjuvant setting after radiation therapy, have not significantly increased response rates.[10]

In an effort to increase response rate, many novel agents and methods of delivery have been tried. Methods that have undergone clinical trials include intra-arterial delivery, bioerodable polymers, blood–brain barrier disruption, bone marrow transplantation, and biological response modifiers.

INTRA-ARTERIAL CHEMOTHERAPY. The purpose of this trial was to increase delivery of the drug to the tumor while limiting systemic toxicity. Initial studies involved placing catheters in the internal carotid arteries with direct instillation of several agents (most commonly BCNU and CCNU). These initial studies resulted in severe ophthalmological toxicities, because the drug streamed into the first branch of the carotid, the ophthalmic artery.[11,12] Subsequent studies have been completed placing the catheter above the ophthalmic artery.[13] Unfortunately, a phenomenon known as "streaming" occurred. This occurs when the drug is unable to mix with the pulsatile arterial blood, resulting in most of the drug entering the first branch reached off of the artery. Severe toxicity occurred if this branch entered normal brain, with necrosis of tissue and resultant neurotoxicity. This was found to occur in 20% of patients in one study.[13] A randomized trial revealed no apparent benefit of intra-arterial BCNU versus intravenous BCNU.[14]

BIODEGRADABLE POLYMERS. The purpose of this trial was again to deliver high concentrations of drug to the tumor with reduced systemic toxicity. During craniotomy, polyanhydride compounds impregnated with BCNU were placed into the tumor cavity. Initial studies were promising. However, a phase III study comparing BCNU impregnated versus plain polymers showed a survival benefit to the BCNU group of only 8 weeks.[15]

BLOOD–BRAIN BARRIER DISRUPTION. Disruption of the blood–brain barrier is another technique attempted to improve drug delivery directly to the tumor. This technique uses intra-arterial mannitol to open transiently the blood–brain barrier, in combination with either intra-arterial or intravenous chemotherapy. Clinical trials have shown modest tumor responses with a high incidence of neurotoxicity. Neuwalt et al. (1986) described a 56% incidence of seizures, a 58% incidence of transient neurological deficit, and an 8% incidence of permanent neurological deficit.[16]

BONE MARROW TRANSPLANTATION. Initial studies using autologous bone marrow transplantation with nitrosureas as a preparatory regimen were limited by severe systemic toxicity, in particular, pulmonary and hepatic fibrosis. Other agents, such as VP-16 have also been tried, but with modest response rates (19% partial response rate).[17] More recent studies are underway using Thiotepa as a preparative regimen. These studies are still underway, and the impact is uncertain.

BIOLOGICAL RESPONSE MODIFIERS. Immunotherapy has been used in an attempt to help the body fight tumors that are often treatment resistant. Local delivery of interleukin-2 and LAK cells into the brain tumor bed showed little effect.[18] Other immunotherapies, such as gamma-interferon, beta-inteferon,

and antiglioma antibody treatment, have shown little survival benefit over conventional chemotherapy.[19]

Future Directions. Current clinical trials are focusing on chemotherapy or gene therapy as "up-front" treatment of glial tumors. Agents currently being used include continuous infusion chemotherapy, paclitaxel (Taxol), phenylacetic acid, and the thymidine-kinase gene. How these novel agents and approaches will affect standard treatment is unclear.

Prognosis

For patients with malignant brain tumors who are treated with surgery alone, the median survival rate is 17 weeks. If surgery and radiation therapy are combined, the median survival is 37.5 weeks. The addition of BCNU chemotherapy does not increase median survival, but it does increase the number of survivors from 4% to 19% at 18 months. These data have become the standard for judging other clinical trials.

Patients with extracerebral brain tumors and low-grade gliomas have varied cure, remission, and survival rates (see Table 25-2).

NURSING MANAGEMENT OF THE PATIENT WITH A BRAIN TUMOR

An Overview

It is difficult to be specific about the nursing management of the patient with a brain tumor. The basis for nursing management is the nursing history and neurological assessment. Physical care will depend on the deficits experienced by the patient. The patient is monitored for changes that indicate deterioration in neurological function. Modifications in the plan of care reflect the changing needs of the patient.

The responses of the patient and family to a brain tumor are influenced by the type, grade, location, and presenting symptoms of the tumor. They are also influenced by the age, disabilities, family dynamics, and coping skills of the patient and family. Patients and families have an ongoing need for information and emotional support, which should be addressed by the nurse as part of the management plan.

Knowledge Deficit is the appropriate nursing diagnosis for addressing informational needs. The nursing intervention for Knowledge Deficit is an individualized teaching plan for the patient and family. It includes information about the medical plan of care, management of present deficits and disabilities, and future needs. Helpful information concerning brain tumors in general, treatment of brain tumors, coping with brain tumors, and other related topics is available in publications from the Association for Brain Tumor Research. In addition, the U.S. Department of Health and Human Services and the National Institutes of Health provide brochures on brain tumors.

The nurse can provide ongoing support for the emotional needs of the patient and family members. Common nursing diagnoses related to emotional needs include the following:

- Fear
- Anxiety
- Personal Identity Disturbance
- Anticipatory Grieving
- Dysfunctional Grieving
- Altered Role Performance
- Social Isolation
- Impaired Social Interaction
- Altered Family Processes
- Impaired Adjustment
- Ineffective Individual and Family Coping
- Ineffective Denial

Nursing interventions are based on individual needs. In addition, referrals are made to appropriate and available resources. Patients and family members should be made aware of brain tumor support groups.

In medical and nursing management of the patient with a brain tumor, quality of life for the patient is an ongoing concern. The *Karnofsky Performance Status Scale* (KPS) is a widely used scale to quantify the functional status of cancer patients.[20] Functional status is an indicator of quality of life. The KPS is an 11-point rating scale that ranges from normal functioning (100) to dead (0). The increment from one category to another is 10 points (*e.g.*, 10, 20, 30). Loss of function is viewed as being related to the cumulative physical, physiological, and psychological effects of the illness. The KPS is helpful for monitoring the patient's quality of life over time.

Nursing Management During Diagnosis

Although one of the nurse's main responsibilities during this diagnostic period is to provide information about the tests to be conducted, the possibility of a brain tumor can subject the patient to extreme emotional stress. The impact of such a diagnosis depends on the patient's ability to comprehend what the diagnosis means and how it will affect his or her life. A patient who has an altered level of consciousness or impaired mental functions may not grasp the total impact of the situation but may react merely to the strangeness of the hospital environment, confinement to bed, or loneliness. However, patients who can comprehend their situation are most apt to demonstrate profound behavioral responses.

The patient who understands what is happening may initially deny the diagnosis. If this is the case, the patient will refuse to consider treatment, so informed consent is impossible. If the patient does accept the diagnosis, he or she may react with anger and hostility. Fear of death, vegetation, and mutilation and loss of independence and mental functions are terrifying concerns. Mental images of other people with similar diagnoses may loom in the patient's mind and threaten body image and self-concept. A sense of powerlessness can overwhelm the patient.

A positive, supportive approach on the part of the nurse can help the patient cope with the reality of the condition. The patient should be encouraged to ask questions and express his or her feelings about the situation. The nurse should provide realistic reassurance for the patient's prospects as an intact, total person. At the same time, the patient should be included in the decision-making process as often as possible.

Several organizations provide information related to treatment options and support. Several of these organizations are listed below:

- National Brain Tumor Foundation, 800-934-CURE
- American Brain Tumor Association, 800-886-2282
- American Cancer Society, 800-ACS-2345
- Cancer Information Service, 800-4-CANCER

Nursing Management Before and After Surgery

Nursing management specific to the surgery is the same as that outlined for other intracranial surgical procedures in Chapter 18.

Nursing Management During Irradiation

As the patient's advocate, the nurse facilitates obtaining satisfactory answers to the patient's questions. If the patient's level of consciousness or mental functions have been impaired, the family will be afforded help so that informed consent can be ensured. The nurse's role during radiation therapy is to provide emotional support to the patient and family, assess patient needs, manage side effects of treatment, and provide general comfort and hygienic needs.

The specific nursing responsibilities during radiation therapy include the following:

1. Prior to the start of treatment, inform the patient and family of the various activities that will occur in the radiation therapy department. As with most patient preparation of this kind, informing the patient of what to expect will help allay any fears caused by unfamiliarity with the procedure.
2. Provide proper skin care of the irradiation site. Radiation dermatitis can be anticipated (the epidural layer is denuded in a 4- to 6-week period). The skin becomes reddened, tanned, and desquamated. Because the skin is sensitive, do not rub, apply tape, expose to sunlight, or apply alcohol, powder, cream, or cosmetics. The skin markings used to localize radiation exposure should not be washed off.
3. If the patient suffers from nausea, vomiting, or diarrhea, administer antiemetics and antidiarrheal agents as necessary.
4. To manage anorexia, offer small portions of food that are easy to digest and liked by the patient.
5. For general malaise, schedule activities to allow for rest periods.
6. Note the results of complete blood counts, with special attention to white blood cell and platelet counts. Bone marrow depression decreases platelets, which in turn increases the possibility of hemorrhage (petechiae, purpura, nosebleeds, or most critical, intratumoral hemorrhage).

CHART 25-1
Summary of Common Nursing Diagnoses Made for Patients Undergoing Irradiation or Chemotherapy for Treatment of a Brain Tumor

Nursing Diagnosis	Nursing Interventions	Expected Outcome(s)
Knowledge Deficit related to (R/T) purpose, method, and goals of treatment protocol	• Ask the patient to tell you his or her understanding of the treatment protocol. • Clarify misconceptions. • Expand on areas of partial understanding. • Introduce new information as necessary. • Encourage the patient to ask questions. • Refer questions to a resource person, as necessary. • Develop a written teaching plan.	The patient will be able to verbalize and describe the purpose, goals, and method of administering the prescribed protocol.
Anxiety R/T approaching or current treatment	• Observe the patient for verbal and nonverbal cues indicating anxiety. • Provide emotional support. • Anticipate the needs of the patient.	The patient's anxiety will be reduced or controlled.
Altered comfort: acute nausea/vomiting R/T chemotherapy	• Assess the patient for nausea. • Provide small, frequent feedings that are easy to digest. • Administer antiemetics as ordered (prophylactically and as necessary). • Give nothing by mouth if vomiting occurs. • Offer mouth care frequently	Nausea will be controlled or minimized; vomiting will be absent or controlled.
Altered Nutrition: Less than body requirements, R/T nausea and vomiting	• Assess the patient's nutritional intake on a 24-hour basis. • Assess the patient's dietary likes and dislikes. • Offer small meals frequently (choose easy-to-digest foods).	The patient will maintain adequate nutritional intake.
Altered Oral Mucous Membrane, R/T stomatitis	• Provide frequent mouth care. • Administer a soothing oral rinse or topical solution for oral comfort, such as glycerin swabs or viscous Xylocaine suspension, as directed. • Avoid irritating foods, such as citrus fruits. • Provide a soft, bland diet.	Discomfort from stomatitis will be eliminated or controlled.
Body Image Disturbance R/T hair loss	• Discuss the cause of alopecia, as well as the regrowth process. • Provide for meticulous personal hygiene. • Encourage female patients to use make-up and wear attractive head coverings. • Suggest the use of wigs when the patient is able to wear one. • Correct any misconceptions. • Allow the patient to verbalize feelings.	The patient will accept altered body image.
Fatigue R/T chemotherapy or irradiaion	• Allow the patient to express his or her feelings about general malaise. • Encourage and plan a schedule that allows for frequent rest periods. • Assess the patient's ability to perform activities of daily living (ADLs). • Provide for frequent rest periods. • Adjust the patient's schedule as necessary to conserve energy.	The feeling of fatigue will be minimized by frequent rest periods.

(continued)

CHART 25-1 Summary of Common Nursing Diagnoses Made for Patients Undergoing Irradiation or Chemotherapy for Treatment of a Brain Tumor (Continued)

Nursing Diagnosis	Nursing Interventions	Expected Outcome(s)
Altered Cerebral Perfusion R/T cerebral edema	• Assess the patient's neurological signs periodically. • Identify any signs of neurological deterioration; report any such changes to the physician, and document findings in record. • Elevate the head of the bed 30 degrees. • Administer drugs and other protocols as ordered. • Continue to monitor the patient.	Neurological changes will be identified early and definitive action taken to control deterioration.
Risk for Infection R/T bone marrow depression	• Protect the patient from exposure to infections. • Monitor the patient for signs and symptoms of infection. • Teach the patient and family the meaning of a decreased white blood cell count and nadir.	The patient and family will verbalize an understanding of preventive measures.
Risk for Injury R/T thrombocytopenia	• Monitor the complete blood count (white blood count, platelet count) and coagulation study results. • Be aware of and discuss with the patient delayed onset of bone marrow suppression (after 3 wk). • Assess the patient for occult bleeding (stools, urine, gastric). • Assess the patient for easy bruising, pretechial bleeding, nosebleeds, and bleeding from the gums.	The patient and family will verbalize an understanding of the precautions against and the risk factors for injury.
Risk for Impaired Skin Integrity R/T radiation-induced dermatitis (With radiation dermatitis, the skin becomes reddened, tanned, desquamatized, and sensitive.)	• Institute special precautions for skin care at the site of irradiation. • Protect the skin from rubbing, application of tape, and exposure to sunlight. • Do not use alcohol, powder, cream, or cosmetics on this area. • Do not wash off the skin markings used to localize the radiation exposure site.	Skin integrity will be maintained.
Knowledge Deficit R/T discharge and follow-up care	• Develop a written teaching plan for discharge. • Stress the importance of follow-up care. • Provide a written list of signs and symptoms that should be reported to the physician. • Caution against use of any drugs (*e.g.,* aspirin) without prior approval of the physician. • Help the patient understand that some side effects of the treatment have a delayed onset. • Arrange for a follow-up appointment.	The patient will verbalize an understanding of the discharge plans and care.

* Note: Some of the nursing diagnoses listed may not apply to all patients; however, those identified are inclusive of major nursing concerns.

7. Monitor neurological signs for indications of increased ICP.
8. Provide emotional support by reassuring the patient that side effects will resolve once the treatment is completed.

See Chart 25-1 for a summary of common nursing diagnoses.

Nursing Management During Chemotherapy

As previously discussed, the role of chemotherapy is increasingly at the forefront of treatment for patients with metastatic CNS tumors, especially malignant gliomas. The nurse should know what drugs the patient is receiving and the common side effects that are related to specific drugs.

University of Pittsburgh Medical Center

<u>Clinical Pathway Name:</u> 1st Cycle BCNU/Cisplatin for Primary
Brain Tumors

Admission Date _____ Time _____ Discharge Date _____
Expected Length of Stay ___ 4 __ days Actual Length of Stay _____ days
Pre-Admission Call Made By: _____ Date: _____
Care Manager _____ Primary Nurse _____

The clinical pathway is a collaborative care plan and is not intended to be construed or to
serve as a standard of medical care. Rather, it is intended to serve as a guideline to promote coordination and communication with respect to patient care, and may be modified to
meet individualized care needs. Individualized care needs are to be noted on the appropriate portion of the form.

Imprint Patient Identification Plate Here

Collaborative Care Plan	Date: Pre-Admission	*	Date: Day 1, Unit: _____	*	Date: Day 2, Unit: _____	*
1. Consults Initials:	a) Surgery (line placement) b) Social work		a) Notify Case Manager b) Home Health Coordinator c) Check if ordered: PT ___ OT ___ PMR ___		a) Check if ordered: PT ___ OT ___ PMR ___	
2. Tests Initials:	a) MRI of head b) Lytes, Bun, Creatinine, Ca, Mg, Alk, Phos c) Bilirubin (total & direct) d) SGOT, GGTP, LDH, TP/Alb, UA e) Anticonvulsant level f) CBC, diff, platelets, PT, PTT g) EKG, Chest x-ray				a) Lytes, Bun, Creatinine b) Ca, Mg c) Anticonvulsant level (pre-dose)	
3. Treatments Initials:			a) Double lumen implanted port inserted b) Double lumen port accessed in OR c) I & O		a) I & O d) PT if ordered b) AM weight e) OT if ordered c) PM weight f) PMR if ordered	
4. Medications Initials:	a) Anti-convulsant _____ 24˙ dose _____ b) Dexamethasone _____ mg c) H-2 blocker po BID		a) Begin IV hydration b) Anticonvulsant and 24˙ dose as per pre-admission c) Dexamethasone as per admission d) H-2 blocker po BID		a) IV hydration b) Cisplatin 40 mg/m^2 c) Carmustine (BCNU) 40 mg/m^2 d) Zofran IV 10 mg q 8˙ e) Lasix IV given for AM weight gain f) Lasix IV given for PM weight gain g) Anticonvulsant and 24˙ dose as per pre-admission h) Dexamethasone as per admission i) H-2 blocker po BID	
5. Nutrition Initials:			a) Baseline diet _____ _____		a) Nutrition High Risk Assessment b) Baseline diet	
6. Activity/Safety Initials:			a) Activity as per baseline _____ _____		a) Activity as per baseline b) Excretion safety	
7. Assessment Initials:	a) Outpatient assessment b) Communication form completed c) History and physical		a) No evidence of DVT b) Neurological deficits: _____ _____ _____ c) WBC > 3.0 and platelets > 100,000 d) Port site without redness e) Port site without edema f) Steri-strips intact to port pocket g) Steri-strips intact to neck h) Blood return from both lumens of port		a) Nausea and vomiting controlled b) No evidence of DVT c) No change in neurological deficits d) Port site without redness e) Port site without edema f) Steri-strips intact to port pocket g) Steri-strips intact to neck h) Blood return from both lumens of port	
8. Discharge Planning Initials:	a) Insurance coverage for neupogen available b) Supply and delivery of neupogen avail.		a) No discharge problems anticipated b) Patient and family aware of LOS c) Patient and family aware of treatment schedule d) Patient and family reviewed clinical path		a) No discharge problems anticipated b) Treatment plan reviewed with patient and family c) Patient and family understand clinical path	
9. Psycho/Social Initials:			a) Patient/family able to verbalize feelings associated with diagnosis/treatment			
10. Patient Education Patient/Significant Other to understand: Initials:			a) Definition, action, individual nature, and rationale for treatment b) Symptoms to report during chemotherapy administration		a) Standard of care for patients experiencing nausea & vomiting followed b) Standard of care for patients receiving cytotoxic agents followed c) Symptoms to report during chemotherapy administration	

˙ Indicates Individualized Care Needs (ICN)   Indicates Completion   Initial(s)/Signature(s) On Back
FORM   ITEM   PAGE 1

FIGURE 25-4

Clinical pathway for patients with malignant gliomas undergoing continuous infusion of carmustine and
cisplatin. *(continued)*

University of Pittsburgh Medical Center

Clinical Pathway Name: 1st Cycle BCNU/Cisplatin for Primary Brain Tumors

Patient Name _____

Social Security Number _____

Imprint Patient Identification Plate Here

The clinical pathway is a collaborative care plan and is not intended to be construed or to serve as a standard of medical care. Rather, it is intended to serve as a guideline to promote coordination and communication with respect to patient care, and may be modified to meet individualized care needs. Individualized care needs are to be noted on the appropriate portion of the form.

Collaborative Care Plan	Date: Day 3, Unit: _____	*	Date: Day 4, Unit: _____	*	Date: Day 5, Unit: _____	*
1. Consults Initials:	a) Check if ordered: PT ___ OT ___ PMR ___		a) Check if ordered: PT ___ OT ___ PMR ___		a) Check if ordered: PT ___ OT ___ PMR ___	
2. Tests Initials:	a) Lytes, BUN, Creatnine b) Ca, Mg c) Anticonvulsant level (pre-dose)		a) CBC, diff, platelets b) Lytes, BUN, creatnine c) Ca, Mg d) Anticonvulsant level (pre-dose)		a) Lytes, Bun, creatnine b) Ca, Mg c) Anticonvulsant level (pre-dose)	
3. Treatments Initials:	a) I & O b) AM weight c) PM weight d) PT if ordered e) OT if ordered f) PMR if ordered		a) I & O b) AM weight c) PM weight d) PT if ordered e) OT if ordered f) PMR if ordered		a) I & O b) AM weight c) Both lumens of port irrigated and deaccessed d) PT if ordered e) OT if ordered f) PMR if ordered	
4. Medications Initials:	a) IV hydration b) Cisplatin 40 mg/m^2 c) Carmustine (BCNU) 40 mg/m^2 d) Zofran IV 10mg q 8* e) Lasix IV given for AM weight gain f) Lasix IV given for PM weight gain g) Anticonvulsant and 24* dose as per pre-admission h) Dexamethasone as per admission i) H-2 blocker po BID j) Haldol IV 1 mg q 8 hours k) Ativan IV 0.5mg q 8 hours prn		a) IV hydration b) Cisplatin 40 mg/m^2 c) Carmustine (BCNU) 40 mg/m^2 d) Zofran IV 10mg q 8* e) Lasix IV given for AM weight gain f) Lasix IV given for PM weight gain g) Anticonvulsant and 24* dose as per pre-admission h) Dexamethasone as per admission i) H-2 blocker po BID j) Haldol IV 1 mg q 8 hours k) Ativan IV 0.5mg q 8 hours prn		a) Post-chemo hydration b) Zofran IV q 8* c) Lasix IV given for AM weight gain d) Anticonvulsant and dose as per pre-admission e) Dexamethasone f) H-2 blocker po BID g) Haldol IV 1 mg q 8 hours h) Ativan IV 0.5mg q 8 hours prn	
5. Nutrition Initials:	a) Baseline diet b) Nutrition screening completed		a) Baseline diet		a) Baseline diet	
6. Activity/Safety Initials:	a) Activity as per baseline b) Excretion safety		a) Activity as per baseline b) Excretion safety		a) Activity as per baseline b) Excretion safety	
7. Assessment Initials:	a) Nausea and vomiting controlled b) No evidence of DVT c) No change in neurological deficits d) Port site without redness e) Port site without edema f) Steri-strips intact to port pocket g) Steri-strips intact to neck h) Blood return from both lumens of port		a) Nausea and vomiting controlled b) No evidence of DVT c) No change in neurological deficits d) Port site without redness e) Port site without edema f) Steri-strips intact to port pocket g) Steri-strips intact to neck h) Blood return from both lumens of port		a) Nausea and vomiting controlled b) No evidence of DVT c) No change in neurological deficits d) Port site without redness e) Port site without edema f) Steri-strips intact to port pocket g) Steri-strips intact to neck h) Blood return from both lumens of port	
8. Discharge Planning Initials:	a) Patient and family understand clinical path		a) Home health services verified b) Patient and family understand clinical pathway c) Patient and family prepared for discharge		a) Patient discharged with individualized calendar b) Arrangements made for outpatient labs	
9. Psycho/Social Initials:	a) Significant other involved in care b) Patient/family adjusting to neuro. deficits				a) High risk Social Work assessment completed _____ (date)	
10. Patient Education Patient/Significant Other to understand: Initials:	a) Standard of care for patients experiencing nausea & vomiting followed b) Standard of care for patients receiving cytotoxic agents followed c) Symptoms to report during chemotherapy administration		a) Standard of care for patients experiencing nausea & vomiting followed b) Standard of care for patients receiving cytotoxic agents followed c) Symptoms to report during chemotherapy administration		a) Standard of care for patients experiencing nausea & vomiting followed b) Standard of care for patients receiving cytotoxic agents followed c) Excretion safety precautions d) When to remove steri-strips e) Signs of bone marrow depression f) Symptoms to report to health care team	

* Indicates Individualized Care Needs (ICN)   Indicates Completion   Initial(s)/Signature(s) On Back

FORM   ITEM   PAGE 2

FIGURE 25-4 *(Continued)*

The patient and family should also be aware of this information. The most common side effects of intravenous chemotherapy include nausea, vomiting, diarrhea, stomatitis, anorexia, alopecia, and bone marrow depression (see Chart 25-1). Novel approaches to delivering chemotherapy result in individualized side effects. These are reviewed in the discussion of treatment.

In addition, some collaborative activities involve the nurse and physician. These include monitoring of vital signs and specific laboratory data and monitoring of the patient's response to the chemotherapy. The specific laboratory data will depend on the toxicity of the drug, which may involve the kidney, liver, blood, or lungs. The use of clinical pathways to streamline care delivery is at the forefront of care today. Figure 25-4 is a clinical pathway developed specifically for patients with malignant gliomas undergoing an intravenous chemotherapy protocol. This pathway has several advantages: Care is standardized and streamlined; a cost savings of $500 per patient has been obtained; and areas of high resource use (such as urokinase administration for central lines with withdrawal occlusion) have been realized.

Summary

The nursing management for the patient with a brain tumor spans a wide variety of circumstances, situations, and treatment modalities. Perhaps no role is more important than that of providing sensitive, supportive care of the patient and family.

References

1. Murphy, G. (Ed.) (1995). Cancer Statistics, 1995. *CA: A Cancer Journal For Clinicians, 45*(1), 12–13.
2. Walker, A. E., Robins, M., & Weinfeld, F. D. (1985). Epidemiology of brain tumors: The national survey of intracranial neoplasms. *Neurology, 35,* 219–226.
3. Barr, M. L., & Kiernan, J. A. (1988). *The human nervous system: An anatomical viewpoint* (5th ed.) (p. 4). Philadelphia: J.B. Lippincott.
4. Adams, R. D., & Victor, M. (1993). *Principles of neurology* (5th ed.). New York: McGraw-Hill.
5. Burger, P. C. (1986). Malignant astrocytic neoplasms: Classification, pathologic anatomy, and response to treatment. *Seminars in Oncology, 13*(1), 16–26.
6. Gilbert, M., & Armstrong, T. (1995). Management of seizures in the adult patient with cancer. *Cancer Practice, 3*(3), 143–149.
7. Nelson, D. F., Urtasum, R. C., Saunders, W. M., Gutin, P. H., & Sheline, G. (1986). Recent and current investigations of radiation therapy of malignant gliomas. *Seminars in Oncology, 13*(1), 46–55.
8. Shapiro, W. R., & Shapiro, J. R. (1986). Principles of brain tumor chemotherapy. *Seminars in Oncology, 13*(1), 56–69.
9. Upchurch, C., Goodwin, W., Brown, T., Selby, G., Vogel, F., & Eyre, H. (1993). Assessment of response to new agents for CNS malignancies. *Proceedings Annual Meeting American Society Clinical Oncology, 12*(abstract), 176.
10. Levin, V., Wara, W., Davis, R. et al. (1985). Phase III comparison of BCNU and the combination of procarbazine, CCNU and vincristine administered after radiotherapy with hydroxyurea for malignant gliomas. *Journal of Neurosurgery, 63,* 218–223.
11. Elsas, T., Watne, K., Fostad, K., & Hager, B. (1989). Ocular complications after intracarotid BCNU for intracranial tumors. *Acta Ophthalmology (Copenh), 67,* 83–86.
12. Maiese, K., Walker, R., Gargan, R., & Victor, J. (1992). Intracranial-arterial cisplatin-associated optic and otic toxicity. *Archives of Neurology, 49,* 83–86.
13. Foo, S., Choi, I., Berenstein, A., Wise, A., Ransohoff, J., Koslow, M., George, A., Lin, J., Feigin, I., Budzilovich, G. et al. (1986). Suraophthalmic intracarotid infusion of BCNU for malignant glioma. *Neurology, 36,* 1437–1444.
14. Shapiro, W., Green, S., Burger, P., Selker, R., VanGilder, J., Robertson, J., Mealey, J., Ransohff, J., & Mahaley, M. (1992). A randomized comparison of intra-arterial versus intravenous BCNU, with or without intravenous 5-flourouracil, for newly diagnosed patients with malignant glioma. *Journal of Neurosurgery, 76,* 772–781.
15. Brem, H., Mahaley, M., Vick, N., Black, K., Schold, S., Burger, P., Friedman, A., Ciric, I., Eller, T., Cozzens, J. et al. (1991). Interstitial chemotherapy with drug polymer implants for the treatment of recurrent gliomas. *Journal of Neurosurgery, 74,* 441–446.
16. Neuwalt, E., Howieson, J., Frenkel, E., Sprecht, H., Weigel, R., Buchan, C., & Hill, S. (1986). Therapeutic efficacy of multiagent chemotherapy with drug delivery enhancement by blood-brain barrier modification in glioblastoma. *Neurosurgery, 19,* 573–582.
17. Giannone, L., & Wolff, S. (1987). Phase II treatment of central nervous system gliomas with highdose etoposide and autologous bone marrow transplantation. *Cancer Treatment Report, 17,* 759–761.
18. Merchant, R., McVicar, D., Merchant, L., & Young, H. (1992). Treatment of recurrent malignant glioma by repeated intracerebral injections of human recombinant interleukin-2 alone or in combination with systemic interferon-alpha. Results of a phase I clinical trial. *Journal of Neurooncology, 12,* 75–83.
19. Jaeckle, K. (1994). Immunotherapy of malignant gliomas. *Seminars in Oncology, 21,* 249–259.
20. Mor, V., Laliberte, L., Morris, J. N., & Wiesmann, M. (1984). The Karnofsky performance status scale. *Cancer, 53,* 2002–2007.

Bibliography

Books

Salmon, S. F., & Bentino, J. (1996). Principles of cancer therapy. In J. C. Bennett & F. Plume (Eds) *Cecil Textbook of Medicine* (2nd ed.) Philadelphia: W. B. Saunders, pp. 1036–1054.

Zulch, K. L. (1986). *Brain tumors, their biology and pathology* (3rd ed.). New York: Springer Verlag.

Periodicals

Adams, B. A., Clancey, J. K., & Eddy, M. S. (1991). Malignant glioma: Current treatment perspectives. *Journal of Neuroscience Nursing, 23*(1), 15–19.

Amato, C. A. (1991). Malignant glioma: Coping with a devastating illness. *Journal of Neuroscience Nursing, 23*(1), 212–223.

Ammirati, M., Vick, N., Youlian, L., Ciric, I., & Mikhael, M. (1987). Effect of the extent of surgical resection on survival and quality of life in patients with supratentorial glioblastomas and anaplastic astrocytomas. *Neurosurgery, 21,* 201–206.

Baumann, C. K., & Zumwalt, C. B. (1989). Intracranial neoplasms. *AORN, 50*(2), 240–257.

Baumann, C. K., & Zumwalt, C. B. (1989). Volumetric interstitial hyperthermia. *AORN, 50*(2), 258–274.

Burgess, K. E. (1983). Neurological disturbance in the patient with an intracranial neoplasm: Sources and implications for nursing care. *Journal of Neurosurgical Nursing, 15*(4), 237–241.

Campbell, C. (1991). Acoustic neuroma: Nursing implications related to surgical management. *Journal of Neuroscience Nursing, 23*(1), 50–56.

Cress, N. B., Owens, B. M., & Hill, F. H. (1991). Imuvert therapy in the treatment of recurrent malignant astrocytomas: Nursing implications. *Journal of Neuroscience Nursing, 23*(1), 29–33.

Edwards, D. K., Stupperich, T. K., & Welsh, D. M. (1991). Hyperthermia treatment for malignant brain tumors. *Journal of Neuroscience Nursing, 23*(1), 34–38.

Fickel, V. D. (1991). Acoustic neuroma: Postoperative deficits and the role of the neuroscience nurse. *Journal of Neuroscience Nursing, 23*(1), 57–60.

Freidberg, S. R. (1986). Tumors of the brain. *Clinical Symposia, 38*(4), 1–35.

Hochberg, F. H., & Miller, D. C. (1988). Primary central nervous system lymphoma. *Journal of Neurosurgery, 68*, 835–53.

Krause, E. A., Lamb, S., Ham, B., Larson, D., & Gutin, P. H. (1991). Radiosurgery: A nursing perspective. *Journal of Neuroscience Nursing, 23*(1), 24–28.

Leahy, N. M. (1986). Intraarterial cisplatin infusion: Nursing implications. *Journal of Neuroscience Nursing, 18*(5), 296–301.

Lichter, A. S., & Lawrence, T. S. (1995). Recent advances in radiation oncology. *New England Journal of Medicine, 332*(6), 371–379.

Loftus, C. M., Copeland, B. R., & Carmel, P. W. (1985). Cystic supratentorial gliomas. Natural history and evaluation of modes of surgical therapy. *Neurosurgery, 17*, 19–24.

Lord, J., & Coleman, E. A. (1991). Chemotherapy for glioblastoma multiforme. *Journal of Neuroscience Nursing, 23*(1), 68–70.

Ransohoff, J., Kelly, P., & Laws, E. (1986). The role of intracranial surgery for the treatment of malignant gliomas. *Seminars in Oncology, 13*(1), 27–37.

Sorenson, S. C., Eagan, R. T., & Scott, M. (1984). Meningeal carcinomatosis in patients with primary breast or lung cancer. *Mayo Clin Proc, 59*, 91.

Willis, D. (1991). Intracranial astrocytoma: Pathology, diagnosis, and clinical presentation. *Journal of Neuroscience Nursing, 23*(1), 7–14.

CHAPTER 26

Spinal Cord Tumors

Joanne V. Hickey
Terri S. Armstrong

OVERVIEW

Primary spinal cord tumors constitute approximately 0.5% of newly diagnosed tumors and 10% to 15% of primary central nervous system neoplasms. The incidence of primary spinal cord tumors is 1 case per 100,000 per year.[1] The ratio of primary spinal cord to primary brain tumors is 1:4 to 1:8. Spinal tumors occur about equally in males and females, generally affecting those in the 20- to 50-year age range, although they can occur in other age groups. Rarely are spinal tumors found in children younger than 10 years old or in the elderly.

Classification of Spinal Cord Tumors

Spinal cord tumors can be classified according to cellular origin (primary or secondary), anatomical location on cross section, specific tumor type, and location in relation to the vertebral column.

Cellular Origin. Spinal cord tumors may be classified as either primary spinal cord tumors or secondary spinal cord tumors. **Primary tumors** arise from tissues that press upon or invade the spinal cord or surrounding spinal meninges, spinal nerves, fat, bone, or blood vessels. The cause of primary spinal cord tumors is unknown. **Secondary tumors** are metastatic tumors attributable to lesions from other parts of the body. The most common primary sites include the lung, breast, prostate, colon, and uterus.

Anatomical Location. Spinal cord tumors may be classified according to anatomical location:

Extramedullary: outside the spinal cord (about 90%)
  Extradural: outside the spinal dura; within the epidural area
  Intradural: within or under the spinal dura but not within the spinal cord
Intramedullary: within the substance of the spinal cord (about 10%)

The locations of primary spinal cord tumors are shown on cross section in Figure 26-1 and in lateral longitudinal section in Figure 26-2.

Specific Tumor Type. Extramedullary tumors account for approximately 90% of primary spinal cord tumors. In adults, extramedullary tumors are neurofibromas and meningiomas, which constitute 55% of all spinal tumors. Other tumors include sarcomas, vascular tumors, chordomas, and epidermoids. When intramedullary tumors are considered, the most common tumors are ependymomas and various grades of astrocytomas.

Location in Relation to the Vertebral Column. The distribution of spinal cord tumors by location is as follows: cervical, 30%; thoracic, 50%; and lumbosacral, 20%. It is not enough to know the general location of a tumor. Knowing the precise level helps one to correlate the dermatome with specific functional assessment for that level (see Chaps. 5 and 22). Conversely, identifying sensory deficits on examination can help to diagnose a spinal cord tumor and identify its location according to the involved dermatome.

Pathophysiology

The pathophysiological changes associated with spinal cord tumors result from *compression* and, much less frequently, *invasion* of the cord. Extramedullary tumors affect the spinal cord by compression, which can cause traction on or irritation of the spinal nerve roots, displacement of the spinal cord, interference with the spinal blood supply, or obstruction of cerebrospinal fluid (CSF) circulation. Intramedullary tumors affect the spinal cord by invasion and destruction of the spinal cord itself.

Cord compression alters the normal physiology involved in providing an adequate blood supply, maintaining stable cellular membranes, and facilitating afferent and efferent impulses for specific sensory, motor, and reflex functions of the spinal cord and related spinal nerves. Cord compression results in *edema*, which can ascend the spinal cord, causing ad-

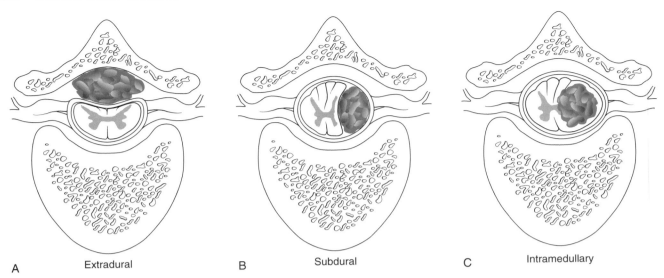

FIGURE 26-1
Location of intramedullary and extramedullary (subdural and extradural) tumors on cross-section.

ditional deficits to the sensitive cord. Control of edema is a major focus in management.

Focal (localizing) signs depend on the spinal level, the cross-section location, and the rate of growth and density of the spinal tumor.

SPINAL LEVEL

Spinal level refers to the specific location of the tumor in the cervical, thoracic, or lumbosacral area. Sensory distribution from the spinal nerves at each level is mapped via dermatome levels (see Chaps. 5 and 22). Loss of sensation will depend on the level of the tumor and correlate with dermatome levels. Motor deficits can also be related to the level of the tumor.

Motor components of various spinal nerves come together to innervate specific areas.

LOCATION OF CROSS SECTION

The major sensations conveyed by the spinal cord are light touch, pain and temperature, and position and vibration. Each sensation is carried by specific tracts located in specific areas on cross section (see Chap. 5). The **posterior columns** (fasciculus gracilis and fasciculus cuneatus) convey *position and vibration sensations*. A tumor compressing the cord from the posterior area would interfere with these modalities. The **lateral spinothalamic tracts** convey *pain and temperature*. The **anterior spinothalamic tract** conveys *light touch*. On cross section, the

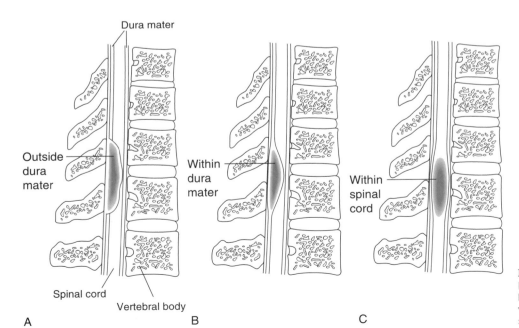

FIGURE 26-2
Locations of spinal tumors in a lateral longitudinal section of the vertebrae and spinal cord. The shaded area indicates tumor sites.

spinothalamic tracts are located in the anterolateral area of the spinal cord. Therefore, the location of the tumor on cross section will help to determine functional loss.

RATE OF GROWTH AND DENSITY

The time required for the development of neurological deficits is directly related to the tumor's rate of growth and its density (soft or hard). Slow-growing tumors allow the spinal cord to accommodate itself to the neoplasm. Many cord tumors grow very slowly over a period of years, compressing the cord into a thin, ribbon-like substance with minimal neurological deficits. However, with rapid-growing tumors, such as malignant or metastatic lesions, the cord fares poorly. The physiological response is substantial edema with major compression of the cord, possibly resulting in rapid paralysis (within a few hours).

A soft tumor can be of a consistency similar to that of the spinal cord. If soft tumors grow slowly, they cause gradual compression of the spinal cord. However, the cord's blood supply is able to respond to this alteration and adequately supply the vascular needs without interruption. The tumor adjusts to the available space for growth, becoming elongated. Neither movement of the spinal column nor normal alterations in blood flow to the cord will produce injury by contusion or ischemia. By contrast, a hard tumor will respond to movement or vascular changes with spinal contusion, ischemia, and irreversible cord damage. Hard tumors do not conform to the available space, so that encroachment of neurological function is apparent earlier than with soft tumors.

The morphological appearance of spinal cord tumors is described as encapsulated or sharply outlined. Soft tumors are irregularly elongated and can extend for two or more segments. Some tumors are cystic, requiring drainage of fluid.

Metastatic Spinal Cord Tumors

Metastatic spinal cord tumors are fairly common, and their incidence is primarily related to three factors: incidence of the primary tumor; propensity to spread to bone; and overall duration of survival for that tumor type. As mentioned previously, the most common primary sites are the lungs, breast, prostate, colon, and uterus. The malignant lesion tends to spread proximal from the primary organ affected. For example, lung and prostatic cancers tend to spread to the thoracic spine. Prostatic cancer tends to spread to the region of T-8 to T-10. Most metastatic lesions are located in the epidural space, affecting the cord by direct compression from the tumor itself or from collapse of the eroded vertebra. Edema, as a consequence of compression, increases the degree of the deficit. Infiltration of the cord does not usually occur.

Early signs and symptoms include localized back pain and radicular pain. In the intermediate stage, there will be localized tenderness over the affected vertebra, muscle weakness, sensory deficits (*e.g.*, paresthesia and decreased pain, temperature, vibration, or position sensation), possible ataxia, decreased deep tendon reflexes, absent cutaneous reflexes, sexual dysfunction (impotence), and bladder (urinary retention, urinary dribbling) and bowel (constipation) dysfunction. In the late stages, paralysis and loss of sphincter control are seen. Because most metastatic lesions affect the lower thoracic area, most signs and symptoms are related to the lower torso and lower extremities. Rapid onset of paraplegia, inability to void (urinary retention), and severe pain often bring the patient to the emergency room.

General Signs and Symptoms

The signs and symptoms experienced by the patient will depend on the anatomical location of the tumor (extramedullary or intramedullary, location on cross section), the specific tumor type, its location in relation to the vertebral column, and the specific spinal nerves involved. Focal signs and symptoms aid in determining the level of the lesion; however, they can also be indistinct, misleading, and intermittently variable.

The general signs and symptoms of spinal cord tumors can be divided into the following areas: pain, sensory deficits, motor deficits, sphincter dysfunction, and other signs.

PAIN

Ninety-five percent of patients with metastatic tumors have pain without neurological deficits as the *initial* symptoms, and 75% have neurological deficits at time of diagnosis. Pain is attributable to compression of the spinal cord or the meninges, tension/traction on the spinal nerve roots and cord, or tumor attachment to the proximal dura. The pain, which may be the only symptom of a slow-growing tumor for months or years, can be described as localized or radicular. *Localized pain and tenderness* are common over the involved area when pressure is applied to the spinous process. This is particularly true with metastatic lesions that can involve the vertebra. **Radicular pain** is described as pain within the distribution of a spinal nerve root. It is caused by compression, irritation, or tension/ traction of the nerve root. Pain can vary from mild to severe and from dull to piercing.

Any activity that increases intraspinal pressure, such as the Valsalva maneuver (as occurs with coughing, sneezing, or straining), may cause intensification and radiation of the pain. Pain can also be exaggerated by reclining, as this position stretches the spinal nerves. Because of the overlap of dermatomes supplying a particular area of the body, pain can be diffuse, mimicking such conditions as angina, an acute abdominal lesion, or intercostal neuralgia.

SENSORY DEFICITS

The specific sensory deficits will depend on the presentation of the tumor on cross section. A lateral presentation will affect pain and temperature sensation, with coldness, numbness, and tingling appearing as early symptoms. Awareness of vibration and proprioception of body parts are affected if the posterior columns are involved. Light touch sensation is preserved in the presence of a unilateral tumor because of the uncrossed and crossed components to the tract. Because the compression of a tumor will affect function below the lesion, it is important to determine the highest level of function. Sensory assessment begins at the toes and moves upward in order to determine the level at which function is intact, which is also the level of the tumor. The tumor level is often accompanied by a narrow band of hyperesthesia (abnormally increased sensitivity to stimuli) directly above it.

MOTOR DEFICITS

Paresis and paralysis develop in conjunction with sensory loss below the level of the lesion. Motor deficits are the result of involvement of the corticospinal tracts of the spinal cord. Symptoms may be overlooked in the early stages, but eventually, paresis, clumsiness, spasticity, and hyperactive reflexes become evident. If spasticity is present in the upper extremities, it may present as clumsiness. If unilateral or bilateral spasticity of the lower extremities is present, it may contribute to difficulty in ambulating and be demonstrated as ataxia. The back and spine should be palpated to note any localized tenderness, spasms, or stiffness, which can indicate the location of a tumor. A positive Babinski sign will be present. A combination of sensory and motor deficits may be seen, signifying Brown-Sequard syndrome (motor loss on the side of the lesion; loss of light touch, vibration, and position sense on the side of the lesion; and contralateral loss of pain and temperature sense).

BOWEL AND BLADDER DYSFUNCTION

The patient may have deficits involving the bowel, bladder, or both. Constipation and, later, paralytic ileus are common deficits in the bowel. Early urinary deficits may take the form of urgency or difficulty in initiating urination. Symptoms gradually progress to urinary retention.

With a cervical intramedullary tumor, *sacral sparing* may occur. Because perineal sensation is controlled by the spinothalamic tracts that are located on the periphery of the spinal cord, sensation to the perineum may be spared. With some tumors, decreased sensation and motor function of the perineum can occur, and impotence and other sexual dysfunctions are possible.

OTHER FINDINGS

As a tumor grows, it consumes all of the space around the spinal cord, thus isolating the CSF below the tumor from normal CSF circulation. Examination of the CSF reveals xanthochromia, an increased protein count, few or no cells, and immediate clotting. Collectively, these findings are called **Froin's syndrome**.

Some types of spinal cord tumor cause a syringomyelic syndrome. A fluid-filled cystic cavity (*syrinx*) is found in the central intramedullary gray matter. This syndrome causes a chronic degenerative disorder of the spinal cord accompanied by motor weakness, spasticity, and pain.

Signs and Symptoms by Tumor Location

Signs and symptoms of spinal tumors can also be considered based on the location of the tumor. Table 26-1 summarizes findings according to location of the tumor on or within the spinal cord.

DIAGNOSIS

The most critical initial component to diagnosis of a spinal cord tumor is an accurate history and physical examination. By demonstrating existing neurologic deficits, the location of spinal involvement can be ascertained and the time necessary for diagnostic testing reduced. This can be of critical importance if there is a threat of spinal instability or rapid deterioration of neurological function.

The diagnostic test of choice for patients suspected of having a spinal cord lesion is currently magnetic resonance imaging (MRI) with paramagnetic contrast enhancement (gadolinium). Other diagnostic tests such as myelography, computed tomography (CT), or plain radiograph are occasionally used to evaluate the patient. These latter tests have been most helpful in evaluating patients with suspected spinal cord compression from metastatic cancer to the spine. This is in direct contrast to patients with primary spinal cord tumors, in whom 80% to 85% of plain radiographs are normal.[2,3] CT scanning is superior to the plain radiograph or myelography for imaging the thecal sac and paraspinal soft tissue.

MRI offers the advantages of being a noninvasive, versatile procedure that allows for multiple axial and midsaggital views without radiological exposure (Fig. 26-3) and for views demonstrating intramedullary pathology (Fig. 26-4).[4] In addition, MRI is the most sensitive technique for detection of tumors in the vertebral bodies.[5] MRI of the spine is a lengthy procedure, often taking several hours if the entire spine is to be visualized. Optimal imaging requires that the patient remain motionless during the procedure, and lying flat for this amount of time can be difficult if the patient is in pain. If the patient is unable to lie still, other diagnostic tests may be ordered to obtain an accurate assessment of the spinal cord. In addition, if the patient has had prior surgery for placement of metal plates or rods, artifact produced by these devices can obscure visualization of the cord.

Spinal cord tumors are often associated with spread into the CSF and can develop from drop metastasis (Fig. 26-5). Furthermore, spread of systemic cancer into the CSF can mimic the signs and symptoms of a spinal cord tumor. Therefore, analysis of CSF by lumbar puncture is necessary to evaluate seeding of tumor cells into the CSF or to obtain a cytological diagnosis. Unfortunately, cytological evaluation is not very sensitive. Most studies report that cytology is positive on initial lumbar puncture in only 50% of cases in which there has been systemic spread. A series of three lumbar punctures increases the detection rate to 85%, and a series of five samples increases the diagnostic yield to 95%.

History and Neurological Examination

The patient will usually provide a history of progressive spinal cord involvement, as evidenced by varying degrees of motor, sensory, bowel/bladder, sexual, and reflex deficits. The progression of symptoms may be gradual or abrupt, as discussed in the previous section.

PRINCIPLES OF TREATMENT

The primary goal of treatment of patients suspected of or diagnosed with spinal cord tumors is preservation of neurological function. A combination of surgical, medical, and radiological approaches is often required. The urgency of care is determined by the degree of neurological dysfunction and the location of the lesion. For example, if a patient presents with

TABLE 26-1
Signs and Symptoms of Spinal Cord Tumors by Vertebral Level

LOCATION	SIGNS AND SYMPTOMS	COMMENTS
CERVICAL LEVELS		
C-4 and above • Especially dangerous because of innervation to the diaphragm (C1–4) and the potential effect on respirations. • High cervical tumors can affect the lower cranial nerves (VIII to XII).	• Possible respiratory difficulty • Quadriparesis or quadriplegia • Paresthesia • Occipital headache • Stiff neck • CN VIII: downbeat nystagmus • CNs IX to X: dysphagia; dysarthria • CN XI: difficulty shrugging shoulders; atrophy of shoulder and neck muscles • CN XII: deviation of tongue; difficulty speaking; unilateral tongue atrophy	Difficult surgical access; may consider proton beam therapy or another nonsurgical modality Downward gaze is controlled by pathways that extend from the brain stem to the upper cervical cord.
Below C-4	• Pain in shoulders and arms • Paresthesia • If the C5 to C6 root is involved, there will be pain along the medial aspect of the arm. • If C7 to C8 is involved, there will be pain along the outer side of the forearm and hand. • Weakness follows pain. • Atrophy of the shoulder, arm, and intrinsic hand muscles is often associated with fasciculation. • Horner's syndrome (ptosis, miosis, and anhidrosis on the affected side) • Hyperactive reflexes	Attributable to interference with sympathetic innervation
THORACIC LEVELS		
T1–12 • Most metastatic lesions involve the thoracic region.	• Pain in chest/back • Use of motor deficits to localize the lesion is difficult; spastic paresis may be evident • Sensory deficits are more accurate in identifying the lesion level: —Know landmark areas, such as T-4 (nipple line) and T-10 (umbilicus). —A band of hyperesthesia is often found above the level of the lesion. • A positive Babinski sign is noted. • Bowel and/or bladder dysfunction • Sexual dysfunction	See Chapter 22 for an explanation and illustration of dermatomes.
LUMBOSACRAL		
L-1 to S-5	• Pain in lower back, which often radiates to legs; may also be felt in the perineal area • Paresis/spasticity of lower extremities, usually in one leg and later in the other • Sensory loss in legs and/or saddle area • Bowel and/or bladder dysfunction • Sexual dysfunction • Reflexes—ankle and knee jerk reflexes are diminished or absent	• Footdrop is common. • Atrophy may affect certain muscle groups.

a mild degree of right upper extremity weakness but is found to have a cervical spine lesion, immobilization of the neck is mandatory until stability has been ascertained.

There are several goals of treatment that must be considered in patients with spinal cord tumors. These goals include preservation of neurological function; control of pain, and initiation of a treatment plan directed at tumor removal or control.

Preservation of Neurological Function

Spinal cord tumors are often associated with edema. The spinal canal is narrow and provides little space for swelling without accompanying neurological dysfunction. Extensive pressure can compromise either venous or arterial blood flow, potentially resulting in irreversible destruction of the spinal cord. The immediate institution of corticosteroids,

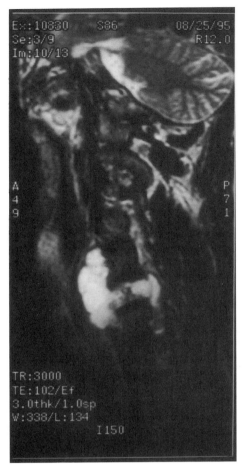

FIGURE 26-3
MRI of chondrosarcoma.

search for tumor was undertaken. A meta-analysis of over 1,300 cases of patients with metastatic spinal cord compression clearly suggests that patients' neurological function at the time of diagnosis was the most important factor in predicting treatment outcome. Patients who were ambulatory at the time of diagnosis remained ambulatory at the end of treatment, whereas patients who were paraplegic rarely regained function. This study underscores the importance of early diagnosis of spinal cord lesions.

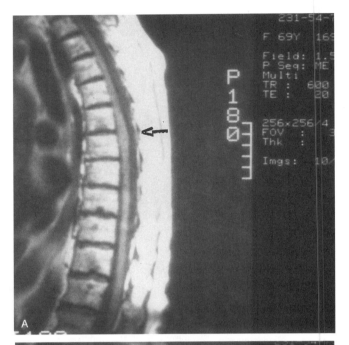

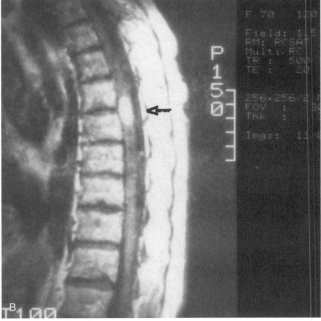

FIGURE 26-4
(*A*) MRI without contrast: metastatic breast cancer. (*B*) MRI with contrast: metastatic breast cancer.

most commonly dexamethasone (Decadron), can rapidly reverse this edema. The dosage and schedule of administration are controversial, with some experts recommending a bolus of Decadron 100 mg followed by 96 mg daily in divided doses with a taper schedule of 4 mg daily every other day.[6] Others recommend a loading dose of 10 mg Decadron followed by 6 mg every 6 hours.[7] No controlled studies in humans have been undertaken to establish efficacy of either dose regimen.

If stability of the spinal cord is in question or a cervical spine lesion is involved, the patient should be immobilized with a cervical collar until surgical stabilization can be undertaken. Also, in patients with a high cervical tumor, respiratory support may be necessary. If there is difficulty with swallowing, a feeding tube will be inserted. For the patient with urinary retention, an indwelling catheter is ordered. As soon as possible, an intermittent catheterization program is started. The patient may also need physical therapy to assist with ambulation or to counteract muscle wasting.

In the case of metastatic tumors, prompt diagnosis has been shown to be imperative to preserve function. Most patients diagnosed with metastatic tumors had pain for an average of 3 months before neurological deficits occurred and a

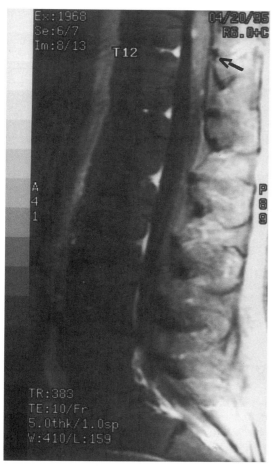

FIGURE 26-5
Drops metastatis from a glioblastoma.

Treatment Options

Treatment of a specific spinal cord tumor depends on the type of tumor, its location, and the rapidity with which signs and symptoms develop. The general medical condition of the patient is also an important consideration in treatment planning. Intradural–extramedullary tumors such as neurofibromas, meningiomas, vascular tumors, chordomas, and epidermoid tumors are usually treated with surgical excision alone.[8] The management of intramedullary tumors such as astrocytomas, ependymomas, and metastatic lesions is much more difficult. These tumors often require a combination of surgery and radiotherapy and, occasionally, chemotherapy.

SURGERY

Surgical intervention is the primary treatment for most types of spinal cord tumors. Surgery is undertaken to establish a diagnosis and to partially or completely remove the tumor. In addition, the rapid loss of motor, sensory, and bowel/bladder function indicates the need for *immediate surgery*, in an attempt to preserve or restore neurological function. Advances in sur-

gical technique have improved operative outcomes. Some of the improvements include intraoperative spinal cord–evoked potential monitoring, intraoperative ultrasound localization, microneurosurgical instrumentation, and surgical lasers.[9] If a laminectomy is performed involving two or more levels, spinal fusion may be necessary.

For rapidly growing metastatic lesions, surgical decompression may be advised to maintain bowel, bladder, or motor function, thus preserving a reasonable quality of life for the time remaining, even though the prognosis is poor. The outcome of surgery is good if extradural metastatic lesions are diagnosed early (when only back pain is present and no neurological deficits have occurred). A poor outcome is likely if neurological deficits are already present.

Extramedullary tumors, such as meningiomas or neurofibromas, can often be completely removed by surgical intervention. Recurrence is rare after complete resection of both of these tumor types.[10] For patients with neurofibromatosis with multiple spinal cord tumors, tumor removal is limited to symptomatic lesions.

Intramedullary tumors are more frequently malignant and often have microscopic infiltration of spinal cord parenchyma. Attempts at complete surgical excision often risk loss of neurological function. Therefore, the goals of surgery are to establish a diagnosis and decompress the spinal cord before embarking on additional treatment.

RADIATION

Radiation therapy is the mainstay of treatment for patients with malignant spinal cord tumors (malignant gliomas, malignant ependymomas, and metastatic lesions). In addition, radiation therapy is utilized (1) for patients with low-grade tumors that are not completely resected; and (2) at the time of recurrence when further surgical intervention cannot be performed.[11]

The spinal cord is less tolerant of radiation therapy than other organs. Varying schedules of radiation doses have been developed. Emergency radiotherapy is often given as large doses that limit subsequent radiotherapy. Most studies suggest that the spinal cord can tolerate a maximum of 4,500 cGy. Higher doses are associated with an increased risk of radiation myelopathy. This is a complication of radiation exposure that begins insidiously at least 6 months after completion of radiation therapy and, more frequently, 12 to 15 months after therapy. At radiation doses exceeding 6,500 cGy, the incidence of myelopathy is 50%.

Radiation myelopathy is a chronic, progressive condition (developed over a period of weeks to months) that initially is seen as sensory impairment to the areas supplied by the affected cord. Pain is not present initially. Motor deficits and changes in pain and temperature sense develop, so that a Brown-Sequard syndrome is observed. This eventually converts to a transverse myelopathy with spastic paraplegia, loss of sensation in the affected areas, and loss of bowel and bladder control. A recent study has shown the benefit of reirradiation of the spinal cord for symptomatic control in patients with recurrent spinal cord compression. These patients achieved symptomatic relief and did not develop myelopathy before succumbing to their systemic cancer.

CHART 26-1
Assessment Parameters for a Patient With a Spinal Cord Tumor

Sensory Assessment

- With patient's eyes closed, assess the following sensory modalities:
  —Light touch
  —Pain (pinprick)
  —Position
- Beginning at the feet and working upward systematically, assess each side of the body and compare findings; often, sensory loss is asymmetrical. (See Chap. 7 for technique.)
- Note the highest level of sensation recorded in relation to an anatomical marking (*e.g.,* umbilicus) or dermatome level. (See Chaps. 5, 7, and 22.)
- If pain is present, describe the characteristics of pain using standard pain assessment criteria.
- Assess progression/change in pain over time.
- Assess for cervical vertebral, thoracic vertebral, and lumbar vertebral pain for *tenderness* while palpating vertebrae.
- Identify highest level of intact sensory function on each side of body.
- Document highest level of function for pain so pain level can be monitored over time.

Motor Assessment

- Systematically assess each side of the body for muscle strength and muscle tone; compare findings. (See Chap. 7 for technique.)
- Observe the patient's gait pattern, if ambulatory.
- Note the presence of spasticity or other abnormal movement.

Motor Assessment (continued)

- Assess deep tendon reflexes and coordination.

Bowel Assessment

- Assess the normal bowel evacuation pattern for the patient (frequency, consistency, time of day, etc.).
- Assess for any changes in bowel habits.
- Assess use of any home remedies for regularity (food, drugs).
- Auscultate the abdomen for bowel sounds and distention.

Bladder Assessment

- Assess the patient's normal voiding pattern.
- Assess the patient for any changes or discomfort in voiding pattern.
- Palpate the suprapubic area for distention or pain.

Respiratory Assessment (for cervical tumors)

- Assess rate, depth, and rhythm of respirations.
- Observe chest movement for asymmetry, abdominal breathing, or abnormal chest movement.
- Auscultate the chest bilaterally for breath sounds.

Other Notations

- Assess the patient for orthostatic hypotension.
- Note any absence of perspiration (*e.g.,* Horner's syndrome).

CHEMOTHERAPY

The role of chemotherapy for spinal cord tumors is very limited. No reports of controlled clinical trials of chemotherapy for primary spinal axis tumors exist. There are certain systemic cancers, such as lymphoma and germ cell tumors, that can be treated effectively with chemotherapy. For most primary tumors, such as astrocytomas and ependymomas, there are chemotherapy regimens that are known to be effective when there is involvement of the brain, but the role of these treatment regimens for spinal cord tumors is unknown.

Adjunctive therapy such as hormonal manipulation may be useful for specific tumors. For example, tamoxifen (Megace) may be helpful for breast cancer, and androgen inhibition, either through chemical means (*i.e.,* diethylstibestol) or orchiectomy, may be beneficial in prostate cancer.[12]

Intrathecal chemotherapy for patients with known leptomeningeal involvement may be instituted. This involves direct administration of chemotherapy into the CSF either by lumbar puncture or an Ommaya reservoir. Unfortunately, there is a very limited selection of suitable drugs and results are often disappointing.

Prognosis and Discharge Planning

Prognosis will vary greatly, depending on the type of tumor and the neurological deficits present. With primary tumors, some resolution of neurological deficits may occur gradually over a period of approximately 2 years, especially with physiotherapy. Levy and colleagues and McCormick and colleagues both showed overall improvement in neurological function in patients undergoing surgery for neurofibromas and benign ependymomas, respectively.[13,14] Each patient should be evaluated to identify individual rehabilitation needs. Most patients with neurological deficits will benefit from a short-term, aggressive rehabilitation program.

Patients with metastatic lesions do not fare as well because of the advanced stage of the primary tumor. For these
(text continues on page 538)

CHART 26-2
Summary of Nursing Management of the Patient With a Spinal Cord Tumor

Nursing Diagnoses	Nursing Interventions	Expected Outcome(s)
Pain Related to (R/T) Spinal Cord and/or Spinal Nerve Compression and Muscle Spasms	• Monitor pain at least every 4 hours. —Monitor quality (dull, piercing), location, and other characteristics. —Monitor the severity of pain by asking the patient to use the Visual Analogue Scale (VAS) to report pain severity on a scale of 1 to 10. —Monitor nonverbal signs of pain (*e.g.*, facial expression, emotional control). —Monitor the effect of pain on activities of daily living (ADLs).	The patient will • Accurately describe pain phenomena. • Identify changes in pain intensity using the VAS.
	• Identify activities/factors that aggravate pain. • Administer analgesics and steroids as ordered, and before the pain intensity has escalated. • Provide physical comfort measures. —Reposition the patient every 1 to 2 hours. —Maintain proper body alignment. —Administer massage (*e.g.*, a back rub). • Apply a special mattress based on any limitations (*e.g.*, a water mattress, an alternating pressure mattress).	The patient will • Participate in controlling activities/factors that aggravate pain. • Report the patient's response to analgesics using the VAS. • Identify measures that facilitate comfort.
	• Teach stress-reducing techniques for pain control (*e.g.*, relaxation, imagery, distraction activities). • Assist the patient to plan individual pain control strategies that are most effective.	The patient will • Learn and use stress-reducing techniques to control pain. • Participate in developing an overall pain control plan. • The comparison of data to baseline data will identify any changes.
Impaired Physical Mobility R/T muscle weakness, paralysis, spasticity, and pain	• Monitor motor function every 8 hours (muscle strength, muscle tone, gait, ability to move in bed). • Teach the proper use of assistive devices. • Provide assistance, as necessary, in transfer and ambulation once spinal cord is stabilized. • Administer range-of-motion exercises every 4 hours. • Position the patient in proper body alignment every 2 hours; use supportive devices as necessary.	

(continued)

CHART 26-2 Summary of Nursing Management of the Patient With a Spinal Cord Tumor (Continued)

Nursing Diagnoses	Nursing Interventions	Expected Outcome(s)
Related Nursing Diagnosis: • Self-Care Deficits • Risk for Impaired Skin Integrity • Risk for Disuse Syndrome	• Monitor the effect of impaired mobility on ADLs. • Develop specific interventions to compensate for deficits. • If spasticity is present, keep the involved extremity warm; reposition periodically; seek suggestions from the physical therapist. • Provide analgesics at least 30 minutes before a planned activity. • If bedrest is ordered, consider protocols to counter the effects of immobility (deep breathing exercises, skin care, turning schedule, etc.) • Request physical therapy (PT) and occupational therapy (OT) consults once patient's spinal cord is stabilized.	• Any ADLs that the patient cannot do independently will be provided for by the nurse, or an alternative way of doing the activity with an adaptive device will be developed. • The patient will report a decrease in pain and an increase in activity tolerance. • Interventions will be in place to prevent the development of disuse syndrome.
Sensory/Perceptual Alterations: Tactile and Kinesthetic, R/T neurological sensory deficits (spinal cord compression, edema) Related Nursing Diagnosis: • High Risk for Injury	• Monitor sensory function; identify the highest level of intact sensory function. • Teach the patient to compensate for any deficits by checking the position of the involved area visually. • Protect the involved area from injury (*e.g.*, burns, bruising). • Monitor ability to ambulate secondary to sensory deficits.	• Comparison of data to baseline data will identify any changes. • The patient will find ways to compensate for the lost sensory modality so that the effect on performance of ADLs will be minimized.
Urinary Retention R/T spinal cord compression and edema	• Monitor the patient's voiding pattern and amount per voiding. • Maintain an accurate intake and output record. • Monitor the patient for suprapubic distention or pain. • Explain the rationale for treatment and management. • Insert indwelling catheter or establish intermittent catheterization schedule.	The patient will • Accurately report his or her former voiding pattern. • Verbalize an understanding of the treatment regimen and the underlying rationale.
Related Nursing Diagnosis: • Risk for Urinary Tract Infection	• Remove the indwelling catheter as soon as possible. • Develop a bladder retraining program: —Teach the Credé and stretch maneuvers. —Measure postvoid residuals after attempts to empty the bladder. —Teach intermittent catheterization. —Set a catheterization time schedule to obtain about 500 mL of urine each time.	• The patient will establish a regular pattern of urinary elimination. • The patient will learn self-catheterization technique.
Constipation R/T decreased peristalsis secondary to spinal cord compression/edema	• Establish the patient's previous bowel elimination pattern. • Auscultate the abdomen for bowel sounds. • Palpate the abdomen for distention.	• The patient will accurately report the previous bowel elimination pattern. • Presence of peristalsis will be monitored.

(continued)

CHART 26-2 Summary of Nursing Management of the Patient With a Spinal Cord Tumor (Continued)

Nursing Diagnoses	Nursing Interventions	Expected Outcome(s)
	• Increase bulk in diet. • Encourage an adequate fluid intake. • Begin a bowel protocol that will provide for satisfactory bowel elimination.	• A diet high in bulk and fluids will be encouraged unless contraindicated by the medical plan. • A bowel protocol will be established that ensures bowel movements (with stools of soft consistency) every 1 to 2 days.
Risk for Injury R/T sensory/perceptual alterations and impaired physical mobility	• Teach the patient to: —Check the position of the affected limbs visually. —Check the integrity of the skin daily, especially affected parts, for evidence of injury. —Check the temperature of the unaffected limb before applying heat to affected areas. —Use heating devices very cautiously. • Assist the patient with ambulation.	• The patient and family will recognize the patient's high-risk status secondary to neurological deficits. • Strategies will be developed to prevent injury. • The patient will seek assistance in ambulation.
Anxiety R/T pain, uncertainty about the disease process, and outcome	• Allow the patient to express his or her feelings. • Correct misinformation and clarify information as necessary. • Refer the patient to appropriate resource people, as necessary. • Help the patient set realistic goals. • Be supportive. • Help the patient find ways to reduce anxiety (*e.g.,* relaxation techniques; diversion).	• Anxiety will be reduced to a manageable level.

Other Possible Nursing Diagnoses General:
• Knowledge Deficit R/T
  —Disease process
  —Treatment modalities (surgery, irradiation, chemotherapy)
• Sexual Dysfunction
• Functional Incontinence
• Fatigue
• Fear
• Ineffective Individual Coping
• Ineffective Family Coping
• Powerlessness
For patients with cervical tumors:
• Ineffective Breathing Pattern
• Ineffective Airway Clearance
• Impaired Swallowing

patients, further treatment of the primary cancer may be planned. For others, hospice care or placement in a chronic care facility may be chosen.

NURSING MANAGEMENT OF THE PATIENT WITH A SPINAL CORD TUMOR

Some commonalties in nursing management exist in the care of patients with spinal cord injuries and those with spinal cord tumors (see Chap. 22). Specifics of care depend on the segmental level of the tumor and the presenting signs and symptoms. If the patient is treated surgically, nursing management follows that outlined for a laminectomy patient (see Chap. 23). Some patients will have metastatic lesions to the spinal cord as a complication of a primary cancer. The nurse will need to consult a text on oncological nursing for specific management and treatment that should be integrated into the plan of care.

The objectives of care for the hospitalized patient with a spinal cord tumor include early recognition of neurological change through ongoing monitoring; control of pain; management of sensory and motor deficits and their impact on activities of daily living (ADLs); and management of bowel and bladder dysfunction. See Chart 26-1 for a summary of assessment parameters.

Assessment

The nurse should conduct a baseline assessment of vital and neurological signs. (Neither the level of consciousness nor pupillary signs are apt to be affected unless the sympathetic innervation of the cervical spinal nerves is involved. In this instance, Horner's syndrome will be seen.) The key areas of assessment include pain and motor, sensory, bowel, and bladder function.

Pain. Assess the quality (on a scale of 1 to 10), location, and type (*e.g.,* dull, piercing) of pain present using the Visual Analog Scale. Note any circumstances that exacerbate the pain.

Motor Function. Motor function is assessed by palpating muscles, asking the patient to move various parts of the body, and comparing findings. Palpate the muscles for signs of atrophy. Assess movement of various muscles. The extremities are graded using a numerical system (see Chap. 7). The hand grasps and pronator drift should be assessed in the upper extremities. If the patient is able to walk, assess the gait. Note any abnormal motor tone (hypotonia or spasticity).

Sensory Function. To assess sensory function, all sensory modalities must be evaluated, including light touch, pain and temperature, and vibration and position sensations) (see Chap. 7). With the patient's eyes closed, begin at the toes and work your way up the body, assessing each side of the body and comparing findings. Determine which modalities are absent or diminished. A band of hyperesthesia often exists over the level of sensory loss. Note any abnormal sensations, such as burning.

Bowel Function. Determine the normal frequency of bowel movements for the patient. Determine whether there has been a change in bowel patterns such as constipation, diarrhea, or incontinence of stool. Auscultate the abdomen for bowel sounds in all four quadrants.

Bladder Function. Note the urinary voiding pattern. Determine whether there is evidence of urinary retention (a common problem with spinal cord tumors) or incontinence. Urinary retention will place the patient at high risk for urinary tract infection.

Management

Once assessment data have been collected, nursing diagnoses and interventions are developed (Chart 26-2).

In preparation for discharge, the nurse will do a complete assessment of the patient to determine the level of independence in performing ADLs, home activities, and activities within the community. Working collaboratively with other health team members, a discharge plan will be developed. As mentioned previously, some patients will benefit from a short-term rehabilitation program at a rehabilitation facility. Others may need only outpatient services or may require no rehabilitation. For the patient with a metastatic lesion, contacting the primary physician managing the cancer and any community resources previously involved in the patient's care will help ensure continuity of care. Hospice care or nursing home placement may be an option for patients in the terminal stages of illness.

References

1. Simeone, F. A. (1990). Spinal cord tumors in adults. In J. R. Youmans (Ed.), *Neurological surgery* (3rd ed.) (pp. 3531–3547). Philadelphia: W. B. Saunders.
2. Raffel, C., & Edwards, M. (1990). Intraspinal tumors in children. In J. R. Youmans (Ed.), *Neurological surgery* (3rd ed.). Philadelphia: W. B. Saunders.
3. Simeone, op. cit.
4. Newton, H., Newton, C., Gatens, C., Hebert, R., & Pack, R. (1995). Spinal cord tumors: Review of etiology, diagnosis, and multidisciplinary approach to treatment. *Cancer Practice, 3*(4), 207–218.
5. Sze, G. (1991). Magnetic resonance imaging in evaluation of spinal tumors. *Cancer, 15*(Suppl.), 1229–1241.
6. Gilbert, M. (1990). Epidural spinal cord compression and carcinomatous meningitis. In B. C. Decker, *Current therapy in neurologic disease* (3rd ed.) (pp. 232–236). Washington, DC: B. C. Decker.
7. Vecht, C., Haaxma-Reiche, H., van Putten, M., de Visser, M., Vries, E., & Twijnstra, A. (1989). Initial bolus of conventional versus high-dose dexamethasone in metastatic spinal cord compression. *Neurology, 39,* 1255–1257.
8. Adams, R., & Victor, M. (1993). *Principles of neurology* (5th ed.). New York: McGraw-Hill.
9. Newton et al., op. cit.
10. Solero, C., Fornari, M., Giombini, S., Lasio, G., et al. (1989). Spinal meningiomas: Review of 174 operated cases. *Neurosurgery, 25,* 153–160.
11. Simeone, op. cit.
12. Gilbert, op. cit.
13. Levy, W., Latchaw, J., Hahn, J., Sawhny, B., May, J., & Dohn, D. (1986). Spinal neurofibromas: A report of 66 cases and a comparison with meningiomas. *Neurosurgery, 18*(3), 331–334.
14. McCormick, P., Torres, R., Kalmon, D., Post, D., & Stein, B. (1990).

Intramedullary innervate of the spinal cord. *Journal of Neurosurgery, 72,* 523–532.

Bibliography

Books

Ogilvy, C. S., & Heros, R. C. (1993). Spinal cord compression. In A. H. Ropper (Ed.), *Neurological and neurosurgical intensive care* (3rd ed.) (pp. 437–452). New York: Raven.

Rengachary, S. S., & Wilkins, R. H. (Eds.). (1994). *Principles of neurosurgery.* New York: McGraw-Hill.

Periodicals

Liskow, A., Chang, C. H., DeSanctis, P., et al. (1986). Epidural cord compression in association with genitourinary neoplasms. *Cancer, 58,* 949–954.

Portenoy, R. K., Lipton, R. B., & Foley, K. M. (1987). Back pain in the cancer patient: An algorithm for evaluation and management. *Neurology, 37,* 134.

Raney, D. J. (1991). Malignant spinal cord tumors: A review and case presentation. *Journal of Neuroscience Nursing, 23*(1), 44–49.

Wilkowski, J. (1986). Spinal cord compression: An oncologic emergency. *Journal of Emergency Nursing, 12,* 9–12.

Section 7

Nursing Management of Patients With Cerebrovascular Problems

CHAPTER 27

Stroke and Other Cerebrovascular Diseases

Joanne V. Hickey

Stroke is the third leading cause of death in the United States after coronary heart disease and cancer. There are approximately 500,000 cases of stroke each year; of these, 150,000 are fatal.[1] From 1980 to 1990, the death rate from stroke declined by 32%.[2] Stroke leaves about 25% of its victims with mental and physical disabilities resulting in the need for assistance with activities of daily living (ADLs). Although stroke is common in Americans 65 years and older, 28% of victims are under the age of 65 years, and women account for 40% of the new cases.[3] There are over 3 million persons with stroke alive in the United States.[4] The annual cost for acute and long-term stroke care is approximately $30 billion.[5] In recent surveys, the prevalence, incidence, and hospitalization rates for stroke are higher among blacks than whites.[6]

Management of stroke is undergoing a fundamental transformation due to research and technological advances, including new pathophysiological models of stroke to understand changes on the biochemical and cellular level; superior diagnostic equipment and technology such as magnetic resonance angiography and improved computed tomography (CT) scanning techniques; the introduction of new pharmacological neuroprotective agents; the definitive role of thrombolytic agents in early treatment; the addition of more interventional therapies, such as angioplasty and stents, to the treatment options; the North American Symptomatic Carotid Endarterectomy Trial studies which delineate the role of surgical management in stroke; and other studies which have provided the scientific basis for patient management guidelines and algorithms.[7]

The term *brain attack* has become more popular in describing stroke, as appreciation has grown of the timeline associated with the development of neurological deficits and the window of opportunity that exists for reversal of neurological deficits with new interventions. Cardiac resuscitation training programs in basic life support (BLS) and advanced cardiac life support (ACLS) have been revamped with a focus on saving brain tissue as well as saving cardiac muscle. The previous dismal view of stroke outcome has been replaced by optimism for better outcomes for stroke victims.

Research is the foundation for both primary and secondary prevention of stroke and the management of stroke victims along a continuum of care with emphasis on early rehabilitation. Several recent research-based guidelines and consensus reports, such as the guidelines for the management of transient ischemic attacks, acute ischemic stroke, and carotid endarterectomy, are now available to guide health care providers in making informed decisions about treatment options.[8–11] In addition, the Agency for Health Care and Policy Research (AHCPR) published in 1995 clinical guidelines for poststroke rehabilitation which set a national standard for management of stroke patients.

With more and more care being provided in managed care environments, many institutions have developed interdisciplinary clinical pathways for stroke. The emphasis is on providing cost-effective care with measurable outcomes. This has resulted in frequent outcomes assessment, which has contributed to further refinement of care along the continuum. Nurses and other health care providers will continue to be challenged to demonstrate efficacy and cost effectiveness of interventions and care.

DEFINITION AND CLASSIFICATION OF STROKE

Stroke is a heterogeneous, neurological syndrome characterized by the gradual or rapid, nonconvulsive onset of neurological deficits that fit a known vascular territory and that last for 24 hours or more. Stroke includes cerebral infarction (ischemic stroke) and intracerebral hemorrhage and subarachnoid hemorrhage (hemorrhagic stroke). The two categories are further subdivided, as discussed later (Fig. 27-1). The type and severity of neurological deficits encompass a wide range and gradation of signs and symptoms. The severity and permanence of symptoms are the factors that differentiate between the so-called minor stroke and major stroke.

Classification of stroke is based on the underlying problem created within the cerebral artery and the blood supply to the brain. An analogy to home plumbing pipes can be made. Only two events create problems with household plumbing: plugging of the pipe so that drainage cannot proceed to its destination; and bursting or rupturing of the pipe so that fluid within the pipe flows into the surrounding areas. In the brain, plugging by atherosclerosis or a clot creates a narrow lumen, preventing adequate flow of blood to cerebral tissue. Alternatively, rupture resulting from a weakened vessel causes leakage of blood into the brain or subarachnoid space.

Thus, stroke is divided into the two major categories of ischemic stroke and hemorrhagic stroke. The ischemic stroke category has been refined from the previous classification of thrombotic and embolic stroke to include additional categories.

Ischemic Stroke

Ischemic stroke accounts for 85% of all strokes and is subdivided into atherosclerotic cerebrovascular disease (20%); penetrating artery disease, or "lacunes" (25%); cardiogenic embolic (20%); cryptogenic (30%); and other (5%). Atherosclerosis of large and small cerebral arteries which results in thrombosis is the most common cause of ischemic stroke in North America and Europe and accounts for 45% of strokes in United States.

TERMS RELATED TO ISCHEMIC STROKE

Transient ischemic attacks (TIAs) are temporary focal brain or retinal deficits, caused by vascular disease, that fit a known vascular territory and clear completely in less than 24 hours.

Most TIAs are much shorter; the majority reverse completely within 1 hour. TIAs are classified into TIAs associated with the carotid and vertebrobasilar vascular territories.

TIAs of the carotid (anterior circulation) cause lateralizing signs. When the carotid territory is involved, the symptoms reflect ischemia to the ipsilateral eye or cerebral hemisphere. A common eye symptom is temporary monocular blindness (TMB). Hemispherical ischemia usually causes weakness or numbness of the contralateral face or limb; language deficits and cognitive and behavioral changes may also occur.

TIAs of the vertebrobasilar (posterior) circulation cause diffuse signs. When the vertebrobasilar territory is involved, the symptoms often include dysarthria, vertigo, dizziness, ataxia, abnormalities of eye movement resulting in diplopia, and unilateral or bilateral motor and sensory deficits (Table 27-1).

A **penumbra** is a zone of compromised neuronal cells that are unable to function but remain viable and are located around an area of lethal injured cells; such a zone is amenable to reversal from ischemia (Fig. 27-2).

A **watershed or border zone infarction** is an infarcted area that occurs between the terminal distributions of two adjacent arteries such as the anterior cerebral and middle cerebral arteries. Because the terminal distributions are at the end of the pipeline, they are subject to low, marginally adequate arterial pressure under normal circumstances (Fig. 27-3). They are also the first to fail when systemic blood pressure drops further. If systemic hypotension occurs, there is failure to maintain adequate cerebral perfusion.

ATHEROSCLEROTIC CEREBROVASCULAR DISEASE STROKE

The large extracranial and intracranial arteries are subject to atherosclerosis with an associated atheroma that narrows the lumen of the vessel. The atheroma can also be the site for thrombus formation. Both conditions can lead to hypoperfusion, ischemia, and ischemic stroke. About 40% of patients will have TIAs before a large-vessel ischemic stroke.

The patient typically awakens with neurological deficits or is sedentary when the symptoms occur. During sleep or at

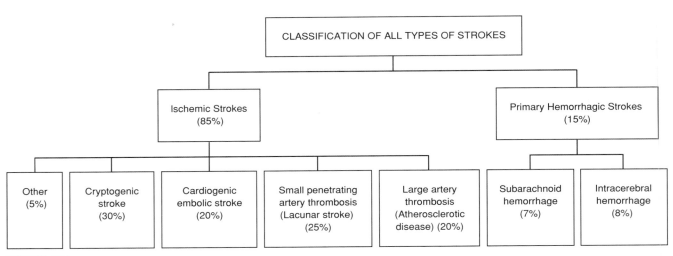

FIGURE 27-1
Classification of all stroke types.

TABLE 27-1
Comparison of Signs and Symptoms of Carotid and Vertebrobasilar TIAs

CAROTID TERRITORY	VERTEBROBASILAR TERRITORY
Related to Ophthalmic Artery	**Related to Posterior Cerebral Artery**
Amaurosis fugax (temporary monocular blindness)	Dysarthria
Transient graying, fogging, or blurred vision	Dysphagia
A "shade" descending over line of vision	Diplopia
	Bilateral blindness
Related to Middle Cerebral Artery	Unilateral or bilateral motor and sensory weakness
	Quadriparesis
Hemiparesis (more arm than leg weakness)	**Related to Cerebellar Arteries**
Hemianesthesia	Ataxia
Contralateral motor or sensory deficits to face or limbs	Vertigo
	Dizziness
Related to Anterior Cerebral Artery	
Hemiparesis (more leg than arm weakness)	

rest, the blood pressure tends to be lowered, and there is less pressure to push the blood through the narrowed arterial lumen. Systemic hypoperfusion, decreased cerebral perfusion, ischemia, and ischemic stroke can develop. The area of cerebral ischemia depends on the vascular territory involved and the location within the vascular territory (proximal or distal) of the thrombus.

If a major artery is involved, large areas of both gray and white matter become ischemic, infarcted, and necrotic. Neuronal ischemia causes changes in the cell membrane, resulting in intracellular edema and compression of the capillaries, further compromising adequate blood supply. Cerebral edema peaks approximately 2 to 5 days after the stroke. Symptoms of ischemic stroke often develop in a stepwise progression relating to cerebral edema and infarction, reaching a peak in 1 to 3 days before stabilizing.

SMALL PENETRATING ARTERY STROKE (LACUNAR STROKE)

The term **lacune** describes the small cavity remaining in the brain tissue that develops after the necrotic tissue of a small, deep infarct has been removed. A **lacunar stroke** is a type of ischemic stroke caused by microatheroma and thrombosis of a small penetrating artery resulting in a small, softened area in the deep white matter structures of the brain. As the softened tissue sloughs away, a small cavity or lake remains called a lacune (diameter of 0.5 mm or less). Lacunar strokes are seen predominately in the basal ganglia, especially the putamen, the thalamus, and the white matter of the internal capsule and pons; they occur occasionally in the white matter of the cerebral gyri. They are rare in the gray matter of the cerebral sur-

face, in the corpus callosum, visual radiations, or medulla (Fig. 27-4). Most lacunes occur in the lenticulostriate branches of the anterior cerebral artery and middle cerebral artery, the thalamoperforant branches of the posterior cerebral arteries, and the paramedian branches of the basilar artery.[12]

There are distinct signs and symptoms associated with a number of recognized lacune syndromes that include pure motor hemiplegia, pure sensory stroke, homolateral ataxia and crural paresis, dysarthria, clumsy hand syndrome, sensorimotor stroke, and basilar branch syndromes. Even though a lacunar stroke is small, it can cause considerable deficits if a critical area, such as the internal capsule, is involved. Patients may have several lacunes, as evidenced on CT or magnetic resonance imaging, and have diffuse white matter changes associated with dementia.

CARDIOGENIC EMBOLIC STROKE

About 20% of ischemic strokes are due to cardiogenic embolism from atrial fibrillation (the most common), valvular disease, ventricular thrombi, and other cardiac problems. Atherosclerosis and atherogenic plaques of the proximal aorta are another source of cardiac emboli detectable with the use of transesophageal echocardiography. The atherogenic plaques commonly found in coronary vessels, in the heart, and at the bifurcation of the aorta are precursors for hypertension and atrial fibrillation. Unstable plaques can break off and become microemboli to the brain, causing stroke. Microemboli from the heart are mobilized and enter the cerebral system most often through the carotid arteries, flowing until the vessel is too narrow to allow further passage of the embolus and the vessel becomes occluded. The left middle cerebral artery is

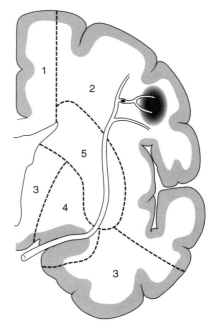

FIGURE 27-2
See distribution of middle cerebral artery and occlusion of a branch. Note area of infarction and surrounding penumbra with viable but nonfunctional cells. These cells will either become infarcted or recover depending on treatment.

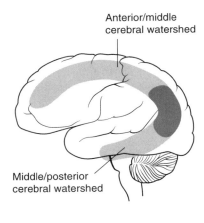

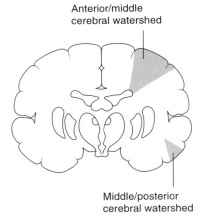

FIGURE 27-3
Location of watershed.

affected most often because it is a relatively straight vessel and provides the path of least resistance for the embolus. Cardiogenic strokes are seen in younger patients and usually occur when the patient is awake and active. The development of the ischemia is very rapid with maximal deficit present within minutes.

CRYPTOGENIC STROKE

About 30% of ischemic strokes are cryptogenic in origin, which means that no cause of the stroke could be found after diagnostic evaluation.

STROKE FROM OTHER CAUSES

About 5% of ischemic stroke is due to coagulopathies, arteritis, migraine/vasospasm, and drug abuse such as cocaine.

Hemorrhagic Stroke

Hemorrhagic stroke is divided into two categories based on the underlying mechanism. **Intracerebral stroke**, also called **intraparenchymal stroke**, is caused by bleeding into the brain tissue as a result of rupture of a small artery, most often a deep, penetrating vessel. **Subarachnoid hemorrhagic stroke** or simply **subarachnoid hemorrhage** is the result of bleeding into the subarachnoid space, most often in relation to a ruptured aneurysm or arteriovenous malformation—in both cases, the result of hemorrhage. In this chapter, only intracerebral hemorrhagic stroke will be discussed. Cerebral aneurysms and arteriovenous malformations are addressed in Chapters 28 and 29.

INTRACEREBRAL HEMORRHAGIC STROKE

The cause of intracerebral hemorrhagic stroke, also called intraparenchymal stroke or primary hypertensive stroke, is a spontaneous hemorrhage related to hypertension. The typical profile is that of an older person with a long history of poorly controlled hypertension. At the moment of hemorrhage, the person is active and has not experienced any warning signs. A typical story is one of a patient straining at stool, and then developing a severe headache, decreased consciousness, hemiplegia, and possible focal seizures and vomiting. Hemorrhagic stroke occurs rapidly, with steady development of symptoms over a period of minutes to hours (1 to 24 hours). The most common sites of intracerebral hemorrhage, each of which has distinguishing signs and symptoms, are the following:

- Putamen (part of the basal ganglia) and adjacent internal capsule (50%)
- Thalamus (30%)

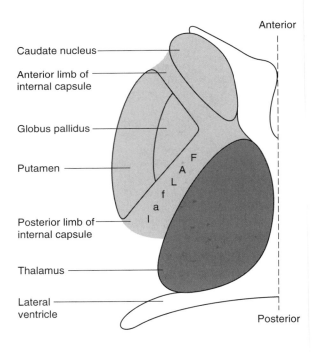

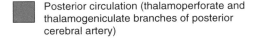

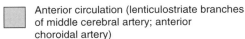

FIGURE 27-4
Primary location of lacunar strokes.

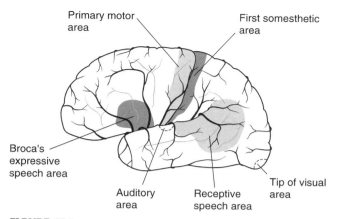

FIGURE 27-5
Distribution of the middle cerebral artery (lateral surface of the brain).

- Cerebellum (10%)
- Pons (10%)

ANATOMY, ATHEROGENESIS, AND PATHOPHYSIOLOGY RELATED TO STROKES

Anatomical Basis for and Correlations Related to Stroke

There are four major cerebral arteries that supply the brain: two internal carotid arteries (ICAs) that constitute the anterior circulation, and two vertebral arteries (VAs) that constitute the posterior circulation. The ICAs ascend from the common carotid bifurcation, enter the cranium at the petrous portion of the temporal bone between the layers of dura, and then begin to branch. The first major small branch is the ophthalmic artery, which supplies the eye. Temporary ischemia to this vessel results in transitory monocular blindness in one eye (also called amaurosis fugax). The major cerebral arteries arising from the ICAs are the middle cerebral artery (MCA), the anterior cerebral artery (ACA), the anterior communicating artery, and the posterior communicating arteries. The MCA supplies the lateral portion of the cerebral hemisphere (Fig. 27-5). The ACA supplies the frontal pole and medial surface of the frontal and parietal lobes (Fig. 27-6).

The two VAs enter the cranial vault through the foramen magnum. They then unite to form the basilar artery (Fig. 27-7). The basilar artery then divides to form the posterior cerebral artery (PCA), which supplies the medial and inferior surfaces and lateral portions of the temporal and occipital lobes (see Figs. 27-5 and 27-6). The basilar artery also gives off a number of cerebellar and brain stem arteries. The circle of Willis, at the base of the skull, joins the anterior and posterior circulation. Collateral circulation for an occluded vessel is possible owing to anastomosis between the vessels. However, anomalies of cerebral vessels are common, so it is difficult to predict if a patient will receive collateral circulation to an oc-

cluded area. Chapter 5 provides further details regarding cerebral circulation.

Atherogenesis and Ischemic Stroke

Atherogenesis is the pathological process of the development of atherosclerosis. Stroke due to atherosclerosis remains the most common neurologic disorder among adults in America. There are two dominant theories of atherogenesis: reaction to injury and the lipid hypotheses. Regardless of the specific mechanism of injury, the arterial wall undergoes a series of morphological changes that result in structural alteration and pathogenesis.

PATHOGENESIS IN LARGER ARTERIES

The earliest lesion of atherosclerosis is seen as a yellowish, fatty streak of the intimal surface of large- to medium-sized arteries which are widely distributed throughout the arterial vasculature and may be seen as early as late childhood or early adolescence. On microscopic examination, the fatty streaks consist of lipid-laden macrophages know as foam cells (some foam cells are smooth muscle cells and some come from circulating monocytes) and extracellular lipid.

Over the course of years, the fatty streaks progress, and by middle to old age, fibrosis plaques (atheromas) begin to develop in more localized sites than fatty streaks, typically occurring at arterial branches or opposite arterial bifurcation of extracranial vessels. The maturated fibrous plaque consists of an intact endothelial lining overlaying a fibrous cap (containing foam cells, transformed smooth muscle cells, lymphocytes, a connective tissue matrix, and a central necrotic core of cellular debris, free extracellular lipid, and cholesterol crystals) extruding from the intima and producing varying degrees of alterations in blood flow. Small arterioles, commonly observed at the plaque periphery, may be the genesis of possible hemorrhagic transformation in some fibrous plaques which contain hemosiderin, areas of intraplaque calcification, and disruption of the endothelial lining. The plaque destabi-

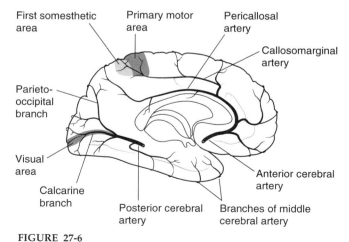

FIGURE 27-6
Distribution of the anterior and posterior cerebral arteries on the medial surface of the cerebral hemisphere.

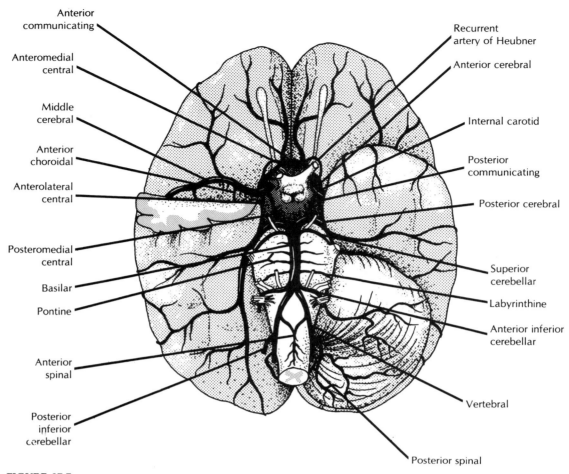

FIGURE 27-7
Arteries that supply the brain, as seen from the ventral surface. The right cerebral hemisphere and the tip of the right temporal lobe have been removed.

lization and luminal thrombi result in endothelial injury and clinical symptoms.[13,14]

Plaque enlargement occurs slowly over decades and the person is asymptomatic until the plaque intrudes on a substantial percentage of the arterial lumen diameter. Typically, luminal thrombi are associated with luminal surface disruption or ulceration of the endothelial lining, leading to arterial obstruction. Blood within the plaque or intraplaque hemorrhage appears to be secondary to the luminal disruption, with dissection of luminal blood into the plaque.

PATHOGENESIS IN SMALLER ARTERIES

The underlying pathological process for smaller penetrating arteries such as the lenticulostriate arteries, basilar penetrating arteries, and medullary arteries that supply deep cerebral white matter is probably different than the atherosclerosis found in the larger arteries. The underlying pathological changes in the small penetrating arteries are attributable to a process called **lipohyalinosis**, in which a hyaline-lipid material coats the small penetrating arteries, causing thickening of the walls. Eventually, the vessel thromboses create a lacunar stroke.

Pathophysiology of Ischemic Stroke

The pathophysiology of ischemic stroke due to atheromas, thrombi, or emboli is the same. The lumen of the blood vessel becomes narrowed or occluded, resulting in ischemia in that vascular territory (Fig. 27-8).

Ischemia can cause primary cellular injuries from no blood flow and secondary cellular injury due to the effects of biochemical and molecular cascades precipitated from ischemia. Ischemia severe enough to kill cerebral cells is called **cerebral infarction**. Consider the injured cerebral area that occurs with ischemic stroke. A core of necrotic tissue often exists from a lack of oxygen and nutrients. However, around the necrotic core is another circumscribed area called the *ischemic penumbra* (see Fig. 27-2). Although the neuronal cells of the penumbra are unable to function, they remain viable and may be amenable to reversal from ischemia with pharmacological agents. Neuroprotective agents are being used in clinical trials

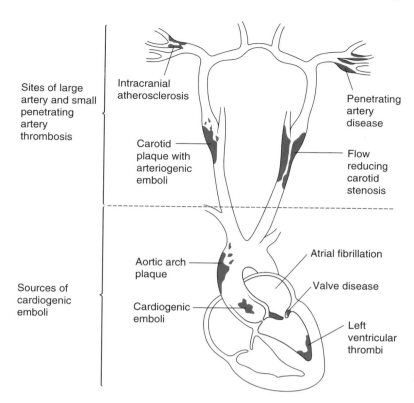

Sites of large artery and small penetrating artery thrombosis

Intracranial atherosclerosis

Carotid plaque with arteriogenic emboli

Penetrating artery disease

Flow reducing carotid stenosis

Sources of cardiogenic emboli

Aortic arch plaque

Cardiogenic emboli

Atrial fibrillation

Valve disease

Left ventricular thrombi

FIGURE 27-8
Major sites and sources related to ischemic stroke.

to protect the cells from the secondary injury associated with the ischemic cascade.

The blood supply to the brain can be compromised due to a no-flow phenomenon (*e.g.*, following cardiac arrest) or a low-flow phenomenon (*e.g.*, following stroke). Low-perfusion states can result in more tissue damage than no-perfusion states because the presence of glucose in an inadequately oxygenated area enhances lactate production.[15] Brain tissue lactate causes severe tissue necrosis and extracellular acidosis which results in infarction. In addition, low-flow states also provide a continued supply of both water, which exacerbates edema, and activated white blood cells, platelets, and coagulation factors, which contribute to tissue damage by further impeding the microcirculation.

Secondary cellular injury associated with ischemia occurs in response to deprivation of oxygen and cessation of oxidative metabolism. Complex biochemical and molecular cascades result in ischemic damage to neurons. Two to five minutes of complete oxygen deprivation is the general benchmark for irreversible neuronal damage. However, extreme hypothermia can significantly increase the viability time, and hypothermia has been used therapeutically to save neurons. Without oxygen, ATP energy-dependent cell functions such as the cellular respiratory chain, lipid metabolism, and maintenance of the transmembrane ion channels rapidly cease. Impairment of the respiratory chain results in anaerobic glycolysis of remaining available glucose. Anaerobic glycolysis proceeds only to pyruvate, which reduces to lactate. Lactic acid and free fatty acid accumulation causes intracellular acidosis, further inhibiting mitochondrial function.

Concurrently, other cell destruction processes occur that include *excitotoxicity, increased intracellular calcium, and gen-*

eration of free radicals. Hypoxia impairs the reuptake of the excitatory neurotransmitter glutamate at the presynaptic membrane. The excessive extracellular glutamate opens sodium, chloride, and calcium channels, resulting in an influx of sodium and chloride ions with water into the cell, causing acute cellular swelling; the voltage-dependent calcium channels allow influx of calcium into the cytosol and efflux of potassium. (Intracellular calcium is normally maintained at a low level by active transport mechanisms.) The high intracellular calcium activates calcium-dependent degradative enzymes (proteases, phospholipases, and endonucleases) that attack the cell membranes and DNA and further inhibit mitochondrial function. Oxygen free radicals with resultant lipid peroxidation occur in inadequately perfused areas and during reperfusion of previously ischemic areas. Oxygen free radicals, superoxide peroxide, and hydroxyl ions destroy fatty acids and disrupt calcium homeostasis, further contributing to cellular demise. Approximately 8 to 12 hours after the insult, the neuron becomes smaller and more angular. The cytoplasm and nucleus shrink, followed by complete dissolution of the cell and cell death.[16]

The ischemic cascade and cellular changes that follow oxygen deprivation were outlined earlier. Another type of injury to neurons results from reperfusion to previously ischemic areas. The cellular injury due to activated oxygen free radicals that occurs after the blood supply to the ischemic area has been restored is called **reperfusion injury**. Oxygen free radicals, partially reduced oxygen molecules which are highly reactive with other molecules, are implicated in postischemic membrane injury. The buildup of adenosine diphosphate (ADP) and pyruvate during ischemia results in rapid production of electrons when the oxygen supply is reestablished. The oxygen free radicals are formed when the electrons are transferred to oxygen. They allegedly injure the cell membrane by stealing hydrogen molecules and by forming abnormal molecular bonds.[17,18] As a result of reperfusion injury, additional injury to neuronal cells is incurred.

When thrombolytic therapy is used, the patient may manifest new or identical stroke symptoms after a successful recanalization. One nursing implication of postthrombolytic therapy is to observe the patient for reperfusion injury.[19] Another example of perfusion injury is the natural break-up of an embolic thrombus and the onset of expanded deficits.

Pathophysiology of Hemorrhagic Stroke

The pathophysiology of hemorrhagic stroke is associated with an immediate rise in intracranial pressure (ICP), ischemic cellular responses, cerebral edema, compromised cerebral perfusion pressure, and possible herniation. With intracerebral hemorrhage (ICH), the usual hemorrhage sites are small, deep cortical arteries or subarachnoid hemorrhage due to aneurysmal rupture (see Chap. 28). At the time of ICH, blood is forced into the surrounding cerebral parenchyma, creating a hematoma. The hematoma displaces and compresses the adjacent cerebral tissue, and ischemic cellular responses and cerebral edema occur, resulting in increased ICP. A major ICH can cause midline displacement and herniation syndromes and has a high mortality rate of about 50%.

SIGNS AND SYMPTOMS OF STROKE SYNDROMES ACCORDING TO THE INVOLVED VESSEL

The presenting signs and symptoms of stroke depend on the extent and location of the insult. When a cerebral artery is occluded by a thrombus or embolus, classical syndromes are said to develop. In reality, syndromes frequently overlap one another rather than appearing in their pure form.

Carotid Region

INTERNAL CAROTID ARTERY SYNDROME

Symptoms of the typical ICA syndrome include the following:

- Paralysis of the contralateral face, arm, and leg
- Sensory deficits of the contralateral face, arm, and leg
- Aphasia, if the dominant hemisphere is involved
- Apraxia, agnosia, and unilateral neglect, if the nondominant hemisphere is involved
- Homonymous hemianopsia

MIDDLE CEREBRAL ARTERY SYNDROME

MCA syndrome is by far the most common of all cerebral occlusions. If the main stem of the MCA is occluded, a massive infarction of most of the hemisphere results. Initially, there may be vomiting and a rapid onset of coma, which may last a few weeks. Cerebral edema is extensive.

Symptoms of MCA syndrome include the following:

- Hemiplegia (involving the face and arm on the contralateral side; the leg is spared or has less deficits than the arm)
- Sensory impairment (same area as hemiplegia)
- Aphasia (global aphasia if the dominant hemisphere is involved)
- Homonymous hemianopsia

ANTERIOR CEREBRAL ARTERY SYNDROME

The ACA is least often occluded. If the occlusion occurs proximal to a patent anterior communicating artery, the blood supply will not be compromised. If the occlusion is distal, or if the communicating artery is inadequate, there will be infarction of the medial aspect of one frontal lobe. Bilateral medial frontal lobe infarction occurs if one ACA is occluded and the other artery is small and dependent on blood flow.

Symptoms of ACA syndrome include the following (note that aphasia and hemianopsia are not part of the profile):

- Paralysis of the contralateral foot and leg (footdrop is a consistent finding)
- Impaired gait
- Sensory loss over the toes, foot, and leg
- Abulia (slowness and prolonged delays to perform acts voluntarily or to respond)
- Flat affect, lack of spontaneity, slowness, distractibility, and lack of interest in surroundings
- Cognitive impairment, such as perseveration and amnesia
- Urinary incontinence

Vertebrobasilar Region

Occlusion of the vessels within the vertebrobasilar system produces unique syndromes. The vertebral and basilar arteries and their branches supply the brain stem and cerebellum. The posterior cerebral arteries are the terminal branches of the basilar artery and supply the medial temporal and occipital lobes, as well as part of the corpus callosum.

VERTEBRAL ARTERY SYNDROME

The following signs and symptoms are characteristic of VA occlusion:

- Wallenberg's syndrome (lateral medullary syndrome)
- Dizziness
- Nystagmus
- Dysphagia and dysarthria
- Pain in face, nose, or eye
- Ipsilateral numbness and weakness of face
- Staggering gait and ataxia
- Clumsiness

BASILAR ARTERY SYNDROME

The following signs and symptoms are characteristic of basilar artery occlusion:

- Quadriplegia
- Possibly, the "locked-in" syndrome
- Weakness of facial, tongue, and pharyngeal muscles

ANTERIOR INFERIOR CEREBELLAR ARTERY SYNDROME

Occlusion of the anterior inferior cerebellar artery is also known as the lateral inferior pontine syndrome.

Symptoms of the anterior inferior cerebellar artery syndrome include vertigo, nausea, vomiting, tinnitus, and nystagmus.

Ipsilateral Side

- Paresis of lateral conjugate gaze
- Horner's syndrome
- Cerebellar signs (ataxia, nystagmus)

Contralateral Side

- Impaired pain and temperature sensation in trunk and limbs (may also involve face)

POSTERIOR INFERIOR CEREBELLAR ARTERY SYNDROME (WALLENBERG'S SYNDROME)

Posterior inferior cerebellar artery syndrome involves the lateral portion of the medulla as a result of the occlusion of the posterior inferior cerebellar artery.

Symptoms include the following:

- Nausea and vomiting
- Dysphagia and dysarthria
- Horizontal nystagmus
- Ipsilateral Horner's syndrome
- Cerebellar signs (ataxia and vertigo)
- Loss of pain and temperature sensation on contralateral side of trunk and limbs

POSTERIOR CEREBRAL ARTERY SYNDROME

Few strokes involve the PCA. The usual consequence of the superficial occlusion (peripheral areas) of a PCA is contralateral homonymous hemianopsia. If the penetrating branches (central areas) are occluded, the cerebral peduncle, thalamus, and upper brain stem are involved. There is wide variation in the manifestations of the syndrome.

Symptoms of PCA syndrome include the following:

Peripheral Area

- Homonymous hemianopsia
- Memory deficits
- Perseveration
- Several visual deficits (cortical blindness, lack of depth perception, failure to see objects not centrally located, visual hallucinations)

Central Area

- If the thalamus is involved, there is sensory loss of all modalities, spontaneous pain, intentional tremors, and mild hemiparesis.
- If the cerebral peduncle is involved, Weber's syndrome (oculomotor nerve palsy with contralateral hemiplegia) occurs.
- If the brain stem is involved, there are deficits involving conjugate gaze, nystagmus, and pupillary abnormalities, with other possible symptoms of ataxia and postural tremors.

Deep Cortical Syndromes

Four syndromes are associated with intracerebral hemorrhagic stroke. In addition to an altered level of consciousness (confusion to coma), headache, nausea, vomiting, nuchal rigidity, hypertension, and bradycardia related to increased ICP, each syndrome has its own distinguishing characteristics.

Putamenal Hemorrhage (often involves the internal capsule)

- Contralateral hemiplegia
- Contralateral hemisensory deficits
- Hemianopsia
- Slurred speech

Thalamic Hemorrhage

- Contralateral hemiplegia
- Contralateral hemisensory deficits
- Deficits of vertical and lateral gaze

Pontine Hemorrhage

- "Locked-in" syndrome
- Deficits in lateral eye movement

Cerebellar Hemorrhage

- Occipital headache
- Dizziness
- Ataxia
- Vertigo

General Comparison of Left-Sided and Right-Sided Stroke

Some generalizations can be made about the deficits incurred with left-sided and right-sided stroke (Table 27-2).

Summary of Deficits Incurred With Stroke Syndrome

A stroke syndrome is a form of cerebral injury. The injury to the brain results from a ruptured blood vessel, in the case of hemorrhagic stroke, or from ischemia that develops over time or suddenly, as may be the case in thrombotic or embolic strokes. In all cases of stroke syndrome, areas of the brain are deprived of an adequate oxygen supply. If the blood supply is cut off for an extended period, the involved cerebral tissue may become necrotic, resulting in permanent neurological def-

TABLE 27-2
Comparison of Signs and Symptoms Associated With Right-Sided and Left-Sided Hemiplegia

STROKE SYNDROME ON LEFT SIDE OF BRAIN (RIGHT-SIDED HEMIPLEGIA)	STROKE SYNDROME ON RIGHT SIDE OF BRAIN (LEFT-SIDED HEMIPLEGIA)
• Expressive aphasia or • Receptive aphasia or • Global aphasia • Intellectual impairment • Slow and cautious behavior • Defects in right visual fields	• Spatial–perceptual deficits • Denial and the deficits of the affected side require special safety considerations • Tendency for distractibility • Impulsive behavior; apparently unaware of deficits • Poor judgment • Defects in left visual fields

icits. In instances of ischemia, temporary neurological impairment may result. Similar hemodynamic changes occur with other forms of cerebral injury, such as head injuries, cerebral aneurysms, or cerebral edema.

The particular type and degree of neurological deficits depend on the particular area of the brain involved. Because the brain is composed of the most highly specialized tissue in the body, the deficits incurred will depend on the area compromised. (The common deficits seen in the stroke patient are summarized in Chart 27-3. The rehabilitation and management of these deficits are discussed in Chapter 14.)

DIAGNOSIS OF STROKE

A patient seen with a question of TIAs or stroke must be carefully evaluated. A complete medical history and comprehensive physical and neurological examination begin the database. In addition to the neurological examination, a neurovascular examination that includes the following components is necessary:[20]

- Blood pressure measurement in both arms and in the reclining and standing positions; especially important when vertebral-basilar ischemia is suspected
- Cardiac auscultation and rhythm check
- Auscultation of the head and neck for bruit
- Palpation of the neck and facial pulses; palpation of superficial temporal arteries for tenderness and edema
- Funduscopic examination for platelet or fibrin, cholesterol, or calcific emboli

A thorough cardiac examination including a search for a carotid bruit (a marker of generalized atherosclerosis and a source of atherogenic microemboli) is important because of the possibility of cardiogenic emboli. Many patients who have significant extracranial occlusive ideas will not have a bruit. In patients with cervical bruits, about 50% have significant carotid stenosis. About 70% of persons who have bruits located near the jaw angle, especially when they extend into

diastole, have carotid stenosis. Ocular bruit may signify high-grade carotid stenosis or a vascular anomaly.[21]

Onset of neurological deficits are not necessarily signs and symptoms of TIAs or stroke, so a detailed history about the onset, signs and symptoms, frequency, progression, and other characteristics is important. Although the clinical presentation of TIA/stroke is heterogeneous, the symptoms are dictated by three key variables: affected vascular territory; duration and severity of ischemia; and underlying mechanism of cerebral hypoperfusion.[22] A review of the history and physical examination is helpful in identifying risk factors for stroke (Table 27-3). A comparison of signs and symptoms related to carotid and vertebrobasilar TIAs is found in Table 27-1. An understanding of the vascular territories and related functional levels is critical in helping the care provider to relate presenting symptoms to vascular territories.

Transient Ischemic Attacks

If a person is having TIAs, by definition, the signs and symptoms clear completely in less than 24 hours. The TIAs should be understood to be forewarnings of possible stroke. The focus of care includes diagnosis of TIAs versus other problems; prevention of stroke by modification of risk factors; treatment with antiplatelet drugs or surgical intervention if indicated; ongoing monitoring for change in risk factors or condition; and patient education.

The person needs to be aggressively worked-up and treated *before* a stroke occurs. Diagnostic evaluation proceeds in a stepwise progression. Initially, the following tests are generally ordered: complete blood cell count, platelets, electrolytes, blood urea nitrogen, creatinine, glucose, fasting lipid panel (total cholesterol, low-density lipoproteins, high-density lipoproteins), prothrombin time, activated partial thromboplastin time, and sedimentation rate. Other studies include an electrocardiogram (EKG), a CT scan (particularly in hemispheric TIAs), noninvasive computed imaging, and transcranial Doppler (TCD). Further investigation to resolve persistent diagnostic uncertainty may include transthoracic echocardiography (TTE), transesophageal echocardiography (TEE), TCDs if not already completed, magnetic resonance angiography, cerebral arteriography, and antiphospholipids. In addition, when continuing to pursue cardiogenic source (for silent myocardial ischemia), an ambulatory EKG, an exercise EKG, or a thallium perfusion may be ordered. Other tests for prothrombotic states are listed in Table 27-4; this table also includes a description of all diagnostics.

TABLE 27-3
Major Risk Factors for Stroke

• Hypertension • Atrial fibrillation • Hyperlipidemia • Diabetes mellitus • Stress • Excessive alcohol use	• Clinical symptoms of CHD • EKG or radiographic evidence of CHD • Sedentary lifestyle • Smoking • Obesity • Valvular disease (*e.g.,* mitral valve)

TABLE 27-4
*Stroke and TIAs: Diagnostics**

CT scan without contrast	Important immediate diagnostic to differentiate between ischemic and hemorrhagic stroke; if hemorrhagic, antiplatelets or anticoagulants are not given because of the increased risk of more bleeding; important for treatment decisions.
CT scan with contrast	Useful to rule out lesions that many mimic a TIA, especially when symptoms are related to hemispheric deficits; hypodense areas on CT scan suggest infarction.
Magnetic resonance imaging (MRI)	Offers excellent soft tissue contrast discrimination with superior demarcation of mass lesion from surrounding structures including areas of ischemia and infarction; good visualization of vascular structures when questioning a vascular lesion; useful for diagnosis of stroke in first 72 hours; a diffusion weighted MRI can show ischemia in first few hours.
Magnetic resonance angiography (MRA)	Less available and higher cost; noninvasive imaging of the carotid, vertebral, basilar, and major intracranial and extracranial arteries to determine occlusion; useful for clot visualization.
Carotid ultrasonography	Noninvasive imaging; widely used initial diagnositic in patients with carotid territory symptoms for whom CEE is considered; cervical carotid artery imaging often required to exclude high-grade stenosis, which is an exclusion for CEE; less sensitive in assessing mild to moderate stenosis.
Transcranial Doppler (TCD)	TCDs are now part of standard work-up for stroke, especially when CEE is considered; useful to detect severe intracranial stenosis, evaluate the carotid and vertebrobasilar vessels, assess patterns and extent of collateral circulation in patients with known arterial stenosis or occlusion, and detection of microemboli.†
Blood flow studies	The PET, SPECT, and Xenox CT are used to determine global and focal blood flow; used mostly for clinical research.
Cerebral angiography	Ordered for patients considered candidates for CEE to precisely define the percentage of occlusion and in patients with unusual presentation with aneurysm, vasculitis, high-grade stenosis.
Transthoracic echocardiography (TTE)	Helpful in search for cardioemboli sources; TTE is particularly helpful for diagnosing of left ventricular thrombi, left atrial myxomas, and thrombi that protrude into the atrial cavity; they are less reliable for small tumors, laminated thrombi, and thrombi limited to the left or right atrium.‡
Transesophageal echocardiography (TEE)	Benefit of TEE is in greater sensitivity for source of cardioemboli (except ventricular disease); TEE provides better visualization of cardiac structures, especially those at greater depth from chest wall and lesions of the atria (atrial appendage thrombi associated with atrial fibrillation, interarterial septum defects (patent foramen ovale, atrial septal defects), mitral valvular vegetation, and atherosclerotic disease of ascending aortic arch.§
Electrocardiogram (EKG)	Useful when cardiogenic embolic stroke or concurrent coronary artery disease is suspected.
Ambulatory EKG monitoring	Reserved for patients who have suspicious palpitations, arrhythmias, or enlarged left atrium.
Prothrombotic states	Protein C, protein S, antithrombin III, thrombin time, Hgb, electrophoresis, anticardiolipin antibody, lupus anticoagulant, and syphilis serology.

CT = computed tomography, CEE = carotidendarterectomy, PET = positron emission tomography, SPECT = single photon emission computed tomography.

* *Feinberg, W. M., Albers, G. W., Barnett, H. J. M., Biller, J., Caplan, L. R., Carter, L. P., Hart, R. G., Hobson, R. W., Kronmal, R. A., Moore, W. S., & Robertson, J. T. (1994). Guidelines for the management of transient ischemic attacks. Stroke, 25(6), 1320–1335.*

† *Tong, D. C., Bolger, A., & Albers, G. W. (1994). Stroke, 25, 2138–2141.*

‡ *Reeder, G. S., Khandheria, B. K., Seward, J. B., & Tajik, A. J. (1991). Transesophageal echocardiography and cardiac masses. Mayo Clinic Proceedings, 66:(11) 1101–1109.*

§ *Ibid.*

Stroke

In the patient who has neurological deficits consistent with a stroke, there are a number of diagnostics that are helpful in determining the type of stroke, which then determines treatment options (see Table 27-4). The most important initial diagnostic is a CT scan without contrast medium to differentiate between ischemic and hemorrhagic stroke. Early treatment for ischemic stroke includes anticoagulation therapy or possible thrombolytic therapy, both of which are contraindicated if hemorrhagic stroke is present. Therefore, differentiating between ischemic and hemorrhagic stroke is critical to treatment decisions.

Once a patient has been stabilized from acute stroke, further diagnostic investigation may follow to determine primary problems related to the stroke (*e.g.*, cardiac disease, carotid or vertebrobasilar occlusion) which will need to be addressed to prevent future strokes.

TREATMENT OF TIAs AND ISCHEMIC STROKE

In the following section, management of stroke will be discussed according to stroke preventive therapy including medical management and treatment, surgical interventions, and interventional neuroradiological treatment; hypervolemic-hemodilution therapy; reperfusion therapy; neuroprotective agents; and rehabilitation.

Paradigm Shift to Prevention

The overall approach to patients with risk factors for stroke—TIAs, stroke, and poststroke—is toward prevention of a first stroke or, in the person who has already had a stroke, prevention of another stroke. Prevention is geared toward identification of all risk factors; modification of modifiable risk factors; drug therapy; surgical interventions, when appropriate; and education of the patient and families. Education is directed at helping the person understand his or her risk factors and the need to make a commitment to lifestyle changes and adherence to treatment plans to prevent stroke. Mass general education directed at educating all people to understand a "brain attack" as a medical emergency that warrants immediate emergency department care must be undertaken. The general public understands that a heart attack is a medical emergency that requires a call to 911 for emergency help to save lives and heart muscle. People need to apply the same sense of urgency to a brain attack. Educating the public about the signs and symptoms of a brain attack and the definitive action to be taken is very cost-effective and can save human potential and quality of life.

Medical Management and Treatment

Antiplatelet and other antithrombotic therapy are the mainstay of medical management. Guidelines for antithrombotic therapy, which have been outlined by expert consensus based on clinical research, include the recommendations shown in the table below.[23]

As noted, the mainstay of drug therapy is aspirin and ticlopidine. Combination of both drugs is not uncommon, but this increases the risk of adverse drug responses such as bleeding. In one study, ticlopidine was shown to be more effective than aspirin for secondary stroke prevention in patients with noncardioembolic TIA or minor stroke. It may also be more effective in blacks, women, and patients with a vertebrobasilar event.[24]

An intravenous heparin infusion for 3 to 5 days during acute care management of progressive ischemic stroke is common. Use of warfarin for anticoagulation is now generally reserved for high-grade artery stenosis, large vessel disease, and cardioembolic sources, especially atrial fibrillation. Low molecular weight heparin, given subcutaneously, is now being used in some centers rather than IV heparin; this has the added advantage of requiring a reduced length of stay.[25] It is also given at the beginning of warfarin therapy to aid in reaching therapeutic international normalizing ratio (INR) levels faster.

There has been much written in the literature to support the use of the INR to monitor anticoagulation therapy rather than prothrombin time (PT). Because of laboratory variability in reagents used to perform PT, the use of INR is recommended nationally.[26]

Surgical Interventions

Selected patients with extracranial or intracranial atherosclerotic disease that is located in accessible sites (areas previously mentioned) may be good candidates for surgery.

PROBLEM	RECOMMENDED	ACCEPTABLE	COMMENT
TIAs or minor ischemic stroke	Aspirin (ASA) 75–1300 mg/d	• ASA 75–1300 mg/d • Ticlopidine (Ticlid) 250 mg bid	Ticlid if ASA intolerant (allergy, GI upset/bleeding); monitor for diarrhea, rash, and CBC q 2 wk for 3 months for neutropenia
TIAs with ASA	Ticlid 250 mg bid		
Carotid bruit and asymptomatic carotid artery stenosis	ASA 325 mg/d Modify risk factors (HPT, smoking, diet)	ASA 75–1,300 mg/d	Evaluate for percent of carotid occlusion; if 70% or greater, consider carotid endarterectomy (CEE)
Symptomatic carotid artery stenosis	Consider CEE ASA, Ticlid, or both	ASA, Ticlid, or both	
Atrial fibrillation	Warfarin international normalizing ratio (INR) 2–3	• Warfarin INR 1.5–3 • ASA 325 mg/d if can't take warfarin	With secondary prevention, warfarin INR 2–4.5
Progressing ischemic stroke	Heparin (IV) anticoagulation for 3–5 d; then to warfarin	Low molecular weight heparin (SC) being used more frequently	Low molecular weight heparin may be given before warfarin therapy to reach therapeutic INR faster
Completed thrombotic stroke	ASA or Ticlid	ASA, Ticlid, or both	
Complete embolic stroke	Heparin followed by warfarin to INR 2–3 for small–moderate stroke if no evidence of hemorrhagic transformation	Anticoagulation Rx usually postponed 5–14 days with large stroke or uncontrolled hypertension because high risk for hemorrhagic transformation	Note hemorrhagic transformation can occur, making the patient high risk for hemorrhage
Lacunar stroke	ASA, Ticlid, or both	ASA, Ticlid, or both	

The goal of the surgical procedures is to prevent TIAs or stroke. Carotid endarterectomy or extracranial graft may benefit the patient with narrowing of the extracranial artery. A bypass grafting procedure may be of value for the patient with an intracranial occlusion, such as of the internal carotid or middle cerebral artery. The procedure often used for intracranial involvement is superior temporal artery/middle cerebral artery (STA-MCA) anastomosis. For patients who have an identified thrombus, a thrombectomy may be done to restore circulation.

CAROTID ENDARTERECTOMY

The North American Symptomatic Carotid Endarterectomy Trial (NASCET) clearly demonstrated that carotid endarterectomy (CEE) is superior to medical therapy alone for stroke prevention in patients with 70% or greater symptomatic internal carotid artery stenosis. Patients with 70% or greater carotid stenosis, without major operative risk factors, have a relative reduction of about 60% and absolute risk reduction of 5% to 10% per year within the subsequent 2 years.[27] The role of CEE as compared to medical management in patients with carotid stenosis in the range of 30% to 69% is still under investigation. Currently, most patients with symptomatic stenosis of less than 70% are managed medically.

The "hot spots" for atheroma buildup are noted in Fig. 27-8. A CEE consists of careful removal of the atherosclerotic plaque and intraluminal clot, if present from the artery after a temporary bypass shunt has been created to provide adequate cerebral perfusion. The plaque is removed after the artery is temporarily occluded both above and below the atheroma. In some instances, a bypass graft is used to improve circulation. The major danger during surgery is embolization of atherogenic plaque and thrombi from excessive manipulation of the carotid bifurcation. Upon completion, a Jackson-Pratt drain may be inserted at the operative site to prevent development of a hematoma.

The major postoperative concerns are blood pressure instability, stroke or transient neurological deficits, cranial nerve injury (facial, vagal), wound hematoma and suture line rupture, TIAs, and hyperperfusion syndromes.[28] After surgery, patients experience a period of postoperative blood pressure instability that lasts for approximately 12 to 24 hours, probably due to a carotid sinus malfunction and loss of effective baroreceptor action. Once blood flow has been restored, maintenance of the systolic pressure at a constant level of approximately 150 mm Hg is critical. The sudden restoration of high flow, especially after removal of a tight stenosis and in the presence of heparin (used during surgery) or antiplatelets, can lead to intracerebral hemorrhage. Hypotensive episodes are just as disastrous and can result in ischemic stroke or TIAs. The potential for cranial nerve injury results from the proximity of these nerves to the operative site.

Hyperperfusion syndromes are related to the marked increase in cerebral blood flow after CEE. Patients often have paralysis of autoregulation ipsilaterally to the surgical site so that the profound increase in blood flow is not blunted. When this occurs, blood pressure must be meticulously maintained in the 120 to 130 mm Hg range. Patients may experience vascular headaches or catastrophic intracerebral hemorrhage. Seizures may occur about 7 to 10 days

postoperative. Finally, a leading cause of death after CEE is myocardial infarction, either immediately or delayed. The patient should be monitored carefully for evidence of myocardial ischemia or infarction.

STA-MCA Anastomosis. Extracranial/intracranial anastomosis, most often of the superficial temporal artery to the MCA, is a microsurgical bypass procedure used to provide collateral circulation to the areas of the brain supplied by the MCA. Currently, it is used infrequently because of the negative results reported in the EC/IC Bypass Trial.[29]

Thrombectomy. An emergency thrombectomy may have some dramatic results. Major concerns are the development of severe cerebral edema due to reperfusion of necrotic tissue. Thrombectomy has been replaced by thrombolytic therapy.

INTERVENTIONAL NEURORADIOLOGICAL TREATMENT

Percutaneous transluminal angioplasty (PTA) and stent placement are experimental interventional neuroradiological options for intracranial large-artery stenosis. Clinical trials with small numbers of patients suggest angioplasty can be done relatively safely by experienced hands without a high rate of distal embolism, dissection, or stroke. Currently, angioplasty for stroke patients is being refined.

HYPERVOLEMIC-HEMODILUTION THERAPY

Intravenous anticoagulation therapy with intravenous heparin is used to decrease further development of thrombi and occlusion. As noted earlier, some centers are now using low molecular weight heparin (LMWH), given subcutaneously, instead of an intravenous heparin drip. The use of LMWH has the added advantage of decreasing the length of hospital stay, with associated cost savings. It is expected that the use of LMWH will be expanded and become a standard approach in stroke management.

To support cerebral hemodynamics, hypervolemic-hemodilution therapy is used (see Chap. 28). This therapy helps to maintain a stable, slightly higher blood pressure, which increases and maintains cerebral perfusion pressure by lowering blood viscosity. The hematocrit is reduced to 33 to 35 mg/dL, and hypervolemia is achieved with saline and albumin.

REPERFUSION

Both intravenous recombinant tissue plasminogen activator (t-PA) and intra-arterial (urokinase and streptokinase) thrombolytic agents have been used in acute ischemic stroke to restore cerebral blood flow, reduce ischemia, and limit neurological disability. The recanalization of an occluded cerebral artery may assist the recovery of ischemic tissue within a brief time span after onset of stroke. The major concern with these therapies is cerebral edema and hemorrhage associated with reperfusion of necrotic tissue. Risk for hemorrhage is further increased by systemic fibrinolytic drug effects. For these reasons, it is necessary to use these therapies very early, before tissue necrosis develops.

Intravenous t-PA. The European Cooperative Acute Stroke Study (ECASS) has provided the first definitive study on the efficacy and safety of intravenous thrombolysis using t-PA in patients with acute ischemic stroke. They found that intravenous thrombolysis in acute ischemic stroke effective improves some functional measures and neurological outcomes in a defined subgroup of stroke patients with moderate to severe neurological deficit and without extended infarct signs on the initial CT scan.[30] In another study, treatment with intravenous t-PA within 3 hours of the onset of ischemic stroke improved clinical outcome at 3 months.[31] Although there are optimistic reports on the use of intravenous t-PA, it is only appropriate for selected patients within 3 to 6 hours of ischemic stroke onset. The most serious adverse effect is intracerebral hemorrhage. (See the Appendix for an algorithm and selection criteria.)

NEUROPROTECTIVE AGENTS

A number of investigational neuroprotective agents designed to protect the brain from delayed injury by interfering in the steps of the ischemic cascade of neuronal injury and reperfusion injury are undergoing clinical trials. The disturbance in calcium flux and calcium-activated enzyme systems, production of free radicals, membrane destruction, and disturbance in protein synthesis are being investigated. NMDA antagonists, calcium antagonists (nimodipine), opiate antagonists, free radical scavengers (Trilazad), superoxide dismutase (a naturally occurring scavenger), and lazaroids are currently in clinical trials. What is known is that they must be given within a brief (several hours) window of opportunity to be effective.

REHABILITATION

Early rehabilitation is important to making optimal recovery; rehabilitation needs to be addressed immediately. Figure 27-9 provides a flow diagram for stroke rehabilitation from the clinical practice guidelines, *Post-Stroke Rehabilitation.*[32] This is an outstanding resource that sets the national standard for stroke rehabilitation and should be familiar to all care providers of stroke patients (see Chap. 14 for rehabilitation content).

ACUTE MANAGEMENT OF INTRACEREBRAL HEMORRHAGIC STROKE

For persons who sustain an intracerebral hemorrhagic stroke, acute management is directed toward management of increased ICP as outlined in Chapter 17. To control increased ICP, a ventriculostomy may be necessary. Vasospasms are not considered a problem with an intracerebral hemorrhage. Chapter 28 also provides guidance for patient management.

For patients that survive, rehabilitation is necessary. In addition, identification and modification of risk factors needs to be undertaken. Nursing management is outlined in Chapters 17 and 28.

GENERAL NURSING MANAGEMENT OF THE STROKE PATIENT

Nursing management of patients with stroke varies according to the specific stroke syndrome and neurological and functional deficits. However, there are a number of areas to consider, including primary and secondary prevention of stroke; initial management during the acute phase; early focus on rehabilitation; discharge planning and continuity of care; and patient education. Assessment and nursing diagnosis guide nursing management.

Primary and Secondary Prevention of Stroke

The paradigm shift from treatment to prevention has redefined the nurse's role in identification of risk factors and working with the patient not only to modify risk factors, but also to promote a healthier lifestyle. The major risk factors for stroke are listed in Table 27-2. These major risk factors are the same for stroke and heart disease, the number one and number three causes of death in the United States. Nurses are particularly effective in helping patients to think through how they can modify risk factors within the context of their lifestyles. Secondary prevention becomes the focus after a stroke to prevent another stroke, regardless of whether the patient is followed in a stroke prevention clinic or by the primary care provider. Along with education and motivation, the patient must be monitored collaboratively by the nurse and physician. Prevention is cost effective and results in cost savings.

Possible nursing diagnoses related to stroke prevention include the following:

- Knowledge Deficit
- Noncompliance
- Ineffective Management of Therapeutic Regimen

Initial Management During the Acute Phase

Early treatment of stroke is recognized as a key factor in optimizing outcomes. Care may be rendered in a neuro ICU or special acute care unit. Once stabilized, the patient may receive therapies to protect the brain from secondary injury related to the ischemic cascade. The brief window of opportunity to use thrombolytic or neuroprotective agents is approximately 3 to 6 hours after onset of ischemic stroke. The acute care management goals for intracranial occlusive disease include maintaining the following:

- An adequate airway and oxygenation to avoid hypoxia
- Stable, slightly higher blood pressure to maximize cerebral perfusion pressure
- Serum glucose in a range below 150 mg/dL with insulin as necessary to avoid the increased risk of cerebral edema and hemorrhage
- Aseptic technique, following procedures to prevent infections (*e.g.,* aspiration pneumonia, urinary tract infection)[33]

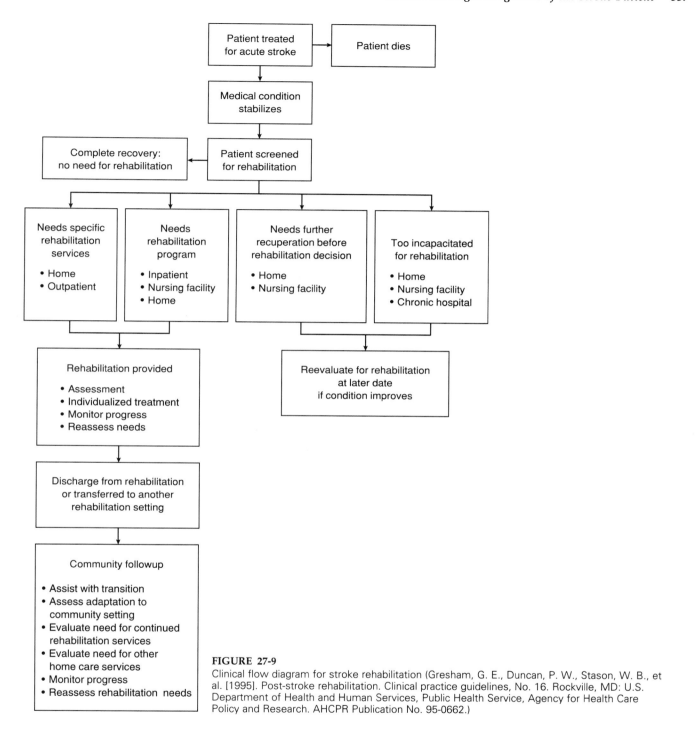

FIGURE 27-9
Clinical flow diagram for stroke rehabilitation (Gresham, G. E., Duncan, P. W., Stason, W. B., et al. [1995]. Post-stroke rehabilitation. Clinical practice guidelines, No. 16. Rockville, MD: U.S. Department of Health and Human Services, Public Health Service, Agency for Health Care Policy and Research. AHCPR Publication No. 95-0662.)

The treatment options include antiplatelet agents, anticoagulation with heparin, thrombolysis, hypervolemia-hemodilution, and calcium channel blockers.[34]

Many patients will be managed in ICU settings to monitor closely for effects from therapies such as thrombolytics. The nurse works collaboratively with the physician to achieve the goals listed above.

The following nursing diagnoses and collaborative problems may be made in the acute phase of illness:

Possible Nursing Diagnoses

- Ineffective Airway Clearance
- Risk of Aspiration
- Impaired Swallowing
- Altered Cerebral Tissue Perfusion
- Risk of Infection
- Ineffective Breathing Pattern
- Sensory Perceptual Alterations

- Impaired Physical Mobility
- Impaired Verbal Communication

Possible Collaborative Problems

- Hypoxemia
- Hypo/hyperglycemia
- Increased intracranial pressure
- Stroke
- Paresis/paresthesia/paralysis
- Gastrointestinal bleeding
- Hypertension
- Reperfusion injury
- Electrolyte imbalances
- Dysrhythmias
- Anticoagulant therapy adverse effects

Frequent neurological, hemodynamic, and respiratory monitoring is necessary to determine early changes and need to adjust management. Cerebral edema develops with all ischemic strokes, but cerebral edema is a major concern with a large stroke. Severe hypertension increases the risk of hemorrhage. Both cerebral edema and hemorrhage are associated with increased ICP. Increased ICP may be due to the original hemorrhage, but hemorrhage can also occur 2 to 4 days after massive infarction of the cerebral hemisphere. The development of edema is heralded by a gradual deterioration in neurological signs, such as drowsiness and sluggish pupillary response. Increased ICP is treated with osmotic diuretics and hyperventilation. Supportive therapy depends on the extent of the deficits and complications present. For the conscious patient, assess for fluent and nonfluent aphasia.

Careful cardiac monitoring is necessary to determine the need to adjust therapy to maximize hemodynamic parameters. It is also necessary to observe for secondary insult such as myocardial infarction. The level of the head of the bed will depend on hemodynamics and ICP, but it is generally elevated to 30 degrees. Respiratory parameters are also monitored closely for evidence of secondary problems such as neurogenic pulmonary edema, atelectasis, and pneumonia. For patients on ventilatory support, weaning should begin as soon as possible. The awake patient should be maintained at "nothing by mouth" until a swallowing study has been conducted and problems of aspiration have been ruled out.

Both hypoglycemia and hyperglycemia are detrimental to the injured brain. Hyperglycemia above 150 mg/dL increases infarct size in experimental stroke models and contributes to poorer outcomes. Serum glucose should be monitored and kept in the normal range with regular insulin. In addition, intravenous solutions should be **saline and not glucose.** For patients receiving anticoagulants such as heparin, monitor the activated partial thromboplastin time and observe for bleeding. Electrolytes, creatinine, and blood urea nitrogen are monitored. Electrolyte imbalance, particularly sodium, is common and should be managed.

For details about the key points in acute care nursing management of stroke patients after treatment with special interventions see Chart 27-1. Chart 27-2 summarizes the common nursing diagnoses associated with stroke. See also Chapter 16 for management of the unconscious patient and Chapter 17 for ICP management. Once the patient's condition has sta-

bilized, nursing management is refocused on rehabilitation and prevention of another stroke (Chart 27-3).

Early Focus on Rehabilitation

Rehabilitation begins as soon as the patient is stabilized. Figure 27-9 provides an overview of stroke rehabilitation. The nurse collaborates with other health professional to develop a plan of care. The case manager is an integral part of the interdisciplinary team who can facilitate access to rehabilitation resources and community based rehabilitation services. Nursing responsibilities in the rehabilitation process are outlined in Chart 27-4. See Chapter 14 for information about rehabilitation.

The following nursing diagnoses are often seen in stroke patients and are related to the need for early rehabilitation:

Possible Nursing Diagnoses

- Self Care Deficits
- Sensory Perceptual Alterations
- Impaired Verbal Communication
- Impaired Physical Mobility
- Altered Urinary Elimination
- Disuse Syndrome
- Altered Thought Processes
- Impaired Adjustment
- Altered Role Performance
- Unilateral Neglect

Possible Collaborative Problems

- Antiplatelet therapy adverse effects

Discharge Planning and Continuity of Care

Discharge planning is taken into account early in the rehabilitative program. The plans for discharge are made with the assistance of the case manager, who assists with continuity and facilitates access to the next level of care, be it rehabilitation or home care. The patient and family should be made aware of community resources (see Chap. 15). A critical point in discharge planning is to be sure that the patient has an appointment for follow-up so that recovery, new problems, and drug therapy can be monitored (see the earlier section on rehabilitation and the *Post-Stroke Rehabilitation* clinical practice guidelines).

Once in the community, integration back into community life and roles is important. Rehabilitation continues and is monitored. Depression is common after stroke and is seen in 40% to 50% of patients. Patients and family need to be prepared for this possibility. Pharmacotherapy is quite effective in the treatment of depression. Related nursing diagnoses are listed in the following section.

Patient Education

Patient and family education takes place within a compressed period of time. It is unrealistic to expect that all education can be completed during this short period. Patient education must be viewed along a continuum that extends through the next

CHART 27-1
Key Points in Acute Care Nursing Management of Stroke Patients After Treatment With Special Interventions

Nursing Management of Patients Who Have Undergone Thrombolytic Therapy

- Monitor vital signs for evidence of extracranial bleeding (*e.g.*, gastric hemorrhage).
- Monitor neurological signs for evidence of deterioration and increased intracranial pressure (ICP) that may be caused by intracerebral hemorrhage or increasing cerebral edema.
- Monitor for reperfusion injury.*
- Monitor for bleeding at catheter site; bleeding may also be noted in urine or stool, or from mouth.
- Monitor coagulation studies and maintain in therapeutic parameters.
- Protect femoral catheter, which is left in place for 24 hours.

Nursing Management of Patients Who Have Undergone Cerebral Angiography/Stent Placement

- Monitor vital signs for hemodynamic instability.
- Monitor for bleeding at catheter site; bleeding may also be noted in urine, stool, GI tract, or mouth.
- Monitor neurological signs for evidence of intracerebral hemorrhage and reperfusion injury.*
- Monitor coagulation studies and maintain in therapeutic range using international normalizing ratio (INR) parameters.

Nursing Management of Patients Who Have Undergone a Carotid Endarterectomy

- Monitor blood pressure and rigorously maintain within set parameters, usually about 150 mm Hg systolic (hypertension predisposes to intracerebral hemorrhage, and hypotension to ischemic stroke); instability of blood pressure is common particularly in the first 12 to 24 hours postoperatively so expect to monitor and manage blood pressure frequently.
- Monitor for cardiac arrhythmias and evidence of myocardial ischemia (myocardial infarction is not uncommon).
- Monitor neurological signs frequently and observe for early signs of deterioration.
  - Monitor for cranial nerve deficits (especially facial and vagal) as a result of surgery.
  - Monitor for signs of intracerebral hemorrhage (increased ICP, new onset of neurological deficits).
  - Monitor for vascular headache and seizures (hyperperfusion syndrome).
- Monitor for reperfusion injury.*
- Maintain head of bed according to physician orders; because of vascular instability, the head of the bed may be flat for the first 24 hours.
- Observe operative site for hemorrhage, hematoma, or tearing of suture site.

Nursing Management of Patients Who Are Receiving Intravenous Heparin Administration

- Monitor neurological signs for evidence of deterioration and increased ICP that may be caused by intracerebral hemorrhage or increasing cerebral edema.
- Monitor coagulation studies and maintain in therapeutic range using INR parameters.
- Adjust intravenous heparin infusion according to coagulation parameters.
- Monitor for bleeding at catheter site and from urine, stool, GI tract, or mouth; note evidence of bruising easily.
- Monitor for reperfusion injury.*

* **Reperfusion injury:** observe for signs and symptoms of cerebral edema, increased ICP, and recurrence stroke symptomology or expansion of neurological deficits after successful recanalization.

---

level of care and in the community by the health provider. Decide what is critical for the patient to know.

Possible Nursing Diagnoses

- Knowledge Deficit
- Caregiver Role Strain
- Altered Family Processes
- Sexual Dysfunction

Possible Collaborative Problems

- Depression

MEDICATIONS

The most common drugs for patients being discharged with medications are antiplatelets and anticoagulants. Both require

(text continues on page 565)

CHART 27-2

Summary of Common Nursing Diagnoses for Stroke Patients in Acute Phase

Nursing Diagnoses (Potential or Actual)	Nursing Interventions	Expected Outcomes
Ineffective Airway Clearance related to (R/T) unconsciousness or ineffective cough reflex	• Position the patient to facilitate drainage of oropharyngeal secretions; turn the patient from side to side every 2 hours. • Elevate the head of the bed to 30 degrees. • Clear secretions from the airway using suction, as necessary; provide for pulmonary hygiene. • Provide for chest physical therapy. • Provide for coughing and deep breathing exercises. • If the patient is receiving oxygen therapy, be sure that it is adequately humidified.	• The airway will be patent, allowing for increased air exchange. • The risk of aspiration will be decreased. • The risk of elevated CO_2, which contributes to cerebral hypoxia and cerebral edema, will be decreased.
Risk of Aspiration R/T inability to protect airway or unconsciousness	• Maintain nothing-by-mouth status. • Swallow studies needed to evaluate swallowing function before oral intake is tried. • When oral intake is resumed, take precautions to prevent aspiration (elevate head of bed, hold head up, etc.).	• Aspiration and aspiration pneumonia will not develop.
Altered Tissue Perfusion, cerebral, R/T ischemia, cerebral edema, or increased intracranial pressure (ICP)	• Monitor vital and neurological signs. • Maintain venous outflow from the brain by elevating the head of the bed 30 degrees. • Maintain the patient's head in a neutral position. • Avoid positions that increase intra-abdominal/ intrathoracic pressure (hip flexion, prone position, etc.; see Chap. 17). • Maintain normothermia. • Avoid activities known to increase ICP (clustering activities, etc.; see Chap. 17).	• Vital signs will be maintained within normal limits. • Cerebral perfusion pressure will be maintained.

(continued)

CHART 27-2 Summary of Common Nursing Diagnoses for Stroke Patients in Acute Phase (Continued)

Nursing Diagnoses (Potential or Actual)	Nursing Interventions	Expected Outcomes
Risk of Infection	• Maintain the patient's blood pressure within the range set for sufficient cerebral perfusion pressure. • Aseptic technique will be followed. • Urinary catheter will be removed as soon as possible. • Measures will be taken to prevent respiratory infections.	• Infections will not develop in lungs, urinary tract, catheter sites.
Sensory/Perceptual Alterations: • Kinesthetic • Tactile • Visual R/T altered consciousness, impaired sensation, or impaired vision	• Provide appropriate stimulation to involved areas of sense. • Monitor the level of sensation. • Patch the patient's eye and alter the patch for diplopia. • Place materials on and approach the patient from the unaffected side if homonymous hemianopia is present. • Provide tactile stimulation to hands and limbs affected by decreased sensation. • Protect the patient from injury. • Develop compensatory strategies to meet particular patient needs.	• Optimal sensory input will be received and interpreted accurately. • Safety will be maintained.
Impaired Verbal Communication R/T cerebral injury/altered level of consciousness	• Assess type of communication deficit present. • Develop appropriate methods for communications.	• An alternative method of communication will be established. • The patient's attempts to communicate will be supported.
Impaired Physical Mobility R/T neurological deficts	• Assess the type and degree of impairment. • Provide slings, braces, support shoes, and so forth, as necessary. • Teach the patient alternative methods of mobility. • Provide for range-of-motion exercises four times per day.	• Alternative methods of mobility will be used. • Passive movement will be provided to prevent the negative effects on the nervous system that are associated with immobility.

CHART 27-3
Common Deficits and Emotional Reactions to Stroke and Related
General Nursing Interventions

Common Motor Deficits

1. Hemiparesis or hemiplegia (side of the body opposite the cerebral episode)
2. Dysarthria (muscles of speech impaired)
3. Dysphagia (muscles of swallowing impaired)

Nursing Interventions

1. Position the patient in proper body alignment; use a hand roll to keep the hand in a functional position.
   - Provide frequent passive range-of-motion exercises.
   - Reposition the patient every 2 hours.
2. Provide for an alternative method of communication.
3. Test the patient's palatal and pharyngeal reflexes before offering nourishment.
   - Elevate and turn the patient's head to the unaffected side.
   - If the patient is able to manage oral intake, place food on the unaffected side of the patient's mouth.

Common Sensory Deficits

1. Visual deficits (common because the visual pathways cut through much of the cerebral hemispheres)
   a. Homonymous hemianopia (loss of vision in half of the visual field on the same side)

Left   Right

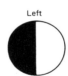 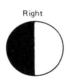

   b. Double vision (diplopia)
   c. Decreased visual acuity
2. Absent or diminished response to superficial sensation (touch, pain, pressure, heat, cold)

3. Absent or diminished response to proprioception (knowledge of position of body parts)
4. Perceptual deficits (disturbance in correctly perceiving and interpreting self and/or environment)
   a. Body scheme disturbance (amnesia or denial for paralyzed extremities; **unilateral neglect syndrome)**

Nursing Interventions

1. Be aware that variations of visual deficits may exist and compensate for them.

   a. Approach the patient from the unaffected side; remind the patient to turn the head to compensate for visual deficits.

   b. Apply an eye patch to the affected eye.
   c. Provide assistance as necessary.
2. Increase the amount of touch in administering patient care.
   - Protect the involved areas from injury.
   - Protect the involved areas from burns.
   - Examine the involved areas for signs of skin irritation and injury.
   - Provide the patient with an opportunity to handle various objects of different weight, texture, and size.
   - If pain is present, assess its location and type, as well as the duration of the pain.
3. Teach the patient to check the position of body parts visually.
4. Compensate for the patient's perceptual–sensory deficits.

   a. Protect the involved area.
   - Accept the patient's self-perception.
   - Position the patient to face the involved area.

(continued)

Common Sensory Deficits

b. Disorientation (to time, place, and person)

c. Apraxia (loss of ability to use objects correctly)

d. Agnosia (inability to identify the environment by means of the senses)

e. Defects in localizing objects in space, estimating their size, and judging distance

f. Impaired memory for recall of spatial location of objects or places

g. Right–left disorientation

Nursing Interventions

b. Control the amount of change in the patient's schedule.
  - Reorient the patient as necessary.
  - Talk to the patient; tell him or her about the immediate environment.
  - Provide a calendar, clock, pictures of family, and so forth.

c. Correct misuse of objects and demonstrate proper use.

d. Correct misinformation.

e. Reduce any stimuli that will distract the patient.

f. Place necessary equipment where the patient will see it, rather than telling the patient "It is in the closet" and so forth.

g. Phrase requests carefully, like "Lift this leg." (Point to the leg.)

Language Deficits

1. Non-fluent aphasia (difficulty in transforming sound into patterns of understandable speech)—can speak using single-word responses
2. Fluent aphasia (impairment of comprehension of the spoken word)—able to speak, but uses words incorrectly and is unaware of these errors
3. Global aphasia (combination of expressive and receptive aphasia)—unable to communicate at any level
4. Alexia (inability to understand the written word)
5. Agraphia (inability to express ideas in writing)

Nursing Interventions

1. Ask the patient to repeat the individual sounds of the alphabet as a start at retraining.
2. Speak clearly and in simple sentences; use gestures as necessary.
3. Evaluate what language skills are intact; speak in very simple sentences, ask the patient to repeat individual sounds, and use gestures or any other means to communicate.
4. Point to the written names of objects and have the patient repeat the name of the object.
5. Have the patient write words and simple sentences.

Intellectual Deficits

1. Loss of memory
2. Short attention span
3. Increased distractibility
4. Poor judgment
5. Inability to transfer learning from one situation to another
6. Inability to calculate, reason, or think abstractly

Nursing Interventions

1. Provide information as necessary.
2. Divide activities into short steps.
3. Control any excessive environmental distractions.
4. Protect the patient from injury.
5. Repeat instructions as necessary.

6. Do not set unrealistic expectations for the patient.

Emotional Deficits

(Recognize that pattern is often inconsistent; patient may have good days and bad days or even good hours and bad hours.)
1. Emotional lability (exhibits reactions easily or inappropriately)
2. Loss of self-control and social inhibitions (may speak inappropriately or swear or may expose self or make sexual advances toward nurse)

Nursing Interventions

1. Disregard bursts of emotions; explain to the patient that emotional lability is part of the illness.
2. Protect the patient as necessary so that his or her dignity is preserved; recognize the involuntary bases of this behavior and set limits; anticipate needs.

(continued)

CHART 27-3 Common Deficits and Emotional Reactions to Stroke and Related General Nursing Interventions (Continued)

Emotional Deficits

3. Reduced tolerance for stress

4. Fear, hostility, frustration, anger
5. Confusion and despair

6. Withdrawal, isolation

7. Depression

Nursing Interventions

3. Control the environment and maintain routines as much as possible; remove stimuli that are upsetting to the patient.
4. Be accepting of the patient; be supportive.
5. Clarify any misconceptions; allow the patient to verbalize.
6. Provide stimulation and a safe, comfortable environment.
7. Provide a supportive environment; consider pharmacotherapy.

Explain behavior to family as a manifestation of brain injury. Be supportive.

Bowel and Bladder Dysfunction

Bladder: Incomplete Upper Motor Neuron Lesion

1. The unilateral lesion from the stroke results in partial sensation and control of the bladder, so that the patient experiences frequency, urgency, and incontinence. (Cognitive deficits affect control.)
2. If the stroke lesion is in the brain stem, there will be bilateral damage, resulting in an upper motor neuron bladder with loss of all control of micturition.

Nursing Interventions

Do not suggest insertion of an indwelling catheter immediately after the stroke; intermittent catheterization is better than an indwelling catheter.

---

1. Observe the patient to identify characteristics of the voiding pattern (frequency, amount, forcefulness of stream, constant dribbling, etc.).

2. Maintain an accurate intake and output record.

Nursing note: Incontinence after regaining consciousness is usually attributable to urinary tract infection caused by use of an indwelling urinary catheter.

---

3. Possibility of establishing normal bladder function is excellent.

3. Try to allow the patient to stay catheter-free:
   - Offer the bedpan or urinal frequently.
   - Take the patient to the commode frequently.
   - Assess the patient's ability to make his or her need for help with voiding known.
   If a catheter is necessary, remove it as soon as possible and follow a bladder training program (see Chap. 8).

Bowel

1. Altered bowel function in a stroke patient is attributable to:
   - Deterioration in the level of consciousness
   - Dehydration
   - Immobility
2. Constipation is the most common problem, along with potential impaction.

1. Develop a bowel training program:
   - Give foods known to stimulate defecation (prune juice, roughage).
   - Initiate a suppository and laxative regimen.

2. Institute a bowel program. Enemas are avoided in the presence of increased intracranial pressure.

CHART 27-4
Rehabilitation Strategies Following Stroke

Nursing Responsibilities	Rationale
1. Encourage the patient to do as much of his or her own personal hygiene as possible.	1. Increases independence
2. Teach activities of daily living (ADLs) with respect to ways to compensate for the patient's disability. (ADLs include dressing, toileting, bathing, eating, gait training, and so forth.)	2. Provides for alternative methods to overcome disabilities and increases the patient's level of independence
3. Instruct the patient in bed exercises, such as quadriceps and gluteal setting.	3. Improves muscle tone
4. Teach the patient transfer techniques (*e.g.*, bed to chair, chair to bed).	4. Increases independence and provides for a greater number of environmental settings for the patient
5. Provide special skin care, such as lubrication and protection from extremes in temperature, for trophic skin areas.	5. Trophic skin changes are possible with flaccidity.
6. Have the patient dress in his or her own clothes rather than a hospital gown.	6. Improves the patient's self-image and dispels image of the "sick role"
7. Provide for the patient's privacy by screening when he or she is learning new skills (such as relearning to feed self).	7. Preserves the patient's self-esteem and decreases embarrassment if "accidents" happen
8. Provide emotional support and encouragement.	8. Helps to motivate the patient
9. Encourage the patient to express feelings.	9. Decreases anxiety and allows for correction of misinformation
10. Be empathetic with the patient's feelings.	10. Increases the nurse's sensitivity to patient needs
11. Know what the physiotherapist is doing with the patient.	11. Activities can be reinforced by the nurse.
12. Encourage the family to participate (*e.g.*, demonstrate range-of-motion exercises to the family).	12. Allows family members to feel that they are "doing something to help"

special teaching and follow-up. Monitor for obvious and occult bleeding. All patients will need periodic monitoring of coagulation and INR to adjust drug dosage. For patients on ticlopidine, a complete blood cell count every 2 weeks for 3 months is necessary to monitor for neutropenia. If the patient has not received the drug while in the hospital, he or she needs to be alerted to the possibility of diarrhea or rash. Other medications previously taken before the episode need to be evaluated for continuation. Giving written instructions about drugs including time and dosage, side effects to expect, adverse reactions, contacting the health provider, and monitoring the schedule increases adherence to the plan of care.

WHAT TO EXPECT

Both the patient and family need to know what to expect upon discharge. The nurse can provide some anticipatory guidance based on the particular needs of the patient. However, the patient and family cannot be prepared for every contingency. It is helpful to plan a time for the nurse to call to assess adjustment to the community and any special problems or concerns. The nurse can triage some problems and manage others completely.

The patient and family need to be aware of community and hospital resources such as stroke support groups, counseling centers, outreach groups, and publications. Some helpful booklets from the American Heart Association include *Caring for a Person with Aphasia* and *Stroke: Why Do They Behave That Way?* Patients and families should be aware of the services of the following organizations:

American Heart Association
7272 Greenville Avenue
Dallas, TX 75231-4596
(800) 242-8721

National Stroke Association
8480 East Orchard Road
Suite 1000
Englewood, CO 80111-5015
(800) 787-6537

Stroke Clubs International
805 12th Street
Galveston, TX 77550
(409) 762-1022

Recovery

Patients who survive a stroke have some potential for recovery of function. The extent of the stroke and preexisting disease influence the degree of recovery. Most of natural recovery in motor function and speech occurs in the first 3 to 6 months. However, recovery continues at a slower pace up to a year and beyond with therapy.

References

1. *Heart and stroke facts.* (1991). Dallas: American Heart Association.
2. *Heart and stroke facts.* (1993). Dallas: American Heart Association.
3. *Stroke facts.* (1988). Dallas: American Heart Association.
4. *Heart and stroke facts.* (1992). Dallas: American Heart Association.
5. Matcher, D. B., & Duncan, P. W. (1994). Cost of stroke. *National Stroke Association Newsletter, 11*(2), 1.
6. Saunders, E. (1991). *Cardiovascular diseases in blacks.* Philadelphia: F. A. Davis, p. 9.
7. Hock, N., MSN, RN, Nurse Coordinator, Stanford Stroke Center, Stanford University Medical Center, Palo Alto, CA. Personal communication, January 2, 1996.
8. Adams, H. P., Brott, T. G., Crowell, R. M., Furlan, A. J., Gomez, C. R., Trotta, J., Helgason, C. M., Marler, J. R., Woolson, R. F., & Zivin, J. A. (1994). Guidelines for the management of patients with acute ischemic stroke. *Circulation, 90*(3), 1588–1601.
9. Feinberg, W. M., Albers, G. W., Barnett, H. J. M., Biller, J., Caplan, L. R., Carter, L. P., Hart, R. G., Hobson, R. W., Kronmal, R. A., Moore, W. S., & Robertson, J. T. (1994). Guidelines for the management of transient ischemic attacks. *Stroke, 25*(6), 1320–1335.
10. National Institute of Neurological Disorders and Stroke, National Institutes of Health, Department of Health and Human Services. (1994). Clinical advisory: Carotid endarterectomy for patients with asymptomatic internal carotid artery stenosis. *Stroke, 25*(12), 2523–2524.
11. Sherman, D. G., Dyken, M. L., Gent, M., Harrison, J. G., Hart, R. G., & Mohr, J. P. (1995). Antithrombotic therapy for cerebrovascular disorders: An update. *Chest, 108*(Suppl. 4), 444S–456S.
12. Mohr, J. P. (1992). Lacunes. In H. J. M. Barnett, J. P. Mohr, B. M. Stein, & F. M. Yatsu (Eds.), *Stroke: Pathophysiology, diagnosis, and management* (2nd ed.) (pp. 539–541). New York: Churchill Livingstone.
13. DeGraba, T. J., Fisher, M., & Yatsu, F. M. (1992). Atherogenesis and strokes. In H. J. M. Barnett, J. P. Mohr, B. M. Stein, & F. M. Yatsu (Eds.), *Stroke: Pathophysiology, diagnosis, and management* (2nd ed.) (pp. 29–48). New York: Churchill Livingstone.
14. Fisher, M. (1991). Atherosclerosis, cellular aspects and potential interventions. *Cerebrovascular Brain Metabolism Review, 3,* 114.
15. Hossman, K. (1985). Post-ischemic resuscitation of the brain: Selective vulnerability versus global resistance. *Progress in Brain Research, 63,* 3–13.
16. Dutka, A. J., & Hallenbeck, J. M. (1991). Pathophysiology of anoxic-ischemic brain injury. In W. G. Bradley, R. B. Daroff, G. M. Fenichel, & C. D. Marsden (Eds.), *Neurology in clinical practice* (Vol. 2) (p. 1354). New York: Butterworth-Heinemann.
17. Banasik, J. (1995). Cell injury, aging, and death. In L. C. Copstead (Ed.), *Perspectives on pathophysiology* (p. 66). Philadelphia: W. B. Saunders.
18. Hallenbeck, J. M., & Dutka, A. J. (1990). Background review and current concepts of reperfusion injury. *Archives of Neurology, 47,* 1245–1254.
19. Hock, op. cit.
20. Furlan, A. J. (1992). Transient ischemic attacks: Recognition and management. *Heart Disease and Stroke, 1*(1), 33–38.
21. Ibid.
22. Yatsu, F. M., Grotta, J. C., & Pettigrew, L. C. (1995). *100 Stroke maxims: Stroke.* St. Louis: Mosby, p. 1.
23. Sherman et al., op. cit.
24. Grotta, J. C., Norris, J. W., & Kamm, B. (1992). Prevention of stroke with ticlopidine: Who benefits most? *Neurology, 42,* 111–115.
25. Kay, R., Wong, K. S., & Woo, J. (1994). Pilot study of low-molecular weight heparin in the treatment of acute ischemic stroke. *Stroke, 25,* 684–685.
26. Hirsh, J., & Poller, L. (1994). The international normalized ratio. *Archives of International Medicine, 154*(3), 282–288.
27. North American Symptomatic Carotid Endarterectomy Trial Collaborators. (1991). Beneficial effect of carotid endarterectomy in symptomatic patients with high-grade carotid stenosis. *New England Journal of Medicine, 325*(7), 445–453.
28. Yatsu, F. M., DeGraba, T. J., & Hanson, S. (1992). In H. J. M. Barnett, J. P. Mohr, B. M. Stein, & F. M. Yatsu (Eds.), *Stroke: Pathophysiology, diagnosis, and management* (2nd ed.) (pp. 1008–1016). New York: Churchill Livingstone.
29. Barnett, H. J. M., Sackett, D., Taylor, D. W., Haynes, B., Peerless, S. J., Meissner, I., Hachinski, V., & Fox, A. (1987). Are the results of the extracranial-intracranial bypass trial generalizable? *New England Journal of Medicine, 316*(13), 800–824.
30. Hacke, W., Kaste, M., Fieschi, C., Toni, D., Lesaffre, E., von Kummer, R., Boysen, G., Bluhmki, E., Hoxter, G., Magagne, M., & Hennerici, M. (1995). Intravenous thrombolysis with recombinant tissue plasminogen activator for acute hemispheric stroke: The European cooperative acute stroke study (ECASS). *JAMA, 274*(13), 1017–1025.
31. National Institute of Neurological Disorders and Stroke rt-PA Stroke Study Group. (1995). Tissue plasminogen activator for acute ischemic stroke. *New England Journal of Medicine, 333(24),* 1581–1587.
32. Gresham, G. E., Duncan, P. W., Stason, W. B., et al. (1995). *Poststroke rehabilitation* (Clinical Practice Guideline No. 16). Rockville, MD: U. S. Department of Health and Human Services, Public Health Service, Agency for Health Care Policy and Research (AHCPR Publication No. 95-0662).
33. National Stroke Association. (1995). Atherosclerotic intracranial occlusion disease diagnosis, prognosis, and treatment: Part II. *National Stroke Association Stroke Clinical Updates, VI*(4), 13–16.
34. Ibid.

Bibliography

Books

Barnett, H. J. M., Mohr, J. P., Stein, B. M., & Yatsu, F. M. (Eds.). (1992). *Stroke: Pathophysiology, diagnosis, and management* (2nd ed.). New York: Churchill Livingstone.

Fisher, M. (Ed.). (1995). *Stroke therapy.* Boston: Butterworth Heinemann.

Periodicals

Adams, H. P., Brott, T. G., Crowell, R. M., Furlan, A. J., Gomez, C. R., Trotta, J., Helgason, C. M., Marler, J. R., Woolson, R. F., & Zivin, J. A. (1994). Guidelines for the management of patients with acute ischemic stroke. *Circulation, 90*(3), 1588–1601.

Albers, G. W. (1993). Laboratory monitoring of oral anticoagulant therapy: Are we being misled? *Neurology, 43,* 468–470.

Blank-Reid, C. (1996). How to have a stroke at an early age: The effects of crack, cocaine, and other illicit drugs. *Journal of Neuroscience Nursing, 28*(1), 19–27.

Barsan, W. G., & Brott, T. (1990). Early treatment of acute ischemic stroke. *Stroke: Clinical Updates, 1*(2), 5–8.

Bronner, L. L., Kanter, D. S., & Manson, J. E. (1995). Primary prevention of stroke. *New England Journal of Medicine, 333(21),* 1392–1400.

Bussey, H. I., Force, R. W., Bianco T. M., & Leonard, A. D. (1992). Reliance on prothrombin time ratios causes significant errors in anticoagulation therapy. *Archives in Internal Medicine, 152*(Feb), 278–282.

Caplan, L. R. (1991). Diagnosis and treatment of ischemic stroke. *JAMA, 266*(17), 2413–2418.

Chimowitz, M. I. (1995). Atherosclerotic intracranial occlusion disease. Diagnosis, prognosis and treatment. Part II. *Stroke: Clinical Updates, 4*(4), 13–16.

Clark, W. M., & Bamwell, S. L. (1995). Interventional neurovascular therapy in cerebrovascular disease. *Stroke: Clinical Updates, 4*(2), 5–8.

Davis, L. L., & Grant, J. S. (1994). Constructing the reality of recovery: Family home care management strategies. *Advanced Nursing Science, 17*(2), 66–76.

Fearon, M., & Rusy, K. L. (1994). Transcranial doppler: Advanced technology for assessing cerebral hemodynamics. *Dimensions of Critical Care Nursing, 13*(5), 241–248.

Feinberg, W. M., Albers, G. W., Barnett, H. J. M., Biller, J., Caplan, L. R., Carter, L. P., Hart, R. G., Hobson, R. W., Kronmal, R. A., Moore, W. S., & Robertson, J. T. (1994). Guidelines for the management of transient ischemic attacks. *Stroke, 25*(6), 1320–1335.

Furlan, A. J. (1992). Transient ischemic attacks: Recognition and management. *Heart Disease and Stroke, 1*(1), 33–38.

Ginsberg, M. D., & Pulsinelli, W. A. (1994). The ischemic penumbra, injury thresholds, and the therapeutic window for acute stroke. *Annals of Neurology, 36*(4), 553–554.

Goldstein, L. B. (1995). Common drugs may influence motor recovery after stroke. *Neurology, 45,* 865–871.

Grotta, J. C. (1993). Acute stroke management. Diagnosis. Part I. *Stroke: Clinical Updates, 3*(5), 17–20.

Grotta, J. C. (1993). Acute stroke management. Part II. *Stroke: Clinical Updates, 3*(6), 21–24.

Grotta, J. C. (1993). Acute stroke management. Part III. *Stroke: Clinical Updates, 4*(2): 13–16.

Gwynn, M. (1993). tPA in acute stroke—risk or reprieve? *Journal of Neuroscience Nursing, 25*(3), 180–186.

Hacke, W., Kaste, M., Fieschi, C., Toni, D., Lesaffre, E., & von Kummer, R. (1995). Intravenous thrombolysis with recombinant tissue plasminogen activator for acute hemispheric stroke. *JAMA, 274*(13), 1017–1025.

Hafsteinsdottir, T. B. (1996). Neurodevelopment treatment: Application to nursing and effects on the hemiplegic stroke patient. *Journal of Neuroscience Nursing, 28*(1), 36–47.

Hilton, G. (1994). Secondary brain injury and the role of neuroprotective agents. *Journal of Neuroscience Nursing, 26*(4), 251–255.

Hinkle, J. L., & Forbes, E. (1996). Pilot project on functional outcome in stroke. *Journal of Neuroscience Nursing, 28*(1), 13–18.

Hirsh, J. (1992). Substandard monitoring of warfarin in North America. *Archives of Internal Medicine, 152*(2), 257–258.

Ikeda, Y., & Long, D. M. (1990). The molecular basis of brain injury and brain edema: The role of oxygen free radicals. *Neurosurgery, 27*(1), 1–11.

Kay, R., Wong, K. S., & Woo, J. (1994). Pilot study of low-molecular-weight heparin in the treatment of acute ischemic stroke. *Stoke, 25,* 684–685.

Kay, R., Wong, K. S., Yu Y. L., Chan, Y. W., Tsoi, T. H., & Ahuja, A. T. (1995). Low-molecular-weight heparin for the treatment of acute ischemic stroke. *New England Journal of Medicine, 333*(24), 1588–1593.

Kilpatrick, L. (1995). Brain attack: Survival and rehabilitation of stroke. *Duke Health, Summer,* 20–24.

Leonard, A. D., & Newburg, S. (1992). Cardioembolic stroke. *Journal of Neuroscience Nursing, 24*(2), 69–78.

Lugger, K. E. (1994). Dysphagia in the elderly stroke patient. *Journal of Neuroscience Nursing, 26*(2): 78–84.

Matchar, D. B., & Duncan, P. W. (1994). The cost of stroke. *National Stroke Association Newsletter, 11*(2), 5–15.

Mayberg, M. R., Batjer, H. H., Dacey, R., Diringer, M., Haley, C., Heros, R. C., Sternau, L. L., & Torner, J. (1994). Guidelines for the management of aneurysmal subarachnoid hemorrhage. *Circulation, 90*(5), 2592–2605.

McDowell, F. H., Brott, T. G., Goldstein, M., Grotta, J. C., Heros, R. C., & Latchaw, R. E. (1993). Stroke: The first six hours—emergency evaluation and treatment. *Stroke: Clinical Updates, 4*(1), 1–12.

National Institute of Neurological Disorders and Stroke, National Institutes of Health, Department of Health and Human Services. (1994). Clinical advisory: Carotid endarterectomy for patients with asymptomatic internal carotid artery stenosis. *Stroke, 25*(12), 2523–2524.

Olsen, T. S. (1989). Improvement of function and motor impairment after stroke. *Journal of Neurological Rehabilitation, 3*(4), 187–192.

Palmer, J. B., & DuChane, A. S. (1991). Rehabilitation of swallowing disorders due to stroke. *Physical Medicine and Rehabilitation Clinics of North America, 3*(3), 529–546.

Patrono, C. (1994). Aspirin as an antiplatelet drug. *New England Journal of Medicine, 330*(18), 1287–1293.

Reeder, G. S., Khandheria, B. K., Seward, J. B., & Tajik, J. (1991). Transesophageal echocardiography and cardiac masses. *Mayo Clinic Proceedings, 66,* 1101–1109.

Sammaritano, L. R., & Gharavi, A. E. (1992). Antiphospholipid antibody syndrome. *Clinics in Laboratory Medicine, 12*(10), 41–59.

Segatore, M. (1996). Understanding central post-stroke pain. *Journal of Neuroscience Nursing, 28*(1), 28–35.

Shepard, T. J., & Fox, S. W. (1996). Assessment and management of hypertension in the acute ischemic stroke patient. *Journal of Neuroscience Nursing, 28*(1), 5–12.

Sherman, D. G., Dyken, M. L., Gent, M., Harrison, J. G., Hart, R. G., & Mohr, J. P. (1995). Antithrombotic therapy for cerebrovascular disorders: An update. *Chest, 108*(Suppl. 4), 444S–456S.

Shuaib, A. (1994). The role of transcranial Doppler in the study of cerebral vasculature. *Stroke: Clinical Updates, 4*(5), 25–28.

Tong, D. C., Bolger, A., & Albers, G. W. (1994). Incidence of transcranial Doppler-detected cerebral microemboli in patients referred for echocardiography. *Stroke, 25*(11), 2138–2141.

Wojner, A. W. (1996). Optimizing ischemic stroke outcomes: An interdisciplinary approach to poststroke rehabilitation in acute care. *Critical Care Nursing Quarterly, 19*(2), 47–61.

CHAPTER 28

Cerebral Aneurysms

Joanne V. Hickey
Mary L. Ryan

OVERVIEW

A **cerebral aneurysm** is a saccular outpouching of a cerebral artery. Rupture of a cerebral aneurysm usually results in a **subarachnoid hemorrhage (SAH)**, which is defined as bleeding into the subarachnoid space. It is estimated that approximately 10 to 15 million Americans have an intracranial aneurysm, most of which are small, innocuous, and do not bleed throughout life.[1] Each year in the United States, there are approximately 30,000 new cases of subarachnoid hemorrhage secondary to rupture of an intracranial aneurysm.[2] Despite considerable advances in diagnostic, surgical, anesthetic, and perioperative techniques, the outcome for patients with ruptured aneurysms remains poor, in fact, only about one third of people who experience aneurysmal SAH will recover without major disability.[3] Cerebral aneurysm rupture is most prevalent in the 35- to 60-year age group, with 50 years being the mean age of occurrence. Aneurysmal SAH occurs more often in women than in men at a ratio of 3:2.[4] Approximately 15% to 20% of people harboring aneurysms will have multiple aneurysms.

Etiology

Although the precise etiology of cerebral aneurysms remains unclear, many extrinsic, congenital, and genetic factors have been implicated in the formation and rupture of intracerebral aneurysms. One theory suggests that a congenital/developmental defect exists in the medial and adventitial layers of the artery in the circle of Willis. There is little scientific basis for this theory, as these defects are commonly found postmortem in persons without aneurysms.[5]

Another theory—the degenerative theory—is strongly supported by current research and ascribes causation to hemodynamically induced degenerative vascular disease.[6] According to this theory, the intima, covered only by the adventitia, bulges from a local weakness. By late midlife, stress causes vessel ballooning and rupture. There may be a predisposition to aneurysm formation in individuals with hypertension and in those in whom connective tissue disease promotes

fragility of the arterial wall.[7] More recently, research has demonstrated an association between the presence of specific human leukocyte antigen alleles and the genetic role they may play in aneurysm formation.[8] There are some families in which a number of individuals are found to have aneurysms. When this occurs, other close family members should be monitored for vascular lesions.

Although the etiology of most aneurysms is as yet unknown, there are types of intracerebral aneurysms in which the etiology has been well demonstrated. Head trauma can result in traumatic intracranial aneurysms due to a localized arterial tear. Bacterial and fungal infections have also been known to cause infectious (mycotic) aneurysms. Infectious aneurysms form when bacteria, usually from septic emboli, break off and actually invade and destroy the vessel wall. Atherosclerotic aneurysms can form in vessel walls that have been damaged by deposits of atheromatous material, resulting in fusiform aneurysms. Fusiform aneurysms are rarely associated with subarachnoid hemorrhage.

Classification

Cerebral aneurysms have a variety of sizes, shapes, and etiologies. When classified by size, the following categories are used:

- **Small:** to 15 mm
- **Large:** 15 to 25 mm
- **Giant:** 25 to 50 mm
- **Super-giant:** >50 mm

Classification by shape and etiology yields the following categories:

Berry aneurysm—most common type; berry-shaped with a neck or stem (Fig. 28-1)
Saccular aneurysm—any aneurysm having a saccular outpouching

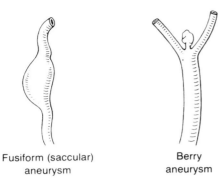

Fusiform (saccular)   Berry
      aneurysm   aneurysm

FIGURE 28-1
Berry and fusiform (saccular) aneurysms.

Fusiform aneurysm—an outpouching of an arterial wall, but without a stem (see Fig. 28-1)

Traumatic aneurysm—an aneurysm resulting from traumatic head injury (accounts for a small number)

Mycotic (infectious) aneurysm—rare; caused by septic emboli from infections, such as bacterial endocarditis; may lead to aneurysmal formation

Charcot-Bouchard aneurysm—microscopic aneurysmal formation associated with hypertension; involves the basal ganglia and brain stem

Dissecting aneurysm—related to atherosclerosis, inflammation, or trauma; an aneurysm in which the intimal layer is pulled away from the medial layer and blood is forced between the layers

Location

Cerebral aneurysms usually occur at the bifurcations and branches of the large arteries at the base of the brain at the circle of Willis. Eighty-five percent of aneurysms develop in the anterior part of the circle of Willis. The remaining 15% are found in the posterior circulation, known as the vertebrobasilar system.

The most common sites of aneurysms are the following:

- Internal carotid artery (ICA) at the bifurcation with the anterior communicating artery (ACoA)
- ICA and origin of the posterior communicating artery (PCoA)
- First major bifurcation of the middle cerebral artery (MCA)
- Bifurcation of the ICA into the MCA and anterior cerebral artery (ACA)
- Junction of the PCoA and the posterior cerebral artery (PCA)
- Bifurcation of the basilar artery
- Origins of three cerebellar arteries

Pathophysiology

At the time of aneurysmal rupture, blood under high pressure is forced into the subarachnoid space at the base of the brain (circle of Willis area), spreading by way of the Sylvian fissures into the basal cisterns. Less often, the aneurysm ruptures into one of the following areas of the brain, resulting in formation of a hematoma: the brain parenchymal tissue (intracerebral hematoma); the ventricles (intraventricular hematoma); the subarachnoid space (subarachnoid hematoma); or the subdural space (subdural hematoma). When rupture occurs, it usually occurs at the thin-walled dome of the aneurysm, causing blood to enter into the subarachnoid space. Tissue pressure surrounding the aneurysm stops the bleeding, and fibrin, platelets, and fluid form a plug which seals off the site of bleeding. The resulting clot can occlude the area or interfere with cerebrospinal fluid (CSF) absorption. The released blood is an irritant to the brain tissue, setting up an inflammatory response that enhances cerebral edema.

Concurrent with the time of rupture, significant subarachnoid hemorrhage occurs, raising intracranial pressure (ICP) toward the mean arterial pressure and lowering cerebral perfusion pressure. These hemodynamic changes probably account for the transient loss of or altered level of consciousness.

Clinically, a stroke syndrome, with associated increased ICP, develops. The specific signs and symptoms associated with the event depend on the location of the hemorrhage and the degree of increased ICP.

SIGNS AND SYMPTOMS

Signs and symptoms arising from an aneurysm can be divided into two phases: those presenting before rupture or bleeding; and those appearing after rupture or bleeding.

Before Rupture or Bleeding

Most patients are completely asymptomatic until the time of bleeding. In approximately 40% of cases, there are warning signs, often called prodromal signs, that are either ignored or attributed to other causes. Prodromal signs may suggest the location of an aneurysm or enlargement of the lesion. Localizing signs and symptoms include the following:

- Oculomotor nerve (cranial nerve III) palsy
- Dilated pupil (loss of light reflex)
- Possible ptosis
- Extraocular movement deficits with possible diplopia
- Pain above and behind the eye
- Localized headache
- Extraocular movement deficits of the trochlear (IV) or abducens (VI) cranial nerves
- Small, intermittent, aneurysmal leakage of blood that may result in generalized headache, neck pain, upper back pain, nausea, and vomiting

After Rupture or Bleeding

At the time of rupture or bleeding, blood is forced into the subarachnoid space. The patient experiences a violent headache, often described by the patient as "explosive" or the "worst headache of my life." Immediate loss of consciousness may occur, or the level of consciousness may decrease. Vomiting is common. Other signs and symptoms include the following:

- Cranial nerve deficits (especially cranial nerves III, IV, and VI)
- Those related to meningeal irritation, including nausea, vomiting, stiff neck, pain in the neck and back, and possible blurred vision or photophobia. Signs of meningeal irritation usually appear 4 to 8 hours after the SAH.[9] Mild temperature elevation may also accompany SAH.
- Those related to a stroke syndrome, including signs and symptoms related to the vascular territory involved and intracerebral hemorrhage (*e.g.,* hemiparesis, hemiplegia, aphasia, cognitive deficits)
- Those related to cerebral edema and increased ICP (mass effect), including seizures, hypertension, bradycardia, and widening pulse pressure
- Those related to pituitary dysfunction secondary to irritation or edema resulting from the proximity of the gland to the common locations of aneurysms and causing possible diabetes insipidus and hyponatremia.

Diagnosis

The diagnosis of a cerebral aneurysm is based on the following criteria:

- History and neurological examination
- Computed tomography (CT) scan, without contrast media, within the first 48 hours of aneurysmal rupture
- Cerebral angiography
- Magnetic resonance imaging or magnetic resonance angiography
- Lumbar puncture (examine CSF for blood); used selectively

COMPUTED TOMOGRAPHY

A plain CT scan, obtained within 48 hours of aneurysmal rupture, is usually the initial diagnostic procedure ordered and is the cornerstone of SAH diagnosis. If the scan is performed within 24 hours of the initial SAH, a high-density clot in the subarachnoid space can be demonstrated in 92% to 95% of cases; if done within 48 hours, the clot can be demonstrated in 75% to 85% of cases.[10–12] A CT scan also aids in establishing the extent and location of subarachnoid bleeding and is useful for identifying patients at high risk for the development of vasospasm and for pinpointing the potential vascular territory of the vasospasm. The plain scan is recommended initially because a CT scan with contrast media may show enhancement of the basal cisterns, a finding that could be mistaken for a clot. A later CT scan with contrast media is performed after 48 hours to determine the location of the aneurysm or an unsuspected arteriovenous malformation. The later scan also demonstrates the presence or absence of hydrocephalus. If an arteriogram is ordered and multiple aneurysms are seen, the CT scan is helpful in identifying which aneurysm has bled, based on the presence of a clot.

When a contrast CT scan yields negative results and there is no indication of increased ICP, the physician usually orders a lumbar puncture to rule out subarachnoid hemorrhage (see the earlier discussion for indications and contraindications for lumbar puncture).

ANGIOGRAPHY

Cerebral angiography is still the mainstay of diagnosis for cerebral aneurysm and should provide visualization of all four major cerebral vessels and their branches. Panangiography is usually done to assess for multiple aneurysms and will definitively demonstrate the precise site and anatomy of the aneurysm that has ruptured. Angiography is usually done immediately following diagnosis of SAH by CT scan in patients that are deemed clinically stable, usually clinical grade I, II, or III. Early angiography allows for definitive diagnosis and enables the surgeon to plan surgical treatment (Fig. 28-2). In addition, early identification will allow for proper surgical treatment should the aneurysm rebleed prior to the time of planned surgery. In addition to the specific location of the aneurysm, the following can be identified using angiography:

- The particular characteristics of the aneurysm (shape, size, etc.)
- Any anomalies of cerebral vasculature (*e.g.,* involving the circle of Willis) that will affect the surgical approach
- The presence of vasospasm, in which case surgery may be postponed

Repeat Angiography. Repeat angiography may be performed for the following reasons:

- Confirmation of the diagnosis when no aneurysm is found on early angiography (small aneurysms can be missed, particularly in the posterior circulation)
- Monitoring the patient for reversal of previously observed vasospasm
- Detection of possible vasospasm when there is a deterioration in neurological function (change in the level of consciousness is the most common situation)

Small aneurysms may obliterate themselves after rupture, leaving no aneurysm to be found on angiography. This type of aneurysm may be referred to as a cryptic aneurysm. If present, vasospasm may hide the presence of an aneurysm. As a rule, when angiography is initially negative, an angiogram is repeated 2 to 3 weeks after aneurysmal rupture, when the high risk period for vasospasm (days 4 to 14) has passed.

OTHER DIAGNOSTICS

Magnetic resonance angiography is an excellent aneurysm screening technique in patients having a positive family history or presenting with chronic headache, but it has not achieved the high resolution necessary to meet the requirements of presurgical evaluation of an aneurysm.[13]

Lumbar puncture is used only if a CT scan is unavailable, if there is no evidence of increased ICP (*e.g.,* papilledema) and the CT scan results are negative, or if the CT scan results are negative and there is need to establish evidence of subarachnoid hemorrhage. A lumbar puncture is contraindicated in the

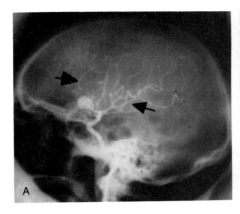

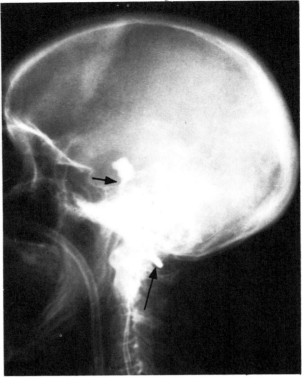

FIGURE 28-2
Carotid angiography indicates a large aneurysm of the anterior communicating artery. (*A*) The anterior cerebral artery (*large arrow*) and the middle cerebral group (*small arrow*) are also illustrated. (*B*) Catheter angiography demonstrates the vertebral artery (*long arrow*), the basilar artery (*short arrow*), and a large, lobulated basilar artery aneurysm.

presence of increased ICP because of the risk of brain stem herniation; it also increases the risk of rebleeding.

CSF analysis usually reveals blood; **xanthochromia** (discoloration of the CSF) is noted when the CSF is centrifuged.

The *transcranial Doppler (TCD)* series is a newer technology that is becoming more important in monitoring flow velocities in major cerebral arteries. A baseline and a series of six or more scans are obtained at given times, such as every other day, for the purpose of monitoring for change and identifying a pattern consistent with vasospasm.

Hunt and Hess Classification System

The Hunt and Hess classification system of clinical grades of aneurysms is a helpful tool to guide the physician in diagnosing the severity of subarachnoid hemorrhage secondary to an aneurysmal bleed, as well as in timing surgical intervention if surgery is an option.[14] The patient is assigned to a category on admission (Table 28-1). Changes in the patient's condition are then monitored according to this baseline.

INITIAL APPROACH TO MEDICAL MANAGEMENT

The patient who survives the initial rupture of a cerebral aneurysm is beset by a number of potential problems and complications that can lead to additional mortality and morbidity. The treatment of choice for a cerebral aneurysm is surgery. However, careful medical management maintains the patient until a decision about surgery is made.

TABLE 28-1
Hunt-Hess Classification of Clinical Grades for Cerebral Aneurysms

GRADE	DESCRIPTIVE CRITERIA
I	Alert, oriented, asymptomatic
II	Alert, oriented, headache, stiff neck
III	Lethargic or confused, minor focal deficits such as hemiparesis
IV	Stupor, moderate to severe focal deficits such as hemiplegia
V	Comatose and severe neurological deficits such as posturing

Adapted from Hunt, W. E., & Hess, R. M. (1968). Surgical risk as related to time of intervention in the repair of intracranial aneurysm. Journal of Neurosurgery, 28, 14–19.

Initial medical management includes the following:

- Complete bed rest and institution of aneurysm precautions (Chart 28-1)
- Application of elastic hose and/or sequential compression boots
- Maintenance of normal fluid volume
- Blood pressure control
- Drug therapy (anticonvulsants, stool softeners, steroids, analgesics, sedatives, and calcium channel blockers)
- Monitoring of neurological signs for changes and/or development of complications.

COMPLETE BED REST AND ANEURYSM PRECAUTIONS

The patient is placed on complete bed rest and aneurysm precautions are instituted. The purpose of aneurysm precautions is to prevent elevations in blood pressure, which could lead to rebleeding, by maintaining a quiet environment. The consensus of medical opinion has changed in the last few years, allowing these precautions to be greatly liberalized. The current thinking is that strict aneurysm precautions (no television, radio, reading, feeding of the patient, etc.) only add to patient stress, thus increasing the risk of rebleeding and nullifying the intended purpose of the precautions. Indeed, strict precautions may lead to sensory deprivation. With strict precautions, it is difficult to determine whether confusion or agitation is attributable to sensory deprivation or to a deterioration in the patient's neurological condition. Most patients fare better if more liberal aneurysm precautions are instituted. Placing the patient in a single quiet room and permitting such activities as watching television, listening to the radio, reading, and visiting with family members is therapeutic.

A more serious concern in preventing rebleeding is prevention of straining at stool. Institution of a bowel management program using stool softeners is critical in preventing rebleeding.

ELASTIC HOSE AND SEQUENTIAL COMPRESSION BOOTS

As a result of immobility from bed rest, the risk for deep vein thrombosis and pulmonary embolus is increased. Thigh-high elastic hose and/or sequential compression boots are applied to decrease the incidence of these problems. Once the aneurysm is secured by clipping, low-dose heparin may be safely instituted 3 to 4 days postoperative.

FLUID VOLUME CONTROL

One of the goals of medical management is to maintain fluid volume within a normal range (euvolia). The underlying reason for this is that dehydration increases hemoconcentration, which is thought to increase the incidence of cerebral vasospasm. If cerebral edema is present, a regimen of a moderate fluid restriction and steroids is usually ordered. Mannitol may be ordered to decrease cerebral edema. If a mass effect is present from a subdural, intracerebral, or other hematoma, early surgical evacuation is usually necessary. Surgery may safely be delayed for a short time if mannitol is used (discussed in the next section).

BLOOD PRESSURE CONTROL

In the early hours/days after rupture, blood pressure is commonly elevated, probably reflecting a physiological response to a rise in ICP. As ICP is decreased, the blood pressure also decreases. If the blood pressure continues to be elevated owing to increased ICP from the mass effect of cerebral edema or a hematoma, mannitol may be administered. The drug is beneficial for two reasons: (1) it decreases cerebral edema and neurological deficits; and (2) it improves cerebral blood flow. Decreased cerebral edema lowers the ICP and blood pressure.

Hypertension is controlled to prevent rebleeding. The goal of therapy is to maintain the systolic blood pressure at about 150 mm Hg. Systolic pressures above this level are usually treated with drugs, such as labetolol and nicardipine. These drugs effectively lower the pressure without sudden drops in the systolic pressure and are easily titrated.

DRUG THERAPY

The following drugs are usually ordered for the patient with an aneurysmal rupture/bleed:

- The calcium channel blocker nimodipine is routinely given for 21 days following SAH. Nimodipine has been shown to enhance collateral blood flow and improve long-term outcome of patients with SAH from aneurysmal rupture.
- Anticonvulsants are given as prophylaxis against seizures.
- Stool softeners prevent constipation and straining at stool, which results in initiation of Valsalva's maneuver, increased ICP, and increased blood pressure, which, in turn, can cause rebleeding of the aneurysm.
- Use of steroids is controversial; however, some believe that it is beneficial for treatment of cerebral edema and the inflammatory effect of meningeal irritation.
- Analgesics (acetaminophen or codeine) are administered to control headache.
- Sedatives may be prescribed, as the agitated patient is at risk for elevated blood pressure. A mild sedative, such as phenobarbital, may be ordered.

MONITORING FOR COMPLICATIONS

In the acute phase, most patients will be managed in the ICU where they can be observed frequently and monitored with invasive hemodynamic monitoring equipment by a well-trained and knowledgeable nursing staff. The rationale for monitoring of neurological signs and other parameters is early detection of complications. The major complications of aneurysmal rupture/bleeding are rebleeding, cerebral vasospasm, and hydrocephalus, which will be discussed in a later section. Other problems associated with aneurysmal rupture/bleed are reflected in laboratory studies and the results of an electrocardiogram (EKG). The following are pertinent data.

CHART 28-1
Typical Aneurysm Precautions

PURPOSE: To provide a quiet environment that controls and minimizes physiological and psychological stress and promotes rest and relaxation

DESIRED OUTCOME: Prevention of aneurysmal rebleeding

PATIENT SELECTION: Patients with rupture/bleeding from cerebral aneurysms who have not undergone surgical intervention to prevent rebleeding (*e.g.,* clipping of aneurysm or endovascular balloon therapy)

INSTITUTED BY: Written order of the physician.

NOTE: The physician may modify or delete parts to meet the therapeutic needs of the patient.

Care/Nursing Responsibilities	**Rationale**

1. Admit to a quiet, single room; remove telephone.
   • The door should be kept partially closed.
2. Control natural and artificial light.
   • Turn blinds or pull shades to prevent direct light from shining into the room.
   • Avoid direct, bright, artificial lights.
3. Reading, watching television, and listening to the radio are allowed, provided they do not upset or overstimulate the patient.
4. Maintain the patient on bed rest with the head of the bed at 30 degrees at all times. The degree of bed rest will be determined by the physician. (Some physicians order complete bed rest whereas others allow bathroom privileges.)
5. Visitors are limited to immediate family/significant others.
   • Limit visitors to two at a time for short visits.
   • Exclude visitors that might upset the patient.
   • Instruct visitors to avoid discussions/topics that may upset the patient.
6. Place an ''Aneurysm Precautions'' sign on the door. (See sample below.)
	1. A private, quiet room minimizes environmental stimuli.
	2. Controlling natural and artificial light decreases environmental stimuli, as well as noxious stimuli to the eyes if photophobia is present.
	3. In the patient who is conscious, selected programs and/or reading can promote relaxation, thus helping to control the blood pressure.
	4. Maintaining bed rest keeps the patient quiet and reduces blood pressure; elevating the head of the bed promotes venous drainage from the brain and helps to decrease increased intracranial pressure (ICP).
	5. Visitors are restricted to keep the patient quiet and calm. (Even this limitation is contingent on the patient's response.)
	
	6. A sign limiting visitors is posted on the door. A simple explanation, both to the patient and the family, is provided.

> ANEURYSM PRECAUTIONS
> • Visitors and non-unit personnel should check with the nurse before entering the room.
> • Only close family members may visit the patient.
> • No more than two visitors may visit at a time.
> • Keep the door partially closed.
> • Avoid exciting or upsetting the patient.
> • Check with the nurse before offering food or drink to the patient.

7. Monitor and document neurological signs and vital signs as ordered. The frequency of assessment will depend on the patient's acuity and stability; assessments may be ordered every 15 minutes on admission, and then increased as the patient improves.*	7. The initial assessment establishes a baseline; subsequent assessments aid in monitoring trends to determine subtle and obvious deterioration. Subtle changes in neurological function may indicate vasospasm, whereas rapid deterioration may indicate rebleeding. In addition, monitoring of vital signs may reflect increased ICP; monitoring of blood pressure is useful in regulating vasopressor and antihypertensive therapy.

(continued)

CHART 28-1 Typical Aneurysm Precautions (Continued)

Care/Nursing Responsibilities	Rationale
8. Provide diet as ordered. • Alert patients may feed themselves unless contraindicated by physician's order.	8. Alert patients are usually allowed to feed themselves, as feeding patients, as was common with strict aneurysm precautions, created anxiety in most patients.

9. Constipation and straining at stool should be prevented.
  • Establish a bowel program according to a bowel protocol (*e.g.,* stool softeners, gentle laxatives)
  • A bedside commode may be ordered or bathroom privileges may be allowed.
  • Avoid enemas.
	9. Straining at stool initiates the Valsalva's maneuver, thus increasing the possibility of rebleeding. It is the nurse's responsibility to establish a bowel program on admission; enemas, just like straining, increase intra-abdominal pressure and subsequently increase ICP.

10. Apply thigh-high elastic hose.
  • Apply air boots (sequential compression boots).
  • Observe the legs for signs/symptoms of deep vein thrombosis (DVT).
  • Report abnormal findings immediately.
	10. The immobility of bed rest and some drug therapy increase the risk of DVT and pulmonary emboli; decrease stasis and improve blood return to the heart with TEDs and air boots.

11. Assist with hygienic care as necessary. (Some protocols allow alert patients to bathe themselves, whereas others require that all care be administered to the patient.)	11. In the alert patient, self-care is less stressful to the patient than when the nurse administers care.
12. Administer care gently (*e.g.,* gentle back care, range-of-motion exercises).	12. Prevent/control any activity that stimulates the patient, thereby increasing blood pressure and increasing the risk of rebleeding.
13. Discourage/control any activity that initiates the Valsalva's maneuver (*e.g.,* coughing, straining at stool, pushing up in bed with the elbows, turning with the mouth closed).	13. Initiating the Valsalva's maneuver increases blood pressure and the risk of rebleeding.
14. Administer analgesics for headache as ordered.	14. Pain activates the sympathetic nervous system, thus increasing blood pressure and the possibility of rebleeding; analgesia provides comfort.
15. Maintain an accurate intake and output record.	15. In order to maintain normothermia, an accurate intake and output record must be kept; hypovolemia is avoided because it increases the risk of vasopasm.
16. The physician may modify the precautions as necessary.	16. Depending on the clinical grade (based on the Hunt and Hess scale) and the patient's level of anxiety, the precautions can be modified by the physician; the nurse assesses the response of the patient to the restrictions and communicates this information to the physician.

*Controversy centers on the use of rectal temperatures in patients who have increased ICP. The crux of the issue relates to concern about vasovagal stimulation as a result of the insertion of a rectal thermometer in a confused or comatose patient. It is known that vasovagal stimulation does increase ICP. However, some believe that is minimal, and of little clinical consequence. Follow the physician's (or institution's) policy on the use of rectal thermometers.

Blood Studies

• White blood cell count: often elevated (15,000 to 18,000) as a result of meningeal irritation
• Hematocrit, fibrinogen, and platelet levels, bleeding time, and osmolality: indicators of the development of cerebral vasospasm

• Electrolytes: hyponatremia often develops as a result of the syndrome of inappropriate secretion of antidiuretic hormone (SIADH) or salt-wasting (see Chap. 10)
• Blood gas levels: monitor adequacy of oxygenation

Electrocardiogram. Changes related to hypothalamic dysfunction result in elevated serum catecholamine levels. Catecholamines stimulate alpha-adrenergic receptors in the myocardium, possibly causing ST changes, prolonged QRS, prolonged Q-T interval, and tall T waves). EKG changes may be consistent with subendocardial damage and, sometimes, myocardial ischemia.

SURGICAL INTERVENTION

Surgery is the treatment of choice for a ruptured or bleeding cerebral aneurysm. A number of factors influence the selection of surgical candidates and the timing of surgery. The goal of surgery is to prevent rebleeding by sealing off the aneurysm so that the aneurysm is totally obliterated with a clip or other method such as muslin wrapping.

Timing of Surgery

The timing of surgery is critical to patient outcome. In the past, the practice had been to wait approximately 2 weeks before scheduling surgery.[15] The rationale for this was that the patient was a better surgical candidate once cerebral edema had subsided and he or she had been medically stabilized. Also at this point, the slackness of the brain allowed for relatively easy dissection. However, the time delay spanned the peak times for occurrence of rebleeding and vasospasm. Since then, multicenter studies have been conducted to determine the optimal time for surgery. As a result of studies demonstrating improved outcomes from earlier surgery, there has been a definite trend toward early (within 48 to 72 hours after hemorrhage) surgery for those patients who are in good neurological condition based on the Hunt and Hess classification system. Patients with clinical grades I and II, and some with clinical grade III, are selected for early surgery. The remaining patients with grade III aneurysms and those with grades IV and V aneurysms are deferred for later surgery, if at all. The following are the benefits of early surgery:

- Results in superior management in patients with anterior circulation aneurysms and some basilar tip aneurysms
- Eliminates the problem of rebleeding
- Allows for removal of basal cistern clots associated with vasospasm
- Permits institution of hypervolemic/hypertensive treatment for postoperative vasospasm without the risk of rebleeding

Surgical Approaches and Considerations

Microsurgical techniques and improved anesthesia offer new options for a precise surgical approach and clipping of aneurysms. The surgical approach and method of aneurysmal obliteration depends on the location and characteristics of the aneurysm. An aneurysm with a stem or neck is usually managed with a surgical clip on the stem/neck (Fig. 28-3). Depending on the location of the aneurysm, more than one clip may be necessary to obliterate it. The surgeon may choose from a wide selection of commercial clips of different sizes, shapes, and angulations. For aneurysms that are difficult to reach, the surgeon may have to modify a clip to accommodate the vessels and structures at the aneurysmal site. Before permanent clips are positioned, a temporary clip is applied to assess the effect of clipping on the blood supply to other areas. Temporary clips are softer and are gold-tipped. When the adequacy of vascular territory circulation is verified, the per-

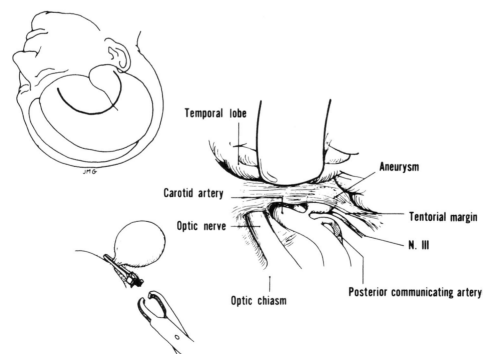

Temporal lobe

Carotid artery

Optic nerve

Optic chiasm

Aneurysm

Tentorial margin

N. III

Posterior communicating artery

FIGURE 28-3
Clipping or a ligation of the aneurysmal neck provides the best protection against rebleeding, although the initial risk may be slightly higher.

manent clips are then applied. Intraoperative cerebral angiography, digital subtraction angiography, or cerebral blood flow studies may be conducted to verify the adequacy of circulation and the security of the clip or other method of aneurysmal obliteration.

Some aneurysms, such as fusiform aneurysms, are not amenable to clipping because of their shape or location. In these situations, the aneurysm may be surgically wrapped in muslin, which provides support to the weakened arterial wall and also induces scarring. Use of glue has fallen out of favor because many surgeons believe that it is associated with more risks than benefits. Another possible approach is ligation of the aneurysm, with subsequent aspiration. If multiple aneurysms are present, it may not be possible to obliterate all lesions at one surgery. The priority site is the aneurysm that has bled, identified by CT scan and angiography. A second surgical procedure may be planned for a later date, if indicated.

Certain situations require special considerations by the neurosurgeon. For example, with an aneurysm involving the ACA, special precautions must be taken to prevent injury to the small perforating vessels emitting from this area. If these vessels are compromised, the patient will either not awaken or memory deficits and personality changes will be prominent, depending on the degree of compromise.

Special considerations are also warranted with a mycotic aneurysm. Usually located at the distal end of a vessel, these rare lesions may result from an infection, such as subacute bacterial endocarditis. Management is controversial. Treatment with antibiotics may result in disappearance of the lesion. However, if the aneurysm remains and enlarges, surgical excision is necessary.

Asymptomatic and Obliterated Aneurysms

Current information suggests that asymptomatic aneurysms that are less than 10 mm in diameter have a low risk of rupture, whereas those with diameters of greater than 10 mm have a much greater risk of rupture. Therefore, asymptomatic aneurysms with diameters of 10 mm or more should probably be treated surgically. Patients whose aneurysms have been obliterated at the time of rupture need to be monitored because these aneurysms may recur.

ENDOVASCULAR BALLOON THERAPY

A relatively new treatment modality, called endovascular balloon therapy, is being used for the treatment of selected cerebral aneurysms and arteriovenous malformations (see Chap. 29). A new subspecialty in radiology, interventional neuroradiology, offers this treatment option. The technology requires new knowledge and skills and uses new catheters. These catheters, which are passed into the vascular lesion by a percutaneous transfemoral approach, are called *superselective catheters* because of their ability to enter vessels that are inaccessible with normal catheters.

The traditional gold standard for treatment of cerebral aneurysms remains intracranial surgical clipping or, less frequently, occlusion of the parent vessel supplying the aneurysm by application of a clamp. New treatment options offered by interventional neurovascular techniques for selected cerebral aneurysms include balloon occlusion of the aneurysm and balloon occlusion of the parent vessel.

Patient Selection

Patients are generally referred for endovascular balloon therapy because they are poor surgical candidates. This group includes patients with aneurysms that are anatomically unclippable (having no neck or a thick or sclerotic neck, or a giant aneurysm) or that are located in inaccessible areas, such as the cavernous sinus or posterior circulation (vertebrobasilar system).

Materials

The mainstay of endovascular balloon technology is a variety of special superselective and supersmall catheters. The diameter of the inflated balloon is about one eighth to one sixth that of a dime. Balloons used for giant aneurysms may be somewhat larger.

Catheters are categorized by *materials* (silicone or latex) and by type (having detachable or nondetachable balloons). A detachable balloon catheter is a double-lumen catheter with a balloon capacity of 0.5 to 2.0 mL or more depending on the specific type.

Techniques

The techniques used for occlusion of an aneurysm and for occlusion of the parent vessel differ. However, the goal of treatment—thrombosis of the aneurysm—is the same.

ANEURYSM OCCLUSION

When a detachable balloon is selected for treatment of an aneurysm, the catheter is inserted into the femoral artery and advanced to the aneurysm. Once in position, the balloon is inflated within the aneurysm by means of a liquid polymerizing agent, such as silicone or HEMA (material similar to that used for soft contact lenses) that solidifies and hardens within approximately 45 minutes. The material remains permanently solidified within the balloon. By providing gentle catheter traction, an internal self-sealing valve ties itself off; the catheter is then detached from the balloon.

A newer, ultra-small catheter is available which does not have to be removed. This catheter extends from the cranial vault to the femoral artery and is left in place permanently.

PARENT VESSEL OCCLUSION

Another treatment approach involves occluding the parent vessel that supplies blood to the aneurysm. Before occlusion of a vessel is considered, it is important to establish whether the vessel can be sacrificed without neurological impairment. The patient is first heparinized. Testing parameters include continuous electroencephalographic (EEG) monitoring and ongoing neurological assessment; it is, therefore, necessary for the patient to be responsive. After baseline data have been collected, the vessel is occluded. Monitoring of parameters continues. Occlusion is maintained for approximately 20 minutes unless neurological deficits occur. In addition, hypotension is deliberately induced for about 5 minutes to assess the patient's response to this condition. Again, the patient is carefully monitored for neurological deficits.

If the patient passes this series of tests, permanent occlusion of the vessel may proceed. If the patient does not pass the test, then a surgical extracranial–intracranial bypass procedure is undertaken to provide an adequate blood supply to the area. Later, an endovascular balloon procedure may be performed to occlude the lesion. This two-step procedure may be necessary for treatment of a giant aneurysm.

Special Considerations and Complications

Regardless of whether an aneurysm or the parent vessel is occluded, the patient receives anticoagulation therapy to prevent emboli. Complications can arise from this therapy. Moreover, cerebral vasospasm may occur during occlusion. Symptoms of ischemia secondary to vasospasm include various neurological deficits related to the cerebrovascular territory. The complications that can arise as a result of endovascular balloon therapy include rupture of the aneurysm, hemorrhage, vasospasm, ischemia, infarction, and stroke. A complication that is associated with aneurysms of the cavernous sinus is a carotid-cavernous fistula.

Future of Interventional Endovascular Treatment

Interventional endovascular technology has great potential for the future. Some believe that endovascular balloon therapy will become a major treatment modality for aneurysms. Early data suggest that use of coils and balloons can promote aneurysm thrombosis in a majority of cases; long-term occlusion, however, remains undetermined.[16]

Balloon cerebral angioplasty is an investigational treatment for the management of vasospasm that is resistant to medical management, including drug therapy. In this procedure, an intravascular balloon catheter technique is used to dilate a cerebral vessel in spasm.

COMPLICATIONS OF ANEURYSMAL RUPTURE/BLEEDING

The major complications of aneurysmal rupture/bleeding, which can lead to significant mortality and morbidity, include rebleeding, cerebral vasospasm, and hydrocephalus.

Aneurysmal Rebleeding

Of the 18,000 persons who survive the initial rupture of an aneurysm annually, 3,000 either die or are disabled from rebleeding. Some believe that the incidence of rebleeding is as high as 30%. The highest incidence occurs in the first 2 weeks after initial hemorrhage. Peaks in the incidence of rebleeding occur in the first 24 to 48 hours and at days 7 to 10. Rebleeding within the first 24 to 48 hours is the leading cause of death in persons surviving the initial bleed. Peaking of rebleeding episodes at about days 7 to 10 appears to correlate with normal clot dissolution by natural fibrinolysis or from hypertension. Approximately 70% of patients who rebleed will die.[17]

SIGNS AND SYMPTOMS

The onset of rebleeding is usually accompanied by sudden, severe headache, often with associated severe nausea and vomiting; a decrease in or loss of consciousness; and new neurological deficits. Death may occur. A question of rebleeding can only be confirmed by a CT scan.

TREATMENT

Systolic blood pressure is maintained at about 150 mm Hg. Dramatic and rapid changes in blood pressure should be avoided at all cost. Current literature indicates that rebleeding may be related to variations in blood pressure rather than to absolute blood pressure.[18] A more direct approach is the use of antifibrinolytic drugs. These drugs are controversial and they are used infrequently because of the serious risks associated with them. **Antifibrinolytics** are drugs that delay the lysis of the clot surrounding the aneurysmal rupture by preventing the dissolution of the fibrin that forms the foundation of the clot. Fibrin is normally broken down by plasmin, a proteolytic enzyme resembling trypsin. Plasmin is converted from naturally occurring plasminogen by various enzyme activators. Such activators are believed to be present in thrombin, CSF, and the meninges. Those present in the meninges prevent fibrinolysis of the clot in the subarachnoid space, including the basal cisterns. Antifibrinolytics inhibit these activators, thereby preventing plasminogen from being converted into plasmin.

Antifibrinolytics that are used clinically include epsilon aminocaproic acid (Amicar) and tranexamic acid. Of the two, Amicar is used more often. It is administered as a continuous infusion at a rate of 30 to 60 g per day from admission to the day of surgery or for no longer than 3 weeks. Although Amicar is also supplied in tablet and liquid form for administration by the oral or feeding tube route, the need to maintain constant blood levels suggests that the intravenous route should be used. Studies indicate that antifibrinolytics are associated with significant increases in the incidence of vasospasm, ischemia, stroke, deep vein thrombosis, and pulmonary embolism. The drug is not given to patients who have been identified by CT scan as being at high risk for vasospasm.

Early surgery for the clipping of the aneurysm is the most effective method of preventing rebleeding. In those patients for whom surgery is deferred (those with grade IV and V aneurysms), the benefits of antifibrinolytics may outweigh the risks. However, the current trend is to use antifibrinolytics less frequently than previously.

Cerebral Vasospasm

Of the 18,000 persons annually who survive initial aneurysmal rupture, 3,000 either die or are disabled from cerebral vasospasm. Vasospasm occurs in approximately 30% of patients.

By definition, **cerebral vasospasm** is narrowing of a cerebral blood vessel. This, in turn, can decrease cerebral perfusion to an area, causing ischemia and perhaps infarction, and can lead to further deterioration of neurological function. The etiology of vasospasm is unknown, although many hypotheses have been proposed. Current hypotheses range from the suggestion that spasmogenic agents are released as the clot breaks down, to the more recent hypothesis that an endothelium relaxing factor known as nitric oxide is somehow inhibited from exerting its relaxing effect due to changes in the endothelial cells which produce nitric oxide. These cellular changes may be induced by the release of blood into the extravascular compartment.

Vasospasm may be differentiated as either angiographic or symptomatic. **Angiographic vasospasm** refers to narrowing of a cerebral arterial territory, as noted on angiography, without clinical symptoms. **Symptomatic vasospasm** is the clinical syndrome of delayed cerebral ischemia associated with angiographically documented narrowing of a major cerebral arterial territory. Vasospasm develops 4 to 14 days after initial hemorrhage (peaking at 7 to 10 days).

SIGNS AND SYMPTOMS

Vasospasm is characterized by a gradual neurological deterioration related to a vascular territory. The neurological deficits may be specific to a particular vascular territory, such as the ACA or MCA, or they may be multifocal or diffuse, as when the cortical areas and boundary zones are involved. Most patients will have an impaired level of consciousness. Deficits may include paresis/paralysis of a limb or side of the body, cranial nerve deficits, and aphasia. As a consequence of the severity and location of the ischemia caused by the vasospasm, cerebral infarction may develop, thus contributing to increased permanent neurological deficits or death.

PREDICTION OF VASOSPASM AND VASCULAR TERRITORY

An initial plain CT scan taken within 1 to 2 days after hemorrhage has gained credibility as a predictor of the incidence, location, and severity of vasospasm. The extent and location of clots in the basal cisterns of the subarachnoid space and cerebral fissures are the specific determinants considered. Patients who have subarachnoid clots larger than 5 × 3 mm in the basal cisterns or who have layers of blood 1 mm thick or greater in the cerebral fissures have a high incidence of vasospasm. Fisher has demonstrated that the amount of blood in the basal cisterns, as shown by the initial CT scan, can reliably predict which patients will develop symptomatic vasospasm, with the amount of blood directly related to the incidence and severity of vasospasm.[19] Bleeding into the brain or ventricles does not result in vasospasm.

Information concerning the probability and location of vasospasm can be helpful to the physician and nurse. Correlation of the vascular territory supplied by the artery at risk with the specific neurological functions of that territory helps to focus attention on those specific functions during neurological assessments. A decreased level of consciousness, the presence of focal signs, or both, together with a CT scan correlated to the cerebral territory, are indicative of vasospasm *when no other changes can explain the neurological deterioration.* When subtle or significant deficits occur, the nurse can quickly alert the physician to these findings so that prompt interventions can prevent extension of the neurological deficits or even death.

HIGH RISK FACTORS: HYPONATREMIA AND FLUID RESTRICTION

A common electrolyte imbalance found after aneurysmal rupture is hyponatremia. This is an important clinical finding because hyponatremia and decreased fluid volume are recognized *high risk factors* for the development of vasospasm. In aneurysmal hemorrhage, hyponatremia can be caused by SIADH or salt-wasting (Table 28-2). If hyponatremia is caused by true SIADH, an expanded blood volume is present that requires fluid restriction. If hyponatremia is attributable to salt-wasting (in which case there is also hypernatriuria), blood volume is decreased. The treatment for salt-wasting is fluid replacement.

Wijdicks and colleagues measured plasma volume, fluid and sodium balance, and serum vasopressin (ADH) levels in patients with ruptured saccular aneurysms. They found that vasopressin values were elevated at the time of the patient's admission, but declined in the first week, regardless of the presence of hyponatremia. By definition, **SIADH** is associated with an increased serum ADH level. The conclusion drawn was that the natriuresis and hyponatremia were the result of **primary salt-wasting**, rather than SIADH. Further, they suggested that the natriuresis and hyponatremia should be corrected by fluid replacement rather than by fluid restriction, which is the treatment for SIADH.[20]

TREATMENT

The result of vasospasm is decreased cerebral perfusion (blood flow) to the clinically affected arterial territory. Currently, treatment for symptomatic vasospasm is directed at the primary goal of increasing cerebral perfusion pressure using hypervolemic/hypertensive therapy. Crystalloids and colloids are used to expand the intravascular volume. Central venous pressure is maintained at approximately 10 mm Hg, and the pulmonary capillary wedge pressure is 14 to 18 mm Hg. Therapy is also aimed at maintaining a hematocrit of 30% to 34%,

TABLE 28-2
Comparison of Cerebral Salt-Wasting and SIADH

CEREBRAL SALT-WASTING (CAUSE UNCLEAR)	SIADH (CAUSED BY CONTINUOUS SECRETION OF ADH)
Hyponatremia (true)	Hyponatremia (dilusional)
Decreased plasma volume	• Increased plasma volume
Loss of fluid from extracellular space	Increased fluid in extracellular space
Decreased body weight	• Increased body weight
Hypernatriuria	• Natriuria not prominent

SIADH = syndrome of inappropriate secretion of antidiuretic hormone; ADH = antidiuretic hormone.

a heart rate of greater than 70 beats per minute, and a 30% rise in mean arterial blood pressure (130 to 150 mm Hg) for the duration of the vasospasm. To maintain the hematocrit in the desired range, albumin and packed red blood cells may be used as volume expanders, or blood may be removed and mannitol may be administered (to decrease volume). If necessary, hypertension can be induced with vasopressors—dopamine (Intropin) or phenylephrine (Neo-Synephrine). The level of hypertension must be carefully controlled in the case of an unclipped aneurysm because of concern for rebleeding. If vasospasm occurs after surgical clipping of the aneurysm, systolic blood pressure is often maintained at between 180 and 200 mm Hg.

Previous drug protocols to prevent or to treat vasospasm have been disappointing. Reserpine, kanamycin, isoproterenol, aminophylline, nitroprusside, and others have been tried with little success. Current research in the area of vasospasm is now taking place at the basic science level and is focusing on changes at the cellular level.

Communicating Hydrocephalus

Hydrocephalus is a condition in which there is either an obstruction to the flow of CSF within the ventricular system or subarachnoid space (noncommunicating) or a problem with reabsorption of CSF (communicating). The type of hydrocephalus that occurs with SAH is communicating hydrocephalus. Hydrocephalus can be classified as either acute, subacute, or delayed. The profiles for each are different and are briefly discussed later. With SAH, hydrocephalus develops as a result of blood in the CSF, which plugs the arachnoid villi, interfering with the reabsorption of CSF. Diagnosis is established on the basis of a CT scan, which will reveal dilated ventricles with blood within the ventricles.

SIGNS/SYMPTOMS AND TREATMENT

The following summarizes the signs and symptoms of the three types of hydrocephalus, as well as the appropriate treatment for each.

Acute

- Occurs within the first 24 hours after hemorrhage
- Associated with intraventricular hemorrhage or excessive blood in the basal cisterns of posterior fossa
- Characterized by the abrupt onset of stupor or persistence of coma
- Management: immediate ventriculostomy to drain the CSF periodically, especially when ICP is elevated above a predetermined level such as 20 mm Hg

Subacute

- Occurs within the first few days to 7 days after hemorrhage
- Associated with blood in the CSF secondary to subarachnoid hemorrhage
- Characterized by drowsiness, the onset of which is usually gradual, although an abrupt onset is possible
- Management: ventriculostomy, or serial lumbar puncture or lumbar drainage of CSF

Delayed

- Occurs 10 or more days after hemorrhage
- Associated with blood in the CSF secondary to subarachnoid hemorrhage
- Characterized by a gradual onset of symptoms when the patient is recovering from surgery; symptoms include gait difficulty and behavioral changes (dull, quiet, and blunted animation)
- Management: surgical placement of a ventriculoperitoneal shunt

Because the signs and symptoms of hydrocephalus are nonspecific, changes in responsiveness may be attributed to other problems, thus delaying appropriate treatment.

NURSING MANAGEMENT OF THE PATIENT WITH AN ANEURYSM

Nursing management of the patient with a cerebral aneurysm can be divided into three areas: management before surgery, management during complications, and management after surgery.

Nursing Management Before Surgery

The patient who has sustained aneurysmal rupture/bleeding requires ongoing assessment, supportive care, implementation of specific protocols (*e.g.,* aneurysm precautions, drug therapy), and management of increased ICP.

ASSESSMENT/MONITORING

The initial and ongoing assessment of the patient includes evaluation of the following parameters:

- Level of consciousness
- Pupillary size, shape, and reaction to light
- Motor function (*e.g.,* hand grasps, pronator drift) of extremities
- Other cranial nerve deficits (blurred vision, extraocular movement deficits, ptosis, facial weakness)
- Aphasia
- Headache and facial pain (*e.g.,* pain behind the eyeball)
- Nuchal rigidity (stiff neck, pain in the neck or back, pain with flexion of the neck, photophobia)

Neurological assessments are conducted periodically. The frequency of assessments depends on the acuity and stability of the patient. Assessments may be conducted every 15 minutes or every 4 hours. Any changes in data are compared to previous findings to determine trends. Accurate documentation and intershift sharing and reporting of information are essential in identifying trends in neurological function.

Upon diagnosis of a cerebral aneurysm, the patient is assigned a grade category according to the Hunt and Hess classification system. The classification gives the nurse information about the acuity of the patient and some indication of the probable medical treatment. Usually, patients are placed on bed rest and are maintained in a controlled and quiet environment. Monitoring and support devices also physically immobilize the patient.

Altered consciousness diminishes the patient's ability to comprehend the significance and implications of events happening around him or her. Environmental information is reduced by alterations of sensory/perceptual input. Motor deficits reduce or prevent voluntary movement.

Because there may not be one clear cause to which altered consciousness can be attributed, determining the etiology of a deterioration in level of consciousness, restlessness, or agitation may be difficult. Such alterations may be the result of rebleeding, ischemia, vasospasm, hydrocephalus, hypoxia, or increased ICP. Alterations may also be caused by the psychological effects of immobility, sensory deprivation, powerlessness, or other responses to hospitalization and the reduced sensory environment associated with aneurysm precautions. The common nursing diagnoses made in the acute phase of nursing management are found in Chart 28-2. Many of these patients also have increased ICP; nursing management of this problem is discussed in Chapter 17.

The following are major medical and neurological complications of SAH:

- Rebleeding
- Secondary brain injury
- Vasospasm
- Cardiac injury
- Hydrocephalus
- Deep vein thrombosis (DVT)
- Hyponatremia
- Infections
- SIADH
- Diabetes insipidus
- Pulmonary complications (neurogenic pulmonary edema, pneumonia)

Most of these have been discussed briefly. Hyponatremia is very common for unknown reasons. The patient is also more prone to DVT and related pulmonary emboli, also for unknown reasons. The nurse needs to keep these potential problems in mind when caring for the patient.

ANEURYSM PRECAUTIONS

General nursing management is modified to incorporate the points of care included in aneurysm precautions. These precautions, along with the underlying rationale, are described in Chart 28-1.

Nursing responsibilities in preventing complications are listed. However, two responsibilities are singled out as being extremely important because they are within the purview of the nurse to monitor and control. First, initiating a bowel program to prevent straining at stool is very important. Most patients received codeine for control of headache. A side effect of this drug is decreased peristalsis, which can result in constipation if action is not taken to counteract this trend. In addition, bed rest and the subsequent immobility also contribute to constipation. A bowel management program must be instituted immediately

upon hospitalization. By the time constipation becomes a problem, the peak time for high incidence of rebleeding is reached. Straining at stool (initiating Valsalva's maneuver) is dangerous because it can cause rebleeding.

The second concern is that the patient who is maintained on extended bed rest is at high risk for deep vein thrombosis (DVT). Drug therapy may also compound the risk of DVT and pulmonary emboli. This risk factor can be controlled by the nurse through the use of elastic (TED) hose and sequential compression boots. It is the nurse's responsibility to be sure that the elastic hose and compression boots are on at all times. The patient's legs should be monitored periodically for the development of DVT. In addition, use of minidoses (5,000 units) of heparin subcutaneously every 12 hours may be started if there are no contraindications.

ADDITIONAL POINTS OF CARE

Fluid Restriction. The practice of fluid restriction has been abandoned by many physicians because it is thought that vasospasm and cerebral ischemia are increased with hemoconcentration (see the earlier discussion of fluid restriction in the section on cerebral vasospasm). If the physician chooses to restrict the patient's fluid intake, the restriction will be specified in terms of the number of milliliters of fluid the patient may be given in a 24-hour period. For example, the patient may be restricted to a daily intake of 1,800 mL. This means that, regardless of the route of administration, the total intake in a 24-hour period should not exceed 1,800 mL. The nurse is responsible for maintaining an accurate intake and output record.

- A large sign placed over the head of the bed indicating that the patient is having fluids restricted is helpful in reminding the entire staff and the family that the patient is not allowed fluids as desired.
- A notation should also be made on the intake and output record sheet.
- A simple explanation will help the family to understand the rationale and importance of this restriction.

Fluid balance may also be followed by monitoring the central venous pressure, weight, and serum osmolality. Use of a central venous line or a pulmonary catheter is common for monitoring patients who are in the ICU.

Seizure Precautions. As a precaution in the event of seizure activity, aspiration, or a deterioration of the patient's condition, a standby suction setup is kept in readiness at the bedside, along with a padded bite stick and oral airway. Padded siderails are also in place to protect the patient from injury.

Protective Devices. The use of wrist and ankle protective devices is avoided as much as possible, as the patient may be inclined to strain against them. Should such measures become necessary to protect the patient from injury, a vest or jacket is usually effective in keeping the patient in bed. Full siderails at the top and bottom of the bed should be pulled up at all times, and the bed should be kept low when the nurse is not at the bedside. At times, to prevent a confused patient from pulling on tubes or the intravenous line, it may be necessary

CHART 28-2

Summary of Nursing Diagnoses Associated With Cerebral Aneurysms

Nursing Diagnosis	Nursing Interventions	Expected Outcomes
Pain (headache, neck/back pain) related to (R/T) meningeal irritation	• Assess the type, location, and specific characteristics of the headache. • Assess the patient for pain and other signs and symptoms of meningeal irritation. • Reposition the patient gently, avoiding any unnecessary movement of the neck or head. • Administer analgesics as ordered. • Darken the patient's room. • Apply a cold, wet cloth or ice cap to the patient's head for comfort.	• The characteristics of the headache will be noted and recorded. • Analgesics and comfort measures will be administered. • The patient will provide objective evidence that the pain has been relieved.
Sensory/Perceptual Alterations, Visual, R/T photophobia secondary to meningeal irritation	• Note any evidence of discomfort when assessing direct light response of the pupils. • Maintain a darkened room by drawing the blinds or shades and avoiding direct light.	• Photophobia will be controlled by maintaining a darkened room.
High Risk for Injury R/T seizure activity secondary to cerebral irritation	• Maintain seizure precautions. • Monitor the patient for any signs of seizure activity and document in the chart. • Administer anticonvulsant drugs prophylactically, as ordered.	• Seizure activity will be prevented. • If a seizure does occur, the patient will not be injured.
Anxiety (mild, moderate, or severe) R/T illness and/or restrictions of aneurysm precautions	• Assess the patient for objective and subjective evidence of anxiety. • If anxiety is present, try to identify the specific causes. • Attempt to clarify, control, or change the circumstances surrounding the anxiety. • Make appropriate referrals, as necessary. • Reassure the patient. • Depending on the patient's level of consciousness, use imagery, relaxation techniques, and so forth to control anxiety. • Administer sedatives, if ordered.	• Depending on the patient's level of consciousness, he or she will demonstrate an understanding of the purpose of the aneurysm precautions. • The patient will be informed of the plan of care and reassured. • The specific causes of anxiety will be identified. • Anxiety will be minimized or controlled.
High Risk for Secondary Brain Injury R/T rebleeding or cerebral vasospasms	• Assess neurological signs frequently for evidence of neurological deterioration. • Report immediately any significant changes in the patient's condition. • Recognize the peak times of occurrence of rebleeding and vasospasms. • If deterioration occurs, implement nursing protocols and standing orders so that ischemic response is treated.	• The patient will be carefully monitored so that any signs or symptoms of neurological deterioration will be identified quickly. • If there is evidence of deterioration, the physician will be notified immediately. • Nursing interventions and standing orders will be implemented quickly.

to apply wrist restraints. The wrist must be properly padded to prevent skin irritation and must be inspected at least every 4 hours.

Drug Therapy. In addition to the nursing care outlined, the nurse is responsible for administering the drug therapy prescribed by the physician and for being aware of the action, toxicity, and interactions of the various drugs used. In this way, pertinent observations can be made in assessing the patient's response to the drug therapy.

PSYCHOLOGICAL SUPPORT

Considering the restrictions placed on the patient's activity, it is important to monitor the patient's psychological and emotional response. A calm and reassuring approach to the patient is most therapeutic.

The following are general suggestions to prevent adverse behavioral or psychological responses secondary to immobility, sensory deprivation, and powerlessness:

- Orient the patient frequently to time, place, and person.
- Familiarize the patient with the environment.
- Be alert for cues from the patient indicating areas of concern.
- Provide information to clarify any concerns in a simple manner. Clarify any misconceptions and quickly reorient the patient.
- As the patient's condition improves, allow the patient to make simple decisions (*e.g.*, "Which way is it easiest to turn?").
- Report any severe responses to the patient's restrictions that might indicate the need for modification by the physician.
- Be supportive and helpful to the family throughout the hospitalization period.

Nursing Management After Surgery/Endovascular Therapy

Nursing management following a craniotomy for aneurysm clipping follows that outlined in Chapter 18. Because there is some incidence of vasospasm even after surgery, the nurse must monitor the patient for any neurological deterioration that may herald the onset of vasospasm. (*Note:* The onset may be gradual, as evidenced by slight pronator drift or confusion.) Cerebral angiography is often ordered after surgery to reassess the placement of the clip. A CT scan is also done to determine the presence of blood or cerebral edema.

For the patient who has undergone endovascular balloon therapy, nursing management focuses on monitoring vital signs and neurological signs for evidence of hemorrhage or vasospasm. In addition, the femoral puncture site is monitored for evidence of bleeding, and the pedal pulses are assessed for evidence of occlusion. The patient is maintained on bed rest with the involved leg extended for a period of time.

Discharge Planning

Even with the technological advances that have been made in the management of patients with aneurysms, the outcome for many patients is significant neurological deficits. Throughout

hospitalization, there is need for interdisciplinary patient management to address the patient holistically and to ensure early diagnosis and treatment of deficits. Many patients will need further rehabilitation after discharge from the acute care setting. Discharge planning should begin at admission or shortly thereafter and should address the individual needs of the patient. Much patient and family teaching is often necessary to assist them in making decisions and coping with the multiple problems that may arise.

FUTURE TRENDS

Future advances in the management of cerebral aneurysms are likely to include early diagnosis and treatment of patients before rupture and hemorrhage. With the dawn of preventative medicine and managed care, aneurysm screening in high-risk patients may be more cost effective since acute medical care and long-term care for patients with aneurysmal SAH costs millions of dollars annually. Continuing research for new and better drugs to prevent rebleeding and vasospasm and further development of endovascular treatment options for more patients may help to decrease the morbidity and mortality associated with this disease.

References

1. McCormick, W. F., & Acousta-Rua, G. J. (1980). The size of intracranial saccular aneurysms: An autopsy study. *Journal of Neurosurgery, 33,* 422–427.
2. Mayberg, M. R., Batjer, H. H., Dacey, R., Diringer, M., et al. (1994). Guidelines for the management of aneurysmal subarachnoid hemorrhage. *Stroke, 25*(11), 2315–2328.
3. Herrick, I. A., & Gelb, A. W. (1992). Anesthesia for intracranial aneurysm surgery. *Journal of Clinical Anesthesia, 4,* 73–82.
4. Heiserman, J. E., & Bird, C. R. (1994). Cerebral aneurysms. *Neuroimaging Clinics of North America, 4*(4), 799–821.
5. Camarata, P. J., Latchaw, R. E., Rufenacht, D. A., & Heros, R. C. (1992). Intracranial aneurysms. *Investigative Radiology, 28*(4), 373–382.
6. Stebhens, W. E. (1989). Etiology of intracranial berry aneurysms. *Journal of Neurosurgery, 70,* 823–831.
7. Ibid.
8. Ryba, M., Grieb, P., Iwanska, K., et al. (1992). HLA antigens and intracranial aneurysms. *Acta Neurochirurgica, 116,* 1–5.
9. Camarata et al., op. cit.
10. Davis, K. R., Kistler, J. P., Heros, R. C., & Davis, J. M. (1982). Neuroradiologic approach to the patient with a diagnosis of subarachnoid hemorrhage. *Radiology Clinics of North America, 20,* 87–94.
11. Mayberg, M. R., Batjer, H. H., Dacey, R., Diringer, M., et al. (1994). Guidelines for the management of aneurysmal subarachnoid hemorrhage. *Stroke, 25*(11), 2315–2328.
12. Fleischer, A. S., Patton, J. M., & Tindall, G. T. (1975). Cerebral aneurysms of traumatic origin. *Surgical Neurology, 4,* 233–239.
13. Camarata et al., op. cit.
14. Hunt, W. E., & Hess, R. M. (1968). Surgical risk as related to time of intervention in the repair of intracranial aneurysm. *Journal of Neurosurgery, 28,* 14–20.
15. Kassell, N. F., Torner, J. C. L., Haley, E. C., et al. (1990). The international cooperative study on the timing of aneurysm surgery. Part 1. Overall management and results. *Journal of Neurosurgery, 73,* 18–36.

16. Mayberg et al., op. cit.
17. Ibid.
18. Ibid.
19. Fisher, C. M., Kistler, J. P., & Davis, J. M. (1980). Relation of cerebral vasospasm to subarachnoid hemorrhage visualized by computerized tomographic scanning. *Neurosurgery, 6,* 1–9.
20. Wijdicks, E. F. M., Vermeulen, M., ten Haaf, J., Hijdra, A., Bakker, W. H., & van Gijn, J. (1985). Volume depletion and natriuresis in patients with a ruptured intracranial aneurysm. *Annals of Neurology, 18,* 211–216.
21. ●●●

Bibliography

Books

Kistler, J. P., Gress, D. R., Crowell, R. M., Pile-Spellman, J., & Heros, R. C. (1993). Management of subarachnoid hemorrhage. In A. H. Ropper (Ed.), *Neurological and neurosurgical intensive care* (3rd ed.) (pp. 291–308). New York: Raven.

Periodicals

Foley, P. L., Caner, H. H., Kassel, N. F., & Lee, K. S. (1994). Reversal of subarachnoid hemorrhage-induced vasoconstriction with an endothelin receptor antagonist. *Neurosurgery, 34*(1), 108–113.

Kassell, N. F., Torner, J. C., Haley, E. C., et al. (1990). The international cooperative study on the timing of aneurysm surgery. Part 1. Overall management and results. *Journal of Neurosurgery, 73,* 18–36.

Kassell, N. F., Torner, J. C., Haley, E. C., et al. (1990). The international cooperative study on the timing of aneurysm surgery. Part 2. Surgical results. *Journal of Neurosurgery, 73,* 37–47.

Manifold, S. L. (1990). Aneurysmal SAH: Cerebral vasospasm and early repair. *Critical Care, 10*(8), 62–69.

Mayberg, M. R., Batjer, H. H., Dacey, R., Diringer, M., Haley, E. C., Heros, R. C., et al. (1994). Guidelines for the management of aneurysmal subarachnoid hemorrhage. A statement for health care professionals from a special writing group of the Stroke Council, American Heart Association. *Stroke, 25*(11), 2315–2328.

Mayer, S. A. (1995). Fluid management in subarachnoid hemorrhage. *Neurologist, 1,* 71–85.

McDonald, E. (1989). Aneurysmal subarachnoid hemorrhage. *Journal of Neurosurgery Nursing, 21*(5), 313–321.

Rutledge, B. (1989). Aneurysm wrapping: Principles applicable to the neuroscience nurse. *Journal of Neuroscience Nursing, 21*(6), 370–374.

Sivakumar, V., Rajshekhar, V., & Chandy, M. J. (1994). Management of neurosurgical patients with hyponatremia and natriuresis. *Neurosurgery, 34*(2), 269–274.

Stebhens, W. E. (1989). Etiology of intracranial berry aneurysms. *Journal of Neurosurgery, 70,* 823–831.

Wijdicks, E. F. M., Vermeulen, M., Hijdra, A., & van Gijn, J. (1985). Hyponatremia and cerebral infarction in patients with ruptured intracranial aneurysms: Is fluid restriction harmful? *Annals of Neurology, 17,* 137–140.

CHAPTER 29

Arteriovenous Malformations and Other Cerebrovascular Anomalies

Joanne V. Hickey
Deidre Buckley

Cerebrovascular malformations are believed to be developmental vascular anomalies that result from failure of the embryonic vascular network.[1] The incidence of cerebrovascular malformations is unclear because many lesions are asymptomatic and are found only incidentally at autopsy.

CLASSIFICATIONS OF VASCULAR MALFORMATIONS

Cerebrovascular malformations are classified into four major categories: capillary telangiectases, cavernous malformations, venous malformations, and arteriovenous malformations.[1] The term *malformation* is preferable to the previously used *angioma*. *Angioma* has the connotation of neoplasia which does not occur in these lesions. The incidence of vascular malformations varies from 0.1% to 4% in various autopsy studies. Because some of these lesions do not have direct arterial vessel input, they may not be visible on angiography.[2-4]

Telangiectases

Telangiectases are small (0.3 to 1.0 cm) capillary lesions that are composed of clusters of vessels that have the appearance of somewhat dilated capillaries separated by normal-appearing parenchyma. These lesions have little clinical significance because they rarely cause hemorrhage; they are not apparent on radiological examination. Telangiectases are an incidental finding at autopsy, and are most commonly located in the brain stem.

Cavernous Malformations

Cavernous malformations, also called cavernous hemangiomas, are nodular lesions composed of sinusoidal-type vessels that are not separated by normal-appearing parenchyma (neural tissue). These low-flow lesions are not apparent on angiography, but may be visualized on computed tomography (CT) scan and magnetic resonance imaging (MRI). Cavernous malformations are well-defined, purple lesions that may reach an appreciable size and may be mistaken for a brain tumor on CT scan. Other cavernous malformations are found incidentally at autopsy. Microscopic examination often reveals small hemorrhages with numerous, hemosiderin-laden macrophages and gliotic tissue in the adjacent parenchyma. Calcification within the lesion is common. Some cavernous malformations may cause seizures and intracerebral hemorrhage. With larger, clinically significant lesions, surgical removal is indicated.

Venous Malformations

Venous malformations, also referred to as venous anomalies, are composed of anomalous veins, separated by normal parenchyma, that drain into a dilated venous trunk. They are the most common vascular anomaly of the brain. These lesions have no recognizable direct arterial input. Calcification within the lesion is rare. The predominant location of venous malformations is in the cerebrum, although some are found in the cerebellum (3:1 ratio). Clinically, the patient may present with seizures. Venous malformations may be evident on CT scan, MRI, or angiography. Those found in the cerebrum rarely cause hemorrhage and are treated conservatively. However, cerebellar venous malformations are associated with an increased incidence of intracerebral hemorrhage; affected patients are, therefore, considered for surgery.

Arteriovenous Malformations

An **arteriovenous malformation** (AVM) is composed of a tightly tangled collection of abnormal-appearing, dilated blood vessels that directly shunt arterial blood into the venous system without the usual connecting capillary network. The blood vessels of the AVM are thin-walled and tortuous and lack the normal characteristics of veins or arteries. The three morphologic components of an AVM are the nidus, the feeding arteries, and the draining veins. (The literature often refers to the nidus when discussing AVMs; a **nidus** is defined as the focus of the AVM—that is, the tangle of abnormal vessels.) The vessels of the AVM vary greatly in diameter, but the veins are generally larger than the arteries. The arterial vessels, also called feeder arteries, supply the AVM. The lesion is drained by dilated veins without the usual intervening capillary network. As a result of the absence of the capillary network, the blood flow is accelerated and the pressure is elevated within the fragile vessels of the AVM. These conditions predispose the lesion to hemorrhage.

AVMs may be small and focal, or they may be large, involving an entire hemisphere. Some are cone-shaped, with the apex pointing inward and the base positioned on the surface of the cerebral cortex. In rare instances, the lesion is so deep that the ventricles and choroid plexus are involved, thus predisposing the person to intraventricular hemorrhage. The parenchyma between the vessels of the AVM is usually abnormal, with nonfunctional gliotic tissue (proliferation of neuroglia [supporting tissue] in the brain). Frequently, there is evidence of old hemorrhage and **hemosiderin** deposits (iron-containing glycoprotein pigment found in tissue, excessive amounts of which occur in pathological conditions). Patients may have a radiographic hemorrhage without clinical signs or symptoms of hemorrhage.

The AVM is the most common cerebrovascular lesion that causes symptoms and is, therefore, clinically significant. AVMs are found in both children and adults. AVMs in adults constitute the focus of the remainder of this chapter.

ARTERIOVENOUS MALFORMATIONS IN THE ADULT: AN OVERVIEW

Several points can be made about AVMs including the following:

- AVMs account for 8.6% of subarachnoid hemorrhages; this means that 1% of strokes are attributable to ruptured AVMs.
- The Harvard Cooperative Stroke Registry did a 3-year study documenting 9 AVM cases among 494 cases of stroke from all causes in a population of 100,000. This yields an incidence of about 3 per 100,000 annually.[5,6]
- The ratio of AVMs to intracranial aneurysms is 1:10.[7,8]

- Approximately 90% of AVMs are located in the supratentorial area and involve the cerebral hemispheres; only 10% of this group are located in the deep subcortical areas (*e.g.*, basal ganglia, thalamus, corpus callosum).
- The location of 10% of AVMs is within the cerebellum and brain stem. Of the patients with AVMs, 80% develop symptoms between the ages of 20 and 40 years of age; the remaining 20% develop symptoms before the age of 20 years.

Pathophysiology and Pathological Characteristics

There are two pathophysiological characteristics related to AVMs. The first is the effect of shunting of blood from the arterial to the venous system without the intervening capillary network. Normally, the capillary network provides capillary resistance to blood flow, thus decreasing the intravascular pressure. However, when an AVM is present, blood is shunted from the high-resistance normal vascular bed to the low-resistance vessels within the AVM, thus exposing the draining venous channels to elevated intravascular pressure. These dynamics predispose the vessels to rupture and hemorrhage.

The second is the effect of impaired perfusion of the cerebral tissue adjacent to the AVM. The elevated intravascular pressure and the elevated venous pressure impair cerebral perfusion pressure. When the AVM is large and high flow, the diversion of blood to the AVM may cause ischemia to the adjacent normal tissue. Clinically, this is evidenced by slowly progressive neurological deficits. The diversion of blood to the AVM is called the *vascular steal phenomenon*.

AVMs are circumscribed vascular lesions that displace, rather than encompass, normal functioning brain tissue. They are separated from normal tissue by abnormal and nonfunctional gliotic parenchyma. Evidence of microscopic or gross hemorrhage is very common. This is true even in patients who have clinically manifested hemorrhage. Partial thrombosis of an AVM is not uncommon and can occur spontaneously. This may explain why some AVMs appear smaller on repeat angiography than on a previous study. This may also explain why some AVMs that are classified as "occult" are not seen on angiography.

Clinical Manifestations

The major clinical manifestations of AVMs are hemorrhage, seizures, headache, and progressive neurological deficits. The following provides a brief discussion of each.

Hemorrhage. Hemorrhage is the most common initial manifestation of AVMs. Approximately 50% of clinically evident AVMs present with intracranial hemorrhage. When an AVM ruptures, it usually causes intraparenchymal hemorrhage.[9,10] If the AVM is superficial, a subarachnoid hemorrhage can occur. In the rare instance of an AVM that involves the choroid plexus, rupture can result in intraventricular hemorrhage. Mortality associated with initial AVM rupture is between 6% and 30% with an average of about 15%. There is a serious morbidity rate reported that ranges from 15% to 80% with an average of about 30%. The combined morbidity and mortality rates from an AVM bleed may be as high as 15% to 80%.[11–14]

The chance of rebleeding during the first year is approximately 6%.[15] Afterwards, the incidence of recurrent hemorrhages decreases to 4% per year. This is the same as the rate of hemorrhage from AVMs that have never bled. The hemorrhage associated with rupture of an AVM is not as devastating as that associated with a ruptured cerebral aneurysm. In addition, the vasospasm and acute rebleeding (20% to 40% rebleed within 14 days) that are associated with aneurysms are not characteristic of AVMs.[3] Vasospasm does not occur within the AVM because there is not blood in the basilar subarachnoid cistern around the major intracranial arteries that is common with aneurysmal rupture.

Seizures. Seizures are the second most common manifestation of AVMs.[16,17] It has been suggested that approximately 70% of patients with AVMs will have seizures at some time.[10] Of the patients who have seizures, about 50% have focal seizures. The natural history of a patient with an AVM presenting with seizures is still not certain.

The etiology of seizures in patients with AVMs is not clear, but two explanations have been suggested. First, cortical injury from hemorrhage into areas adjacent to the AVM may cause foci for seizure activity. Second, chronic ischemia from the vascular steal phenomenon may also cause abnormal cells that may become the foci for seizure activity.[18]

In patients who present with seizure, there is a 25% chance of hemorrhage within 15 years, or 4% per year.[19] It is thought that medical therapy is generally successful in the control of seizure activity. The prognosis for patients who have surgery or embolization/surgery to resect the AVM is favorable in that the frequency of seizures lessens in the majority of cases.[20] It is also thought that seizures improve after radiosurgery.[21]

Headache. Recurrent headache that does not respond to usual drug therapy may be the only symptom of an AVM. Some patients experience migraine-like headaches. A headache work-up with an MRI scan may suggest the presence of an AVM. It is important to note that some types of headaches are related to AVMs. Some AVMs in the occipital lobe cause migraine-like headaches. Often after the removal of the AVM, the patient's headaches are resolved.[22] Because of the high frequency of headaches in the population, the relationship of AVM to headache is difficult to define. As technology improves and becomes more readily available, MRI scans are being ordered by physicians for headaches or other complaints and an AVM or other lesion may be found incidentally. In certain circumstances, headaches are clearly related to an underlying AVM, but in other situations, there is a much less defined relationship. In cases where differentiation of symptoms to lesions is less clear, it would be dangerous to assume the headaches are caused by the malformation and will be relieved by treatment—either partial or complete. The patient must understand that symptoms may be incidental to the lesion.

Progressive Neurological Deficits. The development of progressive neurological deficits is primarily attributed to cerebral ischemia resulting from vascular steal. The signs and symptoms will depend on the specific area of cerebral tissue deprived of adequate blood supply. Progressive deficits may also be related to repeated small hemorrhages that have not been clinically apparent.

Venous hypertension from arterialization of the venous system may also account for neurological deterioration. Hydrocephalus is another mechanism that plays a role in progressive neurological deficits caused by ventricular compression from dilated veins.

Neuropsychiatric Manifestations. AVMs may cause neuropsychiatric manifestations. The incidence has been estimated at approximately 10%. The vascular steal syndrome is thought to be responsible for such symptoms.[23]

Diagnosis

DIAGNOSTIC PROCEDURES

CT Scan. The CT scan is one of the initial screening tools for AVMs. It is a diagnostic test in which cross sections of the brain are examined through the use of an x-ray and computer. The picture of the various layers produced by the scan accurately reflects anatomical structures inside the brain, such as the ventricles, basal ganglia, and thalamus. A CT scan without infusion of contrast material is often ordered to rule out the presence of an acute hematoma. If the AVM has hemorrhaged, it is particularly helpful in monitoring clot and observing for resolution of blood over time.

MRI/MRA. MRI is a diagnostic scan which examines various areas of the body through the use of a large, doughnut-shaped magnet and a computer. Magnetic signals from the part of the body being examined are seen through a computer as radio waves. The computer transforms these radio waves into images. MRI is also an initial diagnostic tool and is ordered more commonly than a CT scan for such complaints as headaches. MRI is critical in defining the treatment plan of the AVM in order to determine the site of its nidus, as well as its relationship to other critical anatomical structures in the brain. It is also better than CT scanning in demonstrating subtle changes in tissue composition (*e.g.*, edema and old hemorrhage).

Magnetic resonance angiography (MRA) is the same procedure as MRI with the only difference being that blood vessels are examined instead of body tissue. MRI and MRA are both noninvasive studies.

Angiography. Cerebral angiography is the definitive diagnostic procedure for AVMs. It demonstrates the feeding arteries, the nidus, and the draining veins. This information is important for making decisions about the advisability of surgery, endovascular therapy, or radiosurgery. Cerebral angiography is also useful for following the progress and development of the AVM over time.

As mentioned earlier, a small number of AVMs are angiographically occult lesions. These lesions are discovered in the diagnostic work-up of patients presenting with intracranial hemorrhage or in patients with seizures.

Treatment

Decisions regarding the best approach to management of AVMs are difficult. Among the factors that influence the outcome for the patient, two are critical—the reputation of the hospital and, in particular, the neurosurgeon's experience with AVMs. The natural history of the lesion for hemorrhaging, along with the specific characteristics of the lesion in the particular patient, are carefully weighed. The physician must compare the long-term risk presented by an untreated AVM with the more immediate risk of surgery or other treatment options.

NATURAL HISTORY OF ARTERIOVENOUS MALFORMATIONS

The biological behavior or natural history of AVMs is helpful in weighing treatment approaches. The following provides statistics about the natural history of AVMs.

Unruptured AVM

- There is approximately a 3% risk of bleeding per year, with about a 1% risk of death per year.

Ruptured AVM

- The mortality rate for the first hemorrhage is about 10%.
- The risk of rebleeding is approximately 6% during the first year; it then declines to approximately 3% per year after that, up to about 15 years.
- The mortality associated with a second hemorrhage is approximately 13%; subsequent hemorrhages carry a mortality rate of about 20%.

With wider use of MRI scanning for screening of patients for a number of neurological signs and symptoms, asymptomatic AVMs are being detected more frequently. The risk of hemorrhage is about 4%.[24] Of all patients with AVMs who have no previous clinical history of hemorrhage, 25% to 33% demonstrate evidence of previous hemorrhage.[25]

The natural history of AVMs suggests a high probability for hemorrhage at some time. Statistics also suggest that the incidence of rebleeding is the same regardless of whether the AVM is unruptured or ruptured. Although the physician makes the decisions about medical management, it is important for the nurse to understand the basis for the decision. This information is helpful in patient and family teaching situations and in reinforcing the information provided to the patient and family by the physician.

GRADING OF ARTERIOVENOUS MALFORMATIONS

Spetzler and Martin have developed a grading system for AVMs according to their degrees of surgical difficulty.[26] The scale is based on three variables and subscales:

- **Size of the AVM:** 1 = small (<3 cm); 2 = medium (3 to 6 cm); and 3 = large (>6 cm)
- **Pattern of AVM venous drainage:** 1 = deep veins; 0 = superficial cortical veins
- **Eloquence of adjacent brain:** 1 = eloquent; 0 = noneloquent

Eloquence refers to areas of the brain that have readily identifiable neurological function; if injury to any of these

areas occurs, a disabling neurological deficit will be noted. According to this grading system, the eloquent areas are the sensorimotor, language, and visual cortex; the hypothalamus and thalamus; the internal capsule; the brain stem; the cerebellar peduncles; and the deep cerebellar nuclei.

Each of these three variables becomes a subscale that is assigned a numerical value. The scores of each subscale are added together, and the total score indicates an AVM grade from I to V. Angiographic findings are used to collect data for each subscale.

TREATMENT OPTIONS

The treatment options available for AVMs include surgery, embolization, radiosurgery, and conservative treatment.

Surgery. With rare exceptions, surgery for an AVM is always elective. Only if there is an intracerebral hematoma or subdural hematoma is early surgery considered. Even when surgery is anticipated after hemorrhage, it is usually delayed for about 3 weeks. This timetable allows for the patient to be stabilized and for the brain to recover from the effects of hemorrhage.

Applying the grading system for AVMs discussed earlier, the experienced neurosurgeon is able to assess the degree of surgical difficulty. The physician considers the age of the patient along with the anatomical location of the lesion and other characteristics that influence the technical approach to the lesion. The goals of surgery are (1) complete excision of the AVM to prevent hemorrhage completely, and (2) excision of the lesion without causing hemorrhage or injury to adjacent tissue during the surgery. Ligation of the feeder vessels does not provide protection from hemorrhage.[27] The lesion may have to be treated in stages with a combination of embolization and surgery (Figs. 29-1 through 29-5; Case Study 29-1).

A special concern related to surgery for large AVMs (larger than 4 to 5 cm) is normal perfusion pressure breakthrough.[28] **Normal perfusion pressure breakthrough** is a rare occurrence and is described as severe, protracted, and unexplained brain edema accompanied by diffuse hemorrhage or focal deep hemorrhage in the parenchyma immediately adjacent to the area of resection. To prevent this occurrence, the interventional neuroradiologist plans one, two, or more stages of endovascular treatment to reduce the blood supply to the AVM.

Embolization. Embolization of brain AVMs is a subspecialty of interventional neuroradiology which has made tremendous strides over the past few years. Improvement in catheters and embolic material, as well as imaging equipment, have led to safer, more efficacious treatment. Depending on size, location, symptoms, hemodynamics, and anatomical vasculature of AVMs, embolization may be curative, palliative, or adjunctive to surgery or radiosurgery.[29]

As with surgery, the interventional neuroradiologist's experience with embolization procedures greatly influences outcome for the patient. Improvements in microcatheter technology have allowed for superselective catheterization of distal vessels as well as intranidal aneurysms. Digital subtraction angiography and the development of "road mapping" technique are essential to endovascular treatment. The use of hep-

Case Study 29-1

This is a 45-year-old woman who presented with a generalized seizure on 6/24/92. Figure 29-1 shows the arteriovenous malformation (AVM) on magnetic resonance imaging; the arrow points to the lesion, which is approximately 3 × 4 × 2 cm. Figure 29-2 is an angiogram showing the size and location of the AVM as well as pertinent feeding vessels which come from the posterior cerebral artery, as well as feeders from the middle cerebral artery and anterior cerebral artery. The patient was treated with two sessions of embolization followed by surgery. Figure 29-3 is the angiogram pre-embolization, Figure 29-4 is an angiogram taken post-embolization, and Figure 29-5 is an angiogram taken after surgery. Patient discharged on anticonvulsant drugs.

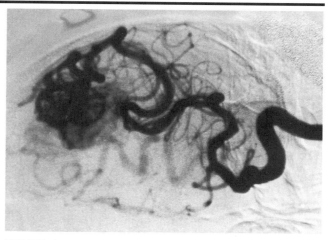

FIGURE 29-3

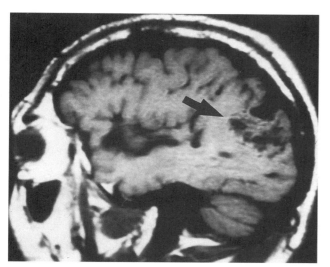

FIGURE 29-1

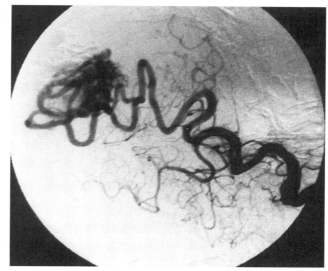

FIGURE 29-4

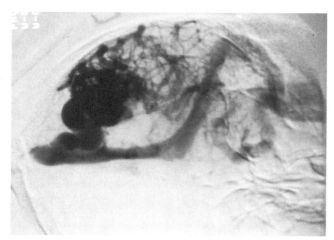

FIGURE 29-2

Follow-up on 1/95: Patient had one seizure in June 1994. She has remained on anticonvulsants and has been seizure free. Neurologically, she is intact and enjoys a very good quality of life.

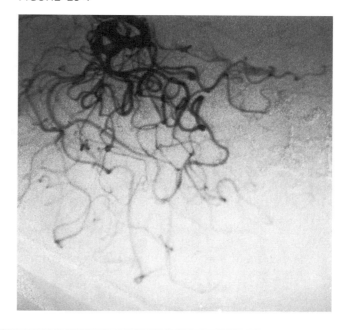

FIGURE 29-5

arin during the procedure has been proven to minimize thromboembolic complications and is a necessary adjunct to embolization.

Some of the embolic materials include n-butyl-cyanoacrylate (NBCA), which is a short-acting liquid polymerizing agent. It is a permanent agent which is not widely available. In its solidified form, it is relatively soft, making it easy for the surgeon to resect.[30] Polyvinyl alcohol (PVA) and gelfoam particles are easier to use but are nonpermanent embolic agents. Alternative materials include microcoils and silk thread, which is highly thrombogenic, though not permanent. The goal of embolization for definitive or palliative treatment is permanent occlusion of the nidus and feeding vessels.

Radiosurgery. The underlying goal of radiation therapy for AVMs is to induce an inflammatory response in the vessel walls of the lesion that will result in permanent thickening of pathological vascular channels, with ultimate thrombosis and obliteration of the lesion.[31] The success in achieving this goal is determined, in part, by the ability to provide partial or total radiation to the lesion. If obliteration is incomplete, the patient is at risk for hemorrhage.

Various types of ionizing radiation have been used in the treatment of AVMs, including x-rays (produced by x-ray tubes or megavoltage linear accelerators); gamma rays (produced by cobalt); and Bragg peak therapy (proton beam and helium beam).[32] A delayed complication common to all types of radiation therapy is radionecrosis of healthy neural tissue. This can occur in a matter of months (3 to 11 months) or years (1 to 8 years) after radiation therapy. It is evidenced by development of new neurological deficits or worsening of previous deficits.

CONVENTIONAL RADIATION THERAPY. Conventional radiation therapy is defined as orthovoltage or megavoltage external beam radiation or cobalt-60 gamma rays without stereotactic technique. Its use has generally not been considered effective in treating AVMs. However, recent publications recommend a reexamination of the use and patient selection criteria for conventional radiation therapy. The literature suggests that desirable changes within the wall of lesions are induced by this type of radiosurgery.

GAMMA KNIFE RADIOSURGERY. Stereotactically directed gamma radiation has been pioneered by Leksell.[33] This so-called bloodless surgery is used to treat surgically inaccessible lesions that are 2 to 3 cm in diameter. For larger lesions, only partial radiosurgery can be offered.

BRAGG PEAK PROTON BEAM THERAPY. For surgically inaccessible AVMs, proton beam radiosurgery has been useful as an ablative approach to shrink the lesion.[13] This is a noninvasive procedure that utilizes the radiation emitted by protons that have been accelerated in a cyclotron. Stereotactic technique controls the focus of the beam to the target area.

The major advantage of proton beam radiosurgery is that, once the diagnostic work-up is completed, the radiation therapy is administered on an outpatient basis or during a brief hospitalization. There is no immediate risk to the patient from the irradiation. The major drawback is the possibility of hemorrhage before the effect of the therapy is realized. Radiosurgery effects develop gradually, requiring 12 to 24 months to reach a therapeutic level that provides protection against hemorrhage. As a result of radiosurgery, the walls of the lesion thicken, and there may be some obliteration of the lesion and reduction in its size. Complications related to proton beam therapy are uncommon, although radiation-induced necrosis has been reported. The physician attempts to keep the risk below 3% to 5%. The possibility of complications in a patient reflects the location of the AVM relative to brain structures.

Conservative Management. In some instances, the treatment of choice may be conservative management. A discussion of any restrictions on activities, such as contact sports, is necessary. For patients who present with seizures, seizure activity can be well controlled with anticonvulsant therapy.

SUMMARY OF TREATMENT

Regardless of the treatment approach recommended to a particular patient, it is necessary to monitor the patient over time. In addition to follow-up appointments, periodic cerebral angiography, MRI, or both are ordered to check the progress of the lesion.

AVMS AND PREGNANCY

The incidence of hemorrhage from brain AVMs during pregnancy has been a controversial topic over the years. Earlier studies suggested a high incidence of hemorrhage during pregnancy when a patient had a true high flow AVM.[33,35] The implication is that when the AVM did present in a pregnant woman, it did so in the form of a hemorrhage.

A more recent retrospective study by Horton and associates found the incidence of hemorrhage in pregnant women with unruptured AVMs during the interval of time during and immediately after gestation to be 3.5% annually.[36] These women had no previous history consistent with hemorrhage. In women with a previous clinical history of hemorrhage, the risk was increased to a 5.8% chance of hemorrhage during pregnancy. In nonpregnant patients, the incidence of hemorrhage is 4% per year. It was therefore concluded by the investigators that pregnancy was not a significant risk factor for hemorrhage in women with unruptured AVMs.

Studies have shown that there is no increase in the rate of hemorrhage during labor or the immediate postpartum period. Therefore, when a woman presents during pregnancy with an AVM, the recommendation is that the pregnancy be brought to term. The patient can also be reassured that the risk of hemorrhage during delivery is very small, as is the case throughout the entire pregnancy. Data suggest in most cases that vaginal delivery is safe, but caesarean section may decrease the already low incidence of hemorrhage during delivery. There are no data to support or deny this statement.[37] The patient, neurosurgeon, and obstetrician need to discuss the safety and efficacy of the mode of delivery carefully on a case-by-case basis. All must be comfortable with the decision. According to the statistics, the actual incidence of problems encountered during pregnancy is low.

If the woman presents with a hemorrhage during pregnancy, care should proceed as in the nonpregnant patient. The nurse plays an important role in reassuring the patient while anticipating potential neurological problems. If a hematoma is present causing significant mass effect, it should be evacuated. Ogilvy and associates recommend removal of the clot only and operating on the AVM at an elective time.[33] Early angiography is often done. This is preferable and is used to define the anatomy of the lesion. If possible, the angiogram should be done during the second or third trimester to avoid added risk to the fetus. As with nonpregnant patients, the treatment modality—either surgery, embolization, radiosurgery, or a combination—is decided based on size, location, and surgical accessibility of the lesion.

Women with known AVMs should be carefully counseled prior to conception. If possible, the lesion should be treated before pregnancy. As previously stated, the risk of hemorrhage in a pregnant woman with an unruptured AVM is very low, but it is not *zero*. Safe management of pregnant patients with neurological diseases such as an AVM requires close collaboration of the health care team—neurosurgeon, neurologist, obstetrician, anesthesiologist, and nurses.[38] Reassuring the patient and reinforcing the information given to her by her physicians is an important role of the nurse during this critical time. Provision of written information is most helpful.

Nursing Management

The patient who is suspected of having a cerebral AVM is at risk for hemorrhage. If hemorrhage has not occurred, management is directed toward preventing hemorrhage by controlling hypertension, preventing seizures, and modifying the patient's lifestyle (*e.g.,* avoiding contact sports and lifting) to prevent surges in blood pressure. In the hospital environment, the nurse can expect to perform the following:

- Conduct a baseline neurological assessment as well as ongoing monitoring of neurological signs
- Monitor vital signs for evidence of hypertension
- Assess and monitor characteristics of headache, if present
- Monitor the patient for evidence of seizure activity
- Administer drug therapy as necessary

If the AVM has ruptured, the patient will be managed in a similar manner to other patients who have had a cerebral hemorrhage (see Chap. 28). The severity of the hemorrhage and the patient's clinical presentation will determine the medical treatment selected and the related nursing management. Hemorrhage is usually intracerebral. However, less frequently, subarachnoid hemorrhage, a subdural hematoma, or an intraventricular hematoma may occur. Unlike patients with ruptured aneurysms, vasospasm is not a concern after hemorrhage. There is some risk of rebleeding, and the patient should be monitored for evidence of rapid neurological deterioration. If surgery, embolization, or both are intended, they are usually delayed for about 3 weeks to allow for planning and for recovery of the brain from hemorrhage.

In addition to carrying out baseline and ongoing monitoring of neurological and vital signs, a major role of the nurse is providing emotional support and teaching to the patient and family. Most patients with AVMs are young, and the thought of having a serious lesion within the brain is very frightening to them. These patients undergo various diagnostic procedures to collect data about the lesion, and they are given much information, including the advantages and disadvantages of each treatment option. Finally, a decision is made regarding the appropriate course of treatment. The nurse is very much involved in the related patient teaching, as well as in reinforcing the information provided by the physician. Anxiety and fear are common responses of the patient and family. Nursing interventions are directed at alleviating these responses and supporting effective coping strategies. A support group specific to patients with brain AVMs may be helpful to both the patient and family members.

PERIOPERATIVE NURSING MANAGEMENT

If surgery is planned, the nurse will be responsible for providing basic preoperative teaching (see Chap. 18). Postoperative nursing management for patients with AVMs is similar to that outlined for a craniotomy patient (see Chap. 18). If a large lesion has been resected, there is the concern that normal perfusion pressure breakthrough can occur, as discussed previously. Clinically, there would be evidence of significant neurological deterioration.

The management of the patient after endovascular therapy includes continuous use of intravenous heparin, which will decrease the possibility of a thromboembolic complication while being carefully monitored in the neuro ICU. The arterial sheath will remain in place for a period of 12 to 24 hours. The patient is kept well hydrated, with tight blood pressure control. Mild systemic hypotension may be helpful in allowing flow changes to occur gradually in the brain tissue surrounding the AVM during the first 24 hours after the procedure. Sometimes the patients will complain of headache. This can be attributed to changes in flow dynamics in the brain. The nature of the headache should be documented, and the physician should be notified. If the indication of embolization is adjuvant to surgery, the patient is prepared for surgery 24 to 48 hours after endovascular treatment.[39]

After recovery from surgery, the patient is discharged with orders for anticonvulsant therapy. Depending on the presence of neurological deficits, there may be need for rehabilitation. For some patients, a neuropsychological evaluation may be ordered after a few months to evaluate the presence of cognitive deficits. The patient's progress is followed by the physician. If the lesion has not been obliterated completely, the patient remains at risk for hemorrhage.

Future Trends

Advances in functional imaging, microsurgical technique, neuroanesthesiology, endovascular therapy, and stereotactic radiosurgery have contributed to the ongoing therapeutic care and management of vascular malformations. Also important have been advances in biological knowledge, which form the foundation for modern success in treatment.[40]

Research continues on various interventional materials including glue (NBCA), PVA, and other liquid agents which are injected into the feeders of these complex lesions. Fractionated radiation is currently being researched as a mode to treat larger AVMs which were once deemed untreatable.

Although technology and knowledge of vascular malformations has increased tremendously over the years, and will continue to do so, one cannot dismiss the importance of individual patient characteristics such as age, medical condition, vocation, and psychological factors in the process of evaluating management options and coming to treatment decisions.

References

1. Tatter, S. B., & Ogilvy, C. S. (1995). Vascular malformations: General considerations. In C. W. Mitchell (Ed.), *Surgical management of neurovascular disease* (pp. 387–403). Baltimore: Williams & Wilkins.
2. Mohr, K., Caplan, L., Melski, J. W., et al. (1978). The Harvard Cooperative Stroke Registry: A prospective registry. *Neurology, 28,* 754.
3. Guidetti, B., & Delitala, A. (1980). Intracranial arteriovenous malformations: Conservative and surgical treatment. *Journal of Neurosurgery, 53,* 149–152.
4. McCormick, W. F. (1978). Classification, pathology, and natural history of angiomas of the central nervous system. *Neurology and Neurosurgery Weekly Update, 1,* 3–7.
5. Mohr et al., op. cit.
6. Ondra, S. L., Troupp, H., George, E. D., & Schwab, K. (1990). The natural history of symptomatic arteriovenous malformations of the brain: A 24 year follow-up assessment. *Journal of Neurosurgery, 73,* 387–391.
7. Guidetti & Delitala, op. cit.
8. McCormick, op. cit.
9. Parkinson, D., & Bachers, G. (1980). Arteriovenous malformations: Summary of 100 consecutive supratentorial cases. *Journal of Neurosurgery, 53,* 285–299.
10. Pertuiset, B., Sichez, J. P., Philippon, J., Fohanno, D, & Horn, Y. (1979). Mortality and morbidity after complete surgical removal of 162 intracranial arteriovenous malformations. *Review of Neurology, 135,* 319–327.
11. Brown, R. D., Jr., Weibers, D. D., & Forbes, G. S. (1990). Unruptured intracranial aneurysms and arteriovenous malformations: Frequency of intracranial hemorrhage in relation to lesions. *Journal of Neurosurgery, 73,* 859–863.
12. Fults, D., & Kelly, D. L., Jr. (1984). Natural history of arteriovenous malformations of the brain: A clinical study. *Neurosurgery, 15,* 658–662.
13. Kjellberg, R. N., Hanamura, J., Davis, K. R., Lyons, S. L., & Adams, R. D. (1983). Bragg Peak proton-beam therapy for arteriovenous malformations of the brain. *New England Journal of Medicine, 308,* 269–274.
14. Luessenhop, A. J., & Rosa, L. (1984). Cerebral arteriovenous malformations: Indications for and results of surgery, the role of intravascular techniques. *Journal of Neurosurgery, 60,* 14–22.
15. Graf, C. J., Perret, G. E., & Torner, J. C. (1983). Bleeding from cerebral arteriovenous malformations as part of their natural history. *Journal of Neurosurgery, 58,* 331–337.
16. Parkinson & Bachers, op. cit.
17. Graf et al., op. cit.
18. Ondra et al., op. cit.
19. Forster, D. M., Steiner, L., & Hakanson, S. (1972). Arteriovenous malformations of the brain: A long term clinical study. *Journal of Neurosurgery, 37,* 562–570.
20. Piepgras, D. G., Sundt, T. M., Jr., Ragoowanse, A. T., & Stevens, L. (1993). Seizure outcome in patients with surgically treated cerebral arteriovenous malformations. *Journal of Neurosurgery, 78,* 5–11.
21. Pollock, B. E., Lunsford, L. D., Kandziolka, D., Maitz, A., & Flickinger, J. C. (1994). Patient outcomes after stereotactic radiosurgery for "operable" arteriovenous malformations. *Neurosurgery, 35,* 1–8.
22. Heros, R. C., & Tu, Y. K. (1986). Unruptured arteriovenous malformations: A dilemma in surgical decision making. *Clinical Neurosurgery, 33,* 187–236.
23. Ondra et al., op. cit.
24. Ibid.
25. Heros & Tu, op. cit.
26. Hacien-Bey, L., Pile-Spellman, J., & Ogilvy, C. S. (1995). Embolization of brain arteriovenous malformations. In C. W. Mitchell (Ed.), *Surgical management of neurovascular disease* (pp. 404–418). Baltimore: Williams & Wilkins.
27. Purdy, P. D., Batjer, H. H., Risser, R. G., & Samson, D. (1992). Arteriovenous malformations of the brain: Choosing embolic materials to enhance safety and ease of excision. *J Neurosurgery, 77,* 217–222.
28. Robinson, J. L., Hall, C. S., & Sedzimir, C. B. (1972). Subarachnoid hemorrhage in pregnancy. *Journal of Neurosurgery, 36,* 27–33.
29. Hacien-Bey, Pile-Spellman, & Ogilvy, op. cit.
30. Purdy et al., op. cit.
31. Ondra, J. L., Doty, J. R., Mahla, M. E., & George, E. D. (1988). Surgical excision of a cavernous hemangioma of the rostral brainstem: Case report. *Neurosurgery, 23,* 490–493.
32. Ibid.
33. Ogilvy, C. S., & Tatter, S. B. (1995). Surgical management of vascular lesions and tumors associated with pregnancy. In H. H. Schmidek & W. H. Sweet (Eds.), *Operative neurosurgical techniques, indications, methods and results* (pp. 1163–1173). Philadelphia: W. B. Saunders.
34. Martin, N. A., & Vinters, H. V. (1995). Arteriovenous malformations. In L. P. Carter & R. F. Spetzler (Eds.), *Neurovascular surgery* (pp. 875–903). New York: McGraw-Hill.
35. Robinson, Hall, & Sedzimir, op. cit.
36. Horton, J. C., Chambers, W. A., Lyons, S. L., et al. (1990). Pregnancy and the risk of hemorrhage from cerebral arteriovenous malformations. *Neurosurgery, 27,* 867–871.
37. Ogilvy & Tatter, op. cit.
38. Ibid.
39. Hacien-Bey, Pile-Spellman, & Ogilvy, op. cit.
40. Martin & Vinters, op. cit.

Bibliography

Books

Edwards, M. S. B., & Hoffman, H. J. H. (Eds.). (1989). *Cerebral vascular disease in children and adolescents.* Baltimore: Williams & Wilkins.

Lunsford, E. D. (Ed.). (1988). *Modern stereotactic neurosurgery.* Boston: Martinus Nijhoff.

Ojemann, R. G., Ogilvy, C. S., Crowell, R. M., & Heros, R. C. (1995). *Surgical management of cerebrovascular disease* (3rd ed). Baltimore: Williams & Wilkins.

Rengachary, S. S., & Wilkins, R. H. (Eds.). (1994). *Principles of neurosurgery.* Baltimore: Wolfe.

Periodicals

Barrow, D. L., & Reisner, A. (1993). Natural history of intracranial aneurysms and vascular malformations. *Clinical Neurosurgery, 40,* 3–39.

Batjer, H. H., Devous, M. D., Seibert, G. B., et al. (1989). Intracranial arteriovenous malformation: Relationships between clinical factors and surgical complications. *Neurosurgery, 24,* 75–79.

Chyatte, D. (1989). Vascular malformations of the brain stem. *Journal of Neurosurgery, 70,* 847–852.

Friedman, W. A., & Bova, F. J. (1993). Radiosurgery for arteriovenous malformations. *Clinical Neurosurgery, 41,* 446–464.

Harbaugh, K. S., & Harbaugh, R. E. (1994). Arteriovenous malformations in elderly patients. *Neurosurgery, 35*(4), 579–584.

Heros, R. C., Morcos, J., & Korosue, K. (1993). Arteriovenous malformations of the brain: Surgical management. *Clinical Neurosurgery, 40,* 139–173.

Lunsford, L. D., Kondziolka, D., & Flinckinger, J. C. (1992). *Clinical Neurosurgery, 38,* 405–444.

McNair, N. (1988). Arteriovenous malformations. *Critical Care Nursing, 8*(4), 35–40.

Ogilvy, C. S. (1990). Radiation therapy for arteriovenous malformations: A review. *Neurosurgery, 26,* 725–735.

Ogilvy, C. S., Heros, R. C., Ojemann, R. G., & New, P. F. (1988). Angiographically occult arteriovenous malformations. *Journal of Neurosurgery, 69,* 350–355.

Willis, D., & Harbit, M. D. (1990). Transcatheter arterial embolization of cerebral arteriovenous malformations. *Journal of Neuroscience Nursing, 22*(5), 280–284.

Section 8

Nursing Management of Patients With Headaches, Seizures, Infections, Degenerative Processes, and Cranial Nerve Diseases

CHAPTER 30

Headaches

Joanne V. Hickey

The purpose of this chapter is to provide an overview of the most common of human ailments, headaches. The focus is on primary headaches, as described later. However, discussion of headaches and how they are associated with neurological problems is included.

Headache has been defined in a number of ways including pain located above the orbitomeatal line.[1] Headache is a very common problem experienced by up to three fourths of the population each year, but of these, only 5% seek medical attention. Slightly more than 1% of all office visits and emergency room visits are primarily for headache.[2] About 18 million patients visit health care facilities each year for headache, and about half of these patients have migraine headaches.[3]

Headaches can be generally categorized as primary or secondary headaches.

A **primary headache** is a headache for which no organic cause can be consistently identified. The headaches included in this classification include migraine, tension-type, cluster, and miscellaneous headaches unassociated with structural lesions. Most headaches fall into this category.

A **secondary headache** is associated with a variety of primary organic etiologies, such as a tumor or an aneurysm.

The impact of a headache on a person's life varies greatly. A headache may be an incidental occasional event, accompanied by mild discomfort and relieved by an over-the-counter analgesic. For others, a headache is a frequent and severe event resulting in disability and a decreased quality of life and often interfering with interpersonal relationships, work productivity, and family life. Lastly, a headache may be a primary symptom of a serious underlying condition requiring immediate intervention.

HEADACHE: ANATOMICAL CONSIDERATIONS AND PATHOPHYSIOLOGY

Anatomical Considerations

Not all anatomical structures of the head and intracranial space are pain-sensitive. Those structures that do have pain receptors (nociceptors) and are capable of causing pain include the following:

- Extracranial: skin, scalp, muscles, fascia, mucous membranes, and parts of the eye and ear
- Nasal cavity: the nasal mucosa and sinuses
- Extracranial: part of the dura mater, arteries at the base of the brain and their major artery/vein branches, and intracranial afferent veins
- Meninges: parts of the dura mater at the base of the brain near large vessels
- Cranial nerves: trigeminal, facial, glossopharyngeal, and vagus
- Other nerves: second and third cervical nerves

Those structures that lack nociceptors and are not pain-sensitive include the skull, the pia-arachnoid, parts of the dura mater, the cerebral and cerebellar (parenchyma) tissue, and the ependymal lining and choroid plexuses of the ventricles.

Pathophysiology

Headache is experienced when there is traction, pressure, displacement, inflammation, or dilation of nociceptors in areas sensitive to pain. The **ascending pain pathways** from the supratentorial space (the anterior and middle fossa) are carried by the trigeminal nerve, and those from the infratentorial space (posterior fossa) are carried by the glossopharyngeal and the vagus nerves and the second and third cervical nerves. The pain pathways ascend through the brain stem to neurons in the midbrain raphe area and then onto the thalamus, the hypothalamus, and the parietal lobe via the posterior limb of the internal capsule. Serotonin is the primary neurotransmitter in the ascending raphespinal tract.

The **descending pain-modulating pathways** originate in the periacqueductal gray region in the midbrain and synapse in the nucleus raphe magnus in the medulla and the dorsal horn. The descending pathways are modulated by norepinephrine, serotonin, and opiates (enkephalins), which produce analgesia by inhibiting pain transmission.

What is the role of serotonin in headaches? Serotonin is widely distributed throughout the body, and high concentrations are found in the gastrointestinal tract, platelets, and brain. Platelets contain all of the serotonin normally present in blood. At the onset of a migraine, there is a significant rise in plasma serotonin normally present in the blood. This is followed by an increase in urinary 5-hydroxyindoleacetic acid, a breakdown product of serotonin which requires platelet aggregation for its release. The platelets of migraine sufferers, even between attacks, contain less monoamine oxidase than normal, and a further decrease occurs with a headache.[4]

During a migraine headache, serotonin within platelets is decreased, although it remains in the normal range between attacks. Platelet serotonin content is also low in persons with chronic tension-type headaches. These findings form the basis for supporting the classification of chronic tension-type headache as a variant of migraine headaches.[5]

MIGRAINE HEADACHES

Controversy continues about the pathophysiology of migraines. It is believed that abnormal extracranial and intracranial vascular reactions occur in migraine and other vascular headaches. Narrowing of the blood vessels supplying the brain and surrounding tissue results in reduced blood flow or **oligemia**. This phase is followed by vasodilation and swelling and noninfectious inflammation of the blood vessels. Concurrently, platelets clump together during an attack, probably due to exposure to several vasoactive amines such as serotonin. The role of other vasoactive amines continues to be the subject of research.

CLASSIFICATION OF HEADACHES

The International Headache Society (IHS) published the first international headache classification including operational diagnostic criteria for all headache disorders in 1988.[6] It has been translated into many languages and is widely accepted throughout the world. Many of the formerly used terms to classify and describe headaches have been changed in the interest of clarity. The classification system of the IHS is included in its entirety as Table 30-1 to provide a framework for this chapter. Identifying the specific type of headache is key to appropriate treatment and patient education.

The following section will describe the major types of primary headaches which include migraine, tension-type, cluster, and miscellaneous headaches unassociated with structural lesions. The reader is directed to the complete IHS classification and diagnostic criteria if more detail is desired.

Primary Headaches

MIGRAINE HEADACHES

Almost half of all patients who have headaches suffer from migraines. Recent estimates suggest that 23 million Americans currently suffer from migraine headaches, and more than 11 million experience significant headache-related disability.[7] Heredity is a factor in 70% to 80% of sufferers. Migraines affect more than 17% of women and 6% of men in the United States.[8] Economic estimates suggest that the cost of migraine in the United States ranges from $1 billion to $17 billion per year.[9] The most surprising information is that most migraine sufferers are neither diagnosed by physicians nor treated with prescription drugs.[10]

Migraine Triggers. There are a number of triggers for migraine headache. For women who suffer from migraines, the menstrual cycle is a trigger in about 65%. Migraines can occur immediately before, during, or immediately after menstruation. Complete cessation of headaches during pregnancy occurs in 75% to 80%. Use of oral contraception also affects headaches; 50% have an increase in headaches, 40% report no change, and 10% report improvement.

Stress and depression are powerful conditions in causing migraine headaches. Other triggers include bright lights, sunlight, fluorescent lights, and watching television or movies; sleep deprivation or altered sleep-wakefulness cycles; fatigue; fever; and hunger. Some drugs, such as overuse of ergotamine, and foods, such as red wine and strong cheese, can also trigger a headache. Patients must be educated to avoid circumstances associated with headaches. Chart 30-1 provides a list of foods to avoid.

Subtypes of Migraines. Under the broad heading of migraine headaches are seven subtypes including **migraine without aura** (previously called common migraine) and **migraine with aura** (previously called classic migraine). Most patients have migraines without an aura. The characteristics of migraines can vary widely even within the same subtype. Migraines with and without aura are similar except for the obvious absence of the *aura* in **migraine without aura**. The time frame for migraines is up to 3 days; when they last longer than 3 days, the term **status migrainosus** is used. Migraine classification, along with subtypes and descriptions, is included in Table 30-2.

MIGRAINE ATTACKS: FIVE PHASES

One way to consider a migraine attack is through a five-phase framework as outlined by Blau.[11] The five phases of migraine headache include prodrome (premonitory symptoms); aura; the headache itself; the headache termination; and the postdrome. Patients may have some or all of the phases in their migraine presentation.

TABLE 30-1
*International Headache Society Classification of Headache**

1. **Migraine**
   - Migraine without aura
   - Migraine with aura
     - Migraine with typical aura
     - Migraine with prolonged aura
     - Familial hemiplegic migraine
     - Basilar migraine
     - Migraine aura without headache
       - Migraine with acute onset aura
   - Ophthalmoplegic migraine
   - Retinal migraine
   - Childhood periodic syndromes that may be precursors to or associated with migraine
     - Benign paroxysmal vertigo of childhood
     - Alternating hemiplegia of childhood
   - Complications of migraine
     - Status migrainosus
     - Migrainous infarction
   - Migrainous disorder not fulfilling above criteria

2. **Tension-type headache**
   - Episodic tension-type headache
     - Episodic tension-type headache associated with disorder of pericranial muscles
     - Episodic tension-type headache unassociated with disorder of pericranial muscles
   - Chronic tension-type headache
     - Chronic tension-type headache associated with disorder of pericranial muscles
     - Chronic tension-type headache unassociated with disorder of pericranial muscles
   - Headache of the tension-type not fulfilling above criteria

3. **Cluster headache and chronic paroxysmal hemicrania**
   - Cluster headache
     - Cluster headache periodicity undetermined
     - Episodic cluster headache
     - Chronic cluster headache
       - Unremitting from onset
       - Evolved from episodic
   - Chronic paroxysmal hemicrania
   - Cluster headache-like disorder not fulfilling above criteria

4. **Miscellaneous headaches unassociated with structural lesion**
   - Idiopathic stabbing headache
   - External compression headache
   - Cold stimulus headache
     - External application of a cold stimulus
     - Ingestion of a cold stimulus
   - Benign cough headache
   - Benign exertional headache
   - Headache associated with sexual activity
     - Dull type
     - Explosive type
     - Postural type

5. **Headache associated with head trauma**
   - Acute post-traumatic headache
     - With significant head trauma and/or confirmatory signs
     - With minor head trauma and no confirmatory signs
   - Chronic post-traumatic headache
     - With significant head trauma and/or confirmatory signs
     - With minor head trauma and no confirmatory signs

6. **Headache associated with vascular disorders**
   - Acute ischemic cerebrovascular disease
     - Transient ischemic attack (TIA)
     - Thromboembolic stroke
   - Intracranial hematoma
     - Intracerebral hematoma
     - Subdural hematoma
     - Epidural hematoma
   - Subarachnoid hemorrhage
   - Unruptured vascular malformation
     - Arteriovenous malformation
     - Saccular aneurysm
   - Arteritis
     - Giant cell arteritis
     - Other systemic arteritides
     - Primary intracranial arteritis
     - Carotid or vertebral artery pain
   - Carotid or vertebral dissection
     - Carotidynia (idiopathic)
     - Post endarterectomy headache
   - Venous thrombosis
   - Arterial hypertension
     - Acute pressor response to erogenous agent
     - Pheochromocytoma
     - Malignant (accelerated) hypertension
     - Pre-eclampsia and eclampsia
   - Headache associated with other vascular disorder

7. **Headache associated with nonvascular intracranial disorder**
   - High cerebrospinal fluid pressure
     - Benign intracranial hypertension
     - High pressure hydrocephalus
   - Low cerebrospinal fluid pressure
     - Post-lumbar puncture headache
     - Cerebrospinal fluid fistula headache
   - Intracranial infection
   - Intracranial sarcoidosis and other noninfectious inflammatory diseases
   - Headache related to intrathecal injections
     - Direct effect
     - Due to chemical meningitis
   - Intracranial neoplasm
   - Headache associated with other intracranial disorders

8. **Headache associated with substances or their withdrawal**
   - Headache induced by acute substance use or exposure
     - Nitrate/nitrite induced headache
     - Monosodium glutamate induced headache
     - Carbon monoxide induced headache
     - Alcohol induced headache
     - Other substances
   - Headache induced by chronic substance use or exposure
     - Ergotamine induced headache
     - Analgesics abuse headache
     - Other substances
   - Headache from substance withdrawal (acute use)
     - Alcohol withdrawal headache (hangover)
     - Other substances
   - Headache from substance withdrawal (chronic use)
     - Ergotamine withdrawal headache
     - Caffeine withdrawal headache
     - Narcotics abstinence headache
     - Other substances
   - Headache associated with substances but with uncertain mechanism
     - Birth control pills or estrogen
     - Other substances

9. **Headache associated with noncephalic infection**
   - Viral infection
     - Focal noncephalic
     - Systemic

(continued)

TABLE 30-1
International Headache Society Classification of Headache* Continued

- Bacterial infection
  - Focal noncephalic
  - Systemic (septicemia)
  - Headache related to other infection
10. **Headache associated with metabolic disorder**
  - Hypoxia
    - High altitude headache
    - Hypoxic headache
    - Sleep apnea headache
  - Hypercapnia
  - Mixed hypoxia and hypercapnia
  - Hypoglycemia
  - Dialysis
  - Headache related to other metabolic abnormality
11. **Headache or facial pain associated with disorder of cranium, neck, eyes, ears, nose, sinuses, teeth, mouth or other facial or cranial structures**
  - Cranial bone
  - Neck
    - Cervical spine
    - Retropharyngeal tendinitis
  - Eyes
    - Acute glaucoma
    - Refractive errors
    - Heterophoria or heterotropia
  - Ears
  - Nose and sinuses
    - Acute sinus headache
    - Other diseases of nose or sinuses
  - Teeth, jaws, and related structures
  - Temporomandibular joint disease

12. **Cranial neuralgias, nerve trunk pain, and deafferentation pain**
  - Persistent (in contrast to tic-like) pain of cranial nerve origin
    - Compression or distortion of cranial nerves and second or third cervical roots
    - Demyelination of cranial nerves
      - Optic neuritis (retrobulbar neuritis)
    - Infarction of cranial nerves
      - Diabetic neuritis
    - Inflammation of cranial nerves
      - Herpes zoster
      - Chronic postherpetic neuralgia
    - Tolosa-Hunt syndrome
    - Neck–tongue syndrome
    - Other causes of persistent pain of cranial nerve origin
  - Trigeminal neuralgia
    - Idiopathic trigeminal neuralgia
    - Symptomatic trigeminal neuralgia
      - Compression of trigeminal root or ganglion
      - Central lesions
  - Glossopharyngeal neuralgia
    - Idiopathic glossopharyngeal neuralgia
    - Symptomatic glossopharyngeal neuralgia
  - Nervus intermedius neuralgia
  - Superior laryngeal neuralgia
  - Occipital neuralgia
  - Central causes of head and facial pain other than tic douloureux
    - Anaesthesia dolorosa
    - Thalamic pain
  - Facial pain not fulfilling criteria in groups 11 or 12
13. **Headache not classifiable**

Headache classification committee of the International Headache Society. (1988). Classification and diagnostic criteria for headache disorders, cranial neuralgias and facial pain. Cephalalgia, 8(Suppl. 7), 13–17.

Prodrome. **Premonitory symptoms**, experienced by 60% of patients, are symptoms that occur hours to a day or two before a migraine headache. Examples of common premonitory symptoms are depression, irritability, mental slowness, fatigue, sluggishness, yawning, feeling cold, craving special foods, increased thirst, increased urination, anorexia, diarrhea, constipation, and change in one's activity level (hypoactive or hyperactive). An individual usually experiences the same prodrome.

Aura. Only about 20% of migraine suffers have an aura. An **aura** is the constellation of focal neurological symptoms which initiates or accompanies an attack. Most auras develop over 5 to 20 minutes and usually last less than 1 hour.[12] Visual disturbances (bright spots, dazzling zigzag lines), often hemianopic, are the most common aura. The most common somatosensory phenomena include unilateral or bilateral numbness or tingling of the lips, face, or hand; slight difficulty in cerebration; paresis of an arm or leg; mild aphasia; slight incoordination of gait; confusion; and drowsiness.

Headache Phase. The headache phase begins with vasodilation, a decline in serotonin levels, and the onset of a throbbing headache. The headache is often unilateral at onset, but may be bilateral (40% of patients) either at onset or as the headache

intensifies over the next several hours. The headache can begin at any time but most often occurs on arising in the morning. The onset is usually gradual, with the pain peaking and then subsiding. The headache lasts from 4 to 72 hours in adults and 2 to 48 hours in children. The headache is moderate to severe, and the pain is described as "throbbing" in the vast majority of victims. Simple physical activity or even moving the head can intensify the pain.

In addition to the pain, a number of other features accompany migraine. Nausea occurs in up to 90% of patients, and vomiting occurs in about one third of patients.[13] Many patients experience sensitivity to light, sound, and smell; they seek a dark, quiet room. Other symptoms that may occur are blurry vision, nasal stuffiness, anorexia, hunger, diarrhea, abdominal cramps, polyuria, facial pallor, sensations of heat or cold, and sweating.[14] Local tenderness of the scalp, periarterial edema of the temporal area, and stiffness or tenderness of the neck may occur. Impaired concentration, depression, fatigue, anxiety, and irritability are common.

Headache Termination and Postdrome. In the termination phase, the pain gradually subsides. Scalp or neck tenderness, feeling of exhaustion, irritability, listlessness, impaired concentration, mood change, and depression are common. In the postdrome, some persons feel refreshed or euphoric while others note depression and malaise.[15]

CHART 30-1
Common Triggers That May Precipitate Migraine Headaches

The following are common triggers that may precipitate migraine headaches in some people:

Foods and Beverages

- Caffeine (coffee, tea, cola)
- Alcoholic beverages, especially red wine and beer (contain tyramine)
- Chocolate
- Foods containing tyramine (strong and aged cheeses, pickled foods, canned figs)
- Nitrites (cured meats)
- Sulfites
- Monosodium glutamate
- Yeast products
- Dairy products

Other Conditions

- Stress (a strong precipitator of headache)
- Hormonal changes associated with the menstrual cycle
- Certain drugs such as estrogen and nitroglycerin
- Weather changes
- Decreased sleep or sleep deprivation
- Bright lights
- Fatigue
- Fever

TENSION-TYPE HEADACHES

Tension-type headaches, previously called tension headache, muscle contraction headache, stress headache, and ordinary headache, is the second major category of primary headaches. Some physiological evidence suggests that the tension-type headache is a variation of a migraine headache and, as such, it may be reclassified in the future.

Tension-type headaches are subdivided into episodic (acute) and chronic headaches. An **episodic tension-type headache** is defined as a recurrent episodic headache that lasts from 30 minutes to 7 days. The bilateral pain is of mild to moderate intensity; the quality is typically described as a feeling of aching, tightness, pressure, or constriction or a viselike feeling around the head. In contrast to migraines, it is not accompanied by nausea nor does it intensify with routine physical activity. A tension-type headache may be accompanied by sensitivity to light or sound.

A **chronic tension-type headache** is a headache similar to the episodic tension-type headache except that the time element is different. In chronic tension-type headache, headache is present for at least 15 days a month during at least 6 months. The bilateral pain is of mild to moderate intensity and is usually pressing or tightening in quality. The pain is neither in-tensified by routine physical activity nor accompanied by vomiting.

Further breakdown of episodic and chronic tension-type headaches includes a distinction between both association with and lack of association with disorders of muscles around the cranium such as in the temples and neck. Muscle contraction can be a part of the discomfort experienced in a headache.

In some patients, only slight muscle contraction will result in pain and headache if, concurrently with muscle contraction, there is also vasoconstriction of the arteries supplying the area. Muscle contraction can be reflexively induced secondary to noxious stimuli from diseases of the eyes, ears, paranasal sinuses, or cervical vertebrae. Anxiety and psychic tension are also common causes of muscle contraction that plague every person living in this complex society to a greater or lesser degree.

CLUSTER HEADACHES

The third major category of primary headache is cluster headaches (previously called Horton's headache, histaminic cephalalgia, and migrainous neuralgia), which are seen primarily in men between 20 and 40 years of age. A **cluster headache** is an extremely severe, unilateral, burning pain located behind or around the eye. The headache lasts from 15 to 180 minutes and comes in groups, or "clusters," of one to eight daily, lasting up to several weeks or months, followed by a period of remission of months to years. Autonomic phenomena are associated with the headache and can include any one or more of the following symptoms: tearing; conjunctival injection; nasal congestion or runny nose; forehead and facial sweating; miosis; ptosis; and eyelid edema. The headache begins during the night without prodromal signs or aura awakening the person. Cluster headaches can be triggered by alcoholic beverages or other vasodilating agents such as nitroglycerin.

MISCELLANEOUS HEADACHES UNASSOCIATED WITH STRUCTURAL LESION

This miscellaneous category includes headaches associated with activity such as coughing, exertion, or sexual activity; environmental factors such as cold; and external compression as experienced when wearing swimming goggles. These types of headaches are not discussed in this chapter.

Secondary Headaches

There are a number of headaches classified as secondary headaches. Selected secondary headaches are included in Table 30-3. Recall that headache can be a *symptom* of an underlying organic problem. Therefore, the health care provider must determine whether the headache is part of a primary headache disorder or a sign of another illness. Chronic headaches may be benign or a sign of a serious, life-threatening illness such as a brain tumor, a cerebral hemorrhage, or meningitis. The intensity of headache can be just as great with a benign or life-threatening illness. Correct diagnosis of the specific headache type is the foundation for selecting appropriate treatment.

(text continues on page 604)

TABLE 30-2
Migraine Headache With Its Seven Subtypes of Headaches

SUBTYPE OF MIGRAINE	SUBDIVISIONS AND DESCRIPTIONS
1. **Migraine without aura**	No subtypes
2. **Migraine with aura**	• Category has been further subdivided into six categories. Only two are mentioned: • **Familial hemiplegic migraine:** a migraine headache with an aura that includes hemiparesis; there is also a history of at least one first-degree relative who has identical attacks. • **Migraine aura without headache:** previously called migraine equivalents, is described as a migrainous aura unaccompanied by a headache.* This headache classification meets the diagnostic criteria for "migraine with aura," but the headache is absent.
3. **Ophthalmoplegic migraine:** repeated attacks of headache associated with paresis of one or more ocular cranial nerves in the absence of demonstrable intracranial lesion.	No subtypes
4. **Retinal migraine:** repeated attacks of monocular scotoma or blindness lasting less than an hour and associated with headache without any other ocular or structural vascular disorder found on examination.	No subtypes
5. **Childhood periodic syndromes**	Not discussed in this adult-focused text.
6. **Complications of migraine**	**Status migrainosus:** migraine with the headache phase lasting more than 72 hours despite treatment. The headache is continuous or interrupted by headache-free periods lasting 4 hours or less. Interruption of headache during sleep is not counted. **Migrainous infarct** (previously called complicated migraine) is one or more migrainous aura symptoms not fully reversible within 7 days and/or associated with neuroimaging confirmation of ischemic infarction; no other causes of infarction have been ruled out.
7. **Migrainous disorder not fulfilling above criteria**	This criteria provides a heading for migraine headaches that do not completely fulfull criteria of other migraines.

* Headache classification committee of the International Headache Society.

TABLE 30-3
Selected Secondary Headaches From the International Headache Society

CLASSIFICATION—HEADACHE ASSOCIATED WITH:	DESCRIPTION OF CAUSES OF HEADACHE
1. Head trauma	Acute and chronic post-traumatic headache with minor or significant head trauma
2. Vascular disorders	Acute ischemic cerebrovascular disease (transient ischemic attacks; thromboembolic stroke), intracranial hematomas, subarachnoid hemorrhage, unruptured vascular malformation (arteriovenous malformation; aneurysm), arteritis, carotid or vertebral artery pain, venous thrombosis, arterial hypertension, and headaches associated with other vascular disorders
3. Nonvascular intracranial disorders	High cerebrospinal fluid (CSF) pressure (benign intracranial hypertension; high pressure hydrocephalus), low CSF pressure, intracranial infections, headache related to intrathecal injections, and intracranial neoplasms
4. Substances or their withdrawal	Acute or chronic substance use (ergotamine induced), acute or chronic substance withdrawal (hangover, caffeine or ergotamine withdrawal, and oral contraceptives and estrogens)
5. Noncephalic infection	Viral, bacterial, and other focal or systemic infections
6. Metabolic disorder	Hypoxia, hypercapnia, hypoglycemia, dialysis, and other metabolic abnormalities
7. Disorder of cranium, neck and other	Disorders of cranial bones, cervical neck, eyes (glaucoma), ears, nose, sinuses, teeth, and temporomandibular joint disease
8. Cranial neuralgias	Compression or distortion of cranial nerves and second or third cervical roots and demyelination, infarction, or inflammation of cranial nerves
9. Headache not classified	All other headaches that do not meet criteria for other classifications are placed in this category.

CHART 30-2
Headache History

General History

- Were any injuries noted at birth?
- Did you have encephalitis or meningitis, either as a complication of childhood disease or as a separate entity?
- Any history of abnormal nervous system development, such as bed-wetting, sleep disturbances, anxiety reactions (nail biting, untoward fear, and so forth), or fainting?
- Have you had middle ear infections, sinusitis, or surgical procedures involving the ears or sinuses?
- Have you had any injuries to the head, neck, or upper spine?
- Is there evidence now or in the past of cardiovascular disease, such as hypertension, heart disease, or orthostatic hypotension?
- Have you ever had kidney disease, pheochromocytoma, tuberculosis, or tropical infections?
- Have you ever had visual problems, such as astigmatism, dysconjugate gaze, or eye strain? Have you had any eye surgery?
- Have you ever had nervous system disease, such as a seizure disorder, vertigo, visual disturbances (diplopia), or psychiatric or emotional problems?
- Do you see the dentist periodically? Have you had any dental problems?
- Have you ever had arthritis or arthropathies of the neck, shoulder, or upper back?
- Do you have any difficulty with chewing?
- Do you use alcohol, tobacco, or any drugs? What kind? How much?
- Do you have any food, drug, or environmental allergies?
- (With women) Are there any particular symptoms associated with menstruation, pregnancy, childbirth, or menopause that are troublesome?

Familial History

- Does anyone in your family suffer from headaches? If so, what is their relationship to you? Describe their headaches.
- Is there a history of seizure disorders, allergies, emotional problems, or depression in your family?

Occupational History

- What kind of work do you do?
- Describe the physical environment in which you work.
- Are chemicals or fumes present? What kind?
- Do your co-workers complain of headaches?

Personal and Family Relationships

- What in your life concerns you? (Most often anxiety is associated with loss—death, divorce, separation, independence, and so forth.)
- Describe your overall emotional makeup.
- What do you do to relax? Hobbies? Sports?
- Describe how you react to stress. What body signals tell you that you are in a stressful state?
- How do you get along with family members?
- Are you able to discuss problems with family members?
- What would you most like to change about your life?

Specific Headache History

- At what age did the headaches start?
- Where is the headache located (generalized, focal, unilateral, bilateral, frontal, occipital)?
- Describe the type of pain (severe, mild, throbbing, aching, constant or intermittent, and so forth).
- How frequent are the attacks?
- How long do they last?
- What factors are associated with the onset of headache (emotions, intoxication, specific foods, temperature, trigger points, menstruation, stress)?
- What relieves the headache?

(continued)

CHART 30-2 Headache History (Continued)

Specific Headache History

- What aggravates the headache?
- What is the usual course of events with the headache?
- What symptoms accompany the headache (nausea, vomiting, visual disturbances, vertigo, watering eyes, flushing, sweating, hemiparesis, numbness, fainting, facial tic)?
- How incapacitating is the headache in terms of your normal activities?
- Are all of your headaches the same in character?
- What do you do to treat the headache? Does it help?

APPROACH TO MANAGEMENT OF HEADACHES

General Considerations

In the current managed care environment, those patients who seek care for their headaches are usually first seen and evaluated by the primary care provider. If there is indication that the headache is secondary to some underlying problem, a referral may be made to a neurologist, or possibly a neurosurgeon, depending on the underlying problem. For persons with primary headaches such as migraines that are intractable to treatment offered by the primary care provider, a referral may be made to a headache clinic. The level of care provided depends, of course, on the managed care environment in which the person receives health care.

Diagnosis

Accurate diagnosis of headache type is paramount to selecting the appropriate treatment. The primary purpose of the physical examination is to rule out systemic causes for headache. The patient evaluation includes a complete medical history, a family history, a headache history, and a complete physical and neurological examination. The patient's history is the single most important component in diagnosis. In collecting a headache history, the frequency, onset, duration, character, and severity of headache pain guide diagnosis (Chart 30-2). Patients who have difficulty recalling details of their headaches should be encouraged to keep a headache diary (Chart 30-3).

What diagnostic procedures should be ordered? An exhaustive headache work-up is very expensive and most often (99% of cases) identifies no underlying cause for the headache. Clinical judgment and common sense guide the diagnostic work-up. The diagnosis of primary headaches is usually made on clinical grounds (headache history) and negative findings on both the physical and the neurological examinations. No specific diagnostic tests are available to confirm the diagnosis.

Table 30-4 lists headache "serious signs" that suggest the need for further evaluation. Tests that may be ordered include a CT scan or MRI and laboratory studies such as complete blood cell count, erythrocyte sedimentation rate, antiphospholipids, glucose, electrolytes, creatinine, and thyroid panel. Based on the findings and laboratory data, a referral may be made to other specialists or more diagnostic procedures may be scheduled. Once the underlying etiology or type of headache is diagnosed, the appropriate treatment can be instituted. The specific treatment protocols will be discussed under the specific type of headache.

Treatment

GENERAL CONSIDERATIONS

The treatment of primary headaches involves a combination of nonpharmacological and pharmacological therapies. **Nonpharmacological therapies** include patient teaching about headaches, control of precipitating factors, stress management, biofeedback, and relaxation techniques. In migraine and tension-type headaches, stress is a frequent cause; thus, causes of stress must be identified and controlled with stress management interventions. In addition, in tension-type headache, identifying postures assumed throughout the day can often uncover sources of prolonged muscle contraction that can lead to headache. Students, office workers, and those engaged in occupations that require prolonged sitting at a desk or computer are prime targets. Slouching while reading or watching television can also lead to prolonged muscle contraction. Abnormal posture, muscle contraction, and spasms may be the sequelae of previous injury. So-called trigger areas, resulting from previous injury elsewhere in the body, can relay impulses to the central nervous system, producing referred pain to the head. Treatment is directed toward using nonpharmacological interventions such as developing coping mechanisms, engaging in exercise programs, and using ergonomics in workplace design.

Pharmacological therapies are directed toward prevention with prophylactic therapy and acute (symptomatic) treatment during an attack that includes abortive therapy for prompt relief of the headache. Acute therapy also includes drugs given to manage symptoms related to the headache, such as nausea.

MIGRAINE HEADACHES

Pharmacological Basis for Migraine Management. Serotonin (5-HT), a potent vasoconstrictor, is an important factor in the migraine cascade. At the molecular level, there are at least three distinct types of 5-HT receptors—gaunine nucleotide G protein-coupled receptors, ligand-gated ion channels, and

CHART 30-3
Headache Diary

Date	Onset: exact time AM or PM	Ending: exact time AM or PM	Triggers (1)	Prodromal signs (2)	Severity of headache (3)	Location (4)	Quality of headache (5)	Other symptoms	Medication taken, frequency, and route	Pain relief (6)

A series of codes are listed for each numbered heading, such as Triggers. Include all the codes that apply in that category.

(1) Triggers
1. Emotional stress/family related
2. Emotional stress/work related
3. Fatigue
4. Anxiety
5. Menstruation
6. Sleep deprived
7. Fasting
8. Missing a meal
9. High altitude
10. Physical illness
11. Major life change
12. None

(1) Triggers: Food/Beverage
A. Caffeine (coffee, tea, cola)
B. Chocolate
C. Strong/aged cheese
D. Pickled foods
E. Canned figs
F. Yeast products
G. Dairy products
H. Cured meats
I. Monosodium glutamate
J. Wine
K. Beer
L. None

(2) Prodromal Signs
1. Depression
2. Irritability
3. Mental slowness
4. Fatigue
5. Sluggishness
6. Yawning
7. Feeling cold
8. Craving special foods
9. Anorexia
10. None

(3) Headache severity scale (rate headache)

1	2	3	4	5	6	7	8	9	10

slight   moderate   very severe

(4) Location of headache (mark location)

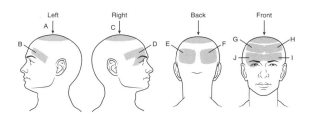

(5) Qualities of headache (include all that apply)
1. Unilateral
2. Bilateral
3. Throbbing
4. Piercing, constant
5. Gradual onset
6. Worse with head movement
7. Worse in lighted room
8. Accompanied by visual changes

(6) Pain relief from drugs scale (rate headache)

1	2	3	4	5	6	7	8	9	10

no relief   moderate   complete relief

TABLE 30-4
Headache "Serious Signs" That Suggest the Need for Further Evaluation

- "Worst" headache of my life
- Onset of headache after the age of 45 years
- Onset of a different kind of headache
- Headache with findings on the neurological examination
  - Altered level of consciousness
  - Altered cognition
  - Motor weakness, ataxia, or altered coordination
  - Altered sensation associated with headache such as tingling or numbness
  - Cranial nerve deficits such as asymmetrical pupils, extraocular palsies, or decreased hearing
  - Progressive visual deficits
  - Abnormal reflexes
  - Signs of meningeal irritation
  - Abnormal findings on physical examination
    - Fever
    - Hypertension
    - Tenderness or pulsation of temporal arteries

transporters—and a number of 5-HT receptor subtypes.[16] Headaches similar to migraine can be triggered by serotonergic drugs such as reserpine (5-HT releaser and depletor). Two drugs effective in the acute treatment of migraine, dihydroergotamine (DHE, an ergot derivation) and sumatriptan (a serotonin analogue) are agonists at selected 5-HT receptor sites. It is believed that these drugs block the development of neurogenically induced inflammation by activating prejunctional 5-HT heteroreceptors on the trigeminal nerve. This, in turn, blocks the release of neuropeptides, including substance P and calcitonin gene-related peptide, preventing neurogenic inflammation. Nonsteroidal anti-inflammatory drugs (NSAIDs) are also thought to prevent neurogenic inflammation, possibly by inhibiting prostaglandin synthesis.[17] These data and others suggest that ergot alkaloids, ergotamine and DHE, and possibly sumatriptan, exert their antimigraine effect by a receptor-mediated neural pathway in both the central nervous system and the trigeminal nerve, where they block neurogenic inflammation.

Drugs and principles of pharmacological therapy for migraine headache are divided into acute (symptomatic) and prophylactic therapy.

Acute Therapy. Acute therapy is directed toward abolishing or significantly limiting a headache that is just beginning or is in progress. There are several drugs that can be used. The effectiveness of any drug is highly individual to the patient, so that the health care provider has a number of different drugs to prescribe and for which to determine patient response. The most common acute therapy drugs are listed in Table 30-5.

Ergotamine tartrate, administered orally, sublingually, rectally, subcutaneously, or intramuscularly at the first sign a migraine headache, may abort the headache. Rectal suppositories are useful if nausea or vomiting occur. The ergot preparations are therapeutic in two ways: (1) they are alpha-adrenergic agonists and antagonists causing vasoconstriction or vasodilation, depending on the state of the vessel; and (2) they block the uptake of serotonin by platelets, which is known to reduce the precipitous decline of serotonin, a mechanism triggering a migraine attack. One side effect of ergot preparations is rebound headache, which may occur if the drug is administered for 2 consecutive days or if a certain dosage is exceeded. Ergotism is also a result of drug overdose.

Once a migraine headache is fully developed, the ergot derivatives are not helpful. When a migraine headache is fully developed, the use of codeine sulfate or meperidine is useful in controlling the pain.

Migraine Prophylaxis. There are no clear guidelines for the indications of migraine prophylaxis. However, in general, prophylaxis is warranted if migraines occur two or more times per month; the headaches are disabling; and the symptomatic drugs are ineffective or contraindicated. The major drug groups used for prophylactic migraine headaches are beta adrenergic blockers, serotonin antagonists, and anticonvulsants. The action of many of these drugs is to interact with serotonergic neural systems, either by binding to 5-HT2 or 5-HT2c receptor sites, "down-regulating" the 5-HT2 receptor, or modulating the discharge of serotonergic neurons.[18]

Propranolol (Inderal), a beta blocker, is the first-choice drug for prophylaxis because it is effective and inexpensive. However, it may not be tolerated well because of its bradycardic effect. There are other beta blockers that can be tried if propranolol is not well tolerated. Another inexpensive and well-tolerated drug choice is amitriptyline (Elavil). See Table 30-6 for a listing of common prophylactic drugs for migraines.

TENSION-TYPE HEADACHES

Pharmacological management of episodic and chronic tension-type headaches is directed toward rapid treatment of the attack. The secondary goal is to prevent or reduce the occurrence of headaches. Most tension-type headaches are caused by anxiety, stress, and associated muscle tension. Less often, headache can be attributed to the effects of former injury or poor posture. Stress-reduction, exercise programs, relaxation technique, meditation, topical heat or cold packs, ergonomic principles for work environment, biofeedback, and possible counseling are important nonpharmacological strategies that should be addressed along with drug therapy.

Drug Therapy. Treatment of the mild to moderate pain of episodic headache may include mild analgesics and muscle relaxants. Antidepressants along with counseling many be beneficial for others. For control of pain, aspirin, acetaminophen, or ibuprofen are helpful. Narcotics should be avoided because of the concern for addiction. Amitriptyline (Elavil) is helpful for muscle contraction pain.

Since pain is interpreted as the presence of a serious problem, headaches may make a person fearful that a life-threatening condition is present. Reassurance helps to relieve the anxiety.

CLUSTER HEADACHES

Treatment of cluster headache is directed at elimination of triggers (*e.g.,* alcohol consumption, sleep cycle disturbances, smoking), drug treatment to prevent headaches, and acute therapy to ameliorate the attack.

TABLE 30-5
Pharmacotherapy for Acute (Symptomatic) Treatment of Migraine Headaches

DRUG	DAILY DOSAGE (DIVIDED)	TYPE/ACTION	MOST COMMON SIDE EFFECTS
Non-narcotic analgesics		For mild to moderate headache; take early in the attack; monitor for overuse.	Rebound headache with frequent use
• Aspirin (ASA)	• PO: 650–1,300 mg	• Analgesic and anti-inflammatory effect	• Bleeding disorder; GI distress
• Acetaminophen	• PO: 650–1,300 mg	• Analgesic	• Does not cause GI upset or bleeding; hepatic necrosis
Nonsteroidal anti-inflammatory drugs (NSAIDs)		NSAIDs prevent prostaglandin synthesis by inhibiting cyclooxygenase, a critical element in prostaglandin synthesis; prostaglandin modulates components of inflammation, pain transmission, and platelet aggregation; useful for abortive and preventive therapy.	• Limited by GI, liver, and renal side effects
• Ibuprofen	• PO: 400–800 mg		• Better tolerated than ASA
• Naproxen	• PO: 1,000 mg		• Better tolerated than ASA
Narcotic analgesics		For severe headache not controlled by non-narcotics; addictive; use with caution and do not overuse.	
• Codeine/ASA	• PO: 30–60 mg		• Sedation, confusion, and constipation for both codeine and meperidine
• Meperidine	• IM: 75–100 mg		
• Butorphanol	• Transnasal: 1 mg followed by 1 mg 1 hour later	• Narcotic agonist–antagonist analgesic; very addictive; use cautiously	• Sedation, nausea, sweating, vertigo, lethargy, confusion
Antiemetics		Often administered to control associated nausea; taken early in the attack.	Drowsiness, dizziness, confusion, hypotension, insomnia, vertigo
• Promethazine	• PO, PR: 25–150 mg	• Adjunct antiemetic therapy	
• Prochlorperazine	• PO, IM 5–20 mg; PR 25 mg	• Adjunct antiemetic therapy	
		• Parenteral treatment for established headache	
• Metoclopramide	• IM: 25–50 mg PO, IM: 10 mg	• Adjunct antiemetic therapy; give 15–30 minutes before DHE or meperidine	
Ergots			
• Ergotamine tartrate	• PO, SL, PR: 1–4 mg stat, then 1–2 mg q 30 minutes (total of 6 mg/attack or 10/mg/wk).	• Abortive treatment for headache unresponsive to nonnarcotic treatment.	Ergots have a cumulative action so must be taken sparingly and as ordered or ergotism (numbness and tingling of fingers and toes, muscle pain, weakness, gangrene, and blindness) will develop. Nausea is a common side effect; need to premedicate with antiemetics.
		• Take usual effective dose at first sign of attack.	
		• Causes cerebral vasoconstriction, which decreases pulsation of cranial arteries.	
• Dihydroergotamine (DHE)	• IM, IV: 1 mg; may repeat in 30–45 minutes; may take up to 3 mg/24 hours or 6 mg/wk	• Parenteral treatment for an established headache	*Contraindications:* Diabetes mellitus, sepsis, hepatorenal disease, peripheral vascular disease (PVD), coronary artery disease, hypertension, and pregnancy.
			• Nausea and vomiting; premedicate 10–15 minutes before with prochlorperazine 5–10 mg PO, IM, or IV; or metoclopramide 10–20 mg PO or 10 mg IM/IV

(continued)

TABLE 30-5
Pharmacotherapy for Acute (Symptomatic) Treatment of Migraine Headaches Continued

DRUG	DAILY DOSAGE (DIVIDED)	TYPE/ACTION	MOST COMMON SIDE EFFECTS
Other			
• Sumatriptan	• SC: 6 mg, PO: 100 mg; take early in the attack.	• First-line abortive therapy; elective agonist for vascular serotonin receptors; causes vasoconstriction of cranial arteries.	• Both drugs contraindicated in pregnancy, coronary artery disease, PVD, ischemia, and stroke; decreases blood pressure and heart rate
• Isometheptene (Midrin)	• PO: 2 tabs at onset then q 1 hour until relief; do not exceed 5/24 hours.	• Sympathomimetic acts as a vasoconstrictor; mild sedative providing tranquilizing effect.	

TABLE 30-6
Pharmacological Therapy for Prophylaxis of Migraine Headaches

DRUG	DAILY DOSAGE	TYPE/ACTION	SIDE EFFECTS
Beta blockers		• Blocks serotonin receptors; prevents vasodilation; propranolol is first drug of choice for prophylaxis; if it is not tolerated, try others in this class as listed.	Bradycaria, fatigue, lethargy, sleep disorders, and depression. Common complaints are gastrointestinal complaints and orthostatic hypotension.
• Propranolol	• PO: 80–320 mg		
• Nadolol	• PO: 40–240 mg		
• Atenolol	• PO: 50–200 mg		
• Timolol	• PO: 10–60 mg		
• Metoprolol	• PO: 50–250 mg		
Tricyclic antidepressants			
• Amitriptyline	• PO: 25–150 mg	• Blocks uptake of serotonin and catecholamines centrally and peripherally. • Most effective for migraine associated with tension-type headache. • Alternative if beta blockers cannot be taken.	May cause dry mouth, urinary retention, and sedation. *Contraindications:* benign prostatic hypertrophy and glaucoma
• Methysergide	• 4–8 mg with meals; must have a drug-free period q 6 months for 3–4 weeks	• Blocks serotonin to prevent early ischemic phase and vasodilation. • Stabilizes platelets against release of serotonin. • Inhibits release of histamine from mast cells. • Potentiates norepinephrine to produce vasoconstriction.	• Nausea and vomiting; fibrotic changes in the retroperitoneal and pleuropulmonary tissue, although uncommon, are the most serious complications; monitor creatinine. • *Contraindications:* PVD, coronary artery disease, and pregnancy
Calcium channel antagonist			
• Verapamil	• 240–640 mg	• Alters calcium flux across smooth muscle. • Prevents vasospasm and reactive vasodilation. • Drug of choice.	*Contraindications:* • Severe left ventricular dysfunction, hypotension, or second- or third-degree heart block • Constipation
Anticonvulsant			
• Valproic acid (divalproex)	• PO: 250–1,000 mg	• Turns off the firing of serotonin neurons of dorsal raphe which controls pain; particularly useful for chronic headache.	• May alter liver function; may cause sedation, hair loss, tremor, and change in cognitive performance.

Drug Therapy. Sumatriptan has been found to be very effective in prompt relief of acute pain. Other acute episode treatments are breathing 100% oxygen for 10 to 15 minutes or subcutaneous dihydroergotamine (DHE). Other drugs used in the treatment of migraines that are also used for cluster headaches are ergotamine, methysergide, and calcium channel blockers.

For preventive therapy, high-dose calcium channel blockers, lithium carbonate (300 mg t.i.d.), methysergide, or a short-term course of corticosteroids may be effective. For corticosteroids, prednisone is given for 1 week (40 to 80 mg/d) and is then tapered over the next week. Ergotamine by rectal suppository or DHE by subcutaneous route at bedtime may be helpful for nocturnal headaches.

NURSING MANAGEMENT OF THE PATIENT WITH HEADACHES

In this section, the nursing management of patients with headache is discussed generally, with emphasis on the role of the nurse in patient education. More specific detail is included on migraine and tension-type headaches. Cluster headaches are not discussed further because patient education is very similar to migraine headaches.

Nurses care for patients who have a variety of headaches. Most patients with primary headaches are managed in the community by a primary care provider or self-managed. For those persons who have primary headaches that are difficult to control, a neurologist or a multidisciplinary team at a headache center may be necessary. Occasionally, primary headache sufferers go to the emergency department because of a severe headache that is intractable to usual acute drug therapy. These persons need to be referred for reevaluation. The major role of the nurse working with primary headache patients is patient education for self-management.

In a hospitalized population, secondary headaches are often symptoms associated with other health problems. Nurses caring for these patients manage the headache with analgesics administered on an "as necessary" basis. Patients admitted for other problems may also be migraine or cluster headache sufferers. In these circumstances, it may be necessary to consider continuing with headache prophylactic therapy. In addition, the possibility of drug interactions between headache drugs and drugs ordered to treat other health problems should be considered.

Nursing Assessment

A detailed nursing assessment and nursing history are the foundation for planning care. Chart 30-2 provides a sample headache history. The patient is key to providing a detailed history; take the time to listen and to collect this information. Based on this database, indications for further assessment may be evident.

Nursing Intervention

Once the diagnosis of the specific type of headache has been established, the nurse can develop a patient teaching plan to educate the person about how to limit the number of attacks and treat acute attacks with both nonpharmacological and pharmacological methods.

Regardless of the type of headache, headaches are most apt to occur when the patient is physically ill, overworked, tired, or under stress. Stress is the major trigger in migraines. Therefore, the nurse should encourage proper diet, adequate rest and exercise, and effective stress management techniques to control stress. Helping the patient to conduct a self-assessment of stressors and circumstances that precipitate headaches may provide the self-awareness to explore alternatives and lifestyle changes to minimize these triggers. Appropriate referrals can be very helpful (Chart 30-4).

Patients should be encouraged to keep a headache diary for reference (see Chart 30-3). The purposes of a headache diary are as follows:

CHART 30-4
Teaching Plan for Persons With Migraine Headaches

The following includes the major points of a teaching plan for persons with migraine headaches:

1. Educate the person about what migraine headaches are and what they are not.
2. Help the person to identify triggers for migraine headache and develop a plan to avoid or ameliorate the triggers (see Chart 30-3).
3. Help the person develop a format for a headache diary.
4. Provide a copy of a tyramine-free diet.
5. Teach stress reduction, stress management, behavioral strategies, and lifestyle changes to minimize the number of headaches.
6. Teach the person about his or her medications including action, how to take the drug, side effects, and how to avoid complications of overuse; include a caution about new drugs included for comorbidity and the possibility of interactions.
7. Teach the person about comfort measures during an attack such as lying down in a dark and quiet room with cold compresses to the head.
8. Suggest resources to help the migraine sufferer become educated about migraines, such as:

National Headache Foundation
5252 North Western Avenue
Chicago, IL 60625   (312) 878-7715

CHART 30-5
Common Nursing Diagnoses Associated With Headache

Nursing Diagnoses (Actual or Potential)	Nursing Interventions	Expected Outcomes
Pain related to (R/T) headache	• Document the characteristics and circumstances of the painful experience. • Help the patient identify factors that precipitate headache. • Manipulate the environment to control or prevent headache.	• Pain will be reduced or abolished. • Factors that precipitate headache will be identified and reduced.
Ineffective Individual Coping R/T lifestyle stress	• Develop techniques to identify the causes of ineffective coping. • Establish a therapeutic nurse–patient interpersonal relationship. • Assist the patient to gain insight into the cause–effect relationship of ineffective coping. • Assist the patient in developing adaptive coping skills.	• The causes of ineffective coping will be identified. • The patient will gain insight into the effects of ineffective coping. • Effective adaptive coping skills will be developed.
Fluid Volume Excess (Fluid Retention) R/T premenstrual fluid retention	• Help the patient to understand why fluid retention can contribute to the onset of headaches. • Identify the signs and symptoms of fluid retention. • Identify any dietary patterns that contribute to fluid retention. • Discuss the purpose of any medications and stress the importance of taking the medications as ordered.	• Fluid retention will be eliminated or controlled.
Sensory/Perceptual Alterations R/T paresthesia and visual alterations	• Document the type and characteristics of sensory/perceptual alterations. • Develop strategies to control or eliminate these signs and symptoms, if possible. • Institute measures to prevent injury. • Collaborate with the physician to provide a therapeutic protocol for treating the problem.	• Sensory–perceptual alterations will be identified and controlled or eliminated. • Precautions for the prevention of injury will be implemented.
Sleep Pattern Disturbance R/T stress and serotonin disorder	• Document the sleep–wakefulness pattern. • Identify factors that prevent adequate sleep. • Develop strategies to overcome obstacles to adequate sleep.	• A satisfactory sleep–wakefulness pattern will be established.
Knowledge Deficit R/T lack of understanding of headache dynamics and treatment protocol	• Identify the specific areas of knowledge deficits or misinformation. • Develop a teaching plan to correct these deficits. • Evaluate the acquisition of new knowledge by the patient.	• The patient will demonstrate a knowledge of headache type, precipitating factors, and treatment.
Anxiety R/T the possibility of headache and the disruption of lifestyle routines.	• Assess the reason for the anxiety. • Help the patient to set realistic goals. • Develop anxiety and stress-reduction strategies.	• Anxiety related to headache or the potential of headache onset will be reduced or eliminated.

- Collect data for analysis to demonstrate causal relationships between diet, drugs, physiological activities, emotional responses/states, and lifestyle to headache
- Identify the specific characteristics of the headache
- Document the *individual's* headache pattern and triggers
- Provide a tool to document and alert the patient to the overall circumstances and characteristics of the headache
- Provide the health professional with data for diagnosis and patient education

This diary can be very enlightening to the patient. For example, the chart may reveal that headaches occur mostly on weekends when the entire family is home. Or, headaches may be noted to occur around the time of menstruation. It is most important to identify any rhythm or pattern in the occurrence of headaches.

For patients who experience fluid retention and weight gain around menstruation, a salt-restricted diet 1 week prior to menstruation should be encouraged. If this is not helpful, diuretics may be prescribed. Other elimination diets should be encouraged for those patients who have identified relationships between the ingestion of certain foods and beverages and the occurrence of headaches. The major nursing diagnoses associated with headaches are found in Chart 30-5.

Nursing Management of Patients With Migraine Headaches

Nursing management of the patient with migraine headache is directed toward treatment of the acute attack and prevention. If a migraine headache appears to be developing, abortive drug therapy should be instituted immediately. If the migraine headache becomes fully developed before abortive therapy is instituted, intervention is directed toward acute management, including the following:

- Providing a darkened, quiet environment
- Elevating the head
- Administering analgesics, antiemetics, and specific migraine drugs

Patient education can be very effective in helping patients to avoid triggers and to adhere to the medication protocol. In addition, because stress is the major trigger for migraine headaches, stress management and relaxation are a necessary part of patient management. The specific stress management plan will depend on the patient's personal inventory of stressors and the development of stress reduction strategies. Referrals may be helpful to achieve this goal.

Nursing Management of Patients With Tension-Type Headaches

Most people treat their own tension-type headaches independent of a nurse or other health professionals. Often, it is within the guise of primary care that tension-type headaches are acknowledged and discussed. Fear that the headaches may be "something serious" prompts discussion of the headaches with the primary care provider for reassurance. The nurse should be aware of the serious signs of headaches (see Table 30-4) because a change in the headache pattern can herald a new, possibly serious, condition.

Several of the same principles suggested for migraine headaches are applicable to tension-type headaches. Health promotion through proper diet, rest, exercise, and relaxation should be encouraged. Many people either say that they do not have time for relaxation or do not know how to relax. Understanding that the marvelous machine called the human body has limits of physical and emotional endurance is helpful. Exceeding limits results in danger signals, such as irritability, fatigue, gastrointestinal upset, or headache.

Stress management includes learning new problem-solving skills. This approach requires honest self-evaluation and motivation to alter established behavioral patterns of dealing with stress. Keeping a headache history to note associations of stress and headache is helpful. Even the patient who is certain that no correlations exist may be surprised when confronted with hard data. Encourage the patient to start with one situation that leads to headache and develop alternatives to avoid the usual outcome.

Enrolling in adult education or college courses that focus on self-awareness, self-assertiveness, and stress adaptation is one approach that can help develop support systems for behavioral change. Many self-help books, audiotapes, and videotapes address similar subjects. Biofeedback, relaxation therapy, yoga, and counseling may be necessary for persons who have more than the occasional tension-type headache.

Nursing Management of Patients With Cluster Headaches

Patient education about cluster headaches, triggers, and drug therapy is the foundation to prepare persons for self-management of their headaches. The same principles that apply to migraine headaches also apply to cluster headaches (see Chart 30-4).

References

1. Headache Classification Committee of the International Headache Society. (1988). Classification and diagnostic criteria for headache disorders, cranial neuralgias and facial pain. *Cephalalgia, 8*(Suppl. 7), 1–96.
2. Silberstein, S. D., & Silberstein, M. M. (1990). New concepts in the pathogenesis of migraine headache. *Pain Management, 3,* 297–302.
3. Rapoport, A. M. (1994). Update on severe headache with a focus on migraine. *Neurology, 44*(Suppl 3), S5.
4. Campbell, J. K., & Caselli, R. J. (1991). Headache and other craniofacial pain. In W. G. Bradley, R. B. Daroff, G. M. Fenichel, & C. D. Marsden (Eds.), *Neurology in clinical practice: The neurological disorders* (pp. 1525–1527). Boston: Butterworth-Heinemann.
5. Ibid., p. 1527.
6. Headache Classification Committee, op. cit., pp. 13-17.
7. Stewart, W. F., Lipton, R. B., Celentano, D. D., et al. (1992). Prevalence of migraine headache in the United States. *JAMA, 267,* 64–69.
8. Lipton, R. B., & Stewart, W. F. (1993). Migraine in the United States: Epidemiology and healthcare utilization. *Neurology, 43*(Suppl. 3), 6–10.
9. Osterhaus, J. T., Gutterman, D. L., & Placheka, J. R. (1992). Healthcare resources and lost labour costs of migraine headaches in the U.S. *Pharmaco Economics, 2,* 67–76.

10. Lipton, R. B., Stewart, W., Celentano, D. D., et al. (1992). Undiagnosed migraine: A comparison of symptom-based and self-reported physician diagnosis. *Archives of Internal Medicine, 156*, 1–6.
11. Blau, J. N. (1980). Migraine prodromes separated from the aura: Complete migraine. *British Medical Journal, 281*, 658–660.
12. Headache Classification Committee, op. cit., pp. 1–96.
13. Lipton, Stewart, Celentano, et al., 1992.
14. Silberstein, S. D., & Lipton, R. B. (1994). Overview of diagnosis and treatment of migraine. *Neurology, 44*(Suppl. 7), S6–S16.
15. Ibid.
16. Humphrey, P. P. A., Feniuk, W., & Perren, M. J. (1990). Antimigraine drugs in development: Advances in serotonin receptor pharmacology. *Headache, 30*(Suppl. 1), 12.
17. Silberstein, S. D., & Lipton, R. B. (1994). Overview of diagnosis and treatment of migraine. *Neurology, 44*(Suppl. 7), S6–S16.
18. Ibid.

Bibliography

Books

Cady, R. K., & Fox, A. W. (Eds.). (1995). *Treating the headache patient.* New York: Marcel Dekker.

Dalessio, D., & Silberstein, S. D. (Eds.). (1993). *Wolff's headache and other head pain* (6th ed.). New York: Oxford University Press.

Diamond, S., & Dalessio, D. J. (Eds.). (1992). *The practicing physician's approach to headache* (5th ed.). Baltimore: Williams & Wilkins.

Olesen, J. (Ed.). (1994). *Headache classification and epidemiology* (Vol. 4). New York: Raven Press.

Robbins, L. D. (1994). *Management of headache and headache medications.* New York: Springer-Verlag.

Periodicals

Baumel, B. (1994). Migraine: A pharmacologic review with newer options and delivery modalities. *Neurology, 44*(Suppl. 3), S13–S17.

Breslau, N., Merikangas, K., & Bowden, C. (1994). Comorbidity of migraine and major affective disorders. *Neurology, 44*(Suppl. 7), S17–S22.

Dalessio, D. (1994). Diagnosing the severe headache. *Neurology, 44*(Suppl. 3), S6–S12.

Diener, H.-C. (1993). A personal view of the classification and definition of drug dependent headache. *Cephalalgia, 13*, 68–71.

Lipton, R. B., Ottman, R., Ehrenberg, B. L., & Hauser, A. (1994). Comorbidity of migraine: The connection between migraine and epilepsy. *Neurology, 44*(Suppl. 7), S28–S32.

Markley, H. G. (1994). Chronic headache: Appropriate use of opiate analgesics. *Neurology, 44*(Suppl. 3), S18–S24.

Post, R. M., & Silberstein, S. D. (1994). Shared mechanisms in affective illness, epilepsy, and migraine. *Neurology, 44*(Suppl. 7), S37–S47.

Rapoport, A. M. (1994). Update on severe headache with a focus on migraine. *Neurology, 44*(Suppl. 3), S5.

Rapoport, A. M. (1994). Recurrent migraine: Cost-effective care. *Neurology, 44*(Suppl. 3), S25–S28.

Raskin, N. H. (1993). Acute and prophylactic treatment of migraine. *Neurology, 43*(Suppl. 3), S39–S42.

Sammartino, L. R., & Gharavi, A. E. (1992). Antiphospholipid antibody syndrome. *Clinics in Laboratory Medicine, 12*, 41–59.

Sandler, M. (1995). Migraine to the year 2000. *Cephalalgia, 15*, 259–264.

Stevens, M. B. (1993). Tension-type headaches. *American Family Physician, 47*(4), 799–805.

Stewart, W., Breslau, N., & Keck, P. E. (1994). Comorbidity of migraine and panic disorder. *Neurology, 44*(Suppl. 7), S23–S27.

Weiss, J. (1993). Assessment and management of the client with headaches. *Nurse Practitioner, 18*, 44–57.

Welch, K. M. A. (1994). Relationship of stroke and migraine. *Neurology, 44*(Suppl. 7), S33–S36.

Whitney, C. M. (1990). New headache classification: Implications for neuroscience nurses. *Journal of Neuroscience Nursing, 22*, 385–388.

Wilkinson, M., Pfaffenrah, V., Schoenen, J., Diener, H.-C., & Steiner, T. J. (1995). Migraine and cluster headache—their management with sumatriptan: A critical review of the current clinical experience. *Cephalalgia, 15*, 337–357.

CHAPTER 31

Seizures and Epilepsy

Joanne V. Hickey

There is a large body of knowledge now available about epilepsy and the management of persons with seizure disorders. The purposes of this chapter are to provide nurses with a basic framework for understanding how to assist persons with epilepsy with self-management and how to manage the hospitalized patient with a seizure problem. Although seizures and epilepsy are common in children, the adult person is the focus of this book and this chapter. Other resources, some of which are listed in the bibliography, can be consulted for more in-depth information.

Most persons with a seizure disorder are managed in the community by a primary care physician or a neurologist. Some persons with epilepsy that is difficult to manage may be followed at an epilepsy center for comprehensive management by epileptologists and a multidisciplinary team. Advanced practice nurses with a focus in seizure management may be available to patients and families or as a consultant to other nurses. Almost all nurses who practice in a hospital environment will see patients who have a seizure secondary to a primary condition such as metabolic imbalance. Other nurses may see persons with intractable epilepsy admitted for surgical intervention. Regardless of the setting in which care is delivered, nurses play an important role in the management and education of patients and their families.

BACKGROUND AND DEFINITIONS

References to epilepsy date back to ancient times, and mystical explanations about seizures continued until the 1870s when Jackson theorized that seizures originated from a localized, discharging focus in the brain. The introduction of the electroencephalogram (EEG) by Berger in 1929 provided the first recordings of epileptic discharge from the brain. This was followed in the 1930s by Gibbs, who correlated the clinical evidence of epilepsy with EEG findings. The development of international classification systems for both epilepsies and seizures have paved the way for better understandings. International research of the clinical and cellular basis for seizures,

new drugs, and comprehensive protocols all have contributed to overall improved outcomes for patients.

Part of the difficulty in understanding epilepsy and seizures in the past has been the imprecise definitions of terms. The following are definitions of common terms based on the current accepted terminology:

Seizure: a single (finite) event that results in an altered state of brain function.
Epilepsy: a chronic disorder of abnormal, recurrent, excessive, and self-terminating discharge from neurons. Periods between seizures can vary widely and can be measured in minutes, hours, days, weeks, months, or even years. However, there is repetition of seizure activity at some time in the future, regardless of the interval. Clinically, epilepsy is recurring seizures in which there is a disturbance in some type of behavior (*i.e.*, motor, sensory, autonomic, consciousness, or mentation).
Seizure disorder: a term adopted by some clinicians when referring to epilepsy. Although this has led to some confusion, the terms *epilepsy* and *seizure disorder* are used interchangeably.
Epileptic syndrome: an epileptic disorder characterized by a cluster of signs and symptoms customarily occurring together.

Epidemiology

The prevalence and incidence of seizures and epilepsy are difficult to establish because of problems of diagnosis and reporting. In *Facts About Epilepsy*, the following statistics are cited for the United States:[1]

- Over 2 million people are currently affected by epilepsy (active epilepsy).
- Each year, 120 per 100,000 individuals (300,000 people) will seek medical attention because of a newly recognized seizure. Of this group, 40% will be under the age of 18 years. The majority of the 40% (75,000 to 100,000) will have had a fever related to a convulsive seizure.

- Each year, 50 per 100,000 individuals (125,000) will be diagnosed with epilepsy. Of this number, 30% will be under the age of 18 years.
- The greatest number of people with newly diagnosed epilepsy will be among children under the age of 2 years and the elderly (over the age of 65 years).
- Trends over time suggest an increase in frequency of epilepsy in the elderly.
- The prevalence of active epilepsy in the over 65-year age group is 1% (300,000 cases).

Some readers may be surprised by the number of persons over the age of 65 years with epilepsy. This has implications for overall management, especially for education in self-management.

Etiology and Risk Factors

No specific cause of epilepsy has been identified in 70% of all cases of epilepsy; thus, the term **idiopathic epilepsy** may be used. Any condition that causes cerebral irritation, either directly or by altering the biochemical milieu of the neurons, may precipitate seizure activity. Given the right circumstances (created by electric shock, certain drugs, or alterations in the metabolic state), anyone can have a seizure, although the threshold for seizures varies among the population. In some types of epilepsies, genetics plays a role. Over 150 different gene traits increase the possibilities of seizures. In a person with epilepsy, parents, siblings, and offspring are more likely to have epilepsy as compared with the general population.

In adults and the elderly, the *major risk factors* for developing epilepsy are as follows:

- Head trauma (contusion; laceration; epidural, subdural, or intracerebral hematoma)
- Central nervous system (CNS) infections (*e.g.*, meningitis, encephalitis, abscess)
- Cerebral tumors (primary and metastatic)
- Cerebral vascular disease (stroke, arteriovenous malformation, cerebral aneurysm)

A seizure may occur at the time of injury or cerebral event; however, this is not epilepsy. The onset of recurrent seizures, epilepsy, may not occur for months or years, if ever. If epilepsy develops, there is a definite pattern of onset. Few people develop epilepsy before 2 months or later than 5 years posttrauma. The highest incidence of onset is 6 months to 2 years following the injury.

In addition to the major risk factors for seizures and possible epilepsy in adults and older adults, there are a number of situations that can result in seizures: alcohol ingestion; drug overdose; seizure-inducing drugs, such as pentylenetetrazol (Metrazol); inorganic substances such as lead; electrolyte imbalance such as hyponatremia; vitamin deficiency; diabetes mellitus and other metabolic disorders; and endocrine disorders caused by pregnancy and menstruation.

Precipitating Factors: Triggers

In patients with epilepsy, seizures can be triggered by a variety of stimuli called triggers. Sometimes the trigger is very specific for a particular person. Common triggers include particular odors or photo stimuli and certain types of music or a specific piece of music. If a specific stimulus can be identified, then the pattern is called **reflex epilepsy**. Of generic stimuli, sleep deprivation and missing medications are the most common causes of seizures. Other generic triggers of seizures in epileptic patients are fatigue, hypoglycemia, emotional stress, electrical shock, febrile illness, alcohol consumption, certain drugs, drinking too much water, constipation, menstruation, and hyperventilation.

Terminology

A few terms that define or describe general signs and symptoms are encountered repeatedly when considering seizures:

Tonus is the degree of tone or contraction present in muscle when it is not undergoing shortening.

Clonus is a term used to describe spasms in which a continuous pattern of rigidity and relaxation is repeated. In the second phase of a generalized seizure, called the clonic phase, rhythmic movements are followed by muscle relaxation. In the clonic phase, the process is repeated again and again.

Aura is a premonitory sensation or warning experienced at the beginning of a seizure, which the patient remembers. An aura may be a gustatory, visual, auditory, or visceral experience such as a metallic taste or flashing lights. If a patient has an aura, it usually is the same experience each time.

Prodromal refers to symptoms, such as a headache or feeling of depression, that herald a seizure by hours.

Ictus refers to an actual seizure; a seizure may be referred to as an ictal event.

Postictal refers to the period immediately after a seizure has occurred.

Todd's paralysis is a temporary, focal weakness or paralysis following a partial or generalized seizure that can last 24 to 48 hours. The deficit can be correlated with a epileptic foci on the motor strip. Temporary neuronal exhaustion is probably the physiological basis for the deficit.

SEIZURE CLASSIFICATION AND OBSERVATION/IDENTIFICATION

Classification of epilepsies has undergone a number of revisions. Currently there are two distinct classification systems widely used and accepted by clinicians. The first is the International Classification of Epilepsies and Epileptic Syndromes (ICE), which represents mostly a classification of epileptic syndromes rather than diseases.[2] Syndromes are delineated by seizure type, age at presentation, and association with recognized illnesses. A classification of epileptic syndromes rather than seizures provides a better identification of homogeneous populations with seizure disorders. As a result of this classification, diagnosis is improved, treatment can be more specific, and prognosis is more accurate. The ICE is divided into two major headings: generalized and localization-related. Each category is further subdivided into primary (idiopathic) and secondary (symptomatic) epilepsy. Those epilepsies that do not fit into either category are placed in a third category (Table 31-1).[3]

The second classification, the International Classification of Epileptic Seizures (ICES), is based on the clinical observation of the seizure and ictal EEG pattern.[4] This classification system divides seizures into the two major categories of partial seizures and generalized seizures (Tables 31-2 and 31-3). The following definitions describe the differences between these two ICES categories of seizures.[5]

Partial Seizures

Partial seizures are seizures in which the first clinical and EEG changes indicate initial activation of a system of neurons limited to part of one cerebral hemisphere. Loss or maintenance of consciousness is the basis for the determination of the type of partial seizures. When consciousness is not impaired, the seizure is classified as a **simple partial seizure**; if consciousness is impaired, the seizure is classified as a **complex partial seizure**. In complex partial seizures, impaired consciousness may be the first clinical sign. Simple partial seizures may evolve into complex partial seizures. In patients with impaired consciousness, aberrations of behavior (automatisms) may occur. Either type of partial seizure may terminate on its own or progress to a generalized motor seizure. On EEG, simple partial seizures usually have unilateral hemispheric (rarely bilateral) involvement; complex partial seizures usually have bilateral hemispheric involvement.

Generalized Seizures

Generalized seizures are seizures that begin with the first clinical change reflecting initial involvement of both cerebral hemispheres. Consciousness may be impaired, and this may be the initial clinical sign. Motor manifestations are bilateral, as evidenced by bilateral, diffuse EEG patterns. The most common type of generalized seizure is the **generalized tonic–clonic seizure**, formerly called the *grand mal seizure*. It is discussed here in some detail because it is so common.

GENERALIZED TONIC–CLONIC SEIZURE

A prodromal period of irritability and tension may precede the seizure by several hours or days. Some persons experience an aura, while in others, the seizure begins without warning. Characteristically, the tonic–clonic seizure begins with a sudden loss of consciousness. In the **tonic phase,** there is a major tonic contraction (increased tonus) of the voluntary muscles so that the body stiffens with legs and arms extended. If standing, the person will fall to the ground. The jaw snaps shut and the tongue may be bitten in the process. A shrill cry may be heard because of the forcible exhalation of air through the closed vocal cords as the thoracic muscles initially contract. The bladder and, less often, the bowel may empty. The pupils dilate and are unresponsive to light. During the tonic phase the person is apneic and may appear pale and dusty. The tonic phase lasts less than 1 minute (average of 15 seconds).

The **clonic phase** begins with a gradual transition from the tonicity of the tonic phase. The clonic phase is characterized by violent, rhythmic, muscular contractions accompanied

---

TABLE 31-1
International Classification of Epilepsies and Epileptic Syndromes

1. Localization-related (focal, local, partial) epilepsies and syndromes
   1.1 Idiopathic with age-related onset (at present, there are two syndromes)
      • Benign childhood epilepsy with centrotemporal spike
      • Childhood epilepsy with occipital paroxysms
   1.2 Symptomatic (includes syndromes of great individual variability)
2. Generalized epilepsies and syndromes
   2.1 Idiopathic, with age-related onset, listed in order of age
      • Benign neonatal familial convulsions
      • Benign neonatal convulsions
      • Benign myoclonic epilepsy in infancy
      • Childhood absence epilepsy
      • Juvenile myoclonic epilepsy
      • Epilepsy with grand mal seizures (GTCS) on awakening
   2.2 Idiopathic and/or symptomatic, in order of age of appearance
      • West syndrome (infantile spasms, Blitz-Nick-Salaam Krampfe)
      • Lennox-Gastaut syndrome
      • Epilepsy with myoclonic-astatic seizures
      • Epilepsy with myoclonic absences
   2.3 Symptomatic
      • Nonspecific etiology
         • Early myoclonic encephalopathy
      • Specific syndromes
         • Epileptic seizures may complicate many disease states (including diseases in which seizures are a presenting or predominant feature)
3. Epilepsies and syndromes undetermined as to whether they are focal or generalized
   3.1 With both generalized and focal seizures:
      • Neonatal seizures
      • Severe myoclonic epilepsy in infancy
      • Epilepsy with continuous spikes and waves during slow wave sleep
      • Acquired epileptic aphasia (Landau-Kleffner syndrome)
   3.2 Without unequivocal generalized or focal features
4. Special syndromes
   4.1 Situational-related seizures
      • Febrile convulsions
      • Seizures related to other identifiable situations, such as stress, hormones, drugs, alcohol, or sleep deprivation
   4.2 Isolated, apparently unprovoked epileptic events
   4.3 Epilepsies characterized by specific modes of seizure precipitation
   4.4 Chronic progressive epilepsia partialis continua of childhood

From Commission on Classification and Terminology of the International League Against Epilepsy. (1985) Proposal for classification of epilepsies and epileptic syndromes. Epilepsia, 26(3), 268–278.

---

by strenuous hyperventilation. The face is contorted, the eyes roll, and there is excessive salivation with frothing from the mouth. Profuse sweating and a rapid pulse are common. The clonic jerking gradually subsides in frequency and amplitude over a period of about 30 seconds, although it may be longer. After the clonic phase, the person is unconscious for about 5 minutes. The extremities are limp, breathing is quiet, and the pupils, which may be equal or unequal, begin to respond to the light reflex. With awakening, confusion and disorientation are common; the person is amnesic with respect to the event.

TABLE 31-2
International Classification of Epileptic Seizures

I. Partial seizures (seizures with a focal, local origin)
  A. Simple (consciousness not impaired)
    1. Focal motor (with and without Jacksonian march)
    2. Somatosensory or special sensory symptoms (simple hallucinations such as tingling, light flashing, buzzing)
    3. Autonomic symptoms or signs such as epigastric sensation, pallor, sweating, flushing
    4. With psychic symptoms (disturbances of higher cerebral function)
  B. Complex (symptoms usually include loss of consciousness)—temporal lobe seizures (psychomotor seizures)
    1. Simple partial onset followed by impairment of consciousness
    2. With impairment of consciousness at onset
  C. Partial seizures evolving into secondary generalized seizures
II. Generalized seizures (generalized bilateral without focal onset)
  A. Absence seizures
  B. Myoclonic seizures
  C. Clonic seizures
  D. Tonic seizures
  E. Tonic–clonic seizures
  F. Atonic seizures
III. Unclassified epileptic seizures (including all seizures that cannot be classified due to inadequate or incomplete data and some that defy classification)

From Commission on Classification and Terminology of the International League Against Epilepsy. (1981) Proposal for revised clinical and electroencephalographic classification of epileptic seizures. Epilepsia, 22, 489–501.

Headache, generalized muscular aching, and fatigue are common. If undisturbed, the person may fall into a deep sleep for several hours.

Because the seizure frequently occurs without warning, it is possible for injury to be sustained from falls or other accidents related to the seizure. Head injury, fracture of the limbs or vertebral column, and burns are examples of serious injuries that may be sustained. Tonic–clonic seizures may occur at any time of the day or night, whether the patient is awake or asleep. The frequency of recurrence can vary from hours to weeks, months, or years.

STATUS EPILEPTICUS

Status epilepticus is defined as "more than 30 minutes of (1) continuous seizure activity or (2) two or more sequential seizures without full recovery of consciousness between seizures."[6] Status epilepticus can occur with both convulsive and nonconvulsive seizures. Therefore, status epilepticus has several forms: (1) repeated generalized convulsive seizures with persistent postictal depression of neurological function between seizures; (2) nonconvulsive seizures that produce a continuous or fluctuating "epileptic twilight" state; and (3) repeated partial seizures manifested as focal motor convulsions, focal sensory symptoms, or focal impairment of function such as aphasia not associated with altered consciousness.[7] The most common type of status epilepticus is **tonic–clonic status**

epilepticus. Convulsive seizures can be easily observed clinically, but partial seizures are less obvious and more difficult to identify. Therefore, an EEG is required for any patient with significant alterations in consciousness when seizures are suspected. Status epilepticus constitutes a medical emergency and is associated with significant morbidity and mortality.

Epileptic Versus Nonepileptic Seizures

Another way of classifying seizures is using the general heading of epileptic and nonepileptic seizures. Epileptic seizures are divided into partial and generalized seizures, as discussed earlier. **Nonepileptic seizures or nonepileptic events** (previously called pseudoseizures) account for about 20% of referrals to epilepsy centers. They can look like seizures clinically, but there is no epileptogenic origin. Nonepileptic seizures can be divided into physiological events, psychogenic events, and malingering.[8]

Physiological Nonepileptic Events. Physiological nonepileptic events occur most often after age 6 years and before middle life. Cardiac, respiratory, and metabolic effects and toxicity can disturb consciousness as a result of decreased oxygen tension to the brain. Perfusion problems as a result of transient ischemic attacks, stroke, or Stokes-Adams syndrome account for underlying cardiac or cerebrovascular problems. A respiratory basis for decreased oxygen tension from poor saturation can result from pneumonia, pulmonary emboli, shunting, or coma. Metabolic causes such as hypoglycemia and electrolyte imbalance can cause nonepileptic events. Toxicity due to street drugs or prescription drugs, including antiepileptic drugs; alcohol toxicity; and environmental exposures to toxic substances such as lead can also result in nonepileptic seizures.

Psychogenic Nonepileptic Events. Differentiation between nonepileptic psychogenic seizures and epileptic seizures can be made only through analysis of simultaneous EEG tracings and audiovideo monitoring during a seizure. The audiovideo portion records the behaviors of the peri-ictal events and the EEG demonstrates the presence or absence of abnormal tracings associated with epileptic seizures. The behavior is triggered by psychogenic internal or external factors. The basis for psychogenic nonepileptic events is secondary gains.

Malingering. Again, secondary gain is the basis for persons claiming seizures. Simultaneous EEG and audiovideo monitoring are necessary for diagnosis.

OBSERVATIONS/IDENTIFICATION

Physiological reasons must be ruled out as possible causes of nonepileptic seizures. A thorough history and physical examination form the basic diagnostic work-up, along with laboratory screening.

With nonepileptic psychogenic seizures, the onset is often dramatic, bizarre, gradual, and in the presence of witnesses. By comparison, epileptic seizures are sudden, paroxysmal, and orderly. Emotional upset usually precipitates nonepileptic

TABLE 31-3
Types of Clinical Seizures

	EEG FINDINGS

I. PARTIAL SEIZURES

A. Simple Partial Seizures

1. With motor signs
   - Any portion of the body may be involved depending on the site of origin of the cortical motor strip epileptic foci.
   - May remain focal or spread to other areas on the motor strip referred to as "march"; seizure called Jacksonian seizures. For example, the seizure may begin in the fingers of one side, and "march" to the hand, wrist, forearm, and arm on the same side of the body. The particular sequence of involvement is helpful in locating the epileptic foci on the motor strip in the hemisphere opposite the convulsive movement.
   - Consciousness usually preserved, but foci may spread to become a generalized seizure.
   - Focal motor attack may be versive and involve head turning to the side opposite the epileptic foci.
   - Todd's paralysis may result, lasting minutes to hours.
   - Continuous focal motor seizure is called epilepsia partialis continua.

   *For **all** simple partial seizures: sharp discharge in 40%–80%; focal paroxysmal, rhythmic activity in 50%*

2. With somatosensory or special sensory symptoms
   - Arise from cortical sensory strip.
   - Usually feels like "pins and needles" or numbness; sometimes, spatial disorientation.
   - May march to other areas or may become a complex partial or generalized tonic–clonic seizure.
   - Special sensory symptoms may include visual seizures such as flashing lights or visual hallucinations, auditory seizures with various sounds, gustatory sensations such as metallic taste or primary tastes (salty, sweet, sour, or bitter), or vertigo and floating sensations.

3. With autonomic symptoms or signs (epigastric sensation, pallor, sweating, flushing, piloerection, pupillary dilation)
   - May occur as simple partial seizures.

4. With psychic symptoms
   - Disturbance in a higher-level function (*i.e.,* distortion of memory), distorted time, feeling of déjà vu, illusions, depersonalization, or hallucinations
   - Usually occur with impairment of consciousness and become complex partial seizures.

B. Seizures With Complex Symptomatology

1. Simple partial seizure followed by impairment of consciousness resulting in a complex seizure with motor, sensory, autonomic, or psychic symptoms as described above.

   All complex seizures: 4–6 Hz, 50–100 microvolt, flat-topped waves throughout cortex

2. Impaired consciousness at onset; the only symptoms may be impaired consciousness or it may progress to include automatisms; note automatisms may occur in partial or generalized seizures. **Automatisms** are described as "more or less coordinated adapted involuntary motor activity occurring during the state of clouding of consciousness either in the course of, or after an epileptic seizure, usually followed by amnesia for the event." * The behavior may be a continuation of the preseizure activity or a new activity. The activity during the seizure is usually a common activity such as pacing or stroking the head. The patient is amnesic of the event.

C. Partial Seizures Evolving to Secondary Generalized Seizures

The following types of seizures may evolve into generalized seizures: simple partial, complex partial, or simple partial evolving into complex and then to generalized seizures.

II. GENERALIZED SEIZURES (CONVULSIVE AND NONCONVULSIVE)

A. Absence Seizures

1. Common in children; characterized by a sudden onset and interruption of activity with a momentary lapse of consciousness lasting 3 to 30 seconds. If talking, the speech stops or slows; if eating the hand and mouth stop, and if called, does not respond.
   - During an attack, the eyes may become vacant, stare, or roll upward; the eyelids may twitch.
   - Seizures occur a few times to hundreds of times per day; person may not be aware of them.
   - Persons who have several attacks daily most often experience difficulty in learning because of inattention.
   - Other forms are absence with impaired consciousness only; mild clonic components; atonic components; tonic components; or automatisms.

   Symmetrical, 3 cycles/sec spikes; wave patterns with abrupt starts and stops.

2. Atypical absence seizures; may be noted as change in tone that are greater that the typical absence seizure.

(continued)

TABLE 31-3
Types of Clinical Seizures Continued

	EEG FINDINGS
B. Myoclonic Seizures • Myoclonic jerks (single or multiple) are sudden, brief, shock-like contractions that may be generalized or isolated. When confined to one area it may be the face and trunk; one or more extremities; an individual muscle; or a muscle group. • Myoclonic jerks are rapidly repetitive or relatively isolated. • Common around time of sleep or awakening; must be differentiated from myoclonic jerks of nonepileptic myoclonus. **C. Clonic; D. Tonic; and F. Atonic Seizures** These are alterations in tone as indicated in the name (common in infants and children; see pediatric text for more details). **E. Tonic–Clonic Seizures** • Most common of the generalized seizures (see p. 627 for detailed description).	Generalized discharge of poly spike and wave or spike wave discharge Fast high-voltage spikes seen in all leads

III. UNCLASSIFIED EPILEPTIC SEIZURES
This group indicates all seizures that cannot be classified because of inadequate or incomplete data. This self-explanatory category is a catch-all for seizures that do not conform to any of the other headings

* Gastaut, H. (1973). *Definitions.* In: *Dictionary of Epilepsy, Part 1. Geneva: World Health Organization.*

seizures, and the episode lasts longer than a true seizure. The dramatic, violent flinging of the extremities, wiry movements, and inconsistent pattern of development are a sharp contrast to the tonic–clonic, orderly, repetitive movements of true seizures. If a scream is heard with a true seizure, it is at the onset of the event. With nonepileptic seizures, screams are usually heard throughout the course of the episode. Observing the features, development, and finale of seizure activity can be most helpful in differentiating between epileptic and nonepileptic seizures.

PATHOPHYSIOLOGY

Epilepsy is due to alterations in membrane potential that predispose certain hyperactive and hypersensitive neurons to respond abnormally to changes in the cellular environment. The hypersensitive neurons have lowered thresholds for firing and can fire excessively, creating an **epileptogenic focus** from which the seizure emanates. The epileptogenic focus generates large numbers of autonomous paroxysmal discharges that can be enhanced or minimized depending on the neurotransmitter that is active on the postsynaptic membrane. The frequency of cell firing can reach 1,000 per second during a seizure. An epileptogenic focus can induce secondary epileptogenic foci in a synaptically related area and between the same anatomical areas in opposite cerebral hemispheres through connecting pathways.

Depolarization is associated with ionic imbalances that alter the chemical environment of the neurons with an intracellular accumulation of sodium, as well as a depletion of intracellular potassium. At the onset of neuronal stimulation, depolarization is followed by a period of hyperpolarization, which is probably caused by an inhibitory postsynaptic potential. The hyperpolarization is soon replaced by depolarization, which rapidly increases in amplitude. The cell begins to fire repeatedly, thereby producing sustained membrane depolarization and seizure activity.

During a seizure, there is a drastic increase in cellular respiration and glycolysis. This markedly increases the demand for adenosine triphosphate (ATP), the major direct source of energy for the brain. The brain relies chiefly upon the metabolism of glucose for the production of the phosphate bonds necessary for ATP. During a seizure, the demand for ATP is increased by approximately 250%. Cerebral blood flow increases to meet increased oxygen demands.

The cerebral blood flow can respond to the metabolic demands as long as hypoxemia, hypoglycemia, and cardiac irregularities do not develop. Increased metabolic activity in contracting skeletal muscles and apnea can result in hypoxemia and hypoglycemia, particularly during status epilepticus. The brain may require more energy than it can produce from the limited oxygen and glucose supply in the blood. A rapid decrease in ATP, phosphocreatine, and glucose occurs concurrently with increased levels of lactate, producing an energy debt. Cellular exhaustion and selected cellular destruction can result as serious consequences.

Variations in the course of a seizure are of interest. **Tonic–clonic generalized seizures** can be divided into the tonic, the clonic, and the postictal phases. In the **tonic phase**, neuronal hyperexcitation spreads to the subcortex, thalamus, and upper brain stem, and consciousness is lost. There are also concurrent signs of autonomic nervous system overactivity, such as salivation, pupillary dilation, tachycardia, and increased blood pressure. Apnea lasts for only a few seconds. Occasionally, death can result from associated cardiac arrhythmias. In the **clonic phase**, inhibitory neurons of the cortex, anterior thalamus, and basal ganglion nuclei become active, intermittently interrupting the tonic seizure discharge with clonic activity. The clonic bursts gradually subside until they cease altogether. The involved cells are left exhausted.

In the **postictal phase**, the high-voltage spikes and waves gradually decrease. The involved cells cease firing. The patient is initially in a deep sleep, which is followed by a period of confusion and lethargy. There may also be temporary paresis, aphasia, or hemianopsia.

Following a seizure of any kind (generalized or partial), focal weakness, called **Todd's paralysis**, can last up to 24 hours. This weakness is important in localization of a focal epileptogenic site and is probably due to neuronal metabolic exhaustion.

DIAGNOSIS

When a seizure occurs, an aggressive search must be undertaken to determine if the seizure is secondary to an underlying cause or is related to epilepsy. The diagnostic process requires a careful history of the clinical presentation of the seizure and surrounding events, a medical history and a physical and neurological examination, and diagnostic testing. Data pertaining to prenatal history and achievement of developmental milestones are very important in infants, children, and adolescents. In adults, a history of trauma, drug use, and toxic environmental exposure are critical. Detailed descriptive information about the seizures is collected, including age of onset; surrounding events such as fever or withdrawal of alcohol, prodromal or aura experiences; precipitating factors; frequency; loss of consciousness; subjective and objective characteristics of the event; postseizure behavior; and any injuries associated with seizures. In addition to the usual baseline blood chemistries other helpful data are as follows:

- Toxicology screen (drug levels, barbiturates, street drugs, lead, etc.)
- EEG
- Computed tomography scan or magnetic resonance imaging
- Lumbar puncture (if not contraindicated)

Some patients will not require all of the procedures listed, whereas others may require additional studies. The objective of the studies is to identify systemic or CNS processes that are manifested, in part, by seizure activity. For many patients, an extensive search for an underlying etiology will yield negative results. The diagnosis of epilepsy may be made after ruling out other possible causes (discussed later). The clinical presentation and EEG findings will help to classify the particular type of epilepsy. Accurate diagnosis of seizure type is important because selection of appropriate drug therapy is seizure-specific in many cases. The EEG is a vital diagnostic procedure because it identifies patterns of abnormal electrical activity that can be correlated with particular types of seizure patterns. An EEG can also aid in lateralization and localizing of an epileptogenic trigger focus. However, in about 50% to 60% of persons with confirmed epilepsy, the interictal EEG can be normal.

There are several special techniques that are useful in augmenting the data from an EEG. A sleep study, in which there is continuous EEG monitoring, is helpful because sleep activates anterior temporal spike discharges and bitemporal discharges in 80% to 90% of persons with complex partial seizures. The increase in interictal epileptiform abnormalities is noted most in non–rapid eye movement (non-REM) sleep. Sleep deprivation also increases the frequency of interictal abnormalities. Extra scalp electrodes, nasopharyngeal electrodes, and sphenoid electrodes help to increase the detection of mesial temporal discharges. The diagnostic ability to detect and localize abnormal ictal discharges in complex partial seizures is greatly enhanced with the use of invasive procedures such as depth, subdural, and cortical electrodes. Surface electrodes often provide false localization.[9] Simultaneous EEG and audiovideo recordings of the patient can provide a total picture to distinguish seizure from nonseizure activity as well as assist in the classification of seizure type.

Differential Diagnosis

With the plethora of causes of seizure activity, diagnosis can become very difficult. Differentiation between epileptic and nonepileptic seizures (discussed earlier) must be made. Brain tumor; cerebral aneurysm; cerebral arteriovenous malformation; transient ischemic attacks; stroke; migraine headaches; syncope; sleep disorders; myoclonus; cardiac sources; drug and alcohol abuse; drug toxicity; metabolic disorders; breath holding; and psychogenic problems such as anxiety attacks, hysterical responses, and psychosis are some of the possibilities that must be excluded. In addition, accurate classification of seizure type is important to specific treatment choices.

The Electroencephalogram and Seizures

The EEG is a diagnostic tool in which the amplified electrical potential of the brain is recorded by placing 14 to 21 electrodes on the patient's scalp. Leads may also be placed on the cortical surface through invasive placement of electrodes. The tracings of electrical activity reflect the combined electrical activity of several neurons, rather than only one. The basic resting electrical pattern of the brain is altered by opening the eyes, focusing attention on a problem, hyperventilation, photic stimulation, drugs, or sleep. Therefore, recordings are taken at rest, after hyperventilation, during stimulation with a strobe light, and during sleep. The patient must be quiet, relaxed, cooperative, able to follow directions, and seated comfortably in a chair with the eyes closed, although not asleep. The testing room must be shielded from extraneous electrical interference and noise. Often, the preparation for the EEG includes keeping the patient awake all night before the recordings. The stress of sleep deprivation is more apt to result in the recording of abnormal EEG tracings than if the patient had a good night's sleep.

Even though the EEG is important in diagnosing seizures, these data must be considered in conjunction with other information, including the history, physical examination, and other laboratory studies. Between seizures, normal EEGs are often recorded in patients with epilepsy. In addition, EEGs that are considered to be borderline by one interpreter may be read as normal by another, indicating some subjectivity in interpretation.

The tracings for the EEG are made with special ink on electromagnetic paper. The recorded tracings signify the electrical potential difference from the scalp to the ear electrodes, and from the scalp to the scalp electrodes. The average EEG consists of 150 to 300 or more pages of recordings, with each page accounting for 10 seconds of tracings. In the **normal adult,** the most characteristic, normal tracings noted at rest are as follows:

Alpha waves—8 to 12 Hz (Hz = cycles per minute)
Beta waves—18 to 30 Hz, a faster wave, seen in the anterior areas of the brain

Both the alpha and beta waves are bilaterally symmetrical, with their own characteristic shapes and amplitudes. Changes occur in the EEG pattern normally with various activities. For example, when the eyes are opened, there is an immediate decrease in the amplitude of the brain waves; in the early stages of sleep, the waves slow (lower voltage); and in the later stages of sleep, "sleep spindles," occurring at a rate of 14 to 16 Hz, develop with subsequent high voltage and slow waves.

ABNORMAL ELECTROENCEPHALOGRAPHIC WAVES

Abnormal EEG waves include the following:

Delta waves—less than 4 Hz with high amplitude; they are often associated with destruction of brain tissue, such as occurs with infarction, tumor, or abscess (localized over abnormal area)
Theta waves—4 to 7 Hz (not always abnormal)
Spikes or sharp waves—high-voltage, faster waves; asymmetry of frequency and amplitude from one side to the other

On an abnormal EEG, slow and fast waves may be combined in paroxysmal runs, thereby interrupting the normal pattern. These paroxysmal waves are highly suggestive of epilepsy. Recordings taken between seizures in the epileptic patient often include isolated spikes without evidence of a clinical seizure.

OTHER CONSIDERATIONS

A clinical seizure will not necessarily occur each time a few epileptogenic cells become hyperactive. Much more seizure activity is noted on EEG than ever develops into clinical seizures.

There are times when a patient who usually experiences generalized seizures may experience only a part of the usual manifestations of a seizure. This configuration of a seizure is termed abortive epilepsy. The change may be due to incomplete control of seizures by an anticonvulsant drug.

TREATMENT

The underlying problem responsible for seizures will determine the treatment instituted. For example, if the diagnostic work-up has revealed a brain tumor as being the cause of seizures, treatment is directed toward management of the primary problem, the brain tumor. Seizures related to the brain tumor can be managed with antiepileptic drugs (AEDs). If the diagnosis is epilepsy, then the specific type of epilepsy is imperative in developing an effective treatment plan.

About 75% of patients with epilepsy can be managed satisfactorily with AEDs. For a small group of patients, surgery is considered if an epileptogenic focus can be identified or if seizures are intractable even with drug therapy. Drug therapy is only part of the management plan. The behavioral, social, and economic consequences of having uncontrolled seizures are significant and need to be addressed. Patient education for self-management is critical for successful adaptation to this chronic problem, along with counseling and support.

Medical Management: Drug Therapy

The first goal of drug therapy is to completely control or reduce the frequency of seizures so that the person can live a normal life. AEDs are not a cure for epilepsy but a chemical means of controlling seizures. As with any drug, there are side effects, such as sedation, which may interfere with daily living. The second goal of medical management is the development of an individualized drug program that minimizes side effects and supports compliance.

In considering drug therapy, the following principles should be followed:[10]

- Establish an accurate diagnosis of seizure type or type of epilepsy
- Select the primary drug that is the most effective for the seizure type
- Titrate the dose to achieve appropriate blood concentrations
- Consider the pharmacokinetics of AEDs and free AED concentrations
- Provide patient education
- Consider the length of time on AEDs

Establishing an Accurate Diagnosis. The importance of an accurate and specific type of epilepsy or seizure syndrome is discussed earlier in the chapter.

Selecting the Primary Drug Most Effective for the Seizure Type. The classifications of epileptic seizures and epilepsies/epileptic syndromes has made it easier to select the drug of choice for the given seizure problem. Table 31-4 outlines seizure types and drug of choice plus an alternate drug. Selection of the correct drug is very important. For example, absence seizures are different that other seizure types. Phenytoin, phenobarbital, and carbamazepine, which are effective in controlling generalized tonic–clonic seizures and partial seizures, are ineffective for absence seizures and may actually precipitate an increase in their incidence.[11]

With a drug that can be used for a variety of seizure types, the therapeutic range may be different for specific seizure types. For example, blood concentrations for complex partial seizures may need to be higher than the concentration for tonic–clonic generalized seizures.

Titrating the Dose to Achieve Appropriate Blood Concentrations. The following are important points to keep in mind:[12,13]

- Begin with a single drug that is the drug of choice for the particular seizure type. Previously, using two drugs simultaneously was a common practice, but because numerous studies have demonstrated that seizure control can be achieved with a single drug, single-drug therapy is the current standard.

TABLE 31-4
Epilepsy/Seizure Disorder Types and Approved Drugs for Adults

EPILEPSY/SEIZURE	DRUG OF CHOICE	USUAL DAILY DOSE	ALTERNATE DRUGS	USUAL DAILY DOSE
Primary generalized tonic–clonic	• Phenytoin or • Carbamazepine or • Valproate	• 300–400 mg (increase slowly) • 800–1,600 mg • 1,000–3,000 mg	• Phenobarbital • Primidone • Lamotrigine • Felbanate • Gabapentin	• 90–150 mg • 750–1,250 mg • 100–500 mg • 1,200–3,600 mg • 1,800–3,600 mg
Secondary generalized	• Carbamazepine • Phenytoin • Valproate	• 800–1,600 mg • 300–400 mg • 1,000–1,600 mg	• Phenobarbital • Primidone • Lamotrigine • Gabapentin	• 90–150 mg • 750–1,250 mg • 100–500 mg • 900–2,400 mg
Absence	• Ethosuximide or • Valproate	• 750–1,250 mg • 1,000–3,000 mg	• Clonazepam • Lamotrigine	• 1.5–20 mg • 100–500 mg
Atypical absence, myoclonic	• Valproate	• 1,000–3,000 mg	• Clonazepam • Felbamate	• 1.5–20 mg • 1,200–3,600 mg
Partial, simple	• Phenytoin • Carbamazepine • Lamotrigine • Phenobarbital	• 300–400 mg • 800–1,600 mg • 100–500 mg • 90–150 mg	• Primidone • Clonazepam • Gabapentin • Felbanate	• 750–1,250 mg • 1.5–20 mg • 900–2,400 mg • 1,200–3,600 mg
Partial, complex	• Phenytoin • Carbamazepine • Lamotrigine • Gabapentin	• 300–400 mg • 800–1,600 mg • 100–500 mg • 1,800–3,600	• Phenobarbital • Primidone • Valproate • Clonazepam • Felbanate	• 90–150 mg • 750–1,500 mg • 1,000–6,000 mg • 1.5–20 mg • 1,200–3,600

- Other considerations when choosing a drug include previous history of drug allergies, age, tolerance of side effects, cost, other drug therapy and potential interactions, and childbearing potential.
- Increase the drug gradually over 3 to 4 weeks until seizure control is achieved, intolerable side effects occur, toxicity develops, or the maximum therapeutic range has been reached.
- Recognize that AEDs are CNS depressants and that drowsiness, lethargy, and tiredness are common in the beginning of therapy; however, these effects will usually subside in 7 to 10 days.
- Because of pharmacokinetics (cited later) and variations in requirements for specific seizure types with the same drug, expect to make individual adjustments in dosage.
- Some patients may need more or less than the recommended therapeutic range for a particular drug.
- Titrate a single drug until maximum benefit is achieved or intolerance or serious side effects occur. If a therapeutic blood concentration has been achieved and seizure control has not been achieved, a second drug may be added. A second drug may be used in combination with the first or will replace the first. If replacement of the first is planned, it should be gradually tapered after the second drug has been titrated to the desired dosage. This practice is necessary because the sudden withdrawal of a drug can cause status epilepticus, even though a new drug has been introduced in its place.
- Check concentration of drug blood levels after 5 to 8 half-lives or a period of 3 to 4 weeks if seizure free. (See Table 31-5 for therapeutic serum concentrations, half-life, and steady state data.)

- The drug half-life is important to note because drugs of long duration (phenytoin, phenobarbital) may be taken once a day in some circumstances.
- Have the patient keep a drug diary routinely, but especially when a new drug is introduced. The diary should include dosage and side effects. The diary is helpful in evaluating the effectiveness of the drug therapy.

Considering Pharmacokinetics and Free AED Concentrations. The pharmacokinetics of AEDs are important to keep in mind. Many AEDs are highly bound to plasma protein. It is the unbound, or "free," concentration that is the active drug capable of penetrating the blood–brain barrier and interacting with receptor sites. For example, patients on high-protein tube feeding will require a higher drug dosage to maintain adequate drug blood levels.

Conditions known to alter AED protein binding capacity are malnutrition, older age, pregnancy, hypoalbuminemia, burns, liver disease, and chronic renal failure.

Plasma Protein Binding Capacity of Selected AEDs

- Phenytoin and valproic acid (high protein binding)
- Carbamazepine (variable binding)
- Phenobarbital and primidone (minimal binding)
- Ethosuximide (not bound)

Although therapeutic ranges are cited for each drug, there are large variations among patients in pharmacokinetics. Therefore, dose requirements for individual patients vary. For determining dosage, use as the gold standard that the patient should become seizure free or experience the onset of serious

TABLE 31-5
Therapeutic Serum Concentration Levels, Half-Life, and Steady State for AEDs

DRUG: GENERIC AND TRADE NAMES	THERAPEUTIC SERUM CONCENTRATION LEVELS	SERUM HALF LIFE (hours)	TIME TO STEADY STATE (days)
Carbamazepine (Tegretol)	6–12 mcg/mL	5–25 on chronic therapy	2–4
Clonazepam (Klonopin)	20–80 mcg/mL	20–35	4–5
Ethosuximide (Zarontin)	40–100 mcg/mL	60	6–12
Felbanate (Felbatol)	Not established	14	3
Gabapentin (Neurontin)	Not established	5–7	1.5
Lamotrigine (Lamictal)	Not established	14	2
Phenobarbital (Luminal)	15–35 mcg/mL	46–136	14–21
Phenytoin (Dilantin)	10–20 mcg/mL	10–34	7–28
Primidone (Mysoline)	6–12 mcg/mL	4–19	1–4
Valproate (Depakene, Depakote)	50–120 mcg/mL	8–20	1–3

AED = antiepileptic drug.

side effects or intolerance. Clinical judgment must be used and patient response and blood levels must be monitored to determine the ideal dose and blood concentration for a patient.

Providing Patient Education. Patient education is the cornerstone of drug therapy and promotes a partnership that supports compliance. Patients who understand the purpose of drug therapy and the drugs that they are taking are more compliant. Patient education must be an ongoing process with reinforcement and updates at each appointment. Because many patients are on long-term or possibly lifelong therapy, education must also be anticipatory to prepare persons for developmental changes and changes in normal life routines.

Serious consideration about how to teach persons initially and how to provide ongoing education must be undertaken by health providers who care for persons with seizures if they are to provide comprehensive management for their patients.

Considering Length of Time on AEDs. Is AED therapy lifelong? It depends on many factors.

If a person has been seizure free for a long period of time (the time period varies among experts, but the range is at least 2 to 4 years, and preferably 5 to 10 years), the possibility of withdrawal should be explored (Table 31-6).

Although Table 31-7 has been developed to consolidate pertinent data about AEDs, a few commonly ordered drugs are discussed to emphasize the associated nursing management. These drugs include phenytoin, phenobarbital, carbamazepine, and valproic acid.

PHENYTOIN

Phenytoin (Dilantin), introduced in 1938, is a synthetic drug that is classified as a hydantoin. It is used in any generalized seizure type except absence epilepsy; it can actually increase the number of absence seizures. Patients with partial seizures have also responded well to phenytoin. Phenytoin blocks posttetanic potentiation by influencing synaptic transmission and therefore spread of potentials. The proposed mechanism of action is stabilization of the membrane potential by ionic and neurotransmitter stabilization.

Pharmacokinetics. Phenytoin is primarily absorbed through the duodenum, and absorption is almost complete. There is

TABLE 31-6
Possibility of AED Withdrawal

	PROMOTE COMPLETE AED WITHDRAWAL	SUGGEST POOR PROBABILITY OF AED WITHDRAWAL
Complete seizure (sz) control within 1 year of onset	yes	no
Combined sz types	no	yes
Sz onset after 2 years and before 35 years	yes	no
Repeated status epilepticus	no	yes
Normal EEG	yes	continued epileptiform activity
Normal MRI	yes	no
Abnormal cognitive function	no	yes

AED = antiepilepsy drug; EEG = electroencephalogram; MRI = magnetic resonance imaging.

TABLE 31-7
Drugs Used for Epilepsy and Seizure Disorders

DRUG: GENERIC AND TRADE NAMES	INDICATIONS	ADJUNCT DRUG FOR:	CONTRAINDICATIONS	SIDE EFFECTS ON MONOTHERAPY	AVERAGE ADULT DAILY DOSE (mg)
Carbamazepine (Tegretol)	Simple partial, complex partial, or generalized tonic–clonic seizures	None	History of bone marrow depression	Rash, drowsiness, blurred vision, diplopia, ataxia, nausea, vomiting; can interfere with cognitive function in learning situations	800–1,600 **only oral form available**
Clonazepam (Klonopin)	Myoclonic seizures	Complex partial seizures and tonic seizures	Severe liver disease; glaucoma	Drowsiness, ataxia, behavior disturbance; 50% of patients on long-term therapy have transient seizures	1.5–20
Ethosuximide (Zarontin)	Drug of choice for uncomplicated absence seizures	None	None	Nausea, vomiting, drowsiness, headache, dizziness, rash; rarely leukopenia, aplastic anemia, or Stevens-Johnson syndrome	750–1,250
Felbanate (Felbatol)	Complex partial, drop attacks, tonic–clonic, and atypical absence seizure	Children with partial and secondary generalized tonic–clonic seizures	None	Insomnia, weight gain, headache, decreased appetite, dizziness, fatigue, and possible rash	1,200–3,600
Gabapentin (Neurontin)	Partial and/or secondary generalized tonic–clonic	None	None	Somnolence, fatigue, dizziness, ataxia	900–2,400
Lamotrigine (Lamictal)	New drug for FDA approval	Partial complex and/or secondary generalized tonic–clonic seizures	None	Drowsiness, dizziness, headache, and nausea	100–500
Phenobarbital (Luminal)	Partial; generalized tonic–clonic seizures	May be given in combination with phenytoin	Absence and atypical absence seizures and drop attacks	Drowsiness, difficulty thinking, ataxia, hyperactivity, anemia	90–150
Phenytoin (Dilantin)	Alternate drug for partial, complex partial, and generalized tonic–clonic seizures	None	Absence seizures	Hirsutism, dizziness, ataxia, hypertrophy of gingiva, nystagmus	300–400
Primidone (Mysoline)	Partial motor, complex partial, and drop attacks	Secondary generalized tonic–clonic seizures	Absence and atypical absence seizures and drop attacks	Drowsiness, difficulty thinking, nausea, psychotic reaction	750–1,500
Valproate (Depakene, Depakote)	Absence, generalized tonic–clonic seizures	Complex partial seizures			1,000–3,000

no first-pass metabolism. Oral absorption is affected by the particle size of the particular brand formulation so that *there can be variations among brands.* The brand of phenytoin that a patient is receiving should not be switched without careful monitoring.[14]

Phenytoin enters the brain quickly and it is then redistributed to other body tissues including breast milk. It crosses the placenta and reaches a state of equilibrium with the mother and fetus. Phenytoin is bound to serum and tissue protein. In the serum, the drug binds primarily to albumin in a predictable, linear fashion provided that the albumin level is normal (see the exceptions in the previous section). Phenytoin is metabolized in the liver and excreted in the urine. At an often unpredictable concentration level, no additional drug can be metabolized because of saturability of metabolism. Any change in dosage at this point will result in significant changes in serum concentrations. In addition, serum concentration does not decline at a predictable linear rate when phenytoin is discontinued. Therefore, serum monitoring is necessary after any dosage change. Because the half-life of phenytoin is 10 to 34 hours (average equals 22 hours), it may be given once a day. However, only the extended-release should be given for once-a-day dosing.

Administration. Administration is by the oral or intravenous route. Intramuscular injection should be avoided because the pH of phenytoin is about 12, so that phenytoin is very irritating to the tissue. Oral phenytoin comes in three dosage forms. The tablets and suspension contain phenytoin acid, whereas the capsules contain phenytoin sodium. Phenytoin sodium is 92% phenytoin. The parenteral form is phenytoin sodium. Given in equal amounts of phenytoin acid, tablets, capsules, and suspension have the same bioavailability. Phenytoin capsules are designated as immediate-release or extended-release. Only the extended-release should be used for once-a-day dosing. The suspension form comes in two different strengths; either can settle and thus deliver doses of unequal concentration.

Because of the high protein binding of phenytoin, the dosage will probably need to be increased when the patient is on enteral feeding to maintain the same blood level. Once enteral feeding is discontinued, the dosage of phenytoin must be decreased. Monitoring phenytoin blood levels provides a guide for adjusting the drug dosage.

If the drug is administered by the intravenous (IV) route, phenytoin must be administered slowly, at a rate no faster than 50 mg/min in *a solution of normal saline.* Proper rate is very important because rapid administration depresses the myocardium and can cause cardiac arrhythmias and cardiac arrest. If given in solution such as 5% dextrose in water, the drug will precipitate into crystals in the solution. If phenytoin is given by IV push, it must be given slowly (no more than 50 mg/min); the effect of rapid administration of phenytoin on the myocardium is dangerous arrhythmias. Patients receiving IV phenytoin should also be observed for the development of phlebitis at IV site.

Drug Interactions. Various drugs in common use can interact with phenytoin:

- Drugs that *potentiate* the action of phenytoin include aspirin, phenylbutazone, chloramphenicol, cycloserine, iso-

niazid, estrogens, disulfiram (Antabuse), chlordiazepoxide (Librium), sulfonamides, and anticoagulants (especially dicumarol).
- Drugs that *decrease* the action of phenytoin include alcohol, antihistamines, barbiturates, glutethimide (Doriden), hypnotics, and sedatives.
- Phenytoin *potentiates* the action of many antihypertensives such as propranolol, folic acid antagonists, methotrexate, quinidine, and tubocurarine.
- Phenytoin *decreases* the action of oral contraceptives, corticosteroids, and digitalis.

Adverse Effects. Lethargy, fatigue, incoordination, visual blurring, higher cortical dysfunction, and drowsiness are related to CNS depressant effects. When serum concentrations exceed 20 mcg/mL, patients may experience nystagmus, ataxia, and slurred speech. A morbilliform rash may occur 7 to 14 days after beginning the drug in some patients. The appearance of such a rash indicates that the drug should be discontinued. A lupus-like syndrome has also been reported and is reversible when phenytoin is withdrawn.

Effects seen with long-term, chronic use include gingival hyperplasia (about 50% of patients), decreased cognitive ability, osteomalacia, hirsutism, hypothyroidism, peripheral neuropathy, megaloblastic anemia, blood dyscrasias, and low serum folate concentrations. Periodic complete blood cell counts (CBCs) are important to monitor the development of anemia or dyscrasias. The low folic acid levels respond to folic acid therapy. There is an increased incidence of malformations in children born of women who are taking AEDs.

PHENOBARBITAL

Phenobarbital, introduced in 1912, was one of the first drugs available for the control of seizures and is still widely used. It is an alternative for generalized seizures, except absence seizures, and also partial seizures. It is the drug of choice for seizures in infants, but its adverse effect on cognitive performance and sedative-hypnotic effect has made it less than ideal for children and adults. Phenobarbital is a CNS depressant; it elevates the seizure threshold by decreasing postsynaptic excitation, possibly by stimulating postsynaptic GABA inhibitor responses.[15] It has been given in combination with phenytoin in some patients.

Pharmacokinetics. Phenobarbital is rapidly and completely absorbed by all routes (oral, intramuscular, rectal). The biphasic distribution includes initial penetration of highly perfused organs, including the brain, followed by even distribution to all body tissues, including fat. By the IV route, peak cerebral concentration is achieved in 3 to 20 minutes. Drugs affecting liver enzymes may alter phenobarbital metabolism. The elimination pattern of phenobarbital is linear. About 20% to 40% of a dose is excreted by the kidneys unchanged. The urine pH affects tubular absorption of phenobarbital and the amount of excreted drug can be increased by administering diuretics and urinary alkalizing drugs. The binding of phenobarbital to protein is 50%.

Administration. The routes of administration are oral and parenteral. In an emergency, phenobarbital can be given by

IV loading. The half-life of phenobarbital is so long that it can be given as a single daily dose. Because it takes about 3 to 4 weeks to reach steady state, changing doses rapidly is not recommended.

Drug Interactions. Phenobarbital decreases the efficacy of oral contraceptives.

Adverse Effects. The chief adverse effects are sedation, drowsiness, and fatigue. In addition, impairment of higher cortical function and depression of cognitive performance such as learning are found with the use of phenobarbital, as discussed earlier.

CARBAMAZEPINE

Carbamazepine (Tegretol) is a safe and relatively side-effect–free drug used in the management of partial and secondary generalized tonic–clonic seizures. It is the drug of choice for partial seizures, especially complex partial seizures; it can make absence and myoclonic seizures worse. The mechanism of action is depression of transmission of the nucleus ventralis anterior thalamus, which acts to decrease the spread of seizure discharge. In addition, it has some depressive effect on post-tetanic potentiation, but to a lesser degree than in phenytoin.

Pharmacokinetics. Carbamazepine has an absorption rate greater than 75%; the dose peak is reached in 6 to 24 hours. It has a high affinity for lipids which bind to body fat; it also binds to albumin. Carbamazepine is metabolized by the liver. Humidity affects its action.

Administration. Carbamazepine is available only in oral form. It is given in divided doses two to four times a day. Dosage should be adjusted gradually. Because the suspension form of the drug may adhere to the nasogastric tube if not diluted, it is recommended that the suspension form be diluted in an equal amount of diluent before administration via enteral tube.

Drug Interactions. Some drugs, such as phenytoin and phenobarbital, may interact with carbamazepine by enzyme induction, thus decreasing the concentration of carbamazepine. Other drugs—erythromycin, cimetidine, and isoniazid—interact by enzyme induction; these drugs increase the concentration of carbamazepine. Carbamazepine interacts with other drugs by inducing their metabolism; these drugs include valproic acid, theophylline, warfarin, and ethosuximide.

Adverse Effects. The major dose-dependent side effects are diplopia, nystagmus, ataxia, unsteadiness, dizziness, and headache. Cognitive deficits are minimal, although present. Carbamazepine has been associated with neural tube defects.

VALPROATE

Valproate, which is marketed as valproic acid (Depakene) or divalproex sodium (Depakote) is approved for management of absence seizures or multiple seizure types that include absence. It is also used for generalized tonic–clonic, myoclonic, and atonic seizures and especially for persons with more than one type of generalized seizure. The drug has low toxicity and is well tolerated. Its mechanism of action is unclear.

Pharmacokinetics. Valproic acid is completely absorbed by the oral route when taken on an empty stomach. Its peak concentration is achieved between 1 and 3 hours. Food delays the time of absorption but does not interfere with the amount absorbed. Valproic acid distributes widely; it is about 90% bound to albumin. The liver is the site of metabolism. There are at least 10 metabolites of valproic acid that have been identified.

Administration. Valproic acid is available in capsule, syrup, and "sprinkle" forms. The tablet form contains divalproex sodium, which must be metabolized in the gut to valproic acid; it is enteric coated to reduce gastrointestinal symptoms.

Drug Interactions. Valproic acid is altered by salicylates, which increase its free concentration. The addition of phenobarbital or phenytoin will decrease the concentration of valproic acid.

Adverse Effects. Mild transient drowsiness and minimal cognitive effects are seen with valproate. Hepatic dysfunction to liver failure and pancreatitis have been reported. The more common adverse effects include nausea and vomiting, which can be controlled by using enteric-coated Depakote or by taking the drug with food. Weight gain, transient hair loss, tremor, and dose-related thrombocytopenia are common. Menstrual disturbances and hyperandrogenism may occur in women. Neural tube defects and congenital abnormalities have been reported in the infants of mothers on the drug.

SUMMARY OF DRUG THERAPY

In summary, any patient receiving long-term drug therapy should be monitored carefully for the development of side effects or toxicity. Most drugs are metabolized by the liver and excreted by the kidneys. Periodic drug blood levels should be monitored. If anemia or blood dyscrasias are common side effects, a CBC should be done routinely. Folic acid deficiency has also been reported with some AEDs; therefore, folic acid assay should be monitored.

Surgical Management

The goal of complete control of seizures guides the presentation of treatment options. For those patients who have been given a reasonable trial on AEDs and still continue to have seizures, a surgical evaluation is a reasonable next step. There are a variety of surgical options available for epilepsy that include resection, callosotomy, vagal stimulation, and subcortical intracranial stimulation of lesions. Among them, resective surgery is the only one that results in a significant proportion of cases with seizure-free results.[16] An NIH Consensus Conference on surgery for epilepsy in 1990 supported the efficacy of surgery for selected persons with epilepsy.[17]

About half of all resected cases become seizure free. The selection criteria are important. Persons who have not responded to medical management of seizure, who have a unilateral focus that will not cause a major neurological deficit if excised, and who have had a significant alteration in their quality of life are good candidates for resective surgery. An extensive diagnostic work-up precedes surgery including electrophysiology, neuropsychology, and imaging studies which should all suggest an epileptogenic focus. The purpose of surgery is to locate and excise as much of the epileptogenic area as possible without causing neurological deficits. A large number of the patients with partial complex seizures and a localized focus have the focus in the temporal lobe. Thus, temporal lobe resections are the most common resective epilepsy procedures.

There are two general surgical approaches to temporal lobe surgery: the first assumes that all patients have uniform anatomical locations of eloquent areas (speech, motor function) and that the purpose of the surgery is removal of the epileptogenic focus; the second approach is one of tailoring the resection to the pathophysiology and location of eloquent areas in each case. The information for the tailoring can be acquired intraoperatively or postoperatively with placement of intracranial recording electrodes that localize the epileptogenic focus. The resection is designed to remove the epileptogenic focus while sparing the individualized eloquent areas. This approach is based on the assumption that there is considerable individual variation in the extent of the epileptogenic lesion and the location of eloquent areas. Selection criteria for this group of approaches require only that the exposure for **intraoperative mapping** or placement of intracranial electrodes be in the general region of seizure onset.[18] Mapping is the procedure for identifying eloquent areas. Data about seizures can also be used to tailor a resection. Scalp ictal recordings do not usually provide sufficiently precise localization for detailed surgical planning. Therefore, intracranial electrodes provide the best data and are required.

Local anesthesia is used for adolescents and adults unless they have behavioral problems. In that case, a light general anesthetic is given. The patient *must* be able to follow commands and answer questions during the EEG and cortical stimulation portion of the lengthy surgical procedure. After surgical exposure of the brain surface and depth, electrodes are applied so that an EEG can be taken to identify the epileptogenic focus. Cortical stimulation is used to identify sensory, motor, and speech areas. Once the tissue to be excised has been identified, cortical resection is undertaken. Following excision, the electrodes are reattached to determine the presence of any other epileptogenic activity that would require any further resection. If the EEG pattern is satisfactory, the patient is anesthetized so that the incision can be closed. Postoperatively, the patient is managed in the same way as any craniotomy patient (see Chap. 18).

Postoperatively and upon discharge, the patient continues on an AED, often carbamazepine. EEG recordings are obtained to determine the presence of seizure activity. The decision to discontinue drug therapy after 2 to 4 years is based on an individual evaluation of the patient.

Complications of Surgery. The mortality from a temporal resection is less than 1%. The complications of surgery include infection; hydrocephalus; cerebral edema, ischemia, or hematoma; hemiparesis or hemiplegia; aphasia; alexia; or visual field deficits. Higher-level functions of cognition, memory, attention, concentration, or language may be affected. In addition, psychosocial impairment such as family interpersonal dynamics, self-esteem, response to treatment failure, and vocational/education disruption are possible.[19]

MANAGEMENT OF SEIZURES AND STATUS EPILEPTICUS IN AN ACUTE CARE SETTING

Most nurses who provide care in an **acute care setting** will manage a patient who has a seizure regardless of whether they are assigned to neuroscience or other types of units. Seizures may also occur in community based settings where persons are being seen for management of seizure disorders. Nurses need to know how to manage seizures and status epilepticus. The following is designed to provide that information.

Managing the Patient During a Seizure in an Acute Care Setting

When a patient has a seizure, the nurse's role is to protect the patient from injury, care for him or her after the seizure, and document the details of the event. In the hospital environment, persons who are at risk for having a seizure are placed on seizure precautions. This means that (1) the siderails of the bed are up and padded; (2) a suction setup and airway are available at the bedside; and (3) the bed is kept in low position.

Management of the patient during a seizure is directed toward prevention of injury and observing for complications. The following points should be observed:

Before and During a Seizure

- If the patient is seated when a major seizure occurs, ease him or her to the floor, if possible.
- Provide for privacy by pulling the bed curtains or screen or closing the door.
- If the patient experiences an aura, have him or her lie down to prevent injury that might occur from falling to the floor.
- Remove glasses and loosen any constricting clothing.
- Do not try to force anything into the mouth.
- Guide the movements to prevent injuries; do not try to restrain the person.
- Stay with the patient throughout the seizure to ensure safety.

After a Seizure

- Position the patient on the side to facilitate drainage of secretions.
- Provide for adequate ventilation by maintaining a patent airway; suctioning may be necessary to prevent aspiration.
- Allow the patient to sleep after the seizure.
- Upon awakening, orient the patient (he or she will probably be amnesic of the event).

Nursing Assessment and Documentation

Collecting data about the seizure requires well-developed observational skills and an understanding of what to look for and how to document observations. It may be helpful to verbalize the observations as events occur. Verbal reinforcement provides for better recall.

The following are several points to consider when organizing information about a seizure:

- Was the seizure witnessed or unwitnessed?
- Were there any warning signs or was there an aura?
- Where did the seizure begin and how did it proceed?
- What type of movement was noted and what parts of the body were involved?
- Were there any changes in the size of the pupils or conjugate gaze deviation?
- What was the duration of the entire attack and of each phase?
- Was the patient unconscious throughout the seizure?
- Was there urinary or bowel incontinence?
- What was the person's behavior after the seizure?
- Was there any weakness or paralysis of the extremities after the seizure?
- Were there any injuries noted?
- Did the patient sleep after the seizure? How long?

The observations can be recorded in narrative form in the nurse's notes or on a separate seizure activity sheet which becomes a part of the patient's permanent record. A sample of a seizure activity sheet for generalized tonic–clonic seizures is found in Fig. 31-1. Observations would be the same for a seizure that was witnessed in a community setting.

Managing a Person During a Seizure in a Community Setting

Seizures may occur in the community in settings such as ambulatory clinics, work and recreational environments, and the home. The same **first aid principles** taught to the person and family should be followed by the bystander nurse who comes upon the person having a seizure. Gumnit (1995) outlines first aid for epilepsy in his book. The first aid management of both generalized tonic–clonic seizures and complex partial seizures are addressed.

First Aid for Generalized Tonic–Clonic Seizures. First aid for generalized tonic–clonic seizures that occur in a community

SEIZURE ACTIVITY CHART FOR GENERALIZED TONIC-CLONIC SEIZURES

Patient's Name _____

_____ Age _____

Date	Time	Before		During							After				Nurse's Initials
		Warning Signs	Part of Body Where Seizure Began	General or Localized	Type of Movement	Duration of Each Phase — Tonic	Clonic	Level of Consciousness	Pupils	Other	Behavior	Paralysis	Location of Paralysis	Sleep	

FIGURE 31-1
A sample of a seizure activity chart for generalized tonic-clonic seizures.

setting is similar to the management of this type of seizure in an acute care setting.

Before and During a Seizure

- The person may fall to the ground, become stiff, and make clonic movements.
- If the person is seated, help him or her to lie down.
- Remove glasses and loosen any constricting clothing.
- Do not try to force anything into the mouth.
- Guide the movements to prevent injuries; do not try to restrain the person.
- Stay with the person throughout the seizure.

After a Seizure

- Position the person on the side to facilitate drainage of secretions.
- Have someone stay with the person until he or she is fully awake.
- Upon awakening, orient the person.

First Aid for Complex Partial Seizures. The person may not seem quite right, engaging in such behaviors as lip-smacking or making chewing motions, walking aimlessly, or not responding to questions (symptoms of automatism).

Before and During a Seizure

- Remove harmful objects from the person's environment or try to coax the person away from anything that could be harmful.
- Demonstrate a calm manner that does not agitate the person.
- Do not try to restrain the person.
- If alone, do not try to approach an angry or agitated person.

After the Seizure

- Do not leave the person alone.
- Have someone stay with the person until consciousness is fully regained; reorient the person.

When Should You Call for Medical Assistance? Call for emergency help if

- The person does not begin breathing after the seizure (CPR should be activated).
- A generalized tonic–clonic seizure lasts for more than 2 minutes.
- The person has one seizure right after another.
- The person is injured.

Managing Status Epilepticus in an Acute Care Setting

Status epilepticus is defined as more than 30 minutes of (1) continuous seizure activity or (2) two or more sequential seizures without full recovery of consciousness between seizures. The most common cause of status epilepticus is an abrupt discontinuation of AEDs. Other causes include withdrawal from alcohol, sedatives, or other drugs, or fever.

Status epilepticus presents itself in many forms: (1) repeated generalized convulsive seizures with persistent postictal depression of neurological function between seizures; (2) nonconvulsive seizures that produce a continuous or fluctuating "epileptic twilight" state; and (3) repeated partial seizures manifested as focal motor convulsions, focal sensory symptoms, or focal impairment of function (*e.g.*, aphasia) not associated with altered consciousness.[20] Generalized tonic–clonic status epilepticus is the most common type of status epilepticus. In over 50% of cases, status epilepticus is the patient's first seizure.[21]

Although there are many types of status epilepticus, the following discussion focuses on the management of convulsive status epilepticus because this form constitutes a medical emergency associated with substantial morbidity and mortality.

CONVULSIVE STATUS EPILEPTICUS (GENERALIZED TONIC–CLONIC STATUS EPILEPTICUS)

Over half of the patients with status epilepticus will respond to therapy with a single AED. Those that remain in status epilepticus present a continuing emergency. For those who present with refractory status epilepticus, a search for an acute or progressive neurological cause should be undertaken.[22]

The initial management of generalized convulsive status epilepticus includes the ABCs of life support (supporting respirations, maintaining blood pressure, supporting circulation), administering an AED, finding and treating the underlying cause, and preventing or treating medical complications.

Supporting the ABCs of Life Support. Position the patient to avoid aspiration or inadequate oxygenation. A soft, plastic oral airway may be inserted if it is possible to do so without forcing the teeth apart. The airway will need to be suctioned to remain patent. Oxygen, often at 100%, administered by mask or nasal prongs is often necessary. If respiratory assistance is needed, it is imperative to control seizures for the insertion of an endotracheal tube. Intravenous access should be secured, and vital signs and neurological signs should be monitored frequently. Extreme cerebral hypoxia can result in severe, irreversible neurological deficits. Support of adequate oxygenation and cerebral perfusion are critical to preventing these serious problems. Monitor glucose by finger stick, because hyperglycemia followed by hypoglycemia is common and needs to be treated. Give 50 mL of 50% glucose for hypoglycemia.

Administering AEDs. The goal of drug therapy is rapid termination of clinical and electrical seizure activity. There is controversy about the best drug treatment protocol for status epilepticus. The following are outlines of common protocols:[23]

Initially, a Fast-Acting Drug is Given to Stop the Seizures

- **Lorazepam (Ativan):** 4 to 8 mg (0.1 mg/min) IV at 1 to 2 mg/min; may repeat 4 to 8 mg every 5 to 10 minutes (maximum 80 mg per 24 hours)

- **Diazepam (Valium):** 5 to 20 mg IV slowly at 1 to 2 mg/min; repeat 5 to 10 mg every 5 to 10 minutes to a maximum of 100 mg per 24 hours

Then, Definitive Seizure Control (Using Longer-Acting Drugs) is Begun

- **Phenytoin (Dilantin):** 15 to 20 mg/kg (about 1 g) in normal saline at a rate of no faster than 50 mg/min
    Monitor blood pressure for hypotension. If hypotension occurs, slow rate of infusion.
    Because of the potential for cardiac arrhythmias, attach to a cardiac monitor.
    Monitor for respiratory depression.
    If seizures persist, the patient is intubated and phenobarbital is considered.
- **Phenobarbital:** 120 to 260 mg (10 to 20 mg/kg) IV at 50 mg/min, repeat; if seizures persist, consider pentobarbital coma or general anesthesia.

Diazepam is a relatively short-acting drug with a half-life of 16 to 90 minutes; however, the later half is eliminated at a much slower rate.[3] There can be serious cardiopulmonary effects. Specifically, the danger of repeated doses of diazepam is accumulation of high levels of active diazepam metabolites, which will result in respiratory depression and hypotension. Therefore, diazepam must be given very cautiously.

Treating the Underlying Cause. The caregivers must try to identify the underlying cause of seizures (*e.g.*, brain tumor, arteriovenous malformation) and treat the primary problem. A number of possible causative factors are discussed earlier in the chapter.

Preventing or Treating Medical Complications. The goal of therapy is to stop the seizures and minimize the adverse physiological consequences of status epilepticus which may include hypoxia, hypoglycemia, hypotension, and hypothermia. Severe metabolic acidosis can occur as a result of loss of base reserve. This change may prevent seizure control with anticonvulsants by increasing the amount of potassium in the extracellular space. It may also contribute to cerebral damage. Blood gases should be monitored. Other medical complications that may develop include cardiac arrhythmias, myocardial infarction, and aspiration pneumonia.

Nursing Management of Status Epilepticus

During status epilepticus, the following nursing measures should be taken (see Table 31-8 for nursing diagnoses related to status epilepticus):

- Maintain a patent airway to ensure adequate ventilation.
- Suction as necessary to prevent obstruction of the airway and possible aspiration.
- Provide oxygen as ordered.
- If drugs are being administered intravenously, protect the IV site so that the flow is maintained.
- Maintain seizure precautions to protect the patient from injury.

TABLE 31-8
Nursing Diagnoses Associated With Seizures and Status Epilepticus

NURSING DIAGNOSES ASSOCIATED WITH SEIZURES	ADDITIONAL NURSING DIAGNOSES ASSOCIATED WITH STATUS EPILEPTICUS
• Risk of Injury	• Altered Tissue Perfusion, Cerebral
• Acute Confusion	• Ineffective Breathing Pattern
• Impaired Communication	• Inability to Sustain Spontaneous Ventilation
• Ineffective Airway Clearance	• Risk of Aspiration
• Altered Protection	• Hyperthermia

NURSING MANAGEMENT OF PERSONS WITH EPILEPSY: COMMUNITY BASED CARE

Most persons with epilepsy are managed in the community by their primary care physician or by a neurologist. In a managed care environment, more persons with epilepsy previously managed by a neurologist will now come under the care of the primary care physician. Those with complicated epilepsy or intractable epilepsy will probably still be managed by a neurologist or in an epilepsy center.

The role of the nurse in managing persons with epilepsy will continue to be important, and in some settings, this role will be expanded. Nursing management of persons with epilepsy in the community is initially directed at assisting with the assessment and diagnostic work-up. However, the major role is that of patient education and patient monitoring. Patient assessment and diagnostics are discussed in earlier sections. Since the major role of the nurse is that of patient education, the next section focuses on this aspect of management. The major nursing diagnoses often made for a newly diagnosed patient with epilepsy are included in Chart 31-1.

For patients who have been hospitalized with a seizure problem, discharge planning must address the transition in care to a community based environment by providing appropriate referrals and special educational resources to span the transition period. The nurse in the community based setting will assume the major role in patient teaching to help persons and their families adapt to life with a chronic health problem and to assist persons to make adjustments in self-management of epilepsy across life span changes such as pregnancy, aging, and incidental minor illnesses and other changes in social, educational, and recreational activities.

Framing an approach to patient education assists the nurse in planning and implementing teaching. Self-management is a helpful unifying framework. **Self-management** is defined as a process by which persons with epilepsy and their families live with epilepsy and maximize the quality of their lives.[24] It does not mean that the person manages his or her epilepsy alone. Self-management means that the individual is free to accept or reject the recommendations of health professionals; this places the ultimate responsibility for management

CHART 31-1
Summary of Nursing Diagnoses Associated With Diagnosis of Epilepsy

Nursing Interventions	Nursing Diagnosis	Expected Outcomes
• Develop an individualized, comprehensive teaching plan (see Chart 31-2 for specifics). • Reassess learning needs periodically. • Provide anticipatory guidance. • Address learning needs of family members.	Knowledge Deficit related to (R/T) diagnosis of epilepsy or seizure disorder including need to know about epilepsy, medication needs, need for lifestyle changes, and special adaptations	• The person and family will demonstrate adequate knowledge of epilepsy or seizure disorder, the individualized management plan, drug therapy, and lifestyle changes. • The person will have adequate knowledge to make self-management decisions.
• Allow the person to verbalize need for information. • Answer questions. • Develop a partnership with the person so he or she feels in control of the health problem • Provide written information about epilepsy/management and information about community resources. • Make appropriate referrals. • Make person aware of the Epilepsy Foundation of America (EFA).	Health Seeking Behavior R/T the new diagnosis of epilepsy	• The person will verbalize satisfaction with information given to begin to self-managing his or her epilepsy. Epilepsy Foundation of America 4351 Garden City Drive Landover, MD 20785 (301) 459-3700
• Allow the patient to verbalize concerns. • Clarify misconceptions. • Determine the person's previous coping style. • Help the person determine which coping mechanisms will be most effective. • Support mobilization of effective coping.	Ineffective Individual Coping R/T altered self-concept and lifestyle adaptation secondary to the diagnosis of epilepsy	• The person will verbalize awareness of the new situation and the need to cope with it. • Effective coping skills will be used. • The person will express a sense of control over the situation.

Other Possible Nursing Diagnoses That May Be Applicable

Related to Psychosocial Response	Related to Potential Side Effects From AEDs
• Adjustment, Impaired • Social isolation • Fear • Personal Identity Disturbance • Role Disturbance • Ineffective Family Coping • Family Process, Altered • Management of Therapeutic Regimen, Ineffective • Altered Sexual Patterns • Noncompliance	• Impaired Physical Mobility: Ataxia • Sensory Perceptual Alterations: Dizziness, Visual Blurring, Nystagmus • Altered Thought Processes • Impaired Memory

AED = antiepileptic drug.

with the person. He or she must decide what lifestyle changes will be made to live with epilepsy.

Patient Teaching: General Points

Patient teaching requires a comprehensive teaching plan to help the patient adjust to the problem. Family teaching cannot be excluded because the family needs help to adjust to a chronic condition that can be frightening by its very nature. The family must be instructed about first aid if a seizure occurs. A teaching plan is based on a systematic assessment of patient needs. Physical, social, psychological, and vocational dimensions must be considered along with a drug teaching plan.

Each teaching plan is individualized to the needs of the patient. A patient who is followed over time will face problems that will require help from the nurse or physician. Some of the major points of information that should be presented to the patient are outlined in Chart 31-2. These points must be expanded so that the patient understands the implications as they apply to his or her particular lifestyle. They also must be reevaluated periodically to determine their relevance to the person. At each encounter with the health professional, compliance must be evaluated because noncompliance is a common problem. Repetition of information must be provided each time the person is seen.

Patients may express concerns about how they will cope with certain aspects of their lives. One common concern most adult patients face is whether they should reveal their ailment when applying for a job. Many report that they are discriminated against by employers when they reveal their condition. Those who choose to conceal this information often feel guilty and live in fear that they will experience a seizure on the job or that their seizures will become known to the employer. Information that is deliberately concealed is cause for immediate dismissal in most places of employment. It is the patient's decision to determine whether to disclose the epileptic condition. Regardless of which alternative is selected, the consequences are serious.

PATIENT TEACHING RELATED TO DRUG THERAPY

It is imperative to provide detailed information to the patient and/or a responsible family member about epilepsy and drug therapy. Side effects and signs of toxicity should be discussed. The patient must understand that the drug must be taken as ordered *every day*. The most common cause of seizures in persons who have previously been controlled is failure to take the AEDs. The person should be asked to maintain a drug chart of time, amount taken, and side effects along with a record of the frequency and characteristics of any seizures.

Because seizures represent a chronic condition in that they are usually not completely arrested, the person must understand the nature of the problem, the precipitating factors, and the adaptations in lifestyle that are required.

The following is an outline of the major points of a drug teaching plan:

- The drug must be taken as ordered to maintain a therapeutic blood level, even if there is no seizure activity.
- Anticonvulsant drugs may be necessary for a few years or longer; for some, they may be necessary for a lifetime. There are criteria for when and how a trial of drug discontinuation should be managed; discuss this with the health care provider.
- Discontinuation of drugs is the most common cause of seizure activity; this should not be done.
- Know the signs of toxicity of the drugs prescribed. Symptoms of toxicity should be reported promptly to the physician.
- Keep a drug and seizure chart and bring it with you for your appointment.

- Because there are serious side effects from some drugs, be sure to have any blood work done that has been ordered (*e.g.*, CBC of anemia and blood dyscrasias).
- Because phenytoin is absorbed slowly from the gastrointestinal tract, daily drug schedules can be adjusted for convenience. Missed doses can be "made up" safely.
- Some may enjoy seizure control with the use of extended-release phenytoin allowing once-a-day dosing; discuss this with your health care provider.
- A Medic Alert bracelet or a card should be carried to indicate a chronic condition. The patient is encouraged to carry a card that indicates that he or she is being treated by a particular physician. If the patient is found unconscious or injured, the physician can be notified.
- Keep follow-up appointments with a health provider for periodic monitoring and reevaluation.
- Status epilepticus can be precipitated by abrupt withdrawal of anticonvulsant drugs.

Special Populations: Women and the Elderly

Two patient populations that have unique needs when discussing epilepsy and seizure disorder are women and the elderly.

WOMEN

Some of the special needs of women are included in the teaching plan in Chart 31-2. Women who have a seizure disorder need anticipatory guidance about contraception and the implications of childbearing. The effectiveness of oral contraceptives appears to be decreased by AEDs, which induce liver enzymes and increase the rate of metabolism. A sign of ineffectiveness of the oral contraceptive is breakthrough bleeding; an oral contraceptive with a higher estrogen content needs to be taken.

For women on AEDs who wish to become pregnant, a discussion with the physician is helpful, as is dispelling myths and discussing the effects of teratogenicity from many of the AEDs on the fetus. There is evidence that there is a doubling of the rate of malformations in babies born to mothers who are taking AEDs. Further, it may be dose related. A combination of AEDs, especially carbamazepine, phenytoin, and valproate, causes a much higher risk of neural tube defects.[25] The question arises as what should be done about AEDs if a woman wants to become pregnant. There is no simple answer. The variables include the particular drugs and dosage involved and the severity of the seizure disorder. For some women, discontinuation of the AEDs may be an option. This is a decision that should be made after careful discussion with the physician. Once a woman is pregnant, it does no good to discontinue the AEDs.

During pregnancy, many women notice a change in their seizure patterns which is unpredictable. There is an increased risk of complications during pregnancy, delivery, and the postpartum period, thus requiring close collaborative management of the woman between the neurologist or primary care physician and the obstetrician. If breast feed-

CHART 31-2
Components of a Teaching Plan for Persons With Epilepsy or a Seizure Disorder

Diet/Nutrition/Beverages

- Eat a well-balanced diet; eat on a routine schedule.
- Avoid excesses of sugar, caffeine, or any other food that may trigger seizures.
- Discuss alcohol consumption with your doctor; if you choose to drink, limit your consumption to whatever your physician recommends. Seizures may be precipitated by alcohol consumption, and even small amounts may trigger a seizure in some persons.

General Health

- Any of the following can trigger seizures in some persons and should be avoided: constipation; excessive fatigue; hyperventilation; and stress.
- Regular exercise is good for general well being and stress reduction. Avoid over-fatigue and hyperventilation. Avoid exercise in hot weather; exercise in a climate-controlled environment.
- Regular sleep patterns on a regular schedule are important. Insomnia or awakening tired are indications of insufficient sleep. This may be due to stress, poor sleep hygiene, or a side effect of medication. Determine cause of sleep disturbance and correct it or seek assistance from the health care provider.
- Showers, rather than tub baths, should be taken.
- Good oral hygiene and periodic visits to the dentist are important because gingival hyperplasia can occur from some antiepileptic drugs (AEDs) such as phenytoin.

Fever and Illness

- Fever can trigger seizures; the fever and underlying cause must be treated.
- Any prescription or over-the-counter drugs should be reviewed for interaction.
- If antibiotics are ordered, interactions with the AEDs should be evaluated.

Environmental, Occupational, and Recreational Risk Factors

- Noisy environments should be avoided; control a noisy environment with ear plugs or a portable radio/cassette player with earphones.
- Avoid bright, flashing lights or fluorescent lights, strobe lights, discos, a flickering television, and flashing bulbs on signs or Christmas trees. Tinted glass on the windshield and eyeglasses will help to control glare.
- Use a screen filter on the computer screen to control glare.
- Do not use recreational or street drugs.
- Work or recreational activities that could cause injury if a seizure occurred should be avoided.
- Swim with a "buddy"; help should be available if a seizure occurs.
- Contact sports (*e.g.,* football, boxing) that could lead to unconsciousness should be avoided.

Stress, Anxiety, and Depression

- Emotional stress is a trigger to seizures; measures need to be taken to uncover the basis for the stress and how this can be decreased. Counseling may be helpful.
- Living with a chronic health problem is stressful and can place a varying degree of limitations on lifestyle. Depression may result. Appropriate psychotherapy through counseling and/or drugs should be provided.

Women's Health

- There may be an increase in seizures around the time of menses. This should be discussed with your health care provider; some adjustment may be made in your medications.
- If the occurrence of seizures increases around the menses, control other triggers for seizures.
- AEDs decrease the effectiveness of oral contraceptives; intrauterine devices or other contraceptive devices may be preferred.
- The seizure pattern often changes during pregnancy; discuss this with your health care provider.
- Some AEDs can cause birth defects. If pregnancy is planned, it should be discussed with the gynecologist and health care provider following the epilepsy.

(continued)

CHART 31-2 Components of a Teaching Plan for Persons With Epilepsy or a Seizure Disorder (Continued)

Legislation to Protect Persons With Epilepsy and Seizure Disorder

The following laws protect persons with epilepsy or seizure disorders from discrimination:

- Americans With Disabilities Act
- Rehabilitation Act
- Individuals With Disabilities Education Act

- *Legal Rights of Persons with Epilepsy* (1992) is published by the Epilepsy Foundation of America and is a good resource about epilepsy and the law.
- Driver's licenses are controlled by individual states; information on the laws governing driving can be obtained from the Division of Motor Vehicles.

Other

- Issues related to marriage, childbearing, and parenting need to be discussed. Risk factors and questions related to children having epilepsy need a frank discussion.

---

ing is planned, consideration of the effect of the AED on breast milk needs to be addressed. For details of management, other sources should be consulted.

THE ELDERLY

The highest incidence of new onset of epilepsy in a population other than children under the age of 5 years is noted in the 65-year-old and older age group.[26] The risk factors associated with the increased incidence in this group include stroke, head trauma, dementia, infection, alcoholism, and aging. Of these, stroke that is associated with paresis and cortical involvement is the leading risk factor for the development of epilepsy in the elderly.[27] Although generalized tonic–clonic seizures are easily recognizable, simple and complex seizures may pose a more difficult problem because of the subtle symptoms and other competing diagnoses. The differential diagnosis includes transient ischemic attacks, syncope, drop attacks, transient global amnesia, psychiatric disorders, and sleep disorders.[28]

To make a diagnosis of a seizure disorder and epilepsy, nurses and physicians first have to recognize it as a possibility when evaluating older patients. Raising a level of suspicion will assist the health provider in collecting a detailed history from the person and family member and conducting a complete physical and neurological examination. In addition, computed tomography or magnetic resonance imaging and an EEG may be useful. It is noteworthy that a normal EEG does not necessarily exclude the diagnosis of epilepsy. An EEG with stresses such as sleep deprivation increases the possibility of observing epileptiform abnormalities. Focal or diffuse slowing on EEG may be seen in older persons without being an indicator of epilepsy. Of interest are EEG findings known as periodic lateralized epileptiform discharges (PLEDs). **PLEDs** are abnormal interictal EEG wave patterns characterized by paroxysmal, sharp wave complexes suggestive of an underlying *focal* seizure disorder.[29]

Treatment depends on the underlying diagnosis and choosing the right AED for the seizure type. In choosing an AED for an elderly person, several points should be considered:

1. The pharmacokinetics (absorption, distribution, metabolism, and excretion) are altered in the elderly due to hematological, renal, and liver function changes. Before ordering any AEDs, CBC, clotting factors, albumin, liver function studies, and creatinine values should be evaluated to determine the effect of the AED on the person.
2. Many older people are on a number of drugs for chronic health problems such as cardiac and respiratory problems. Consider drug interactions when choosing an AED.
3. Consider the effect of the drug on cognitive function and balance and how it will affect daily living and patient safety.
4. Consider cost. If the drug is too expensive for the person, compliance will not be maintained.
5. Begin with AED monotherapy starting at a low dose and titrating slowly to seizure control or toxicity. Monitor the patient for side effects such as folate deficiency with phenytoin. Free AED concentrations should be measured in any patient with renal or liver dysfunction who has signs of toxicity when in the therapeutic range.

Lannon's article provides details of management of seizures in the elderly.[30]

Long-Term Management of Persons With Epilepsy

Long-term management and periodic reevaluation are necessary with any chronic condition. All drugs have side effects and toxicity, so the patient must be monitored for signs of toxicity. Medication may need to be adjusted or changed. Periodic reevaluation provides the opportunity for assessment of emotional, psychological, social, and vocational problems that are apt to develop as the patient adjusts to living with a seizure disorder.

References

1. Hauser, W. A., & Hesdorffer, D. C. (1990). *Facts about epilepsy.* New York: Epilepsy Foundation of America.

2. Commission on Classification and Terminology of the International League Against Epilepsy. (1989). Proposal for revised classification of epilepsies and epileptic syndromes. *Epilepsia, 30*(4), 389–399.

3. DeLorenzo, R. J. (1991). The epilepsies. In W. G. Bradleu, R. B. Daroff, G. M. Fenichel, & C. D. Marsden (Eds.). *Neurology in clinical practice: The neurological disorders* (Vol. II) (p. 1462). Boston: Butterworth-Heinemann.

4. Commission of Classification and Terminology of the International League Against Epilepsy. (1981). Proposal for revised clinical and electroencephalographic classification of epileptic seizures. *Epilepsia, 22*, 489–501.

5. Commission of Classification and Terminology of the International League Against Epilepsy. (1981). Proposal for revised clinical and electroencephalographic classification of epileptic seizures. *Epilepsia, 22*, 493–494.

6. Working Groups on Status Epilepticus. (1993). Treatment of convulsive status epilepticus: Recommendations of the Epilepsy Foundation of America's Working Group on Status Epilepticus. *JAMA, 270*, 854–859.

7. Treiman, D. M., & Delgado-Escueta, A. V. (1980). Status epilepticus. In R. S. Thompson & J. R. Green (Eds). *Critical care of neurological and neurosurgical emergencies* (pp. 53–99). New York, Raven.

8. Gumnit, R. J. (1995). *The epilepsy handbook: The practical management of seizures* (2nd ed.). New York: Raven, pp. 124–127.

9. DeLorenzo, R. J. (1991). The epilepsies. In W. G. Bradleu, R. B. Daroff, G. M. Fenichel, & C. D. Marsden (Eds.). *Neurology in clinical practice: The neurological disorders* (Vol. II). Boston: Butterworth-Heinemann, p. 1455.

10. Garnett, W. R. (1993). Seizures. In J. T. DiPiro, R. L. Talbert, P. E. Hayes, G. C. Yee, G. R. Matzke, & L. M. Posey (Eds.), *Pharmacotherapy: A pathophysiologic approach* (2nd ed.) (pp. 883–899). Norwalk, CT: Appleton & Lange.

11. Ibid., p. 884.

12. Gamnit, op. cit., p. 26.

13. Garnett, op. cit., pp. 884–885.

14. Ibid., pp. 886–887.

15. Ibid., p. 890.

16. Ojemann, G. A., & Silbergerld, D. L. (1993). Approaches to epilepsy surgery. *Neurosurgery Clinics of North America, 4*(2), 184.

17. NIH Consensus Conference: Surgery for epilepsy. (1990). *JAMA, 264*, 729–733.

18. Ibid., p. 731.

19. Pilcher, W. H., & Rusyniak, W. G. (1993). Complications of epilepsy surgery. *Neurosurgery Clinics of North America, 4*(2), 312.

20. Treiman, D. M., & Delgado-Escueta, A. V. (1980). In R. A. Thompson & J. R. Green (Eds.), *Critical care of neurological and neurosurgical emergencies* (pp. 53–99). New York: Raven.

21. Hauser, W. A. (1990). Status epilepticus: Epidemiologic considerations. *Neurology, 40*(Suppl.), 9–13.

22. Working Group on Status Epilepticus, op. cit., p. 854.

23. Ibid., p. 856.

24. Shafer, R. O. (1994). Nursing support of epilepsy self-management. *Clinical Nursing Practice in Epilepsy, 2*(1), 5–6.

25. Gamnit, p. 62–64.

26. Lannon, S. (1993). Epilepsy in the elderly. *Journal of Neuroscience Nursing, 25*(5), 273–282.

27. Olsen, T. S., Hogenhaven, H., & Thage, O. (1987). Epilepsy after stroke. *Neurology, 37*(7), 1209–1211.

28. Drury, I., & Beydoun, A. (1993). Seizure disorders of aging: Differential diagnosis and patient management. *Geriatrics, 48*(5), 52–58.

29. Lannon, op. cit., p. 275.

30. Ibid.

Bibliography

Books

Adams, R. D., & Victor, M. (1993). *Principles of neurology* (5th ed.). New York: McGraw-Hill.

DiPiro, J. T., Talbert, R. L., Hayes, P. E., Yee, G. C., Matzke, G. R., & Posey. L. M. (Eds.). (1993). *Pharmacotherapy: A pathophysiologic approach* (2nd ed.). Norwalk, CT: Appleton & Lange.

Engel, J. (1986). *Surgical treatment of the epilepsies.* New York: Raven.

Engel, J. (1989). *Seizures, epilepsy, and the epileptic patient. Vol. 31. Contemporary neurology series.* Philadelphia: F. A. Davis.

Gumnit, R. J. (1995). *The epilepsy handbook: The practical management of seizures* (2nd ed.). New York: Raven.

Periodicals

Dichter, M. A., & Brodie, M. J. (1996). New antiepileptic drugs. *New England Journal of Medicine 334*(24), 1583–1590.

Dupuis, R. E., & Miranda-Massari, J. (1991). Anticonvulsants: Pharmacotherapeutic issues in the critically ill patient. *AACN Clinical Issues in Critical Care Nursing, 2*(4), 639–656.

Lannon, S. L. (1993). Epilepsy in the elderly. *Journal of Neuroscience Nursing, 25*(5), 273–282.

Ojemann, G. A., & Silbergerld, D. L. (1993). Approaches to epilepsy surgery. *Neurosurgery Clinics of North America, 4*(2), 183–191.

Ozuna, J. (1993). Nursing diagnoses in epilepsy: Guidelines for reassessment. *Clinical Nursing Practice in Epilepsy, 1*(1), 11–14.

Ozuna, J. (1994). Nursing assessment of complex partial seizures. *Clinical Nursing Practice in Epilepsy, 2*(1), 4–6.

Pilcher, W. H., & Rusyniak, W. G. (1993). Complications of epilepsy surgery. *Neurosurgery Clinics of North America, 4*(2), 311–325.

Rose, B. A. (1993). Neurologic therapies in critical care. *Critical Care Nursing Clinics of North America, 5*(2), 237–246.

Santilli, N. (1993). The spectrum of epilepsy. *Clinical Nursing Practice in Epilepsy, 1*(1), 4–7, 14.

Santilli, N. (1994). Seizurelike phenomena in children and young adults. *Clinical Nursing Practice in Epilepsy, 2*(1), 7–10.

Shafer, R. O. (1994). Nursing support of epilepsy self-management. *Clinical Nursing Practice in Epilepsy. 2*(1), 5–6.

Working Group on Status Epilepticus. (1993). Treatment of convulsive status epilepticus: Recommendations of the Epilepsy Foundation Of America's Working Group on Status Epilepticus. *JAMA, 270*(7), 854–859.

CHAPTER 32

Selected Infections of the Nervous System

Joanne V. Hickey

Of the many infectious diseases that can affect the central nervous system (CNS), only the most common problems are addressed in this chapter. Infections included are bacterial meningitis, viral encephalitis, and the parameningeal infections of brain abscess and extradural abscess. Other selected nervous system infections are presented in tabular format. Chapter 33 focuses entirely on acquired immunodeficiency syndrome (AIDS).

NOSOCOMIAL INFECTIONS

A **nosocomial infection** is defined as an infection occurring during hospitalization that was not present or incubating at the time of admission. The current nationwide rate of nosocomial infections is about 5%, but the rate is much higher in critical care areas. Although the hospital infection control department has the overall responsibility for the control of infections, this goal cannot be accomplished without the diligent cooperation of every hospital employee.

The single most important method of controlling infections is through preventive measures. The advent of universal precautions in health care facilities is a comprehensive approach to prevent contamination and the spread of organisms that can lead to illness. There are a number of treatment situations that make the neuroscience patient population particularly vulnerable to infections. First, some drug and treatment regimens have the side effect of immunosuppression. Steroid drugs (*e.g.*, dexamethasone) are frequently ordered to decrease cerebral edema. These potent corticosteroids contribute to immunosuppression in the patient. Other patients receive radiation therapy and chemotherapy for the treatment of neoplasms and conditions such as multiple sclerosis. These treatment modalities are known to immunosuppress the patient.

Second, a number of multitrauma patients receive potent antibiotics that decrease flora normally present in the gastrointestinal (GI) tract, predisposing the patient to secondary infections. Moreover, a number of critically ill neuroscience patients are admitted to intensive care units (ICUs) where invasive monitoring (*e.g.*, ICP monitor) and tubes (*e.g.*, ventriculostomy, indwelling catheters) are used. These situations also put the patient at high risk for infections. Finally, some neuroscience patients have a poor nutritional status related to chronic debilitating conditions, such as advanced stages of brain tumors, chronic vegetative state, or stroke. The generalized debilitated condition is a another risk factor for infections.

The nurse plays an important role by decreasing risk factors for nosocomial infections and by following universal precautions, including meticulous handwashing technique. In addition, baseline assessment and monitoring for signs and symptoms of infection are an integral part of nursing management. Immunosuppressed patients do not demonstrate the cardinal signs and symptoms of infection, such as significant elevations in temperature and elevated white blood cell (WBC) counts. Therefore, the nurse must learn to observe for more subtle signs of infection.

CAUSATIVE ORGANISMS

Route of Entry

For any organism to affect the body, an appropriate route of entry for the specific organism must be available. In CNS infections, the routes of entry include the blood stream; direct extension from a primary site; cerebrospinal fluid (CSF); extension along cranial and peripheral nerves; the mouth and nasopharynx; and in utero.

Blood Stream. Perhaps the most common route by which infectious microorganisms reach the CNS is the blood stream. Microorganisms may enter the blood stream as a result of insect bites, spread of infection from primary foci (middle ear infection, mastoiditis, sinusitis, cellulitis), or infection associated with congenital anomalies, such as myelomeningocele.

Direct Extension From a Primary Site. Fracture of the frontal or facial bones may result in seepage of infectious contents, thereby causing contamination of the CNS. Any compound cranial fracture that creates direct communication between the sterile intracranial area and the outside environment is a prime source for infection. Thus, aggressive treatment with antibiotics is absolutely necessary to prevent infection.

Cerebrospinal Fluid. Dural tearing as a result of injury can create a connection between the CSF and the ear or nose. Drainage of fluid from either of these areas is referred to as *otorrhea* and *rhinorrhea,* respectively. If microorganisms are directly extended into the CSF, a major CNS infection develops rapidly. Poor sterile technique during a lumbar puncture or spinal surgery can also contaminate the CSF.

Extension Along Cranial and Spinal Nerves. Some microorganisms reach the CNS by following the peripheral nerves. Rabies is an example of such a disease.

Mouth and Nasopharynx. Certain organisms are transmitted by oral and nasopharyngeal secretions, especially when people are in close contact. An example of a CNS infection transmitted in this way is meningococcal meningitis.

In Utero. The fetus in utero is also subject to CNS infections from the following possible causes: contaminated amniotic fluid from amniocentesis; massive maternal infection that is transmitted across the placenta; viruses, such as rubella or other microorganisms that cross the placental barrier; and microorganisms that come in contact with the fetus as it passes through the vaginal canal. The newborn infant is also subject to contamination of the postnatal environment with organisms that proliferate in the moist, warm environment of an incubator.

Need for Isolation

The need to place a patient on isolation precautions to prevent the spread of disease depends on the type of invading organism and the stage of the illness. For example, in the acute phase of meningococcal meningitis, it is possible to infect others with secretions from the nasopharynx and droplets from the respiratory tract. Meningococci usually disappear within 24 hours of administration of appropriate antimicrobial drugs. Therefore, isolation of the patient to protect the nursing and health care personnel, visitors, and other patients should be maintained until cultures are negative. The hospital infection control department is the best source of information about conditions requiring isolation and specific points regarding type and duration of isolation.

MENINGITIS

Bacterial Meningitis

CAUSES

The most common causes of bacterial meningitis depend on the age of the patient. In newborns, *Streptococcus agalactiae* (Group B), gram-negative bacilli, and *Listeria monocytogenes* are the most common etiologies. In children, the organisms *Hemophilus influenzae, Neisseria meningitidis,* and *Streptococcus pneumoniae* are the organisms usually responsible. As patients get older, *Streptococcus pneumoniae* becomes a more common cause (Table 32-1).

Most bacteria capable of causing bacterial meningitis reach the meninges by way of the blood stream or by extension from cranial structures, such as the paranasal sinuses or the ear. Bacteria can also enter from penetrating head wounds and skull fractures. In many cases, the three major organisms causing bacterial meningitis in children and adults are inhabitants of the nasopharynx. Under conditions not clearly understood, these organisms can enter the blood stream and localize themselves in the meninges. Incidence is fairly constant throughout the seasons with the exception of summer, at which time a decrease in incidence is noted.

PATHOPHYSIOLOGY

Bacterial meningitis is a pyogenic (purulent or suppurative) infection that involves the pia-arachnoid layers of the meninges and the subarachnoid space, including CSF. Because the CSF circulates around the brain and spinal cord, the inflammation spreads quickly. When the ventricles are involved, the accumulation of exudate upon the choroid plexus causes hydrocephalus, and the arachnoid villi become plugged, causing obstruction to CSF absorption.

Initially, when bacteria invade the pia-arachnoid and subarachnoid spaces, the blood supply to the involved area increases rapidly. Neutrophils soon migrate into the subarachnoid space in massive numbers and engulf the bacteria. These phagocytic cells rapidly degenerate and disintegrate, combining with the exudate from tissue destruction to form purulent material within the subarachnoid space. The exudate increases, particularly over the base of the brain, extending into the sheaths of cranial and spinal nerves and even into the perivascular spaces of the cortex. The introduction into the perivascular space leads to a slight encephalitis.

The cortical vessels, especially the veins, become dilated and congested. If the inflammation extends through the walls of the veins (vasculitis), thrombosis or necrosis with possible hemorrhage often develops. Arterial changes within the small and medium vessels of the subarachnoid space begin to occur early in the infection. The irritation from the bacteria and toxins causes swelling and an increase in endothelial cells. Neutrophils and lymphocytes migrate between the layers of the vessel, with resulting fibrotic changes.

In the acute phase of meningitis, the cerebral cortex undergoes little change except for perivascular inflammation with some infiltration into the cortex. In subacute cases, there may be diffuse degenerative changes, with necrosis and glial proliferation within the superficial areas of the brain, spinal cord, or cranial nerves. The optic and acoustic nerves are often affected, although the oculomotor, trochlear, abducens, and facial nerves can also be involved. With meningitis, there is often an associated encephalitis.

The resolution of the meningitis depends on how extensive the infection is and how quickly effective treatment is initiated. If the process is arrested early, resolution may be complete, without any major sequelae. However, fibrotic changes of the arachnoid layer can cause fibrosis and scar

TABLE 32-1
*Causative Organisms of Bacterial Meningitis**

DISEASE	ORGANISM	COMMENTS
Pneumococcal meningitis	*Streptococcus pneumoniae* (gram-positive diplococci)	• Found in the young and those over 40 years of age • Most common meningitis occurring in adults • Predisposing conditions to pneumococcal meningitis include penumonia, sinuistis, alcoholism, head trauma, splenectomy, and sickle cell anemia.
Haemophilus influenzae meningitis	*Haemophilus influenzae* (gram-negative cocci)	• Pediatric problem seen in those 3 months to 8 years of age (6 to 8 months, highest incidence) • Often follows upper respiratory or ear infections
Meningococcal meningitis	*Neisseria meningitidis* (gram-negative diplococci)	• Highest incidence in children and young adults • Petechial rash, purpuric lesions, or ecchymosis develop in 50% of patients. • About 10% of affected patients develop a fulminating infection with overwhelming septicemia (meningococcemia); this can create a medical emergency owing to high fever, purpuric lesions, and circulatory collapse from adrenocortical insufficiency secondary to hemorrhage and necrosis of the adrenals (called Waterhouse–Friderichsen syndrome); disseminated intravascular coagulation may also be evident; death can result hours after onset.
Other less common diseases	*Staphylococcus aureus* Streptococcus group A Streptococcus group B ⎫ *Escherichia coli* ⎤ ⎬ Klebsiella ⎪ ⎭ Proteus ⎬ Pseudomonas ⎦	• Common in neonates • Often introduced during neurosurgical procedures (especially shunting), lumbar puncture, or spinal anesthesia; seen often in hospitalized neurosurgical patients; head-injured patients, particularly those with cerebrospinal fluid rhinorrhea; or debilitated patients.
	Myobacterium tuberculosis	• Secondary infection due to bacterial seeding of the meninges from tuberculosis elsewhere in the body • Most common in children • Incidence reflects the rate of tuberculosis in a country (relatively low in the United States)
	Listeria monocytogenes Salmonella ⎤ Shigella ⎪ Clostridium ⎬ Gonococcus ⎦	• Seen in neonates, the aged, and the immunosuppressed • Rare

* The organisms presented here are responsible for 80% to 90% of the cases of bacterial meningitis worldwide; these organisms are normally found in the nasopharynx of a significant portion of the population. The mechanism by which they cause illness in some people, but not others, is unclear.

tissue formation. Adhesions and effusions can develop in the subarachnoid space, thereby interfering with the normal circulation of CSF. Fibrotic changes in the structures responsible for the production and absorption of CSF may result, contributing to the development of hydrocephalus. Some organisms may produce abscesses. Much of the outcome from bacterial meningitis depends on early and aggressive treatment to prevent the development of the various complications.

SIGNS AND SYMPTOMS

Although many different organisms are capable of producing meningitis, common signs and symptoms are shared by all. In infants and very young children, many of the characteristic signs and symptoms may not be present or may be nonspecific. In such instances, diagnosis can be very difficult. Common symptoms of meningitis in young children include fever, anorexia, vomiting, diarrhea, listlessness, a shrill cry, and bulging fontanels.

In the older child and the adult, the following symptoms are noted:

• Headache
• Fever
• Deterioration in the level of consciousness (LOC)
• Signs of meningeal irritation
• Generalized convulsions
• Increased ICP
• Cranial nerve dysfunction
• Endocrine disorders
• Others (hypersensitivity, hyperalgesia, muscle hypotonia)

Headache and Fever. The headache, which is usually the initial symptom, is described as very severe. This symptom is probably attributable to irritation of the pain-sensitive dura and traction on related vascular structures.

Fever is the rule with bacterial meningitis, and can vary from 38° C to 39.5° C (101° F to 103° F) or higher. The temperature remains high throughout the course of the illness, and can rise to 40.5° C (105° F) and higher in the terminal stages because of decompensation of increased intracranial pressure (ICP) on the brain stem.

Changes in the Level of Consciousness. In the very early stages, a shortened attention span and misinterpretation of environmental stimuli are common. The patient becomes disoriented to time, place, and person, is easily bewildered, has poor memory, and appears to have difficulty following commands. Other patients may become restless, agitated, irritable, and disoriented. The patient is often noisy and combative and is sometimes fearful of personal harm as a result of misinterpretation of environmental stimuli. As the course of the illness progresses, a deterioration in the level of consciousness develops. Affected patients are drowsy, lethargic, and generally unresponsive, except to repeated stimulation. If they speak, they are not coherent. They gradually become more unresponsive and lapse into a deep coma.

Signs of Meningeal Irritation. A stiff neck is an early sign of meningeal irritation. Attempts to flex the neck forward, either actively or passively, prove difficult. This resistance is caused by spasms of the extensor muscles of the neck. Forceful flexion produces severe pain. The extensor position may be so exaggerated that the patient may assume the opisthotonus position in bed.

Two additional signs of meningeal irritation are Kernig's and Brudzinski's signs. **Kernig's sign** is elicited by flexing the upper leg at the hip to a 90-degree angle and then attempting to extend the knee. In the presence of meningitis, there is pain and spasm of the hamstrings when an attempt is made to extend the knee (Fig. 32-1). The pain is caused by inflammation of the meninges and spinal roots. The spasms are a protective mechanism to deter painful flexion. **Brudzinski's sign** is positive when both the upper leg at the hip and the lower leg at the knee flex in response to passive flexion of the neck and head on the chest. This reflex is caused by irritating exudate around the roots in the lumbar region. Photophobia is also a common sign of bacterial meningitis, but the pathophysiology for this symptom is not clear.

Generalized Convulsions. Development of generalized seizures indicates irritation of the cerebral cortex. Following a seizure, transitory paralysis may be noted. A focal motor seizure may be evident if there is an accumulation of exudate over one cortical convexity.

Increased Intracranial Pressure. Increased ICP accompanies meningitis because of purulent exudate, cerebral edema, and hydrocephalus. Papilledema, a sign of increased ICP, is rare with an acute attack of meningitis. If it is apparent, it is most often associated with a brain abscess or venous sinus occlusion. Symptoms of brain stem pressure are reflected in vital sign changes, such as widening of pulse pressure, decreased pulse, and ataxic respirations. Vomiting is a frequent finding. If the infection is not aggressively treated or response to treatment is poor, cerebral herniation can occur.

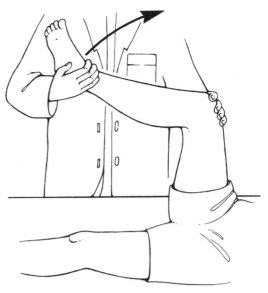

FIGURE 32-1
Testing for Kernig's sign.

Cranial Nerve Dysfunction. Inflammation or vascular changes can cause cranial nerve dysfunction. The major deficits are ocular palsies (involving cranial nerves III, IV, and VI), facial paresis (cranial nerve VII), and deafness and vertigo (caused by involvement of cranial nerve VIII). Pupils are often unequal and sluggishly responsive to light. If the patient's condition deteriorates, the pupils will become dilated and fixed. Other eye symptoms that relate to cranial nerve dysfunction are ptosis and diplopia.

Endocrine Disorders. A small percentage of patients develop hyponatremia (a decrease in serum sodium) and excessive release of the antidiuretic hormone. There are signs and symptoms of water retention, along with oliguria and hypervolemia. ICP is further increased by this situation. Limiting water intake is part of management.

Other Signs. Other signs and symptoms noted include skin hypersensitivity, hyperalgesia, and muscular hypotonia, although motor function is well preserved. Sensory loss does not occur. Toxic effects on the brain or thrombosis of the vascular supply to a cerebral area can cause permanent disability of cerebral function. If such pathological changes do occur, examples of deficits might include hemiparesis, dementia, and paralysis.

One specific complication of meningococcal meningitis should be mentioned. There is a phase of meningococcemia often noted before the meningitis is evident or diagnosed. The combination of signs during this period is referred to as **Waterhouse-Friderichsen syndrome** and includes the following: chills, fever, headache, malaise, and possible joint and muscle pain; petechial hemorrhage or ecchymosis noted on the skin and mucous membranes; and possible adrenal hemorrhage resulting in adrenal insufficiency followed by hypotension, cyanosis, respiratory distress, and circulatory collapse. If this occurs, immediate administration of adrenal corticosteroids is necessary to avoid death.

DIAGNOSIS AND TREATMENT

The diagnosis of bacterial meningitis is based on a history and physical examination, along with laboratory data. In gathering a history, recent infections, such as those involving the ears, sinuses, or respiratory tract, are of particular interest.

Data gathered from lumbar puncture and CSF analysis are vital for accurate diagnosis. Table 32-2 includes the basic CSF criteria for diagnosis of bacterial meningitis and compares these findings with those associated with aseptic (viral) meningitis. Methods of identifying the specific causative organisms include gram stain, smear, or culture. Other laboratory findings that may be of diagnostic value include a blood culture and nose and throat cultures. Radiographs of the patient's chest, skull, and sinuses should be taken for the purpose of noting infection, abscess formations, or fractures. Once the diagnosis of bacterial meningitis is ascertained, treatment is directed at general supportive measures, antibacterial drug therapy, and recognition and management of complications.

General supportive measures include maintaining adequate ventilation and a patent airway, maintaining fluid and electrolyte balance, instituting hypothermia management, and controlling seizures and headache. Because antibacterial drug therapy should not be delayed to obtain final CSF culture results, such therapy is usually directed at the most likely organisms based primarily on the patient's age. For example, newborns, older adults (older than 50 years of age), or immunosuppressed adults will usually be presumptively treated with ampicillin (200 mg/kg per day intravenously [IV]) and cefotaxime (200 mg/kg per day IV). Older children and adults less than 50 years of age can be treated with cefotaxime alone. Patients with meningitis after a craniotomy are usually treated with vancomycin (1 g q 6 hours IV). Antimicrobial therapy is then refined to the drug most effective against the invading organism once it is identified. Dosage will depend on the age of the patient. The administration of dexamethasone (0.15 mg/kg) in infants and children immediately prior to the first dose of cefotaxime has been shown to be beneficial.[1]

COMPLICATIONS

The complications of bacterial meningitis relate to the type of causative organism and the severity of the illness. Postmeningitis sequelae include visual impairment, optic neuritis, deafness, personality change, headache, seizure activity, paresis or paralysis, hydrocephalus, pneumonia, and endocarditis.

PREVENTION

Often, bacterial meningitis can be prevented if the following principles are observed:

- Provide adequate treatment of infections, such as sinusitis, mastoiditis, ear infections, and pneumonias
- Maintain strict aseptic technique during all intracranial, intraspinal, mastoid, and sinus operations
- Maintain strict aseptic technique in dressing changes for these procedures
- Administer prophylactic antibiotics after these procedures
- Administer prophylactic antibiotics with basal skull fractures, compound skull fractures, dural tears, and injuries causing CSF drainage from the ear or nose

Viral Meningitis

Viral meningitis is also known as *acute benign lymphocytic meningitis* and *acute aseptic meningitis*. Any number of viruses, such as mumps, can cause symptoms that correspond to those of meningitis caused by bacteria and other organisms. Viral meningitis is not usually fatal and occurs sporadically or as small epidemics. All age groups are susceptible, but children are most often affected.

SIGNS AND SYMPTOMS

Signs and symptoms include those of the meningitis syndrome, such as headache, fever, and signs of meningeal irri-

---

TABLE 32-2
Comparison of the Classic Cerebrospinal Fluid Findings in Acute Bacterial Meningitis and Acute Aseptic (Viral) Meningitis

CSF CHARACTERISTICS	ACUTE BACTERIAL MENINGITIS*	ACUTE ASEPTIC (VIRAL) MENINGITIS
Appearance	Turbid, cloudy	Clear; sometimes turbid
Cells	Increased white blood cells (1,000 to 2,000 mm^3 or more; mostly polymorphonuclear neutrophils)	Increased white blood cells (300 mm^3; mostly mononuclear)
Protein level	Increased (100 to 500 mg/dL)	Normal or slightly increased
Glucose level	Decreased (<40 mg/dL or about 40% of blood glucose level)	Normal
Smear and culture	Bacterial present on gram stain and culture	No bacteria present on gram stain or culture; the virus may be demonstrated by special techniques
Pressure on lumbar puncture	Elevated (>180 mm of water pressure)	Variable

* All patients do not follow this classic profile; about 30% of patients with bacterial meningitis show some of the findings seen in aseptic meningitis.

tation. A major elevation in CSF lymphocytes is noted, as well as lymphocytic infiltration of the pia-arachnoid layers. Often, perivascular infiltration of the brain and spinal cord develops. Because of the similarities in symptoms, a clear-cut distinction between encephalitis and meningitis is not always possible.

DIAGNOSIS AND TREATMENT

Diagnosis corresponds to that of other forms of meningitis. Lymphocytes are the predominant cell in the CSF. The glucose content is also normal, unlike in bacterial meningitis. The protein level is elevated and the CSF is turbid. Treatment of viral meningitis is symptomatic and supportive. No drug therapy is effective against the virus. Complete recovery is usual, although some paralysis and arachnoiditis have been reported.

Nursing Management of Patients With Meningitis

The nursing management of the patient with meningitis, regardless of etiology, is directed toward assessing the patient's condition, providing supportive care and adhering to specific protocols, preventing complications, and enhancing rehabilitation. Within this framework, nursing management can be divided into acute and convalescent phases.

ASSESSMENT

In the acute stage of meningitis, the patient appears to be seriously ill. The vital signs are assessed and are compared with previous recordings in order to detect changes. Rectal temperatures should be taken because the LOC is usually diminished, making an oral thermometer dangerous. It is not uncommon for the temperature to reach 40.5° C (105° F). The pulse and respiratory rate are also high in response to the fever. If signs and symptoms of increased ICP are present, the pulse may be decreased and systolic blood pressure elevated.

Assess neurological signs frequently and compare with previous findings to determine trends. Monitor for signs and symptoms of meningeal irritation. Check the patient for any signs of nuchal rigidity such as stiff neck, photophobia, pain upon neck flexion, or positive Kernig's or Brudzinski's signs. The LOC characteristically deteriorates from confusion to restlessness, lethargy, stupor, and, finally, coma. As the LOC deteriorates, the nurse should take special precautions to prevent injury. Other neurological signs are also monitored.

An accurate intake and output record should be maintained so that the hydration level and kidney function can be assessed. A patient with an elevated temperature can easily become dehydrated from profuse perspiration and insensible loss from the skin. Profuse perspiration, oliguria, and dry skin indicate dehydration that requires IV fluid replacement. Serum electrolytes are monitored daily for electrolyte imbalances, such as hyponatremia.

Because hydrocephalus is a common complication with meningitis, observe for the following signs and symptoms: deterioration in the LOC, a gradual increase in ICP, incontinence,

dementia, and gait disturbances. The signs and symptoms of hydrocephalus may not occur until after the acute phase has subsided.

NURSING MANAGEMENT

The key points of nursing management of patients with meningitis, as well as the nursing diagnoses appropriate for these patients, are presented in Charts 32-1 and 32-2.

REHABILITATION

The specific rehabilitative needs of the patient depend on the degree of functional disability resulting from meningitis. Minor functional disabilities may not require any special intervention because they will reverse themselves with time. Other functional deficits require an aggressive rehabilitation plan. A comprehensive assessment by the interdisciplinary team is the best means for identifying deficits, determining need for rehabilitation, and setting realistic goals. The nurse works collaboratively with the case manager and other team members to assist in the transition to rehabilitation or home.

ENCEPHALITIS

Encephalitis is an inflammation of the brain caused by viruses, bacteria, fungi, or parasites, although viruses are the most common offending organism. Several of the viruses are endemic to particular geographic areas, as well as to seasons of the year. The list of specific viruses known to cause viral encephalitis is lengthy, but there are only a few that appear with any appreciable frequency in the United States. Table 32-3 includes a list and description of the major viruses capable of causing viral encephalitis. Other less frequent causes of encephalitis include toxic substances, such as ingested lead or arsenic or inhaled carbon monoxide; vaccines for measles, mumps, and rabies, which cause postvaccination encephalitis; and viral infections, such as measles, mumps, infectious mononucleosis, and others. The following section will address encephalitis caused by viruses, because viruses are the most common cause of encephalitis in the United States.

Signs and Symptoms

The list of signs and symptoms of viral encephalitis is long, and it varies according to the particular invading organisms and the area of the brain involved. The basic syndrome of viral encephalitis is characterized by fever, headache, seizures, stiff neck, and a change in the LOC, which varies from disorientation, agitation, restlessness, and short attention span to lethargy or drowsiness, and finally to coma. In addition to the wide diversity of levels of consciousness, the patient may exhibit any combination of the following symptoms: aphasia or mutism; motor deficits such as hemiparesis, involuntary movements (myoclonic), ataxia, nystagmus, ocular paralysis, or facial weakness; or generalized seizures.

Although the basic clinical picture of acute viral encephalitis has been outlined, variations of signs and symptoms are noted with specific groupings of viral organisms that produce

CHART 32-1
Summary of the Nursing Management of Patients With Acute Meningitis/Encephalitis

Nursing Responsibilities	Rationale
Assessment	
• Assess vital signs at frequent intervals.	• Establishes a baseline and provides ongoing data to denote stability, improvement, or deterioration in overall conditions
• Assess neurological signs at frequent intervals.	• Establishes a baseline and provides ongoing data for comparison to determine change
• Assess for signs of meningeal irritation (nuchal rigidity, hyperirritability, hyperalgesia, photophobia).	• Indicates irritation of the covering of the brain and the need for special nursing intervention
• Assess respiratory function (auscultate chest; observe chest movement).	• Alerts the nurse to initiate respiratory support if necessary
Basic Supportive Care	
• Maintain a patent airway. —Position the patient to facilitate drainage. —Suction as necessary.	• Provides for adequate drainage of oral and nasal secretions
• Maintain adequate oxygenation. —Monitor blood gases. —Administer oxygen therapy, as ordered. —Assess the patient for signs and symptoms of dyspnea and cyanosis.	• Provides supplemental oxygen to maintain adequate oxygenation
• Administer basic hygienic care.	• Keeps patient dry and comfortable, especially when diaphoretic
• Provide for mouth care every 2 hours.	• Refreshes and moistens the patient's oral cavity, particularly when the temperature is elevated
• Protect the patient from injury by: —Putting side rails up —Keeping the bed low when the patient is left alone —Observing frequently —Protecting the intravenous site or any tubes	• Prevents physical injury to a patient who has a deteriorated level of consciousness and who is often extremely restless
• If the temperature is elevated, measures should be taken to control the temperature, including: —Administering antipyretic drugs, such as acetaminophen (Tylenol), 650 mg orally or rectally —Removing excess bedclothes —Maintaining a cool room temperature (68°F or 20°C) —Giving tepid baths —Using a hypothermia blanket	• An increase in temperature increases the need for oxygen to support increased metabolism. An elevated temperature also increases ICP.
• Control pain of headache, if present, by: —Elevating the head 30 degrees —Applying an ice cap as necessary —Maintaining a quiet, darkened room —Administering analgesics as necessary (*e.g.,* acetaminophen [Tylenol], 650 mg; or codeine, 15–30 mg q 4 h	• Provides for the patient's comfort and removes a major source of restlessness

(continued)

CHART 32-1 Summary of the Nursing Management of Patients With Acute Meningitis/Encephalitis (Continued)

Nursing Responsibilities	Rationale
• Provide for adequate nutrition. If the patient is not able to tolerate oral intake because of reduced level of consciousness, or if intake is insufficient, the intravenous route will be necessary. —Maintain an intake and output record.	• A patient with an infection and a fever requires additional fluid and calories.
• Monitor laboratory (arterial blood gas levels, electrolytes, creatinine level, osmolalities).	• Provides evidence of the development of complications
• Provide emotional and psychological support to the patient and family.	• The patient and family need emotional support throughout the illness to decrease anxiety and improve their coping skills.

Specific Protocols

• Provide a quiet environment in a darkened room where the patient is maintained on strict bed rest.	• Because the patient with meningitis may be hypersensitive to environmental stimuli such as noise, a quiet environment is provided to eliminate the sensory overload produced by normal environmental noise. The darkened room is necessary to provide a soothing environment, because most patients experience photophobia.
• In the acute stage of meningitis, hyperirritability and hyperalgesia are common. The hyperirritability intensifies the perception of environmental stimuli to such a degree that the sound of running water in the sink is perceived as the noise of Niagara Falls. Touching, even slightly, initiates a startle response. Even the weight of the bed linen is irritating. —Avoid needless stimulation by consolidating nursing activities. —Be careful when touching that the intensity of the stimuli is reduced to the minimal amount necessary to accomplish the required activity. —Loosen any constricting bedclothing. —Adjust the tone of your voice so that it is soft and calm. Communication should be simple and direct. —Control environmental noise. —Control direct light (many patients experience photophobia, making indirect light more comfortable for them).	• Minimizes the effects of hyperirritability and hyperalgesia
• Maintain seizure precautions, which include oral airway; padded side rails; and oropharyngeal suction. (Prophylactic anticonvulsant drugs are routinely ordered.)	• Seizure activity is common in patients with central nervous system infections.
• If seizure activity occurs, a seizure chart should be maintained (see Chap. 31).	• Provides documentation of the frequency, type, and characteristics of seizure activity
• Incorporate nursing protocols to manage the increased intracranial pressure that has resulted from cerebral edema (see Chap. 17).	• Managing increased intracranial pressure is a major responsibility in caring for the patient.

(continued)

CHART 32-1 Summary of the Nursing Management of Patients With Acute Meningitis/Encephalitis (Continued)

Nursing Responsibilities	Rationale
Prevention of Complications	
The duration of the acute and chronic phase of meningitis depends on many variables. However, specific nursing protocols are followed to prevent complications.	
• Provide for skin care every 2 to 4 hours. —If the feverish patient perspires profusely, bed linens may need to be changed to prevent irritation of the skin. —Give special attention to bony prominences.	• Prevents skin breakdown; if unable to change position, lubricate, and inspect the skin
• If the patient is not able to turn spontaneously, turn him or her every 2 hours. —If the patient can follow instructions, facilitate deep breathing exercises every 2 hours.	• Prevents lung congestion, atelectasis, and pneumonia
• Apply elastic hose when maintained on bed rest.	• Improves blood return to the heart and decreases the chances of thrombophlebitis
• Position carefully in good body alignment.	• Prevents development of orthopedic deformities
• Observe for signs of adrenal insufficiency in the patient with meningococcal meningitis (hypotension, respiratory collapse, petichiae).	• Immediate intervention is necessary to preserve the patient's life.

encephalitis. The following is a general summary of specific encephalitis-causing syndromes.

Viral Encephalitis Caused by Arthropod-Borne Viruses

The effects on the brain include degenerative changes in the nerve cells, with scattered areas of inflammation and necrosis. There is also some inflammation of the meninges.

SIGNS AND SYMPTOMS

The clinical picture presented by all arthropod-borne viruses in the United States is essentially the same. In infants, viral encephalitis begins with an acute onset of febrile illness and convulsions. In older children and adults, the onset is gradual and is characterized by a febrile illness, headache, listlessness, drowsiness, and nausea and vomiting for several days. Seizures, confusion and stupor, stiff neck, muscle pain, ataxia, photophobia, and tremors then become apparent. Reflexes are abnormal, and hemiparesis may be present. Residual effects include mental retardation, epilepsy, personality changes with psychosis, dementia, paresis or paralysis, deafness, and blindness.

The mortality rate and the residual effects associated with viral encephalitis from arboviruses vary greatly. Eastern equine encephalitis has a higher mortality rate than the western variety. Approximately 80% to 90% of patients with eastern equine encephalitis develop complications, as opposed to only 5% to 10% of patients with western equine infections.

DIAGNOSIS AND TREATMENT

Diagnosis is based on the clinical picture, rapid serology assays, and CSF analysis. CSF findings often associated with arboviruses include elevated WBC (mononuclear cells), increase in protein, and normal glucose. There is no definitive treatment or drug therapy for viral encephalitis. Treatment is supportive and symptomatic. Drugs often administered include steroids to control cerebral edema, anticonvulsants to prevent seizures, analgesics for headache, and antipyretics to control hyperthermia.

NURSING MANAGEMENT

The nursing management for all patients with viral encephalitis is supportive. The basic points of care are outlined in Charts 32-1 and 32-2.

Herpes Simplex Encephalitis

The most important nonepidemic encephalitis in the United States that affects all age groups is herpes simplex encephalitis. It is caused by herpes simplex virus type 1. Recall that there are two types of herpes simplex virus: type 1, which is associated with the common cold sore and is present in most people in the dormant state, and type 2, which is associated with the sexually transmitted genital disease. The type-2 herpes virus can also cause encephalitis in the neonate, but only if it passes through the birth canal of a mother with a genital herpes infection. Herpes simplex virus type 1, which is responsible for the common herpetic lesions on the oral mucosa, is also capable of producing acute encephalitis in the adult. The

CHART 32-2
Summary of Major Nursing Diagnoses Associated with Meningitis/Encephalitis

Nursing Diagnoses	Nursing Interventions	Expected Outcomes
Pain (headache, backache, photophobia, and neck pain) related to (R/T) swelling of intracranial contents and irritation of pain receptors	• Assess the location, quality, and severity of pain (cognitively impaired patients may not be able to use the visual analog scale [VAS] to rate severity of pain). • Provide comfort measures, such as positioning, turning, and application of cool, wet cloths to the head. • Control direct light; darken the patient's room. • Assess the need for use of prn analgesics and administer medication as necessary. • Monitor the patient's response to pain and analgesics.	• The patient will report relief or amelioration of pain (documented by the VAS, if possible), or will demonstrate signs of enhanced comfort, such as decreased agitation and ability to sleep.
Altered Tissue Perfusion, Cerebral, R/T cerebral edema and increased intracranial pressure (ICP)	• Elevate the head of the bed to a 30 degree angle. • Keep the neck in a neutral position. • Prevent Valsalva's maneuver. • Monitor neurological signs for evidence of neurological deterioration. • If an intracranial pressure (ICP) monitor is in place, monitor cerebral perfusion pressure (CPP). • Monitor blood gas levels. • Use prn measures to support CPP following parameters set by physician.	• If an ICP monitor is in place, CPP will be maintained at > 70 mm Hg pressure. • Neurological signs will reflect stability or improvement.
Hyperthermia R/T infection, inflammation, and pressure on the hypothalamus	• Remove excess bedclothes. • Control room temperature at <70°F. • Apply a cool, wet cloth to the head. • Provide tepid water baths as necessary. • Assess the need for use of prn antipyretic drugs and administer drugs as necessary. • Avoid shivering in the patient.	• Rectal temperature will be maintained at 99°F or lower.
Sleep Pattern Disturbance R/T agitation and/or increased sensitivity to environmental stimuli	• Assess sleep–wakefulness pattern. • Manage the environment to control and decrease environmental stimuli at night. • Make the patient comfortable.	• At least three sleep periods, lasting 2 hours each, will be experienced during the night.

(continued)

CHART 32-2 Summary of Major Nursing Diagnoses Associated with Meningitis/Encephalitis (Continued)

Nursing Diagnoses	Nursing Interventions	Expected Outcomes
High Risk for Injury R/T agitation, seizure potential, altered consciousness, and cognitive impairment.	• Plan nursing care to provide for uninterrupted quiet and rest. • Maintain seizure precautions. • Provide a safe environment (*e.g.,* keep the bed in a low position). • Apply a jacket restraint, as necessary. • Observe the patient frequently. • Assess the need for use of prn orders for sedatives and administer as necessary.	• Physical injury will not be sustained while hospitalized.
Risk for Disuse Syndrome R/T prolonged bedrest	• Develop a turning and repositioning schedule to prevent skin breakdown. • Use supportive devices as necessary. • Apply elastic stockings. • For some patients, alternating compression air boots may be used. • Institute a bowel program. • Position the patient to facilitate breathing and patency of airway. • Provide a urinary elimination program. • Monitor intake and output, electrolytes, blood gas levels, skin integrity, bowel and bladder elimination pattern, and peripheral tissue perfusion.	• The patient will not develop —Pressure ulcers —Contractures —Deep vein thrombosis —Constipation —Urinary stasis —Atelectasis and pneumonia —Dehydration

reason the latent virus becomes activated is not known, although fever, emotional stress, and infectious diseases may be responsible. It is also unclear how the virus enters the CNS, although it is postulated that it may enter through the blood stream or peripheral nerves.

Herpes simplex encephalitis is a severe, life-threatening illness. Death occurs in 70% to 80% of patients if treatment is not begun before the patient becomes comatose. The mortality rate is reduced to 28% if treatment with acyclovir (Zovirax) is begun before coma occurs. For those that survive, morbidity varies from moderate to severe neurological deficits.

PATHOPHYSIOLOGY

The virus attacks the brain and has a particular propensity for the frontal and temporal lobes. The brain or, more specifically, the temporal lobes become edematous, and necrotic areas with or without hemorrhage develop. The cerebral edema, once developed, is pronounced, and ICP is increased, with temporal lobe herniation. The pathophysiology is associated with the cerebral edema and subsequent increased ICP.

SIGNS AND SYMPTOMS

Symptoms evolve over a few days and include fever, nausea and vomiting, headache, confusion, stupor, focal deficits such as hemiparesis, and seizures. Some patients also experience symptoms of temporal lobe–limbic system deficits, such as olfactory and gustatory hallucinations, anosmia, temporal lobe seizures, periodic bizarre behavioral manifestations, and aphasia.

The cerebral edema and hemorrhage cause an abrupt increase in ICP. Temporal or brain stem herniation can result. The marked increase in ICP produces coma, causes changes in vital signs, and affects the respiratory patterns. Death is most apt to occur within the first 72 hours when the cerebral edema is most pronounced. If the disease is allowed to progress, temporal lobe herniation of one or both lobes develops, leading to deep coma, respiratory arrest, and death.

DIAGNOSIS AND TREATMENT

The diagnosis of herpes simplex encephalitis is difficult to establish in its early state. By the time a diagnosis is estab-

TABLE 32-3
Major Viruses Responsible for Viral Encephalitis

TYPE OF VIRUS OR DISORDER	SPECIFIC DISORDER OR CAUSATIVE ORGANISM	COMMENTS

Arboviruses (arthropod-borne)
    Altered cycle of infection of
        mosquito and host
    Mosquito bites infect host,
        which subsequently becomes
        infected
    Infected mosquito infects host
        (including humans)
	Eastern equine encephalitis*
	Western equine encephalitis
	St. Louis encephalitis
	California virus encephalitis
	Venezuelan equine encephalitis
	
	Japanese B encephalitis
	Murray Valley (Australian X) encephalitis
		Early autumn outbreak in Eastern states;
		    year-round incidence throughout
		    country
		Late summer outbreak throughout the
		    U.S. except on the West coast
		Early autumn outbreak in Midwest
		Year-round incidence in southwestern
		    U.S.
		South and Central America

Type of virus	von Economo disease, also called encephalitis lethargica
	    and sleeping sickness
		Epidemic in U.S. following the influenza
		    epidemic of 1918; has not recurred
		    since 1926

Postviral disease resulting in central nervous system infection	Measles Mumps Chickenpox	
Postvaccination encephalitis	Develops within a week after vaccination for measles, rubella, mumps, or rabies	Appears to be an immune reaction
Other viral infections	Poliomyelitis Rabies Herpes simplex Herpes zoster Infectious mononucleosis	

* *Most serious of the arboviruses in the United States; significant mortality rate and serious deficits in many that survive (e.g., retardation, seizures, personality changes, hemiplegia); least frequent arbovirus.*

lished, it may be too late to benefit the patient; therefore, an aggressive approach to diagnosis is essential. The usual diagnostic work-up includes a history and neurological examination; CSF analysis from lumbar puncture; a computed tomography (CT) or, preferably, a magnetic resonance imaging (MRI) scan; and an electroencephalogram (EEG). Pressure during lumbar puncture is markedly elevated. Findings on CSF analysis include increased polymorphonuclear cells (early) and lymphocytes, increased protein, normal glucose (usually), and possible xanthochromia if cerebral hemorrhage has occurred.

Recent advances in molecular biology now allow very early detection of deoxyribonucleic acid (DNA) from the virus in the CSF, and such techniques are routinely used at many centers. Herpes simplex virus is difficult to isolate early; a fourfold elevation in antibody titer may be seen in the convalescent serum, but this is of no help in crucial early diagnosis and may be misleading, so the detection of viral DNA has been an important step in early diagnosis.

Early in the course of the illness, the CT scan results may be normal, but the MRI scan is usually abnormal even in the first week of the disease. Hemorrhagic areas in the inferior frontal–temporal region, together with surrounding edema, are usually evident on both studies later in the disease. The EEG may show focal or generalized slowing. Often, there is evidence of seizure activity in the temporal region.

The drug of choice for treatment of herpes simplex encephalitis is acyclovir (Zovirax). Other drugs that are commonly administered include the following:

- Dexamethasone (Decadron) in tapering doses to reduce cerebral edema
- Cimetidine (Tagamet) to decrease gastric secretion and prevent development of gastric hemorrhage associated with the use of steroids
- Furosemide (Lasix) or mannitol for diuresis
- Phenytoin (Dilantin) to prevent or control seizures
- Acetaminophen (Tylenol) to control hyperthermia and headache

In addition to the drug therapy, treatment is supportive and symptomatic and includes support of respiratory function and an adequate oxygen supply, support of fluid and electrolyte balance, nutrition, and management of increased ICP.

NURSING MANAGEMENT

Charts 32-1 and 32-2 describe basic principles of management and nursing diagnosis. Management is also similar in some instances to the care of the patient with meningitis. Additional nursing interventions include the following:

- Monitor to detect deterioration in consciousness; coma indicates a poor prognosis.
- Isolation is *not necessary*; however, good handwashing technique should be followed.
- Control of rapidly rising ICP with subsequent herniation risk becomes the focus of care.

PROGNOSIS

If the patient survives the acute episode, neurological deficits are common and may include cognitive deficits (*e.g.,* memory, reasoning), personality changes with dementia, seizure disorders, motor deficits, and dysphagia.

OTHER VIRAL ORGANISMS THAT ATTACK THE CENTRAL NERVOUS SYSTEM

A few selected, uncommon diseases caused by viruses are presented in Table 32-4. They include herpes zoster, poliomyelitis, rabies, tetanus, Lyme disease, cysticercosis, and parameningeal infections. **Parameningeal infections** are infections that occur in and around the meninges. Three major localized, suppurative lesions in this area are brain abscesses, subdural empyema, and extradural abscesses.

Brain Abscess

A brain abscess is caused by an infection extending into the cerebral tissue or by organisms carried from other sites in the body. The major sources of primary infections that extend directly into the brain are infections of the middle ear, mastoid, and sinus. Approximately 40% of all brain abscesses result from middle ear and mastoid infections. Sinus infections (frontal and sphenoid) are responsible for another 10%. A few abscesses occur as a result of intracranial surgery, compound skull fractures, or oral surgery. Those remaining (approximately 50%) are carried by the blood throughout the body from infectious sites, such as from lung infection, lung abscess, bronchiectasis, empyema, skin infections, acute bacterial endocarditis, and congenital heart or lung disease with a right-to-left shunt. These abscesses are sometimes called metastatic abscesses.

The location of the abscess depends on the source and method of the spread of the infection. Those infections that spread directly from a primary focus create an abscess directly adjacent to the primary site. Infections around the face spread in retrograde fashion through venous sinuses and can be located at some distance from the primary focus.

PATHOPHYSIOLOGY

Initially, the infected tissue is soft, edematous, congested, and infiltrated with polymorphonuclear leukocytes. The lesion is poorly delineated and may represent a localized, suppurative encephalitis. Within the next 2 weeks, the necrotic tissue liquefies. The abscess becomes encapsulated by a zone of fibroblasts that surrounds the site and progressively thickens. This wall of granulated tissue is replaced by collagenous connective tissue. The wall is not of uniform thickness and tends to be thinner in its deepest portion. The abscess, which can vary in size and shape, usually lies in the white matter. The deepest thin-walled portion of the abscess lying in the white matter can eventually rupture into the ventricles with catastrophic results. One or more poorly encapsulated daughter abscesses may surround the major abscess, with possible direct communication between the two.

SIGNS AND SYMPTOMS

The signs and symptoms of brain abscess can be considered in two stages: (1) the initial, acute invasion, and (2) the enlarging lesion.

Initial Invasion. The initial invasion corresponds to the initial formation of the abscess. The patient may encounter the following symptoms: headache; chills and fever; malaise; elevated WBCs; and neurological deficits such as confusion and drowsiness, focal or generalized seizures, motor or sensory deficits, and speech disorders. Some patients may be asymptomatic during this period. There may be a history of reactivation of an infectious process in a patient who has had a previous ear, sinus, or lung infection. Symptoms of this earlier recurring infection may be superimposed on the symptoms of the brain abscess formation. Symptoms associated with the initial stage may subside for a period in response to drug therapy.

The Enlarging Lesion. In the second stage, the formalized abscess behaves as a rapidly growing, space-occupying lesion. Within a few weeks, depending on the size of the abscess, the following signs and symptoms may be observed: flu-like symptoms; recurrent headache that becomes increasingly severe; confusion, drowsiness, and stupor; focal or generalized seizures; focal deficits; signs of increased ICP; and possible herniation syndromes.

Symptoms According to Abscess Location. Abscesses in particular areas have characteristic signs and symptoms. The following are three common areas of abscess formation with a list of related symptoms:

- **Frontal lobe abscess**—contralateral hemiparesis, expressive aphasia (if the dominant hemisphere is involved), focal or Jacksonian seizure, and frontal headache
- **Temporal lobe abscess**—localized headache, upper quadrant visual deficit, contralateral facial weakness, and minimal aphasia
- **Cerebellar abscess**—postauricular (below the ear) or occipital headache, ipsilateral ataxia and limb paresis, nystagmus and weakness of gaze to the side of the lesion

DIAGNOSIS

The diagnosis of brain abscess is based on the following criteria:

- Identification of a primary infection, such as middle ear, sinus, or lung infection, helps to pinpoint the source of the problem. Chest, skull, and sinus radiographs may be necessary to identify the primary focus of infection.
- On lumbar puncture, the CSF pressure is elevated. Findings on analysis of the CSF include an elevated WBC count from a few to several thousand, with lymphocytes being the predominant cell; elevated protein; and normal glucose. An abrupt onset of coma with a WBC count of 50,000 in the CSF should make one highly suspicious of rupture of an abscess into the ventricles.
- Other laboratory data to localize the lesion include an EEG (area of high voltage over the abscess) and a CT scan.

TABLE 32-4
Other Selected Nervous System Infections

DISEASE/ORGANISM	DESCRIPTION/COURSE	DIAGNOSIS/TREATMENT
Cruetzfelt-Jakob disease; caused by a prion	• Spongiform encephalopathy characterized by progressive dementia, dysarthria, spastic weakness of the limbs, myoclonic jerks, and seizures • Three years is the average incubation period. • Usually occurs in fifth or sixth decade • Vacuolar or spongelike appearance of brain tissue • Death is the final outcome.	• *Diagnosis:* confirmed by brain biopsy • *Treatment:* supportive care
Herpes zoster (shingles) (herpes virus–varicella zoster)	• Latent virus from an attack of chickenpox that remains latent in the sensory ganglia • When the host defenses fail, the virus multiplies within the sensory ganglia and is then transported down the sensory nerve and released to the vesicles at the nerve endings. • Involves the dorsal root ganglia; follows the sensory distribution of dermatome • An extremely painful afflication in which a rash (vesicles and large irregular bullae on the erythematous base) develops; rash develops from papules → vesicles → pustules → scabs. • Some patients may develop post-herpetic neuralgia after an attack; otherwise, it is a self-limiting condition. • Herpes zoster can attack the ophthalmic branch of the trigeminal nerve and can cause scarring of the eye.	• *Diagnosis:* based on clinical findings (vesicles (occurring 2 to 5 days after pain); pain along the peripheral nerve); • *Treatment:* acyclovir, 800 mg 5 times a day for 7 to 10 days; isolation not required
Poliomyelitis (caused by one of three polioviruses)—type 1, 2, or 3	• Attacks the motor cells of the anterior horn cells of the spinal cord • Severity varies from mild to paralysis, with death from paralysis of respiratory muscle • Enters by way of the gastrointestinal (GI) tract • Spread through contact with feces and pharyngeal secretions from infected persons	• *Diagnosis:* based on clinical findings and isolation of the virus • *Treatment:* supportive care; may need ventilation support; most patients require extensive rehabilitation; isolation precautions are maintained for a period of time. • *Note:* With the advent of the effective Salk vaccine, the incidence of this disease has virtually been eliminated because of mass immunization.
Rabies (rhabdovirus) (<10 cases in the U.S./year)	• An acute encephalomyelitis infection • Transmitted to humans from the saliva of infected animals through bite or contact with saliva • Spread from the wound to the central nervous system by the peripheral nerves • Incubation period varies depending on the distance of the wound from the head • Course of disease —*Early phase:* vague flulike symptoms (headache, malaise, vomiting, fever, drowsiness) —*Second phase:* extreme excitement and salivation, deranged behavior, convulsions, severe and painful spasms of the pharyngeal and laryngeal muscles from slight stimuli or sight of food (lasts 2 to 7 days) —*Final phase:* onset of coma, followed by cardiac and respiratory arrest	• *Diagnosis:* based on a history of a bite and isolation of the virus • *Treatment:* administration of antitoxin (causes serious side effects); supportive care; isolation required; death may result. Vaccination used even after disease has begun. • *Note:* Vaccination for those traveling to areas of prevalence is encouraged.

(continued)

TABLE 32-4
Other Selected Nervous System Infections Continued

DISEASE/ORGANISM	DESCRIPTION/COURSE	DIAGNOSIS/TREATMENT
Tetanus (*Clostridium tetani*)	• Spread through horse and cattle feces that contaminate soil and objects within the soil • Enters humans from pentrating and crush wounds • Produces three exotoxins that attack the spinal cord and cranial nerves • Causes severe muscle spasms, extreme sensitivity to stimuli, and convulsions • Death may occur from asphyxia	• *Diagnosis:* based on the history and clinical findings • *Treatment:* administration of antitoxin and supportive care • *Note:* Immunization is available (tetanus toxoid and tetanus immunoglobulin).

Lyme disease (caused by *Borrelia burgdorferi*)—named for Lyme, Connecticut, where an outbreak caused attention	• Spirochete transmitted by the bite of an infected tick of the *Ixodes ricinus* complex
	• Carried on white-tailed deer and other wild animals
	• Course of disease
	  —*Stage 1:* localized erythema migrans, a rash that resembles a bull's-eye; rash fades within 3 to 4 weeks; there may be occurrence of signs of meningitis, radiculitis, and neuritis in an afebrile patient.
	  —*Stage 2:* complications may develop—heart block in 10%; Bell's palsy in 10%; other problems may include meningitis, encephalitis, polyradiculitis, or inflammation of the eyes
	  —*Stage 3:* occurs 4 weeks to years after the bite; characterized by arthritis symptoms affecting the large joints and chronic joint pain
		• *Diagnosis:* based on a history of bite (which the patient may not recall); elevated titer to Lyme disease after 4 weeks
		• *Treatment:*
		  —*Stage 1:* azithromycin, amoxicillin, and doxycycline are recommended for treatment of stage 1 to prevent the development of subsequent stages; ceftriaxone is usually given IV in patients with neurological symptoms and helps to resolve symptoms.
		  —*Stage 2:* intravenous administration of 20 million U of penicillin; others recommend tetracycline 500 mg q.i.d.
		  —*Stage 3:* controversial; antibiotics are used

Cysticercosis of CNS (caused by *Taenia solium*)	• Most common parasite affecting the CNS • In Central and South America, this is the leading cause of epilepsy and neurological disturbances. • Humans who consume raw or undercooked meat from infected animals can become contaminated. • When ingested, cyst forms that contains larva; the cyst can lodge in the brain, as well as in other areas. • May lodge in ventricles	• *Diagnosis:* Based on multiple, calcified lesions in the brain noted on CT scan or radiological studies • *Treatment:* oral praziquantel, for 3 days; symptomatic treatment of cerebral edema with steroids; surgery may be required to remove intracranial cyst

TREATMENT

Early diagnosis and prompt antimicrobial treatment are essential. Because anaerobic streptococci and *Bacteroides* are the predominant causative organisms, penicillin G (20 million U) and chloramphenicol (4 to 6 g daily IV in divided doses) are given. In addition, management of the rapidly rising ICP is achieved with IV mannitol, followed by a course of dexamethasone (Decadron, 6 to 12 mg q 6 hours). If this is not effective, surgery will be necessary to remove or aspirate the abscess. If the abscess is well encapsulated, attempts are made to surgically excise both the abscess and membrane totally. If this is not possible, the abscess is aspirated and drained. Injection of the sac with antimicrobial drugs follows. It may be necessary at some future time to drain the sac again because of a buildup of suppurative material.

The use of drugs has greatly reduced the mortality rate from brain abscess. The aggressive treatment of infections that can lead to the formation of brain abscesses has also been a prophylactic aid. The cause of death from brain abscess is the massive increase in ICP and rupture of the abscess into the ventricles. Of the patients who survive, approximately 30% develop neurological deficits, of which focal seizures are most common.

EXTRADURAL ABSCESS

Extradural abscesses may be caused by osteomyelitis of a cranial bone, or they may be associated with an infection of the sinuses or the ear or a surgical procedure in which the frontal sinus or mastoid has been opened. A pus pocket accumulates between the bone and dura.

Symptoms include localized pain, fever, tenderness, and purulent discharge. Stiffness of the neck is possible. Localized neurological signs are often absent. If they occur, focal seizures, cranial nerve VI palsy, and decreased sensory perception of the face are the most common symptoms. The only abnormalities noted in the CSF are a few lymphocytes and neutrophils and a slightly elevated protein level.

Treatment consists of antibiotics and surgery for removal of the diseased bone at a future date.

Nursing Management of Patients With Parameningeal Infections

The nursing management of the patient with a brain abscess can be viewed in two stages: the acute initial invasion when the infection organizes into an abscess, and the second stage when the abscess behaves like a space-occupying lesion.

During the initial stage, symptoms correspond to a general systemic infection. If neurological symptoms are present, they can be important in localizing the lesion. Often, symptoms are so general that a diagnosis is unclear. Nursing management during this period includes assessing the patient's condition, managing any presenting symptoms, providing supportive care, and administering drug treatment. If signs of increased ICP are present, the basic care outlined in Chapter 17 for increased ICP is followed. Seizure precautions are maintained to prevent injury. Noting how a seizure progresses is helpful for diagnosis. Neurological assessment, including assessment for signs and symptoms of meningeal irritation, is important.

Medications ordered are given through IV. As with meningitis, adherence to the administration timetable is imperative for maintaining therapeutic blood levels. Because the drugs used are potent, the patient must be observed for both drug side effects and the development of secondary infections, which can flourish when antimicrobial therapy is used.

In the second stage, the abscess behaves like a space-occupying lesion. This means that there are signs and symptoms of neurological deficit that are investigated to make a diagnosis. Once the diagnosis is made, appropriate treatment is begun. If surgery is necessary to remove or drain the abscess, nursing management pertinent to the craniotomy patient should be implemented (see Chap. 18).

References

1. Odio, C. M., Faingezecht, I., Paris, M., Nassar, M., Baltodino, A., Rogers, J., et al. (1991). The beneficial effects of early dexamethasone administration in infants and children with bacterial meningitis. *New England Journal of Medicine, 325*(23), 1654–1655.

Bibliography

Books

Adams, R. D., & Victor, M. (1993). Nonviral infections of the nervous system. In R. D. Adams & M. Victor (Eds.), *Principles of neurology* (5th ed.). New York: McGraw-Hill.

Hoeprich, P. D., Jordan, M. C., & Ronald, A. R. (1994). *Infectious diseases: A treatise of infectious processes* (5th ed.). Philadelphia: J. B. Lippincott.

Hopkins, C. C. (1993). Nosocomial infections. In A. H. Ropper (Ed.), *Neurological and neurosurgical intensive care* (3rd ed.) (pp. 121–131). New York: Raven.

Schooley, R. T. (1993). Encephalitis. In A. H. Ropper (Ed.), *Neurological and neurosurgical intensive care* (3rd ed.) (pp. 411–435). New York: Raven.

Periodicals

Alarcon, F., Esclante, L., Duenas, G., Montalvo, M., & Roman, M. (1989). Neurocysticercosis. *Archives of Neurology, 46,* 1231–1236.

Barzaga, R. A., Klein, N. C., & Cunha, B. A. (1992). Herpes simplex meningoencephalitis. *Heart and Lung, 21*(4), 405–406.

Cabellos, C., Viladrich, P. F., Veraguer, R., Pallares, R., Linares, J., & Gudiol, F. (1995). A single daily dose of ceftriaxone for bacterial meningitis in adults: Experience with 84 patients and review of the literature. *Clinical Infectious Diseases, 20*(5), 1164–1168.

Gardner, P., Leipzig, T., & Phillips, P. (1985). Infections of central nervous system shunts. *Medical Clinics of North America, 69*(2), 297–314.

Hart, C. A., Cuevas, L. E., Marzouk, O., Thomson, A. P., & Sills, J. (1993). Management of bacterial meningitis. *Journal of Antimicrobial Chemotherapy, 32*(Suppl. A), 49–59.

Ho, D. D., & Hirsh, M. S. (1985). Acute viral encephalitis. *Medical Clinics of North America, 69*(2), 415–430.

Kaplan, K. (1985). Brain abscess. *Medical Clinics of North America, 69*(2), 345–360.

Lau, D. W., Klein, N. C., & Cunha, B. A. (1989). Brain abscess mimicking brain tumor. *Heart and Lung, 18*(6), 634–639.

Lee, B. C. (1989). Be ready for Lyme disease in your own backyard. *RN, 52*(4), 26–29.

Minnick, A. (1986). Cysticercosis: Etiology and nursing care. *Journal of Neuroscience Nursing, 18*(3), 135–145.

Prendergast, V. (1987). Bacterial meningitis update. *Journal of Neuroscience Nursing, 19*(2), 95–99.

Ratzan, K. R. (1985). Viral meningitis. *Medical Clinics of North America, 69*(2), 399–414.

Roos, K. L. (1992). Management of bacterial meningitis in children and adults. *Seminars in Neurology, 12*(3), 155–164.

Sabeeta, J. R., & Andriole, V. T. (1985). Cryptococcal infection of the central nervous system. *Medical Clinics of North America, 69*(2), 333–344.

Silverberg, A. L., & DiNubile, M. J. (1985). Subdural empyema and cranial epidural abscess. *Medical Clinics of North America, 69*(2), 361–374.

Steere, A. C. (1989). Lyme disease. *New England Journal of Medicine, 321*(9), 586–596.

Vetter, R., Iverson, G. R., & Kuzel, M. D. (1993). Adult meningitis: Rapid identification for prompt treatment. *Postgraduate Medicine, 93*(1), 99–102, 105–106, 109–112.

Zackson, R., Calabro, L., & Cunha, B. (1994). Meningitis in adults: Differentiating the sources. *Emergency Medicine, 26*(4), 113–114, 117–118.

CHAPTER 33

AIDS: Neurological Manifestations

Jane T. Settle
Sherry W. Fox

INTRODUCTION

Neurological disease is now recognized as a frequent cause of mortality and morbidity in patients infected with the human immunodeficiency virus (HIV). Clinical manifestations of central nervous system (CNS) involvement have been found in up to 70% of reported cases. Histologic involvement has been found in 90% of autopsies of patients who have died with acquired immunodeficiency syndrome (AIDS).[1] This chapter is designed to provide readers with general information about HIV, the causative agent of AIDS, as well as detailed information about common opportunistic infections, tumors, neuropathies, myopathies, and AIDS dementia complex, all of which may cause alterations in the function of the nervous system.

Since individuals with HIV-related illnesses may be seen in the acute hospital setting, long-term care facilities, outpatient clinics, and at home, it is important to consider the health–illness continuum and needs these patients may have over a period of months to years. Nursing care of the patient with HIV/AIDS depends on the specific diagnoses, acuity of the current illness, and overall functional level. However, assessment, development of an individualized care plan, coordination of the implementation of the plan with the patient and other care providers, and evaluation of the outcomes remain a constant in nursing practice.[2]

DEFINITION

Infection with HIV leads to a progressive immunosuppression which results in susceptibility to a number of opportunistic infections, malignancies, and neurological disorders. The primary target cell for HIV is the CD4 positive helper lymphocyte; these cells decrease in number over the course of the disease. Since CD4 positive lymphocytes play a major role in initiating and orchestrating other humoral and cell-mediated immune responses, virtually all components of the immune system are affected either directly or indirectly by HIV infection.[3,4]

The HIV glycoprotein mediates binding to the CD4 molecules found on cells, including T helper cells, monocytes, macrophages, and possibly dendritic cells. After binding to the CD4 cell, the lipid bilayers of HIV and the target-cell plasma membrane fuse, resulting in the release of the viral core into the cytoplasm. The events that result in the fusion are not completely understood, but it appears that binding to CD4 alone is insufficient to cause infection and that one or more cellular cofactors is required.[5]

The interaction of HIV with CD4 positive lymphocytes and the immune system is a complex process involving multiple viral regulating products. HIV infection is an evolutionary process marked by characteristic early-to-late changes in viral phenotypes of distinct cellular tropism and cytopathic potential. Early studies of viral load in the peripheral blood lymphocytes showed large volumes of virus present only late in the disease process. More recent studies using improved techniques to detect and quantify the viral burden in lymphoid organs and the peripheral blood stream have shown the HIV load is significantly higher than previously recognized throughout the course of the disease (Staprans & Feinberg, 1995).

HIV can be transmitted by sexual intercourse, contaminated needles used in injecting drugs, transfusion of contaminated blood or blood products, or perinatally. At its entry point, which may be mucous membrane or intravenous introduction into the blood stream, free HIV or HIV-infected cells are presumably cleared from interstitial spaces and delivered into the blood or lymphatic vessels. Entry of free HIV or HIV-infected cells into lymph nodes or other lymphoid tissue, where immune response to antigens occurs, leads to new cycles of HIV replication and infection. The immunologically activated lymphoid tissue perpetuates viral spread to additional T cells and macrophages.[5]

It is unclear why some individuals do not develop HIV infection despite repeated exposure to the virus through unprotected sexual intercourse with an infected partner or repeated use of contaminated needles. For those individuals who do become infected, the primary HIV infection generally becomes evident 2 to 6 weeks after exposure to the virus. For some individuals the illness is subclinical; for others, an acute viral illness including fever, arthralgia, myalgia, and fatigue lasts for 2 to 3 weeks.[6] Most individuals who are infected with the virus will develop a positive HIV antibody test within 6 to 12 weeks after exposure. Once symptoms of the primary illness subside, the individual generally enters an asymptomatic stage which may last for as long as 7 to 11 years before development of significant immunodeficiency. Although the individual may be asymptomatic, viral replication continues to occur in the lymph nodes, indicating that the disease is active and progressive.[5]

Progression of HIV infection to AIDS is evidenced by an increase in the loss of CD4 positive lymphocytes (Table 33-1). Profound immunodeficiency is manifested by opportunistic infections, specific malignancies, and neurologic disorders. Considerable variation exists in the time it takes for clinical disease to develop. A small number of persons develop an accelerated course which results in a diagnosis of AIDS within 1 to 2 years after initial infection. Other individuals continue symptom free with normal CD4 counts more than 10 years after initial infection.[5]

In general, individuals with CD4 counts greater than 500 are asymptomatic and have nearly normal immune systems by standard laboratory assessment. Individuals with CD4 counts in the range of 200 to 500 are often asymptomatic but may have occasional infections related to pathogens that also cause disease in normal hosts. These include pulmonary tuberculosis, pneumococcal pneumonia, herpes zoster, and vaginal candidiasis. Those individuals with CD4 counts of less than 200 are at greatest risk for major complications, but may remain asymptomatic for extended periods of time.[7]

The Centers for Disease Control and Prevention has classified the spectrum of HIV-related clinical manifestations into distinct groups. This provides a standardized way to describe and classify symptoms and diseases (Table 33-2).

EPIDEMIOLOGY

The impact of the HIV/AIDS epidemic has been significant. As of December 1994, approximately 435,000 AIDS cases had been reported in the United States.[8] Individuals in the 25- to 44-year-old age group have been most heavily affected, but individuals at any age are at risk. Initially, AIDS was identified in the early 1980s as a disease of white homosexual men, however it quickly spread into the heterosexual community through intravenous (IV) drug use and sexual intercourse. In recent years, the impact of the epidemic has been greatest on minorities, particularly among African-Americans and Hispanics. Although men continue to account for the majority of AIDS cases, infection in women is increasing at a dramatic rate. Many women do not perceive themselves to be at risk and unknowingly acquire HIV infection through sexual intercourse with infected partners.[9]

HIV TESTING

Patients may present for medical care already aware of their HIV infection, or they may present with a history or symptoms suggestive of HIV. If suspicion for HIV in a individual exists, consent for testing must be obtained from the patient (or family if the patient is unable to participate in the discussion) before the blood is drawn. Government and institutional policies differ from state to state, but in many agencies, signed consent is required for testing. This is to ensure that the patient understands the need for the test and the possible implications of the test results.

When blood is drawn for an HIV antibody test, it may be tested by several procedures. The two most commonly used tests are the enzyme-linked immunosorbent assay (ELISA) and the Western blot.[10] The ELISA test is designed to detect the presence of antibodies to HIV. If this test is negative, no further testing is done as a general rule. If the ELISA test is positive (shows evidence of antibodies), then a Western blot is done. The Western blot is a more specific test for the HIV antibody and is less likely to yield a false positive test. If an HIV test is reported as positive, it is important to confirm that

---

TABLE 33-1
Sequence of Events: Progression of HIV to AIDS

Viral transmission	
Acute HIV infection	2–4 weeks after clearly defined exposure
Seroconversion	Generally occurs approximately 6–12 weeks after transmission
Asymptomatic infection	May have persistent generalized lymphadenopathy and stable to slowly declining CD4 counts; stage generally lasts for several years
Early symptomatic disease	Usual CD4 count 100–300; common problems include bacterial pneumonia, vaginal candidiasis, thrush, hairy leukoplakia, herpes zoster, idiopathic thrombocytopenia purpura, and pulmonary tuberculosis
Late symptomatic disease	CD4 count less than 200; all AIDS defining diagnoses
Advanced HIV disease	CD4 count less than 50; multiple infections and complications.

Adapted from Bartlett, J. G. (1995). Pocket guide of infectious disease therapy. Baltimore: Williams and Wilkins.

TABLE 33-2
Clinical Category

IMMUNOLOGIC CATEGORY	A ASYMPTOMATIC OR ACUTE PRIMARY INFECTION	B SYMPTOMATIC, BUT NOT A OR C*	C AIDS DEFINING CONDITION†
1 CD4 >500	A1	B1	C1‡
2 CD4 200–499	A2	B2	C2‡
3 CD4 <200 (or <14%)	A3‡	B3†	C3‡

* Examples of clinical conditions in category B: thrush, oral hairy leukoplakia, herpes zoster (multidermal or recurrent), fevers, diarrhea, weight loss, persistent vaginal candidiasis which is resistant to treatment, cervical dysplasia, immune thrombocytopenia purpura (ITP), peripheral neuropathy.
† Examples of AIDS defining conditions in category C: Candida esophagitis, invasive cervical cancer, extrapulmonary cryptococcus, cytomegalovirus (CMV), HIV encephalopathy (AIDS dementia complex), Kaposi's sarcoma, lymphoma, Mycobacterium avium complex, Pneumocystis carinii pneumonia, recurrent bacterial pneumonia, toxoplasmosis, and wasting syndrome.
‡ Denotes diagnosis of AIDS.
From Fisher, E. J. (1995). Clinician's guide to therapy of adults with HIV/AIDS (3rd ed.). Richmond: Virginia Commonwealth University HIV/AIDS Center.

both the ELISA and Western blot have been done and determined to be positive. Newer testing techniques including viral cultures and polymerase chain reaction (PCR) are being used but are not yet widely available and are quite expensive.[11]

Although testing techniques for the HIV antibody are both sensitive and specific, there are occasions when test results may be inaccurate. An individual who has recently been exposed to the virus but not yet developed primary HIV infection and seroconverted may have a negative test. A few individuals with advanced AIDS also have negative tests because their immune systems can no longer produce antibodies. It is important to recognize that an occasional patient may have a false positive test, a false negative test, or an indeterminate test. If the individual's medical condition does not match the test results, or the person doubts the test results for any reason, then additional testing should be carried out to confirm or disprove the diagnosis of HIV infection.

HIV AND THE CENTRAL NERVOUS SYSTEM

Prior to the identification of HIV and recognition of AIDS as a distinct disease process, numerous opportunistic infections involving the central nervous system were described. As experience with the disease evolved, it became evident that neurologic disorders were common in HIV-infected patients, and that some of the disorders could not be solely attributed to opportunistic processes.[1] Evidence now suggests that some processes are the direct result of infection of CNS tissue by HIV.[12,13]

Until recently, the CNS was considered to be "immunologically privileged." Factors such as the absence of lymph nodes, lymphatic drainage, and the presence of the blood–brain barrier appeared to limit the immune function of the CNS. Studies have challenged these assumptions and suggested that there is a clear relationship between the CNS and the immune system.[14]

Research suggests that peripherally activated lymphocytes or macrophages infected with the virus may enter the CNS through breaks in the epithelial lining of small capillaries.

Once in the brain, the infected lymphocytes and macrophages may release toxic factors or cease to secrete trophic substances which ultimately impede the functioning of the affected cells.[12] The infected cells may actively release the virus or carry it in a latent state. Owing to the indolent nature of HIV infection, the virus spreads slowly in the brain and eventually causes progressive neurological involvement.[15]

The sites of CNS damage in individuals infected with HIV are numerous. The virus has been isolated in the cerebrospinal fluid (CSF), the cerebrum, the cerebellum, and the spinal cord. Gross examination of brain tissue in these patients reveals marked cerebral atrophy and acquired microcephaly.[16] Histological damage has been noted in the subcortical regions of the cerebrum, consisting of glioses and demyelination. Recent studies have also identified CD4 glycoprotein in the frontal lobes, the perilimbic cortex, and the amygdala (Tables 33-3 and 33-4).[14]

OPPORTUNISTIC DISEASES

Primary Seroconversion

A small percentage of patients undergoing primary HIV infection develop symptoms similar to mononucleosis, including include fever, myalgia, and rash. This presentation is usually self-limiting and occurs as antibodies to HIV are developing. Neurological infection may appear early in HIV infection. Studies have isolated HIV antibodies in the CSF of symptomatic and asymptomatic patients.[14,17]

The most common clinical manifestation of HIV infection of the CNS is an aseptic meningoencephalitis. Other presenting illnesses and symptoms may include myelopathy, peripheral neuropathy, brachial neuritis, facial palsies, and Guillain-Barré syndrome. Some patients report headaches, retro-orbital pain, and photophobia. Symptoms are usually self-limiting but persistent deficits have been reported.[17]

TOXOPLASMOSIS

Toxoplasmosis gondii is an obligate intracellular parasite that may exist in the cyst stage within the tissue of the normal host. The parasite enters the body via the gastrointestinal tract, in-

TABLE 33-3
Common HIV-Related Disorders of the Central Nervous System

INFECTIONS
Primary seroconversion
Toxoplasmosis
Cryptococcoses
Cytomegalovirus (CMV)
Progressive multifocal leukoencephalopathy (PML)
Herpes encephalitis
Meningeal tuberculosis

PERIPHERAL NEUROPATHIES AND MYOPATHIES
Distal symmetrical polyneuropathy (DSP)
Inflammatory demyelinating polyneuropathy (IDP)
Mononeuropathy multiplex
Progressive polyradiculopathy
Autonomic neuropathy
Medication-induced neuropathy
Polymyositis
Zidovudine myopathy

PRIMARY CNS LYMPHOMA

AIDS DEMENTIA COMPLEX

vading the blood stream and ultimately traveling to the brain.[13] Toxoplasmosis is the most frequently seen CNS infection in the AIDS population and is associated with a mortality rate of up to 70% according to some studies.[13]

T. gondii infection (generally referred to as toxoplasmosis) in AIDS patients occurs as a result of immune abnormalities due to HIV infection. The depletion of antigen-specific T-helper cells results in the inability to provide activating signals to CD8 T cytotoxic cells and macrophages. Resting macrophages are susceptible to infection with the *T. gondii* parasite and have reduced ability to function in phagocytosis and antimicrobial killing. The failure to stimulate T cells in the systemic lymphoid tissues results in an inability to detect the parasitic infection in the CNS because activated cells are not available to cross the blood–brain barrier.[14]

If the cyst ruptures in an immunocompromised host, a diffuse meningoencephalitis with cell necrosis may occur. The thrombosis of vessels causes areas of necrosis and may progress to abscess formation).[13] The mass lesions and abscesses are often multifocal and scattered throughout the cerebral hemispheres, with the abscesses having a preference for the basal ganglia.[14]

The clinical presentation of toxoplasmosis varies. The early neurologic signs may consist only of myoclonus and asterixis, indicating a metabolic encephalopathy. More often, the presenting signs, developing over days or weeks, include seizures, confusion, and signs of meningeal irritation. Global neurologic symptoms may be followed by focal deficits including mild hemiparesis, ataxia, limb dysmetria, and cranial nerve palsies. Some patients have a persistent fever along with the neurologic manifestations.[13]

Diagnostic studies such as magnetic resonance imaging (MRI) and computerized tomography (CT) characteristically demonstrate multiple lesions that are typically ring enhancing. Areas of edema often surround toxoplasma lesions, sometimes producing a mass effect and shift of brain structures. Areas affected, in order of frequency, are basal ganglia; frontal, parietal, and occipital lobes; and occasionally the cerebellum.[14] Analysis of CSF is usually abnormal, revealing protein elevations, with varying degrees of pleocytosis and glucose depression. Lumbar puncture may need to be deferred in some patients owing to the mass effect associated with toxoplasmosis. Elevations of immunoglobulin levels have also been reported.[1]

While elevations of IgM toxoplasma serum titers are diagnostic for acute systemic toxoplasmosis, they are not diagnostic for CNS toxoplasmosis. Neither CT nor MRI are absolutely reliable for differentiating toxoplasmosis from lymphoma or other causes of brain abscess. Because a definitive diagnosis of suspected toxoplasmosis is difficult to make on clinical grounds alone, most patients are given a trial of antitoxoplasmosis agents, such as pyrimethamine and sulfadiazine. Clinical improvement and improvement on MRI or CT scan can usually be seen in 1 to 3 weeks. If no improvement occurs or the patient's symptoms worsen, stereotactic brain biopsy may be indicated.[18] Pharmacological maintenance therapy must be continued for life because of the high probability of relapse of the infection. Patients with sensitivity to sulfadiazine may be maintained on a combination of clindamycin and pyrimethamine.[19] Identification of side effects related to drug therapy in patients receiving treatment for toxoplasmosis is critical. Pyrimethamine use may result in folic acid deficiency which may lead to swelling, burning, and tingling of the tongue and changes in taste sensation. Combination drug therapy has also been reported to result in diarrhea, anemia, bone marrow suppression, hemorrhagic complica-

TABLE 33-4
Continuum of HIV-Related Illnesses

ILLNESS	ASYMPTOMATIC	EARLY SYMPTOMATIC	LATE SYMPTOMATIC	ADVANCED
Opportunistic infections			×××××	×××××
Primary CNS lymphoma			×××××	×××××
Neuropathies	×××××	×××××	×××××	
Myopathies		×××××	×××××	×××××
AIDS dementia complex		×××××	×××××	×××××

Adapted from Newton, H. B. (1995). Common neurologic complications of HIV-1 infection and AIDS. American Family Physician, *51,(2), 387–398.*

tions, anorexia, and vomiting. Weight loss, nutritional deficits, infections, and poor wound healing may also be significant problems.[13]

CRYPTOCOCCAL MENINGITIS

Cryptococcus neoformans is a common soil fungus. Individuals are exposed to the fungus when the organisms are inhaled. Initially, the infection develops in the lungs, where it lies dormant. In the immunocompromised host, the fungus may be reactivated, invading the blood stream and eventually lodging in brain meninges.[20]

Currently, cryptococcus is the third leading cause of neurologic disease in the AIDS population. Extraneural cryptococcosis may accompany CNS disease. The lungs are most commonly involved, but sites such as the skin, genitourinary tract, bone marrow, and blood may also be affected.[20]

It is not clear how the fungus enters the cerebral cortex; however, it usually forms cysts and small granulomas in cortical tissue.[13] Although unusual, cryptococcus can also form mass lesions deep within cortical tissue. Generally, this occurs in the basal ganglia where the fungus invades the brain along penetrating arteries to form clumps of organisms that develop into mass lesions.[1]

A majority of patients with CNS cryptococcosis present with symptoms of fever, headache, and malaise.[13,20] Meningismus, with altered mental status and photophobia, may ensue. Focal neurologic deficits, hydrocephalus, and increased intracranial pressure have been reported as clinical manifestations in 20% to 30% of cases. Seizures are uncommon, occurring as a presenting symptom in only 10% of cases.[13] The diagnosis is made by identification of the organism in the CSF. A CT scan or MRI should be done prior to the lumbar puncture to rule out any intracranial masses. The CT scan or MRI may be normal or show evidence of mild atrophy or nonenhancing lesions. CSF cell count, protein, and glucose levels are usually normal. CSF organism-specific antigens and cultures are usually positive. Complete destruction of the organism is unusual and relapse is common; therefore lifelong suppressive therapy is recommended. Antifungal therapy using amphotericin B initially, followed by fluconazole, is the standard approach. Side effects of amphotericin B therapy include anemia, leukopenia, bone marrow suppression, and renal insufficiency.

CYTOMEGALOVIRUS

Cytomegalovirus (CMV) is a viral CNS infection that may cause encephalitis. Both reactivated latent virus and primary CMV infection can cause neurological disease. The inability to develop antigen-specific activation of CD4 helper/inducer cells results in impaired CD8 cell cytotoxicity, which is the primary immune reaction to CMV-infected cells.[14] Untreated CMV infection progresses rapidly and produces diffuse inflammation of the brain and spinal cord, resulting in cerebral atrophy and areas of white matter infarctions. CMV encephalitis generally presents as altered mental status, sensory impairment, and meningismus, progressing to stupor and coma. CT or MRI studies demonstrate periventricular white matter abnormalities and contrastenhancing lesions in the subependymal and

cortical regions. CSF analysis is not diagnostic because viral cultures are typically negative. A brain biopsy is needed for confirmation of the diagnosis. In actual practice it may not be practical, or possible, to obtain a brain biopsy; therefore, when the diagnosis is suspected, treatment with intravenous ganciclovir should be initiated. After initial treatment, ganciclovir must be continued at a maintenance dose for life. The most significant side effect of the drug is leukopenia. Foscarnet is an alternate drug, but it also has significant side effects.[19]

PROGRESSIVE MULTIFOCAL LEUKOENCEPHALOPATHY

Reactivation of papovavirus in the presence of immunodeficiency may lead to progressive multifocal leukoencephalopathy (PML). The reactivated virus affects the hemispheric white matter and causes patchy areas of demyelination. The subcortical areas are usually the first to become involved, but the gray matter or periventricular areas may also be affected. Atypical astrocytes and oligodendroglia with large nuclei are noted.

PML generally presents as focal neurologic deficits that progress over a period of weeks or months to death. Typical focal deficits may include aphasia, ataxia, and hemiparesis.

Diagnosis is usually made by identifying the indolent clinical course. Imaging studies demonstrate multiple nonenhancing areas within the subcortical white matter. CSF studies are nondiagnostic. Brain biopsy may be useful in differentiating PML from toxoplasmosis and other opportunistic infections. Currently, there is no effective treatment for PML. Cytarabine has been noted in some studies to promote limited improvement.

HERPES ENCEPHALITIS

Herpes simplex virus (HSV) is a virus that may lead to encephalitis in the patient who is immunocompromised. A majority of cases are caused by HSV-1, which is found in the trigeminal ganglion. Some cases have also been associated with HSV-2, found in the sacral ganglion. The virus can cause either a mild, diffuse encephalitis or a hemorrhagic necrotizing encephalitis of the temporal and inferior frontal lobes.

Clinical manifestations are nonfocal and may include fever, headache, changes in mental status, and seizures. The mental status changes may range from mild cognitive deficits to coma. Focal deficits may also be seen. A definitive diagnosis is made by brain biopsy and culture, but treatment is generally initiated if clinical suspicion is high.

The treatment for herpes encephalitis is an antiviral agent such as acyclovir. Foscarnet is the drug of choice for treating strains of herpes that are resistant to acyclovir (Fisher, 1995). Patients treated for herpes encephalitis may recover fully or may experience permanent neurologic damage, depending on the timely determination of the diagnosis and initiation of therapy.

MENINGEAL TUBERCULOSIS

Mycobacterium tuberculosis occurs frequently in individuals with HIV infection. Although generally confined to the lungs, extrapulmonary tuberculosis is seen occasionally.

Meningeal tuberculosis is a chronic infection which may be manifested by meningeal signs, cranial nerve impairment, and seizures. CSF analysis may show high protein, low glucose, and lymphocytosis. Late reactivation of meningeal tuberculous foci may produce disease in adults who have no evidence of pulmonary tuberculosis. Tuberculomas of the meninges or brain may become evident many years after primary infection. Acid-fast bacillus (AFB) cultures of the CSF are usually positive.[21,22]

If meningeal tuberculosis is suspected, therapy with four drugs should be initiated. The drugs of choice are isoniazid (INH), rifampin, pyrazinamide (PZA), and ethambutol.[7] The patient should not be considered contagious unless there is evidence of active pulmonary disease. Since most immunocompromised patients are anergic when purified protein derivatives are placed, a skin test may not show evidence of previous exposure to tuberculosis.

Neuropathies and Myopathies

Patients may present with neuropathy or develop neuropathy during the course of their systemic disease.[23] The exact pathogenesis of neuropathies remains unclear; factors such as concurrent infection, use of neurotoxic medications, nutritional deficits, and metabolic disorders may contribute to the process. Other possible mechanisms are direct viral infection or cell-mediated immune attack on various components of peripheral nerves.[24]

DISTAL SYMMETRICAL POLYNEUROPATHY

Distal symmetrical polyneuropathy (DSP) is the most common of the neuropathies seen in patients with HIV/AIDS. The primary symptom of DSP is symmetric burning pain in the soles of the feet which is exacerbated by touch or pressure. Stocking and glove sensory loss, distal weakness, and muscle atrophy may occur later in the course. Physical examination of the lower extremities demonstrates a distal to proximal decrease in sensation to pinprick, cold, and vibration, along with hypoactive Achilles reflexes. Nerve conduction studies show mild slowing of maximal conduction velocity with low amplitude sensory nerve action potentials and minimal denervation on needle electromyography. The CSF is usually normal, although a lymphocytic pleocytosis and increased protein may be seen.

Treatment is symptomatic with tricyclic antidepressants (amitriptyline, nortriptyline), carbamazepine (Tegretol), phenytoin (Dilantin), and topical capsaicin cream (Zostrex-HP).[18]

INFLAMMATORY DEMYELINATING POLYNEUROPATHY

Inflammatory demyelinating polyneuropathy (IDP) is an acute monophasic, relapsing, or chronic progressive process which tends to occur early in the course of HIV infection. Symptoms resemble Guillian-Barré syndrome; patients present with progressive weakness, areflexia, and mild sensory changes. The CSF generally shows pleocytosis. Electrophysiological studies generally indicate features of primary demyelination. Nerve biopsy in IDP reveals segmental demyelination and perivascular lymphocytic infil-

trates. The pathogenesis has not been proven but may be autoimmune. The clinical course is variable; patients with acute onset and rapid progression generally do poorly irrespective of therapy and have more residual disability. Chronic IDP is more common in asymptomatic patients with immune systems that are still partially intact. Steroid therapy, plasmapheresis, or both may be effective in restoring motor function. High-dose intravenous immunoglobulin may also be effective.[24] Treatment with zidovudine has been reported to produce improvement in symptoms in some patients, supporting the hypothesis of an infectious cause.

MONONEUROPATHY MULTIPLEX

The pathogenesis of this syndrome is obscure. Cranial, peripheral, or spinal nerves may be affected. Asymmetric multifocal peripheral and cranial nerve deficits may occur, along with fever, generalized wasting, and CSF pleocytosis. When individual nerve lesions become diffuse and confluent, the course of the disease may resemble IDP. Electrophysiological studies may assist in distinguishing the axonal lesions of mononeuropathy multiplex from primary demyelinating pathology. Treatable etiologies of mononeuropathy such as herpes zoster and CMV must be ruled out. No specific therapy has been identified.[24]

PROGRESSIVE POLYRADICULOPATHY

CMV has been identified as a possible cause of this syndrome. The symptoms of progressive polyradiculopathy are lower extremity and sacral paresthesia followed by rapidly progressive flaccid paraparesis, areflexia, ascending sensory loss, and urinary retention. If untreated, the course is rapidly fatal. The CSF generally reveals marked polymorphonuclear pleocytosis. If CMV is suspected as the causative agent, immediate treatment with intravenous ganciclovir should be initiated, pending outcome of cultures. With early intervention, some patients have significant reversal of symptoms.

AUTONOMIC NEUROPATHY

The autonomic nervous system is affected in an estimated 10% of patients with HIV-related neuropathies. Although CNS impairment and medications may contribute to dysautonomia, the symptoms may be due to small-fiber peripheral neuropathy. Patients may complain of fainting, orthostatic dizziness, impotence, diarrhea, and urinary dysfunction. Autonomic function testing may be helpful in diagnosis. Heart rate variation, mean arterial blood pressure fall to tilting, and arterial blood pressure response to isometric exercise have been reported.[24] The treatment is symptomatic; fludrocortisone, antiarrhythmic agents, and appropriate management of electrolytes and fluid intake may be beneficial.[18]

DIDEOXYINOSINE AND DIDEOXYCYTIDINE NEUROPATHIES

In some studies, neuropathies occurred in as many as 22% of patients on dideoxyinosine (ddI) and 45% of patients on dideoxycytidine (ddC). The specific mechanism by which these two nucleoside analogs cause neuropathy is unclear. This specific toxicity is not associated with the use of zidovudine, the other commonly used antiretroviral. Patients complain of painful neuropathy characterized by tingling, burning, or aching, primarily in their feet. Physical examination shows mild sensory loss and diminished ankle reflexes. The degree of neuropathy appears to be dose related and may continue to intensify for 6 to 8 weeks after discontinuing the drug.

In addition, patients may be taking other neurotoxic drugs such as vincristine, isoniazid, and dapsone, which are known to cause neuropathies. The treatment is to stop the drug for 6 to 8 weeks. Most patients will not tolerate rechallenge, although lower doses can be tried if no other alternative is available.[25]

POLYMYOSITIS

Myopathy may occur as the presenting manifestation of HIV or at any time in the course of the disease. The pathogenesis is unclear; direct infection of myofibers with HIV appears unlikely, and autoimmunity is possible but not proven. Polymyositis is characterized by proximal muscle weakness, myalgia, excessive fatigue, and increased creatine phosphokinase (CPK). It presents with subacute, progressive weakness and is often manifested by difficulty climbing stairs or rising from a chair. Myalgia, most prominent in the thighs, is common. Physical examination reveals symmetrical, predominately proximal muscle weakness, usually involving the legs and neck flexors more than the arms. Weakness progresses over months, with waxing and waning. The diagnosis may be complicated by concurrent disorders such as peripheral neuropathy or dementia. CPK elevation is mild to moderate (plus or minus 2 to 4 times normal values). CPK serum levels in HIV-associated myopathy appear to correlate well with the degree of "activity" (ongoing tissue damage) but poorly with the degree of clinical weakness.

An abnormal electromyogram is reported in about 90% of patients with polymyositis. Muscle biopsy shows fibrous tissue proliferation, necrosis, and phagocytosis of muscle fibers accompanied by an inflammatory infiltrate.[21]

The treatment of choice is prednisone, starting at 60 mg per day and continuing with alternate day dosing, with tapering as tolerated. Although there is some concern over the risk of treating HIV-infected individuals with steroids, experience does not indicate that this therapy accelerates the course of the disease. The risk has not been studied in controlled trials; therefore, the drug should be used carefully and only in patients with progressive and disabling weakness who do not have active systemic disease.

ZIDOVUDINE MYOPATHY

This myopathy tends to occur in patients who have been treated with high doses of zidovudine over long periods of time, but it may be seen at any time. Muscle wasting, particularly of the buttocks muscles, and associated leg weakness have been reported. An increased CPK is expected. If zidovudine myopathy is recognized early and the drug is discontinued, complete resolution of the symptoms should occur.[26]

Primary Central Nervous System Lymphoma

CNS lymphoma is found in 4% to 6% of patients with HIV infection. It is the second most common mass lesion of the brain after toxoplasmosis. The majority of tumors originate in B cells and are usually of small cell, noncleaved, or large cell immunoblastic histologic subtypes.[27] Studies have shown that Epstein Barr virus may serve as an effector of tumorigenesis. CNS lymphoma can present in several ways: (1) solitary or discrete intracranial nodules, (2) diffuse meningeal or periventricular presentations, (3) uveal or vitreous deposits (uveitis/vitreitis), and (4) localized intradural masses.[27]

The clinical presentation is one of confusion, memory loss, hemiparesis, and dysphasia. Cranial nerve palsies, headache, and seizures are also common. The symptoms may occur acutely or evolve over several weeks.

CT or MRI scans of the head typically show single or multiple discrete lesions with contrast enhancement and some degree of mass effect. The CSF may be normal or may show elevated protein, mild pleocytosis, and positive cytology. The differential diagnosis includes toxoplasmosis. If treatment for toxoplasmosis fails, then brain biopsy is indicated.

The primary treatment for CNS lymphoma is radiation therapy and dexamethasone. Radiation to the whole brain improves short-term survival, but most patients die from other AIDS-related infections in a relatively short period of time. Dexamethasone has cytotoxic effects against lymphoma and may reduce tumor size and edema. Chemotherapy is not generally used because of extensive systemic disease and reduced bone marrow reserve.

AIDS Dementia Complex

AIDS dementia complex (ADC), also known as chronic or subacute HIV encephalopathy, is characterized by disturbances in three areas of functioning: cognitive, motor, and behavior. The term ADC was introduced to describe a group of signs and symptoms rather than an established disease. The word *dementia* is used because there is acquired and persistent cognitive decline demonstrated by mental slowing and inattention, which is characteristically not accompanied by decline in alertness. The word *complex* is used to describe the multiple impairments in functioning which may affect the patient. Morbidity of the condition is comparable to that of other AIDS-defining complications of HIV infection.[28]

Although unusual, patients may develop ADC with CD4 counts in the 250 to 500 range. With progression of HIV infection and decline in CD4 count, ADC becomes more common and more severe.

Prior to widespread use of zidovudine, most patients with AIDS were expected to develop some level of dementia. Early and widespread use of zidovudine appears to have decreased the frequency and severity of the diagnosis. The prevalence of ADC is estimated at anywhere from 40% to 90%, depending on the population studied.

The pathogenesis of ADC is not clearly understood. It has been suggested that direct HIV infection of the brain may be responsible. Both CT and MRI have been reported to show cortical atrophy and white matter abnormalities ranging from scattered, periventricular high signal lesions to large, complex lesions. Size and progression of lesions seen on MRI only roughly correlate with the extent and progression of ADC.[29] Cell culture studies have demonstrated low-level infection of astrocytic and other neuroectodermal cells involving a non-CD4 virus cell interaction.[28]

The clinical presentation of ADC must be considered within the context of premorbid functioning, including alcohol and drug abuse. Early cognitive impairment includes difficulty with concentration and performance of complex sequential mental activities and complaints of memory loss, particularly related to tasks requiring concentration. Early motor impairment involves the legs more than the arms, with clumsiness and weakness in gait; if upper-extremity involvement occurs, alterations in handwriting or fine movement are noted. Behavioral changes include apathy, loss of spontaneity, and social withdrawal; some individuals display anxiety, hyperactivity, and inappropriate behavior.[18]

On physical examination, slowness in verbal and motor responses are noted. There is a slowing of rapid movement, including finger opposition, wrist rotation, and toe tapping. Hyperreflexia of deep tendon reflexes in the lower extremities may be noted. With disease progression, mutism, ataxia, paraparesis, and incontinence may occur.[30] Symptoms of motor dysfunction generally lag behind those of intellectual impairment.

The Price/Brew staging scheme (Table 33-5) is widely used for staging ADC. The World Health Organization (WHO) and American Academy of Neurology (AAN) also have staging schemes, but Price/Brew's model is preferred because of its descriptive vocabulary, which is useful for both clinical and investigational purposes.[28]

The diagnostic work-up for ADC is somewhat dependent on the patient's presentation, including other symptoms and results of previous diagnostic studies.

A complete physical examination should be done and changes in motor function and general cognition should be

TABLE 33-6
Medication Side Effects

DRUG	SIDE EFFECTS
Zidovudine (ZDV)	Headache, nausea, malaise, myalgias, anemia, neutropenia, myopathy, nail hyperpigmentation
Dideoxyinosine (ddI)	Dry mouth, altered taste, nausea, vomiting, diarrhea, peripheral neuropathy, pancreatitis, hepatitis, electrolyte imbalance
Dideoxycytidine (ddC)	Rash, fever, mouth ulcers, peripheral neuropathy, pancreatitis, cardiomyopathy, hyperglycemia
Stavudine (D4T)	Headache, nausea, vomiting, confusion, increased serum transaminase, increased creatine phosphokinase

From Fischl, M. A. (1995). Drug interactions and toxicities in patients with AIDS. In M. A. Sande & P. A. Volberding (Eds.), Medical Management of AIDS (4th ed.). Philadelphia: W. B. Saunders.

documented. The patient and/or significant others should be questioned about changes in functional status.

A CT scan or MRI of the brain should be done to rule out masses or other possible causes of symptoms. These will generally show cerebral atrophy, widened cortical sulci, and enlarged ventricles. Basal ganglia are reduced in volume. Some patients have patchy or diffuse T2-weighted abnormalities on MRI in the hemispheric white matter and, occasionally, in the basal ganglia or thalamus.[28]

A lumbar puncture should be done to rule out infectious processes. CSF analysis may reveal nonspecific abnormalities, but significant mononuclear pleocytosis may also be present. This finding may be somewhat dependent on the degree of immunocompromise. Significant cell counts are more likely to be found in patients with relatively intact immune systems.

Neuropsychological testing may support clinical findings and help establish the level of impairment. It can also serially follow the course of the disease and response to therapy.[28] A formal neuropsychological evaluation uses standardized tests with known reliability and validity to measure performance in a series of cognitive domains. The tests come from a variety of sources, and the specific tests used on an individual patient will depend on the patient's specific signs and symptoms. Each test is designed to measure performance representing a specific cognitive area. The results of neuropsychological evaluation must be considered in the same context as the results of other diagnostic studies.[31]

For patients with advanced HIV-related illness and clearcut cognitive decline, comprehensive testing may not be necessary. A brief battery of tests or a mental status evaluation such as the Folstein Mini Mental State Exam may provide adequate information about improvement or decline in function over a period of time.[31]

The only therapy shown to be of benefit in ADC is zidovudine. In studies using dosages of zidovudine at 1000 to 2000 mg per day, a beneficial effect on cognitive function was

TABLE 33-5
Price and Brew's Staging Scheme for AIDS Dementia Complex

STAGE	DESCRIPTION
0	Normal mental and motor function
0.5–1	(Subclinical) Minimal symptoms without impairment of work function or activities of daily living (ADLs)
1	(Mild) Cognitive or motor deficits that compromise more demanding aspects of work or ADLs
2	(Moderate) Cognitive deficit; patient unable to work or perform more demanding ADLs
3	(Severe) Patient can perform only most rudimentary skills
4	(End stage) Patient has no understanding of surroundings and requires complete care

From Brew, J. B. (1992). Central and peripheral nervous system abnormalities. Medical Clinics of North America, 76(1), 63–81.

TABLE 33-7
Nursing Diagnoses

NURSING DIAGNOSIS	INTERVENTION	OUTCOME
Inadequate Nutrition related to (R/T) decreased intake	Determine reasons for inadequate intake: mouth ulcers, dysphasia, nausea, inability to prepare food.	Meets caloric requirements.
	Determine appropriate nutritional needs (refer to dietitian if necessary).	Weight is stable or increased.
	Provide nutritional supplements, meal preparation assistance.	
	Consider alterations in medication schedules.	
	Assess need for feeding tube or total parenteral nutrition.	
Self Care Deficit R/T cognitive/ motor impairment	Assess ability to complete activities of daily living (ADLs).	Patient participates in ADLs at highest possible level of functioning.
	Assist with aids/cues to maintain independence.	
	Provide ADLs which patient cannot do—bathing, dressing, feeding etc.	
	Be sure patient has adequate supervision/assistance at home.	
Risk for Injury R/T impaired cognitive/motor functioning	Regular assessment of level of functioning.	Safe environment is maintained.
	Adequate supervision/assistance with ADLs, meals, medication administration.	Assistance or intervention is provided when appropriate.
	Problem solving and/or direct intervention when unsafe behavior is identified.	
Pain R/T altered sensory perception	Pain assessed regularly using a standard scale.	Pain level is acceptable to patient.
	Skin assessed regularly for pressure areas, breakdown.	Medication side effects are tolerable.
	Clothing, shoes do not cause pressure.	
	Pain medications are taken as prescribed and reassessed regularly for most effective management.	
Impaired Social Interaction/Isolation R/T impaired physical mobility and/or cognitive defects	Assess/determine patient's baseline functioning.	Interactions are appropriate for patient's level of disability.
	Determine types of activities appropriate to current level of functioning.	
	Assist patient/family to plan for activities and outings to stimulate interaction.	
	Encourage patient to be as independent as circumstances allow.	
Risk for Infection R/T immunocompromised state	Skin integrity assessed regularly.	Patient does not acquire preventable infections.
	Catheter sites/IV sites are assessed and dressings changed on schedule.	Infections are identified and treatment initiated promptly.
	Appropriate level of medical care is available to patient.	
	New symptoms: fever, chills, local signs and symptoms of infection are promptly evaluated and treated.	
	Good hand washing.	
	Food prepared under sanitary conditions.	
Impaired Physical Mobility R/T motor weakness	Conduct baseline assessment for motor function and reassess regularly.	Patient does not suffer injuries related to weakness or falls.
	Assess for assistive devices such as canes, walkers, bath aids.	Appropriate aids are available.
	Maintain/increase mobility through planned exercise, activity.	Changes in level of function are consistent with overall condition.
	Consultation with physical therapist, occupational therapist as necessary.	
	Assist patient with activities unable to do for self.	

(continued)

TABLE 33-7
Nursing Diagnoses Continued

NURSING DIAGNOSIS	INTERVENTION	OUTCOME
Altered Coping R/T multiple life stressors	Assess current coping of patient and/or family.	Patient is able to identify positive coping skills.
	Assist patient in identifying specific stressors.	Referrals are made to appropriate resources.
	Assist patient in identifying possible resolutions to problems.	
	Refer to appropriate resources: social worker, social services, community based agencies, mental health professional.	
Alteration in Health Maintenance R/T progression of illness	Provide information to patient/family about disease process and treatment options for specific problems.	Patient will contribute to and comply with treatment plan.
	Encourage patient to be actively involved in decisions related to care.	Patient will make informed decisions about medical care.
	Assist patient in identifying resources to meet needs.	Patient will complete advance directives and power of attorney.
Alteration in Vision and/or Hearing R/T complications of central nervous system disorders	Assess for degree of vision/hearing loss.	Patient remains free of injury.
	Assess environment for hazards and institute measures to ensure safety.	Patient uses compensatory devices to communicate effectively and participate in ADLs.
	Establish alternative means of communication as needed.	
	Use interdisciplinary approach to assist patient with compensatory techniques and devices that promote activities.	
Decreased Level of Arousal R/T changes in intracranial dynamics	Assess neurological status as condition warrants.	Patient will remain free of complications associated with decreased arousal.
	Assess cardiovascular and respiratory status regularly.	Patient will progress to highest level of arousal.
	Manipulate environment to deliver appropriate levels of stimulation.	
	Use interdisciplinary approach to prevent complications of immobility	
	Educate and involve family in care.	

shown. This dose is significantly higher than the usual daily dose of 500 to 600 mg and may not be tolerated because of bone marrow suppression. Since only about 30% of zidovudine crosses the blood–brain barrier, it is reasonable to expect that higher-than-normal doses would be necessary. The time needed for maximum response is not known, but it appears to be in the range of 8 weeks. Since the optimal dose is not known, most physicians recommend the highest tolerable dose—usually 1000 to 1200 mg per day.

The effect of other antiretrovirals on ADC is not as well known. Dideoxyinosine has limited penetration across the blood–brain barrier, and ddC has poor CSF penetration. Several newer antiretroviral agents, including the non-nucleoside analogs and protease inhibitors, are nearing clinical trial stage and may provide new options.[26]

With the limitations in medication options, interventions should focus on assisting the patient in identifying functional deficits and strategies to compensate for the deficits. Interventions such as promoting cognitive stimulation and orientation, promoting independence and self-esteem, and providing for safety are important.[6]

GENERAL PRINCIPLES OF CARE

Although this chapter is primarily concerned with the neurological manifestations of HIV, there are general principles of caring for individuals with HIV infection that are important regardless of the specific symptoms or disease with which a patient presents. HIV is considered incurable; however, there are many interventions that can be initiated over the course of the illness to improve the quality of the individual's life and delay disease progression.

Drug Therapy

There are a number of drugs that are designed to slow viral replication and prolong the period of time before the individual develops HIV-related symptoms. Any patient with a CD4 count of less than 500 may wish to consider taking an antiretroviral drug. The most commonly used drugs in this group include zidovudine, ddI, and ddC. Stavudine (also known as

TABLE 33-8 *Sample Critical Pathway: Cryptococcal Meningitis*	
TIME FRAME	**ACTIVITIES**
Day 1	Diagnosis confirmed by LP and serum cryptoantigen.
	General nursing assessment and identification of a primary nurse and/or case manager.
	Management of headache and other symptoms.
	Monitor vital signs.
	Obtain baseline laboratory tests: CBC with differential, chemistries.
	Initiate amphotericin B therapy.
Day 2	Place secure IV line which will provide access for at least 2 wk.
	Patient education about diagnosis and treatment plan.
	Begin patient education about home IV therapy.
	Monitor for and manage medication side effects.
	Refer for financial and social services support as appropriate.
	Determine home care agency
	Check CBC with differential and electrolytes.
Day 3	Monitor functional status.
	Continue teaching medication administration, including IV care.
	Continue management of symptoms and medication side effects and develop plan for how to manage at home.
	Provide emotional support as appropriate.
	Check CBC with differential and electrolytes.
Day 4	Discharge from hospital with adequate home care arranged.
Days 5–14	IV amphotericin B administered at home.
	Home nursing visits 2–3 times per wk for general assessment, laboratory tests and for followup on psychosocial problems and connection with resources as needed.
Day 14	Convert to oral medication.
	Continue home based or community based services as needed.
Indefinite	Regular medical followup.
	Compliance with medications.
	Labs depending on overall medical condition.

D4T or Zerit) has also recently been approved for use. These drugs may be used individually or in combination. Their benefits include delaying disease progression, increasing the CD4 count, and suppressing viral replication. It is important to recognize that all of these medications have significant adverse effects (Table 33-6).

Prophylaxis

Since one of the goals of HIV treatment is to prevent opportunistic infections or control recurrence, prophylaxis for a va-

riety of infections is recommended. Any patient with a CD4 count of less than 200 is at significant risk for opportunistic infections. It is well documented that pneumocystis pneumonia prophylaxis is valuable. Studies are currently underway to evaluate the value of prophylaxis against Mycobacterium avium complex, cryptococcus, and other infections.[11,19,32]

Ongoing Treatment

Patients developing signs or symptoms of disease progression or a specific opportunistic infection or tumor should be evaluated and offered appropriate therapy. At any given time, there are investigational drug trials in progress to evaluate medications for treatment of a variety of infections and against the virus itself. Patients should be made aware of the availability of these studies and, when appropriate, encouraged to participate.

PATIENT OUTCOMES, CASE MANAGEMENT, AND CRITICAL PATHWAYS

As health care delivery models change and increasing emphasis is placed on cost of care, focusing on patient outcomes becomes a critical element of nursing practice. Case management and critical pathway models both rely on nursing diagnoses, identification of appropriate interventions, and measurable outcomes. Major nursing diagnoses are listed in Table 33-7.

Because HIV/AIDS is a chronic, long-term illness with many complications requiring the services of multiple specialists, a coordinated approach to care is critical. Any individual with an HIV diagnosis should have a primary care provider (physician, nurse practitioner, physician assistant) to coordinate overall medical care. In addition, each individual should have a case manager, a primary nurse, or both to assist in coordinating services. It is ideal if this team can begin to work with the patient before severe illness occurs, in order to assess the patient and family under normal circumstances. Unfortunately, many patients do not present for care until they are acutely ill with an opportunistic infection and in need of crisis intervention.[33]

Although neurological nurses are specialists, they may have long-term contact with HIV/AIDS patients in the acute care setting, for patients needing multiple hospitalizations for CNS infections, or in an outpatient setting, for regular followup. In any setting where a patient receives ongoing care, a primary nurse should be available to work with the patient's case manager and other primary nurses to identify needs and coordinate services.

Much has been written about the use of case management and critical pathway models to monitor individual patient outcomes and provide high-quality, cost-effective care. Experience has shown that critical pathways are valuable for a clearly defined diagnosis in a patient who has no other complications or concurrent illnesses. For example, a patient with newly diagnosed cryptococcal meningitis who is functioning independently and who has no other opportunistic infections or neurological deficits could be tracked on a critical pathway (Table 33-8).

Few HIV/AIDS patients present with a single infection and no complications. Therefore, a case management model in addition to or instead of a critical pathway model is important. The case manager may be based in the hospital or community. The goal is to manage hospital care and coordinate outpatient, home, and community based services to meet the patient's medical and psychosocial needs in the most cost-effective way. Case managers rely heavily on primary nurses to provide information on changes in the patient's condition and need for services. The goals are to prevent repeated hospital admissions for preventable complications and to identify therapies that can be delivered in an outpatient setting or in the home.

QUALITY OF LIFE AND ADVANCE DIRECTIVES

Because of widespread availability of HIV testing, health maintenance, and medical intervention, individuals with HIV are living for years with their illness. An important issue is quality of life during the continuum and planning for death when complications can no longer be managed. From the time of initial contact, it is important to learn how the individual perceives the impact of HIV on his or her life. As the illness progresses and the ability to manage complications becomes more limited, it is important to engage the patient in discussion about interventions desired or not desired. This should include discussion about hospital admissions, admission to an intensive care unit, intubation, and cardiopulmonary resuscitation. It is strongly recommended that patients sign advance directive forms designating someone to make decisions in the event that they cannot communicate their own wishes.

These discussions are best initiated when the patient is not in a crisis. The issues may need to be revisited over a period of time with the primary medical provider, the primary nurse, and the case manager.

Summary

The number of patients with neurological disorders will continue to increase as the HIV/AIDS epidemic evolves, and diagnostic testing and treatment options will continue to expand. Nurses will be challenged to stay current in scientific information and in finding ways to provide compassionate, cost-effective care.

References

1. McArthur, J. (1992). Neurologic manifestations of human immunodeficiency virus infection. In A. Asbury, G. McKhanna, & W. McDonald (Eds.), *Diseases of the nervous system: Clinical neurobiology*. Philadelphia: W. B. Saunders.
2. Ake, J. M., & Peristein, L. M. (1987). AIDS: Impact on neuroscience nursing practice. *Journal of Neuroscience Nursing, 19*(6), 300–304.
3. Zunich, K. M., & Lane, H. C. (1991). Immunologic abnormalities in HIV infection. *Hematology/Oncology Clinics of North America, 5*, 215–228
4. Stein, D. S., Korvich, J. A., & Vermund, S. T. (1992). CD4+ lymphocyte cell enumeration for prediction of clinical course of human immunodeficiency virus disease: A review. *Journal of Infectious Diseases, 165*, 352–363.
5. Staprans, S. I., & Feinberg, J. (1995). Natural history immunopathogenesis of HIV-1 disease. In M. A. Sande & P. A. Volberding (Eds.), *Medical management of AIDS* (4th ed.). Philadelphia: W. B. Saunders.
6. Ungvarski, P. J. (1992). Nursing management of the adult client. In J. H. Flaskerud & P. J. Ungvarski (Eds.), *HIV/AIDS: A guide to nursing care* (2nd ed.). Philadelphia: W. B. Saunders.
7. Bartlett, J. G. (1995a). *Johns Hopkins Hospital guide to medical care of patients with HIV infection* (5th ed.). Baltimore: Williams & Wilkins, pp. 1–9, 16–18.
8. Centers for Disease Control. (1995). *HIV/AIDS Surveillance Report, 6*(2).
9. Buehler, J. W., Peterson, L. R., & Jaffe, H. W. (1995). Current trends in the epidemiology of HIV/AIDS. In M. A. Sande & P. A. Volberding (Eds.), *Medical management of AIDS* (4th ed.). Philadelphia: W. B. Saunders.
10. Saag, M. S. (1995). AIDS testing now and in the future. In M. A. Sande & P. A. Volberding (Eds.), *Medical management of AIDS* (4th ed.). Philadelphia: W. B. Saunders.
11. Bartlett, J, G. (1995b). *Pocket guide of infectious disease therapy*. Baltimore: Williams & Wilkins, pp. 65–66.
12. Elder, G., & Sever, J. (1988). AIDS and neurological disorders: An overview. *Annals of Neurology, 23*(Suppl.), S4–S6.
13. Fisher, E. J. (1995). *Clinician's guide to therapy of adults with HIV/AIDS* (3rd ed.). Richmond: Virginia Commonwealth University HIV/AIDS Center.
14. Houff, S. (1988). Neuroimmunology of human immunodeficiency virus. In M. Rosenblum, R. Levy., & D. Bredesen (Eds.), *AIDS and the nervous system*. New York: Raven.
15. Levy, J. (1988). The biology of the human immunodeficiency virus and its role in neurological disease. In M. Rosenblum, R. Levy, & D. Bredesen (Eds.), *AIDS and the nervous system*. New York: Raven.
16. Tam, D. A., Shapiro, S. M., & Snead, R. W. (1995). Neurologic and psychiatric manifestations of pediatric AIDS. *Immunology and Allergy Clinics of North America, 15*(2), 285–305.
17. Tindall, T., & Cooper, D. (1991). Host responses and intervention strategies. *AIDS, 5*, 1–14.
18. Newton, H. B. (1995). Common neurologic complications of HIV-1 infection and AIDS. *American Family Physician, 51*(2), 387–398.
19. Hilton, G. (1994). Neuroscience nursing and HIV. In E. Barker (Ed.), *Neuroscience nursing*. St. Louis: Mosby.
20. Mocsny, N. (1992). Cryptococcal meningitis in patients with AIDS. *Journal of Neuroscience Nursing, 24*, 265–268.
21. Berger, J. R., & Levy, R. M. (1993). The neurologic complications of human immunodeficiency virus infection. *Medical Clinics of North America, 77*(1), 1–21.
22. Wilson, J. D., Braunwald, E., Isselbacher, K. J., Petersorf, R. G., Martin, J. B., Fauci, A. S., & Root, R. K. (1991). *Harrison's principles of internal medicine* (12th ed.). New York: McGraw-Hill, p. 641.
23. Parry, G. J. (1988). Peripheral neuropathies associated with human immunodeficiency virus infection. *Annals of Neurology, 23*(Suppl.), S49–S53.
24. Simpson, D. M., & Wolfe, D. E. (1991). Neuromuscular complications of HIV infection and its treatment. *AIDS, 5*, 917–926.
25. Kieburtz, K. (1995, May). *Treatment of neurologic complications of HIV infection*. Paper presented at the meeting of the American Academy of Neurologists, Seattle, WA.
26. Brew, J. B. (1992). Central and peripheral nervous system abnormalities. *Medical Clinics of North America, 76*(1), 63–81.
27. Rosenblum, M. L., Levy, R. M., Bredesen, D. E., So, Y. T., Wara,

W., & Ziegler, J. L. (1988). Primary central nervous system lymphomas in patients with AIDS. *Annals of Neurology, 23*(Suppl.), S13–S16.

28. Price, R. W., & Worley, J. M. (1995). Management of neurologic complications of HIV-1 infection and AIDS. In M. A. Sande & P. A. Volberding (Eds.), *Medical management of AIDS* (4th ed.). Philadelphia: W. B. Saunders.

29. Kieburtz, K. D., Ketonen, L., Zettelmaier, A. E., Kido, D., Caine, E. D., & Simon, J. H. (1990). Magnetic resonance imaging findings in HIV cognitive impairment. *Archives of Neurology, 47,* 643–645.

30. Price, R. W., Sidtis, J., & Rosenblum, M. (1988). The AIDS dementia complex: Some current questions. *Annals of Neurology, 23*(Suppl.), S27–S33.

31. Stern, Y. (1994). Neuropsychological evaluation of the HIV patient. *Psychiatric Clinics of North America, 17*(1), 125–134.

32. Levy, R. M., Bredesen, D. E., & Rosenblum, M. L. (1988). Opportunistic central nervous system pathology in patients with AIDS. *Annals of Neurology, 23*(Suppl.), S7–S12.

33. Loder, P. (1993). HIV infections of the central nervous system: What are the nursing implications. *Nursing Clinics of North America, 28*(4), 839–847..

CHAPTER 34

Selected Degenerative Diseases of the Nervous System

Joanne V. Hickey

Although there are several degenerative diseases of the nervous system, only a few of the most common disorders will be discussed in this chapter—namely, dementia and Alzheimer's disease, multiple sclerosis, amyotrophic lateral sclerosis, myasthenia gravis, and Parkinson's disease. Guillain-Barré syndrome is also discussed in this chapter. Although it is not a degenerative problem in the same sense as the other conditions listed, it has many management similarities. The understanding and management of these conditions has seen much progress in the last 10 to 15 years, and a brief overview of changes are reflected in this chapter.

A similar philosophy of care can be applied to most degenerative diseases; that is, the patient is kept as independent and functional as possible for as long as possible within the context of his or her lifestyle. This goal is achieved through a collaborative, multidisciplinary, integrated, holistic approach that includes the patient and family in decisions related to management. Most patients are managed in the community, where care is more cost effective, with the assistance of their families, professional care providers, and community resources. Hospitalization, if necessary, is usually short and limited to serious relapses or complications related to the disease.

PSYCHOSOCIAL CONSIDERATIONS

The very nature of a degenerative disease indicates a process of loss. How quickly functional deterioration occurs depends on the particular disease and the individual course for that patient. The adjustments and ability to cope will depend on how the patient perceives the loss of function. For example, loss of mobility and control of body functions creates various deprivation syndromes and changes in body image and day-to-day living.

Degenerative diseases most often deprive the individual of degrees of independence. Patients need help to cope with this loss, which can take the form of accentuating the positive and identifying those activities in which independence can be maintained. At the same time, it is important to accept those areas of dependence that exist. Patients and families need help to accept the illness and set realistic goals.

The educational needs of the patient and family are met by developing a teaching plan, the objectives of which include knowledge of the illness and therapeutic modalities used, precautions to be taken, and accentuation of the positive aspects of the condition. The patient is helped to modify the environment, lifestyle, and routines to allow for maximal independence. Occupational and vocational counseling can help in the adjustments necessary for gainful employment and life roles, such as homemaking. Recreational activities, hobbies, and other pursuits enjoyed by the patient are encouraged.

Physiotherapy is often important in the management of degenerative diseases. Based on a systematic, individualized assessment and ongoing evaluation, specific exercises and therapeutic regimens are selected for the patient. Regimens can include passive range-of-motion and active, resistive, and stretching exercises to strengthen muscles, reduce spasticity, improve coordination, and control the development of contractures. Physiotherapy might also involve massage; hydrotherapy; gait retraining; prescription of aerobic exercises such as swimming or walking; and selection of assistive devices such as braces, splints, canes, and feeding equipment. Managing patients with nervous system degenerative diseases is a challenge with high stakes—quality of life and independence.

ORGANIC MENTAL DISORDERS

Organic mental disorders is a broad classification applied to a group of mental disorders caused by local or widespread cognitive impairment as listed in the **Diagnostic and Statistical Manual of Mental Disorder III-R.**[1] In this classification, dementia and Alzheimer's disease (AD) are included. There is a wide range of types of dementias.

Dementia is defined as a global deterioration of acquired cognitive function with a clear sensorium. In some instances, dementia may be associated with an underlying primary condition and may be reversible with prompt treatment of the primary problem. Common underlying etiologies are drug toxicity, metabolic disorders, neurological conditions, and dysfunction in other body systems. In other instances, dementia is a chronic, irreversible condition, resulting in progressive loss of overall cognitive function. At times, organic mental disorders are difficult to distinguish from acute, functional psychotic states because of overlapping clinical signs and symptoms. Short- and long-term memory deficits are the most striking symptoms noted. The causes of progressive dementias are numerous and varied and include the following:

- Diffuse parenchyma diseases of the central nervous system (CNS) (*e.g.,* Alzheimer's disease, Pick's disease, Parkinson's disease)
- Metabolic disorders (*e.g.,* hypoglycemia, metachromatic leukodystrophy)
- Vascular disorders (*e.g.,* arteriosclerosis, arteriovenous malformation)
- Normal pressure hydrocephalus
- Hypoxic and anoxic states
- Deficiency diseases (*e.g.,* Wernicke-Korsakoff syndrome)
- Toxins and drug toxicity (metals, organic compounds)
- Brain tumors
- Cerebral trauma
- Infections (meningitis, encephalitis, Creutzfeldt-Jakob disease, AIDS)

Regardless of the cause, the effects on the brain involve interference with cellular metabolism. Management of dementia can be difficult. Three principles guide management:

- Treatment of the underlying cause
- Treatment of the presenting symptoms (*e.g.,* agitation, sleep disorder, wandering)
- Control of environmental or situational factors that precipitate cognitive or behavioral dysfunction

The problematic behavior often presents concerns for safety and must be addressed. For example, if agitation and wandering behaviors are present, then interventions designed to address the underlying cause of these problems must be implemented. Interventions may include cognitive therapy, drug therapy, or a combination of both. Supervision is a twofold responsibility. Controlling the environment is a form of supervision and manipulation of the patient. Supervision of the patient helps to monitor and control the patient to prevent injuries. Providing a stable and controlled environment is helpful in minimizing disorientation, confusion, frustration, agitation, and combative behavior. Too many environmental stimuli, tasks beyond the patient's ability, or unfamiliar surroundings are examples of situations that may precipitate behavioral problems. Management protocols must be individualized according to particular patient needs.

ALZHEIMER'S DISEASE

Alzheimer's disease (AD) is a chronic, progressive degenerative disorder of the brain characterized by profound global impairment of cognitive functions. AD can affect people at any age, but it usually involves people in middle and late life. The Diagnostic and Statistical Manual of Mental Disorders III-R outlines the diagnostic criteria for Primary Degenerative Dementia of the Alzheimer Type as dementia; insidious onset with a generally progressive deteriorating course; and exclusion of all other specific causes of dementia by history, physical examination, and laboratory tests. AD was formerly subdivided into a presenile dementia in persons under the age of 65 and a senile dementia of Alzheimer's type in persons 65 years old and older. This distinction is no longer used because there is no appreciable difference between early and late onset of AD.[2]

Cerebral atrophy and cellular degeneration are the major neuropathological changes noted at autopsy. The cellular degenerative changes include neurofibrillary tangles and amyloidal plaque deposits found chiefly in the temporoparietal and anterior frontal regions. It has been suggested that the pattern of cellular pathology may involve the major projection neurons of the hippocampal formation. The cause of AD is unknown although genetic factors have been implicated in some cases.

Pathophysiology

Intensive study continues on the neurobiology of AD, with much interest focused on the neurotransmitter systems. Abnormalities in the cholinergic system include reduced activity of choline acetyltransferase, the enzyme necessary for acetylcholine synthesis, and a decrease in acetylcholine synthesis. Beta protein, a major component of the amyloid fibrils, has also been located on chromosome 21 in older patients with Down's syndrome and familial AD. All of these pieces of information will someday elucidate a clear understanding of AD and, perhaps, ways to prevent the disease.

Signs and Symptoms

Progressive impairment of short- and long-term memory is a major feature of AD. Beginning with forgetfulness that can be subtle, it can be dismissed easily by the patient and the family. The patient may try to conceal the forgetfulness with excuses, compensating with notes and reminders. There is a deterioration in activities of daily living (ADLs) and instrumental ADLs as noted in work performance and ability to deal with everyday family living and social situations. The progressive course continues until the patient's loss of global cognitive functions includes impaired abstract thinking and impaired judgment, and personality change becomes obvious. In the terminal stage, the patient is bedridden, emaciated, aphasic, and apraxic and lacks control of the body, including sphincters. All cognitive functions and emotional responses are lost. Death is usually caused by infection, such as aspiration pneumonia. Chart 34-1 summarizes the time span and behavior associated with each of the three stages of AD.

Diagnosis

Confirmation of AD is possible only at autopsy. Diagnosis is one of exclusion and based on a clinical and neuropathological pattern. Therefore, a search for a primary underlying cause is conducted before the diagnosis of AD is made. The accuracy of clinical diagnosis is based on the ability of the clinician to predict the presence or absence of the typical neuropathological lesions at autopsy.[3] However, we care for live patients and look to practical ways to diagnose patients. An accurate history (information from family) and a neurological examination, in association with a mental status examination and neuropsychological testing, are critical in suggesting the diagnosis of AD. Serial use of the Mini-Mental Status Examination is an inexpensive way to monitor cognitive function over time.[4–6]

Part of the difficulty in distinguishing the dementia of AD from the dementia associated with other conditions is lack of clarity of definitions. Delirium and depression, which can resemble dementia, must be excluded. **Delirium** is a *transient and potentially reversible condition* in which there is fluctuation in levels of awareness (agitation to stupor), hallucinations, and cognitive impairment, particularly memory. The key defining characteristic of delirium is the pattern of fluctuation in time

---

CHART 34-1
Stages of Alzheimer's Disease

The stages of Alzheimer's disease vary from patient to patient, but a few time approximations, as well as characteristic behaviors, can be identified.

Stage 1: Early Stage—2 to 4 years

- Forgetful—may be subtle, may try to cover up by using lists and notes
- Exhibits a declining interest in environment, people, and present affairs
- Demonstrates vague uncertainty and hesitancy in initiating actions
- Performs poorly at work, may be dismissed from job

Stage 2: Middle Stage—2 to 12 years

- Exhibits a progressive memory loss
- Hesitates in response to questions; shows signs of aphasia
- Has difficulty following simple instructions or doing simple calculations
- Has episodic bouts of irritability
- Becomes evasive, anxious, and physically active
- Becomes more active at night owing to sleep–wakefulness cycle disturbance
- Wanders, particularly at night
- Becomes apraxic for many basic activities
- Loses important papers
- Loses way home in familiar surroundings or loses way in own home
- Forgets to pay bills; lets household chores slip and newspapers pile up; does not dispose of garbage; does not take medications
- Loses possessions and then claims that they were stolen
- Neglects personal hygiene (bathing, shaving, dressing)
- Loses social graces; can cause embarrassment to family and friends, which usually results in social isolation of the family and patient

Stage 3: Final Stage

- Loses much weight because of lack of eating; becomes emaciated
- Is unable to communicate verbally or in writing
- Does not recognize family
- Is incontinent of urine and feces
- Has a predisposition for major seizures
- Grasping, snout, and sucking reflexes are readily elicited
- Finally loses the ability to stand and walk and becomes bedridden
- Death is usually caused by aspiration pneumonia

and in symptoms observed. **Depression** and other psychiatric disorders are potentially reversible and are related to poor performance on the mental status examination or formal neuropsychological testing.

Computed tomography (CT) and magnetic resonance imaging (MRI) are the most helpful diagnostic tools. A positron emission tomography (PET) scan, although sometimes ordered, is controversial and not readily available in all facilities. In the later stages, there is diffuse slowing of the waves on electroencephalogram (EEG). Other laboratory tests should be ordered to rule out conditions that are treatable.

Treatment

Unfortunately, there is no specific treatment for AD. A new drug, tacrine hydrochloride (Cognex), is now available and acts to increase brain acetylcholine levels. Some believe that this drug may slow the mental deterioration process. More longitudinal studies are needed to establish long-term efficacy. In managing AD, the patient and family must be prepared for what lies ahead. This includes awareness of available support services and encouragement and support for the difficult decisions that must be made about home or institutional care, financial arrangements, family caregiver stressors, and other matters.

Nursing Management

Patients with AD are managed in the home with the assistance of family, home services, and health providers. Needs vary depending on the stage of AD. The number of patients diagnosed as having AD is steadily rising, giving nurses increased opportunity to care for these patients. Nurses employed in hospitals have contact with AD patients admitted for other reasons such as a fractured hip related to a fall. Nurses based in clinics or community based AD programs are involved directly in management. Although there is no specific treatment, the patient and family need much sensitivity and emotional support during the course of this devastating disease. Several principles can guide the nurse in working with AD victims and their families and in teaching the family. These include the following:

- Provide supervision to protect the patient from becoming injured, humiliated, or lost.
- Encourage the patient to participate in ADLs for as long as possible.
- Provide for the patient's nutritional needs.
- Provide the family and patient with specific information about the disease.
- Make the patient and family aware of such resources as the Alzheimer's Disease and Related Disorders Association, which has chapters in many states and several family support groups.
- Encourage the family to seek legal advice regarding financial and legal measures to be taken to protect the patient and family.
- Make referrals to social services and community resources that may assist the patient and family.
- Encourage the development of realistic short- and long-term planning.

- Encourage the patient to seek medical supervision for the management of other health problems that may arise and for periodic reassessment of cognitive abilities.
- Help the family understand caregiver stress and develop coping skills. Referral for counseling may be appropriate.
- Help the family or caregiver develop strategies to deal with the specific problems of patient management.
- Help the family in decisions concerning institutionalization.

The nurse is in a position to support the patient and family and assist them in dealing with the various painful and monumental decisions that will need attention as the disease develops. See Chart 34-2 for a summary of major nursing diagnoses associated with AD.

Additional resources on AD are available from the following organizations:

Alzheimer's Disease and Related Disorders Association, Inc.
National Headquarters
919 North Michigan Avenue, Suite 1000
Chicago, IL 60611-1676
(313) 334-8700 or (313) 272-3900

Alzheimer's Foundation
8177 South Harvard M/C-114
Tulsa, OK 74137
(918) 481-6031

MULTIPLE SCLEROSIS

Multiple sclerosis (MS) or disseminated sclerosis is a chronic, progressive, degenerative disease that affects the myelin sheath and conduction pathways of the CNS. The clinical course is variable. The classification of MS is based on the clinical course:

- In **relapsing/remitting disease** (65% of cases), the relapses develop over 1 to 2 weeks, resolve over 4 to 8 weeks, and return to their baseline.
- **Relapsing/progressive disease** (15% of cases) is similar to the relapsing/remitting form, but with less recovery, so that the patient does not return to baseline and is left with significant residual disability.
- **Chronic progressive disease** (20% of cases) is characterized by spinal cord and cerebellar dysfunction; symptoms of the spinal cord and the cerebellum are the initial manifestations. It can also occur as a conversion of the relapsing/remitting form over time.[7]
- The category of **stable MS** is sometimes used for patients who have had no active clinical disease nor any subjective deterioration in their condition in the last year.

Based on long-term follow-up, between 20% and 35% have a very benign form of MS with minimal or no disability. In addition, upon autopsy, characteristic sclerotic lesions may be found in patients who never noticed neurological deficits. The number of sclerotic plaques can be surprisingly high and the patient can still be asymptomatic. About 3% to 12% of patients have a malignant form in which severe disability develops within months to a few years.[8] The majority of patients

CHART 34-2
Summary of Major Nursing Diagnoses Associated With Alzheimer's Disease

Nursing Diagnoses	Nursing Interventions	Expected Outcomes
Altered Cognitive Function: Confusion, Impaired Memory related to (R/T) loss of cells in cerebral cortex	• Maintain intact function for as long as possible. • Provide missing information. • Protect patient from needless embarrassment by structuring the environment.	• Frustration level will be minimized. • Self-care and instrumental ADLs will be provided.
Self-Care Deficit Syndrome R/T dementia, motor weakness, and sensory deficits Self-Care Deficit, Instrumental, R/T loss of cognitive function and loss of independence	• Provide for ongoing assessment of self-care needs and the patient's ability to participate in this activity. • Provide direct care and necessary services as needed.	• Self-care needs will be provided by the patient under supervision or, when this is no longer possible, self-care needs will be provided by caregiver.
Sleep Pattern Disturbance R/T agitation and/or daytime sleeping	• Control the patient's activity so that he or she will stay awake during the daytime. • Provide measures to facilitate sleep at night. • Manipulate the environment to provide an environment conducive to sleep. • Administer medications as ordered.	• An adequate sleep–wakefulness pattern will be established. • The pattern will not be disruptive to others living in the environment.
Impaired Verbal Communications R/T dementia and/or motor deficits	• Develop alternative methods for communication. • Anticipate the patient's needs.	• An alternative method of communication will be established. • The patient's needs will be anticipated.
Altered Thought Processes R/T cognitive deterioration and/or altered consciousness	• Do not ask the patient to perform cognitive skills beyond his or her ability. • Control the patient's stressors. • Develop a daily routine for the patient to follow. • Provide for continuity of care.	• The patient will be protected from being required to participate in cognitive functions beyond his or her ability. • The patient will be protected from stress that leads to behavioral outbursts.
High Risk for Injury R/T impulsive behavior and/or motor or sensory weakness	• Recognize that the patient's impaired cognitive functions can lead to injury. • Provide a safe environment. • Provide for frequent supervision.	• The patient will not be injured.
Caregiver Role Strain R/T physical and mental deterioration of family member and the 24-hour need for care and supervision	• Educate caregiver about role strain. • Support decisions on management of patient. • Refer to support groups. • Encourage self-care of caregiver.	• Caregiver will meet basic needs for rest, nutrition, and respite. • Through education, the caregiver will understand role strain and the need to make decisions for self-care.

(continued)

CHART 34-2 Summary of Major Nursing Diagnoses Associated With Alzheimer's Disease (Continued)

Nursing Diagnoses	Nursing Interventions	Expected Outcomes
Other Related Nursing Diagnoses • Impaired Adjustment • Anxiety • Risk of Aspiration • Ineffective Denial • Compromised Family Coping • Fear • Grieving • Altered Nutrition: Less Than Body Requirements • Total Incontinence • Impaired Social Interactions • Social Isolation		

have a course that is someplace in the middle. Initial symptoms resolve, and periods of relapsing tend to be spaced at longer intervals in the earlier stages. As the illness progresses, the periods of relapsing become closer together and there is progressive residual disability after each relapse that develops over several years.

Etiology and Epidemiology

The etiology of MS is unknown, a viral infection has been suggested as a cause. Immunologic abnormalities are part of the clinical and laboratory picture. MS has been called the disease of young adults because the highest rate of incidence is between the ages of 20 and 40 years. About 20% of patients experience their first symptoms in their 40s and 50s.

There are approximately 500,000 cases of MS in the United States, with women being affected slightly more frequently than men. The incidence of the disease in first-degree relatives of persons with MS is 15 times greater than that of the general population. Many epidemiological studies have reported that MS is more prevalent in the colder northern latitudes, and that it is more common in the northern Atlantic states, the Great Lakes region, and the Pacific Northwest than in southern parts of the United States. In Europe, high-incidence areas include Scandinavia, northern Germany, and Great Britain. However, moving to a warmer climate after diagnosis does not arrest the disease.

Pathophysiology

MS affects the white matter of the brain and spinal cord by causing scattered, demyelinated lesions, preventing conduction of normal nerve impulse through the demyelinated zone. The destruction or demyelination of the fatty substance, called the myelin sheath, that surrounds the axons leaves patches of sclerotic tissue. The remission of symptoms is the result of healing of the demyelinated areas by sclerotic tissue. Eventually, the nerve fibers may degenerate, so that disabilities in-

crease and become permanent. Upon autopsy, multiple sclerotic plaques are scattered throughout the white matter of the brain and cord. The scattering differs from patient to patient, accounting for the various presenting symptoms experienced by the individual. Neurological deficits are apparent during periods of relapse and can completely disappear during remission.

Signs and Symptoms

The signs and symptoms of MS vary greatly from patient to patient. Initial symptoms can occur alone or in any combination. Signs and symptoms may include the following:

- **Sensory symptoms**—numbness; anesthesia; paresthesia (burning, prickling, tingling); pain; decreased proprioception and sense of temperature, depth, and vibration
- **Motor symptoms**—paresis, paralysis, dragging of foot; spasticity; diplopia; bladder and bowel dysfunction (incontinence or retention)
- **Cerebellar symptoms**—ataxia; loss of balance and coordination; nystagmus; speech disturbances (dysarthria, dystonia, scanning speech, slurred speech); tremors (intentional tremors, described as tremors that increase when a purposeful act is initiated); vertigo
- **Other symptoms**—fatigue; optic neuritis; impotence or decreased genital sensation, and sexual dysfunction; neurobehavioral disorders such as depression or euphoria. Rarely, about 5% of patients experience hemiplegia, trigeminal neuralgia, facial paralysis, and deafness.

SENSORY SYMPTOMS

Numbness and tingling on the face or involved extremities are common. Loss of proprioception and joint sensation is frequently accompanied by edema of the limb or feelings of constriction. Fifty percent of patients develop objective sensory loss (position, vibration, shape, texture). Pain is uncommon except with flexor spasms of the limbs.

Lhermitte's sign is described as an electric or shock-like sensation that extends down the arms, back, or lower trunk bilaterally upon flexion of the neck. The sensation probably results from the buckling effect on the dorsal roots of the posterior columns from sclerotic plaques. (Unilateral Lhermitte's sign has been noted in such conditions as cervical spondylosis and narrowing of the cervical spinal canal.)

MOTOR SYMPTOMS

Motor symptoms often begin with weakness in the lower extremities and complaints of a feeling of heaviness or uselessness of the involved limb. Although complaints initially center on one limb, both limbs are usually involved to varying degrees. Spasticity, with its usual concurrent hyperreflexia, is common. Presence of spasticity often interferes with ambulation and ADLs.

The decline in motor function may last from minutes to hours and is, therefore, not always observed by the physician. Motor function can worsen spontaneously, after strenuous exercise, or after a hot shower or hot tub bath. Decline in motor function after exposure to a hot shower or tub bath is known as **Uhthoff's sign**. It can be of diagnostic significance in diagnosing MS.

Incoordination is another frequent symptom. Intentional tremors are noted in the upper extremities. An **intentional tremor** is defined as a tremor occurring when a voluntary act is initiated. The finer the required movement, the greater the tremor. In the lower extremities, the incoordination appears as ataxia. Head tremors are not evident until the terminal stages, when the cerebellum is involved.

Spastic weakness or ataxia of the muscles of speech is responsible for the dysarthria common in MS. Speech, in the early stages, is often slurred. Later, it becomes explosive or staccato and unintelligible. Scanning speech is seen sometimes with late-stage bulbar involvement if cerebellar ataxia is prominent. **Scanning speech** is defined as speech that is slow and measured, with pauses between syllables.

OCULAR, VESTIBULAR, AND AUDITORY SYMPTOMS

Optic neuritis, a common early symptom, is evidenced by visual clouding, visual field (often central) deficits, and pain with eye movement; pallor of the optic disks is noted. Diplopia and nystagmus are common. Internuclear ophthalmoplegia of lateral gaze, when noted, strongly suggests MS. The Marcus Gunn phenomenon, related to reduced light perception in the affected eye, is seen with retrobulbar neuritis.

Vertigo is a common early symptom usually noted as a mild instability. Vomiting and nystagmus can accompany the vertigo. Deafness is a rare finding.

PAROXYSMAL SYMPTOMS

Paroxysmal symptoms, which are less common but can occur in MS, include focal or generalized epilepsy, tonic seizures, trigeminal neuralgia, and, occasionally, tetanus-like spasms. The spasms are described as contractions of the hands or feet into a dystonic, sustained, abnormal position and can be very painful.

NEUROBEHAVIORAL DISORDERS

Neurobehavioral disorders associated with MS include emotional lability, irritability, apathy, inattentiveness, poor judgment, euphoria, dementia, and cognitive impairment. Depression is very common, occurring in 30% to 54% of patients. Less common are extreme anxiety, bipolar disease, and psychosis.

OTHER SYMPTOMS

Fatigue is a very common symptom in MS and can range from mild to severely disabling. The basis for fatigue is unknown. Bladder and bowel dysfunction and impotence are common. Bladder retention or reflex emptying is often seen in later stages of MS.

Course of the Illness

The course of MS is varied and unpredictable, as outlined earlier. Symptom clusters have been noted when a particular area of the brain is involved. For example, **Charcot triad**, which includes nystagmus, intentional tremors, and staccato speech, occurs with brain stem involvement. However, MS is usually not confined to one area, so it is not a particularly useful classification.

Events that may precipitate relapses are menstruation; emotional stress; cold or humid, hot weather; hot baths; overheating; fever; and fatigue. Many relapses last a few days to a few weeks, after which there is complete or incomplete reversal of symptoms. Deficits present after 3 months are usually permanent. Prediction of when the next episode will occur is impossible. Some patients may experience another attack in a few weeks, whereas others may be spared for many years.

Diagnosis

The diagnosis of MS is difficult to make because various symptoms, evident during relapse, may completely disappear during remission. Suspicion is raised when neurological deficits are noted in a relapsing-progressing cycle. Other suspicious circumstances are a familial history and worsening of symptoms during exposure to heat. When the body temperature is raised even slightly by exposure to dry heat, moist heat (as created by soaking in a hot bath), or fever, the affected nerves may stop transmitting impulses. Thus, symptoms become exaggerated.

There is no single reliable diagnostic test for MS. Certain laboratory tests may help to establish the diagnosis, but no test is definitive. The total protein level in the cerebrospinal fluid (CSF) may be elevated to 45 to 75 mg/dL (normal: 15 to 45 mg/dL). CSF immunoglobulin G (IgG), a protein fraction of gamma globulin, is elevated in two thirds of patients, and oligoclonal bands are seen in the gamma globulin region on electrophoresis in 80% to 90% of the patients. In addition, myelin basic protein, the major protein in the myelin sheath, is liberated from the sheath in an acute attack.

MRI is very sensitive to white matter lesions and is therefore helpful in the diagnosis of MS. In addition, evoked potential studies provide information on conduction pathways.

The diagnosis is made on clinical grounds by exclusion of all other neurological disorders that have similar presenting symptoms and by the following **diagnostic criteria**:

- Neurological examination that reveals objective abnormalities attributable to the CNS
- Involvement of two or more parts of the white matter of the brain or spinal cord
- Involvement following one of two possible patterns:
- Two or more relapses, each lasting at least 24 hours and each 1 month or more apart
- Slow, stepwise progression for at least 6 months
- Age at onset of 10 to 50 years

Treatment

There is no specific effective curative treatment currently available. Drug therapy and symptom management are the main methods available to patients.

DRUG THERAPY

Drug therapy is used to treat an acute attack, decrease the number of attacks and subsequent neurological disability, or to stop progression in MS.[9] Some patients do not respond to specific drug therapy, or if they do, the effectiveness decreases over time. The efficacy of many of these drug protocols requires further investigation. Many of the drugs' side effects and their toxicity are significant, and careful patient selection and monitoring are critical in management.

Drug Therapy for Acute Attacks. A short course of corticosteroids may or may not be given to treat acute relapses and accelerate recovery. The determining factor is the presence of functionally disabling symptoms with objective evidence of neurological impairment. Previously, adrenocorticotropic hormone (ACTH) and oral prednisone were primarily used. Currently, the preferred treatment is a short course of **methylprednisolone**, 0.5 g to 1 g intravenously daily for 3 to 7 days, with or without a short prednisone taper.[10] A prednisone taper may begin with 60 mg every day for 3 days followed by decreases in dosage by increments of 10 mg per day. Oral **prednisone** may be used alone following a similar schedule, except the initial 60-mg dose is extended for 5 to 7 days. An alternative treatment for an acute relapse is 25 to 60 U of **ACTH** intramuscularly or infused over an 8-hour period and tapered gradually over a 2- to 4-week course.[11] Selection of appropriate drug therapy will depend on available resources to treat patients with intravenous therapy and also the severity of the relapse.

Drug Therapy to Decrease the Number of Relapses. Interferon is not a single substance but has at least three main subtypes: alpha, beta, and gamma. The alpha and beta forms are produced by cells infected by a virus. These substances "interfere" with subsequent infection of adjoining cells by the same virus. **Beta interferon** (Betaseron) decreases the frequency of relapses in MS and may affect the underlying disease based on fewer lesions observed on MRI. The route of administration includes subcutaneous self-administration every other day as well as intrathecal or intramuscular routes. Beta interferon causes abortion in pregnant women and, therefore, should not be given to a woman planning a pregnancy or to sexually active women of childbearing age without education and a careful review of contraceptive practices. Other side effects include flu-like symptoms, local injection site reaction, and depression. A new interferon Beta-1a, recombinant, sold under the trade name of Avonex, has recently been released for use in the United States. It is used for treatment of relapsing and remitting M. S. The usual adult dosage is 3–9 million IU, administered SC three times per week for 6 months. The major side effects are flu-like symptoms and a reaction at the injection site.

Two other drugs that have been tried to decrease frequency of attacks are Copolymer 1 and azathioprine. **Copolymer 1** is an injectable polymer with an immunological effect that may be useful if started early in the disease course. **Azathioprine** (Imuran) is an anti-inflammatory and immunosuppressive drug that interferes with purine nucleic acid metabolism and protein translation. Current reports of efficacy of both drugs are inconclusive.

Drug Therapy Directed at Halting Disease Progression. Cyclophosphamide (Cytoxan), total lymphoid irradiation (TLI), cyclosporin, methotrexate, and 2-chloro-deoxyadenosine (cladribine) have shown some positive clinical effects in progressive disease by causing immunosuppression.[12] A variety of protocols have been tried with varying results. For example, a monthly dose of Cytoxan is often sufficient to control signs and symptoms of MS. The risk of bone marrow suppression and the increased risk of infection are the major side effects. In addition, hemorrhagic cystitis is common with cyclophosphamide therapy. Periodic blood studies and monitoring for infection are also necessary. As with other protocols, more investigation is necessary to determine value in practice. Oral myelin is in phase III trials in relapsing, remitting M. S., with results expected in 1997.

SYMPTOM MANAGEMENT

The management of symptoms often requires a multidisciplinary approach. The patient and family must be educated to understand the problem, how to prevent relapse of symptoms, and management strategies if relapse occurs. Physical therapy is an important part of management.

The goal of care is to keep the patient as independent as possible for as long as possible. A physiotherapy program is designed to maintain function for as long as possible. Techniques and devices can be employed to allow for ambulation, self-feeding, dressing, and other ADLs.

Although lost motor function usually is not regained, range-of-motion and muscle-strengthening exercises are important to maintain intact function. The physiotherapist can prescribe a brace or support device (cane, walker), as necessary, to maintain ambulation and independence. If leg spasticity develops, gait retraining designed to develop alternative muscles and stretching exercises may be helpful. Stretching exercises are effective for spastic arms also. With severe spasticity, drugs, such as baclofen (Lioresal), diazepam (Valium), and dantrolene sodium (Dantrium), may be beneficial in improving motor function. Baclofen may be given intrathecally via an infusion pump. Surgical procedures may be necessary for some patients.

To prevent muscle shortening and joint contractures, passive range-of-motion exercises must be a daily part of any patient activity. The patient who is ataxic may be helped by means of gait retraining or by use of a weighted cane or walker to widen the base of support. Weighted bracelets on either extremity are also of value.

Patients with sensory loss must be taught to protect themselves from injury by using their eyes to locate the extremities. The body must also be protected from trauma, heat, cold, and pressure. The key to helping the patient to maintain independence is planning by the health care team based on an individualized assessment of the patient's needs.

Nursing Management

Many patients with MS live normal lives between periods of relapses. When relapses occur, most patients are managed at home. Patients who have permanent disabilities can often live independently with the aid of family members and adaptation of the physical environment of the home. Some patients with advanced disease are managed in nursing homes.

Patients with MS are only seen in the acute care setting when severe relapses or complications occur, and those stays are usually short. Most MS patients reside in the community managed by a primary care physician or neurologist in a clinic. Regardless of the setting in which the nurse comes in contact with the patient, it is important for the nurse to assess the patient's understanding of the illness, the factors that cause relapse (Chart 34-3), and the need for lifestyle adaptation to live as independently and normally as possible. A teaching plan should be developed based on the patient's needs.

The major nursing diagnoses associated with MS and the appropriate nursing interventions are presented in Chart 34-4. If permanent disabilities develop, the amount of support necessary from the nurse and other health care professionals increases. Many patients will note a decreased energy level, urinary tract problems, motor deficits, sexual dysfunction, changes in their social and recreational activities, and concerns about roles and employment. Most patients need support in their adjustment process. Some patients need counseling and psychotherapy to deal with behavioral and cognitive deficits. Patients should also be

---

CHART 34-3
Exacerbating Factors in Multiple Sclerosis

The following factors are known to exacerbate symptoms and should be avoided:

- Undue fatigue or excessive exertion
- Overheating or excessive chilling or exposure to cold
- Infections
- Hot baths
- Fever
- Emotional stress
- Pregnancy (should be discussed with the physician to weigh the problems before a decision is made to become pregnant)

---

made aware of the purposes and services offered by the National Multiple Sclerosis Society. Many patients and family members benefit from MS support groups:

Multiple Sclerosis Association of America
601-603 White Horse Pike
P.O. Box 187
Oaklyn, NJ 08107
(609) 858-3211
(800) 833-4MSA

National Multiple Sclerosis Society
733 3rd Avenue, 6th Floor
New York, NY 10017-5706
(212) 986-3240
(800) 344-4867

For the patient with advanced disease, the use of braces and canes and, finally, confinement to a wheelchair may be a reality. These patients need instruction and help in modifying their lifestyles to maintain the greatest level of independence possible. In some instances, the patient will be bedridden. In addition to considering all of the nursing diagnoses in Chart 34-4, the nurse will need to incorporate measures to manage the potential problems associated with immobility.

AMYOTROPHIC LATERAL SCLEROSIS

Amyotrophic lateral sclerosis (ALS) also known as Lou Gehrig disease, is a rapidly progressing, fatal, degenerative disease of the upper and lower motor neurons. It is characterized by destruction of motor neurons in the brain stem and in the anterior gray horns of the spinal cord, along with degeneration of the pyramidal tracts, resulting in wasting of the muscles of the body. Sensory changes are not a part of the disease. Some muscles become weak and atrophy, whereas spasticity and hyperreflexia are noted in others. Various patterns of involvement can develop, but the classic pattern begins with a combination of weakness with increased tone, atrophy, and fasciculations of the limbs.

There are three recognized forms of ALS: sporadic, familial, and Western Pacific. The etiology of ALS is unknown, although there is a genetic component in some families. A high incidence of ALS is found in natives of Guam. In the United States, the incidence of ALS is 4 to 6 per 100,000 people. Men are affected approximately three times more frequently than women.

Pathophysiology

There are marked degenerative changes in the following structures: anterior horn cells of the spinal cord; motor nuclei of the brain stem (especially cranial nuclei of cranial nerves VII [facial] and XII [hypoglossal]); corticospinal tracts; and Betz cells and precentral cells of the frontal cortex. Involvement of the upper motor neurons results in spasticity and reduced muscle strength, whereas lower motor neuron involvement results in flaccidity, paralysis, and muscle atrophy. Functions

(text continues on page 677)

CHART 34-4

Summary of the Major Nursing Diagnoses Associated With Multiple Sclerosis*

Nursing Diagnoses	Nursing Interventions	Expected Outcomes
Impaired Physical Mobility related to (R/T): • Muscle weakness/paralysis • Incoordinated movement	• Maintain proper body alignment when in and out of bed (use support devices as needed). • Teach active and passive range-of-motion exercises. • Involve the family in implementing modifications in activities of daily living (ADLs) and to maintain function. • Focus on developing the continuum of activities from sitting, transferring to a chair, standing, and ambulation; increase activity to the next level as each step is accomplished. • Collaborate with occupational therapists (OTs), physical therapists (PTs), speech therapists (STs), and other health professionals to provide holistic care.	• Optimal range of motion of all joints and muscle mass will be maintained.

Sensory/Perceptual Alterations (visual, auditory, kinesthetic, and tactile) R/T:
• Misinterpretation and/or altered awareness of sensory input
• Visual disturbances (diplopia, hemianopia, blindness)
• Tactile disturbances (burning, tingling, paresthesia)
	• Monitor the function of all senses.
	• For kinesthetic and tactile alterations:
	—Provide tactile stimulation to affected areas.
	—Tell the patient to protect affected parts around cold or heat.
	• For visual alterations:
	—Hemianopia
	  • Arrange personal articles, bedstand, and food tray on the patient's unaffected side.
	  • Teach the patient to scan the environment by moving the head.
	  • Approach the patient from the unaffected side or midline and incorporate stimuli from both sides.
	—Diplopia
	  • Alternate eye patch every 2 hours from one eye to the other.
		• The patient will be able to compensate for sensory/perceptual deficits using techniques that ensure safety and maximize sensory input.

Self Care Deficit syndrome: bathing, hygiene, dressing, grooming, and/or toileting R/T: • Muscle weakness/paralysis • Incoordinated movements • Sensory/perceptual deficits • Fatigue	• Identify factors that limit performance of ADLs (*e.g.,* perceptual/sensory alterations, fatigue). • Identify areas in which assistance is needed; specify the type of assistance needed and the best approach in assisting with ADLs.	• The patient will initiate and complete as much self-care as possible based on endurance, physical strength, and coordination.

(continued)

CHART 34-4 Summary of the Major Nursing Diagnoses Associated With Multiple Sclerosis* (Continued)

Nursing Diagnoses	Nursing Interventions	Expected Outcomes
	• Demonstrate the use of assistive devices. • Encourage the patient to increase ADLs when symptoms of the disease abate. • Provide for basic care that the patient cannot provide for self. • Seek OT, PT, and other referrals as necessary.	
Risk for Injury R/T: • Muscle weakness/paralysis; sensory/perceptual deficits, incoordinated movements, or fatigue	• Teach the patient to identify potential risk factors related to injury. • Assist the patient as necessary. • Follow standards for injury prevention.	• The patient will remain injury free while hospitalized.
Constipation R/T: • Altered peristalsis • Decreased neural innervation	• Monitor bowel movements for frequency and consistency. • Begin with a clean bowel, then institute a bowel program. • Include foods high in fiber in the diet, as well as adequate fluids.	• A bowel evacuation pattern will be established that includes bowel movements every 1 to 2 days and soft and formed stools.
Altered Bladder Function (altered urinary elimination; incontinence; retention) R/T: • Neural innervation changes, atonic bladder or spastic bladder	• Monitor the frequency and amount of urine voided. • Ascertain the type of bladder problem present. • Institute a bladder retraining program. • Monitor postvoid residuals via catheterization.	• An adequate bladder evacuation program will be established that includes minimal postvoid residuals, no urinary tract infections, and no incontinences.
Sexual Dysfunction R/T: • Alterations in neural innervation to sacral segments; decreased sensory perceptual sensation • Misinformation and lack of knowledge	• Discuss the possibility of sexual dysfunction with the patient. • Establish whether dysfunction is present. • Make appropriate referrals for counseling for patient and sexual partner as necessary.	• Sexual dysfunction will be discussed with the patient and appropriate referrals will be made.
Fatigue R/T the disease process	• Assess causative or contributing factors (lack of sleep, poor nutrition, sedentary lifestyle, inadequate stress management). • Explain causes of fatigue. • Assist in identifying energy patterns and scheduling activities. • Assist in identifying tasks that can be delegated. • Explain pacing and prioritizing activities. • Teach energy conservation techniques.	The patient will: • Establish priorities for daily and weekly activities • Participate in a balanced lifestyle

(continued)

CHART 34-4 Summary of the Major Nursing Diagnoses Associated With Multiple Sclerosis* (Continued)

Nursing Diagnoses	Nursing Interventions	Expected Outcomes
	• Explain the effects of stress on energy. • Identify appropriate community resources.	
Self-Concept Disturbance (body image disturbance, self-esteem disturbance, altered role performance, personal identity disturbance) R/T: • Situational crisis • Motor and sensory deficits • Loss of independence • Fatigue and powerlessness • Change in roles (dependency) • Inability to perform activities with previous level of success	• Explore the patient's self-concept to identify particular areas of change. • Allow expression of feelings. • Correct misconceptions. • Be supportive; assist in developing strategies to deal with change. • Make appropriate referrals. • Identify support groups in the community.	• Express feelings about changes; supports will be provided • Have a positive self-concept • Make lifestyle changes to support a positive self-image
Ineffective Individual Coping R/T: • Situational crisis • Inadequate and/or ineffective support systems and/or coping mechanisms • Loss of control and independence • Inability to deal with severity of illness • Change in role and lifestyle, stress, irritability • Unrealistic perception of self or condition	• Review the psychosocial history to anticipate response. • Provide resources regarding coping with deficits or disorders. • Encourage verbalization of concerns. • Identify potential solutions to problems. • Encourage independence and participation in self-care. • Assess the effects of family on the patient. • Ensure accurate information about the illness. • Refer for pastoral care as desired. • Obtain social service and home care consults as necessary.	The patient will: • Adapt effectively to alterations in function • Participate in care within the limitations of illness • Develop positive ways to cope with illness
Impaired Social Interaction/social isolation R/T: • Emotional lability • Decreased mobility • Altered self-concept • Inability to participate in previous activities • Fear of appearing in public with visible deficits	• Communicate empathy for the patient's problems; spend time with the patient. • Explore strengths and resources that may help make socialization more comfortable; emphasize capabilities. • Accept the patient as he or she is. • Be alert to verbal and nonverbal cues indicating increased isolation, withdrawal, or despair.	The patient will: • Maintain social interactions • Retain sense of self
Knowledge Deficit R/T: • Disease process, effect on lifestyle, and community supports	• Establish what the patient knows about the disease and what he or she wants to know. • Develop a teaching plan. • Provide information from Multiple Sclerosis Society publications. • Arrange for appropriate referrals.	The patient will be knowledgable about the illness, able to describe: • Disease process as applies to self • Appropriate lifestyle modifications

(continued)

CHART 34-4 Summary of the Major Nursing Diagnoses Associated With Multiple Sclerosis* (Continued)

Nursing Diagnoses	Nursing Interventions	Expected Outcomes
Impaired home maintenance management R/T: • Difficulty in caring for self or family at home; motor/sensory deficits; fatigue; limited family supports	• Allow the patient to express concerns. • Identify particular areas of difficulty. • Explore possible solutions. • Evaluate the family's ability to participate in care. • Make referrals for assessment of the home environment as necessary. • Identify community agencies that may help. • Consult the social worker as necessary.	The patient will be able to: • Identify problems of home maintenance and suggest solutions • Modify the home environment to optimize care for self and others • Utilize family members to meet home maintenance needs

* This summary was developed with the assistance of Carol Fairfield Johnston, MSN, RN.

that are not affected include intellectual ability, sensory function, vision, and hearing. Bowel and bladder are usually spared until very late in the disease.

Signs and Symptoms

The signs and symptoms of ALS can vary from patient to patient. The initial symptoms are usually weakness and wasting of the limbs. A summary of the signs and symptoms follows:

• Muscle weakness, wasting, and atrophy—the muscles most commonly affected are the intrinsic muscles of the hand, as evidenced by clumsiness. The next-most-commonly affected muscles are the shoulder and upper arm muscles. The lower limbs are affected last; they characteristically feel heavy and are subject to fatigue and easy cramping.
• Muscle spasticity and hyperreflexia
• Fasciculations
• Brain stem signs evidenced by atrophy of the tongue and causing dysarthria. The muscles of speech, chewing, and swallowing may be affected so that dysarthria and dysphagia occur.
• Dyspnea (if the respiratory muscles are involved)
• Fatigue

Diagnosis

The diagnosis of ALS is made primarily on the basis of the history and a neurological examination that demonstrates upper and lower motor neuron disease. An electromyogram (EMG) is helpful because it will demonstrate fibrillations, which are signs of denervation, muscle wasting, and atrophy. The blood creatine phosphokinase (CPK) level is often elevated. A myelogram may be ordered to rule out other diseases.

Treatment and Management

There is no known treatment to cure this fatal disease. The first drug to slow the detorioration from ALS is riluzole (Riluzole), which was approved by the FDA for "early access" in late 1995. Riluzole is generally well-tolerated. Although the effectiveness of Riluzole is not clear, no other treatment is currently available. Patients must be managed with a multidisciplinary approach that includes the following:

• Physical therapy—range-of-motion exercises to control or improve the weakness or spasticity. Support devices, such as a cervical collar, foot brace, splints, or slings, may be ordered. A cane, walker, gait training, or wheelchair may be prescribed to assist the patient in ambulation. Even though the disease is progressive and fatal, therapy optimizes independence for as long as possible.
• Occupational therapy—useful in selecting equipment, such as special eating utensils, and electronic equipment for alternative ways of accomplishing ADLs
• Speech therapy—helpful in giving the patient instruction on projection of the voice
• Gastrostomy tube—if the patient's ability to chew and swallow is limited, a gastrostomy tube may be inserted to facilitate nutrition and prevent aspiration.
• Nutrition assessment—to assess caloric needs and modify diet to meet nutrition goals and patient's nutritional needs as they change; education to prevent aspiration
• Periodic assessment of respiratory function and monitoring of pulmonary function studies including vital capacity; use of respiratory therapy, incentive spirometry, intermittent positive pressure breathing, and suctioning, as necessary
• Long-term assistive ventilation, when necessary
• Ongoing counseling, support, and patient/family teaching—the patient and family need support and help in coping with the problems associated with this debilitating, fatal disease.

- Home health referral and assistance with home equipment and community services
- Management of any other health problems or complications precipitated by the disease
- Drug therapy for various problems
  Spasticity: diazepam (Valium) or dantrolene sodium (Dantrium)
  Cramps: quinidine
  Sialorrhea (increased salivation)
- Frank discussion of planning and making decisions for the future, including advance directives, hospice care, financial arrangements, and other issues.

Course of Illness

Because the onset of ALS is insidious, the early signs and symptoms may be overlooked. Diverse muscle groups gradually become involved, demonstrating weakness, atrophy, muscle wasting, and fasciculations. As the disease progresses, the arms and legs become severely impaired, and spasticity and hyperreflexia are noted. If the frontal lobe cells are involved, emotional lability may be apparent even though intellectual function is not affected. In the advanced stages, when the brain stem is involved, the muscles of speech and swallowing are affected. Speech is thick and hard to understand, and chewing, swallowing, and managing secretions become very difficult. At the terminal stage, the patient has dyspnea and shortness of breath. Speaking may no longer be possible. Death usually occurs as a result of aspiration, infection, or respiratory failure. ALS is a rapidly progressing disease in which 50% of victims are dead 3 years after onset.

Nursing Management

No treatment can currently arrest ALS. The nurse's role is directed toward the following goals:

- Assisting the patient to be as independent and comfortable as possible for as long as possible through symptom management
- Limiting the development of complications
- Assisting the patient to prepare for discharge and crisis
- Providing emotional and psychological support for the patient and family
- Developing and implementing an individualized teaching plan
- Making appropriate referrals to other health professionals and community resources
- Helping the patient to make decisions about advance directives, hospice care, and getting his or her affairs in order
- Preparing for death; reassurance of a comfortable death
- Providing information about support groups

Amyotrophic Lateral Sclerosis Association
21021 Ventura Blvd., Suite 321
Woodland Hills, CA 91364
(818) 340-7500
(800) 782-4747

Muscular Dystrophy Association
3300 East Sunrise Drive
Tucson, AZ 85718
(602) 529-2000
(800) 572-1717

Patient problems are numerous in this rapidly developing disease. The major nursing diagnoses and interventions are included in Chart 34-5.

PREPARATION FOR DISCHARGE AND CRISIS

The patient and family are central for planning for discharge from the hospital. The patient and family need to know what lies ahead so plans can be made to deal with the inevitable. If home discharge is chosen, plans must be made that include the following:

- Patient and family education about treatment protocols and treatment routines
- Home care services and equipment (*e.g.,* suction, oxygen, ventilator, walker)
- Adjustment in household routines
- Arrangement for outpatient services and community resources
- Special therapeutic regimens, such as physical therapy, speech therapy, and occupational therapy
- Spiritual support and counseling
- Awareness of the services offered by the National Amyotrophic Lateral Sclerosis Foundation and community support groups
- Continued follow-up

PATIENT AND FAMILY EMOTIONAL AND PSYCHOLOGICAL SUPPORT

The stresses of coping with the fatal diagnosis of ALS and its effects on roles, relationships, self-concept, self-esteem, body image, finances, and independence are overwhelming. The patient and family need a tremendous amount of support. Depression is commonly seen and needs to be treated. A multidisciplinary collaborative approach is mandatory, and the nurse can contribute to meeting this need as a collaborative group member.

MYASTHENIA GRAVIS

Great strides in the understanding and management of **myasthenia gravis** (MG) have occurred in the last 15 years so that the death rate is almost zero. MG is a chronic disease of the neuromuscular junction in which an autoimmune process destroys a variable number of acetylcholine receptors at the postsynaptic muscle membrane. The hallmarks of the disease are fatigability and muscle weakness of selected voluntary muscle distribution. The weakness tends to increase with repeated activity and improve with rest. The thymus gland may play some role in the autoimmune process of MG, although this is still poorly defined. About 80% of myasthenics have thymic hyperplasia; 15% have thymic tumors.

The prevalence of MG is about 0.5 to 14.5 per million in the population, or approximately 25,000 people in the United

CHART 34-5
Summary of Major Nursing Diagnoses Associated With Amyotrophic Lateral Sclerosis

Nursing Diagnoses	Nursing Interventions	Expected Outcomes
Impaired Physical Mobility related to (R/T) muscle wasting, muscle weakness, and spasticity	• Collaborate with physical therapist (PT) to promote mobility and motor function. • Apply necessary support equipment, teaching the patient to apply correctly. • Teach the use of ambulatory aids. • Control noxious stimuli known to increase spasticity such as cold.	• Motor function and tone will be maintained for as long as possible.
Risk for Disuse Syndrome R/T altered mobility and prolonged bedrest	• Implement a plan of care to prevent the development of the complications of immobility (*e.g.,* skin breakdown, atelectasis)	• Complications of immobility will be prevented.
Fluid Volume Deficit and Altered Nutrition, Less Than Body Requirements, R/T impaired swallowing secondary to weak muscles of swallowing	• Provide a soft diet with small, frequent feedings. • Encourage the patient to eat slowly. • Have suction equipment accessible. • If a feeding tube is in place, provide for feedings. • Teach the patient and family the correct procedure for tube feedings.	• The patient will be provided adequate fluid and nutritional intake. • The patient will not aspirate.
Impaired Verbal Communication R/T weak muscles of speech	• Suggest speech therapy if necessary. • Develop an alternative method of communication if speech is incomprehensible.	• An alternative method of communication will be developed.
Ineffective Breathing Pattern R/T weakness of respiratory muscles and an inability to manage secretions	• Assess for signs and symptoms of respiratory insufficiency. • Provide for proper body alignment and positioning. • Administer oxygen as necessary. • Maintain a patent airway. • If ventilatory support is necessary, provide necessary care.	• Respiratory function will be supported.
Alterations in Bowel and Bladder function R/T muscle weakness/dysfunctional innervation of bowel/bladder	• Assess bowel and bladder function. • Provide a bowel and bladder program.	• The patient's bowel will be evacuated every 1 to 2 days. • Urinary drainage will occur every 8 to 10 hours.
High Risk for Aspiration R/T an inability to manage own secretions or protect airway	• Maintain aspiration precautions. • Have suction ready.	• The patient will not aspirate.

Other Related Nursing Diagnoses:
• Risk for Infection
• Self-Care Deficits
• Fatigue
• Impaired Home Maintenance Management
• Anxiety
• Fear
• Powerlessness
• Knowledge Deficit
• Ineffective Individual Coping
• Caregiver Role Strain

States. The national Myasthenia Gravis Foundation estimates that there are approximately 100,000 patients in the United States with the disease.[13] The peak incidence of MG is age- and gender-related, with one peak in the second and third decades that mostly affects women and a peak in the sixth and seventh decades that mostly affects men.[14]

Pathophysiology

Muscle weakness and fatigability are due to an antibody-mediated autoimmune attack directed against acetylcholine receptors (AChRs) at the neuromuscular junctions which results in a reduction in the number of receptor sites. What factors trigger and maintain the autoimmune response in MG is still unknown. Studies of muscle biopsy specimens of the neuromuscular junction of myasthenia patients demonstrate only about one third as many AChRs as in normal specimens.[15] The degree of severity of MG correlates with the number of AChRs. In MG, there is loss of postsynaptic membrane folds and an increase in the gap between the nerve terminal and the postsynaptic membrane.[16]

Muscle contraction is controlled by effective neuromuscular transmission; the effectiveness of transmission is dependent on the number of interactions between acetylcholine (ACh) molecules and AChRs. When ACh binds to the AChR, the receptor's cation channel opens transiently, producing a localized electrical end-plate potential. If the amplitude of this potential is sufficient, it generates an action potential that spreads along the length of the muscle fiber and triggers the release of calcium from internal stores, leading to muscle contraction. At normal neuromuscular junctions, the end-plate potentials are adequate for generation of action potentials consistently. However, at myasthenia junctions, the decreased number of AChRs results in end-plate potentials of decreased amplitude. This results in a failure to trigger action potentials in some fibers.[17] The strength of a muscle contraction decreases given a sufficient number of junctional failures, and muscle weakness is observed. With repeated stimuli, there is a reduction in the amount of ACh and the muscle becomes fatigued. This is compounded by a concurrent decease in the number of AChRs, resulting in an ACh "run down" phenomenon.[18]

Signs and Symptoms

The onset of MG is usually gradual, although rapid onsets have been reported in association with respiratory infections or emotional upset. The course of the illness is extremely variable. In some patients, the disease is unchanged for months and may or may not progress, whereas in others, there is rapid involvement of other muscle groups. Ptosis and diplopia are early findings in a majority of patients. The levator palpebrae and extraocular muscles are involved. Ptosis may be unilateral or bilateral and becomes intensified when the patient attempts to look upward. Pupillary response to light and accommodation remain normal.

The next series of muscles to be affected are the facial, masticator, speech, and neck muscles. When chewing food, the patient becomes tired and must rest. After a few moments of rest, chewing can be resumed, but muscles fatigue quickly again. Because the facial muscle is affected, the mobility and expression of the face are altered. Any attempt to smile looks like a snarl and there is flattening of the nasolabial fold. The voice is often nasal and weak and fades after talking. There may be problems in managing saliva because of difficulty with swallowing. Food must be eaten very slowly to prevent aspiration.

Generalized weakness develops in approximately 85% of patients.[19] The limb muscles and, often, the proximal muscles, as well as the diaphragm and the neck extensors, are affected. Weakness of the neck extensors tends to cause the head to fall forward. If the shoulder girdle is involved, patients have difficulty keeping their arms above the head when reaching for an object, and combing or fixing the hair is difficult. When the intercostal muscles or the diaphragm are involved and there is weakness of respirations, mechanical ventilation may be necessary. Breathlessness is often an early sign of this involvement. The need for ventilatory support results in myasthenia crisis.

In summary, the muscle groups affected tend to be weaker after use or toward the end of the day when the patient is fatigued. As the disease progresses, muscle fatigue is noted with less exertion and earlier in the day. See Chart 34-6 for the clinical classification of MG.

Diagnosis

The diagnosis of MG is based on history, physical examination, and confirmatory laboratory testing. The patient usually reports that selected muscles become weak with activity and a period of rest improves the motor function. However, the muscle becomes fatigued again quickly. On physical examination, there is muscle weakness. MG does not affect reflexes, coordination, or sensory perception. Confirmation of MG is based on the following tests in the order listed: cholinesterase inhibitor drug test; repetitive nerve stimulation; antibody titer for anti-AChRs; and single-fiber electromyography (if necessary).

Cholinesterase Inhibitor Drug Testing: The drug commonly used is edrophonium (Tensilon) because it has a rapid onset of 30 seconds and a short duration of about 5 minutes. The test is performed by drawing 10 mg of Tensilon into a syringe and administering 2 mg intravenously. If no adverse symptoms appear, the remaining 8 mg is injected. If there is improvement in the muscle strength of a previously weak muscle that lasts 5 to 10 minutes, the test is considered positive.

Repetitive Muscle Stimulation: While electrical shocks are delivered to a nerve at the rate of 3 per second, surface electrodes over the muscle record electrical potentials. A rapid reduction of the amplitude of the muscle potential is considered positive.

Antibody Titer for AChR: This is conducted by assay of blood. In 80% to 90% of patients with generalized myasthenia, the AChR antibody titer is elevated.

Single Fiber Electromyography: This test can detect delay or failure of neuromuscular transmission in pairs of muscle fibers supplied by branches of a single nerve fiber.[20] It is about 99% sensitive in confirming MG.

A mediastinal MRI may be ordered to determine if the thymus gland is enlarged. Respiratory function studies are helpful if respiratory symptoms are present. In summary, the

MG. The goal of treatment is to achieve a quality of life that is as symptom free as possible. Currently, there are four methods of treatment in use: cholinesterase (ChE) inhibitor drugs; long-term immunosuppression; plasma exchange and intravenous immune globulin; and thymectomy.[21]

CHART 34-6
Global Clinical Classification of Myasthenic Severity

Class 0	No complaints, no signs after exertion or at special testing.
Class 1	No disability. Minor complaints, minor signs. The patient knows that he or she (still) has MG, but family members or outsiders do not perceive it. The experienced doctor may find minor signs at appropriate testing, *e.g.,* diminished eye closure, some weakness of the foot extensors or triceps muscles, the arms cannot be held extended for 3 minutes. The patient may have complaints such as heavy eyelids or diplopia only when fatigued, inability to perform heavy work.
Class 2	Slight disability, clear signs after exertion. The patient has some restrictions in daily life, *e.g.,* he or she cannot lift heavy loads, cannot walk for more than half an hour, has intermittent diplopia. Bulbar signs are not pronounced. Family members are aware of the signs but outsiders (inexperienced doctors included) are not. Weakness is obvious at appropriate testing.
Class 3	Moderate disability, clear signs at rest. The patient is restricted in domestic activities, needs some help in dressing, meals have to be adapted. Bulbar signs are more pronounced. Signs of MG can be observed by any outsider.
Class 4	Severe disability. The patient needs constant support in daily activities. Bulbar signs are pronounced. Respiratory function is decreased.
Class 5	Respiratory support is needed.

From Oosterhuis, H. J. G. H. (1984). *Myasthenia gravis.* Edinburgh: Churchill Livingstone.

CHOLINESTERASE INHIBITORS

Drug therapy with ChE inhibitor drugs is the first-line choice in the management of symptoms of MG, but it does not treat the underlying disease. ChE inhibitors enhance the neuromuscular transmission of an impulse by preventing the degradation of ACh by the enzyme ChE. The ACh inhibitor drug that is the mainstay in managing symptoms of MG is pyridostigmine (Mestinon). Neostigmine (Prostigmin), formerly prescribed, is used much less frequently, and many more recent articles do not include it in their discussions of management. Side effects for both drugs are muscarinic and nicotinic types (discussed later). Atropine is the antidote for ChE inhibitor drugs and must be available for any patient receiving ChE inhibitor therapy. There is no standard dosage of Mestinon because there are great variations among patients and in the same patient from time to time.

Pyridostigmine (Mestinon). Mestinon, the drug of choice, is available in tablet, syrup, timed-release, and intravenous forms. Its onset is within 30 to 45 minutes and it peaks in about 2 hours and lasts 3 to 6 hours. The daily dosage and time interval must be carefully adjusted using an affected muscle group as the target muscle to gauge effect, thus producing maximal muscle strength with minimal side effects. For example, if the oropharyngeal muscles are weak, then dosage should be timed to enhance muscle strength optimally at mealtime.[22] The dosage prescribed for most patients falls within the range of 30 to 120 mg every 4 hours orally during daytime hours. Pyridostigmine in 180 mg timed-release tablets is sometimes advisable at bedtime for patients who have nocturnal weakness or weakness on arising in the morning.

If ChE inhibitors become ineffective in treating symptoms, then other forms of therapy may be indicated.

The following are common drug-related side effects:

Muscarinic-Type Side Effects (on smooth muscle and glands)

- Gastrointestinal tract—heartburn, belching, epigastric distress, abdominal cramps, increased peristalsis, diarrhea, nausea, and vomiting
- Genitourinary tract—involuntary micturition, increased tone and motility of uterus
- Cardiovascular—bradycardia
- Vision—blurred vision, constricted pupils
- Respiratory tract—bronchoconstriction/bronchospasm, increased bronchial secretions, wheezing cough
- Other—profuse sweating and increased salivation

Nicotinic-Type Side Effects (on skeletal muscle)

- Skeletal muscle fasciculations (twitching) and spasms, followed by fatigue and weakness.

diagnosis of MG is made based history, physical findings, and confirmatory laboratory testing. The diagnosis may be delayed for a year or two if there is not suspicion about the possibility of MG.

Treatment

Once the diagnosis of MG has been established, an *individualized* management plan is developed because no single treatment is ideal for all patients. The drug protocols are designed to interfere with the autoimmune process that is the basis of

IMMUNOSUPPRESSION: LONG-TERM GLUCOCORTICOSTEROID THERAPY AND OTHER AGENTS

For those who do not respond well to ChE inhibitors, long-term corticosteroid therapy may be tried. Prednisone is the drug of choice, producing marked improvement or remission in about 70% to 80% of cases. There are two protocols for managing patients with corticosteroids: a high-dose protocol and a gradually increasing dosage protocol. Sanders and Scoppetta outline the following daily high-dose protocol:

- In patients with oropharyngeal or respiratory dysfunction, use plasmapheresis until definitive improvement is evident.
- Administer 60 to 100 mg of prednisone daily.
- Maintain the dose for at least 10 days or until definite prednisone-induced improvement has been evident for 3 to 4 days.
- Begin alternate-day dosing schedule of 100 to 120 mg of prednisone QOD.
- Reduce dose *slowly* to minimum necessary level.[23]

About 30% of patients experience some degree of worsening from 1 to 21 days after beginning prednisone; this worsening may last about 6 days.

An alternative approach is to start with a low dose (10 to 25 mg) daily and gradually increase the dose by 10 mg daily until improvement is noted. The dose is maintained until maximum improvement is noted; that dose of maximum improvement is continued for 2 to 4 weeks. After that time, the prednisone is slowly decreased to the smallest dose necessary to maintain an acceptable effect. It may be necessary to begin this protocol with the inclusion of Mestinon. It is often possible to decrease or discontinue the Mestinon as the patient is weaned off the prednisone.[24] With either protocol, consideration of side effects of long-term steroid therapy, such as peptic ulcer prophylaxis, hyperglycemia, and fluid retention, must be kept in mind.

Azathioprine (Imuran) is frequently used with success to treat symptoms of MG. It is the second-line choice after prednisone and a good choice if prednisone is contraindicated. The dosage schedule varies among physicians, but it may be gradually increased to about 150 to 200 mg a day. Onset of improvement is gradual, often occurring over 12 months.[18] After 1 to 2 years of improvement, the drug can be gradually discontinued. Usual precautions and monitoring must be followed with administration. Side effects include bone marrow depression, hepatotoxicity, anorexia, nausea, vomiting, and teratogenic effects. Cyclophosphamide (Cytoxan) is rarely used any more for treatment of MG because of its high toxicity.

PLASMA EXCHANGE AND INTRAVENOUS IMMUNOGLOBULIN

Plasmapheresis removes antibodies from the blood. In the case of MG, plasmapheresis removes the anti-AChR antibodies, resulting in short-term clinical improvement. The indications for plasmapheresis are to stabilize a patient in myasthenia crisis or to serve as a short-term treatment for a patient undergoing thymectomy. The plasmapheresis is done at the bedside with a blood cell separator machine and albumin as the plasma exchanger. An antecubital shunt provides access. The procedure takes 3 to 5 hours, depending on the size of the patient. Three to five exchanges every other day is the usual regimen. An improvement in muscle strength is noted about 24 to 48 hours after the first exchange, but it is temporary. Treatment usually consists of a course of five treatments over a 2-week period.

The indications for the use of **intravenous immunoglobulin (IVIG)** are the same as for plasmapheresis—short-term treatment for a serious relapse of MG. IVIG is useful for immunodeficiency and autoimmune conditions and has been used with success in MG. As with plasmapheresis, improvement occurs within 4 to 5 days.

THYMECTOMY

Although no controlled studies have been conducted, empirically, thymectomy has been helpful for many patients. About 80% of MG patients have hyperplasia of the thymus; about 10% have thymomas. A thymectomy induces improvement in a number of patients and remission of symptoms in approximately 40% if the procedure is done early in the course of the disease. The best results occur in patients between 10 and 40 years of age who have had an onset in the last 3 to 5 years. Some patients enjoy a sustained, drug-free remission after the thymectomy.

Surgery is planned collaboratively by the surgeon and anesthesiologist because the myasthenia patient is prone to have unpredictable responses to drugs and the possibility of respiratory failure is always present. The surgeon has two possible surgical approaches: the suprasternal and the transsternal. The suprasternal approach results in less postoperative pain and morbidity. Its disadvantage is that less of the thymus gland can be removed because of inaccessibility. The transsternal splitting approach continues to be selected by many surgeons because it allows better access to the thymus gland, making complete removal possible. The disadvantage of this approach is that the sternum is split for surgical access, thereby causing more postoperative discomfort.

Cholinergic Crisis Versus Myasthenic Crisis

Two situations can precipitate a crisis that requires respiratory support and intensive care—myasthenic crisis and cholinergic crisis. **Myasthenic crisis** is a sudden relapse of myasthenic symptoms in a patient with moderate to severe myasthenia or generalized myasthenia. A common precipitating event for crisis is infection, although in some instances, there is no apparent cause. Even with an increase in medication, the patient can rapidly develop swallowing and respiratory difficulties that may require intubation and ventilation support. Many physicians will monitor the vital capacity and blood gases and set predetermined values, such as a vital capacity of less than 1,000, at which time an elective intubation is ordered. By following such a protocol, an emergency intubation is avoided. These patients require intensive medical and nursing management.

There are many drugs that may compromise transmission of impulses across the neuromuscular junction and exacerbate myasthenic muscle weakness. These drugs include neuromuscular blocking drugs such as curare-like drugs; local anesthetics and antiarrhythmics (quinine, quinidine, procainamide); aminoglycoside antibiotics (gentamycin, kanamycin, neomycin, streptomycin); clindamycin and lincomycin; trimethadione; morphine; chloroquine; beta blockers; calcium channel blockers; and d-penicillamine. Many other drugs intensify myasthenic weakness. As a rule, MG patients should be observed for deterioration after any new medication is begun. Patient education is critical.

In myasthenic crisis, ChE-inhibitor drugs are usually ineffective for a few days. They are withheld until the patient demonstrates a responsiveness to the drugs. When drug therapy is resumed, the best dosage and combination of drugs must once again be determined. Concurrently, as motor strength and respiratory function improve, the patient is weaned from the ventilator.

Cholinergic crisis is an event precipitated by toxic effects of ChE-inhibitor drugs and the subsequent muscarinic and nicotinic effects described earlier. It is essentially a problem of over-medication. Muscarinic effects develop slowly, with abdominal cramping and diarrhea often being present for some time before the onset of nicotinic effects. The onset of nicotinic symptoms is rapid. Clinical examination reveals profound, generalized weakness; excessive pulmonary secretions; and impaired respiratory function. Management is similar to that for myasthenic crisis—that is, monitoring of respiratory function for difficulty, possible elective intubation, ventilatory support, and temporary withholding of ChE-inhibitor drugs.

The Tensilon test can be used to differentiate myasthenic crisis from cholinergic crisis. An improvement in muscle strength upon injection of the drug suggests myasthenic crisis. If there is no improvement or a deterioration in muscle strength, the patient is probably in cholinergic crisis.

Nursing Management

The myasthenic patient is usually managed in the community. Patient education is key for helping the patient to manage this chronic disease. The more the patient knows, the less apt he or she is to develop complications. Family members must also be knowledgeable so that they will know what to do in the event of respiratory difficulty or the development of crisis. Hospitalization may be necessary during myasthenic crisis regardless of cause (*e.g.,* pneumonia, heat exhaustion), during cholinergic crisis, or if a thymectomy is planned. At these times, an endotracheal tube may be necessary and may be used in conjunction with ventilatory support. Management of the myasthenic patient during complications will depend on the specific presenting complications. However, assessment of muscle weakness, respirations, ability to protect the airway, and drug therapy are major concerns when complications occur.

The following parameters are included in the nursing assessment:

- Assess respiratory function by auscultation and observation and by evaluating respiratory tests for vital capacity and tidal volume.
- Observe the patient for unpredictable responses to any drugs used (*e.g.,* excessive sedation, decreased respirations, or agitation).
- Assess the degree of strength or weakness of all muscles involved:

Respirations: rate, rhythm, quality (labored or smooth), abdominal breathing

Voice: quality of voice (whisper, monotone, normal intensity)

Hand strength and equality: (ability to hold or pick up objects)

Leg movement: ability to move legs freely in bed

Extraocular muscles: full range of extraocular movement; presence of eyelid ptosis

Head: ability to hold up head

- See Chart 34-7 for the major nursing diagnoses associated with MG.

PATIENT TEACHING

While the patient is undergoing diagnostic testing or making adjustments in lifestyle or drug schedule, a teaching plan should be developed as an important part of nursing management. Encourage living as normal a life as possible. The patient must have a comprehensive understanding of the disease. Determine what information the physician has conveyed. Clarify and reinforce this information and allow the patient to ask questions.

The patient and a responsible family member should be familiar with any drugs being taken, as well as the prescribed dosage and potential side effects. They should also know the signs, symptoms, and differences between cholinergic and myasthenic crises. An ambu bag and portable suction device should be available at home for patients who are prone to crisis. The patient should be familiar with the Myasthenia Gravis Foundation. The Foundation is an excellent education and referral resource for patients, their families, and health professionals. The patient education materials are excellent.

Myasthenia Gravis Foundation of American, Inc.
222 S. Riverside Plaza, #1540
Chicago, IL 60606
(312) 258-0522
(800) 541-5454
Fax: (312) 258-0461

The following points should be included in the patient teaching plan:

- Wear a Medic Alert bracelet to identify yourself as having MG, and carry a card stating the name of your primary physician.
- Take medication with bread or a cracker to reduce the risk of nausea and gastric irritation.
- Take the medication in enough time before eating to optimize maximal strength of muscles for chewing and swallowing.
- Do not take any over-the-counter medication without your doctor's permission.
- Eat slowly and select a soft diet if you have difficulty in swallowing.
- Relapses of symptoms can be caused by menstruation, infections, extremes in temperature, extensive exposure to sunlight (ultraviolet light), and emotional stress.
- Provide for adequate rest periods during the day.

CHART 34-7

Summary of Major Nursing Diagnoses Associated With Myasthenia Gravis

Nursing Diagnoses	Nursing Interventions	Expected Outcomes
Impaired Physical Mobility related to (R/T) motor weakness	• Assess the effectiveness of the drug program in supporting motor function. • Note the times of day when weakest. • Consult physician to adjust the drug program. • Help patient pace self and establish realistic goals.	• Voluntary motor function will be supported for optimal physical mobility.
Fatigue R/T muscle weakness	• Develop a daily schedule that allows for periods of rest and activities. • Assess the adequacy of the drug program. • Teach about activities or circumstances that cause increased fatigue. • Teach the patient to pace self. • Encourage identification of stressors and adjustment of lifestyle.	• The patient will follow a daily schedule that will provide for periods of rest and activity. • An adequate energy level will be maintained. • Undue fatigue will be avoided.
Risk for Ineffective Breathing Pattern R/T weakness of the muscles of respiration	• Assess breathing pattern. • If the breathing pattern is not adequate, assess the reasons for the problems. • Take definitive action to support an adequate breathing pattern.	• An adequate, effective breathing pattern will be maintained.
High Risk for Aspiration R/T weakness of the muscles of swallowing	• Develop a teaching plan that includes practices to decrease the possibility of aspiration (*e.g.,* encourage small bites and frequent swallowing, provide a soft diet). • Provide for emergency management if aspiration occurs.	• The patient will not aspirate.
Knowledge Deficit R/T hospitalization and diagnosis	• Teach about the illness and how to adapt lifestyle. • Encourage as normal a life as possible. • Inform the patient about the local chapter of the Myasthenia Gravis Foundation; provide written information about the disease from the organization.	• The patient will demonstrate a knowledge of the disease and the treatment program.

Other Related Nursing Diagnoses:
• Risk for Activity Intolerance
• Ineffective Breathing Pattern
• Impaired Home Maintenance Management
• Impaired Verbal Communication
• Fear
• Anxiety
• Impaired Adjustment
• Ineffective Individual Coping
• Diarrhea (R/T drugs)
• Risk for Injury (falls)
• Altered Family Processes
• Adverse Drug Reaction

- Set priorities and plan ahead so that undue fatigue will not develop. Pace yourself.
- Wear sensible shoes to minimize weakness and loss of balance.

NURSING MANAGEMENT AFTER A THYMECTOMY

The patient will be managed as any patient who has undergone chest surgery. Chest tubes will probably be in place. Special considerations of nursing care include the following:

- Maintain a patent airway by suctioning; encourage the patient to cough. These measures decrease stress on the respiratory muscles and support a patent airway.
- Provide chest physiotherapy, turn the patient frequently, and encourage deep breathing exercises to prevent pulmonary infection.

PARKINSON'S DISEASE

Parkinson's disease (PD) is a chronic degenerative disorder of the basal ganglia of unknown etiology. The disease usually begins insidiously, often unilaterally, and progresses. The major signs and symptoms include tremors, rigidity, akinesia/bradykinesia, and postural deformity (thus the mnemonic, *TRAP*). PD affects people in middle to later adult life, with a mean age of onset of 55 to 60 years of age.

Pathophysiology

Basal ganglia is a collective term for the subcortical motor nuclei of the cerebrum. The structures that compose the basal ganglia include the striatum, globus pallidus, subthalamic nucleus, substantia nigra, and red nucleus. In PD, the major lesion involves degenerative changes in the zona compacta of the substantia nigra, including the locus ceruleus. Depletion of the dopaminergic neurons of the substantia nigra results in reduction of striatal dopamine, the main biochemical abnormality in PD. The motor cells of the motor cortex and pyramidal tracts are not affected.

Signs and Symptoms

Because symptoms may develop slowly, diagnosis is often delayed, with symptoms often attributed to aging. The disease is progressive, so that eventually the patient's ability to perform ADLs and other independent functions is reduced. Some patients become confined to bed.

The signs and symptoms of PD include the following:

Major Manifestations

- **T**remors
- **R**igidity of muscles
- **A**kinesia/bradykinesia
- **P**ostural disturbance and loss of postural reflexes

Secondary Manifestations

- Difficulty with fine motor function such as writing and eating

- Soft monotone voice
- Mask-like face
- General weakness and muscle fatigue
- Cognitive impairments
- Autonomic manifestations

MAJOR MANIFESTATIONS

Tremors. Tremors occur most often in the distal portions of extremities, and especially in the hands. A so-called **"pill-rolling"** motion of the hand is characteristic. Other areas where tremors are seen include the foot, lip, tongue, and jaw. Tremors are present when the hand is motionless, and thus are termed *resting tremors* (Fig. 34-1). Tremors are absent during sleep.

Rigidity of Muscles. Muscle rigidity is associated with slowness of voluntary movement (bradykinesia or akinesia). The muscle feels stiff and requires much effort to move, thus appearing as difficulty in initiating movement. Because the patients move minimally when sitting, edema can develop in the feet, legs, hands, and arms. **Cogwheel rigidity** refers to rigidity or ratchet-like, rhythmic contractions, especially in the hand, upon passive muscle stretching.

Akinesia/Bradykinesia. The patient has difficulty initiating a movement and then moves very slowly. As a result, difficulty in rising from a chair, getting into a car, and performing ADLs are common. Slow or absent movement renders the patient at high risk for pneumonia, deep vein thrombosis, constipation, and pressure ulcers.

Postural Disturbance, Loss of Postural Reflexes. Patients walk in a stooped-over position with small, shuffling steps and a broad base on turns. The forearms are semiflexed, and the fingers are flexed at the metacarpophalangeal joints. The characteristic appearance and posture of the patient with PD are illustrated in Figure 34-2. Once movement is initiated, it fre-

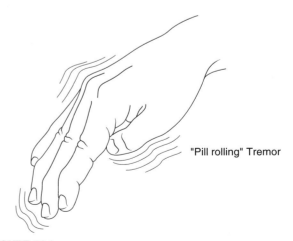

"Pill rolling" Tremor

FIGURE 34-1
The tremor in Parkinson's disease is exaggerated by the resting posture, is often relieved by movement, and usually disappears during sleep. The movement of the thumb across the palm gives it a "pill-rolling" character.

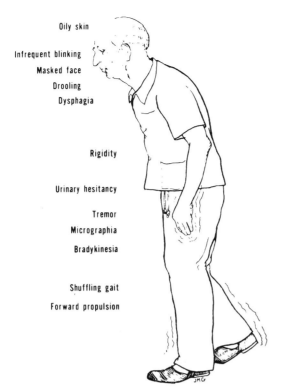

Oily skin
Infrequent blinking
Masked face
Drooling
Dysphagia

Rigidity

Urinary hesitancy

Tremor
Micrographia
Bradykinesia

Shuffling gait
Forward propulsion

FIGURE 34-2
The clinical features of Parkinson's disease.

quently accelerates almost to a trot. The patient may fall forward (propulsion) or backward (retropulsion). If pushed, the patient makes no attempt to brace himself or herself or to reach out and stop the movement. As a result, this patient is at high risk for injury. Patients have difficulty in maintaining balance and sitting erect.

SECONDARY MANIFESTATIONS

Difficulty With Fine Motor Function. Difficulty with fine motor control is seen early in the disease. Handwriting becomes progressively smaller and more difficult to read. Clumsiness and difficulty with ADLs, such as buttoning of clothing, is evident.

Monotonic Voice. The voice gradually becomes soft to whisper-like, monotonic, and muffled. These changes result in impaired verbal communications.

Mask-Like Face. The face is expressionless and the eyes stare straight ahead; blinking is less frequent than normal—5 to 10 times per minute rather than the normal 15 to 20 times.

General Weakness and Muscle Fatigue. Initiation of purposeful movement is slow. During movement, the patient may become momentarily frozen. Fatigue is a common complaint, especially when ADLs are attempted. Muscle cramps of the legs, neck, and trunk are common.

Cognitive Changes. Cognitive decline, such as visuospatial deficits, impaired executive functions, memory deficits, and depression, are common in many patients over the course of the illness. Some have used the term "subcortical dementia" to describe the cognitive changes related to PD. There is currently debate about the nature of cognitive deficits and the underlying cause.

Depression. This is seen in over 50% of persons with PD and may occur before classic symptoms of PD are noted.

Other Common Manifestations. Additional signs and symptoms, many associated with autonomic dysfunction, include the following:

- Drooling—secondary to decreased frequency of swallowing. When the patient awakens, the pillow is wet.
- Seborrhea (oily, greasy skin)—probably attributable to hypothalamic dysfunction, which causes release of an increased amount of sebotropic hormone
- Dysphagia—secondary to the neuromuscular incoordination of the hypopharyngeal musculature. This problem can interfere with normal fluid and dietary intake.
- Excessive perspiration—probably the result of a disorder of the hypothalamic heat regulator mechanism, as well as impairment of perspiration controls. The patient may be diaphoretic even in cold weather and may have a fever in warm weather.
- Constipation—secondary to hypomotility of the gastrointestinal (GI) tract and associated with prolonged gastric emptying time. Decreased fluid intake, lack of roughage, and decreased activity contribute to the development of constipation.
- Orthostatic hypotension—possibly the result of peripheral autonomic failure noted in Parkinsonism. It is also a side effect of levodopa therapy.
- Urinary hesitation and frequency—secondary to autonomic dysfunction. A catheter will rarely be necessary.

Medical Management

The management of the patient with PD is directed toward (1) symptom management with appropriate drug therapy; and (2) supportive and maintenance therapy including a physiotherapy program.

Although PD cannot be cured or arrested, symptoms can usually be controlled with drug therapy. Consideration must be given to timing of drug introduction, selecting the right drug, and adjusting the drug schedule for optimal results. The patient must be educated about the drugs used, side effects, and precautions to be observed while taking the drugs.

Supportive therapy is directed toward managing symptoms that are common in PD, such as constipation, perspiration, and urinary dysfunction. Advisement on adjustments of lifestyle and the prevention of complications and injuries is also important. Speech therapy may be recommended for some patients. A comprehensive physiotherapy program that may include gait retraining, balance maintenance, heat therapy, massage, and an exercise program can be most helpful in slowing the rate of disability.

It is now generally recognized that many individuals with PD experience some form of cognitive decline over the course of their illness. What is not agreed upon is the exact form of cognitive disturbance and whether the pattern of neuropsychological impairment represents a clinically anatomically distinct dementia syndrome.[25] Depression is common, and can be so severe that suicidal ideation develops. In such instances, psychotherapy, with the use of pharmacological and electroconvulsive therapy, may be necessary.

Most patients can be well managed at home with or without home health care or community services depending on the disability associated with the illness and the availability of family assistance. An effective drug program often allows the individual to maintain a near normal lifestyle. In the advanced stages, management in a nursing home may be necessary if adequate arrangements cannot be made at home. Admission to an acute care facility is necessary only for special problems such as surgery or treatment of complications. Individuals with PD are at high risk for injury because of incoordination, loss of postural reflexes, and rigidity. Injuries, such as a fractured hip, head injury, or spinal fracture, can result from a fall.

DRUG THERAPY

Although there is no known treatment that will permanently arrest the degeneration of the basal ganglia, drug therapy offers a means of relieving the many symptoms of PD. There are five drug classes used in management of PD: anticholinergics, antivirals, L-dihydroxyphenylalanine (levodopa), dopamine agonists, and monamine oxidase B inhibitors. These drugs are summarized in Chart 34-8. A few additional comments will be made about drug management.

Once the diagnosis of PD has been made, the severity of symptoms must be assessed and an appropriate management plan developed. The particular treatment plan must be developed with the age, lifestyle, and degree of disability kept in mind. The patient and family need to be involved in decision making and need to be educated about the disease and the drugs used. Selegiline is usually begun because it may slow the progress of PD and postpone the need for levodopa. An important decision is when to begin levodopa therapy. Although levodopa is the mainstay of drug treatment for PD, it has many side effects and a limited time span for effectiveness. This drug is begun in the moderately symptomatic patient. Although most patients deserve a trial on the drug, those with severe cerebral or cardiovascular disease, psychosis, or severe medical problems need to be carefully evaluated.

The long-term use of levodopa can result in toxicity and in unpredictable responsiveness to drug therapy. The signs and symptoms are listed in Chart 34-8. The "on-off" phenomenon, a side effect, is described as a fluctuation in motor function from being ambulatory and active one moment ("on" phase) to being unable to rise from a chair ("off" phase), all within a few minutes.

Patient Teaching for Levodopa. The patient should be made aware of the following limits when taking levodopa:

- Pyridoxine (vitamin B_6) is a cofactor of the enzyme dopa decarboxylase. It increases the decarboxylation of levodopa in the liver, thereby decreasing the amount available to be converted to dopamine in the brain. Therefore, patients on levodopa therapy should not take vitamin B_6 or multivitamin preparations that include vitamin B_6.
- Alcohol may antagonize the effects of levodopa and should be avoided.
- High-protein meals block the effect of levodopa when given alone or in combination. Therefore, intake of the following foods should be controlled: milk, meat, fish, poultry, cheese, eggs, peanuts, nuts, sunflower seeds, whole grains, and soybean products.
- Although levodopa is best absorbed on an empty stomach, it may cause nausea; therefore it should be taken with some food to decrease the side effect of nausea.
- Dryness of the mouth can be combatted by chewing gum or sucking on hard candy.
- Wearing elastic stockings will help to avoid orthostatic hypotension. Changing positions slowly is also helpful.
- Depression is common and may develop into severe depression with suicidal overtones. The physician should be advised if the patient feels depressed.

Dopa Decarboxylase Inhibitors. One might wonder why dopamine is not given rather than its precursor, levodopa. If dopamine were given orally, it would be metabolized before reaching the brain. Levodopa, however, is able to cross the blood–brain barrier and, once there, become converted into dopamine. For this chemical reaction to take place, the enzyme dopa decarboxylase must be present. In its presence, levodopa converts to dopamine and carbon dioxide, both in peripheral tissue and in the brain.

For the symptoms of PD to be controlled, levodopa must be converted to dopamine within the brain. If the reaction occurs in peripheral tissue, side effects of nausea and other symptoms occur. Inhibitors are given to prevent the conversion of levodopa to dopamine in peripheral tissue. The inhibitors selected to block the dopa decarboxylase enzyme do not cross the blood–brain barrier and thus allow dopamine production in the brain. By using levodopa in combination with dopa decarboxylase inhibitors, the dosage of levodopa can be reduced and side effects can be eliminated or greatly diminished. The inhibitor most often used is carbidopa (Sinemet). When given in combination, the dosage often used is carbidopa, 10 to 25 mg, and levodopa, 100 to 250 mg, three or four times daily.

Anticholinergic Drugs. Anticholinergic drugs are used in conjunction with levodopa or singularly if the patient cannot tolerate levodopa or symptoms are mild. The drugs most often used are Artane (2 to 5 mg three or four times daily) and Cogentin (0.5 to 6.0 mg daily).

Summary of Drug Therapy. Drugs provide relief of symptoms only. With the possible exception of selegiline, they do not alter the underlying progressive disease. In the early stages of PD, when only mild resting tremors are present, anticholinergic drugs are helpful for about 6 to 18 months. As the disease progresses, the patient will need drugs that provide dopaminergic stimulation. Levodopa is the mainstay of drug therapy.

CHART 34-8
Drugs Used in Management of Parkinson's Disease

Drug Classes	Purpose	Action	Side Effects	Comments
Anticholinergics: trihexyphenidyl (Artane); benztropin (Cogentin)	Tremors and rigidity	Muscarinic receptor blockers which penetrate the central nervous system (CNS) and antagonize transmission of acetylcholine by striatal interneurons	Result from both peripheral and central cholinergic blockade; **Peripheral:** dry mouth, constipation, urinary retention, and blurred vision **CNS:** lapses in memory, concentration, hallucinations, and confusion	May be given in combination with L-dopa
Antiviral: amantadine (Symmetrel)	Limited effect on akinesia, rigidity, and tremors	Promotes the synthesis and release of dopamine	Edema of legs; can cause psychiatric problems similar to anticholinergic drugs	
Levodopa (often given as Sinemet, a combination of L-dopa and carbidopa, a peripheral decarboxylase inhibitor)	Rigidity and bradykinesia	Immediate natural precursor of dopamine which is converted to dopamine by the amino acid decarboxylase; ↓ response to drug in advanced stages of PD	Nausea and vomiting related to **peripheral** dopamine receptor stimulation; **central** response includes orthostatic hypotension, dry mouth, constipation, dizziness, cough, cardiac arrhythmias, sleep disturbance, and "on-off" phenomenon	Sinemet overcomes peripheral dopamine receptor stimulation. L-dopa associated with fluctuation in hourly motor function; wide variety of dyskinesias; hallucinations or confusion
Dopamine agonists: bromocriptine (Parlodel, analog of dopamine); pergolide stimulates both D1 and D2 receptors	↓ fluctuation in motor response to L-dopa	Directly simulates dopamine receptors. There are two dopamine receptors; D1 (coupled to adenylate cyclase) and D2 (not linked). Most effective agonists stimulate D2 receptors.	Similar to L-dopa, but with lower incidence of dyskinesia and greater incidence of mental dysfunction	
Monoamine oxidase B inhibitor: selegiline (Eldeprenyl)	Slows PD; ↑ response to L-dopa	Blocks the metabolism of central dopamine; *delays need for L-dopa therapy;* slows the underlying degenerative disease process		Given in early stages to delay need for L-dopa; usually given throughout illness

The addition of peripheral dopa decarboxylase inhibitors has helped to control its many side effects (*e.g.,* anorexia, nausea, vomiting). Sinemet combines levodopa and carbidopa into one medication.

Treatment of drug toxicity and unresponsiveness to drugs is problematic. Drug therapy may be changed or dosages altered. So-called "drug holidays" of a few days have been suggested, with hospital supervision. The effect of such an approach may be improved clinical function that lasts weeks to months.

SURGERY

For the patient with severe, medically intractable tremors, rigidity, or bradykinesia, a pallidotomy via stereotactic surgery may be helpful for symptomatic therapy for selected Parkinson's disease patients. In this procedure, part of the globus pallidum of the basal ganglia is destroyed using an electrical stimulator. Only one side of the brain can be operated upon at a given time. If symptoms are bilateral, an interval of approximately 6 months must elapse before a stereotactic procedure on the other side is considered. At the time of pallidotomy, mapping of the area is also conducted. Mapping consists of identification of optic tracts, sensory and motor tracts, and white matter so that these areas will not be injured during the procedure. Follow-up studies document improved control of the symptoms, although the procedure is not a cure for the underlying disease.

Interest in autotransplantation of the adrenal medulla into the caudate nucleus to decrease the debilitating effects of PD waxes and wanes. It is unclear if this surgery will ever be a viable option for patients.

Nursing Management

Individuals with PD are managed in the community. See Chart 34-9 for a summary of nursing diagnoses associated with PD. Nurses provide support, education, and monitoring of patients over the course of illness. In order to determine the degree of disability, a number of instruments can be used to monitor the patient over time. The Unified Parkinson Disease Rating Scale (UPDRS) includes speech, salivation, swallowing, handwriting, cutting food and handling utensils, dressing, hygiene, turning in bed, falling, freezing, walking, tremor, and sensory symptoms. This comprehensive database provides a means to rate the degree of disability in many functional areas commonly affected by PD.

Drug therapy and effective methods of dealing with the symptoms of PD can prolong independence. Patient and family education is key to management. The teaching needs of the patient will depend on the stage of the illness and the symptoms at that time. The following are general considerations that should be addressed by the teaching plan:

- A clear explanation of PD and what to expect
- Explanation of the drugs being used including side effects, toxicity, and precautions (see earlier discussion of patient teaching precautions for levodopa)
- Discussion of the high risk for injury (*e.g.,* falls, spilling hot liquids)

- Helping the patient and family to evaluate the home environment for potential dangers (*e.g.,* scatter rugs, poor lighting, need for hand rails in the bathroom)
- Advising the patient to maintain a weight chart. Weight loss can occur as a result of inadequate nutrition secondary to vomiting and dysphagia. Obesity can also be a problem, particularly with ambulation.
- Dietary alterations for dysphagia should include soft, ground foods and small feedings.
- Constipation can be managed with the use of stool softeners.
- Urinary problems should be evaluated carefully. Incontinence may be caused by an inability to get to the bathroom fast enough; suggest a bedside urinal at night.
- Orthostatic hypotension can be helped by wearing elastic stockings and changing position slowly.
- A bedridden person should change position every 2 hours to prevent skin breakdown, contractures, and pulmonary complications. Deep breathing should be encouraged to avoid lung congestion and pneumonia.
- Range-of-motion exercises prevent stiffness and contractures and are encouraged three to four times a day.
- Speech can be improved by reading aloud, singing, and raising the voice. (Consult with a speech therapist, as necessary.)
- Intolerance to heat is common; temperature control is needed for comfort.
- Using a wide-based (12 to 15 inches) stance helps to maintain balance and improves balance and walking.
- Become aware of the National Parkinson Foundation (educational material, referrals, and community resources):

National Parkinson Foundation, Inc.
1501 NW 9th Avenue
Bob Hope Road
Miami, FL 33136-1494
(305) 547-6666
(800) 327-4545
(800) 433-7022 (in FL)

American Parkinson Disease Association
60 Bay Street, Suite 401
Staten Island, NY 10301
(718) 981-8001
(800) 223-2732

GUILLAIN BARRÉ SYNDROME

Guillain-Barré syndrome (GBS) is an acute inflammatory polyneuropathy with an incidence of 1.7 per 100,000. The etiology is unknown, but it is believed to be an autoimmune response to a viral infection. GBS is a rapidly progressive disorder that primarily affects the motor component of peripheral nerves. (The peripheral nerves include both cranial nerves and spinal nerves.) Most patients give a history of a recent (within the previous 2 weeks) acute infection, such as an upper respiratory infection, viral pneumonia, or GI infection. In a few instances, the patient has received a vaccination prior to the onset of GBS. As a result of improved respiratory management, most patients survive. Approximately 80% to 90% will have little or no residual disabilities.

CHART 34-9
Summary of Major Nursing Diagnoses Associated With Parkinson's Disease

Nursing Diagnoses	Nursing Interventions	Expected Outcomes
Impaired Physical Mobility related to (R/T) muscle rigidity and weakness	• Provide for range-of-motion exercises 4 times/d. • Evaluate the effectiveness of the drug program and adjust as necessary. • Suggest a physical therapy referral to assist in mobility.	• An optimal level of mobility will be supported.
Risk for Injury R/T muscle rigidity, muscle weakness, gait disturbance, and loss of postural reflexes	• Provide assistive devices to support mobility. • Remove environmental objects that could cause falls.	• Physical injury will be avoided.
Body Image Disturbance R/T slow movement, rigidity, and loss of facial animation	• Develop a trusting nurse–patient relationship. • Promote social interaction. • Provide necessary information to adjust to changes brought about by the disease.	• A realistic positive self-concept will be supported. • The patient will demonstrate adoption of a positive altered body image.
Impaired Communication (verbal and written) R/T a monotonic soft voice and poor handwriting	• Suggest a speech therapy evaluation for patients with a verbal deficit. • For writing difficulty, develop an alternative method of communication. • Evaluate drug therapy program to determine need for adjustments.	• Methods of communication will be supported and adapted as necessary.
Knowledge Deficit R/T hospitalization and diagnosis	• Develop a teaching plan. • Make aware of Parkinson's Disease Foundation and services offered.	• The patient will demonstrate a knowledge of the disease and the treatment plan.

Other Related Nursing Diagnoses:
• Altered Urinary Elimination
• Colonic Constipation
• Self-Care Deficits
• Diversional Activity Deficit
• Impaired Home Maintenance Management
• Risk for Disuse Syndrome
• Fluid Volume Deficit
• Nutrition: Less than body requirements, altered
• Fear
• Anxiety
• Social Isolation
• Caregiver Role Strain
• Adverse Drug Reaction

Pathophysiology

In GBS, an immune-mediated response triggers destruction of the myelin sheath surrounding the cranial and spinal nerves. The demyelination process is accompanied by edema and inflammation of the peripheral nerves. Collections of lymphocytes and macrophages are allegedly responsible for the actual stripping of myelin from between the nodes of Ranvier. The demyelination of axons results in loss of saltatory conduction. In addition, the same inflammatory process may result in varying degrees of axonal injury, which is related to a reduction in amplitude of muscle potential and signals a poorer recovery. Demyelination is patchy. The remyelination process occurs slowly.

Syndrome Variants

There are four different variants of GBS that reflect the degree of peripheral nerve involvement: ascending GBS, descending GBS, Miller-Fisher variant, and pure motor GBS.

Ascending GBS

- Most common presentation
- Weakness and numbness begin in the legs, then progress upward to the trunk, arms, and cranial nerves
- Motor deficits: paresis to quadriplegia; deficits are symmetrical
- Sensory deficits: mild numbness which is worse in toes
- Reflexes: diminished or absent
- Respiratory function: respiratory insufficiency occurs in about 50% of patients

Descending GBS

- Motor deficits: initial weakness in the brain stem cranial nerves (facial, glossopharyngeal, vagus, and hypoglossal nerves); then weakness progresses downward
- Sensory deficits: numbness occurs distally, more often in the hands than in the feet
- Reflexes: diminished or absent
- Rapid respiratory involvement

Miller-Fisher Variant of GBS

- Rare
- Seen as a triad of ophthalmoplegia, areflexia, and pronounced ataxia
- Usually no sensory loss
- Rare respiratory involvement

Pure Motor GBS

- Identical to ascending GBS, except sensory signs and symptoms are absent
- May be a mild form of ascending GBS
- Muscle pain is generally not present

In general, GBS is characterized by motor weakness and areflexia. Motor weakness tends to be symmetrical, beginning in the legs and then progressing to the trunk and arms. Respiratory failure is attributable to mechanical failure and fatigue of the intercostals and diaphragm. If the cranial nerves are involved, the facial (VII) nerve is most often affected. Other cranial nerves that are less often affected are the glossopharyngeal (IX), vagus (X), spinal accessory (XI), and hypoglossal (XII). Signs and symptoms of facial nerve dysfunction include an inability to smile, frown, whistle, or drink with a straw. Dysphagia and laryngeal paralysis can develop as a result of cranial (IX and X) nerve paralysis. Vagus nerve deficit, if present, is thought to be responsible for the autonomic dysfunction noted in some patients.

When sensory changes are present, paresthesias and pain may be noted. The paresthesia is frequent and temporary and is described as a tingling, "pins and needles" feeling, a heightened sensitivity to touch, or numbness. Sensory changes are often noted in the hands and feet (glove and stocking distribution). About 25% of patients will experience pain. Pain is underrated in terms of frequency and intensity. The pain may begin as cramping and progress to frank pain in the arms, legs, back, or buttock. Pain is often worse at night and often interferes with sleep. Analgesics are often necessary to keep the patient comfortable. The pain may be so severe that a morphine drip is necessary.

Autonomic dysfunction is much more common than once thought. The signs and symptoms may include any of the following: cardiac arrhythmias, paroxysmal hypertension, orthostatic hypotension, paralytic ileus, urinary retention, or syndrome of inappropriate secretion of antidiuretic hormone (SIADH).

GBS does not affect the level of consciousness, cognitive function, or pupillary signs.

Clinical Course

There are three stages of acute GBS: (1) acute onset, which begins with the onset of the first definitive symptom and ends when no further symptoms or deterioration is noted (lasts from 1 to 3 weeks); (2) the plateau period, which lasts for several days to 2 weeks; and (3) the recovery phase, which is synonymous with the remyelination and axonal regeneration process. In some patients who have sustained secondary axonal injury, recovery may take up to 2 years for maximal improvement, even though permanent deficits may result.

Diagnosis

Guillain-Barré syndrome is distinguished from other forms of polyneuritis by its clinical picture. The course of the illness is as follows: (1) acute onset, (2) rapid development of weakness and paralysis, (3) involvement of both the proximal and distal limbs, (4) absence of, or slight, muscle atrophy; and (5) absence of other causes.

Diagnosis is based on the clinical presentation just described, a history of a recent viral infection, elevated CSF protein levels with a normal cell count, and EMG studies. Nerve conduction velocities are slowed soon after paralysis develops. If denerved potentials (fibrillations) develop, they will occur later in the illness.

Medical Treatment

The medical treatment of GBS includes possible plasmapheresis, respiratory support, and supportive therapy. Steroids are of no benefit although there are anecdotal reports to the contrary. Plasmapheresis may be used for patients with severe GBS that involves the respiratory muscles. Three clinical studies demonstrate beneficial effects of plasmapheresis in patient with severe GBS in terms of shortening the time to recovery. When plasmapheresis is used, timing is important. It must be started 7 to 14 days after onset of the disease to be effective. Three to four treatments, 1 to 2 days apart, are usual. Some patients need a second course of treatments because of deterioration after the first round has been completed.

RESPIRATORY SUPPORT

Respiratory mechanical failure secondary to neuromuscular weakness is common in GBS. Vital capacity decreases, the cough becomes weaker, and ineffective airway clearance results. Peripheral alveoli collapse for longer portions of the respiratory cycle, lose their surfactant coating, and remain collapsed. This creates pulmonary tissue that is unventilated but perfused. Pulmonary vascular shunting develops as the vital capacity declines, causing a diminished CO_2 level. The consequences of a lowered vital capacity are atelectasis and probable hypoxemia. Concurrently, the intercostal muscles and diaphragm become fatigued, causing tachycardia, dyspnea, and diaphoresis to develop rapidly. Some patients will need to be intubated and supported temporarily on a ventilator. To avoid emergency intubation and the increased risk of aspiration, vital capacity is monitored and compared with a predetermined optimal level for the patient (approximately 12 to 15 mL/kg). In a 160-pound person, the target vital capacity is about 1,000 to 1,200 mL. When the patient's vital capacity falls below this level, elective intubation may be indicated. The type of mechanical ventilation usually provided is intermittent positive pressure.[16] Pneumonia related to mechanical respiratory failure is a common complication in these patients.

Some patients require ventilatory support for a short period of time (less than 2 weeks). However, for those who require extended ventilation, a tracheostomy will be necessary. Once the patient's illness is stabilized and respiratory function has improved (as evidenced by a vital capacity of 8 to 10 mL/kg), weaning from the ventilator is begun.

The mainstay of treatment is supportive care. Recovery from GBS is usual, but takes time. Hospitalization in the intensive care unit usually continues for approximately 2 to 3 months. Supportive care is directed toward preventing complications and maintaining the patient in the best condition possible. In addition to the respiratory problems already mentioned, other complications may include **autonomic dysfunction** (*i.e.*, hypotension, hypertension, cardiac arrhythmias, paralytic ileus, bladder retention, and SIADH), **sleep dysfunction**, possible **pain, nutrition,** and **psychological responses** (*i.e.*, fear, depression).

AUTONOMIC DYSFUNCTION

Monitoring of autonomic cardiac responses is required so that tachycardia and arrhythmias can be detected early and treatment instituted as necessary. Placing the patient on a cardiac monitor is helpful in identifying cardiac arrhythmias. If paralytic ileus occurs, a nasogastric tube is inserted for gastric decompression. An intermittent catheterization program is instituted to relieve urinary retention. Fluid and electrolytes are monitored for imbalance caused by SIADH. Restriction of free water is common in the event that SIADH develops.

SLEEP DYSFUNCTION

A disturbed sleep–wakefulness cycle leads to sleep deprivation. The basis for this problem is unclear, but it contributes to the psychological stress experienced by the patient.

PAIN

Pain, the quality of which is described as a "severe charley horse," can be underrated in those 25% of patients who have pain. The pain appears to be worse at night and is not relieved by nonsteroidal agents or non-narcotics. Narcotics may be indicated for some patients. Administering narcotics via a slow IV drip has yielded good results. Pain can interfere with sleep, although the altered sleep pattern common to GBS patients may also have an autonomic basis.

NUTRITION

Patients can rapidly lose weight and muscle mass, leading to weakness, fatigue, and failure to wean from a ventilator. Nutritional support should be aimed toward beginning feeding as soon as possible, with consideration of an appropriate goal for the patient.

IMMOBILITY

Finally, problems related to immobility must be addressed collaboratively with the nursing staff through emphasis on such nursing interventions as proper nutrition and maintenance of skin integrity. Mini-doses of heparin are administered to prevent deep vein thrombosis (DVT) and pulmonary emboli. There is some controversy related to the use of compression boots for the prevention of DVTs. The boots may apply undue pressure to the sensitive demyelinated peripheral nerves of the leg (*e.g.*, peroneal), leading to palsies. This is the basis for choosing heparin rather than compression boots for patients with GBS. In addition, careful positioning and very gradual introduction of limited physical therapy also help to prevent palsies.

Once the patient with GBS is in the rehabilitation phase, care is planned according to the rehabilitation framework. Respiratory rehabilitation may take some time and may limit the progress of the rehabilitation program, which includes extensive physical therapy and occupational therapy. In addition, many patients fatigue easily and have a limited tolerance to activity. Once respiratory function is well established, the patient can proceed with the rehabilitation program. This may be managed best in a rehabilitation facility or on an outpatient basis.

Nursing Management

Nursing management in the acute phase of GBS begins with a comprehensive baseline respiratory and neurological assessment and ongoing monitoring for early recognition of change. Assessment and ongoing monitoring include the following:

Respiratory Focus

- Assess respiratory rate and quality frequently.
- Assess vital capacity frequently; know the predetermined value for intubation.
- Monitor the patient for respiratory insufficiency (*e.g.,* air hunger, abdominal breathing, cyanosis, diaphoresis, dyspnea, confusion, anxiety).
- Monitor arterial blood gas levels.
- Administer oxygen as ordered.
- Be prepared for the possibility of intubation.

Neurological Focus

- Assess motor function frequently.
- Assess sensory function frequently.
- Assess cranial nerve function, especially cranial nerves III, V, VI, VII, IX, X, XI, and XII (most frequently affected).

Other

- Autonomic dysfunction: cardiac arrhythmias; vital signs indicating hypotension or hypertension; urinary retention

CHART 34-10
Summary of Major Nursing Diagnoses Associated With Guillain-Barré Syndrome: Hospitalized Patient

Nursing Diagnoses	Nursing Interventions	Expected Outcomes
Risk for Ineffective Breathing Pattern related to (R/T) neuromuscular weakness of the respiratory muscles (diaphragm and intercostals)	• Monitor the patient's respiratory status (rate, vital capacity, tidal volume), breath sounds, blood gases, and signs of respiratory fatigue. • Use an oximeter to monitor adequate oxygenation. • Position the patient to facilitate respirations. • Administer oxygen as ordered. • If on a ventilator, ensure safe use within the parameters set for the ventilator.	• Adequate ventilation will be maintained. • The patient will be free of respiratory distress.
Ineffective Airway Clearance R/T weakness of the cough reflex and the respiratory muscles (diaphragm and intercostals)	• Monitor ability to manage secretions and clear airway. • Monitor the effectiveness of the cough reflex. • Position the patient on the side to facilitate drainage from airway. • Elevate the head of the bed to facilitate coughing. • Administer chest PT every 2 to 4 hours. • Suction the airway to maintain a patency. • If a tracheostomy tube is present, provide tracheostomy care every 4 to 8 hours.	• A patent airway will be maintained.
Risk for Disuse Syndrome R/T immobility secondary to paralysis and confinement of ventilator	• Maintain a bowel program. • Prevent pressure ulcers (turn the patient periodically, monitor skin, use special bed if needed). • Promote venous return by applying thigh-high elastic (TED) stockings. • Provide for diversional activities. • Promote patient decisions and input about care.	The patient will demonstrate: • Soft, formed stools on a schedule that is adequate to maintain bowel pattern • Intact skin • Maximal peripheral blood flow without development of deep vein thrombosis • Participation in some form of diversional activity appropriate for health status • Participation in making some decisions related to care
Impaired Verbal Communication R/T paralysis of the muscles of speech or intubation	• Develop a method of communication that is appropriate for the patient (*e.g.,* eye blinking, raising a finger, using a computer board). • Teach how to communicate within physical limitations. • Teach family how to communicate with patient.	• A method of communication will be developed that allows the patient to convey needs. • Family members and other health professionals will be aware of the communications system and will use it.

(continued)

CHART 34-10 Summary of Major Nursing Diagnoses Associated With Guillain-Barré Syndrome: Hospitalized Patient (Continued)

Nursing Diagnoses	Nursing Interventions	Expected Outcomes
Urinary Retention R/T autonomic effects on bladder	• Establish a bladder retraining program (*i.e.*, intermittent catheterization) based on established physician protocol. • Monitor the intake and output record. • Palpate the suprapubic area for evidence of distention; monitor patient comfort.	• The bladder will be emptied on a 6- to 8-hour schedule. • When independent voiding is restablished, postvoid residuals will be less than 50 mL.
Pain R/T injury to peripheral nerves	• Establish the character and pattern of pain. • Enhance comfort through positioning/turning. • Teach imagery and relaxation techniques. • Administer analgesics as ordered. • Monitor response to analgesics using the visual analog scale (VAS).	• The patient will convey feeling relief from peripheral pain. • A decrease in pain will be documented by a decrease in intensity on the VAS.
Sleep Pattern Disturbance R/T altered autonomic function and pain	• Reduce or eliminate environmental distractions and sleep interruptions. • Identify factors, such as pain, that interfere with sleep and control.	• The patient will establish an effective sleep pattern that includes blocks of 3 to 4 hours' sleep at a time.
Fear R/T illness, hospitalization, treatment protocols, and death	• Assess factors that contribute to fear. • Control/reduce factors that contribute to fear. • Clarify misconceptions that contribute to fear. • Make appropriate referrals as needed. • Help mobilize effective coping strategies.	The patient will: • Report increased psychological comfort • Differentiate real from imagined concerns • Describe effective and ineffective coping patterns • Identify own effective coping methods.
Knowledge Deficit R/T hospitalization and changes in body function	• Develop a teaching plan to help the patient understand illness, hospital routines and equipment, what to expect, etc. • Answer questions posed by patient/family. • Anticipate need for information in patients unable to communicate freely.	• The patient will demonstrate a knowledge of the illness, hospital routines, equipment, what to expect, etc. • The family will understand same information.

Other Related Nursing Diagnoses:
• Risk for Infection
• Self-Care Deficit
• Constipation
• High Risk for Aspiration
• Nutrition: Less than body requirements, altered
• Impaired Swallowing
• Impaired Gas Exchange
• Sensory/Perceptual Alterations (kinesthetics)
• Fatigue
• Anxiety
• Powerlessness
• Impaired Social Interaction
• Dysfunctional Ventilatory Weaning Response

NUTRITION

These are the initial areas of focus for neurological assessment in the acute phase. As the signs and symptoms of GBS develop, the chief concern is respiratory insufficiency and the top priority is providing appropriate support. Many patients will require intubation and ventilatory support. Nursing interventions are directed toward maintaining adequate respirations, maintaining a patent airway, and preventing pulmonary infections.

The patient is maintained on bed rest for an extended period of time and is, therefore, at high risk for the multiple problems associated with immobility. A major concern is the development of DVT and pulmonary emboli. As discussed earlier, the physician will probably order mini-doses of heparin, rather than compression boots, to prevent DVTs. Special attention to positioning and turning is important to avoid pressure on vulnerable peripheral nerves and to prevent nerve palsies. Other areas of concern include management of paralytic ileus, urinary retention, range-of-motion exercises, and nutritional support.

The quality and quantity of the pain and fear associated with the acute phase of GBS are unique to this illness. As discussed earlier, those patients who have pain can have such severe pain that only a continuous titration of IV narcotics can give them some relief. The pain, described as worse at night, interferes with sleep. There may also be some autonomic changes that alter the sleep cycle. The patient experiences sleep deprivation, which also influences the ability to cope with immobility and the powerlessness associated with the illness.

Most patients with GBS are helpless and very fearful, communicating the ultimate fear, a fear of dying. It is often difficult to convince a patient that recovery from GBS is possible. They need continued support and reinforcement of the fact that the outcome is optimistic. To be fully conscious and cognitively intact yet be on ventilatory support must be an overwhelmingly frightening experience. Some patients are maintained on a ventilator for a few months before weaning is completed; they may need much information and continued support throughout the long months of recovery. The book *Bed Number One*, which is listed in the bibliography, is essential reading for anyone who cares for patients with GBS. It shares the experience and insight of one woman who developed GBS.

As patients move into the plateau and rehabilitation phases of GBS, the nursing focus changes to meet the altered needs of the patient. Many patients will require rehabilitation that extends beyond acute care in the hospital. Multidisciplinary management and planning assist the patient toward an optimal recovery. Chart 34-10 summarizes the nursing management of patients with GBS. Patients and families may also receive information from the Guillain-Barré Syndrome Foundation:

Guillain-Barré Syndrome Foundation International
P.O. Box 262
Wynnewood, PA 19096
(610) 667-0131

Summary

A number of the most common neurological degenerative diseases and their management are discussed in this chapter. There are many other disorders too numerous to cover within the limits of this text. However, common to all chronic degenerative conditions is the fact that rehabilitation, and especially patient and family education, is vital to effective management of the illness. Although there may be no cure, the nurse, along with other health team members, can help the patient maintain the highest level of independence possible at each stage of the illness. As skills and functions are lost, compensation for these deficits helps the patient to adapt. Along with the physical adjustment, there is the need for psychological adjustment and mobilization of effective coping skills. The desired outcome of the comprehensive care and rehabilitation program is to maintain an optimal quality of life for the patient and family.

References

1. American Psychiatric Association. (1987). *Diagnostic and statistical manual of mental disorders III-R.* Washington, DC: Author.
2. Richter, R. W., & Blass, P. J. (1994). *Alzheimer's disease: A guide to practical management, Part I.* St. Louis: Mosby, p. 1.
3. Ibid.
4. Folstein, M. F., Folstein, S. E., & McHugh, P. R. (1975). "Mini-Mental State": A practical method for grading the cognitive state of patients for the clinician. *Journal of Psychiatric Research, 12*: 189–198.
5. Crum, R. M., Anthony, J. C., Bassett, S. S., & Folstein, M. F. (1993). Population-based norms for the Mini-Mental State Examination by age and education level. *JAMA, 69*, 2420–2421.
6. Folstein, M., Anthony, J. C., Parhad, I., Duffy, B., & Gruenberg, E. M. (1985). The meaning of cognitive impairment in the elderly. *Journal of the American Geriatric Society, 33*, 228–235.
7. Mitchell, G. (1993). Update on multiple sclerosis therapy. *Medical Clinics of North America, 77*(1), 231.
8. Matthews, W. B., Compston, A., Allen, I. V., et al. (1991). *McAlpine's multiple sclerosis* (2nd ed.). New York: Churchill Livingstone.
9. Weiner, H. L., Hohol, M. J., Khoury, S. J., Dawson, D. M., & Hafler, D. A. (1995). Therapy for multiple sclerosis. *Neurologic Clinics of North America, 13*(1), 175.
10. Kupersmith, M. J., Kaufman, D., Paty, D. W., et al. (1994). Megadose corticosteroids in multiple sclerosis. *Neurology, 44*, 1.
11. Mitchell, G. (1993). Update on multiple sclerosis therapy. *Medical Clinics of North America, 77*(1), 240.
12. Weiner et al., op. cit., p. 177.
13. Phillips, L. H. The epidemiology of myasthenia gravis. *Neurologic Clinics of North America, 12*(2), 265.
14. Kurtzke, J. F., & Kurland, L. T. (1992). The epidemiology of neurologic disease. In R. J. Joynt (Ed.). *Clinical neurology* (rev. ed.) (pp. 80–88). Philadelphia: J. B. Lippincott.
15. Pestronk, A., Drachman, D. B., & Self, S. G. (1985). Measurement of junctional acetylcholine receptors in myasthenia gravis: Clinical correlates. *Muscle Nerve, 8*, 245–251.
16. Engel, A. G., Tsujihata, M., Lindstrom, J. M., & Lennon, V. A. (1976). The motor end plate in myasthenia gravis and in experimental autoimmune myasthenia gravis: A quantitative ultrastructural study. *Annals of the New York Academy of Sciences, 274*, 60–79.
17. Drachman, D. B. (1994). Myasthenia gravis. *New England Journal of Medicine, 339*(25), 1798.
18. Ibid.
19. Grob, D., Arsura, E. L., Brunner, N. G., & Namba, T. (1987). The course of myasthenia gravis and therapies affecting outcomes. *Annals of the New York Academy of Sciences, 505*, 472–499.
20. Stailberg, E., & Trontelj, J. (1979). Single fiber electromyography. Old Woking, England: Mirvalle.

21. Drachman, D. B. (1993). Myasthenia gravis. In R. T. Johnson & J. W. Griffin (Eds.), *Current therapy in neurologic disease* (4th ed.) (pp. 379–384). St. Louis: Mosby Year Book.
22. Sanders, D. B., & Scoppetta, C. (1994). The treatment of patients with myasthenia gravis. *Neurologic Clinics of North America, 12*(2), 345.
23. Ibid, pp. 343–368.
24. Donohoe, K. M. (1994). Nursing care of the patient with myasthenia gravis. *Neurologic Clinics of North America, 12*(2), 370.
25. Levine, B. E., Tomer, R., & Rey, G. J. (1992). Cognitive impairments in Parkinson's disease. *Neurologic Clinics of North America, 10*(2), 471.

Bibliography

General

Corbin, J. M., & Strauss, A. (1988). *Unending work and care: Managing chronic illness at home.* San Francisco: Jossey-Bass.
Lubkin, I. M. (1990). *Chronic illness: Impact and interventions* (2nd ed.) (pp. 2–42). Boston: Jones and Bartlett.

Alzheimer's Disease

Beck, C., & Heacock, P. (1988). Nursing interventions for patients with Alzheimer's dementia. *Nursing Clinics of North America 23*(1), 95–102.
Richter, R. W., & Blass, P. J. (1994). *Alzheimer's disease: A guide to practical management, Part I.* St. Louis: Mosby.
Whitehouse, P. J. (1990). *Contemporary neurology series: Vol. 33. Dementia.* Philadelphia: F. A. Davis.

Multiple Sclerosis

Francis, G. S., Evans, A. C., & Arnold, D. L. (1995). Neuroimaging in multiple sclerosis. *Neurologic Clinics of North America, 13*(1), 147–172.
Herndon, R. M., & Seil, F. J. (Eds.). (1994). *Multiple sclerosis: Current status of research and treatment.* New York: Demos Publication.
Kupersmith, M. J., Kaufman, D., Paty, D. W., et al. (1994). Megadose corticosteroids in multiple sclerosis. *Neurology, 44,* 1.
Lublin, F. D., & Whitaker, J. N. (1996). Management of patients receiving interferon beta-1b for multiple sclerosis. *Neurology, 46*(1), 12–18.
Lynch, S. G., & Rose, J. W. (1996). Multiple sclerosis. *Disease-A-Month, 42*(1), 1–55.
Matthews, W. B., Compston, A., Allen, I. V., et al. (1991). *McAlpine's multiple sclerosis* (2nd ed.). New York: Churchill Livingstone.
Mitchell, G. (1993). Update on multiple sclerosis therapy. *Medical Clinics of North America, 77*(1), 231–249.
Murray, T. J. (1995). The psychosocial aspects of multiple sclerosis. *Neurologic Clinics of North America, 13*(1), 197–223.
Weiner, H. L., Hohol, M. J., Khoury, S. J., Dawson, D. M., & Hafler, D. A. (1995). Therapy for multiple sclerosis. *Neurologic Clinics, 13*(1), 173–196.
Weinshenker, B. G. (1995). The natural history of multiple sclerosis. *Neurologic Clinics of North America, 13*(1), 119–146.

Amyotrophic Lateral Sclerosis

Kurtzke, J. F. (1991). Risk factors in amyotrophic lateral sclerosis. *Advances in Neurology, 56,* 245–270.
Tidwell, J. (1993). Pulmonary management of the ALS patient. *Journal of Neuroscience Nursing, 25*(6), 337–342.
(1995). Riluzole for amyotrophic lateral sclerosis. *The Medical Letter, 37*(963), 113–114.

Myasthenia Gravis

De Baets, M. H., & Oosterhuis, H. J. G. H. (Eds.). (1993). *Myasthenia gravis.* Boca Raton, FL: CRC Press.
Donohoe, K. M. (1994). Nursing care of the patient with myasthenia gravis. *Neurologic Clinics of North America, 12*(2), 370–385.
Drachman, D. B. (1994). Myasthenia gravis. *New England Journal of Medicine, 339*(25), 1797–1810.
Hohlfed, R., & Wekerle, H. (1994). The thymus in myasthenia gravis. *Neurologic Clinics of North America, 12*(2), 331–341.
Hopkins, L. C. (1994). Clinical features of myasthenia gravis. *Neurologic Clinics of North America, 12*(2), 243–261.
Howard, J. F., Sanders, D. B., & Massey, J. M. (1994). The electrodiagnosis of myasthenia gravis and the Lambert-Eaton myasthenic syndrome. *Neurologic Clinics of North America, 12*(2), 305–329.
Maselli, R. A. (1994). Pathophysiology of myasthenia gravis and Lambert-Eaton syndrome. *Neurologic Clinics of North America, 12*(2), 285–303.
Osserman, K. (1968). *MG.* New York: Grune & Stratton.
Pascuzzi, R. M. (1994). The history of myasthenia gravis. *Neurologic Clinics of North America, 12*(2), 231–242.
Phillips, L. H. (1994). The epidemiology of myasthenia gravis. *Neurologic Clinics of North America, 12*(2): 265–271.

Parkinson's Disease

Dogali, M., Fazzini, E., Kolodny, E., Eidelberg, D., Sterio, D., Devinsky, O., & Beric, A. (1995). Stereotactic ventral pallidotomy for Parkinson's disease. *Neurology, 45*(4), 753–761.
Fitzsimmons, B., & Bunting, L. K. (1993). Parkinson's disease: Quality of life issues. *Nursing Clinics of North America, 28*(4), 807–818.
Goetz, C. G., & Diederich, N. J. (1992). Dopaminergic agonists in the treatment of Parkinson's disease. *Neurologic Clinics of North America, 10*(2): 527–539.
Juncos, J. L. (1992). Levodopa: Pharmacology, pharmacokinetics, and pharmacodynamics. *Neurologic Clinics of North America, 10*(2), 487–509.
Laitinen, L. V. (1995). Pallidotomy for Parkinson's disease. *Neurosurgery Clinics of North America, 6*(1), 105–112.
Lieberman, A. (1992). An integrated approach to patient management in Parkinson's disease. *Neurologic Clinics of North America, 10*(2), 553–551.
Levine, B. E., Tomer, R., & Rey, G. J. (1992). Cognitive impairments in Parkinson's disease. *Neurologic Clinics of North America, 10*(2), 471–485.
LeWitt, P. A. (1992). Treatment strategies for extension of levodopa effect. *Neurologic Clinics of North America, 10*(2), 511–525.
Riley, D., & Lang, A. E. (1988). Practical application of a low-protein diet for Parkinson's disease. *Neurology, 38,* 1026–1031.
Standaert, D. G., & Stern, M. B. (1993). Update on the management of Parkinson's disease. *Medical Clinics of North America, 77*(1), 169–183.
Taira, F. (1992). Facilitating self-care in clients with Parkinson's disease. *Home Healthcare Nurse, 10*(4), 23–27.
Tanner, C. A. (1992). Epidemiology of Parkinson's disease. *Neurologic Clinics of North America, 10*(2), 317–330.

Guillain-Barré Syndrome

Baier, S., & Schomaker, M. Z. (1985). *Bed number ten.* Boca Raton, FL: CRC Press.
Murray, D. P. (1993). Impaired mobility: Guillain-Barré syndrome. *Journal of Neuroscience Nursing, 25*(2), 100–104.
Ropper, A. H. (1993). Critical care of Guillain-Barré syndrome. In A. H. Ropper, (Ed.). *Neurological and neurosurgical intensive care* (3rd ed.) (pp. 363–382). New York: Raven.
Ropper, A. H., Wijdicks, E. F. M., & Truax, B. T. (1989). *Contemporary neurology series: Vol. 34. Guillain-Barré syndrome.* Philadelphia: F. A. Davis.
Ross, A. P. (1993). Nursing interventions for persons receiving immunosuppressive therapies for demyelinating pathology. *Nursing Clinics of North America, 28*(4), 829–838.

CHAPTER 35

Cranial Nerve Diseases

Joanne V. Hickey

Certain cranial nerves are especially vulnerable to injury because of their location within the cranial vault. Others are subject to specific disease processes, including the following cranial nerves: the trigeminal (V), the facial (VII), the glossopharyngeal (IX), and the vagus (X). The major diseases discussed in this chapter are trigeminal neuralgia, Bell's palsy, Meniere's disease, and glossopharyngeal neuralgia.

TRIGEMINAL NEURALGIA

Trigeminal neuralgia, also known as tic douloureux, is a disease affecting the fifth cranial nerve. **Trigeminal neuralgia** is characterized by intense paroxysmal pain in the distribution of one or more branches of the trigeminal nerve. The term **tic**, as used in relation to the disease, refers to the paroxysmal contortions of the face in response to the pain. The pain is abrupt in onset, unilateral, and lasts from a few seconds to a few minutes. There are no motor or sensory deficits found with trigeminal neuralgia. Terms commonly used to describe the pain are paroxysmal, sharp, piercing, shooting, burning, and lightening-like jabs.

Most patients are able to identify trigger zones that initiate a bout of pain when stimulated. The trigger zone is usually a small area on the cheek, lip, gum, or forehead. These trigger zones are sensitive to the simplest of stimuli such as touch, cold, pressure, or a blast of air. Chewing, talking, smiling, shaving, brushing the teeth, or going out of doors on a windy day are common activities that may result in acute pain. Trigeminal neuralgia may occur at any age, although it is most common in middle and later life. Women are affected more frequently than men, at a ratio of 3:2, respectively.

The etiology of trigeminal neuralgia is unknown, although many contributing factors have been identified. It has been suggested that trauma or infection of the teeth or jaw, as well as flu-like illnesses, may precipitate the disorder. In most patients, pressure on the trigeminal nerve as it exits the brain stem by an adjacent, elongated, usually atherosclerotic artery, seems to be the etiology. Compression by an aneurysm or neoplasm, arachnoiditis, or multiple sclerosis can also produce the

symptoms of trigeminal neuralgia. In making a diagnosis, other etiologies must be ruled out in order to initiate appropriate treatment.

The trigeminal nerve emerges from the pons, passing across the petrous ridge to become the gasserian ganglion, which, in turn, separates into the ophthalmic, maxillary, and mandibular divisions (Fig. 35-1). It is the largest of the cranial nerves, possessing both motor and sensory components. The sensory fibers relay touch, pain, and temperature sensations, while the motor component innervates the temporal and masseter muscles used for chewing, jaw-clenching, and lateral movement. The following areas are supplied by each branch:

- *Ophthalmic*—forehead, eyes (including the cornea), nose, temples, meninges, paranasal sinuses, and part of the nasal mucosa
- *Maxillary*—upper jaw, teeth, lip, cheeks, hard palate, maxillary sinus, and part of the nasal mucosa
- *Mandibular*—lower jaw, teeth, lip, buccal mucosa, tongue, part of the external ear, auditory meatus, and meninges.

In trigeminal neuralgia, the second and third branches of the trigeminal nerve are about equally affected. Fortunately, involvement of the first branch is rare, occurring in about 10% of patients. When the ophthalmic or first branch is involved, the corneal reflex, a very important protective mechanism, may be lost.

The diagnosis of trigeminal neuralgia is based on the history. The neurological examination is entirely normal except in the rare patient with multiple sclerosis or a tumor that compresses the trigeminal nerve. The pain is precipitated by stimulation of trigger points; it is also unilateral, paroxysmal, and confined to the distribution of the fifth cranial nerve.

Course of the Disease

Many patients with trigeminal neuralgia experience bouts of pain for several weeks or months, followed by a spontaneous remission. The length of remission varies from days to years. With aging, there is a tendency for these remissions to be

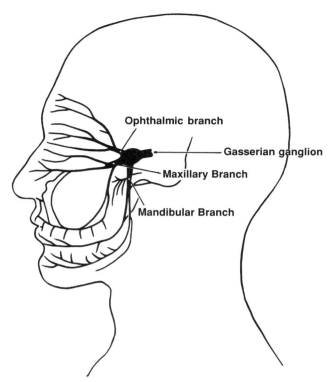

FIGURE 35-1
The main divisions of the trigeminal nerve are the ophthalmic, maxillary, and mandibular. Sensory root fibers arise in the gasserian ganglion.

shorter. The pain causes much suffering and limitation of the activities of daily living (ADLs). Because of the fear of pain, patients may not talk, eat, or attend to personal hygiene, such as washing the face, brushing the teeth, or shaving. Some individuals have become emaciated from not eating in their attempt to keep the face immobilized to prevent triggering pain.

Treatment

The treatment of trigeminal neuralgia includes drug therapy, injection with alcohol or phenol, and surgery. Carbamazepine (Tegretol) is the drug most commonly used to suppress or shorten the bouts of paroxysmal pain. Because carbamazepine can cause myelosuppression and liver damage, patients must be closely monitored with periodic complete blood cell counts (CBCs), liver enzymes, and liver function tests. If carbamazepine is not successful or tolerated, phenytoin (Dilantin), clonazepam, or baclofen can be given.

Injection of alcohol or phenol into one or more branches of the trigeminal nerve for the temporary relief of pain has been used less frequently. The relief of pain usually lasts from 8 to 16 months, with complete anesthesia to the areas supplied by the injected branches. Blocking of the gasserian ganglion provides more permanent control of pain, but the possibility of extraocular palsies, keratitis, blindness, masticator paralysis, and lack of selective cell destruction makes it an unattractive alternative. With both blocking procedures, the complete anesthesia to a portion of the face can be most distressing to the patient.

The patient with severe pain will probably require surgery. The most common surgical approach is stereotactic thermocoagulation of the trigeminal roots using radiofrequency. Radiofrequency percutaneous electrocoagulation provides lasting relief of pain with limited destruction of the trigeminal nerve. The basic principle is that small, poorly myelinated fibers that carry pain impulses are more sensitive to thermal lesions. With a heat-controlled electrocoagulation instrument, the sensory fibers are sufficiently destroyed to relieve pain without compromising touch or motor function.

A state of neuroleptanalgesia is achieved by administering small doses of intravenous diazepam (Valium) and fentanyl citrate (Sublimaze) during the procedure. The patient is comfortable but still able to respond verbally to questions. After each lesion is made, the corneal and ciliary reflexes, as well as facial sensation, are checked. Access to the foramen ovale, an opening from which the third branch of the trigeminal emerges, is gained through the cheek. The needle is advanced until cerebrospinal fluid (CSF) is obtained. Radiographic verification of the location within the foramen ovale follows. The electrode is inserted so that the selective electrocoagulation can proceed. The advantages of the procedure are many, and include long-term, if not permanent, relief of pain; short-term hospitalization (may be discharged the day after the procedure); good toleration by the elderly; no facial paralysis; and intact sensation of touch. Disadvantages include the possibility of puncturing the internal carotid artery and the occurrence of anesthesia dolorosa.

For many patients, a posterior fossa craniotomy, during which any blood vessel that appears to be compressing the trigeminal nerve is padded away from the nerve, is becoming the procedure of choice. If no vessel is seen that appears to be compressing the nerve at surgery, the trigeminal nerve may be partially cut to provide pain relief. If the nerve is sectioned at surgery, some sensory loss of the face may be expected postoperatively.

Nursing Management

The major nursing diagnoses for patients with trigeminal neuralgia who are being managed medically are listed in Chart 35-1. Specific nursing management after surgery is included in the section on postoperative care.

DRUG THERAPY

If drug therapy for the control of pain is ineffective, other treatment options are available. In addition to anticonvulsants for pain control, analgesics and tranquilizers are frequently prescribed. However, prolonged use of such drugs can result in habituation. Poor control of pain may also be a disappointing outcome of surgery. Drug habituation, disappointment from ineffective drug therapy or surgery, and fear that pain will be initiated by any activity all contribute to an elevated anxiety level. In collecting a nursing history, the nurse should carefully question the patient about his or her use of drugs. Sometimes, patients may not wish to speak or move the face in an attempt to prevent pain. This behavior may be interpreted as withdrawal or depression. The goal of nursing care is effective pain control.

CHART 35-1
Summary of Nursing Diagnoses Associated With Trigeminal Neuralgia

Nursing Diagnoses	Nursing Interventions	Expected Outcomes
Pain related to (R/T) stimulation of trigger area(s) on the face	• Assess the patient to identify those activities and circumstances that trigger pain. • Develop strategies with the patient to control precipitating factors. • Discuss with the patient common precipitating factors. • Administer pain medication at the first indication of paroxysmal bouts of pain. • Assess the effectiveness of the pain medication. • Assess and document the characteristics, frequency, and intensity of pain.	• The patient will not experience pain, or if present, the pain will be controlled, brief, and not incapacitating.
Self-Care (bathing/hygiene/ grooming) Deficits R/T fear of triggering pain	• Encourage the patient to take care of hygiene between bouts of pain. • Teach the patient to avoid trigger points and precipitating factors such as extremes in temperature. • Provide the necessary equipment appropriate for the activities. • Discuss the need for semiannual visits to the dentist for examination and care of the teeth.	• Bathing, hygiene, and grooming needs will be met satisfactorily.
Altered Nutrition: Less Than Body Requirements, R/T fear of triggering pain by chewing	• Assess the patient's diet for the proper consistency and temperature of appropriate food. • Consult with the dietitian in planning for nutrition. • Teach the patient to chew on the unaffected side. • Develop a written nutritional plan with the patient. • Discuss alterations in diet with the person who will be reponsible for the patient's food preparation upon discharge. • If adequate nutrition cannot be consumed orally, a nasogastric feeding tube will be necessary. Teach the patient and family the technique for tube feedings. • Teach the patient to maintain a written weekly record of weight.	• Adequate nutrition will be maintained.
Social Isolation R/T fear of engaging in activities that might trigger pain	• Assess the physical and social activities in which the patient engages. • Assess the patient's level of satisfaction with these activities. • Develop specific strategies to deal with the identified problems.	• Satisfactory social interactions will be maintained.

(continued)

CHART 35-1 Summary of Nursing Diagnoses Associated With Trigeminal Neuralgia (Continued)

Risk for Injury (to eye) R/T the rubbing or irritation of the eye	• Assess the patient for a corneal reflex. • Inspect the cornea perodically for signs of irritation. • Teach the patient to avoid rubbing the eye.	• No injury to the eye will be sustained.
Knowledge Deficit R/T the drug regimen and disease process	• Develop and implement a drug teaching program. • Alert the patient to the need for periodic complete blood counts if phenytoin or carbamazepine are being administered. • Provide the patient with written material on the drug, dosage, side effects, toxicity, and so forth. • Discuss with the patient the need to be monitored by the physician. • Review the disease process and lifestyle changes necessary to adjust to the condition.	The patient will be able to: —Demonstrate a knowledge of the disease process —Discuss the use of drugs to control the problem —Outline lifestyle changes that are necessary to accommodate the condition.

POSTOPERATIVE CARE

After surgery, neurological assessments are conducted periodically. Areas of special focus include the corneal reflex, extraocular movement, and facial movement for symmetry. Taste on the anterior two thirds of the tongue may also be assessed. The motor component of the trigeminal nerve is evaluated by asking the patient to clench the teeth. The contracted masseter and temporal muscles are then palpated to feel the bulk and tightness of the contracted muscles. To test the pterygoid muscles, the patient is directed to open the mouth slightly and press the examiner's finger laterally with the jaw. Weakness of the muscle will result in deviation of the jaw toward the weak side.

After surgery that has resulted in dissected sensory tracts, the affected side of the face becomes permanently insensitive to pain. The patient is cautioned against rubbing the eye because the protective mechanism of pain, which warns of injury, is absent. The eye is inspected for redness and conjunctival erythema. Because pain sensation is lost on the affected side, routine visits to the dentist should also be scheduled. Artificial tears are instilled into the eyes on the affected side, and the eye is protected from injury. Chewing is prohibited on the operative side until the paresthesia has diminished. A soft diet is ordered.

FACIAL PARALYSIS OR BELL'S PALSY

Sir Charles Bell of England first described acute paralysis of cranial nerve VII, the facial nerve, in 1821. The facial nerve originates in the pons and emerges from the stylomastoid foramen. It is composed mostly of motor nerves, which supply all the muscles associated with expression on one side of the face. The sensory component innervates the anterior two thirds of the ipsilateral half of the tongue. Because of Bell's interest in this cranial nerve disorder, the disease has been named after him. Bell's palsy may be preceded by symptoms of pain behind the ear or on the face for a few hours or days prior to the onset of paralysis. The disorder is characterized by a drawing sensation on the affected side of the face, followed by paralysis of all ipsilateral facial muscles. The eye does not close and the forehead does not wrinkle (Fig. 35-2). The patient cannot smile, whistle, or grimace. The affected side of the face is mask-like and sags, with constant tearing of the eye and possible drooling. The sense of taste for the anterior two thirds of the tongue may also be affected. The diagnosis is based on the history and clinical picture of seventh cranial nerve unilateral deficits.

Course and Prognosis

Bell's palsy can occur at any age but is most frequent in the 20- to 60-year age group. Both genders are affected about equally. Paralysis may gradually evolve over 24 to 36 hours, or paralysis may be complete upon awakening. Some persons never have complete paralysis but will have weakness. Eighty percent of affected persons will recover completely within a few weeks or a few months. Electromyography studies conducted 10 days after the onset of symptoms can indicate denervation and a prolonged incomplete recovery. Recovery depends on nerve regeneration. Although the etiology of Bell's palsy is unknown, it is believed to be caused by an inflammatory reaction. It may also be secondary to other diseases, such as Guillain-Barré syndrome or the mass effect of a tumor.

Treatment

Prednisone, 60 mg daily, is helpful for the first week after the onset of symptoms. In addition, analgesics are given to relieve pain. Gentle massage, moist heat, and electrical stimulation of

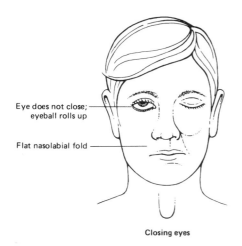

Eye does not close; eyeball rolls up

Flat nasolabial fold

Closing eyes

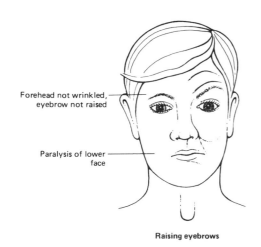

Forehead not wrinkled, eyebrow not raised

Paralysis of lower face

Raising eyebrows

FIGURE 35-2
Manifestations of Bell's palsy.

the nerve are common methods of treatment. Special facial slings have been developed to support the sagging face. Such a device may be suggested for selected patients. As muscle tone improves, grimacing, wrinkling the brow, forcing the eyes closed, whistling, and blowing air out of the cheeks should be practiced three or four times daily for 5 minutes in front of a mirror.

Nursing Management

Nursing management for patients with Bell's palsy focuses on the major deficits and the need to provide psychological and emotional support. Because the eye does not close, the cornea must be protected from injury and from drying to prevent corneal ulceration and blindness. Instruct the patient to close the eyelid manually. Artificial tears are instilled into the eyes four times daily for lubrication. The eyelids may be taped closed, or an eye patch may be worn for protection. Eye strain and sunlight are other stresses that may be avoided by wearing sunglasses.

Eating is problematic because the patient is unable to sip through a straw, chew, or control saliva on the affected side. Frequent, small feedings of soft food can be managed. The problems associated with eating are major sources of anxiety and embarrassment. Mealtime, a time of relaxation and socialization for many, becomes a nightmare unless the patient is helped to cope and adapt to the situation.

The simple techniques of moist heat application, massage, and facial exercise can easily be taught to the patient at home. A patient who develops Bell's palsy without other disorders will be treated in the community. If electrostimulation therapy is ordered, it will be provided on an outpatient basis. Patient education for home care outlines eye care and protection, mechanical adjustments of the diet, and a simple physiotherapy and exercise program.

All patients with Bell's palsy need much emotional support in order to cope with the radical change in self-concept and body image. Fortunately, most patients (80%) will recover completely, but that is of little comfort when patients view the distorted reflection of themselves in the mirror.

MENIERE'S DISEASE

The most common cause of true vertigo is labyrinthine lesions, of which Meniere's disease is a classic variety. Meniere's disease is thought to be the result of fluid accumulation in the endolymphatic space. The disorder affects cranial nerve VIII, involving both the vestibular and cochlear branches. **Meniere's disease** is characterized by recurrent attacks of vertigo associated with tinnitus and deafness. Tinnitus and deafness may not be evident initially, but will gradually become apparent with increased severity as the attacks continue.

The vertigo is of the rotational or whirling variety, lasting from minutes to hours and becoming so severe that the patient is unable to stand or walk. Accompanying symptoms include nausea and vomiting, a feeling of fullness in the ears, tinnitus, and rotational or horizontal nystagmus with the slow movement on the ipsilateral side. In most patients, vertigo ceases with complete deafness, although there are exceptions. The attacks vary in frequency and severity, with a possibility of remission between a series of bouts. Patients with recurrent attacks are apt to be anxious and in a mild state of disequilibrium.

The hearing loss associated with Meniere's disease may begin early, even before the onset of vertigo. Hearing loss occurs gradually until there is complete unilateral deafness. In 10% of patients, the disorder is bilateral. Both sexes are affected with equal frequency. The fifth decade of life is the most frequent time of onset.

Diagnosis

The diagnosis of Meniere's disease is based on the patient's history and the clinical findings of fluctuating, progressive hearing loss leading to deafness; episodes of vertigo; and significant tinnitus. The disease is usually unilateral and is characterized by periods of remission and exacerbation. Diagnostic testing includes caloric testing and audiometry. The audiometric studies reveal depression of air and bone conduction. Brain stem auditory evoked potentials and magnetic resonance imaging are routinely used to rule out other structural lesions outside the labyrinthine that may require specific treatment.

Treatment

During an attack, bed rest is most effective. The patient should be encouraged to try different recumbent positions until one that minimizes the vertigo is found. A salt-restricted diet and drugs are of value in controlling the vertigo. Drug therapy usually involves the use of a diuretic, hydrochlorothiazide (50 mg four times a day), with a potassium supplement; a vestibular suppressant, meclizine (Antivert), in dosages of 25 to 50 mg every 4 hours during acute attacks; and a vasodilator, papaverine (150 mg twice a day). Other drugs of this category may be ordered. Mild sedatives and hypnotics are worthwhile in controlling anxiety in the anxious individual.

If the attacks are frequent and disabling, surgical labyrinthine destruction for the patient with unilateral disease and complete deafness is possible. In patients with bilateral disease or incomplete hearing loss, the vestibular portion of the eighth cranial nerve can be sectioned intracranially or the labyrinth can be destroyed selectively with cryotherapy.

Nursing Management

Most patients with Meniere's disease are treated at home unless they are admitted for surgery or for other conditions. A major concern to the nurse is the prevention of accidents from falls as a result of the vertigo. Suggestions should be made to the patient concerning the prevention of injury, based on an assessment of the home environment and the vertigo pattern. The nurse should also assist the patient in evaluating the efficacy of the prescribed drugs in controlling the symptoms. The patient will require much emotional support throughout the illness.

GLOSSOPHARYNGEAL NEURALGIA

Glossopharyngeal neuralgia is a much rarer syndrome than trigeminal neuralgia. The syndromes resemble each other in many respects. Similar aspects include attacks of intense, paroxysmal pain; certain activities triggering bouts of pain; no sensory or motor loss of the cranial nerve; and unclear etiology. In glossopharyngeal neuralgia, the paroxysmal pain originates in the throat around the tonsillar area. Pain may also be localized in the ear or may radiate to the ear from the throat. A number of different nerves can be responsible in such cases; it is not necessary to distinguish which nerves are involved because the treatment is the same.

The paroxysmal pain patients experience may be initiated most commonly by swallowing, talking, chewing, yawning, laughing, sneezing, coughing, or blowing the nose. With time, more and more activities of this type (requiring less stimulation) will become trigger mechanisms. After an attack, the trigger area is insensitive for a time, but gradually builds up to a state of hypersensitivity.

The diagnosis of glossopharyngeal neuralgia is based on the patient's history.

Treatment

Administering phenytoin (Dilantin) or carbamazepine (Tegretol) or spraying the throat with a topical anesthetic may be of some temporary benefit to the patient. An intracranial surgical procedure, however, is usually required for long-term relief. The surgery includes division of the glossopharyngeal nerve and upper rootlets of the vagus nerve near the medulla. This posterior fossa procedure carries a small risk of cerebellar and brain stem injury, as well as the risk of injury to the cranial nerves located in the area, but it is usually successful at producing pain relief.

Nursing Management

Nursing management of patients with glossopharyngeal neuralgia is directed toward helping the patient evaluate the response to drug therapy in terms of pain control and development of side effects. If drug therapy is unsuccessful, the patient will probably require surgery, for it is unlikely that the patient can function for long if swallowing, blowing the nose, and so forth create pain. These basic activities are necessary to control saliva and maintain nutrition and patency of the upper respiratory tract.

If surgery is performed, nursing management follows the principles outlined for posterior fossa surgery (see Chap. 18).

References

Barker, F. G. Jannetta, P. J., & Bissonnette, D. (1996). The long-term outcome of microvascular decompression for trigeminal neuralgia. *New England Journal of Medicine, 334*(17), 1077–83.

Resnick, D. K., Jannetta, P. J., Bissonnette, D., Jho, H. D., & Lanzino, G. (1995). Microvascular decompression for glossopharyngeal neuralgia. *Neurosurgery, 36*(1), 64–69.

Bibliography

Books

Rovit, R. L., Murali, R., & Jannetta, P. J. (1990). *Trigeminal neuralgia.* Baltimore: Williams & Wilkins.

Wilkins, R. H. (1994). Trigeminal neuralgia. In S. S. Rengachary & R. H. Wilkins (Eds.), *Principles of neurosurgery* (pp. 471–476). Baltimore: Wolfe.

Periodicals

Barker, F. G., Jannetta, P. J., Bissonette, D. J., Shields, P. T., Larkins, M. V., & Jho, H. D. (1995). Microvascular decompression for hemifacial spasm. *Journal of Neurosurgery, 82*(2), 201–210.

Broggi, G., Franzini, A., Giorgi, C., Servello, D., & Brock, S. (1993). Trigeminal neuralgia: New surgical strategies. *Acta Neurochirurgica, 58*(Suppl.), 171–173.

Counsell, C. M., Guin, P. R., & Limbaugh, B. (1994). Coordinated care for the neuroscience patient: Future directions. *Journal of Neuroscience Nursing, 26*(4), 245–250.

Levins, T. T. (1994). Bell's palsy versus trigeminal neuralgia questioned. *Journal of Emergency Nursing, 20*(2), 86–70.

Mauskop, A. (1993). Trigeminal neuralgia (tic douloureux). *Journal of Pain and Symptom Management, 8*(3), 148–154.

McConaghy, D. J. (1994). Trigeminal neuralgia: A personal review and nursing implications. *Journal of Neuroscience Nursing, 26*(2), 85–90.

Tien, R. D., & Wilkins, R. H. (1993). MRA delineation of the vertebral-basilar system in patients with hemifacial spasm and trigeminal neuralgia. *American Journal of Neuroradiology, 14*(1), 34–36.

Weir, A. M., Pentland, B., Crosswaite, A., Murray, J., & Mountain, R. (1995). Bell's palsy: The effect on self-image, mood state and social activity. *Clinical Rehabilitation, 9*(2), 121–125.

Wollenberg, S. P. (1989). Primary care diagnosis and management of Bell's palsy. *Nurse Practitioner, 14*(12), 14–18.

Appendix I
Activase Therapy For Acute Ischemic Stroke

RAPID TREATMENT ALGORITHM

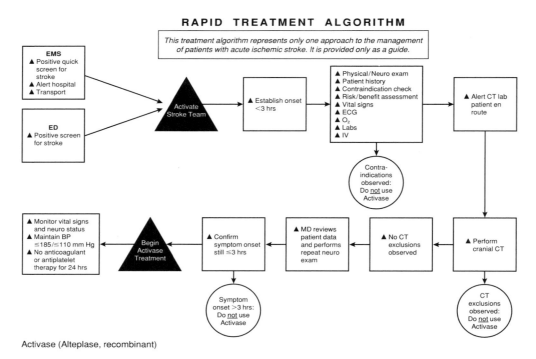

Activase (Alteplase, recombinant)

Activase is indicated for the management of acute ischemic stroke in adults for improving neurological recovery and reducing the incidence of disability. **Treatment should only be initiated within 3 hours after the onset of stroke symptoms, and after exclusion of intracranial hemorrhage by a cranial computerized tomography (CT) scan or other diagnostic imaging method sensitive for the presence of hemorrhage (see CONTRAINDICATIONS).**

CLINICAL PRESENTATION: Focal neurologic deficits, including

▲ Aphasia (expressive, receptive, or global)
▲ Ataxia
▲ Cranial nerve palsies
▲ Diplopia
▲ Dysarthria

▲ Hemianopsia
▲ Hemiparesis
▲ Loss of sensation
▲ Quadriparesis
▲ Visual field disturbances

PATIENT SELECTION:
▲ Patients must present within 3 hours of acute ischemic stroke symptom onset
▲ Obtain baseline CT to exclude intracranial hemorrhage and other risk factors
▲ Review patient history for potential contraindications

CONTRAINDICATIONS:
▲ Evidence of intracranial hemorrhage on pretreatment evaluation
▲ Suspicion of subarachnoid hemorrhage
▲ Recent intracranial surgery or serious head trauma or recent previous stroke
▲ History of intracranial hemorrhage
▲ Uncontrolled hypertension at time of treatment (e.g., >185 mm Hg systolic or >110 mm Hg diastolic)

▲ Seizure at the onset of stroke
▲ Active internal bleeding
▲ Intracranial neoplasm, arteriovenous malformation, or aneurysm
▲ Known bleeding diathesis, including but not limited to:
   — Current use of oral anticoagulants (e.g., warfarin sodium) with prothrombin time (PT) > 15 seconds
   — Administration of heparin within 48 hours preceding the onset of stroke and an elevated activated partial thromboplastin time (aPTT) at presentation
   — Platelet count <100,000/mm^3

WARNINGS:
▲ Patients with severe neurological deficit (e.g., NIH Stroke Scale >22) at presentation. There is an increased risk of intracranial hemorrhage in these patients
▲ Patients with major early infarct signs on a computerized CT scan (e.g., substantial edema, mass effect, or midline shift)
To assist in a full risk/benefit assessment, please see accompanying prescribing information for a complete list of WARNINGS.

DOSING INFORMATION FOR ACUTE ISCHEMIC STROKE:
0.9 mg/kg; maximum dose ≤90 mg
10% of the total dose administered as an IV bolus over 1 minute
Remaining 90% infused over 60 minutes

FOLLOWUP:
▲ Monitor vital signs and neurological status
▲ Maintain blood pressure ≤185/≤110 mm Hg
▲ No anticoagulant or antiplatelet therapy for 24 hours
Please see full prescribing information.

(Courtesy of Genentech, Inc.)

INDEX

Page numbers followed by *f* indicate figures; those followed by *t* indicate tables; those followed by *c* indicate charts.